Atlas of Percutaneous Edge-to-Edge Mitral Valve Repair

Ted Feldman • Olaf Franzen • Reginald Low
Jason Rogers • Khung Keong Yeo
Editors

Atlas of Percutaneous Edge-to-Edge Mitral Valve Repair

Springer

Editors
Ted Feldman, M.D., FESC, FACC, FSCAI
Cardiology Division
Evanston Hospital
Illinois
USA

Olaf Franzen, M.D
Department of Cardiology
Rigshospitalet University Hospital
Copenhagen
Denmark

Royal Brompton Hospital
Royal Brompton and Harefield NHS
Foundation Trust
London
UK

Reginald Low, M.D., FACC
Department of Cardiovascular Medicine
University of California
Davis Medical Center
Sacramento
CA
USA

Jason Rogers, M.D., FACC, FSCAI
Department of Cardiovascular Medicine
University of California
Davis Medical Center
Sacramento
CA
USA

Khung Keong Yeo, M.B.B.S., FACC, FSCAI
Department of Cardiology
National Heart Centre Singapore
Singapore
Singapore

Department of Cardiovascular Medicine
University of California
Davis Medical Center
Sacramento
CA
USA

ISBN 978-1-4471-7203-1 ISBN 978-1-4471-4294-2 (eBook)
DOI 10.1007/978-1-4471-4294-2
Springer London Heidelberg New York Dordrecht

Printed on acid-free paper

Springer is part of Springer Science+Business Media (www.springer.com)

Foreword

Atlas of Percutaneous Edge-to-Edge Mitral Valve Repair

The field of percutaneous therapy for mitral regurgitation has grown dramatically since the first procedures were performed in June and July 2003.

When first performed in patients, the technical and cognitive features of both the device manipulations and procedure goals were not well defined. Each movement of the catheter required some discussion among the procedural team. Optimal imaging planes for transesophageal echo guidance of the procedure had not been developed. Communication between the echocardiographer and the interventional physician was difficult because the two disciplines used completely different nomenclature to describe the left atrial and mitral valve anatomy.

The result of this was that procedures often took several hours. The procedures were tedious and based largely on trial and error. The path from the point of guide catheter entry into the left atrium at the level of the interatrial septum to the mitral valve could easily take more than an hour. The additional steps of orienting the open clip arms perpendicular to the line of coaptation while still in the left atrium were similarly tedious. Three-dimensional transesophageal echocardiography was not widely available at that point, and the necessity to have either a good transgastric short axis or even to switch between transthoracic and transesophageal echo for this step of the procedure added another level of both difficulty and time.

As our experience developed, an understanding of the anatomy that was common to both echocardiographer and interventionalist resulted in improved communication during the procedure. A greater understanding of the orientation and manipulation of the guide catheter in the left atrium ultimately led to the point where we find ourselves today. It typically takes only a few minutes to navigate the clip delivery system from the entry site into the left atrium until it is centered above the mitral orifice. The step of clip orientation perpendicular to the line of coaptation takes only several minutes even with two-dimensional echocardiography due to a more uniform use of intercommissural and left ventricular outflow tract two-dimensional views. The utility of orthogonal planes of two-dimensional images as a by-product of the three-dimensional probes makes this step even easier.

There has been as much learning regarding patient selection. Further developments include understanding the importance of having a one- or two-clip strategy prior to beginning the procedure, so that a first clip can be placed to one side or another of the jet, facilitating rapid progress to an orderly placement of a second clip.

This atlas illustrates the confluence of all of this procedural learning. These cases illustrate the refinements in technique and understanding of the procedure that lead to optimal outcomes from both technical and clinical standpoints. The further recognition that we can treat a wide variety of anatomic variations diverging from the original EVEREST anatomic inclusion criteria is further illustrated in the range of cases seen in the atlas.

The value of case-based learning is shown nowhere better than in a collection of case material such as this. For those interested in learning about the procedure for any purpose, this atlas serves as a wonderful basis. For both the practitioner and the interventional operator, there is a wealth of experience collected here that illustrates the spectrum of treatable disease, the potential for procedural challenges and complications, and the remarkable ability to successfully treat mitral regurgitation with a nonsurgical therapy.

Illinois, USA Ted Feldman M.D., FESC, FACC, FSCAI

Contents

Contributors

Eustachio Agricola, M.D. Cardio-Thoracic-Vascular Department, San Raffaele Institute (IRCCS), Milan, Italy

Juhani Airaksinen, M.D., Ph.D. Department of Medicine, Turku University Hospital, Turku, Finland

Kai A. Andersen, M.D., Ph.D. Department of Cardiothoracic Surgery, Rikshospitalet, Oslo University Hospital, Oslo, Norway

Iryna Arendar, M.D. Cardiothoracic Department, San Raffaele University Hospital, Milan, Italy

Ehrin J. Armstrong, M.D., M.Sc. Division of Cardiovascular Medicine, University of California, Davis Medical Center, Sacramento, CA, USA

Magnus Bäck, M.D., Ph.D. Department of Cardiology, Unit for PCI/GUCH, Karolinska University Hospital, Huddinge, Stockholm, Sweden

Stephan Baldus, M.D. Department of General and Interventional Cardiology, University Heart Center, Hamburg, Germany

Jacek Baranowski, M.D., Ph.D. Seldinger Unit, Heart Center, University Hospital, Linköping, Sweden

Department of Clinical Physiology, Heart Centre, University Hospital, Linköping, Sweden

Stephan Blazek, M.D. Department of Internal Medicine/Cardiology, Heart Centre, University of Leipzig, Leipzig, Germany

Gabriella Boano, M.D. Seldinger Unit, Heart Center, University Hospital, Linköping, Sweden

Department of Thoracic Surgery, Heart Centre, University Hospital, Linköping, Sweden

Steven F. Bolling, M.D. Department of Cardiothoracic Surgery, Section of Cardiac Surgery, University of Michigan Health System, Ann Arbor, MI, USA

Department of Cardiothoracic Surgery, University of Michigan Cardiovascular Center, University of Michigan, Ann Arbor, MI, USA

William J. Bommer, M.D. Division of Cardiovascular Medicine, Department of Internal Medicine, University of California, Davis, Sacramento, CA, USA

Nicholas Boudou, M.D. Pôle CardioVasculaire et Métabolique, Rangueil University Hospital, Toulouse, France

Department of Cardiology, CHU Rangueil, Toulouse, France

Magne Brekke, M.D. Department of Radiology, Ullevål, Oslo University Hospital, Oslo, Norway

Eric Brochet, M.D. Department of Cardiology, AP-HP, Bichat Hospital, Paris, France

Mamta Buch, MBChb, Ph.D., MRCP Department of Cardiology, North West Heart Centre, University Hospital of South Manchester NHS Foundation Trust, Manchester, Lancashire, UK

Valeria Cammalleri Divisione Clinicizzata di Cardiologia, A.O.U. Policlinico Vittorio Emanuele, Ospedale Ferrarotto, Universià di Catania, Catania, Italy

Didier Carrié, M.D., Ph.D. Pôle CardioVasculaire et Métabolique, Rangueil University Hospital, Toulouse, France

Department of Cardiology, CHU Rangueil, Toulouse, France

Paul Toon Lim Chiam, M.B.B.S. Department of Cardiology, National Heart Centre Singapore, Singapore, Singapore

Saqib Chowdhury, M.B.B.S., Ph.D., MRCP Department of Cardiology, North West Heart Centre, University Hospital of South Manchester NHS Foundation Trust, Manchester, Lancashire, UK

Mehmet Cilingiroglu, M.D., FSCAI, FACC, FESC Department of Medicine/Cardiology, UPMC Heart and Vascular Institute, Pittsburgh, PA, USA

Antonio Colombo, M.D. Cardio-Thoracic-Vascular Department, San Raffaele Institute (IRCCS), Milan, Italy

Cardiac Catheterisation Laboratory, EMO-GVM Centro Cuore Columbus, Milan, Italy

Roberto Corti, M.D. Department of Cardiology, University Hospital Zurich, Zurich, Switzerland

Gry Dahle, M.D. Department of Cardiothoracic Surgery, Rikshospitalet, Oslo University Hospital, Oslo, Norway

Giuseppe D'Ancona, M.D., Ph.D. Department of Cardiology, Heart Center Rostock, University Hospital Rostock, Rostock, MV, Germany

Zee Pin Ding, M.B.B.S. Department of Cardiology, National Heart Centre Singapore, Singapore, Singapore

Gregory Ducrocq, M.D. Department of Cardiology, AP-HP, Bichat Hospital, Paris, France

Nicholas Dumonteil, M.D. Pôle CardioVasculaire et Métabolique, Rangueil University Hospital, Toulouse, France

Department of Cardiology, CHU Rangueil, Toulouse, France

Ted Feldman, M.D., FSCAI, FACC, FESC NorthShore University Health System, Evanston, IL, USA

Cardiology Division, Evanston Hospital, Evanston, IL, USA

Olaf Franzen, M.D. Department of Cardiology, The Heart Center, Rigshospitalet, University of Copenhagen, Copenhagen, Denmark

Royal Brompton Hospital, Royal Brompton and Harefield NHS Foundation Trust, London, UK

Christian Frerker, M.D. Department of Cardiology, Asklepios Clinics St. Georg, Hamburg, Germany

Gretchen T. Gary, B.A. Abbott Vascular Structural Heart, Abbott Park, IL, USA

Oliver Gaemperli, M.D. Department of Cardiology, University Hospital Zurich, Zurich, Switzerland

Mathieu Gautier, M.D. Pôle CardioVasculaire et Métabolique, Rangueil University Hospital, Toulouse, France

Cosmo Godino, M.D. Cardio-Thoracic-Vascular Department, San Raffaele Institute (IRCCS), Milan, Italy

Howard C. Herrmann, M.D. Department of Medicine, University of Pennsylvania, Philadelphia, PA, USA

Dominique Himbert, M.D. Department of Cardiology, AP-HP, Bichat Hospital, Paris, France

Mark Hünlich, M.D. Abteilung für Kardiologie und Pneumologie, Herzzentrum, Universitätsmedzin, Georg-August-Universität Göttingen, Göttingen, Germany

Nikolaj Ihlemann, M.D., Ph.D. Department of Cardiology, Rigshospitalet, University Hospital of Copenhagen, Copenhagen, Denmark

Hüseyin Ince, M.D., Ph.D. Department of Cardiology, Heart Center Rostock, University Hospital Rostcok, Rostock, MV, Germany

Bernard Iung, M.D., Ph.D. Department of Cardiology, AP-HP, Bichat Hospital, Paris, France

Per-Herman Jacobsen, M.D. Department of Cardiology, Unit of GUCH, Karolinska University Hospital, Stockholm, Sweden

Jean Michel Juliard, M.D. Department of Cardiology, AP-HP, Bichat Hospital, Paris, France

Saibal Kar, M.B.B.S., M.D. Heart Institute, Cedars-Sinai Medical Center, Los Angeles, CA, USA

Kuck Karl-Heinz, M.D. Department of Cardiology, Asklepios Clinics St. Georg, Hamburg, Germany

Stephan Kische, M.D., Ph.D. Department of Cardiology, Heart Center Rostock, University Hospital Rostcok, Rostock, MV, Germany

Felix Kreidel, M.D. Department of Cardiology, Asklepios Clinics St. Georg, Hamburg, Germany

Tian Hai Koh, M.B.B.S. Department of Cardiology, National Heart Centre Singapore, Singapore, Singapore

Giovanni La Canna, M.D. Cardiothoracic Department, San Raffaele University Hospital, Milan, Italy

Eric Lim, M.B.B.S., M.A. (Cantab) Department of Cardiology, National Heart Centre Singapore, Singapore, Singapore

Scott Lim, M.D. Department of Cardiology, University of Virginia Medical Center, Charlottesville, VA, USA

Soo Teik Lim, M.B.B.S. Department of Cardiology, National Heart Centre Singapore, Singapore, Singapore

Poay Huan Loh, MB, BCh, BAO, MRCP(UK) Department of Cardiology, Rigshospitalet University Hospital, Copenhagen, Denmark

Reginald Low, M.D., FACC Department of Cardiovascular Medicine, University of California, Davis Medical Center, Sacramento, CA, USA

Juha Lund, M.D. Department of Medicine, Turku University Hospital, Turku, Finland

Heart Centre, Rigshospitalet, University of Copenhagen, Copenhagen, Denmark

Matti Luotolahti, M.D., Ph.D. Department of Clinical Physiology, Nuclear Medicine and PET, Turku University Hospital, Turku, Finland

Heart Centre, Rigshospitalet, University of Copenhagen, Copenhagen, Denmark

Philipp C. Lurz, M.D., Ph.D. Department of Internal Medicine/Cardiology, Heart Centre, University of Leipzig, Leipzig, Germany

Anita Macnab, MBChB, FRCP Department of Cardiology, North West Heart Centre, University Hospital of South Manchester NHS Foundation Trust, Manchester, Lancashire, UK

Francesco Maisano, M.D., FESC Cardiothoracic Department, San Raffaele University Hospital, Milan, Italy

Norman Mangner, M.D. Department of Internal Medicine/Cardiology, Heart Centre, University of Leipzig, Leipzig, Germany

Bertrand Marcheix, M.D., Ph.D. Pôle CardioVasculaire et Métabolique, Rangueil University Hospital, Toulouse, France

Department of Cardiovascular Surgery, CHU Rangueil, Toulouse, France

Takashi Matsumoto, M.D. Heart Institute, Cedars-Sinai Medical Center, Los Angeles, CA, USA

David Messika-Zeitoun, M.D. Department of Cardiology, AP-HP, Bichat Hospital, Paris, France

Neil Eric Moat, M.B.B.S., MS, FRCS Department of Cardiac Surgery, Royal Brompton Hospital, London, UK

Niels Erik Nielsen, M.D., Ph.D. Seldinger Unit, Heart Center, University Hospital, Linköping, Sweden

Department of Cardiology, Heart Center, University Hospital, Linköping, Sweden

Eva Nylander, M.D., Ph.D. Seldinger Unit, Heart Center, University Hospital, Linköping, Sweden

Department of Clinical Physiology, Faculty of Health Sciences, Heart Center, University Hospital, Linköping, Sweden

Liliya Paranskaya, M.D. Department of Cardiology, Heart Center Rostock, University Hospital Rostcok, Rostock, MV, Germany

Kian Keong Poh, MBBChir (Camb) Department of Cardiology, National University Heart Centre Singapore, Singapore, Singapore

Susanna Price, M.B.B.S., B.Sc., MRCP, EDICM, Ph.D., FFICM, FESC Department of Cardiology, Royal Brompton Hospital, London, UK

Miriam Puls, M.D. Abteilung für Kardiologie und Pneumologie, Herzzentrum, Universitätsmedzin, Georg-August-Universität Göttingen, Göttingen, Germany

Janne M. Rapola, M.D., Ph.D. Department of Cardiology, Helsinki University Hospital, Helsinki, Finland

Kjell Arne Rein, M.D., Ph.D. Department of Cardiothoracic Surgery, Rikshospitalet, Oslo University Hospital, Oslo, Norway

Jason Rogers, M.D., FACC, FSCAI Department of Cardiovascular Medicine, University of California, Davis Medical Center, Sacramento, CA, USA

Volker Rudolph, M.D. Department of General and Interventional Cardiology, University Heart Center, Hamburg, Germany

Department of Cardiology, Heart Center, University Hospital Cologne, Cologne, Germany

Antti Saraste, M.D., Ph.D. Department of Medicine, Turku University Hospital, Turku, Finland

Markku Saraste, M.D. Department of Medicine, Turku University Hospital, Turku, Finland

Department of Clinical Physiology, Nuclear Medicine and PET, Turku University Hospital, Turku, Finland

Jaydeep Sarma, MA, MB, BChir, Ph.D., FRCP Department of Cardiology, North West Heart Centre, University Hospital of South Manchester NHS Foundation Trust, Manchester, Lancashire, UK

Salvatore Scandura Divisione Clinicizzata di Cardiologia, A.O.U. Policlinico Vittorio Emanuele, Ospedale Ferrarotto, Universià di Catania, Catania, Italy

Ulrich Schäfer, M.D. Department of Cardiology, Asklepios Clinics St. Georg, Hamburg, Germany

Wolfgang Schillinger, M.D. Abteilung für Kardiologie und Pneumologie, Herzzentrum, Universitätsmedzin, Georg-August-Universität Göttingen, Göttingen, Germany

Department of Cardiology and Pneumology, University Medical Center Göttingen, Heart Center Göttingen, Göttingen, Germany

Gerhard Schuler, M.D. Department of Internal Medicine/Cardiology, Heart Centre, University of Leipzig, Leipzig, Germany

Magnus Settergren, M.D., Ph.D. Department of Cardiolog, Unit for PCI/GUCH, Karolinska University Hospital, Stockholm, Sweden

Alpay Sezer, M.D. Department of Cardiology, American Hospital Istanbul, Nisantasi, Istanbul, Turkey

Satya S. Shreenivas, M.D. Department of Medicine, University of Pennsylvania, Philadelphia, PA, USA

Frank E. Silvestry, M.D., FACC, FASE Cardiovascular Division, University of Pennsylvania School of Medicine, Philadelphia, PA, USA

Department of Medicine, Hospital of the University of Pennsylvania, Philadelphia, PA, USA

Thomas W. Smith, M.D. Division of Cardiovascular Medicine, Department of Internal Medicine, University of California, Davis, Sacramento, CA, USA

Lars Søndergaard, M.D., Dm.Sc. Department of Cardiology, Rigshospitalet, University Hospital of Copenhagen, Copenhagen, Denmark

Cardiology Invasive Laboratory, University Hospital of Copenhagen, Copenhagen, Denmark

Martin J. Swaans, M.D. Department of Cardiology, St. Antonius Hospital, Nieuwegein, The Netherlands

Corrado Tamburino Divisione Clinicizzata di Cardiologia, A.O.U. Policlinico Vittorio Emanuele, Ospedale Ferrarotto, Università di Catania, Catania, Italy

Jack Tan, M.B.B.S. Department of Cardiology, National Heart Centre Singapore, Singapore, Singapore

Maurizio Taramasso, M.D. Cardiothoracic Department, San Raffaele University Hospital, Milan, Italy

Edgar L.W. Tay, M.B.B.S. Department of Cardiology, National University Heart Centre Singapore, Singapore, Singapore

Holger Thiele, M.D. Department of Internal Medicine/Cardiology, Heart Centre, University of Leipzig, Leipzig, Germany

Gian Paolo Ussia, M.D. Divisione Clinicizzata di Cardiologia, A.O.U. Policlinico Vittorio Emanuele, Ospedale Ferrarotto, Università di Catania, Catania, Italy

Alec Vahanian, M.D., Ph.D. Department of Cardiology, AP-HP, Bichat Hospital, Paris, France

Jan A.S. Van der Heyden, M.D. Department of Cardiology, St. Antonius Hospital, Nieuwegein, The Netherlands

Ali Vazir, M.B.B.S., MRCP, CCDS, Ph.D. Department of Cardiology, Royal Brompton Hospital, Royal Brompton and Harefield NHS Foundation Trust, London, UK

Department of Cardiology, Royal Brompton Hospital, National Heart and Lung Institute, Imperial College, London, UK

Karsten Tange Veien, M.D. Department of Cardiology, Odense University Hospital, Odense, Denmark

Lars Wallby, M.D., Ph.D. Seldinger Unit, Heart Center, University Hospital, Linköping, Sweden

Department of Cardiology, Heart Centre, University Hospital, Linköping, Sweden

Reidar Winter, M.D., Ph.D. Department of Cardiology, Karolinska University Hospital, Huddinge, Stockholm, Sweden

Raymond Wong, M.B.B.S. Department of Cardiology, National University Heart Centre Singapore, Singapore, Singapore

Khung Keong Yeo, M.B.B.S., FACC, FSCAI Department of Cardiovascular Medicine, University of California, Davis Medical Center, Sacramento, CA, USA

Department of Cardiology, National Heart Centre Singapore, Singapore, Singapore

Wen-Loong Yeow, M.D., M.B. B.S., FRACP Heart Institute, Cedars-Sinai Medical Center, Los Angeles, CA, USA

James Wei Luen Yip, M.B.B.S. Department of Cardiology, National University Heart Centre Singapore, Singapore, Singapore

Genco Yucel, M.D. Department of Cardiology, American Hospital Istanbul, Nisantasi, Istanbul, Turkey

Introduction

Atlas of Percutaneous Edge-to-Edge Mitral Valve Repair

The MitraClip represents a new therapeutic frontier for mitral regurgitation. For the first time in the world, physicians now have the capability of repairing the mitral valve percutaneously without the need for a sternotomy or cardiopulmonary bypass. However, as with all new endeavors, there exists a steep learning curve, not just for the individual operator but also for the entire specialty. Not all mitral regurgitation cases are suitable for percutaneous repair, and not all cases are straightforward. It is therefore crucially important for physicians in this unique specialty to communicate their experience, successes, failures, and complications with each other.

The MitraClip procedure also emphasizes the need for multispecialty teamwork with close collaboration and communication between the interventional cardiologist, cardiac surgeon, echocardiologist, and anesthesiologist. This occurs from the time of patient screening and patient selection to the procedure itself and the post-procedure evaluation. Each subspecialist has to understand and appreciate what the other is doing and respond accordingly.

This atlas aims to assist in this conversation by providing a basic procedural "textbook." Each chapter addresses basic components of the MitraClip procedure. In addition, the atlas also showcases a series of simple and complex cases, which are meant to highlight important learning points. It represents a large body of experience from operators around the world from the United States, Europe, and Asia.

We believe that this atlas will be an important resource for specialists interested in this field. Trainees and junior doctors will find the basic chapters useful in understanding how the procedure is planned for and performed. Operators early in their experience with MitraClip will find the pictures in the atlas more useful than simple text descriptions. Experienced operators will find the unusual and complex cases enriching. We are deeply grateful to our contributors for taking the time to prepare these cases for inclusion in the atlas. It is also very gratifying to see that physicians from around the globe are willing to share their learning experiences with their successful or unsuccessful procedures and complications. It is the hope of the editors that the physicians share their experiences and learn from one another. We are at the cusp of a new era in percutaneous structural heart interventions. We believe that this atlas will be a valuable and meaningful contribution to this exciting new field.

Sacramento, CA, USA — Reginald Low, M.D., FACC
Copenhagen, Denmark — Olaf Franzen, M.D
Sacramento, CA, USA — Jason Rogers, M.D., FACC, FSCAI
Singapore, Singapore — Khung Keong Yeo, M.B.B.S., FACC, FSCAI

1

Mitral Valve Anatomy and Current Surgical and Percutaneous Approaches to Mitral Regurgitation

Jason Rogers, Olaf Franzen, and Steven F. Bolling

Abstract

The mitral valve apparatus consists of numerous anatomic elements which must interact in a coordinated manner to ensure normal leaflet movement and coaptation. Specifically, pathologies of the mitral annulus, chordae tendineae, papillary muscles, left ventricle, and left atrium can all result in mitral regurgitation (MR). In this chapter, we review current surgical and emerging percutaneous approaches for MR correction, with specific attention to anatomic targets for therapy, as well as the challenges faced by percutaneous techniques.

Keywords

Mitral regurgitation • MitraClip • Mitral valve repair • Mitral valve surgery • Percutaneous mitral valve repair

Introduction

The mitral valve apparatus consists of numerous anatomic elements which must interact in a coordinated manner to ensure normal leaflet movement and coaptation. Specifically, pathologies of the mitral annulus, chordae tendineae, papillary muscles, left ventricle, and left atrium can all result in mitral regurgitation (MR). Applying percutaneous or surgical therapies to correct MR depends on an understanding of the key structural elements that can be targeted for mechanical correction. In the case of MitraClip therapy, understanding the anatomic substrate for MR in each patient helps to individualize and guide therapy.

The Mitral Valve Apparatus

The mitral valve consists of anterior and posterior leaflets which are attached at their bases to a fibro-muscular annulus, and the leaflets are suspended by numerous chordae tendineae. These two leaflets are separated by the anterolateral and posteromedial commissures which bracket the mitral valve orifice. Although the anterior leaflet has a larger surface area, the posterior leaflet subtends a larger portion of the mitral annular circumference. The posterior leaflet is divided into three major scallops, named P1, P2, and P3 from lateral to medial. The anterior leaflet does not have formal scallops, and the anterior leaflet sections are named A1, A2, and A3 based on their adjacent positions to the posterior scallops (Fig. 1.1).

The mitral annulus has a three-dimensional "saddle" shape with the highest (farthest from the left ventricular

J. Rogers, M.D., FACC, FSCAI (✉)
Department of Cardiovascular Medicine, University of California, Davis Medical Center, 4860 Y Street, Suite 2820, Sacramento, CA 95817, USA
e-mail: jason.rogers@ucdmc.ucdavis.edu

O. Franzen, M.D.
Department of Cardiology, The Heart Center, Rigshospitalet, University of Copenhagen, Blegdamsvej 9, Copenhagen 2100, Denmark

Royal Brompton Hospital, Royal Brompton and Harefield NHS Foundation Trust, London, UK
e-mail: owfranzen@gmx.de

S.F. Bolling, M.D.
Department of Cardiothoracic Surgery, Section of Cardiac Surgery, University of Michigan Health System, 1500 E. Medical Center Dr. Floor 3, Ann Arbor, MI 48109, USA

Department of Cardiothoracic Surgery, University of Michigan Cardiovascular Center, University of Michigan, Ann Arbor, MI, USA
e-mail: sbolling@umich.edu

T. Feldman et al. (eds.), *Atlas of Percutaneous Edge-to-Edge Mitral Valve Repair*, DOI 10.1007/978-1-4471-4294-2_1,

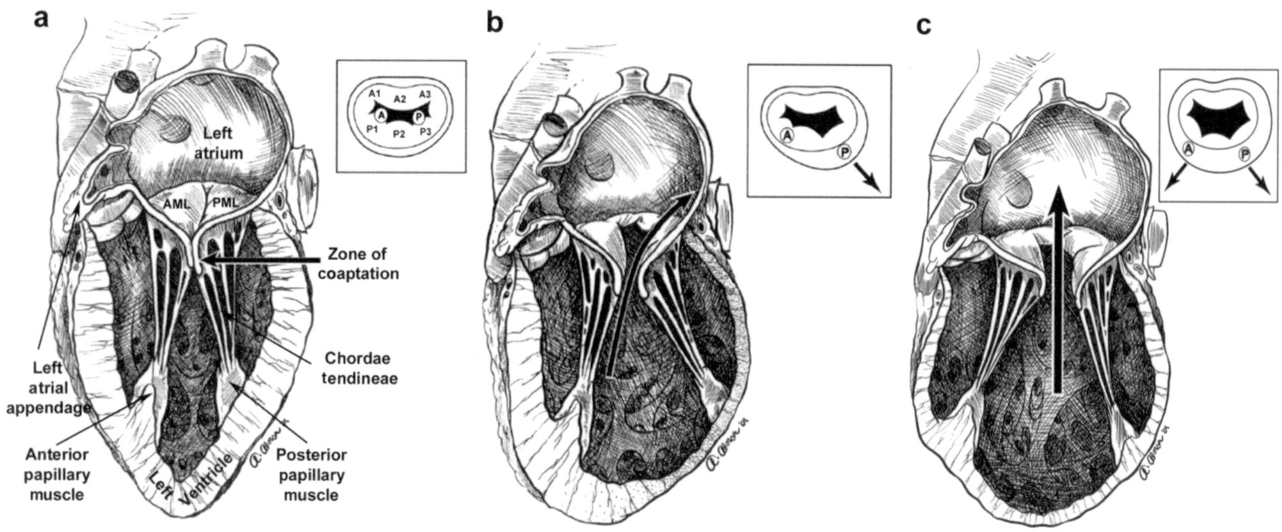

Fig. 1.1 Normal mitral valve anatomy and pathologic changes in functional mitral regurgitation. (**a**) Normal mitral valve anatomy. The zone of coaptation between the anterior and posterior mitral valve leaflets is intact with no mitral regurgitation (MR). Note the named segments of the mitral valve leaflets (A1-A3, P1-P3) and the position of the anterior and posterior papillary muscles within the mitral annular perimeter (*inset*). (**b**) Ischemic MR due to infarction of the infero-posterior wall, with displacement of the posterior papillary muscle outward, tethering of the posterior leaflet, and a posteriorly directed MR jet. (**c**) Functional MR due to global LV enlargement and outward displacement of both papillary muscles, with bileaflet tethering and a centrally directed MR jet. *AML* anterior mitral leaflet, *PML* posterior mitral leaflet

apex) portions located anteriorly and posteriorly, and the lowest portions located near the commissures. As seen from above, the annulus has an elliptical shape with the minor axis (septal-lateral dimension) being normally less than 30 mm [1]. The anterior portion of the mitral annulus contains the right and left fibrous trigones, two collagenous structures which demarcate the intersection of the aortic root with the mitral annulus. Between these fibrous trigones, the anterior mitral leaflet is in direct continuity with portions of the left and noncoronary aortic valve leaflets, forming the aortomitral curtain. This intimate aortic-mitral relationship has implications for percutaneous and surgical interventions on either valve, since maneuvers that alter the geometry of one valve may affect the other.

The chordae tendineae arise from two papillary muscles which are anchored in the left ventricular wall. The anterolateral papillary muscle has a single head, whereas the posterior papillary muscle often has two or more subheads. Both papillary muscles give rise to chordae tendineae which are attached to both mitral leaflets. The papillary muscles are aligned parallel to the intercommissural axis of the mitral valve. Importantly, the papillary muscles are separated from each other by a distance which optimizes leaflet motion and coaptation. With left ventricular enlargement or regional infarction, the papillary muscle position and function can change, applying traction to the leaflets which results in functional MR (FMR) (Fig. 1.1). The chordae that originate from the papillary muscle heads are known as first-order chordae, which then progressively divide into second- and third-order chordae. These chordae then insert either onto the free edge or body of the mitral leaflets. There are also basal chordae which arise directly from the ventricular wall and insert into the base of the mitral leaflets. Rupture of chordae tendineae (as well as primary leaflet prolapse from fibroelastic deficiency or myxomatous degeneration) can result in leaflet prolapse and/or flail with resultant degenerative MR (DMR). In properly selected cases, MitraClip therapy can reapproximate the leaflets and significantly reduce DMR or FMR.

In summary, proper function of the mitral leaflets depends on the complex interaction of the numerous structures that comprise the mitral apparatus, and coordinated left ventricular and left atrial functions are also important contributors to normal mitral leaflet motion.

Classification of Mitral Regurgitation and Surgical Correction

Etiologies of MR fall into several basic categories that have been previously described by Carpentier, Barlow, and others (Fig. 1.2) [2–4]. The classification proposed by Carpentier in 1972 described three classic mechanisms of MR. Type I dysfunction describes MR with normal leaflet motion due to annular dilation or leaflet perforation. Type II dysfunction is due to excessive leaflet motion from degenerative changes of the leaflets or chordae tendineae. Finally, Type III dysfunction is a result of restricted leaflet motion either due to leaflet thickening (rheumatic) or tethering of leaflets from papillary muscle or left ventricular dysfunction.

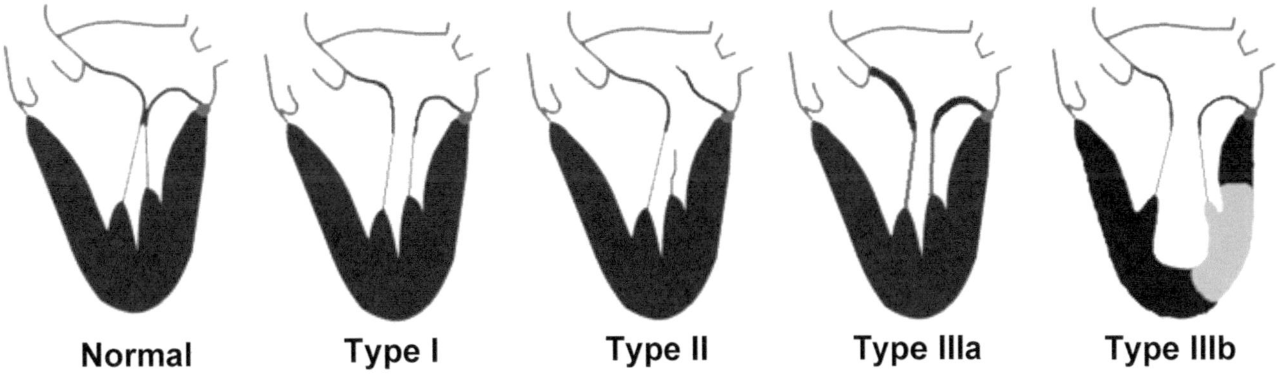

Fig. 1.2 Carpentier classification of mitral valve regurgitation. Type I: normal leaflet motion with annular dilation. Type II: increased leaflet motion (leaflet prolapse or flail). Type IIIa: restricted leaflet motion in systole and diastole, usually associated with leaflet and subvalvular thickening (rheumatic). Type IIIb: restricted leaflet motion in systole, often seen in ischemic cardiomyopathy with history of infarct (light region in left ventricle)

Presently, degenerative mitral regurgitation (DMR, Carpentier Type II dysfunction) is the most common form of MR referred for surgical correction. DMR occurs from fibroelastic deficiency with leaflet prolapse, myxomatous leaflet degeneration, or Barlow's disease with diffuse excess tissue and chordal elongation. The natural history of severe MR due to a flail posterior leaflet is known, with 90 % of patients expiring or requiring an MV operation within 10 years [5]. Compared to replacement, surgical MV repair is generally the preferred treatment for degenerative MR, since it affords improved postoperative outcomes and survival when compared to MV replacement [6]. Exceptions to this advantage may be in elderly subjects with degenerative MR using current valve-sparing techniques. Surgical intervention for degenerative MR consists of multiple techniques including leaflet repair with resection, chordal transfer, use of polytetrafluoroethylene neochordae, and prosthetic ring or band annuloplasty [7].

Functional MR (FMR, Carpentier Type I or IIIb) is far more prevalent than DMR and is due to underlying left ventricular dysfunction and annular dilation in the presence of normal leaflet anatomy. Since these patients universally have left ventricular dysfunction, they often have concomitant heart failure and a poorer prognosis than those with DMR. Surgical correction of FMR has not become the standard of care as it has for DMR. Patients with FMR are generally at higher surgical risk, and although surgical correction of FMR has been shown to improve functional class and left ventricular remodeling [8], there has been no proven survival benefit [9]. A major limitation of current surgical annuloplasty techniques is that up to one-third of treated patients have moderate or greater MR recur within 1 year of surgery [10–12]. Preoperative predictors of recurrent MR and poor outcomes after restrictive annuloplasty for FMR include LV end-diastolic diameter >65 mm [13], posterior leaflet angle ≥45° [14], and MV coaptation depth ≥11 mm [15].

The promise of percutaneous approaches to mitral regurgitation lies within the reduced morbidity of these approaches as compared to surgery and the potential to treat many patients not currently offered surgical correction. As many as 500,000 people in North America alone have clinically significant congestive heart failure–associated MR, most of whom are not offered mitral valve intervention. In Europe, it is estimated that one in three individuals over the age of 55 will develop heart failure [16]. Since even asymptomatic patients with severe MR have higher 5-year rates of death, heart, failure, and atrial fibrillation, consideration of valve repair is clinically warranted in these patients. Many patients with comorbidities and high surgical risk do not undergo surgery because of a failure to refer and perceived excessive morbidity and mortality [17, 18]. Until the advent of percutaneous mitral valve procedures, surgical mitral valve repair or replacement had been the sole option for treating MR.

Categories of Percutaneous Approaches to Mitral Regurgitation

Surgical therapies have evolved over several decades to address derangements of the annulus, leaflets, chordae tendineae, and left ventricle. In cases where repair is not feasible, mitral valve replacement is performed. Although percutaneous approaches have broadly mimicked surgical approaches, exact replication of surgical techniques is not easily attained. Therefore, several novel approaches have been developed, often loosely based on currently utilized or more obscure surgical methods. These percutaneous technologies have been categorized as those acting on or involving the leaflets, annulus, chordal implants, LV remodeling techniques, and percutaneous mitral valve replacement (Table 1.1) [19].

Table 1.1 Transcatheter therapies for mitral valve regurgitation

Target of therapy	Device name (manufacturer)	Mechanism of action
Leaflet repair	MitraClip (Abbott)	Clip-based edge-to-edge repair
	Percu-Pro (Cardiosolutions)	Regurgitant orifice space occupying
	Mobius (Edwards)	Suture-based edge-to-edge repair
Chordal implant	NeoChord (Neochord)	Synthetic chordae tendineae
Indirect annuloplasty	Carillon (Cardiac Dimensions)	Coronary sinus reshaping
	Monarc (Edwards)	Coronary sinus reshaping
	PTMA Device (Viacor)	Coronary sinus reshaping
	Mitral Cerclage (NIH)	Coronary sinus-right atrial encircling
	PS3 System (MVRx)	Transatrial coronary sinus-atrial septal shortening
Direct annuloplasty	Mitralign (Mitralign)	2×2 plicating anchors through posterior annulus
	AccuCinch (Guided Delivery Systems)	Plicating anchors in ventricular side of mitral annulus
	Cardioband (Valtech)	Plicating anchors on atrial side of mitral annulus
	QuantumCor (QuantumCor)	Radiofrequency energy shrinking annular collagen
	Millipede (Millipede)	Semirigid circumferential annular ring
Left ventricular reshaping	iCoapsys (Edwards)	Transventricular reshaping
	BACE (Mardil)	External basal myocardial reshaping
Mitral valve replacement	Endovalve-Herrmann (Endovalve)	Valve replacement
	CardiAQ (CardiAQ)	Valve replacement

Leaflet Repair

MitraClip Therapy

MitraClip therapy is an important therapeutic option for patients with mitral regurgitation, and clinical success with this device has given credence and momentum to the entire field of percutaneous mitral valve repair [20]. MitraClip therapy mimics surgical edge-to-edge repair first described by Ottavio Alfieri [21]. The surgical technique involves the use of suture at the free edge of the leaflets (generally at the A2/P2 interface) to convert a regurgitant mitral orifice into a competent double-orifice valve ("Alfieri" technique). The inspiration for this technique came from intraoperative inspection of a normal function of a congenital double-orifice mitral valve, which was then recreated surgically in subsequent patients [22]. While initially applied to patients primarily with complex degenerative disease involving anterior or bileaflet prolapse without annuloplasty (for fear of inducing stenosis), the technique has since been used in bileaflet prolapse with annuloplasty and also functional MR (Fig. 1.3) [23–26].

Briefly, the MitraClip device (described in detail within another chapter of this book) consists of a percutaneously delivered cobalt chromium implant with two arms and two grippers used to grasp the opposing free edges of the anterior and posterior leaflet in order to improve leaflet coaptation and generate a double-orifice valve. MitraClip therapy is intended for the treatment of MR that has a primarily central origin (A2/P2 interface), based on the original surgical technique described by Alfieri. The MitraClip has been applied successfully to a wide spectrum of degenerative (anterior, posterior, and bileaflet prolapse) and functional pathologies with central regurgitant jets. Regardless of regurgitation etiology, the final common objective of MitraClip implantation is the generation of a double-orifice valve (Fig. 1.4).

Although the surgical edge-to-edge technique has not been widely adopted by surgeons for routine mitral valve repair because of more sophisticated techniques which directly address leaflet pathologies (such as partial leaflet resection and chordal reconstruction or transfer), the simplicity of the edge-to-edge approach has held interest for application in selected patients and for the development of analogous percutaneous techniques such as MitraClip therapy.

Although the initial clinical results with the MitraClip have been encouraging, there has been discussion as to the potential importance of concomitant annuloplasty in edge-to-edge leaflet repair. Annuloplasty has become routine during surgical degenerative mitral valve repair, and it is also an essential component of surgery for functional MR. Failure to perform annuloplasty at the time of degenerative leaflet repair (either with partial leaflet resection techniques or with Alfieri repair) has been shown to adversely affect the repair durability [21, 27–29]. In ischemic MR, the application of edge-to-edge repair without annuloplasty has resulted in significant rates of recurrent MR [23, 24]. Maisano et al. demonstrated reasonable outcomes in a group of patients without concomitant annuloplasty. In a retrospective series of 29 patients with degenerative or functional MR, 5-year freedom from recurrent MR>2+ or reoperation was 90±5 % [30]. However, these patients generally had conditions which precluded ring implantation such as annular calcification, rheumatic disease, or previous failed attempts at repair. Whether or not emerging percutaneous annuloplasty procedures will be complementary to the MitraClip procedure and whether either will have robust stand-alone or long-term efficacy remains to be shown.

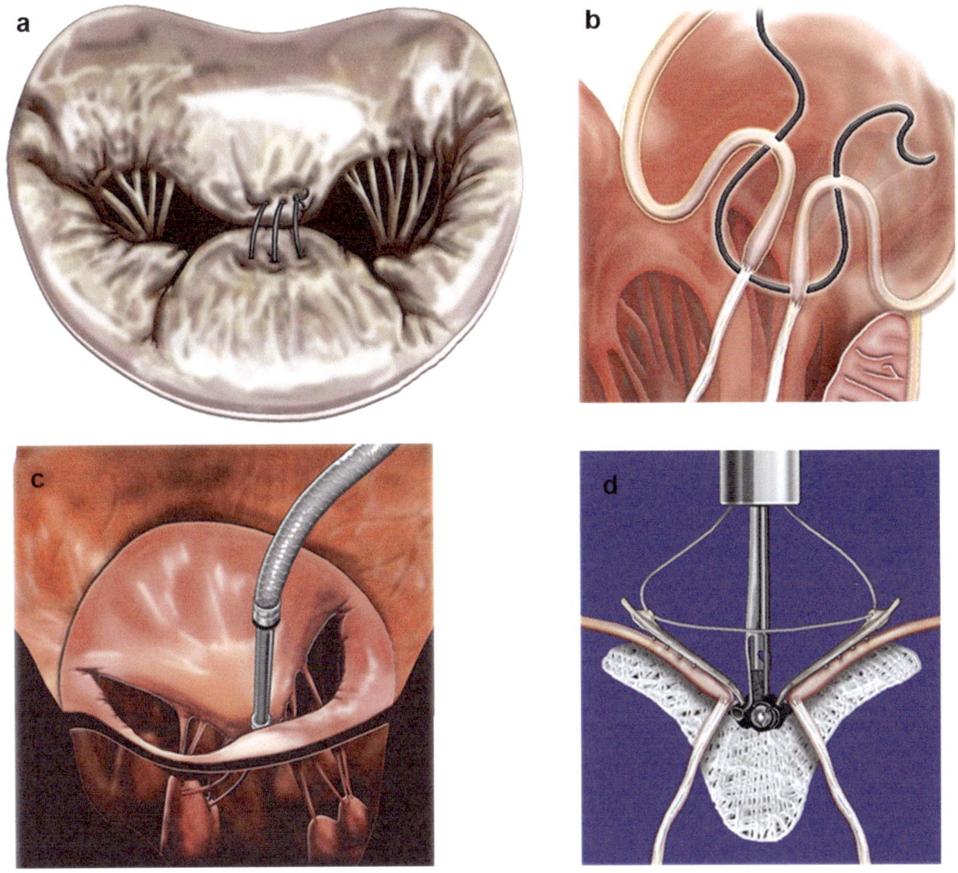

Fig. 1.3 The edge-to-edge approach to mitral valve repair. (**a**) The original surgical technique as described by Alfieri with suture approximation of the A2/P2 interface and creation of a double-orifice valve. (**b**) Detail of technique in which the leading edge of the leaflets are engaged with suture, followed by a second bite to gather redundant leaflet tissue. (**c**) The MitraClip device, which is attached to the delivery catheter, is being implanted in the center of the mitral valve. (**d**) Close-up of leaflets inserted between the MitraClip arms and grippers (Reprinted with permission from Maisano et al. [22], page 2175, Elsevier)

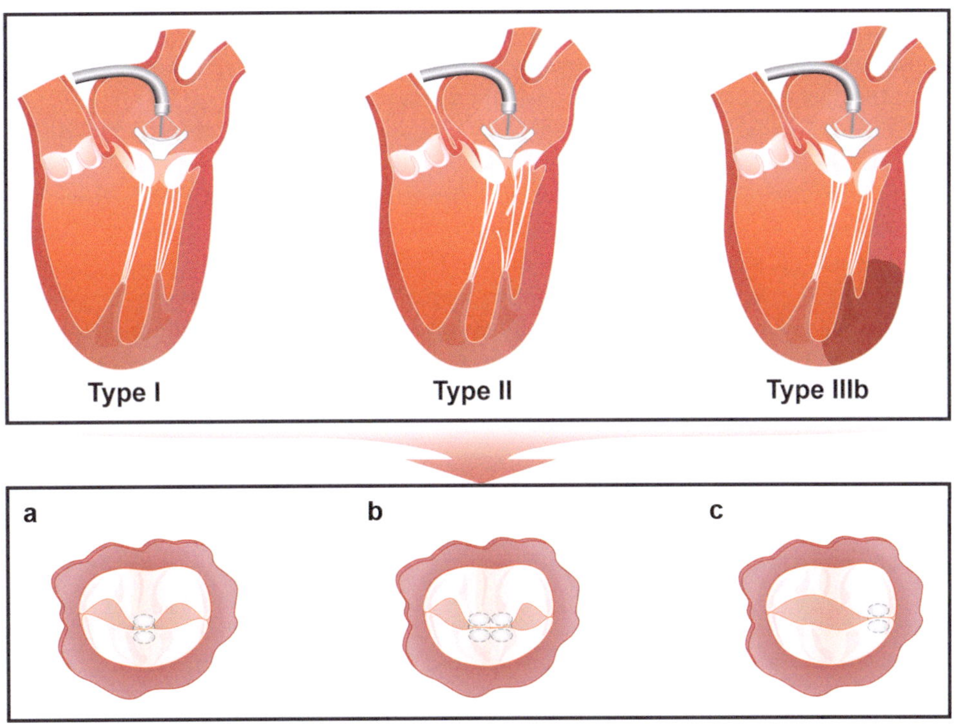

Fig. 1.4 Pathologies treatable with Mitraclip therapy. Multiple Carpentier types of MR can be treated with MitraClip therapy (*top panel*). The *lower panel* illustrates the final common pathway for MitraClip therapy. One or more MitraClips can be placed centrally with generation of a double orifice (**a**, **b**). For lateral jets, a MitraClip can be placed in the commissural region creating a single orifice (**c**) (Reproduced with permission from Rogers and Franzen [20], page 2553, Oxford Journals)

For patients with clinically significant recurrent MR after MitraClip therapy, it is preferred that surgical options for MV repair are preserved. This is most important in low surgical risk patients with DMR. It is debatable whether mitral valve repair after a failed MitraClip procedure in FMR should even be attempted, as a mortality difference has not

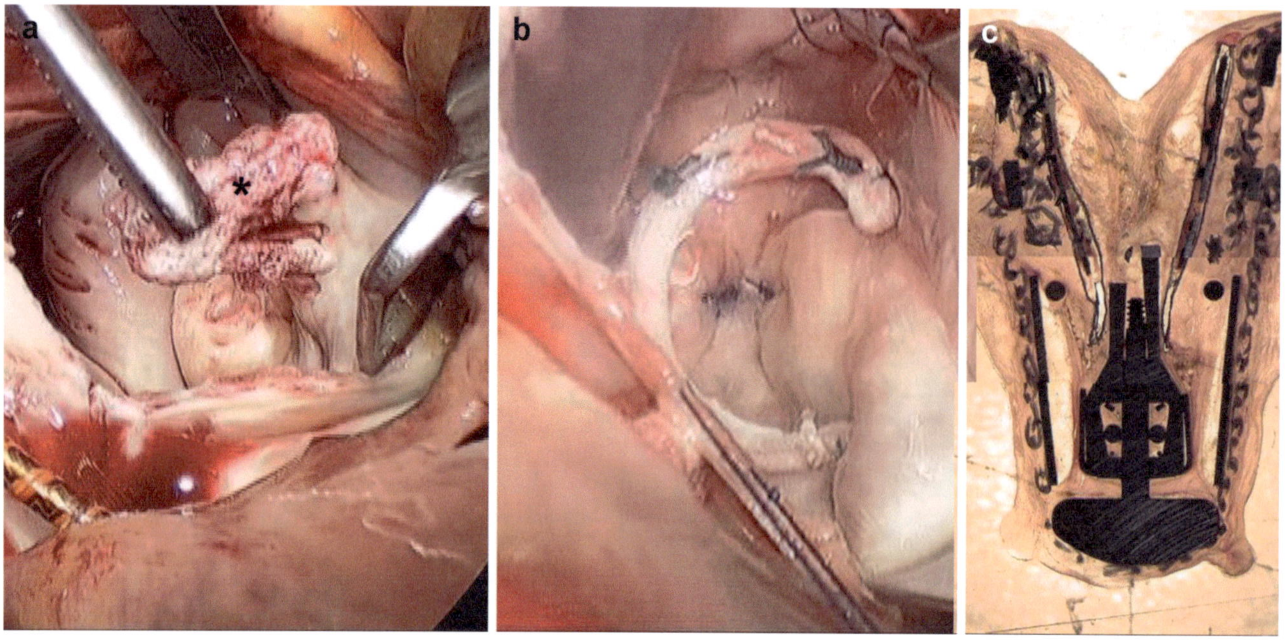

Fig. 1.5 Surgical repair after MitraClip therapy. (**a**) Surgical removal of MitraClip device (*asterisk*) which had been implanted 18 months prior. (**b**) Successful mitral valve repair with annuloplasty after MitraClip removal in the same patient. (**c**) Histologic cross section of the MitraClip 12 weeks after implantation in an animal model showing complete healing

been shown between repair and replacement in patients with ischemic MR up to 6 years after surgery [31]. Surgical repair can nonetheless be performed in many subjects successfully after MitraClip therapy, with successful repair having been reported up to 5 years after implantation [32, 33]. Not every patient will be able to have successful surgical repair after MitraClip therapy, and it is very likely that fibrosis over time will hinder successful clip removal without injuring the leaflets (Fig. 1.5). The degree to which this limitation will be clinically significant requires further study. In an analysis of subjects in the EVEREST II trial undergoing surgery after failed MitraClip therapy, the presence of anterior/bileaflet flail or prolapse was shown to be a significant predictor of the need for MV replacement. Additionally, surgeon experience (defined as the number of surgeries performed annually), duration of implant, or an operative note of valve injury or difficulty removing the device did not have an impact on whether a repair or replacement was performed [34].

Other Leaflet Repair Technologies

The Mobius device (Edwards Life Sciences, Irving, California) uses an innovative transseptal catheter with suction capability to grasp the leaflets and deliver suture to create a double-orifice valve. Despite feasibility, human clinical development was abandoned due to limited clinical benefit [35]. The Cardiosolutions Percu-Pro™ System (Cardiosolutions Inc., Stoughton, MA) is a percutaneously delivered balloon-shaped spacer that occupies the regurgitant mitral orifice and is anchored to the left ventricular apex. Animal studies have shown that the device is nonthrombotic with minimal inflammatory response.

Chordal Implantation

The NeoChord device is a beating-heart transapical approach to implantation of artificial chordae tendineae in patients with leaflet prolapse or flail. The system utilizes a fiber-optic feedback system to ensure the target leaflet is appropriately centered in the jaws of the device. The European TACT (Transapical Artificial Chordae Tendineae) Trial will enroll subjects with severe degenerative mitral regurgitation.

Annular Shape Change Approaches

Percutaneous techniques have been developed to mimic surgical annuloplasty. Whereas earlier approaches attempted to reshape the annulus “indirectly” by reshaping the coronary sinus, more recent techniques achieve more “direct” annuloplasty by attaching a series of anchors near or on the annulus which can be drawn together (plicated). Technology is being developed to replicate a surgical annuloplasty with a semi-rigid implantable circumferential annular ring.

Indirect Annuloplasty

The coronary sinus (CS) travels close to but up to 19 mm superior and external to the posterior mitral annulus [36] and is separated from the mitral annulus by nonfibrous atrial myocardium. Because of this distance, attempts to reshape the coronary sinus often do not effectively reshape the annulus. Several transcatheter devices which can be placed in the CS have been developed. Although these devices can be deployed with relative ease, significant limitations include the lack of robust and reproducible efficacy and the risk of coronary artery compression. A coronary artery (usually the circumflex) travels between the CS and mitral annulus up to 68 % of the time [37].

The Carillon Mitral Contour System (Cardiac Dimensions, Inc., Kirkland, WA) consists of a pair of helical self-expanding nitinol distal and proximal anchors connected by a nitinol bridge. The device is placed percutaneously in the coronary sinus from a right internal jugular vein approach and can be retrieved acutely if positioning or MR reduction is not favorable. The bridge can be shortened after the anchors are deployed in order to plicate posterior annular tissue and create movement of the posterior annulus anteriorly and reduce the septal-lateral dimension (Fig. 1.6).

The AMADEUS (CARILLON Mitral Annuloplasty Device European Union Study) trial was the first investigation into the potential role of a percutaneous CS-based intervention to reduce functional mitral regurgitation (FMR) in patients with heart failure [38], and, on the basis of the findings, the Carillon device was granted CE-mark approval in 2009. The subsequent prospective non-randomized TITAN (Tighten the Annulus Now) trial showed significant reduction in MR grade, favorable LV remodeling, and improved quality of life when compared to the control group of non-implanted subjects. Because of several clinically silent wire-form fractures in the device, a newer Carillon mXE2 device was developed and will be used in future trials. Despite promising early results, the device has limitations related to modest MR reduction and transient coronary compression, and further investigation is ongoing.

The Monarc device (Edwards Lifesciences, Irvine, CA) is a self-expanding device with distal and proximal stent-like anchors, and a connecting spring-like "bridge" with shape memory. The distal anchor is placed near the anterior interventricular vein and the proximal anchor near the ostium of the CS. The bridge has a dissolvable element which results in shortening over 3–6 weeks and improvement in MR. A pilot study in humans with the first-generation Viking device demonstrated acute feasibility, but there were device fractures in follow-up [39]. A second-generation device (Monarc device) has been studied in the prospective non-randomized EVOLUTION I and II trials (Clinical Evaluation of the Edwards Lifesciences Percutaneous Mitral Annuloplasty System for the Treatment of Mitral Regurgitation) [40]. Despite encouraging initial clinical results, the MONARC program is no longer undergoing active investigation.

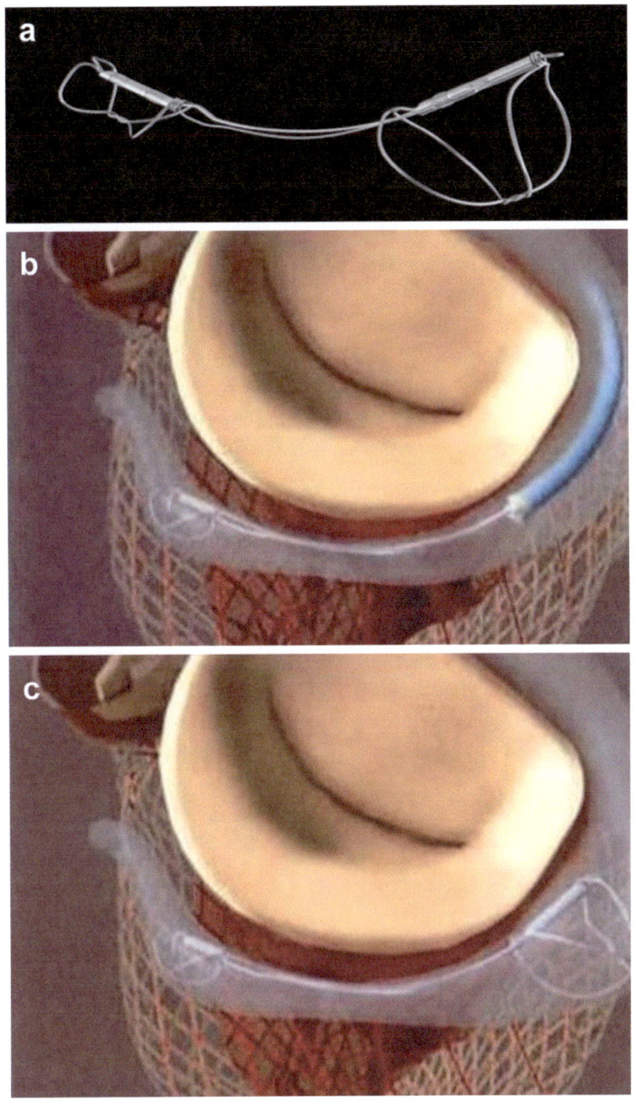

Fig. 1.6 Cardiac dimensions Carillon device. (**a**) The Carillon device. The distal anchor is smaller and deployed first in the distal great cardiac vein (**b**) traction applied, followed by proximal anchor deployment in the proximal great cardiac vein/coronary sinus (**c**)

The Viacor percutaneous transvenous mitral annuloplasty (PTMA) device (Viacor, Inc., Wilmington, Massachusetts) uses a coronary sinus catheter containing up to three nitinol rods of varying length and stiffness that exert a displacement force. The safety and feasibility of this device was reported for 19 subjects who underwent temporary "diagnostic device" implantation to assess acute MR reduction. Although it was feasible to implant this device in humans, further device development has been abandoned due to limited MR reduction and technical issues [41].

Other Coronary Sinus-Based Devices

Cerclage annuloplasty is an investigational technique which uses magnetic resonance imaging fused with fluoroscopy to encircle the annulus by passing a wire from the right atrium, through the coronary sinus, and reentering the right atrium by traversing a short segment of the basal septal myocardium. By tensioning the guidewire in a porcine model of ischemic cardiomyopathy, mitral annular size and MR grade can be decreased. A small curved nitinol tube can prevent coronary artery compression by acting as a miniature arch [42].

The Percutaneous Septal Sinus Shortening System (PS [3] System, MVRx, Belmont, CA) uses magnetic catheters in order to allow accurate placement of an anchor in the CS which is then connected to an anchor on the interatrial septum by a suture "bridge" which spans the left atrium. Tension can be applied to the bridge element, effectively shortening the septal-lateral (SL) dimension. Using an ovine model, the investigators found that device implantation with an average 24 % SL diameter reduction resulted in acute and chronic MR reduction [43]. Since this approach had shown early promise, temporary devices were implanted in a first-in-human study, confirming efficacy and significantly reducing MR [44]. Further studies have not been performed.

Direct Annuloplasty

Surgical closed-ring mitral annuloplasty is the preferred surgical gold approach for the treatment of functional mitral regurgitation. Prior to the advent of rigid rings, suture-based annuloplasty based on the prior work by Paneth and Burr had been used [45]. Although this technique can result in reductions of the septal-lateral dimension and mitral annular circumference, this technique has been abandoned since the durability of suture-based or nonrigid annuloplasty has been shown to be inferior to rigid mitral annular rings [12, 46, 47]. Nonetheless, given the ability to achieve suture-based annuloplasty through percutaneous approaches, several transcatheter approaches have been developed. Other approaches include the application of radiofrequency energy and the development of a percutaneously delivered circumferential mitral annuloplasty ring.

The Mitralign Percutaneous Annuloplasty System (Mitralign, Inc., Tewksbury, MA) is based on surgical suture annuloplasty of the mitral valve. The Mitralign procedure involves a left ventricular approach through retrograde femoral arterial access. A deflectable catheter is placed under the posterior mitral leaflet, beneath the annular tissue under the valve. The procedure is performed under fluoroscopic and echocardiographic guidance. A specially designed catheter carries two crossing wires (the "bident") that are passed from the ventricular aspect of the annulus into the left atrium using a brief application of radiofrequency energy. These wires then serve as the guides over which two sets of paired anchors are placed through the posterior annulus of the mitral valve. These anchors are plicated together, resulting in segmental posterior annuloplasty and reduction in mitral regurgitation (Fig. 1.7). This technology is undergoing safety and feasibility testing in Europe and South America.

The AccuCinch System (Guided Delivery Systems, Santa Clara, CA), which is also based on the suture annuloplasty method, is focused on correction of annular dilation. This procedure uses a retrograde femoral arterial approach to gain access to the ventricular side of the mitral annulus. Using a proprietary catheter, 9–12 anchors can be placed from the

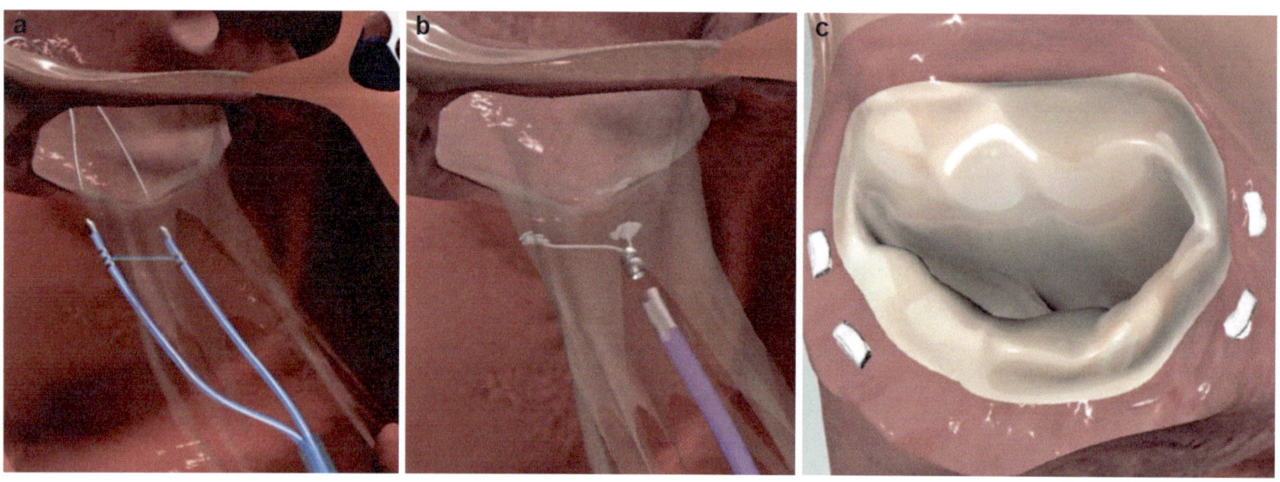

Fig. 1.7 Mitralign Annuloplasty System. (**a**) A deflectable catheter allows passage of the "bident" crossing wires through the mitral annulus from the left ventricle to the left atrium. (**b**) Paired pledgeted sutures are placed on opposite sides of the posterior annulus, and then tensioned. (**c**) Final appearance of 2 x 2 annular plication

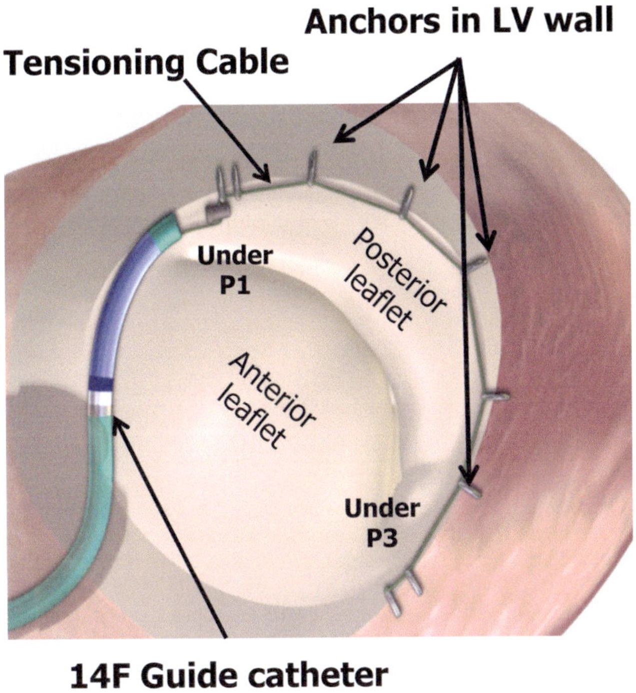

Fig. 1.8 Guided Delivery Systems Percutaneous Ventriculoplasty. Subvalvular placement of anchors are plicated using a tensioning cable along the LV free wall via a retrograde transfemoral approach

anterior to posterior commissures under the posterior mitral annulus. The anchors are then connected by a suture element and tensioned to reduce the mitral annular circumference (Fig. 1.8). Chronic surgical and percutaneous human implants have been performed.

The QuantumCor System (QuantumCor, Bothell, WA) is based on the concept of thermal remodeling of collagen. Since the mitral valve annulus has significant collagen content, catheter-based application of radiofrequency (RF) energy at subablative temperatures to the mitral annulus will heat and contract the collagen fibers, thereby reducing mitral annular circumference. This technology has been proven to reduce mitral annular dimensions and mitral regurgitation in an animal model [48]. The favorable aspects of this technology are that no material is left behind and that repeat applications can be applied. Therapy in humans has not yet been reported.

The Millipede system (Millipede, Inc., Minneapolis, MN) attempts to mimic a surgical circumferential and rigid annuloplasty. This consists of the placement of a novel expandable annular ring with an innovative attachment system via either minimally invasive surgical or percutaneous methods to restore the native mitral annular shape and diameter. The device will be repositionable and retrievable prior to deployment and could be used to treat functional MR or as an adjunct to leaflet repair technologies.

The Cardioband (Valtech Ltd., Or Yehuda, Israel) allows a series of anchors to be placed percutaneously onto the left atrial aspect of the mitral annulus. These anchors are connected by a sleeve which can be tightened, resulting in reduction of the mitral annular circumference.

Ventricular Reshaping Technologies

The iCoapsys system (Edwards, Irvine, CA) is a novel transcatheter method of reshaping the left ventricle. The procedure is based on the surgically placed Coapsys system which has been shown to reduce mitral regurgitation [49]. Under fluoroscopic and echocardiographic guidance, the iCoapsys intra-pericardial anchoring devices are placed on the epicardial ventricular surfaces in an anterior-posterior configuration and are connected by a tethering suture that passes through the left ventricle. By applying tension to the suture, the geometry of the ventricle is made more elliptical with decreased leaflet tethering and improved coaptation. Further development of the device was terminated due to device complexity and other technical issues

The BACE device (basal annuloplasty of the cardia externally, Mardil Inc., Morrisville, North Carolina) requires a mini-thoracotomy and is implanted on a beating heart. It consists of a silicone band with inflatable chambers that is placed around the atrioventricular groove.

Percutaneous Mitral Valve Replacement

Although surgical mitral valve repair is generally preferable to replacement for degenerative MR, many pathologies will not be easily repaired using percutaneous techniques. Therefore, percutaneous mitral valve replacement (PMVR) may be important for several reasons. First, PMVR could result in superior reduction of MR compared to repair. Second, for patients with FMR, replacement may be an attractive option, as there is no proven mortality difference between repair and replacement in patients with FMR [31]. Significant technical challenges must be overcome, including secure anchoring and elimination of paravalvular leaks. Patients with FMR will generally have large mitral annular diameters, and devices should occupy the orifice without paravalvular leak.

The Endovalve-Herrmann Mitral Valve (Endovalve, Inc., Princeton, NJ) is a foldable nitinol-based valve in development with a sealing skirt that attaches to the mitral valve apparatus. It is valve sparing and repositionable before release. The CardiAQ prosthesis (CardiAQ Valve Technologies, Winchester, MA), which is also in development, can be delivered by a transseptal approach. The valve is attached to a self-expanding nitinol frame which centers itself on the mitral annulus (Fig. 1.9).

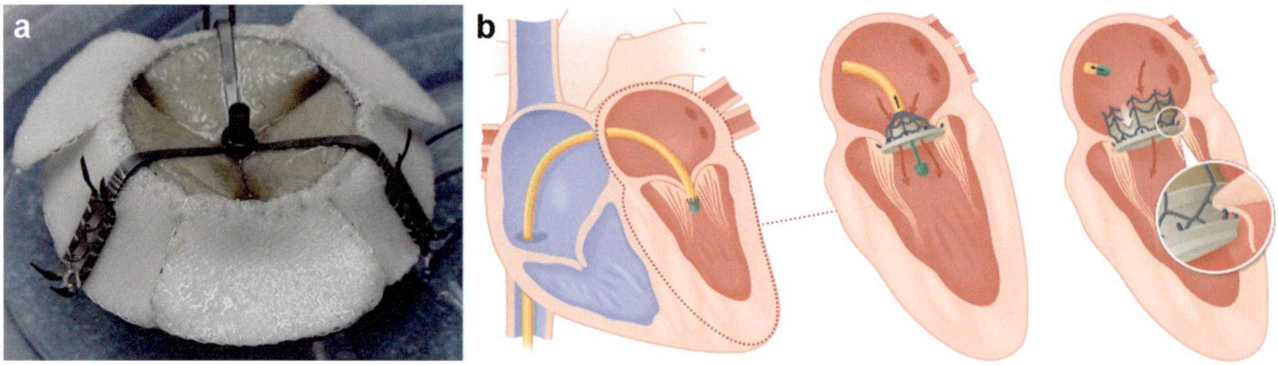

Fig. 1.9 Percutaneous mitral valve replacements. (**a**) The Endovalve-Herrmann prosthesis, shown also in collapsed form (*inset*). (**b**) Schematic of delivery of CardiAQ prosthesis via transseptal route with self-expanding frame

Conclusion

Numerous percutaneous technologies have been developed in an effort to treat mitral regurgitation. To date, the MitraClip device is the only percutaneous mitral valve repair technology to have completed a pivotal trial and to achieve significant adoption, especially in subjects at high risk for surgery. Continued innovation is necessary to develop viable repair and replacement approaches and to expand the population of subjects which can be treated with percutaneous therapies.

References

1. Kaji S, Nasu M, Yamamuro A, et al. Annular geometry in patients with chronic ischemic mitral regurgitation: three-dimensional magnetic resonance imaging study. Circulation. 2005;112(9 Suppl): I409–14.
2. Carpentier A. Cardiac valve surgery – the “French correction”. J Thorac Cardiovasc Surg. 1983;86(3):323–37.
3. Adams DH, Rosenhek R, Falk V. Degenerative mitral valve regurgitation: best practice revolution. Eur Heart J. 2010;31(16):1958–66.
4. Barlow JB, Pocock WA. The significance of late systolic murmurs and mid-late systolic clicks. Md State Med J. 1963;12:76–7.
5. Ling LH, Enriquez-Sarano M, Seward JB, et al. Clinical outcome of mitral regurgitation due to flail leaflet. N Engl J Med. 1996;335(19): 1417–23.
6. Enriquez-Sarano M, Schaff HV, Orszulak TA, Tajik AJ, Bailey KR, Frye RL. Valve repair improves the outcome of surgery for mitral regurgitation. A multivariate analysis. Circulation. 1995; 91(4):1022–8.
7. Seeburger J, Falk V, Borger MA, et al. Chordae replacement versus resection for repair of isolated posterior mitral leaflet prolapse: a egalite. Ann Thorac Surg. 2009;87(6):1715–20.
8. Bax JJ, Braun J, Somer ST, et al. Restrictive annuloplasty and coronary revascularization in ischemic mitral regurgitation results in reverse left ventricular remodeling. Circulation. 2004;110 (11 Suppl 1):II103–8.
9. Wu AH, Aaronson KD, Bolling SF, Pagani FD, Welch K, Koelling TM. Impact of mitral valve annuloplasty on mortality risk in patients with mitral regurgitation and left ventricular systolic dysfunction. J Am Coll Cardiol. 2005;45(3):381–7.
10. Hung J, Papakostas L, Tahta SA, et al. Mechanism of recurrent ischemic mitral regurgitation after annuloplasty: continued LV remodeling as a moving target. Circulation. 2004;110(11 Suppl 1): II85–90.
11. Marwick TH. Restrictive annuloplasty for ischemic mitral regurgitation: too little or too much? J Am Coll Cardiol. 2008;51(17):1702–3.
12. McGee EC, Gillinov AM, Blackstone EH, et al. Recurrent mitral regurgitation after annuloplasty for functional ischemic mitral regurgitation. J Thorac Cardiovasc Surg. 2004;128(6):916–24.
13. Braun J, van de Veire NR, Klautz RJ, et al. Restrictive mitral annuloplasty cures ischemic mitral regurgitation and heart failure. Ann Thorac Surg. 2008;85(2):430–6; discussion 436–7.
14. Magne J, Pibarot P, Dagenais F, Hachicha Z, Dumesnil JG, Senechal M. Preoperative posterior leaflet angle accurately predicts outcome after restrictive mitral valve annuloplasty for ischemic mitral regurgitation. Circulation. 2007;115(6):782–91.
15. Calafiore AM, Gallina S, Di Mauro M, et al. Mitral valve procedure in dilated cardiomyopathy: repair or replacement? Ann Thorac Surg. 2001;71(4):1146–52; discussion 1152–53.
16. Bleumink GS, Knetsch AM, Sturkenboom MC, et al. Quantifying the heart failure epidemic: prevalence, incidence rate, lifetime risk and prognosis of heart failure. The Rotterdam Study. Eur Heart J. 2004;25(18):1614–9.
17. Mirabel M, Iung B, Baron G, et al. What are the characteristics of patients with severe, symptomatic, mitral regurgitation who are denied surgery? Eur Heart J. 2007;28(11):1358–65.
18. O’Brien SM, Shahian DM, Filardo G, et al. The Society of Thoracic Surgeons 2008 cardiac surgery risk models: part 2–isolated valve surgery. Ann Thorac Surg. 2009;88(1 Suppl):S23–42.
19. Chiam PT, Ruiz CE. Percutaneous transcatheter mitral valve repair: a classification of the technology. JACC Cardiovasc Interv. 2011; 4(1):1–13.
20. Rogers JH, Franzen O. Percutaneous edge-to-edge MitraClip therapy in the management of mitral regurgitation. Eur Heart J. 2011;32(19):2350–7.
21. Alfieri O, Maisano F, De Bonis M, et al. The double-orifice technique in mitral valve repair: a simple solution for complex problems. J Thorac Cardiovasc Surg. 2001;122(4):674–81.
22. Maisano F, La Canna G, Colombo A, Alfieri O. The evolution from surgery to percutaneous mitral valve interventions: the role of the edge-to-edge technique. J Am Coll Cardiol. 2011;58(21): 2174–82.
23. Bhudia SK, McCarthy PM, Smedira NG, Lam BK, Rajeswaran J, Blackstone EH. Edge-to-edge (Alfieri) mitral repair: results in diverse clinical settings. Ann Thorac Surg. 2004;77(5):1598–606.
24. De Bonis M, Lapenna E, La Canna G, et al. Mitral valve repair for functional mitral regurgitation in end-stage dilated cardiomyopathy:

role of the "edge-to-edge" technique. Circulation. 2005;112(9 Suppl):I402–8.
25. Maisano F, Schreuder JJ, Oppizzi M, Fiorani B, Fino C, Alfieri O. The double-orifice technique as a standardized approach to treat mitral regurgitation due to severe myxomatous disease: surgical technique. Eur J Cardiothorac Surg. 2000;17(3):201–5.
26. Maisano F, Torracca L, Oppizzi M, et al. The edge-to-edge technique: a simplified method to correct mitral insufficiency. Eur J Cardiothorac Surg. 1998;13(3):240–5; discussion 245–6.
27. Flameng W, Herijgers P, Bogaerts K. Recurrence of mitral valve regurgitation after mitral valve repair in degenerative valve disease. Circulation. 2003;107(12):1609–13.
28. Gillinov AM, Cosgrove DM, Blackstone EH, et al. Durability of mitral valve repair for degenerative disease. J Thorac Cardiovasc Surg. 1998;116(5):734–43.
29. DiBardino DJ, ElBardissi AW, McClure RS, Razo-Vasquez OA, Kelly NE, Cohn LH. Four decades of experience with mitral valve repair: analysis of differential indications, technical evolution, and long-term outcome. J Thorac Cardiovasc Surg. 2010;139(1):76–83; discussion 83–4.
30. Maisano F, Vigano G, Blasio A, Colombo A, Calabrese C, Alfieri O. Surgical isolated edge-to-edge mitral valve repair without annuloplasty: clinical proof of the principle for an endovascular approach. EuroIntervention. 2006;2(2):181–6.
31. Magne J, Girerd N, Senechal M, et al. Mitral repair versus replacement for ischemic mitral regurgitation: comparison of short-term and long-term survival. Circulation. 2009;120(11 Suppl):S104–11.
32. Argenziano M, Skipper E, Heimansohn D, et al. Surgical revision after percutaneous mitral repair with the MitraClip device. Ann Thorac Surg. 2010;89(1):72–80; discussion p. 80.
33. Rogers JH, Yeo KK, Carroll JD, et al. Late surgical mitral valve repair after percutaneous repair with the MitraClip system. J Card Surg. 2009;24(6):677–81.
34. Glower D, Young JN, Alexander J, et al. EVEREST II randomized clinical trial: a critical assessment of anatomical predictors of de novo mitral valve replacement or following the MitraClip procedure. J Am Coll Cardiol. 2010;56(13, Supplement 1):B25.
35. Webb JG, Maisano F, Vahanian A, et al. Percutaneous suture edge-to-edge repair of the mitral valve. EuroIntervention. 2009;5(1):86–9.
36. Maselli D, Guarracino F, Chiaramonti F, Mangia F, Borelli G, Minzioni G. Percutaneous mitral annuloplasty: an anatomic study of human coronary sinus and its relation with mitral valve annulus and coronary arteries. Circulation. 2006;114(5):377–80.
37. Tops LF, Van de Veire NR, Schuijf JD, et al. Noninvasive evaluation of coronary sinus anatomy and its relation to the mitral valve annulus: implications for percutaneous mitral annuloplasty. Circulation. 2007;115(11):1426–32.
38. Schofer J, Siminiak T, Haude M, et al. Percutaneous mitral annuloplasty for functional mitral regurgitation: results of the CARILLON Mitral Annuloplasty Device European Union Study. Circulation. 2009;120(4):326–33.
39. Webb JG, Harnek J, Munt BI, et al. Percutaneous transvenous mitral annuloplasty: initial human experience with device implantation in the coronary sinus. Circulation. 2006;113(6):851–5.
40. Harnek J, Webb JG, Kuck KH, et al. Transcatheter implantation of the MONARC coronary sinus device for mitral regurgitation: 1-year results from the EVOLUTION phase I study (Clinical Evaluation of the Edwards Lifesciences Percutaneous Mitral Annuloplasty System for the Treatment of Mitral Regurgitation). JACC Cardiovasc Interv. 2011;4(1):115–22.
41. Sack S, Kahlert P, Bilodeau L, et al. Percutaneous transvenous mitral annuloplasty: initial human experience with a novel coronary sinus implant device. Circ Cardiovasc Interv. 2009;2(4):277–84.
42. Kim JH, Kocaturk O, Ozturk C, et al. Mitral cerclage annuloplasty, a novel transcatheter treatment for secondary mitral valve regurgitation: initial results in swine. J Am Coll Cardiol. 2009;54(7):638–51.
43. Rogers JH, Macoviak JA, Rahdert DA, Takeda PA, Palacios IF, Low RI. Percutaneous septal sinus shortening. A novel procedure for the treatment of functional mitral regurgitation. Circulation. 2006;113(19):2329–32.
44. Palacios IF, Condado JA, Brandi S, et al. Safety and feasibility of acute percutaneous septal sinus shortening: first-in-human experience. Catheter Cardiovasc Interv. 2007;69(4):513–8.
45. Burr LH, Krayenbuhl C, Sutton MS. The mitral plication suture: a new technique of mitral valve repair. J Thorac Cardiovasc Surg. 1977;73(4):589–95.
46. Aybek T, Risteski P, Miskovic A, et al. Seven years' experience with suture annuloplasty for mitral valve repair. J Thorac Cardiovasc Surg. 2006;131(1):99–106.
47. Nagy ZL, Bodi A, Vaszily M, Szerafin T, Horvath A, Peterffy A. Five-year experience with a suture annuloplasty for mitral valve repair. Scand Cardiovasc J. 2000;34(5):528–32.
48. Heuser RR, Witzel T, Dickens D, Takeda PA. Percutaneous treatment for mitral regurgitation: the QuantumCor system. J Interv Cardiol. 2008;21(2):178–82.
49. Mishra YK, Mittal S, Jaguri P, Trehan N. Coapsys mitral annuloplasty for chronic functional ischemic mitral regurgitation: 1-year results. Ann Thorac Surg. 2006;81(1):42–6.

Device Description and Procedural Overview

2

Mehmet Cilingiroglu, Gretchen T. Gary, and Ted Feldman

Abstract

The MitraClip device has been in US trials since 2003 and in clinical use internationally since 2008. A great deal has been learned about how to perform the procedure since its inception. This chapter details the technique of percutaneous mitral leaflet repair. The mechanics of the procedure and the associated echocardiographic and anatomic imaging necessary to understand the procedure are reviewed in a step-by-step guide. The chapter is of interest to anyone wishing to learn how to perform this novel therapy or for operators who wish to learn more. Cardiologists, cardiac catheterization lab nurses and technicians, and echocardiographic technicians will also find the chapter informative.

Keywords

Mitral regurgitation • MitraClip • Procedure • Technique

Device Description and Procedural Overview

Over the last decade, as significant advances have been made in developing minimally invasive surgical repair of valvular heart disease, several percutaneous catheter-based technologies have been tested for the repair of severe mitral regurgitation (MR). In a surgical technique that was initially described by Dr. Ottavio Alfieri and his group in 1991, the placement of one or more sutures, approximating the edges of the mitral leaflets at the origin of the MR jet, led to the creation of a so-called bow-tie or double orifice with a significant reduction in the MR jet and has immediate and long-term sustainable results. Adapted from this technique, the MitraClip (Abbott Laboratories, Menlo Park, CA) has rapidly evolved as the only percutaneous method to gain wide clinical application for mitral valve repair (MVR) for selected patients. The procedure requires a dedicated team of physicians and is performed under general anesthesia using fluoroscopy and primarily transesophageal echocardiographic (TEE) guidance in the cardiac catheterization laboratory. The main procedure elements are well developed with a significant

M. Cilingiroglu, M.D., FSCAI, FACC
Department of Medicine/Cardiology,
UPMC Heart and Vascular Institute,
Pittsburgh, PA, USA
e-mail: mcilingiroglu@yahoo.com

G.T. Gary, B.A.
Abbott Vascular Structural Heart,
200 Abbott Park Road, AP52-1,
Abbott Park, IL 60064-6214, USA
e-mail: gretchen.gary@av.abbott.com

T. Feldman, M.D., FESC, FACC, FSCAI (✉)
NorthShore University Health System,
Evanston, IL, USA

Cardiology Division, Evanston Hospital,
Walgreen Building 3rd Floor, 2650 Ridge Ave.,
Evanston, IL 60201, USA
e-mail: tfeldman@northshore.org

T. Feldman et al. (eds.), *Atlas of Percutaneous Edge-to-Edge Mitral Valve Repair*,
DOI 10.1007/978-1-4471-4294-2_2, © Springer-Verlag London 2013

learning curve. It is critical that the interventional operator and the echocardiographer have a common vocabulary for the basic procedural TEE views so that clear communication can be maintained during the procedure. The US-based randomized Endovascular Valve Edge-to-Edge Repair Study (EVEREST) clinical trials showed both the safety and efficacy of this therapy. The device is already CE approved and is being used increasingly for the percutaneous repair of both high surgical risk degenerative as well as functional MR patients in Europe, Asia, and Australia. In the USA as of this printing, its use is still under investigation and is not yet FDA approved.

MitraClip Device

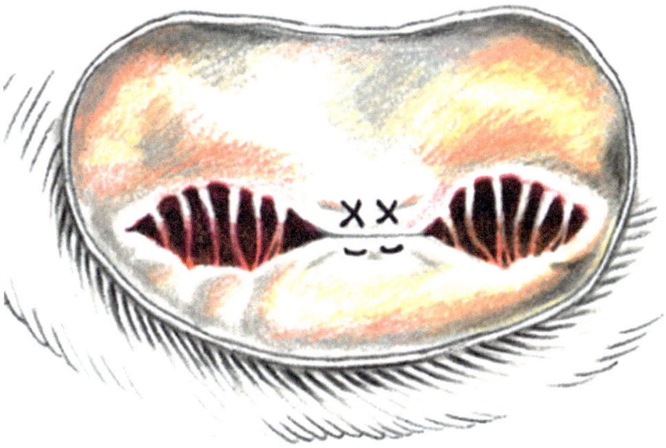

Fig. 2.1 Double-orifice surgical MVR with a suture. Surgical repair of anterior leaflet prolapse using an edge-to-edge technique by opposing the middle scallops of the anterior and posterior leaflets with stitches creating a so-called dual-orifice or double-orifice mitral valve is shown [1–3]. The clinical success and simplicity of this technique prompted interest in development of a catheter-based MitraClip technology that would enable the interventional cardiologist to perform a percutaneous, endovascular valve repair in the cardiac catheterization laboratory

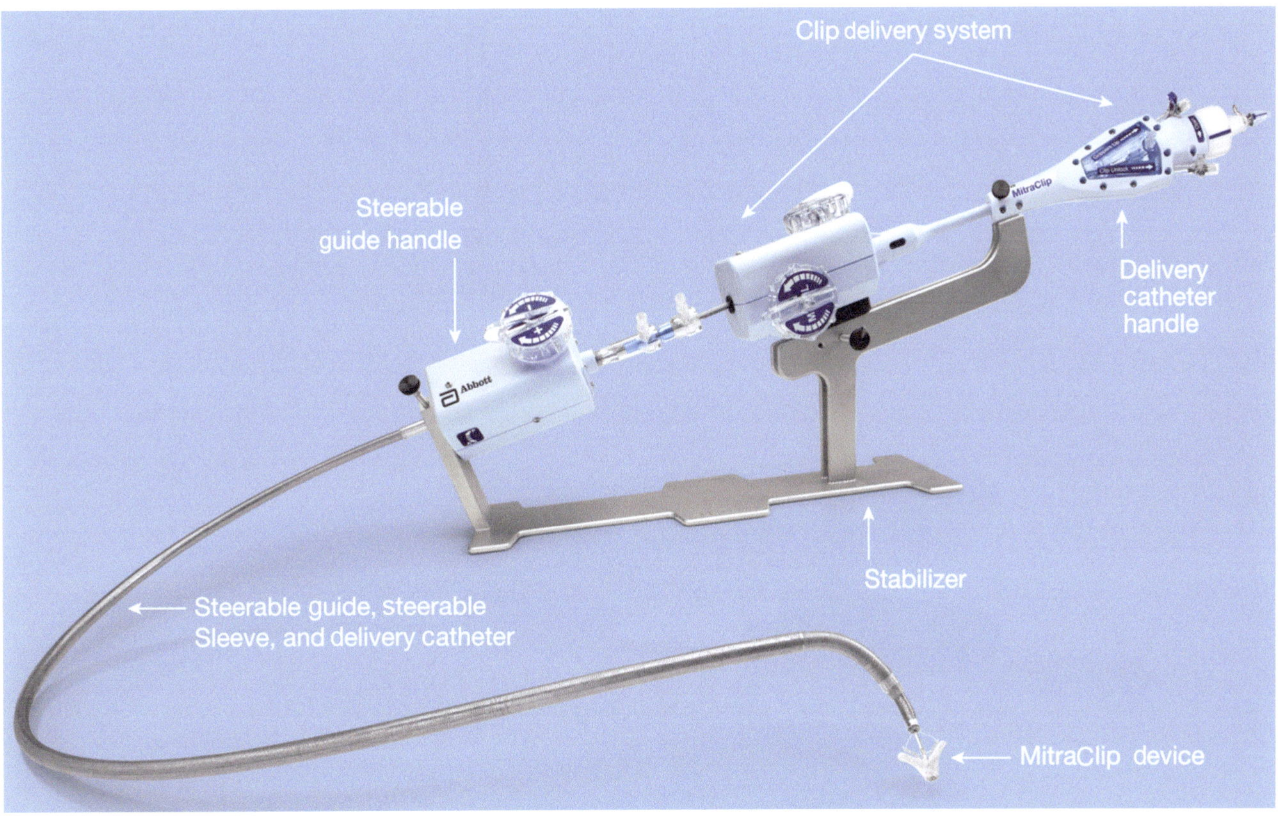

Fig. 2.2 Components of the MitraClip system. The MitraClip system consists of a 24-Fr steerable guide catheter and a clip delivery system (CDS), which includes the detachable clip itself. The guide catheter tapers down to 22 Fr at the point where it crosses the atrial septum. A steering knob on the proximal end of the guide catheter marked as "±"allows for flexion and movement of the distal tip [4–12]

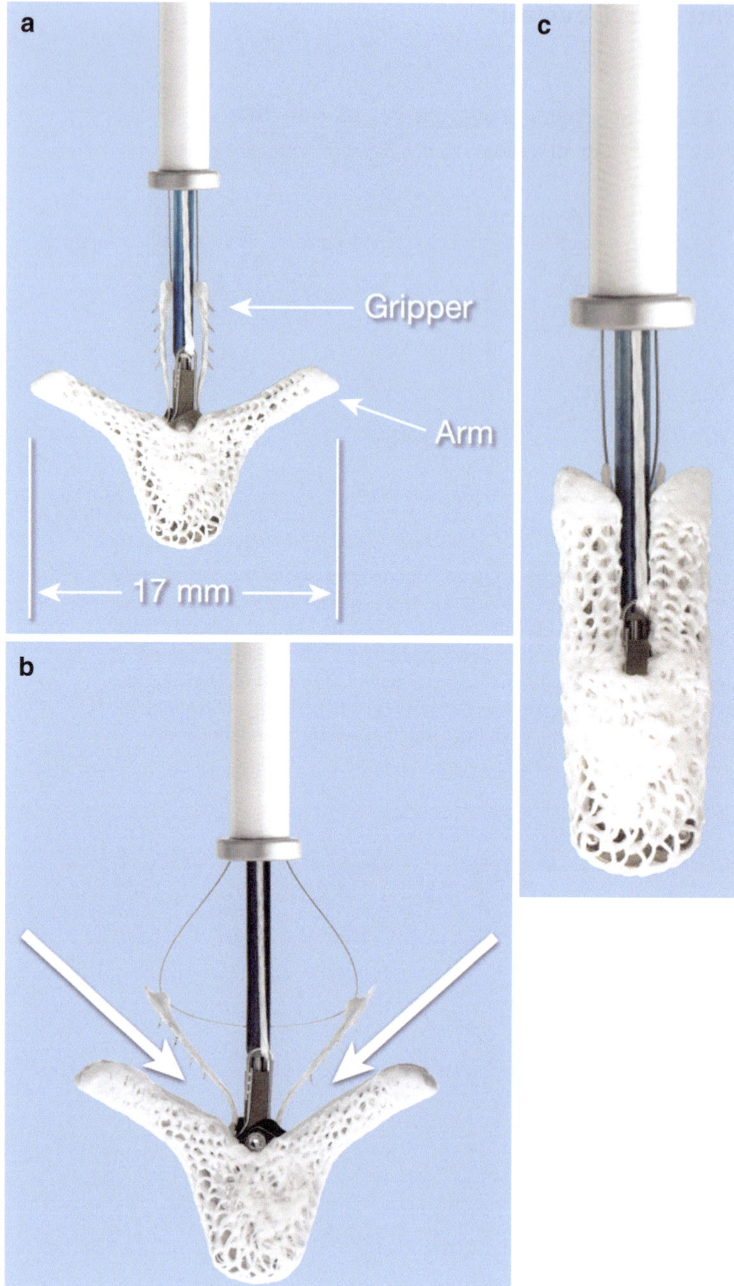

Fig. 2.3 The MitraClip. (**a**) The clip itself is a polyester-covered mechanical device with two arms that are opened and closed by control mechanisms on the CDS. The two arms have a span of approximately 2 cm when opened in the grasping position. On the inner portion of the clip are U-shaped "grippers," as indicated by the *arrows* which appose and stabilize the leaflets from the atrial aspect as they are captured during closure of the clip arms. When closed, the clip has an outside diameter of 15 Fr. It is designed to hold up to 8 mm of leaflet height (*vertically*) and 4 mm of width (*horizontally*). (**b**) Leaflet tissue is secured between the arms and each side of the gripper, and (**c**) the clip is then closed and locked to effect and maintain coaptation of the two leaflets

Procedural Technique

A 6-Fr arterial and an 8-Fr venous sheath are placed in the left femoral artery (LFA) and femoral vein (FV), respectively. Alternatively, radial artery and internal jugular venous access can be obtained to minimize groin access sites. A 14-Fr sheath is placed in the right FV for transseptal access and guide catheter delivery. Using the left femoral access, a 7-Fr balloon-tipped pulmonary artery catheter and a 6-Fr pigtail left ventricular (LV) catheter are placed. Cardiac output, baseline pulmonary capillary wedge, and LV and pulmonary artery pressures are measured. An activated clotting time (ACT) of 250–300 s is maintained throughout the procedure, with ACT measurements taken every 30 min.

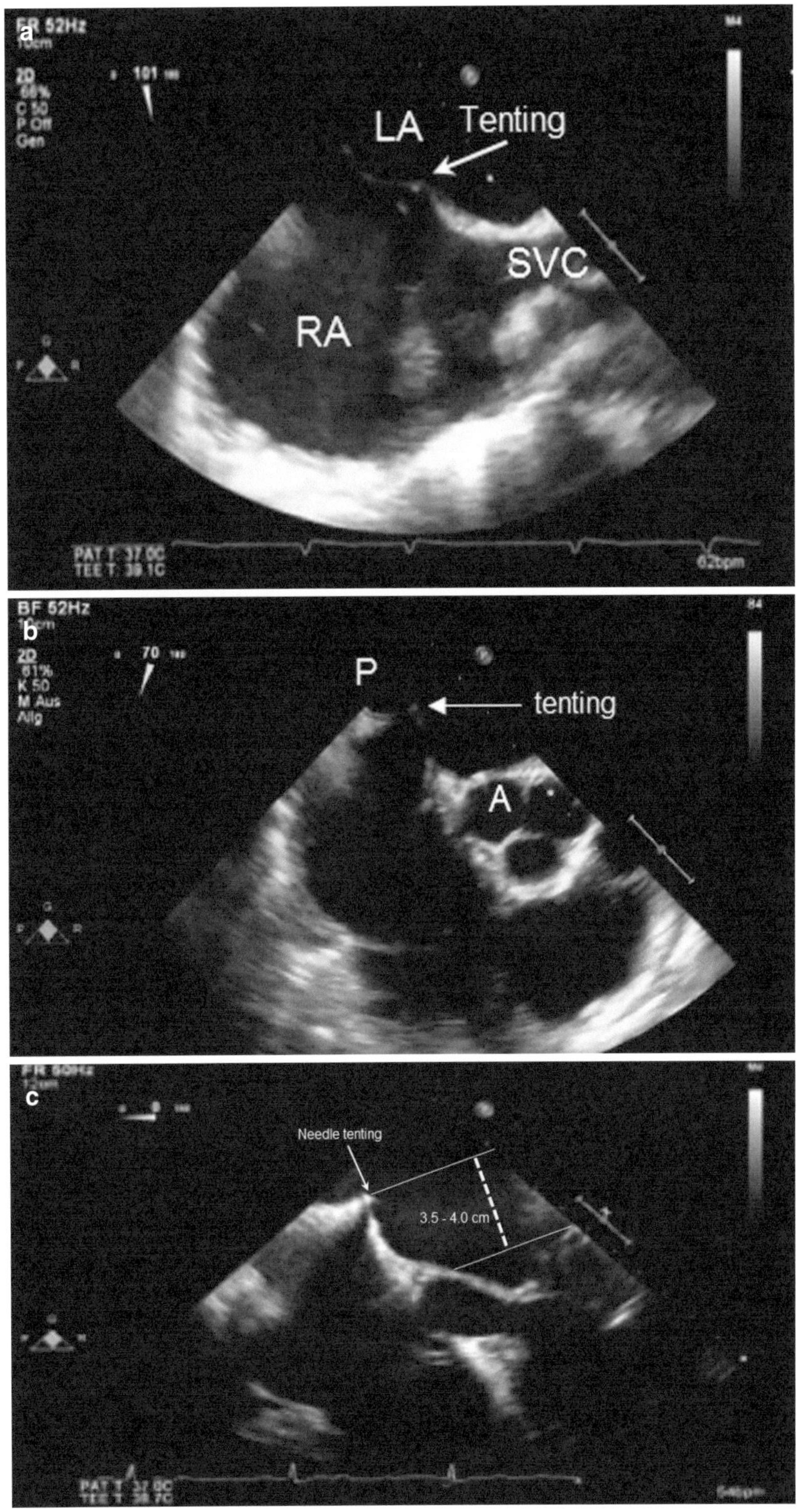

Fig. 2.4 TEE-guided transseptal puncture. Initially, an 8-Fr Mullins sheath and then a transseptal needle are advanced into the right atrium (*RA*). A TEE-guided transseptal puncture is performed in a location, ideally in the superior and posterior part of the interatrial septum with the aim of obtaining adequate working space and distance above the mitral annulus (the ideal height from the annulus should be 3.5–4.0 cm). Using TEE bicaval (**a**) and short-axis views at the base of the heart (**b**) the position of the puncture site is evaluated, and the "tenting" of the atrial septum can be seen as the transseptal needle is pushed against it. In the short-axis view (**b**) the tenting should be close to the posterior edge, and in the bicaval view (**a**) it should be at the junction of the muscular and membranous septum. Afterward, using a long-axis four-chamber view (**c**) the catheter tip should be moved to as "high" a position as possible while remaining in the fossa ovalis. A transseptal puncture should be only performed if such tenting is clearly seen in both of these views (**a**, **b**)

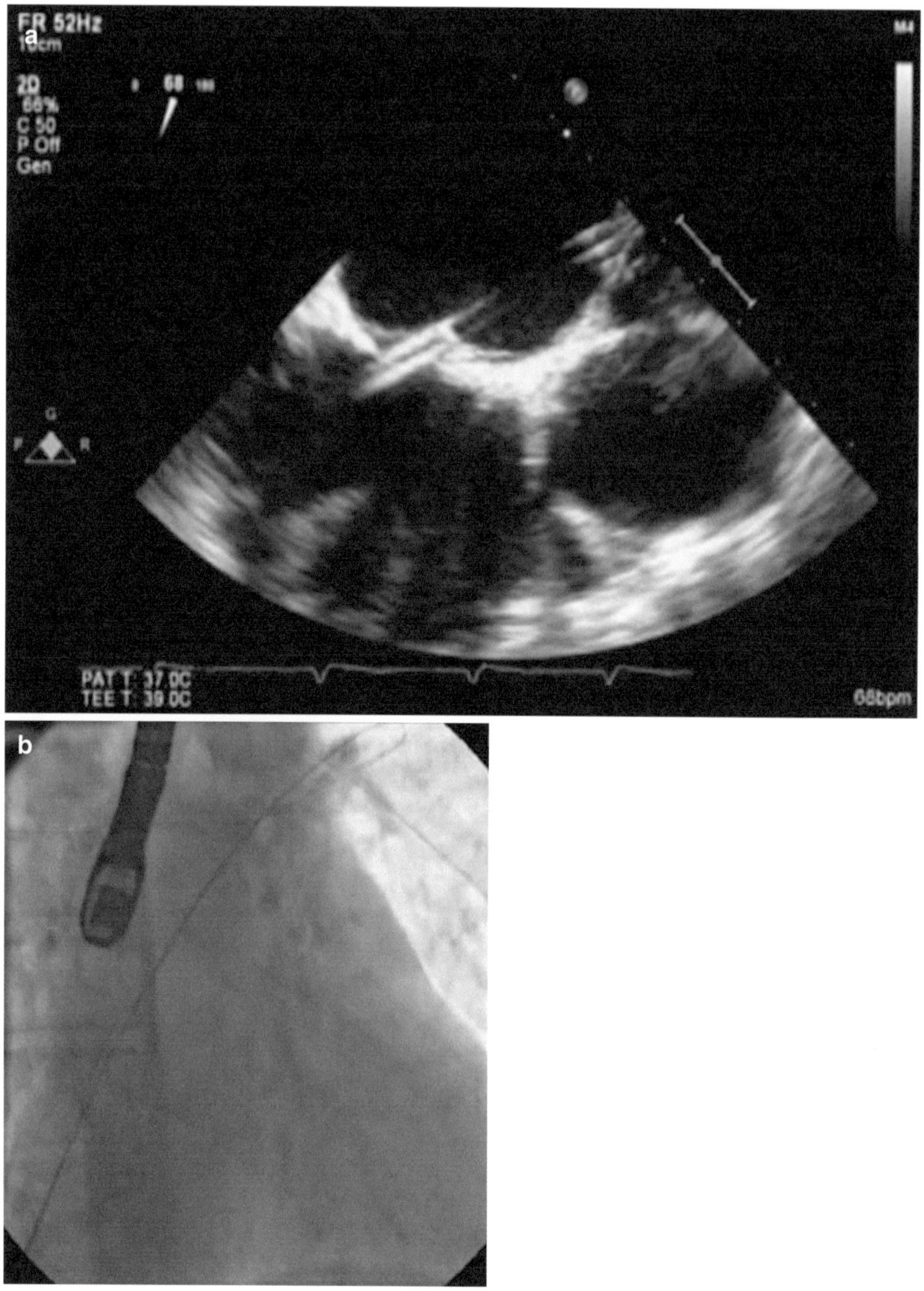

Fig. 2.5 Advancement of Mullins sheath into the LA and placement of guide wire. (**a**) After the appropriate transseptal puncture is achieved, an 8-Fr Mullins sheath is advanced into the LA, and LA–LV pressure is measured at the baseline. (**b**) A 260-cm (0.035-in.), extra-stiff J-tipped Amplatzer guide wire is then placed, ideally in the left superior pulmonary vein or alternatively looped in the LA. Intravenous heparin is given (50–70 units/kg) to achieve ACT greater than or equal to 250 s

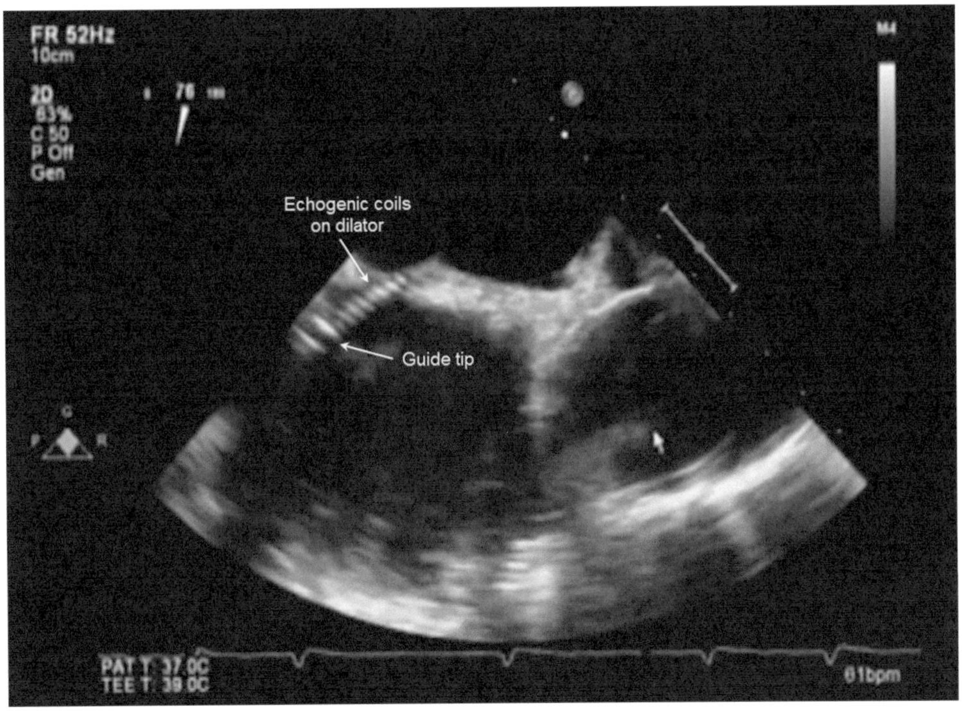

Fig. 2.6 Dilation of the interatrial septum. After removing the Mullin's sheath, the puncture site is dilated to accommodate a 22-Fr guide catheter by gentle and forward movement of the dilator tip, which can be visualized by TEE due to echogenic coils. When the dilator tip is halfway to three-quarters across the septum, waiting a few seconds is often useful to allow the atrial septum to stretch

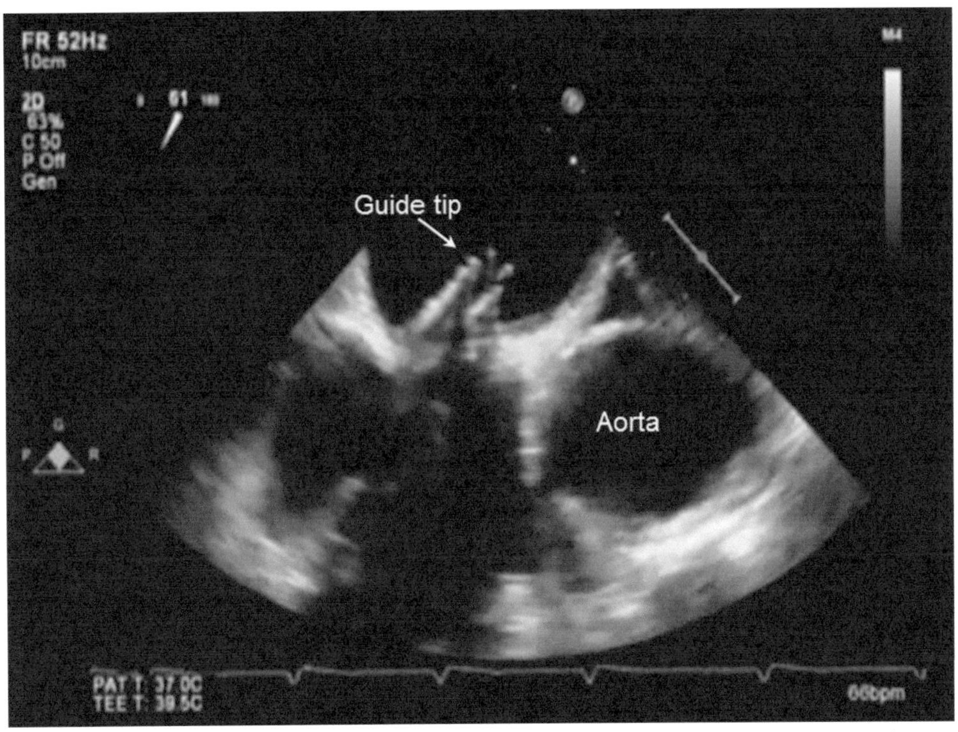

Fig. 2.7 Advancement of the guide catheter into the LA. It is very important not to place the guide catheter tip too far into the LA to avoid contact with LA walls, but rather to aim for a position of its tip about 1 or 2 cm across the atrial septum in the center of the LA in the short-axis view at the base. It is critical to carefully de-air the guide catheter upon removal of the dilator and guide wire assembly once the guide catheter tip is 1–2 cm across the atrial septum prior to advancement of CDS

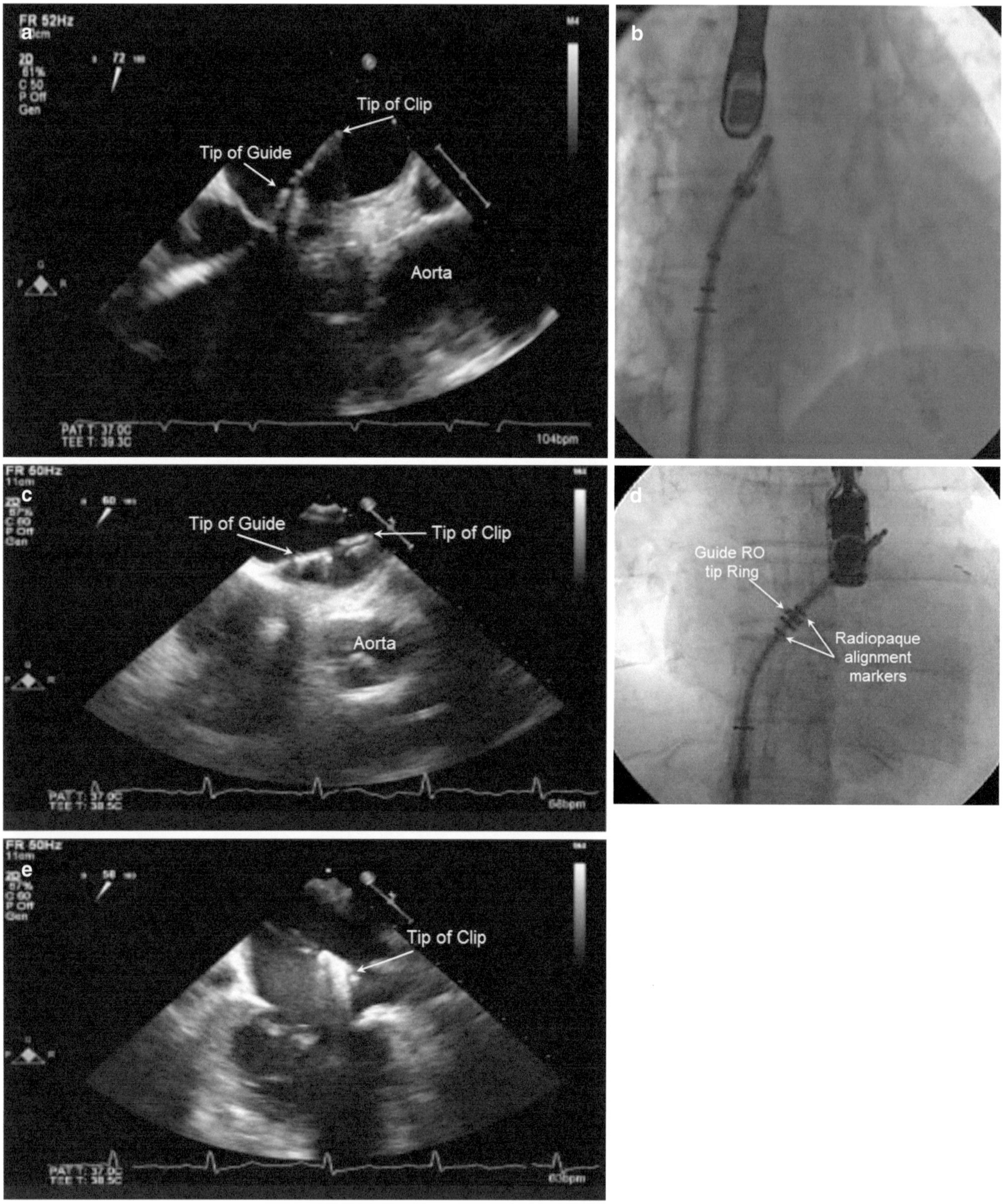

Fig. 2.8 Steering and positioning of the MitraClip CDS in the LA. Once introduced into the guide catheter, the CDS is advanced until its tip is even with the guide tip under fluoroscopic guidance. Then, the CDS is further advanced into the LA while observing the MitraClip device in the short axis at the base or two-chamber intercommissural TEE views to avoid tissue contact (**a**, **b**). The CDS is further advanced until the guide radiopaque (RO) tip ring marker is centered between the sleeve alignment markers with confirmation on fluoroscopy (**c**, **d**). Afterward, the CDS is steered down toward the mitral valve (**e**)

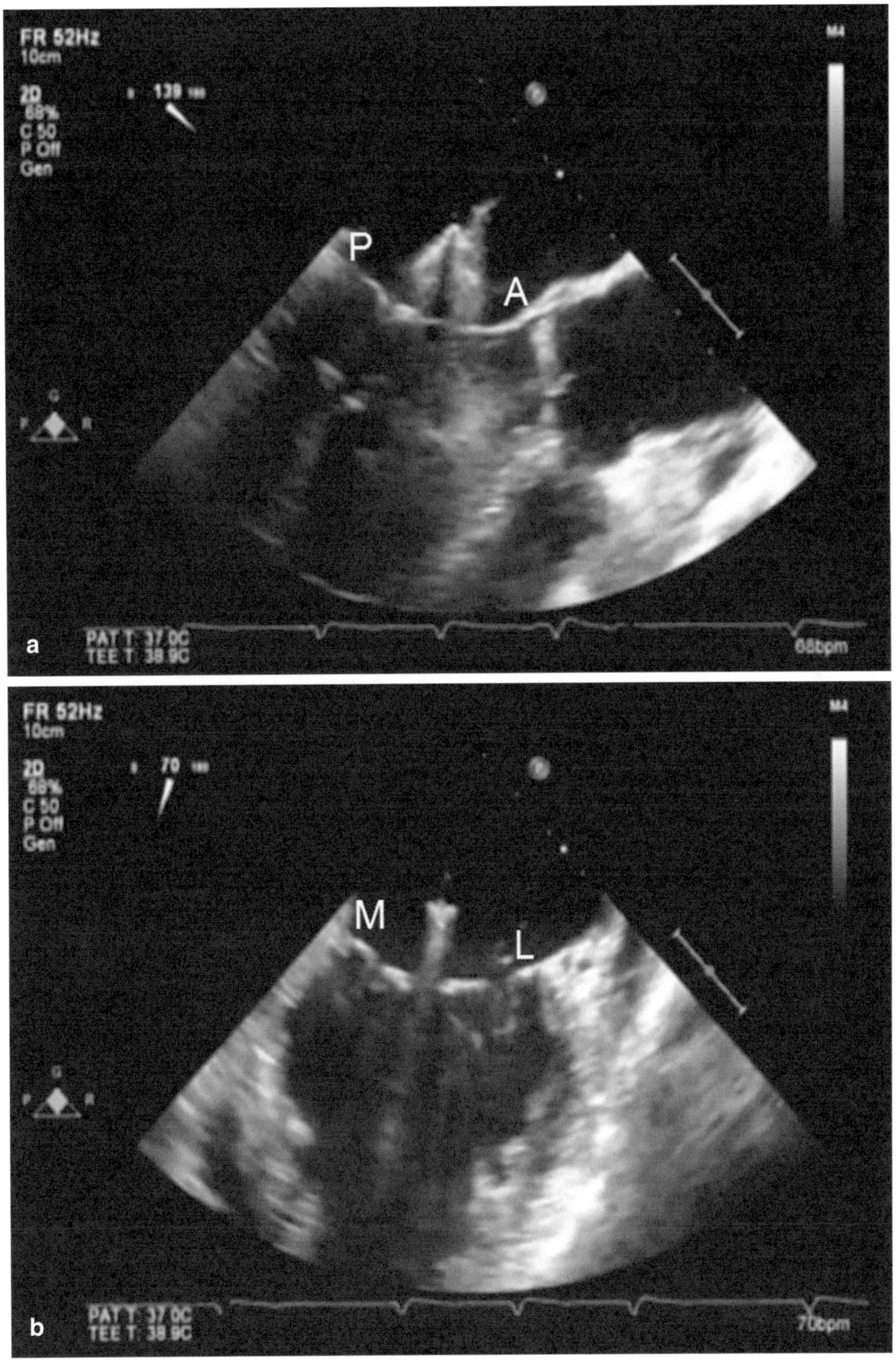

Fig. 2.9 Steering the clip toward the mitral valve. The MitraClip device is then steered down until the trajectory is perpendicular to the line between the annular hinge points of the mitral valve in both the left ventricular outflow tract (LVOT) anteroposterior (*A-P*) alignment and two-chamber intercommisural mediolateral (*M-L*) alignment imaging planes (**a**, **b**). The clip is positioned over the MR jet origin to split the jet (**c**)

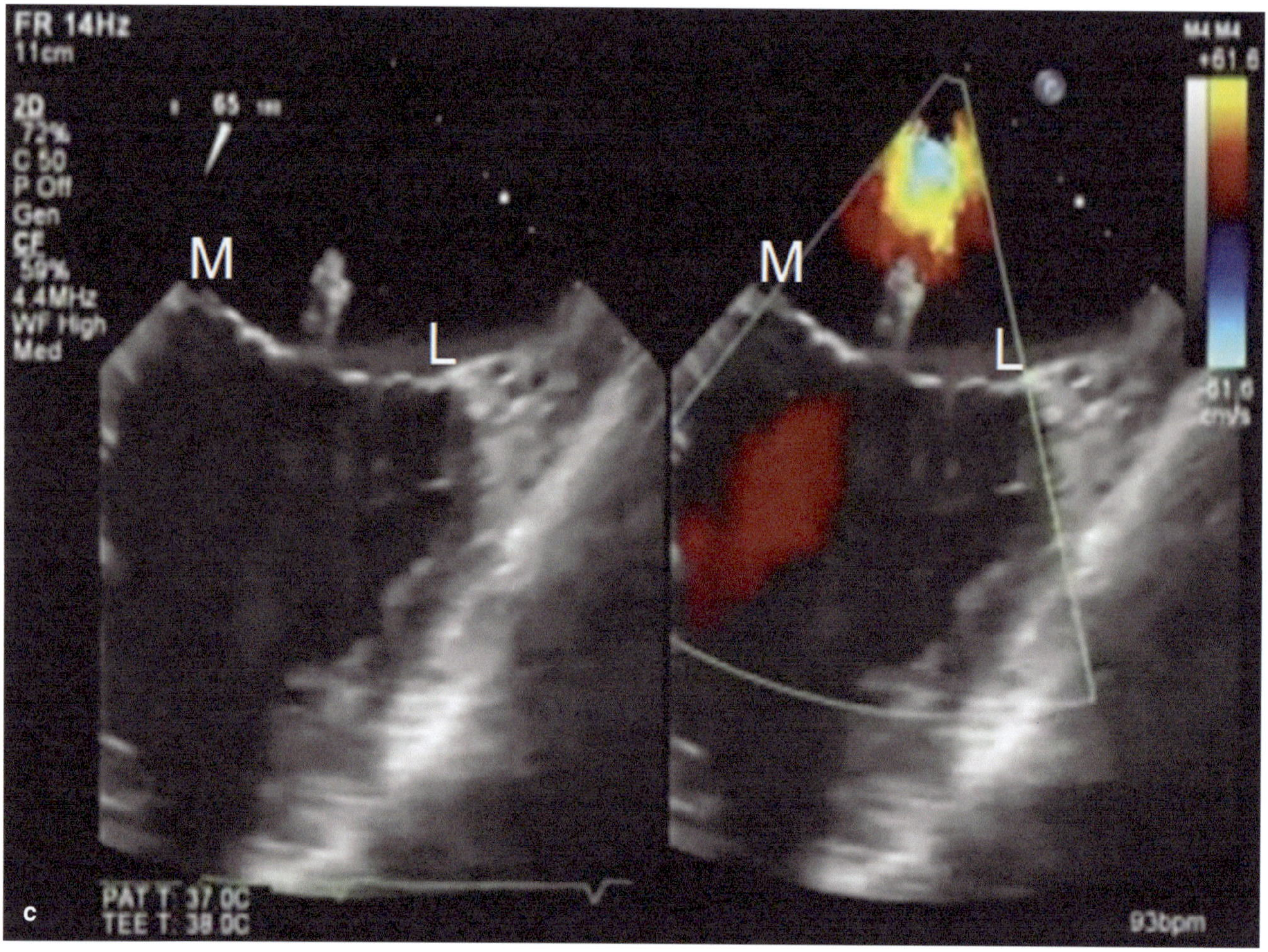

Fig. 2.9 (continued)

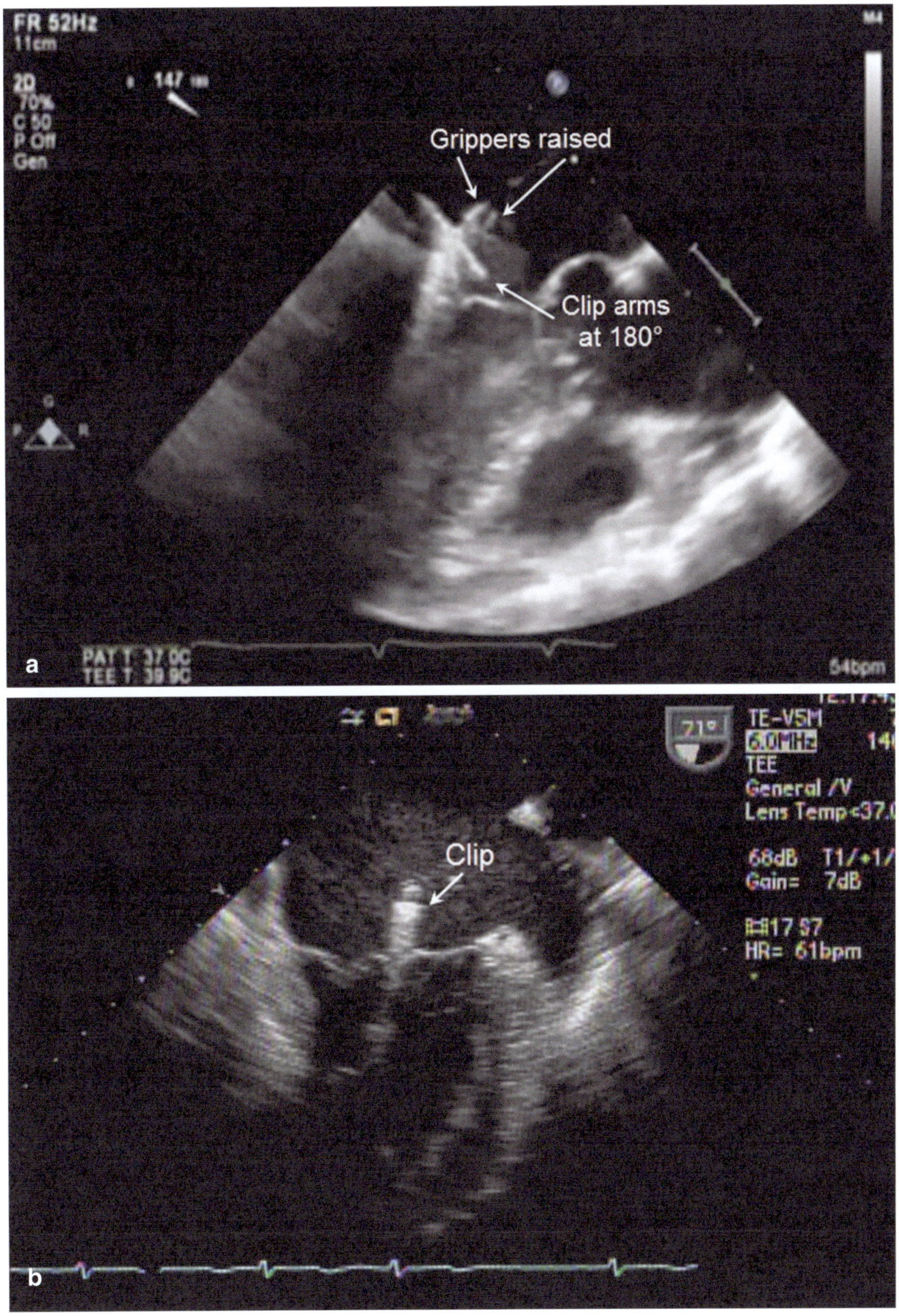

Fig. 2.10 Opening of the clip arms. The clip arms are opened to 180° and aligned perpendicular to the line of coaptation in the LVOT view. In the LVOT view, the open arms should be visible and symmetric (**a**). Arm alignments are checked also in the two-chamber intercommissural and the transgastric short-axis or 3D En Face views (**b**, **c**). *L* lateral, *M* medial

Fig. 2.10 (continued)

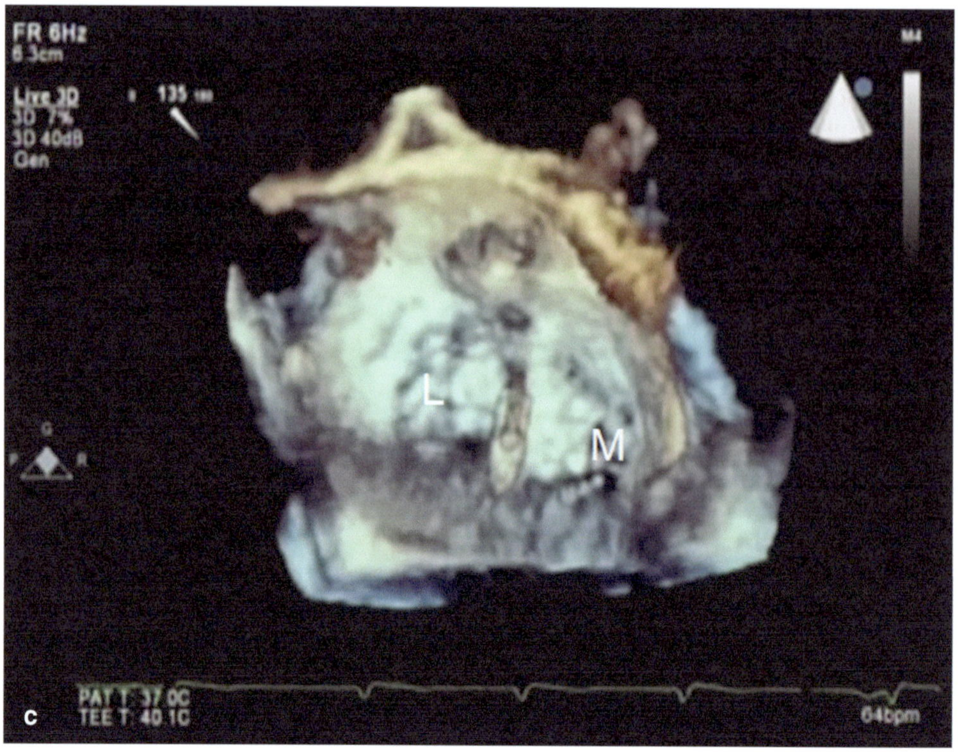

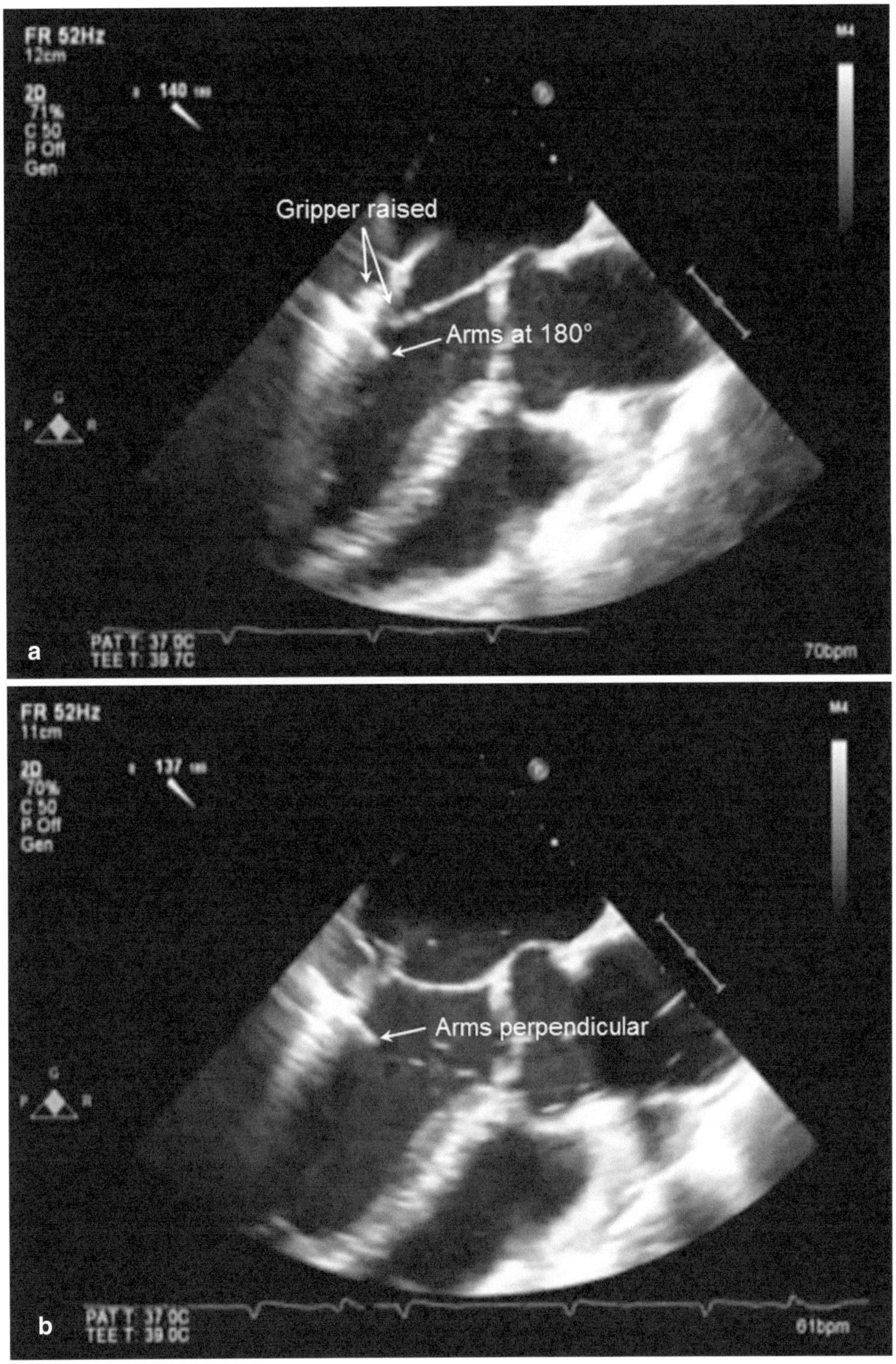

Fig. 2.11 Crossing the mitral valve with the clip. After the proper alignment is achieved, the clip is advanced into the LV so that the clip arms are under the free edges of the mitral leaflets (**a**). Free motion of the leaflet edges is important to note, and restriction of the leaflets by the clip arms means it is not far enough below the free edges to achieve a successful grasp. Using LVOT, two-chamber intercommissural, and short-axis views, a final check of the perpendicular orientation is done with the clip in the LV to be sure there is no deviation of clip orientation to the mitral leaflets (**b–d**)

Fig. 2.11 (continued)

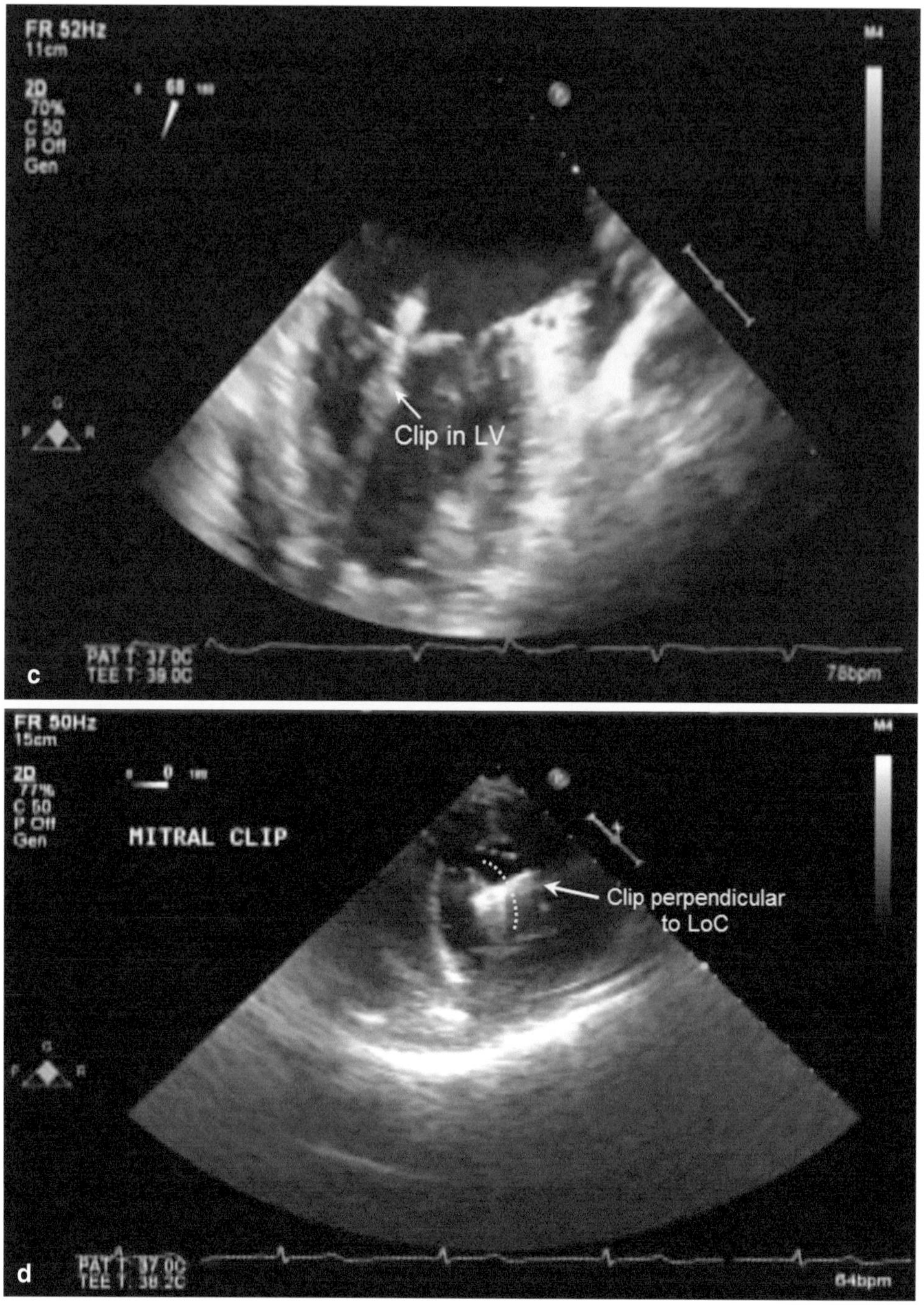

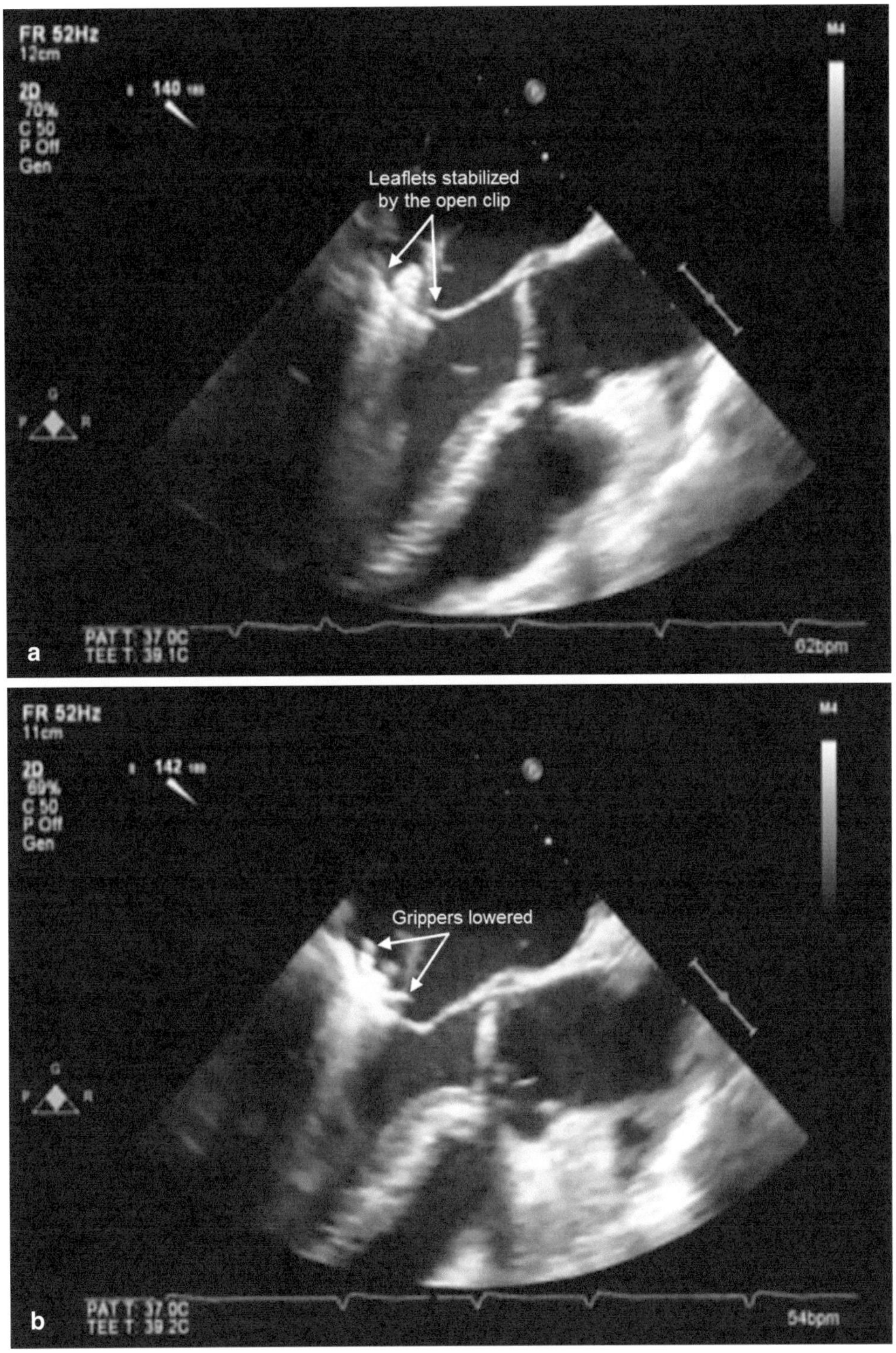

Fig. 2.12 Grasping of leaflets. The leaflets are grasped by retracting the delivery catheter slowly as the mitral leaflets are closing in systole in the LVOT view (**a**). If the leaflets are successfully stabilized by the open clip, then the grippers are quickly lowered, and the clip is closed to about 60° (**b**, **c**). When fully inserted, the leaflets should be stable and immobile at the clip entry point in the LVOT view (**d**). In the two-chamber intercommissural view, the leaflets should enter the center of the clip and be stable medial and lateral to the clip (**e**). This stability can also be confirmed in the four-chamber view (**f**). Finally, once more, the MitraClip device is assessed in the LV to confirm that the clip arms are perpendicular to the line of coaptation in the transgastric short-axis view. There should also be medial and lateral contact between the anterior and posterior leaflets during diastole adjacent to the MitraClip device (**g–h**). Once adequate leaflet insertion has been confirmed at 60°, continue slowing closing the clip just until the leaflets are coapted and MR is sufficiently reduced. Leaflet insertion assessment is repeated using LVOT, two-chamber intercommissural, and transgastric short-axis views

Fig. 2.12 (continued)

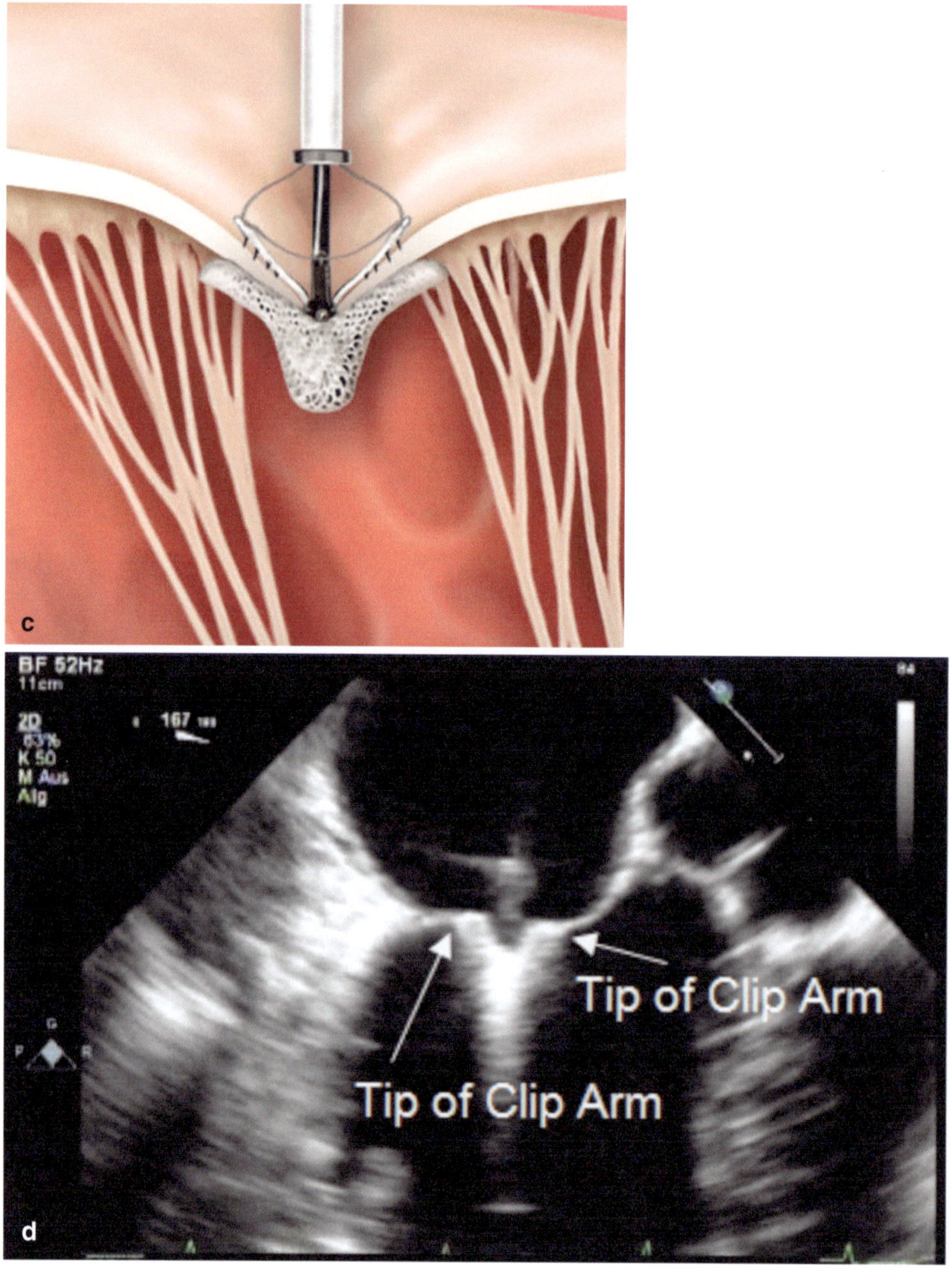

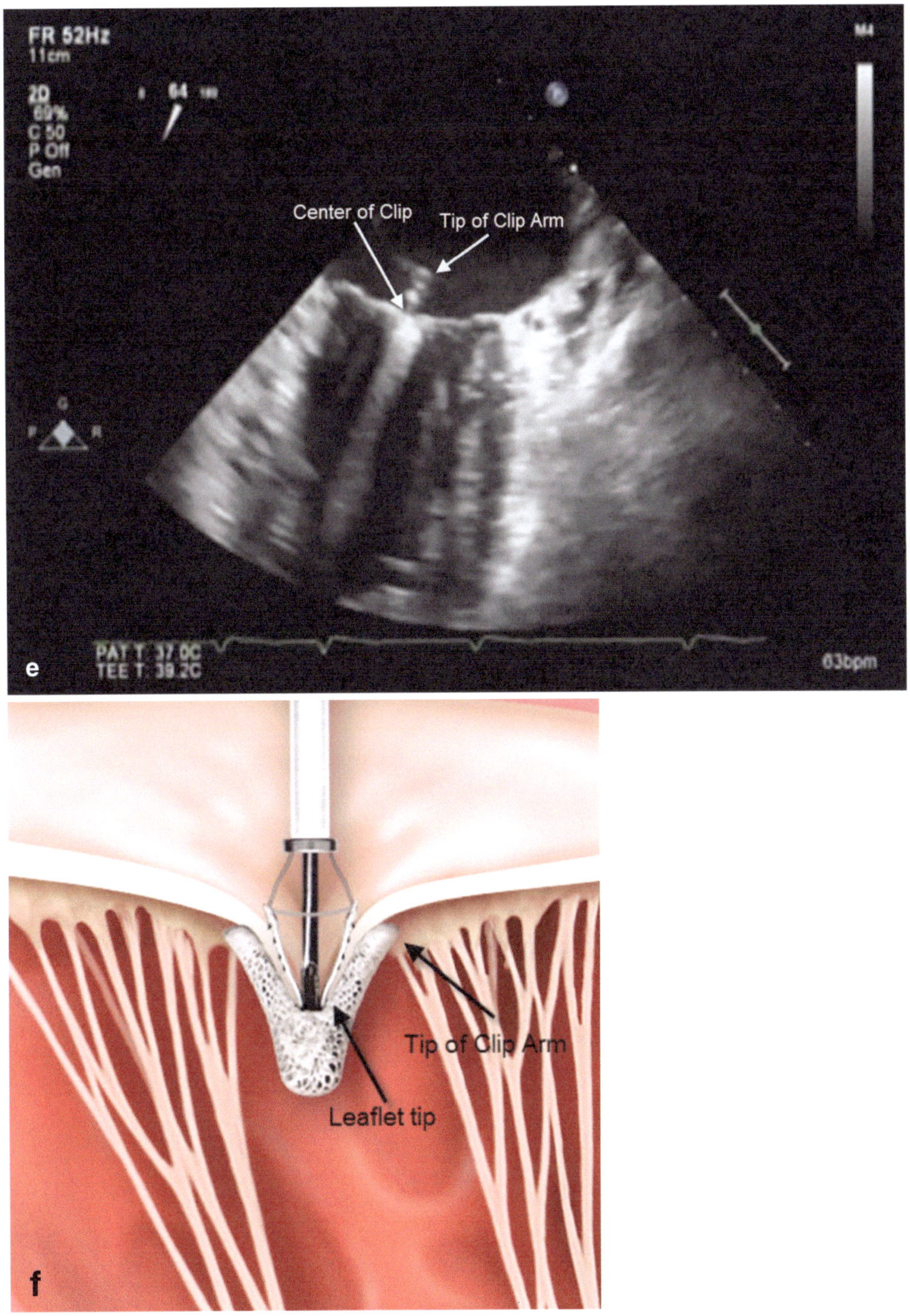

Fig. 2.12 (continued)

Fig. 2.12 (continued)

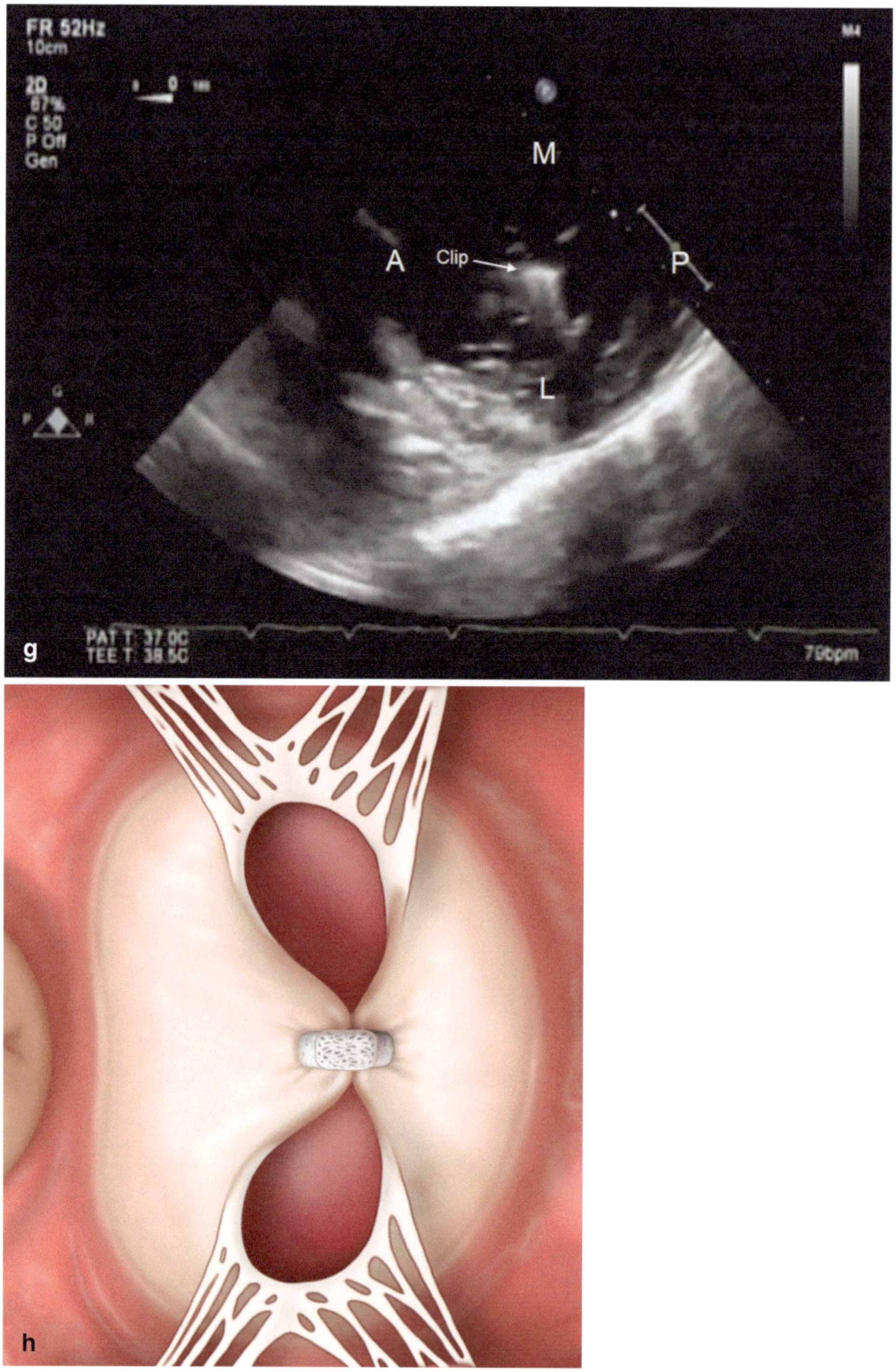

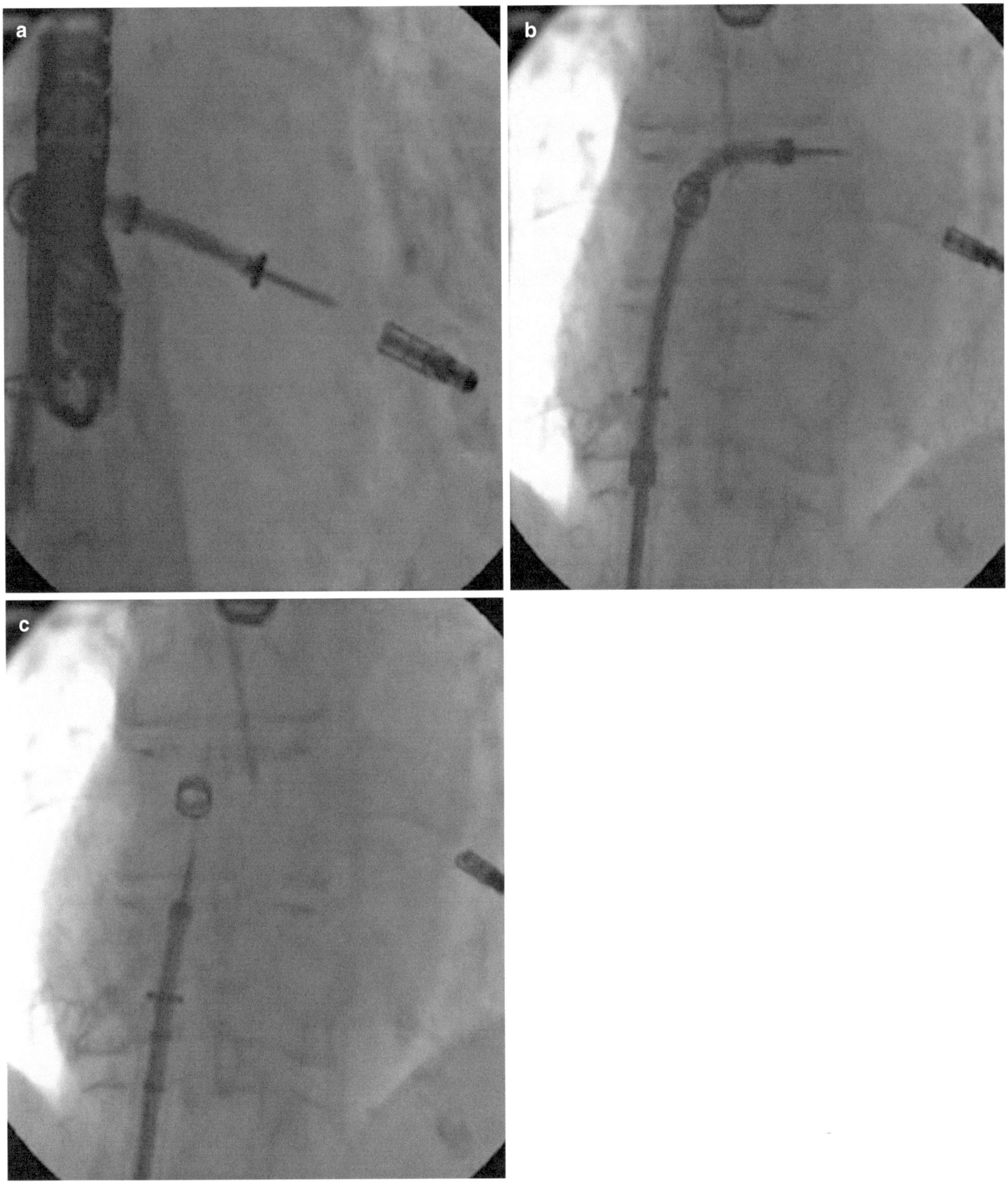

Fig. 2.13 MitraClip device deployment and system removal. Once the optimal reduction in MR jet is achieved, the clip is released using fluoroscopic guidance (**a**). A RAO-caudal or LAO-cranial view may be used for the side view of the clip after its deployment. It is critical that the tip of the delivery catheter is carefully retracted back into the guide catheter to avoid damage to the LA (**b**). Careful and reverse steering with slow retraction of the CDS back into the guide catheter is performed using TEE. Once the CDS is retracted, the guide catheter is withdrawn into the RA and removed (**c**). Hemodynamic measurements, mainly simultaneous LV and PCWP, are repeated after the clip placement. There are several techniques to achieve femoral vein hemostasis which are described in a separate chapter. In one technique, the large-caliber venous access site can be closed using subcutaneous "figure-of-eight" sutures for immediate hemostasis, and they can be removed after several hours [13] (Adapted from Cilingiroglu et al. [14])

References

1. Alfieri O, Maisano F, DeBonis M, et al. The edge-to-edge technique in mitral valve repair: a simple solution for complex problems. J Thorac Cardiovasc Surg. 2001;122:674–81.
2. Maisano F, Torracca L, Oppizzi M, et al. The edge-to-edge technique: a simplified method to correct mitral insufficiency. Eur J Cardiothorac Surg. 1998;13:240–5.
3. Maisano F, Schreuder JJ, Oppizzi M, et al. The double orifice technique as a standardized approach to treat mitral regurgitation due to severe myxomatous disease: surgical technique. Eur J Cardiothorac Surg. 2000;17:201–15.
4. Fann JI, St.Goar FG, Komtebedde J, et al. Beating heart catheter-based-edge-to-edge mitral valve procedure in a porcine model; efficacy and healing response. Circulation. 2004;110:988–93.
5. St Goar FG, James FI, Komtebedde J, et al. Endovascular edge-to-edge mitral valve repair: short-term results in a porcine model. Circulation. 2003;108:1990–3.
6. Feldman T, Wasserman HS, Herrmann HC, et al. Percutaneous mitral valve repair using the edge-to-edge technique: six-month result of the EVEREST Phase 1 Clinical Trial. J Am Coll Cardiol. 2005;46:2134–40.
7. Feldman T, Kar S, Rinaldi M, et al. EVEREST investigators. Percutaneous mitral repair with the MitraClip system: safety and midterm durability in the initial EVEREST (Endovascular Valve Edge-to-Edge REpair Study) cohort. J Am Coll Cardiol. 2009;54(8):686–94.
8. Feldman T, Foster E, Glower DG, et al. Percutaneous repair or surgery for mitral regurgitation. N Engl J Med. 2011;364:1395–406.
9. Feldman TE. Two-year follow-up from EVEREST-II trial. Presented at the American College of Cardiology sScientific Sessions. New Orleans, 2–5 Apr 2011.
10. Perlowski A, Feldman TE. The EVEREST percutaneous mitral leaflet repair trials. Cardiac Interventions Today. 2011;70–5.
11. Franzen O, Baldus S, Rudolph V, et al. Acute outcomes of MitraClip therapy for mitral regurgitation in high-surgical-risk patients: emphasis on adverse valve morphology and severe left ventricular dysfunction. Eur Heart J. 2010;31:1373–81.
12. Franzen O, van der Heyden J, Baldus S, et al. MitraClip therapy in patients with end-stage systolic heart failure. Eur J Heart Fail. 2011;13:569–76.
13. Cilingiroglu M, Salinger M, Zhao D, et al. "Figure-of-eight" sutures to achieve hemostasis after removal of large-caliber femoral venous sheaths. Catheter Cardiovasc Interv. 2011;78(1):155–60.
14. Cilingiroglu M, Gary G, Salinger MH, Feldman TE. Step-by-step guide to percutaneous mitral leaflet repair. Cardiac Interventions Today. 2010;69–76.

Room Setup

3

Khung Keong Yeo, Jason Rogers, and Reginald Low

Abstract

The procedural room setup is an important part of the MitraClip procedure. A well-planned layout not only aids in communication between the operator, echocardiologist, and anesthesiologist, but also can reduce the risk of errors. The procedure may be performed in the cardiac catheterization laboratory or in a hybrid operating room. Key requirements included fluoroscopy, transesophageal echo capability, and sufficient working space.

Keywords

Hybrid operating room • Cardiac catheterization laboratory

MitraClip

The procedural room setup is an important part of the MitraClip procedure and requires advance planning and thinking. A well-planned layout not only aids in communication between the operator, echocardiologist, and anesthesiologist, but also can reduce the risk of errors. A poorly planned room can result in excessive radiation exposure to team members or result in mechanical injury or musculoskeletal strain.

The MitraClip procedure can be performed either in the cardiac catheterization laboratory (CCL) or in a hybrid operating room (OR). There are advantages and disadvantages to using either space, but we feel this will largely be dependent on the logistics and physician preferences in each institution. Table 3.1 indicates some of the practical aspects of choosing either the CCL or hybrid OR as well as pros and cons. These are all relative and will have to be assessed in the context of the individual institution. Importantly, given the number of individuals and equipment present in the room during a MitraClip procedure, the room should be of adequate size.

Table 3.1 Comparison of performing the MitraClip in the CVL or Hybrid OR

		CVL	Hybrid OR
1.	Size	Smaller	Bigger
2.	Sterility	Less	More
3.	Anesthesiologist preference	Less	More
4.	Urgent cardiac surgery	Slight delay	No delay
5.	Interventional cardiologist preference	More	Less
6.	Availability	Dependent on institution	Dependent on institution
7.	Cost	Dependent on institution	Dependent on institution

K.K. Yeo, M.B.B.S., FACC, FSCAI (✉)
Department of Cardiovascular Medicine,
University of California, Davis Medical Center,
4860 Y Street, Suite 2820, Sacramento, CA 95817, USA

Department of Cardiology, National Heart Centre Singapore,
Mistri Wing, 17 Third Hospital Avenue,
Singapore 168752, Singapore
e-mail: yeo_kk@yahoo.com, yeo.khung.keong@nhcs.com.sg

J. Rogers, M.D., FACC, FSCAI • R. Low, M.D., FACC
Department of Cardiovascular Medicine,
University of California, Davis Medical Center,
4860 Y Street, Suite 2820, Sacramento, CA 95817, USA
e-mail: jason.rogers@ucdmc.ucdavis.edu; ptcra@aol.com

T. Feldman et al. (eds.), *Atlas of Percutaneous Edge-to-Edge Mitral Valve Repair*,
DOI 10.1007/978-1-4471-4294-2_3, © Springer-Verlag London 2013

Basic Room Requirements and Setup

The basic room setup is as shown in Fig. 3.1. Essentially, the primary operators work on the patient's right side, while the monitors are on the patient's left. These monitors should display real-time and saved fluoroscopic images, hemodynamics and physiologic data, and echocardiographic images for the primary operator. It is not practical for the echocardiologist and the primary operator to share the same monitor. The echo machine and echocardiologist are on the left side of the patient's head. The fluoroscopy equipment is above the patient's head. The anesthesiologist and the anesthesia equipment are on the right side of the patient's head.

The working tables, upon which the MitraClip equipment is placed, are located behind the operators. Importantly, a long table is required. This allows the MitraClip guide and delivery system to be safely prepared without having any part off the sterile field.

The accompanying figures (Figs. 3.2, 3.3, 3.4, 3.5, 3.6, 3.7, 3.8, 3.9, 3.10, 3.11, 3.12, 3.13, 3.14, 3.15, 3.16, 3.17, 3.18, and 3.19) demonstrate how the room setup may be in the hybrid OR and in the CCL. In general, it is important to ensure clear lines of communication between the operator and the echocardiologist (i.e., no equipment should be in the way). Second, because of the procedure's dependence of TEE, the echocardiologist should be in a comfortable position during the procedure. Since the echocardiologist is in close proximity to the fluoroscopy equipment, the use of lead or plexiglass shielding during the case is essential. Finally, the ergonomics of table height, monitor height, lighting, and room temperature should all be adjusted for maximal comfort and efficiency.

Summary

The MitraClip procedure may be performed safely in the CVL or Hybrid OR. However, careful planning to ensure that the operator, the echocardiologist, and anesthesiologist are able to view the relevant images and screens is crucial. A proper room setup enhances communication between the different team members and will ensure a successful procedure.

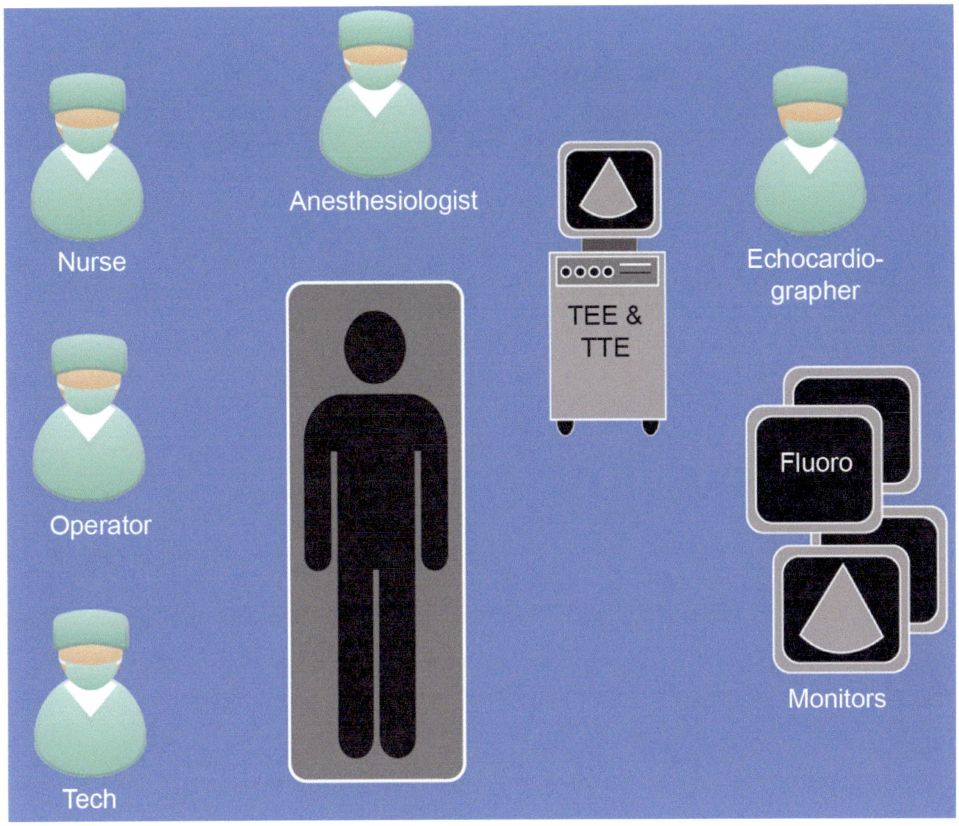

Fig. 3.1 This shows the basic room setup for the MitraClip procedure (Image courtesy of Abbott Vascular. ©2012 Abbott Laboratories. All Rights Reserved)

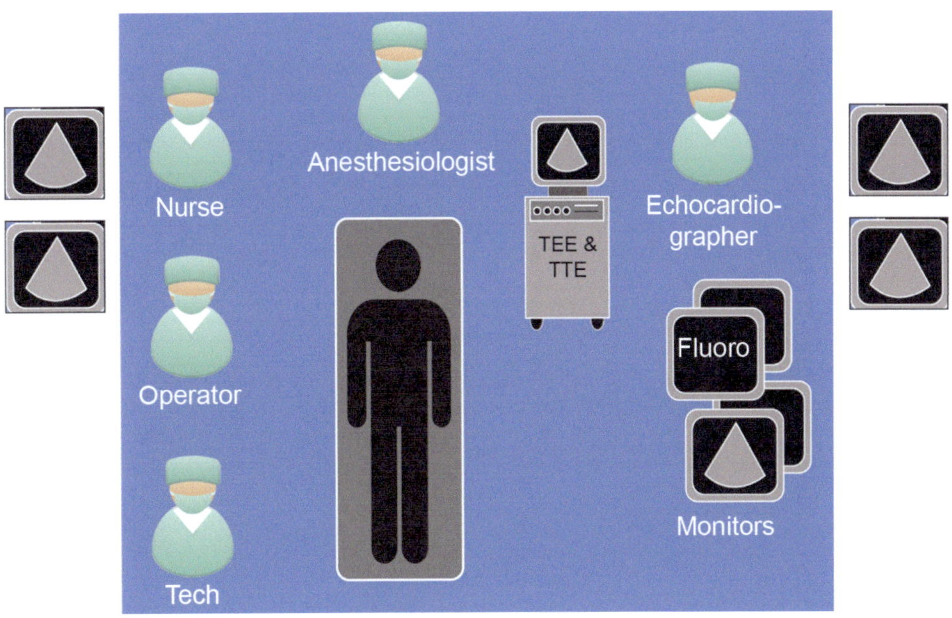

Fig. 3.2 This shows the room setup for the MitraClip procedure with additional monitors on each side wall. The monitors may show hemodynamics or fluoroscopy images. These additional monitors may aid the operator and the echocardiologist (Modified from images courtesy of Abbott Vascular. ©2012 Abbott Laboratories. All Rights Reserved)

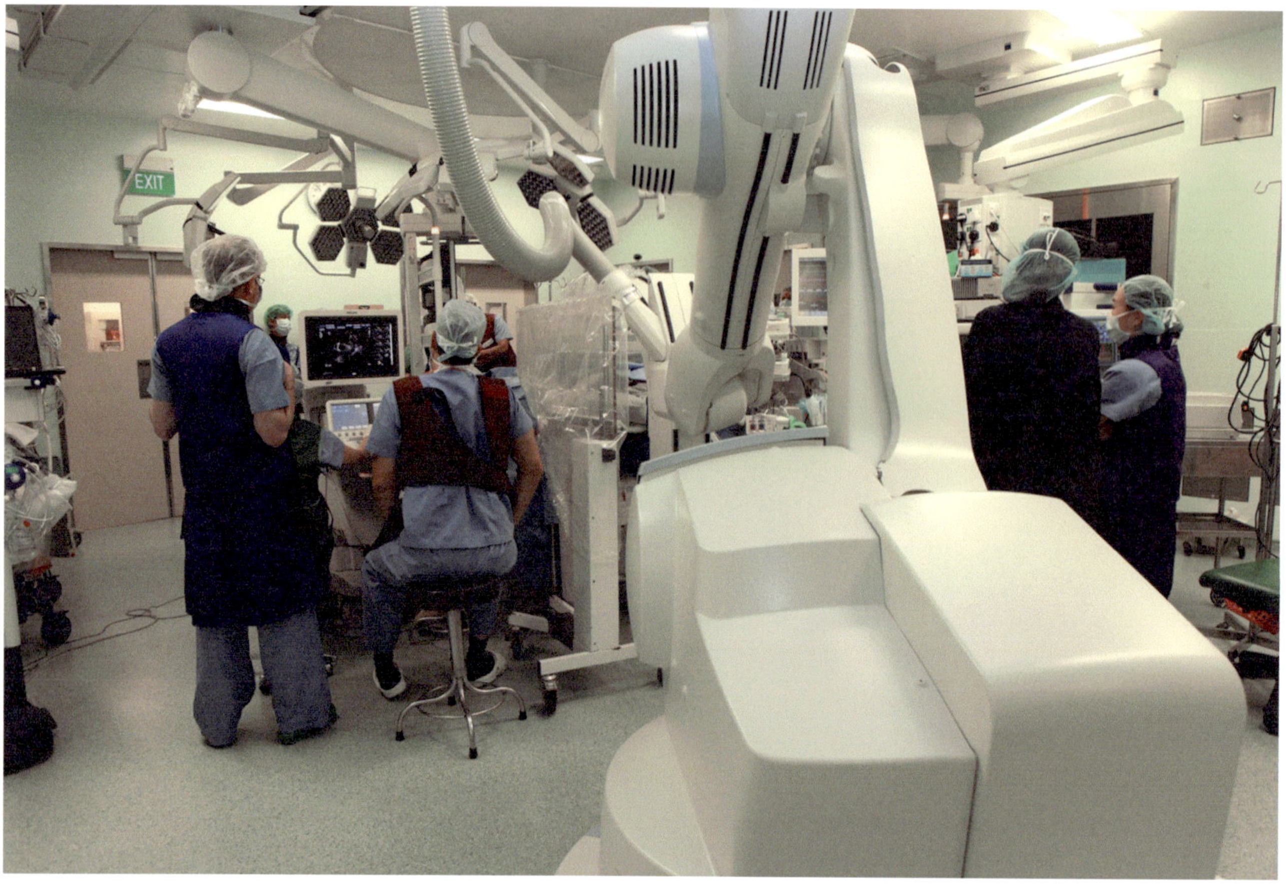

Fig. 3.3 Hybrid OR setup showing the Siemens Artis zee fluoroscopy machine approaching from the *top left side* of the patient. A lead shield is on the patient's left side and protects the echocardiologist

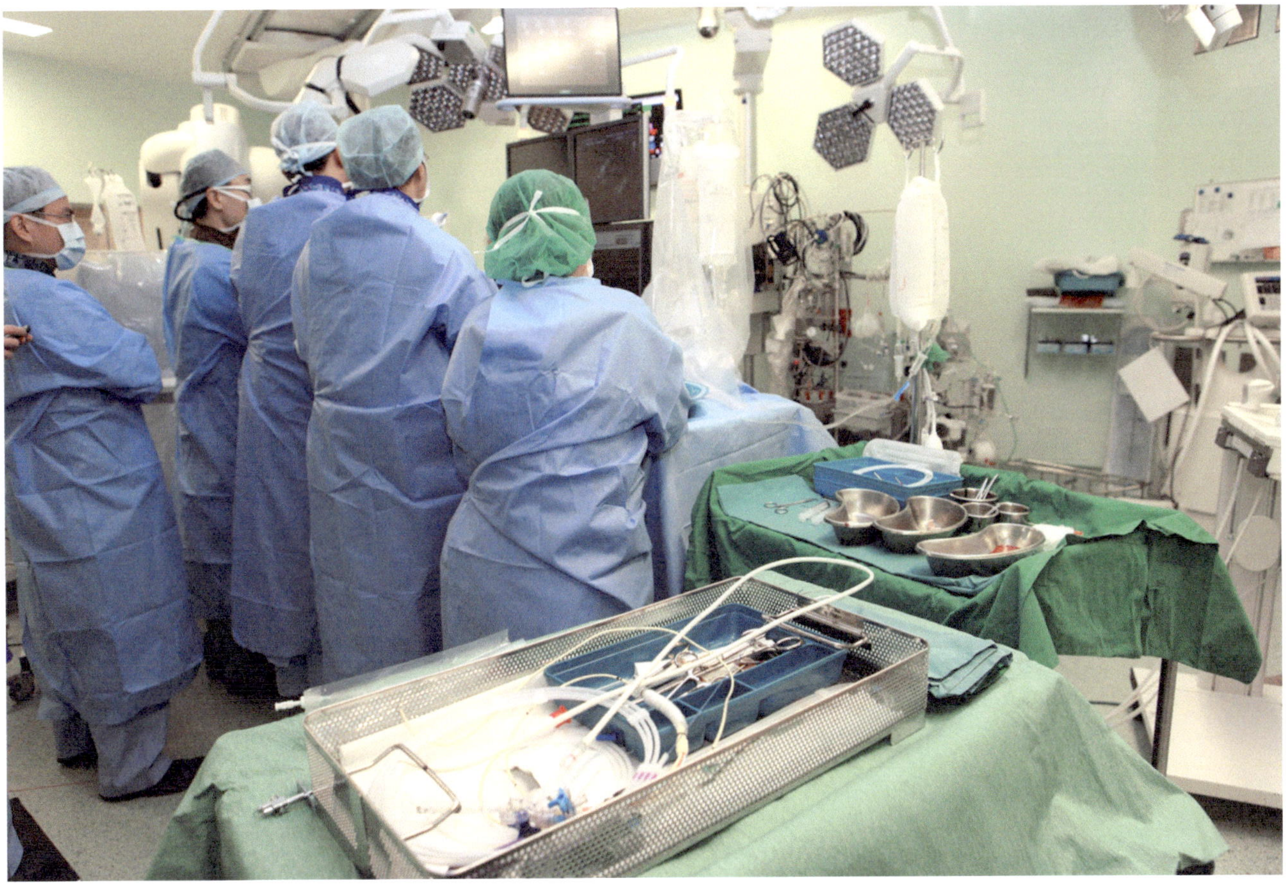

Fig. 3.4 Hybrid OR setup with the view from the back of the table. The operators are looking at the monitors

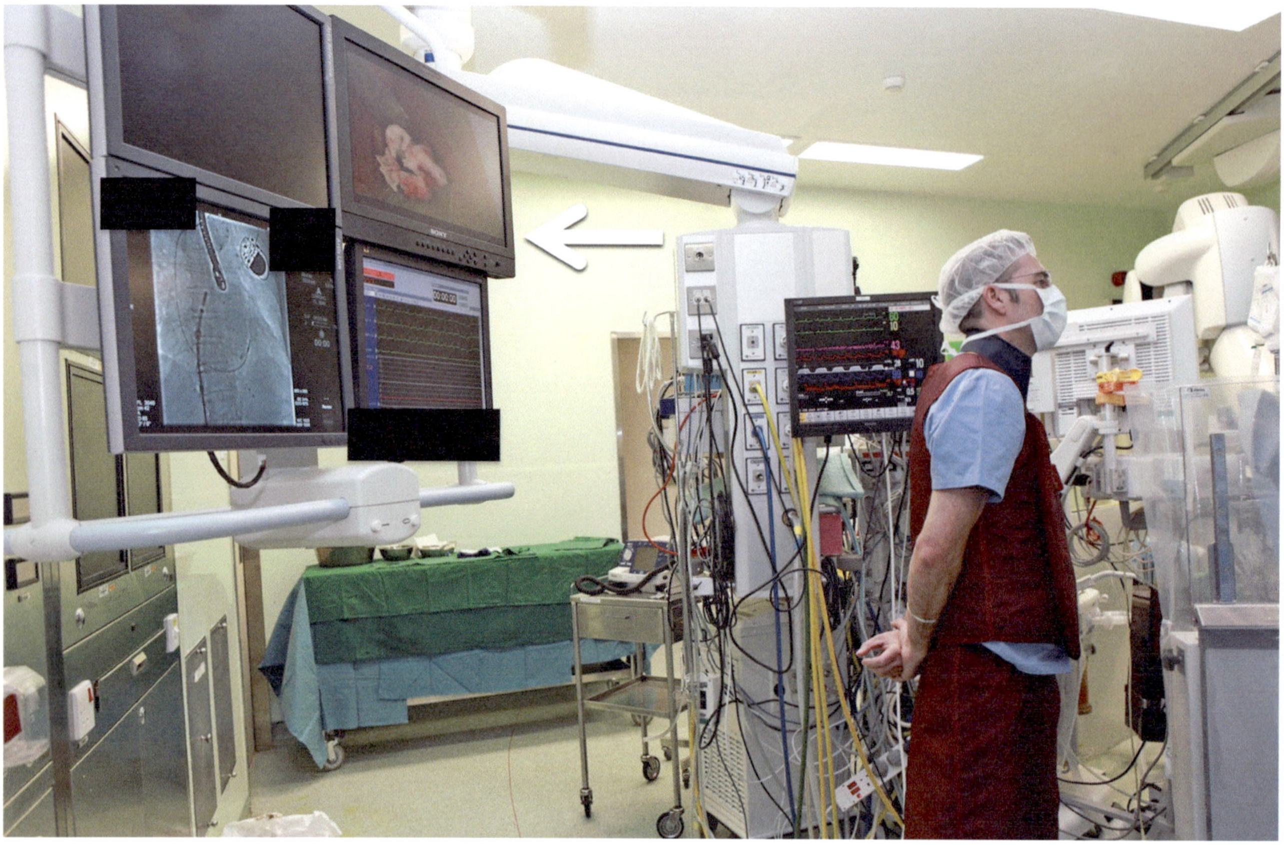

Fig. 3.5 Hybrid OR setup with the additional monitors mirroring fluoroscopy, echo, and hemodynamics (*arrow*)

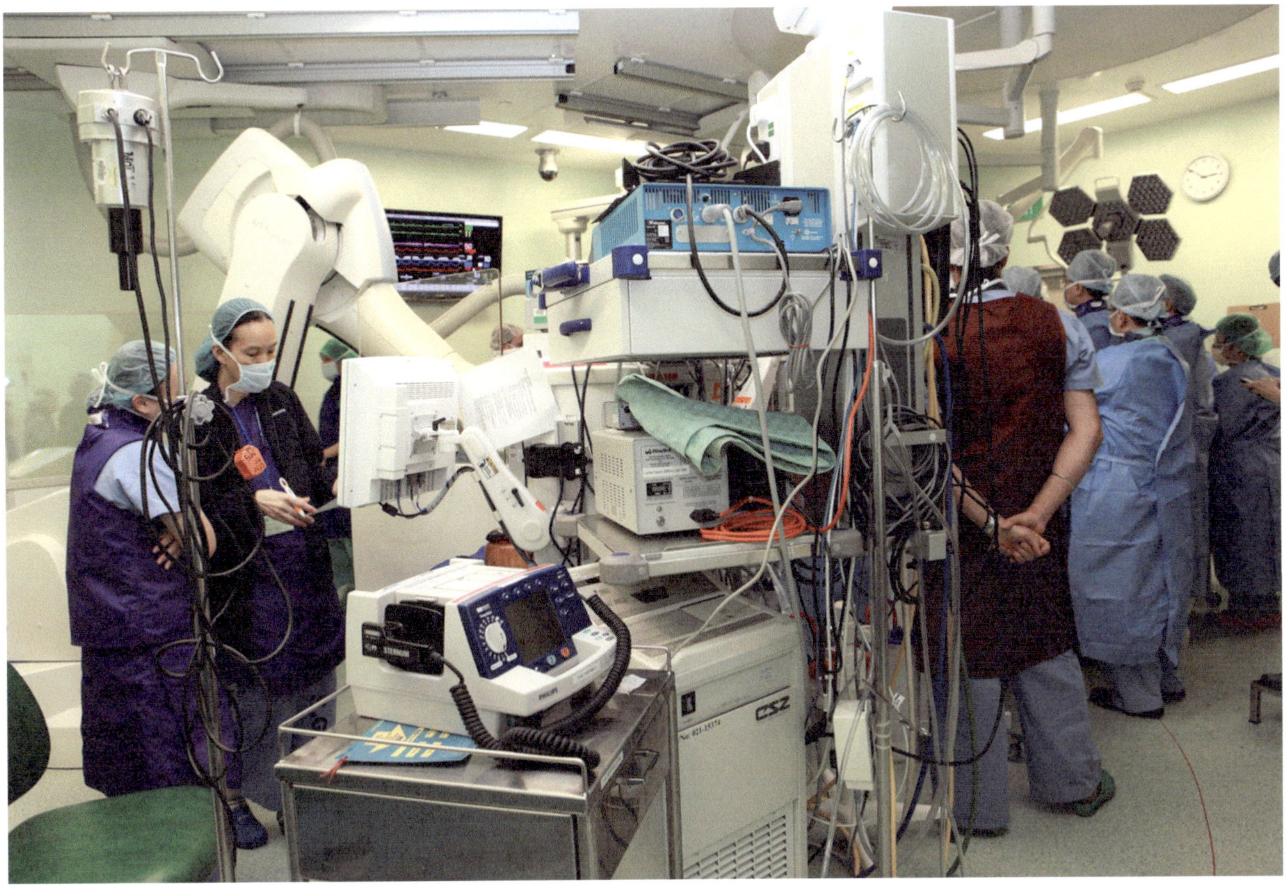

Fig. 3.6 Hybrid OR setup with the anesthesiologists and anesthesia equipment to the right side of the patient's head

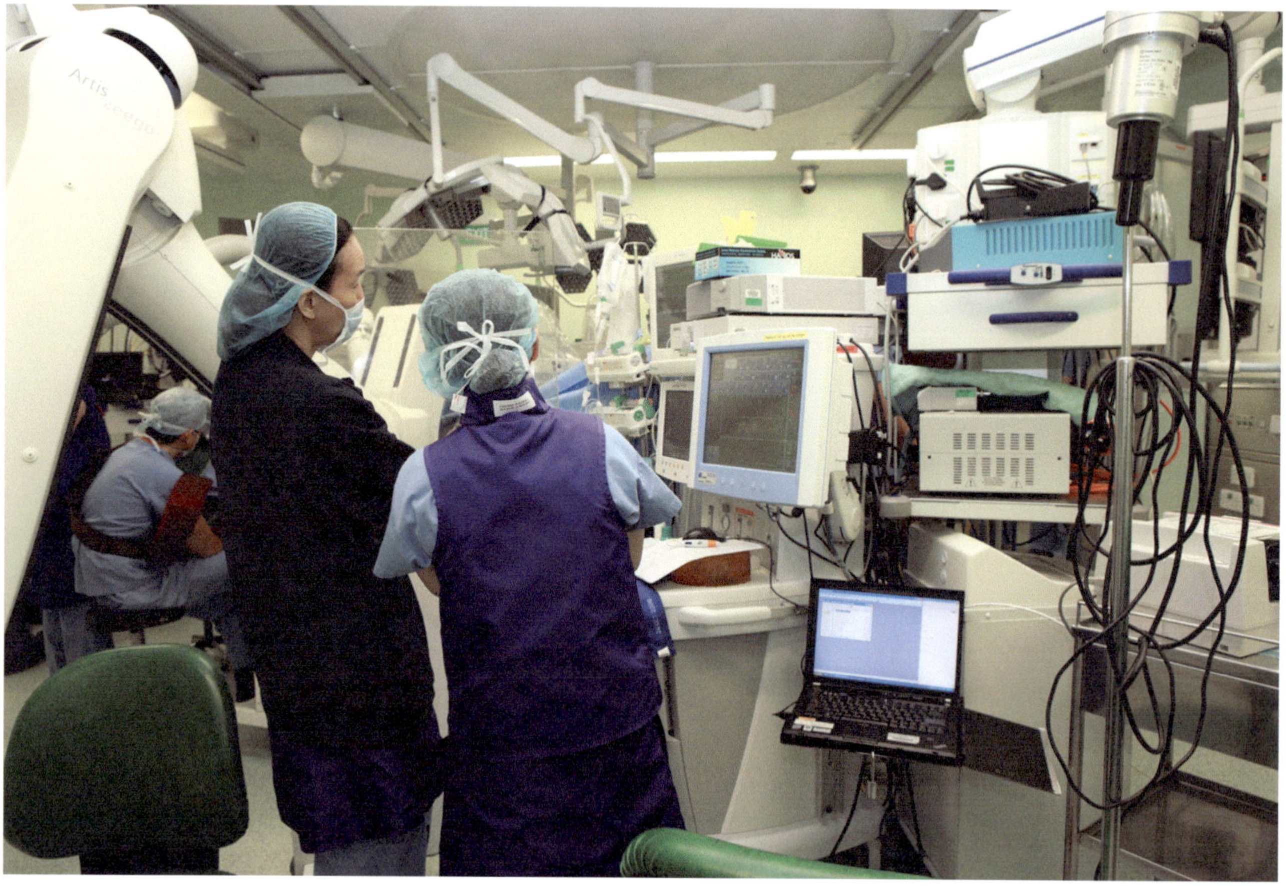

Fig. 3.7 Hybrid OR setup with anesthesia just to the right side of the patient's head. The Siemens Artis zee fluoroscopy arm just to the left of the patient's head

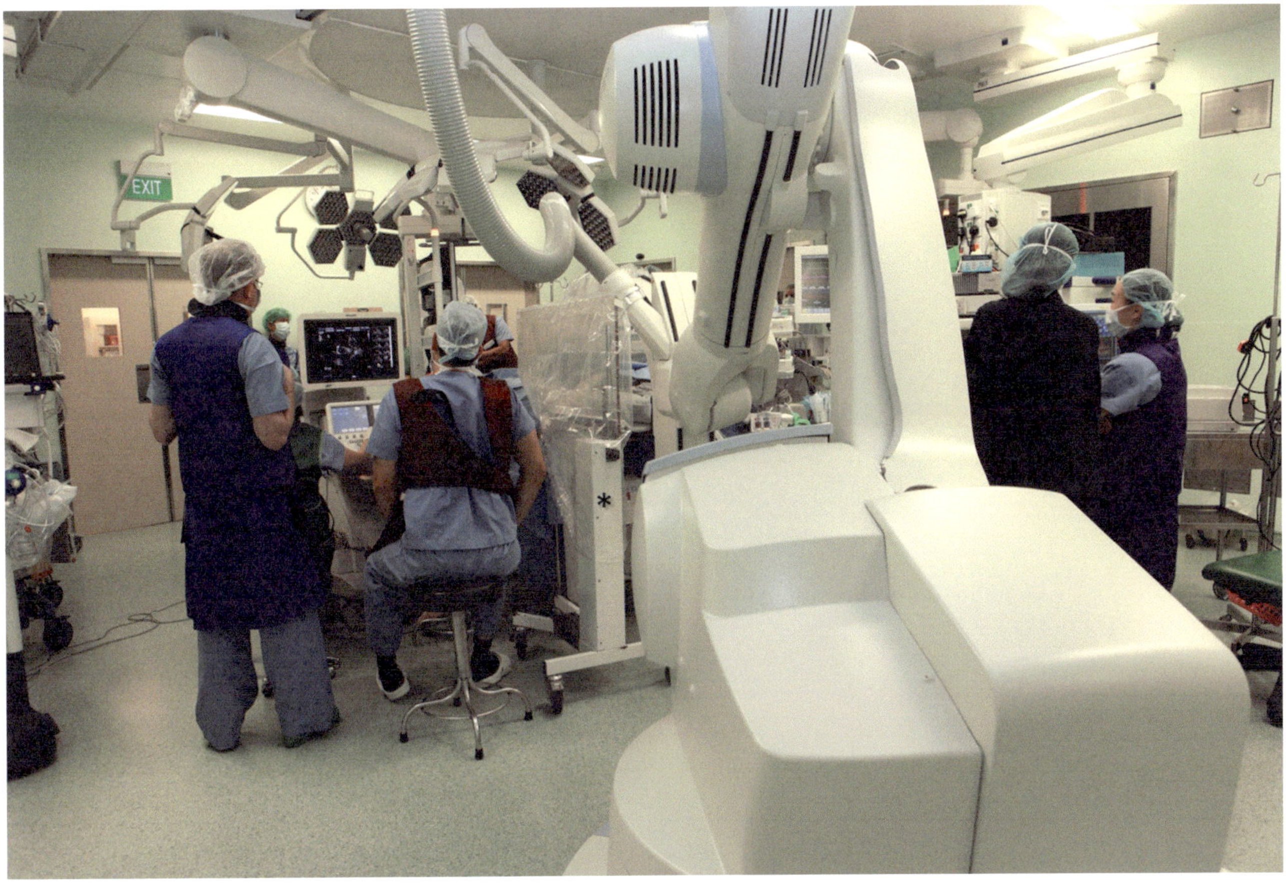

Fig. 3.8 Hybrid OR setup with the Siemens Artis zee fluoroscopy arm approaching from the left side of the patient's head. On the left side of the patient is a lead shield that protects the echocardiologist from radiation during the procedure (*Asterisk* *)

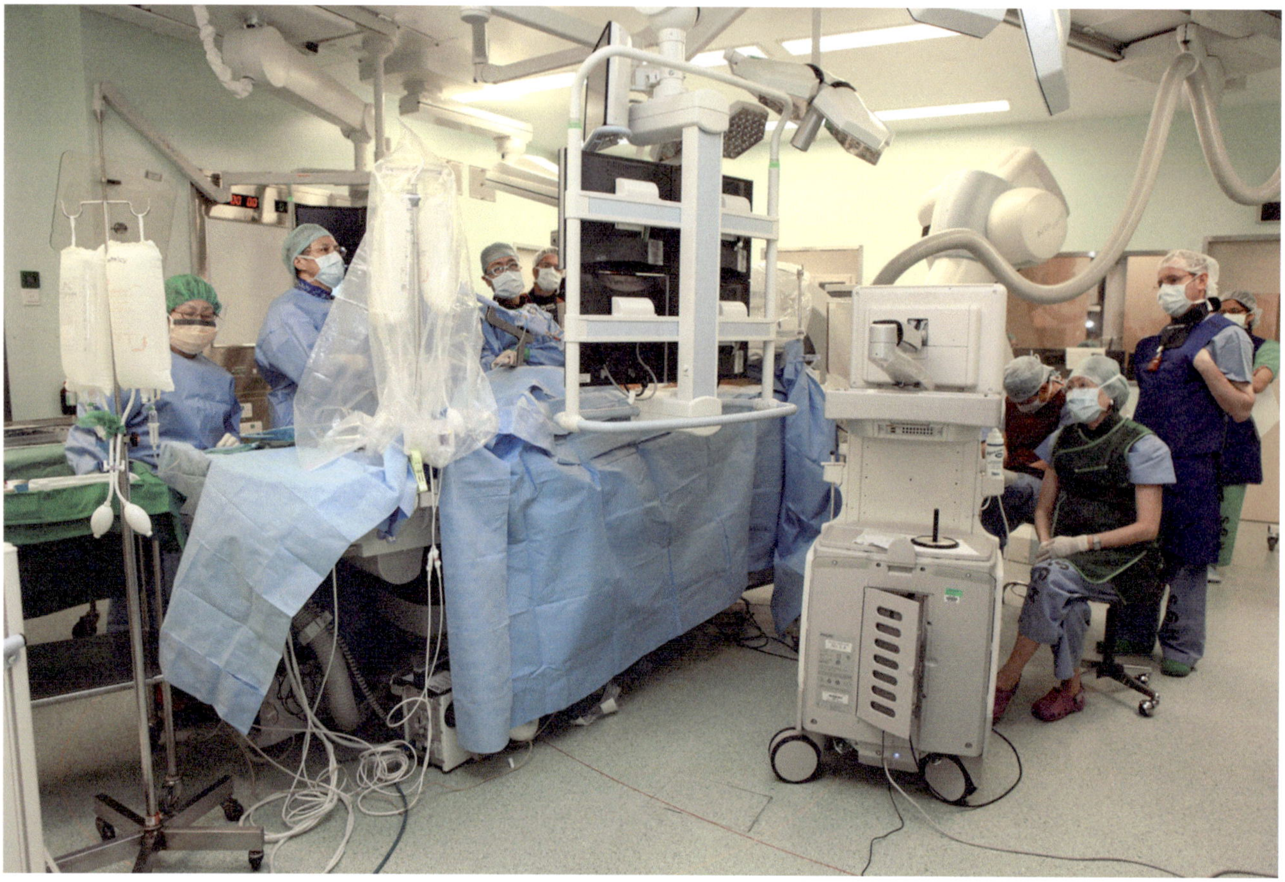

Fig. 3.9 Hybrid OR showing the positioning of the echocardiologist and echo machine

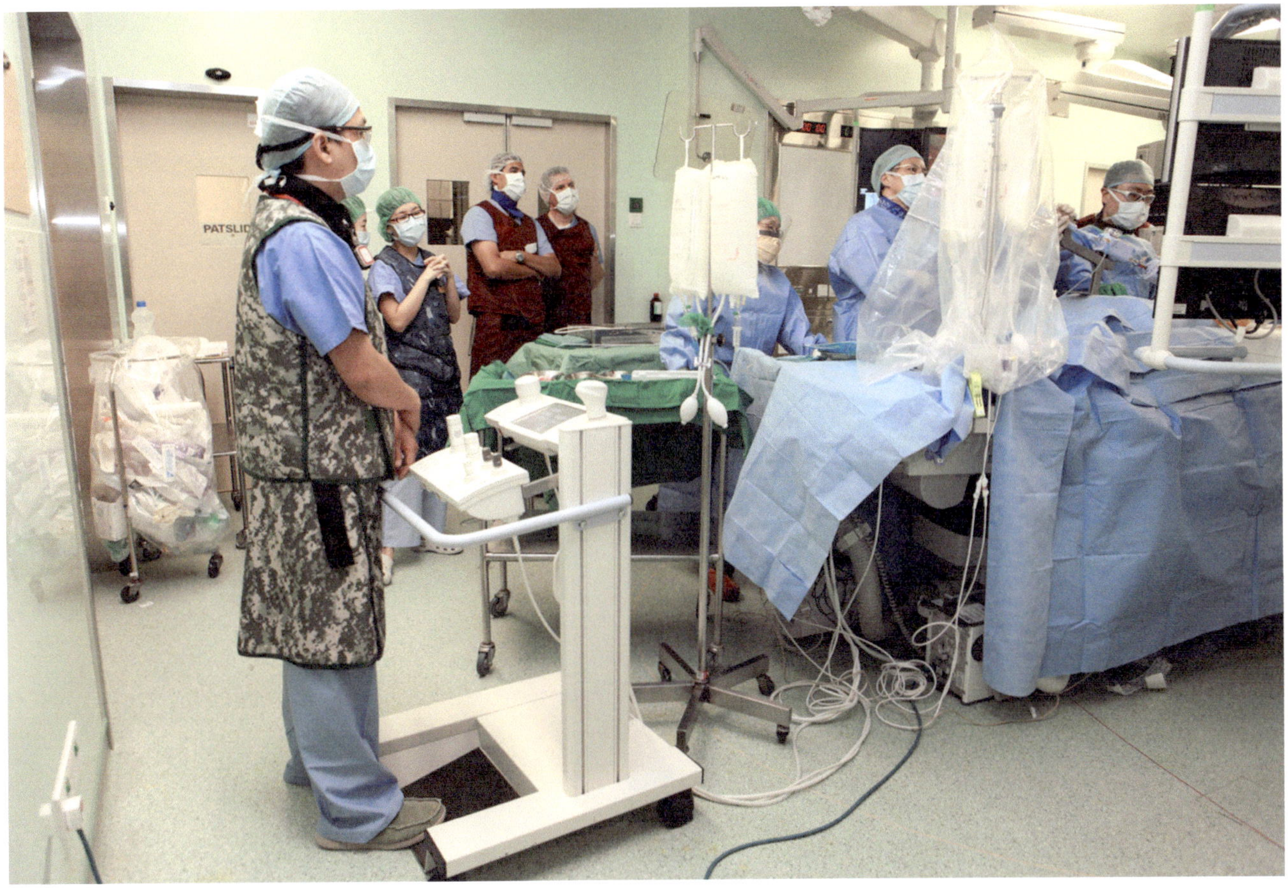

Fig. 3.10 Hybrid OR setup with the radiographer at the foot of the bed. The radiographer may see the fluoroscopic images on the monitors located on left wall of the room

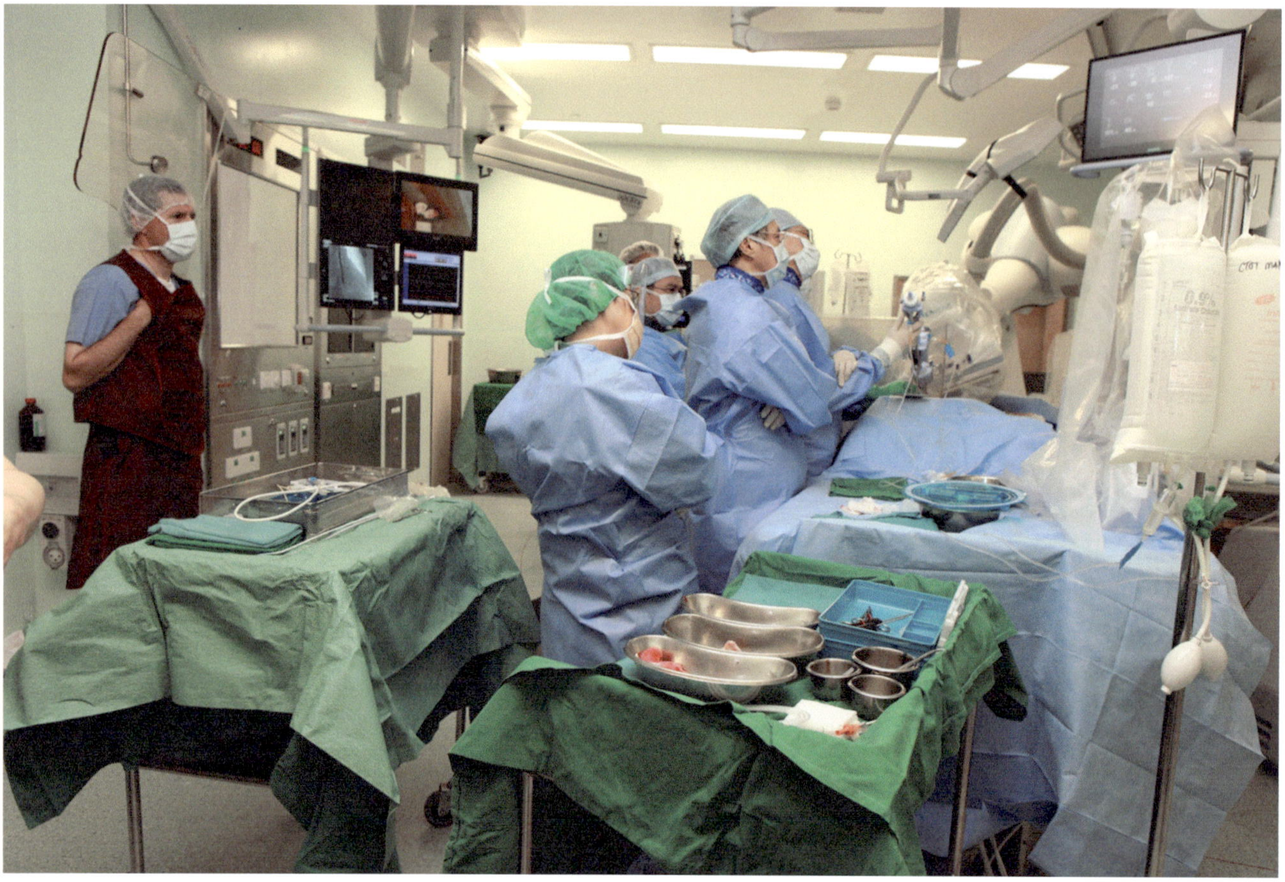

Fig. 3.11 Hybrid OR setup showing the view from the foot of the bed

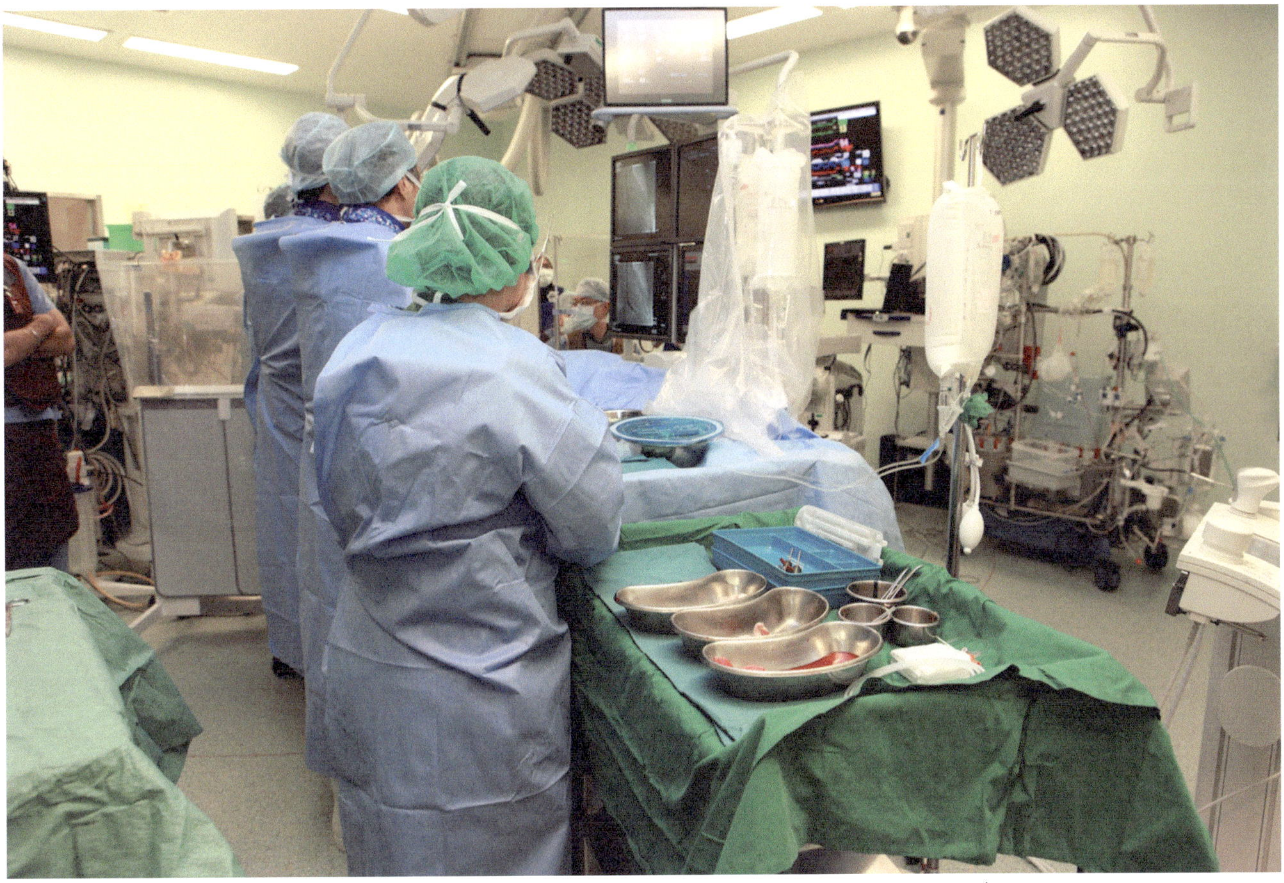

Fig. 3.12 Hybrid OR setup showing the view from the caudal end of the table from the bed. Notice the screens on the right wall of the room showing hemodynamics

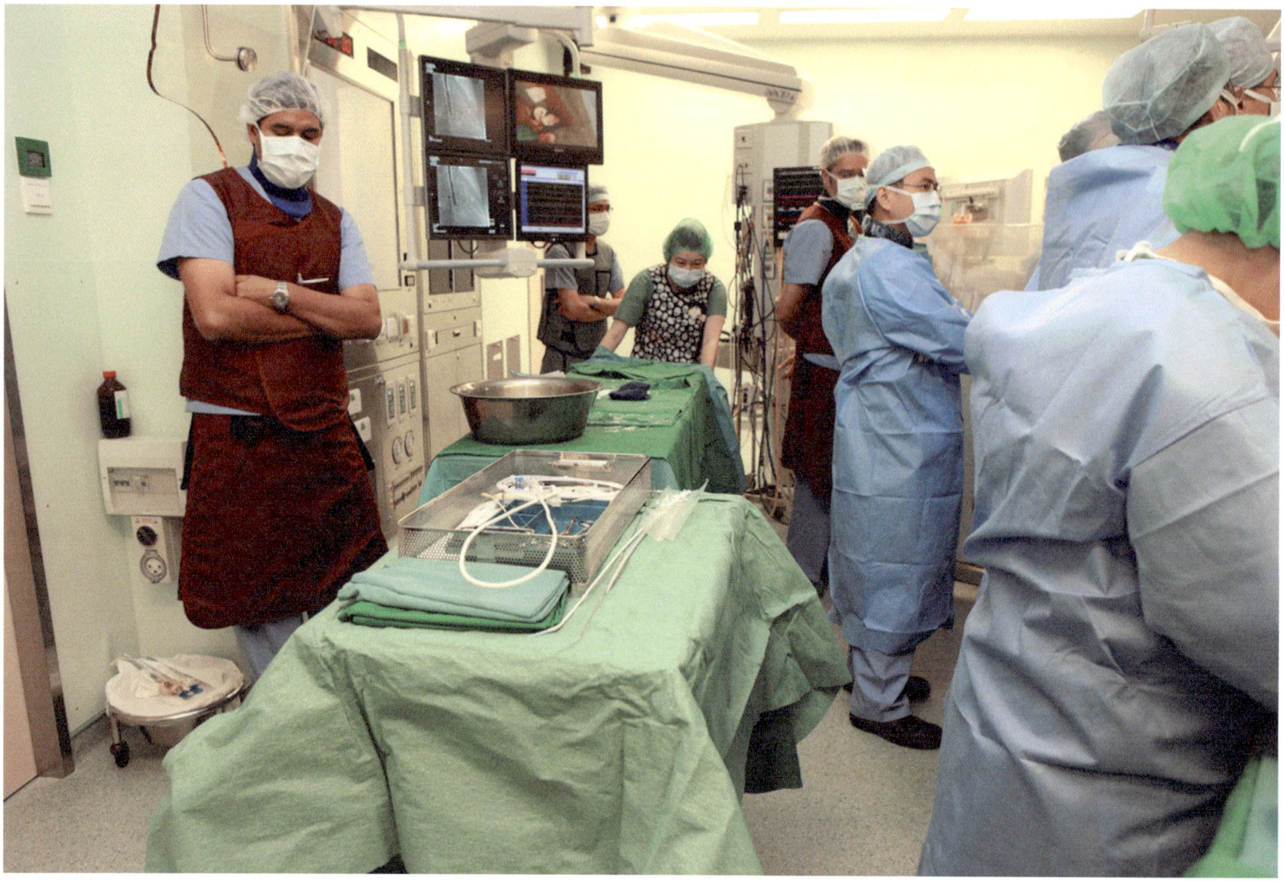

Fig. 3.13 Hybrid OR setup. At least one long table is used

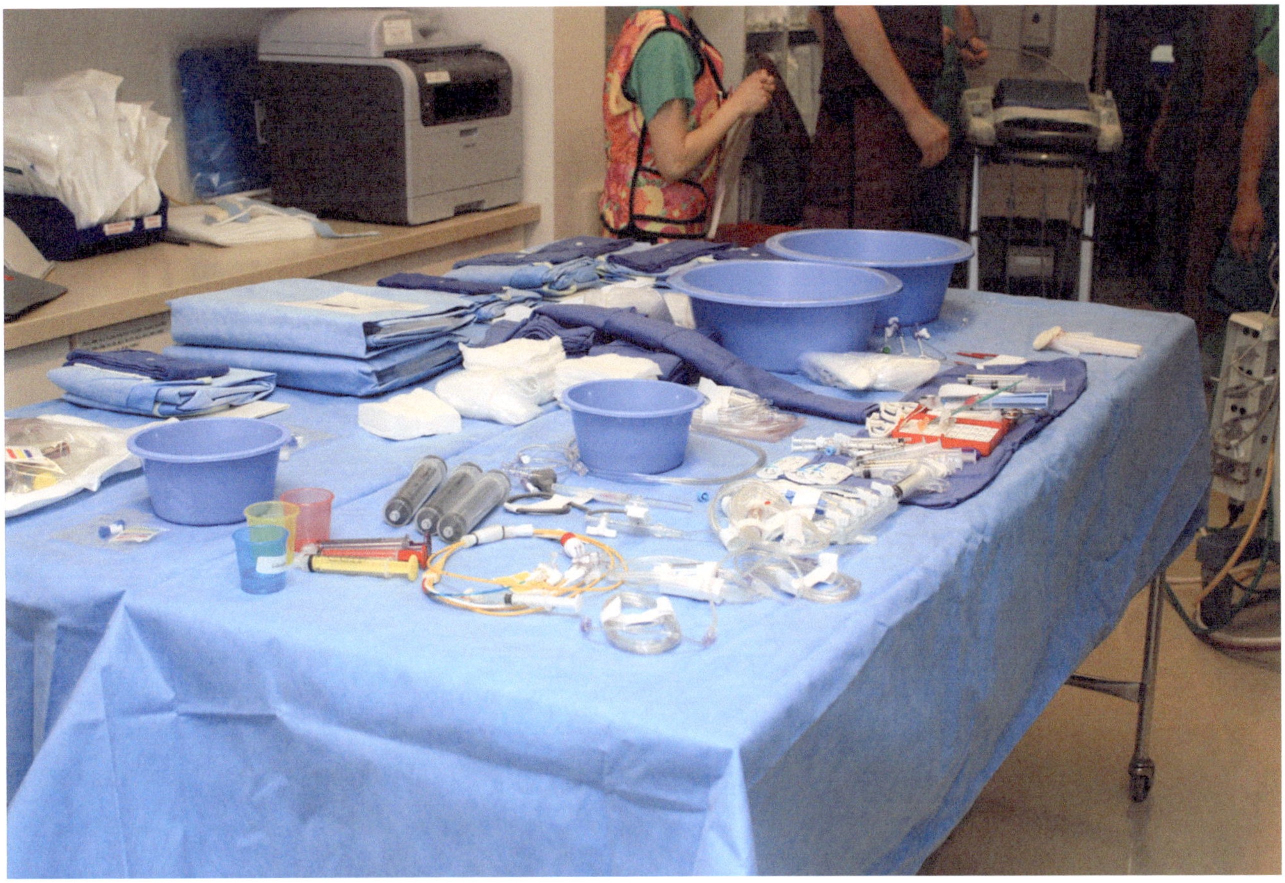

Fig. 3.14 Cath Lab setup with periprocedural equipment prepared for the procedure. In this case, two long tables are used

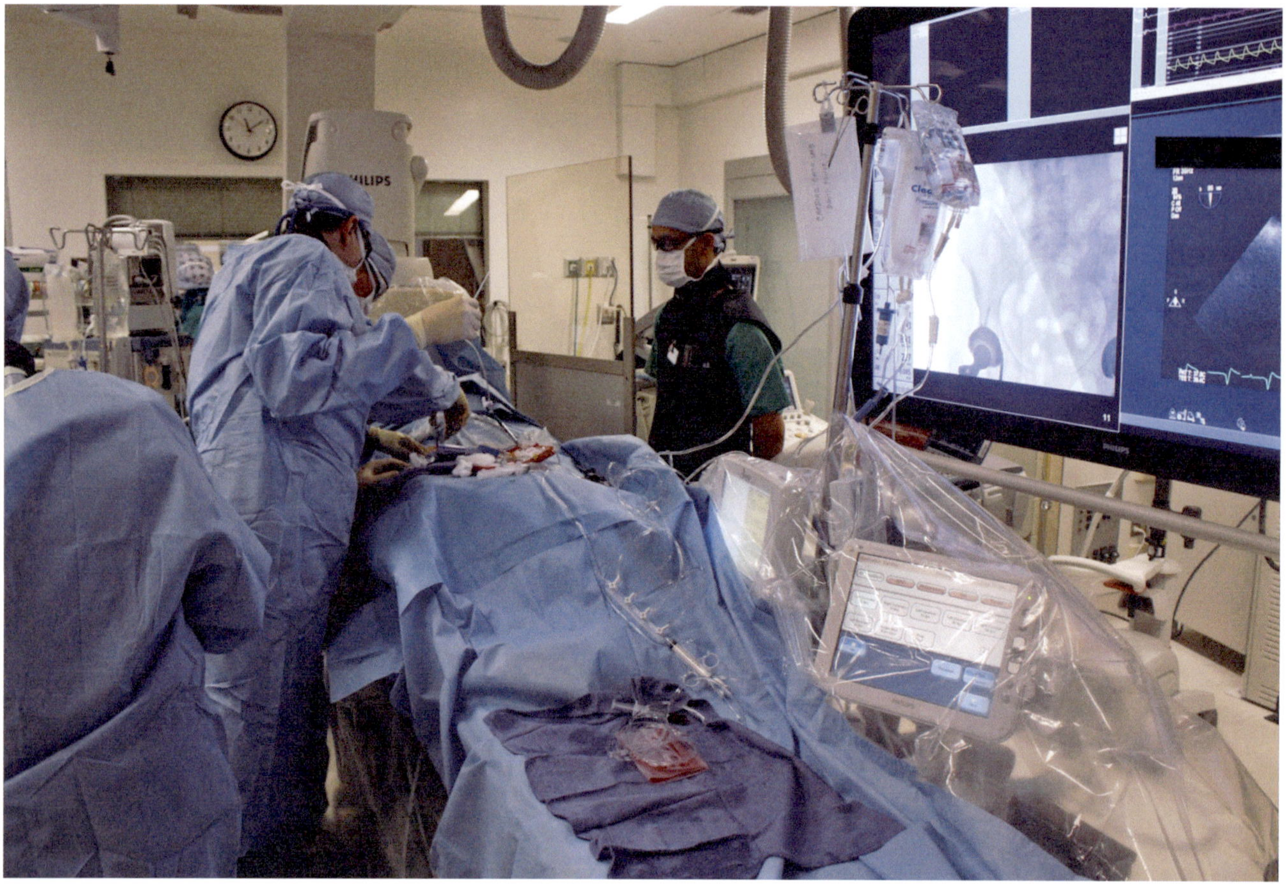

Fig. 3.15 Cath Lab setup with the monitors as shown across the patient from the operator

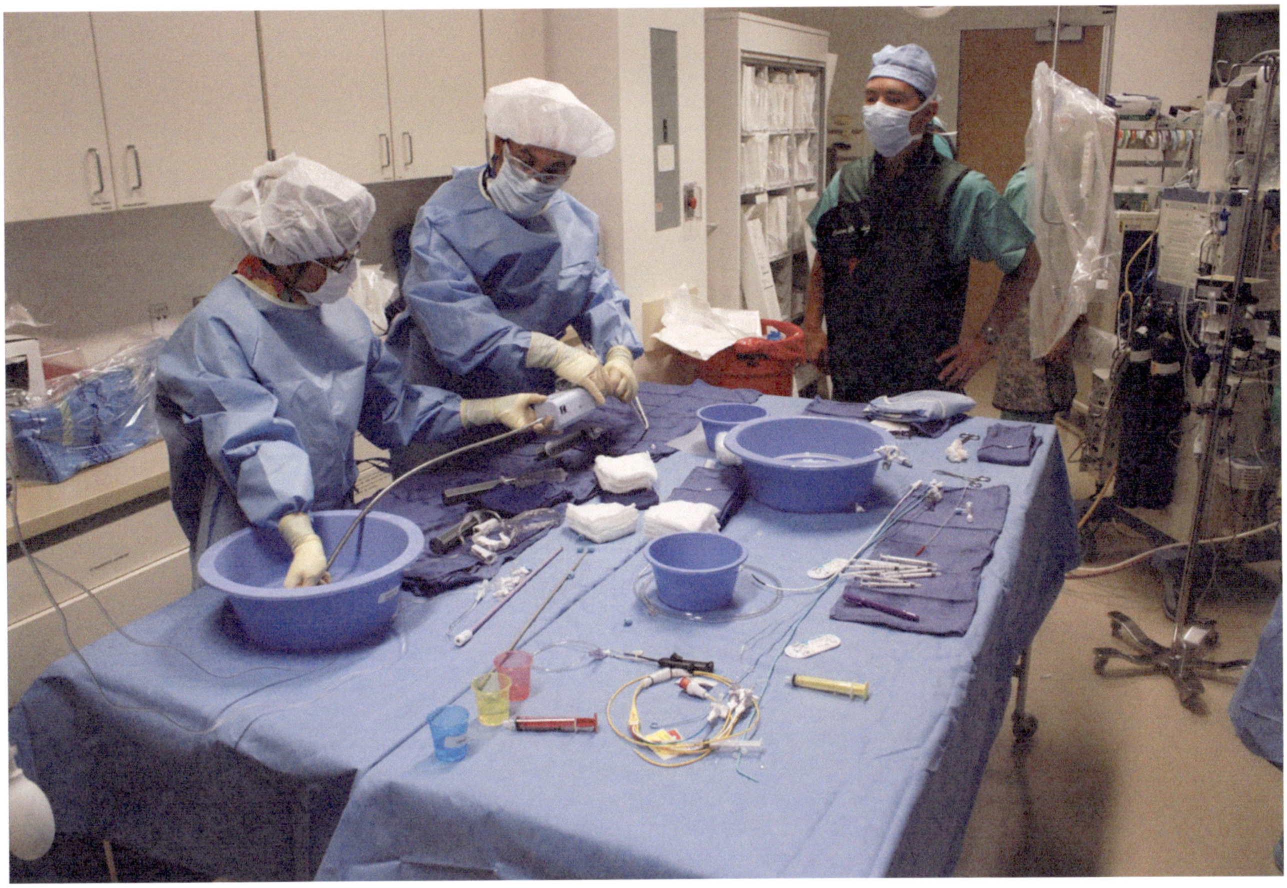

Fig. 3.16 Cath Lab setup with team members preparing the guide

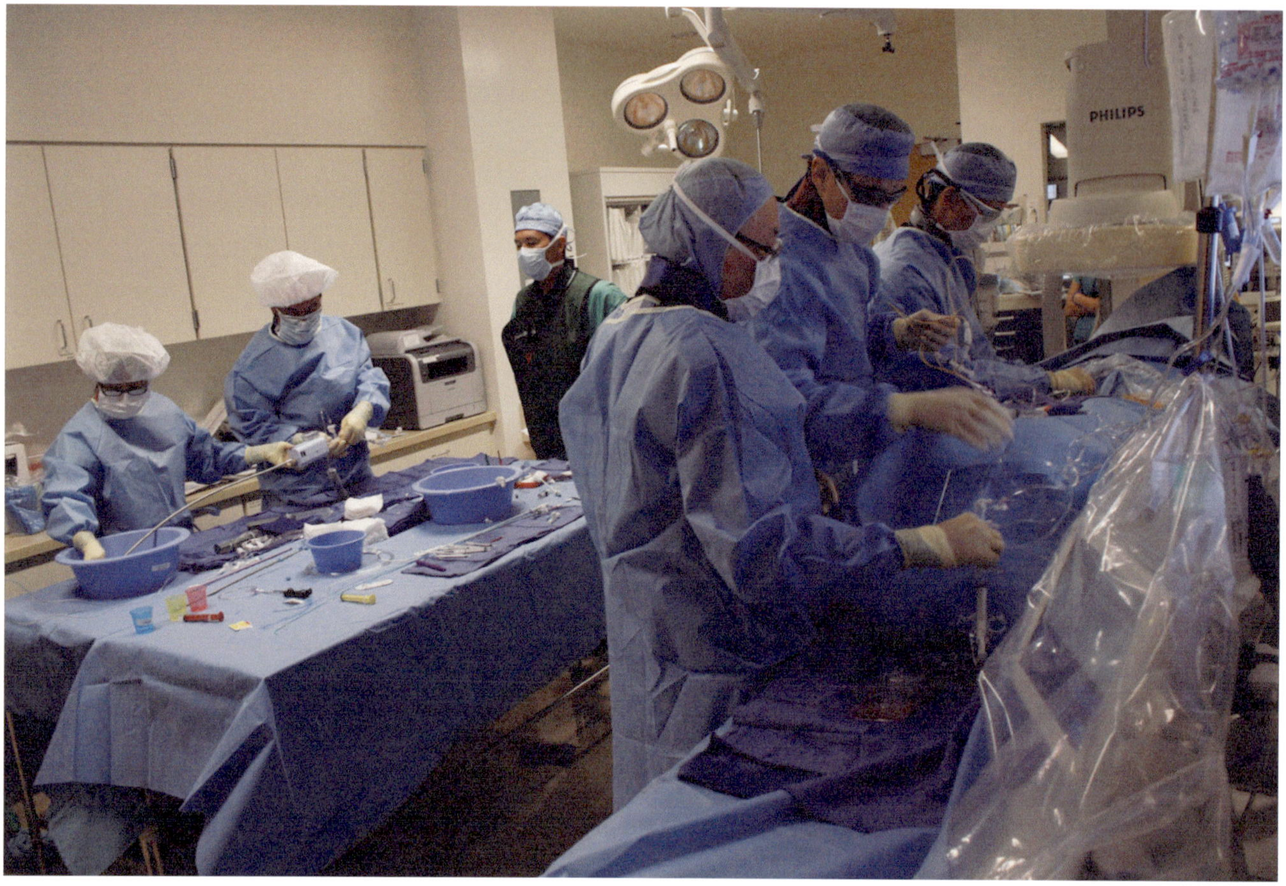

Fig. 3.17 Cath Lab setup with team members preparing the guide, while the rest of the team completes the right heart catheterization and prepares for the transseptal puncture

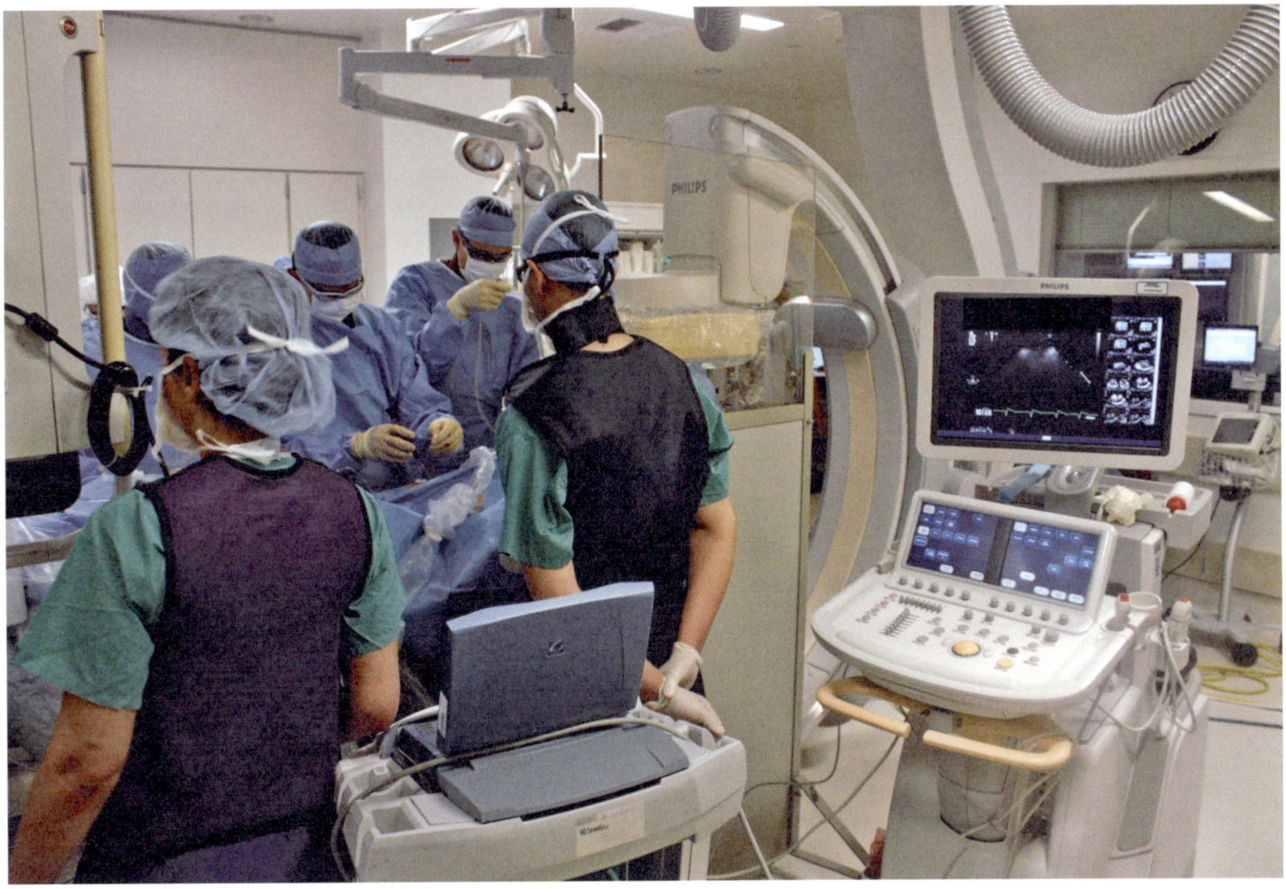

Fig. 3.18 Cath Lab setup the echocardiologist on the left side of the patient, while the fluoroscopy equipment is at the head of the table. The echocardiologist is protected by a lead shield

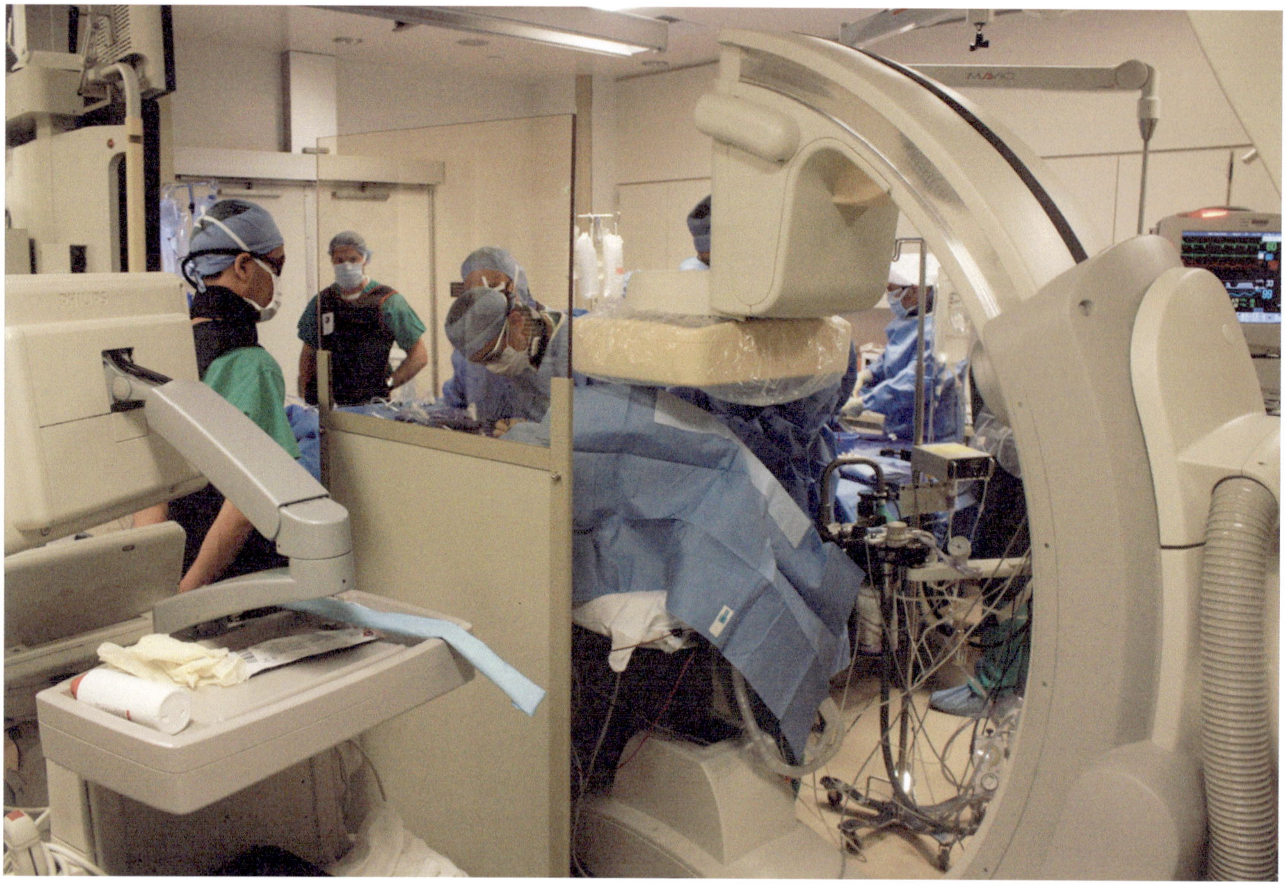

Fig. 3.19 Cath Lab setup with the view from the left side of the patient's head showing the position of the echo machine, the fluoroscopy machine, and the anesthesia equipment seen at the right side of the head

Summary of MitraClip Clinical Data and Approach to Patient Selection

4

Ehrin J. Armstrong and Jason Rogers

Abstract

Since its initial conception as a percutaneous approach to mitral valve repair, MitraClip therapy has undergone extensive clinical testing and refinement. Through these studies, we have gained an increased understanding of the spectrum of patients who benefit from this procedure and the longer-term effects of MitraClip therapy on MR and patient outcomes. In this chapter, we review the major results of the US-based EVEREST studies, including the safety and feasibility trial, the pivotal randomized trial, and the high-risk registry. We then discuss the published experience of case series and registries from Europe. Surgical repair after initial MitraClip therapy is also discussed. Although there have been over 5,000 global implants at the time of publication of this atlas, it is notable that only a single randomized trial has been completed. This chapter concludes with a discussion of high-risk subgroups of patients that may particularly benefit from MitraClip therapy.

Keywords

MitraClip • Clinical trials • EVEREST study • Mitral regurgitation

Introduction

Since its initial conception as a percutaneous approach to mitral valve repair, MitraClip therapy has undergone extensive clinical testing and refinement [1, 2]. Through these studies, we have gained an increased understanding of the spectrum of patients who benefit from this procedure and the longer-term effects of MitraClip therapy on MR and patient outcomes. In this chapter, we review the major results of the US-based EVEREST studies, including the safety and feasibility trial, the pivotal randomized trial, and the high-risk registry. We then discuss the published experience of case series and registries from Europe. Surgical repair after initial MitraClip therapy is also discussed. Although there have been over 5,000 global implants at the time of publication of this atlas, it is notable that only a single randomized trial has been completed (Table 4.1). This chapter concludes with a discussion of high-risk subgroups of patients that may particularly benefit from MitraClip therapy.

E.J. Armstrong, M.D., M.Sc. (✉)
Division of Cardiovascular Medicine,
University of California, Davis Medical Center,
4860 Y Street, Suite 2820, Sacramento, CA 95817, USA
e-mail: ehrin.armstrong@ucdmc.ucdavis.edu

J. Rogers, M.D., FACC, FSCAI
Division of Cardiovascular Medicine,
University of California, Davis Medical Center,
4860 Y Street, Suite 2820, Sacramento, CA 95817, USA
e-mail: jason.rogers@ucdmc.ucdavis.edu

T. Feldman et al. (eds.), *Atlas of Percutaneous Edge-to-Edge Mitral Valve Repair*,
DOI 10.1007/978-1-4471-4294-2_4, © Springer-Verlag London 2013

Table 4.1 Total number of MitraClip procedures performed worldwide as of January 2012

Study	Population	*N*
EVEREST I (feasibility)	Feasibility patients	55
EVEREST II (pivotal)	Pre-randomized patients	60
EVEREST II (pivotal)	Non-randomized patients (high-risk study)	78
EVEREST II (pivotal)	Randomized patients (2:1 clip to surgery)	279 (184 clip, 95 surgery)
REALISM (continued access)	Non-randomized patients	595
Compassionate/emergency use	Non-randomized patients	28
ACCESS Europe phase I	Non-randomized patients	566
ACCESS Europe phase II	Non-randomized patients	53
Commercial use	Commercial patients	2,551
Total		*4,170 + 95 surgery*

EVEREST Trials

All of the major EVEREST (Endovascular Valve Edge-to-Edge Repair Study) trials have been completed and published. These consist of a feasibility study and roll-in phase for the randomized trial, the EVEREST II randomized controlled trial comparing MitraClip therapy to surgery, and the EVEREST high-risk registry.

EVEREST I: Feasibility and Roll-In

The initial experience with the MitraClip device consisted of a phase I feasibility trial and an additional 52 patients treated in the pre-randomization start-up experience (roll-in phase) of the EVEREST II pivotal trial [3]. These data represent the early North American experience with the MitraClip device, with 70 % of these procedures being the first, second, or third procedures at each respective site. Patients were selected if they were candidates for MV surgery, met major ACC/AHA indications for MV surgery, and had specific anatomic criteria including a primary central regurgitant jet associated with the A2/P2 segments, a coaptation length ≥2 mm, a coaptation depth ≤11 mm, a flail gap <10 mm, and a flail width <15 mm. Key exclusion criteria included LVEF ≤ 25 %, LV end-systolic dimension >55 mm, mitral valve orifice area <4 cm^2, or recent myocardial infarction [4]. These EVEREST-specific clinical and anatomic criteria were used for all North American trial and registry data but have not been consistently applied in the European experience.

Of the 107 patients who underwent the MitraClip procedure in this early US experience, 70 (74 %) achieved acute procedural success (APS), defined as a post-procedure reduction of MR to ≤2+. Of subjects who did not achieve APS, 17 (16 %) had MitraClip implantation with acute MR grade >2+, and 11 (10 %) had no MitraClip implanted with post-procedure MR >2+. At 12 months, not including crossover to surgery, 50 of 76 APS patients (66 %) had echocardiographic follow-up and continued with MR ≤2+. A total of 32 patients underwent MV surgery after a clip procedure, and when repair was planned, 84 % were successfully repaired, demonstrating that MV repair is feasible after prior MitraClip attempt or implantation. Freedom from death at up to 3 years follow-up was 90.1 %, and freedom from surgery was 76.3 %. The majority of patients included had degenerative MR (79 %), but patients with functional MR (21 %) had similar acute results and durability.

An important feature of the EVEREST data is that an independent core laboratory assessed all echocardiograms. Mitral regurgitation was graded strictly according to American Society of Echocardiography guidelines using a composite of color-flow Doppler of the regurgitant jet area, pulmonary vein flow, regurgitant volume, and regurgitant fraction. Interobserver variability was low using this methodology, with 84 % concordance in regard to MR severity. This analysis of echocardiograms pre- and post-percutaneous or surgical MV therapy differs from the majority of prior surgical repair studies, which have not used quantitative echocardiographic methods or core laboratories. Analyses of echocardiograms from enrolling EVEREST sites demonstrated that without the use of quantitative methodology, baseline MR grade is often overestimated by using qualitative methods [5].

EVEREST II: Randomized, Controlled Trial

The prospective, randomized EVEREST II study is a landmark trial in that it is the first randomized trial of a percutaneous mitral repair device measured against conventional surgical therapy; it also represents the first echocardiographic core lab-adjudicated follow-up after surgical mitral valve repair [6]. This trial randomized 279 patients with 3–4+ MR prospectively to receive either device therapy with the MitraClip device ($n=184$) or conventional surgical repair or replacement ($n=95$) in a 2:1 ratio. The primary efficacy end point was defined as 12-month freedom from the combined outcome of death, new surgery for mitral valve dysfunction, or the occurrence of >2+ MR. The primary safety end point was the major adverse event rate (MAE) at 30 days, and

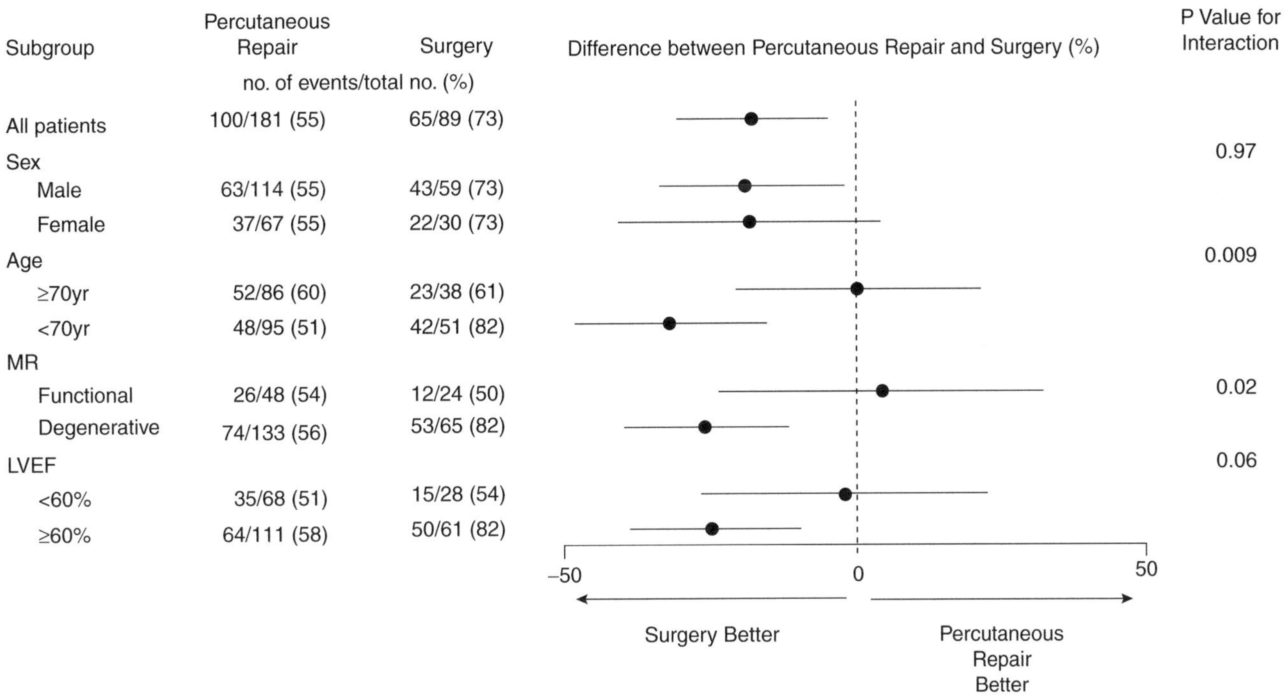

Fig. 4.1 Subgroup analyses for the primary efficacy end point at 12 months from the EVEREST II trial. Displayed are differences in the rates of the primary efficacy end point (freedom from death, from mitral valve surgery, and from grade 3+ or 4+ mitral regurgitation) between percutaneous and surgical randomized patients. Data are displayed for all patients and for four post hoc subgroups. The *horizontal lines* indicate 95 % confidence interval (Reprinted with permission from Feldman et al. [6])

prespecified MAEs were death, major stroke, reoperation of the mitral valve, urgent/emergent CV surgery, myocardial infarction, renal failure, deep wound infection, ventilation >48 h, new onset permanent atrial fibrillation, septicemia, GI complication requiring surgery, or transfusion ≥2 units. Clinical efficacy at 12 months was achieved in 55 % of the MitraClip device patients and 73 % of the surgery group, and this difference was driven by largely by increased need for surgery in the MitraClip arm ($P=0.007$). An important exploratory analysis identified age ≥ 70, functional MR, and LVEF < 60 % as subgroups in which surgery was not superior to percutaneous treatment with regard to efficacy (Fig. 4.1). The 30-day MAE rate was lower in the MitraClip group when compared to the surgery group (9.6 % vs. 57 %, superiority $P<0.0001$). The MAE difference was driven largely by transfusion requirements in the surgical arm; in response to this critique, a modified MAE analysis was also performed, which defined major bleeding as transfusion ≥4 units or significant bleeding requiring surgical intervention. This modified end point still demonstrated a lower MAE rate in the MitraClip group (5.0 % vs. 30.9 %, $P < 0.0001$) [7]. Clinical efficacy at 12 months was achieved in 72.4 % of the MitraClip device patients and 87.8 % of the surgery group (non-inferiority $P=0.0012$).

It is important to emphasize that the EVEREST II trial examined the safety and efficacy of MitraClip therapy as an initial approach to the treatment of patients with MR. Not every procedure was successful in reducing MR, but of these failures at acute procedural success, the majority had successful subsequent mitral valve surgery.

EVEREST II High-Risk Registry

Concomitant with the EVEREST II trial, a single-arm "high-risk registry" (HRR) enrolled 78 patients with MR and an STS or surgeon-estimated surgical procedural mortality risk of ≥12 % [8]. These patients also met echocardiographic-based inclusion criteria for MitraClip therapy similar to the RCT, with the exception that there was no maximum coaptation depth, and the LVEF inclusion criteria were ≥20 %. The enrolled patients were older than those in the EVEREST II RCT (mean age 77 vs. 67 years) and more frequently had a functional etiology of MR (59 % vs. 49 %). All patients in the HRR had a history of congestive heart failure, and more than half had a history of prior cardiac surgery.

Among the 78 patients in the HRR, 75 (96 %) had successful MitraClip implantation, with an acute (in-hospital) reduction of MR by at least one grade in 83 % of these patients. The 30-day mortality of these patients was 7.7 % with none of the deaths occurring intra-procedurally. Among patients alive at 12-month follow-up, MR remained ≤2+ in 78 % of patients. Compared to the year prior to MitraClip implantation, there was also a trend toward reduced hospitalizations for heart failure (rate per patient-year 0.65 at baseline vs. 0.36 at 1 year, $P=0.018$).

A concurrent group of 36 patients who were initially screened for the HRR but who did not undergo MitraClip therapy was also used as a comparator group for clinical outcomes. These patients had similar baseline demographic characteristics but did not undergo device implantation due to mitral valve anatomic exclusion criteria or because the high-risk registry had ended. When compared to this nonintervention group, patients who underwent MitraClip implantation had significantly higher 12-month survival (76.4 % vs. 55.3 %, $P=0.047$). While this is not a randomized comparator group, these data do suggest that MitraClip therapy may have a mortality benefit among patients with severe functional MR who are at high risk for surgery.

European Registry Data

Since CE mark approval in 2008, the majority of MitraClip implants worldwide have been performed in Europe. The European experience with the device reflects real-world practice where application of the MitraClip device has not required the strict control of a randomized trial. The largest reports to date on the European MitraClip experience originate from a single center in Germany [9] and two centers in Italy [10], but a number of other reports have also recently been published, with increasing emphasis on application of this technology to patients at prohibitive risk of surgery and patients with functional MR and heart failure.

German Experience

Franzen et al. reported their initial experience with the MitraClip system in patients who met current guideline criteria for treatment of MR [9]. Their interdisciplinary team of interventional cardiologists and cardiac surgeons treated 51 patients with ≥3+MR who were at high risk for mitral valve surgery based on a logistic EuroSCORE >20, an STS score >12, or other clinical factors which the team felt conferred a high surgical risk (i.e., prior chest radiation therapy, frailty, prior stroke, or prior sternotomy). The exclusion criteria were relatively few and consisted of a mitral valve area ≤2.0 cm^2, active endocarditis, or extensively prolapsed or flail leaflets (prolapse width >25 mm, flail gap >20 mm).

Patients in this series had significantly worse left ventricular dysfunction and more adverse valve morphology than patients enrolled in the EVEREST trials. Specifically, there was no lower limit on LVEF or upper limit on LV size, and there was a broader spectrum of allowable leaflet anatomy and regurgitant jet location (noncentral jet allowed). Among the patients undergoing MitraClip therapy, there were 35 patients (69 %) with LV or leaflet characteristics that would have excluded them from enrollment in the EVEREST trials. These were termed the "EVEREST–" cohort and had a significantly higher logistic EuroSCOREs (33 vs. 18) and larger LV end-systolic volumes (124 vs. 101 mm^3). The remaining patients were defined as "EVEREST+" and would have met enrollment criteria for the EVEREST trials.

MitraClip therapy was performed in 51 consecutive patients with a mean logistic EuroSCORE of 29±22 and a Society of Thoracic Surgeons score of 15±11. MitraClip implantation was successful in 49 patients (96 %), with the majority of patients (34/49, 69 %) treated with a single clip, 14 patients (29 %) receiving two clips, and one patient receiving three clips. All 16 EVEREST+patients had successful MitraClip implantation, whereas 2 of the 35 EVEREST– patients did not have clips implanted. This was due to a 17-cm left atrium in one case and substantial subvalvular calcification in the other case. Procedure-related reduction in MR severity was one grade in 16 patients (31 %), two grades in 24 patients (47 %), and three grades in nine patients (18 %). There was no clinically significant mitral stenosis observed after therapy, and there were no procedure-related major adverse events and no in-hospital mortality. In summary, the authors demonstrated the feasibility and short-term efficacy of the MitraClip in high surgical-risk patients, with a substantial proportion of patients treated that would have been excluded from the EVEREST trials.

A follow-up study from the same group examined the echocardiographic and clinical outcomes up to 1 year among patients at prohibitive risk for surgery [11]. This series of 104 patients had a mean logistic EuroScore of 36, and the majority (66 %) had a functional etiology of MR; all patients were NYHA congestive heart failure class III or IV. Eighty percent of the patients also had one or more EVEREST II exclusion criteria at baseline, with the most frequent reasons being mitral valve area <4.0 cm^2 (43 %) or left ventricular end-systolic dimension >55 mm (38 %). Ninety-two percent of patients had successful device implantation, with 13.5 % of patients experiencing peri-procedural complications. Among patients with successful device implantation, six required repeat clipping for early recurrent MR (performed at a median of 140 days), and two patients underwent mitral valve surgery.

At a median follow-up of 1 year, 69 % of surviving patients were NYHA functional class I or II. The Kaplan–Meier estimated 1-year mortality was 22 %. At follow-up, surviving patients had significant increases in 6-min walk distance, a significant decrease in NT-pro BNP levels, and reduced scores on the Minnesota Living with Heart Failure Questionnaire. The authors concluded that approximately three-quarters of patients with severe MR and prohibitive risk of surgery derived clinical benefit from MitraClip implantation. These results are similar to an initial smaller cohort of patients with systolic heart failure and severe MR reported from seven European centers [12].

Another group in Germany has also recently reported short-term results of 33 patients with moderate to severe MR and logistic EuroScore >15 % who underwent successful MitraClip implantation [13]. The mean patient age was 76 years, all patients were NYHA class III or IV, and 63 % of patients had a functional etiology of MR. The calculated logistic EuroScore for this cohort was 41 ± 7 %, and the STS score was 24 ± 4 %, representing an extremely high-risk group of patients. There were no intra-procedural deaths or deaths at 30 days. At 30 days, the mean NYHA class improved from 3.4 to 2.2 ($P < 0.001$). Patients also had a significant increase in 6-min walk distance and a trend toward decreased NT-pro BNP. These recent studies emphasize the need to better understand long-term clinical outcomes after MitraClip implantation among high-risk patients, as patients in this subgroup are not candidates for surgery and may derive significant benefit from reduction in MR after transcatheter intervention.

Italian Experience

Tamburino et al. reported results from the initial Italian clinical experience with the MitraClip at two centers. Their multidisciplinary teams selected patients who met criteria for mitral intervention based on established guidelines and who were high risk for surgery based on the consensus between cardiologist and cardiac surgeon, logistic EuroSCORE >20, hepatic cirrhosis, autoimmune disease, severe renal failure requiring hemodialysis, or any contraindication to extracorporeal circulation. Anatomic leaflet criteria were similar to EVEREST criteria, with a requirement for primarily central regurgitation (at the A2/P2 interface) and sufficient leaflet tissue for mechanical coaptation. Key exclusion criteria were similar to the EVEREST trials, including mitral valve orifice area <4 cm^2, flail width ≥15 mm, flail gap ≥10 mm, coaptation depth ≥11 mm, and coaptation length <2 mm. Importantly, unlike EVEREST, there was no exclusion for very low LV ejection fraction, nor was there an upper limit on LV size. The primary efficacy end point was acute device success defined as clip placement with reduction of MR to ≤2+. The primary acute safety end point was 30-day freedom from major adverse events, defined as the composite of death, myocardial infarction, nonelective cardiac surgery for adverse events, renal failure, transfusion of >2 units of blood, ventilation for >48 h, deep wound infection, septicemia, and new onset atrial fibrillation.

Thirty-one patients were successfully treated using standard techniques, with 19 patients undergoing single MitraClip implantation and 12 patients having two clips placed. There were no unsuccessful attempts at MitraClip placement and no procedural mortality. At 30 days, there was an intra-procedural cardiac tamponade (treated successfully with pericardiocentesis and subsequent MitraClip implantation) and one noncardiac death, resulting in a primary safety end point of 93.6 %. Acute device success was observed in 96.8 % of patients. At 30 days, there was favorable LV remodeling, with reduction in the diastolic mitral annular septal-lateral dimension. Mitral valve area significantly diminished at 30 days, but this did not result in any clinically significant mitral stenosis.

A follow-up report of 45 patients treated at these centers in Italy reported on quality of life measures before and 6 months after MitraClip implantation [14]. Among these cases (which include temporal overlap with the prior publication), there was no intra-procedural or 30-day mortality. At 6-month follow-up, five patients had died. Among the surviving patients, MR at 6 months was reported as ≤1+ in 86 % of patients. Pre procedure, 85 % of patients were NYHA functional class III or IV; at 6 months, 97 % of surviving patients were functional class I or II. Quality of life measures were also significantly improved at 6 months compared to baseline, with improvement in both physical and psychological parameters of perceived quality of life.

Netherlands Experience

Van den Branden et al. recently reported on a separate single-center cohort of 52 patients at high surgical risk who underwent 55 MitraClip procedures [15]. All patients had baseline MR ≥3+ and were declined for surgery because of a logistic EuroScore ≥20 %. A device was successfully implanted in 96 % of procedures. Three patients had partial clip detachment and therefore required implantation of an additional device. Six-month mortality was 11.5 %, with five of the six deaths due to progressive heart failure. Among patients with 6-month follow-up, 79 % had MR grade ≤2+. Overall, patients also had evidence of left ventricular remodeling at 6 months, with improvements in left ventricular end-diastolic diameter, an increase in ejection fraction, and a reduction in right ventricular systolic pressures.

PERMIT-CARE Registry

Patients with a depressed ejection fraction and functional MR represent a high-risk subset of patients who may derive benefit from MitraClip therapy. Because many of these patients may also be candidates for cardiac resynchronization therapy (CRT), it is important to understand the additive role of MitraClip therapy in this high-risk subset of patients. The PERMIT-CARE registry is an international study of nonresponders to CRT with persistent 2+ or greater MR who subsequently underwent MitraClip implantation [16]. All 51 reported patients were NYHA functional class III or IV; the etiology of cardiomyopathy was ischemic in 37 (73 %) of patients and non-ischemic in the other 14 (27 %). Mean logistic EuroSCORE was 29.7, and the mean STS score was 13.9 %. MitraClip implantation was performed a mean of 33 months after initial CRT. These patients also had significantly dilated left ventricles, with mean LVESD of 60.3 mm and LVEDD of 71.0 mm; the mean baseline ejection fraction was 27.1 %. Two patients died during the procedure—one because of cardiogenic shock and continued need for inotropic support and the other due to chordal rupture and resulting acute heart failure. Overall 30-day mortality was 4.2 %. At 6-month follow-up, 80 % of patients were NYHA functional class I or II, and more than 80 % of patients had MR grade ≤2+. Follow-up echocardiography also demonstrated improvements in LVEDD, LVESD, and EF on serial echocardiography, consistent with reverse remodeling after MitraClip implantation. These initial findings suggest that MitraClip implantation has significant benefit among patients with prior CRT but persistent symptoms of heart failure and functional MR.

MitraClip Efficacy and Surgery After MitraClip Therapy

After MitraClip implantation, the device undergoes fibrous encapsulation and eventually forms a tissue bridge that bolsters device stability [18]. In cases of recurrent MR where surgical intervention may be necessary, the device can often be explanted with minimal disruption of the mitral valve structure, thereby allowing valve repair rather than replacement.

Argenziano et al. have reported on the 32 patients who underwent MV surgery after a MitraClip procedure from the EVEREST and EVEREST II roll-in cohort [19]. Twenty-seven patients underwent the surgical procedure planned before surgery (21 repairs, 6 replacements), one patient without a known pre-procedure strategy had MV replacement, and four planned repairs subsequently underwent MV replacement. The overall repair rate after the MitraClip procedure was 66 %. Glower et al. recently presented data from EVEREST II regarding repairability of the mitral valve after MitraClip placement and found that the repair rate ≤90 days was 52 % (14/27 patients) and the repair rate >90 days after surgery was 60 % (6/10). The presence of bileaflet/anterior flail/prolapse was a significant predictor of the need for MV replacement, but surgeon experience, defined as the number of surgeries performed annually, did not have an impact on whether a repair or replacement was performed [20].

Geidel et al. has reported that mitral valve pathology can be aggravated by MitraClip implantation [21]. However, in this report, complex successful mitral valve repair was still achieved. Rogers et al. reported a series of four patients who underwent successful surgical MV repair up to 5 years and 2 months after MitraClip device implantation, demonstrating that very late MV repair remains possible, including after implantation of two devices [22]. Other than for degenerative MR, it is debatable whether mitral valve repair after a failed MitraClip procedure in ischemic mitral regurgitation should be attempted. Magne et al. did not find a mortality difference between repair and replacement in patients with ischemic MR 6 years after surgery [23].

Approach to Patient Selection

A summary of all published series to date is presented in Table 4.2. Based on the these data, it has been demonstrated that the MitraClip can be safely and successfully applied to a diverse patient population in terms of age, surgical risk, and mitral valve pathologies. The anatomic leaflet criteria for MitraClip patient selection were rigorously defined in the EVEREST trials, but the European experience has shown us proof of principle that the MitraClip can be delivered to more complex (non-EVEREST) leaflet anatomy. Although further investigation will undoubtedly refine our understanding of "acceptable" leaflet anatomy, the main limitations appear to be the ability to grasp both leaflets and the undesired development of mitral stenosis. Despite concerns about possible mitral stenosis, the reported experience from both North America and Europe suggests that the development of clinically significant mitral stenosis is uncommon [17].

Based on adoption patterns in Europe and North America to date, it would appear that patients with functional MR, and those degenerative MR patients at high risk for surgical therapy, will constitute the target population for MitraClip use. Younger low-risk patients with degenerative MR generally have very good surgical outcomes, and MitraClip therapy should not be considered as first-line therapy for these patients [24, 25]. Since functional MR is primarily a ventricular problem, it remains to be seen whether a leaflet intervention will have durable efficacy. Numerous predictors of recurrent MR after restrictive annuloplasty for FMR have been identified, and their relevance to determining patient selection for MitraClip therapy is yet to be determined [26–28]. Future MitraClip and delivery system designs may allow a wider range of valve anatomies to be treated and may simplify leaflet insertion and grasping. In addition, innovations in echocardiographic and intracardiac imaging will increasingly revolutionize this and other structural heart procedures. Studies focused on long-term clinical outcomes, including symptomatic heart failure, quality of life, and reverse remodeling, will continue to refine patient cohorts who derive the greatest benefit from MitraClip therapy.

Table 4.2 Comparative summary of published MitraClip clinical trials

	n (patients)	Degenerative/ functional/mixed etiology	Age, mean	Baseline LVEF (%)	STS score/ logistic EuroSCORE, mean	Baseline NYHA III/ IV (%)	Follow-up NYHA III/IV (%)	Mean MR grade at baseline	MR ≤2+ at follow-up	Echocardiographic core lab	Procedural mortality/ in-hospital death
EVEREST and EVEREST II roll-in registry (USA), Feldman et al.	107	79 %/21 %	71	62	NR/NR	46	8 (At 12 months)	3.3	74 % (Discharge)/66 % (12 months)	Yes	0(0 %)/1(0.9 %)
EVEREST II randomized controlled trial (USA), Feldman et al.	184	73 %/27 %	67	60	NR/NR	52	NR	3.5	79 % (At 12 months)	Yes	Two deaths (1 %) at 30 days
EVEREST II high-risk registry (USA), Whitlow et al.	78	41 %/59 %	77	54	14/NR	90	26 (At 12 months)	77/78 (99 %) with MR grade 3+ or 4+	78 % (12 months)	Yes	0 (0 %)/3 (3.8 %)
German experience Franzen et al.	51	31 %/69 %	73	36	16/28	98	33 (At discharge)	3.6	94 % (At discharge)	No	0(0 %)/0 (0 %)
German experience, Rudolph et al.	104	27 %/66 %/7 %	74	43	NR/36	100	31 (Median 1 year)	3.6	82 % (Median 1 year)	No	0(0 %)/4(4 %)
German experience, Pleger et al.	33	36 %/63 %	76	39	24/41	100	25 (At 30 days)	2.9	75 %	No	0(0 %)/0(0 %)
Italian experience Tamburino et al.	31	42 %/58 %	71	42	10.3/14.3	87	0 (At 30 days)	3.9	97 % (30 days)	No	0(0 %)/NR
Italian experience, Ussia et al.	39	36 %/64 %	72	NR	11/20	85	3 (At 6 month)	3.7	100 % (At 6 months)	No	0(0 %)/0(0 %)
Netherland experience, Van den Branden et al.	52	10 %/90 %	73	37	10/27	98	16 (At 6 months)	4	79 % (At 6 months)	No	1(1.8 %)/2(3.6 %)
PERMIT-CARE registry, Auricchio et al.	51	0 %/100 %	70	27	14/30	100	22 (At 12 months)	100 % with ≥2+	10 % with ≥2+ (12 months)	Yes	1(2 %)/3 (4.2 %)

NR not reported

References

1. Condado JA, Acquatella H, Rodriguez L, Whitlow P, Velez-Gimo M, St Goar FG. Percutaneous edge-to-edge mitral valve repair: 2-year follow-up in the first human case. Catheter Cardiovasc Interv. 2006;67(2):323–5.
2. St Goar FG, Fann JI, Komtebedde J, Foster E, Oz MC, Fogarty TJ, Feldman T, Block PC. Endovascular edge-to-edge mitral valve repair: short-term results in a porcine model. Circulation. 2003; 108(16):1990–3.
3. Feldman T, Kar S, Rinaldi M, Fail P, Hermiller J, Smalling R, Whitlow PL, Gray W, Low R, Herrmann HC, Lim S, Foster E, Glower D. Percutaneous mitral repair with the MitraClip system: safety and midterm durability in the initial EVEREST (Endovascular Valve Edge-to-Edge REpair Study) Cohort. J Am Coll Cardiol. 2009;54(8):686–94.
4. Mauri L, Garg P, Massaro JM, Foster E, Glower D, Mehoudar P, Powell F, Komtebedde J, McDermott E, Feldman T. The EVEREST II Trial: design and rationale for a randomized study of the evalve mitraclip system compared with mitral valve surgery for mitral regurgitation. Am Heart J. 2010;160(1):23–9.
5. Foster E, Wasserman HS, Gray W, Homma S, Di Tullio MR, Rodriguez L, Stewart WJ, Whitlow P, Block P, Martin R, Merlino J, Herrmann HC, Wiegers SE, Silvestry FE, Hamilton A, Zunamon A, Kraybill K, Gerber IL, Weeks SG, Zhang Y, Feldman T. Quantitative assessment of severity of mitral regurgitation by serial echocardiography in a multicenter clinical trial of percutaneous mitral valve repair. Am J Cardiol. 2007;100(10):1577–83.
6. Feldman T, Foster E, Glower DD, Kar S, Rinaldi MJ, Fail PS, Smalling RW, Siegel R, Rose GA, Engeron E, Loghin C, Trento A, Skipper ER, Fudge T, Letsou GV, Massaro JM, Mauri L. Percutaneous repair or surgery for mitral regurgitation. N Engl J Med. 2011;364(15):1395–406.
7. Feldman T, Mauri L, Kar S, Rinaldi M, Fail P, Hermiller J, Smalling R, Gray W, Wang A, Herrmann H, Rogers J, Lasala J, Bajwa T, Grayburn P, Pedersen W, Foster E, Trento A, Glower D. EVEREST II randomized clinical trial: a critical assessment of the safety data in patients treated with the MitraClip. J Am Coll Cardiol. 2010;56(13, Supplement 1):B23.
8. Whitlow PL, Feldman T, Pedersen WR, Lim DS, Kipperman R, Smalling R, Bajwa T, Herrmann HC, Lasala J, Maddux JT, Tuzcu M, Kapadia S, Trento A, Siegel RJ, Foster E, Glower D, Mauri L, Kar S. Acute and 12-month results with catheter-based mitral valve leaflet repair: the EVEREST II (Endovascular Valve Edge-to-Edge Repair) High Risk Study. J Am Coll Cardiol. 2012;59(2):130–9.
9. Franzen O, Baldus S, Rudolph V, Meyer S, Knap M, Koschyk D, Treede H, Barmeyer A, Schofer J, Costard-Jackle A, Schluter M, Reichenspurner H, Meinertz T. Acute outcomes of MitraClip therapy for mitral regurgitation in high-surgical-risk patients: emphasis on adverse valve morphology and severe left ventricular dysfunction. Eur Heart J. 2010;31(11):1373–81.
10. Tamburino C, Ussia GP, Maisano F, Capodanno D, La Canna G, Scandura S, Colombo A, Giacomini A, Michev I, Mangiafico S, Cammalleri V, Barbanti M, Alfieri O. Percutaneous mitral valve repair with the MitraClip system: acute results from a real world setting. Eur Heart J. 2010;31(11):1382–9.
11. Rudolph V, Knap M, Franzen O, Schluter M, de Vries T, Conradi L, Schirmer J, Treede H, Wegscheider K, Costard-Jackle A, Meinertz T, Reichenspurner H, Baldus S. Echocardiographic and clinical outcomes of MitraClip therapy in patients not amenable to surgery. J Am Coll Cardiol. 2011;58(21):2190–5.
12. Franzen O, van der Heyden J, Baldus S, Schluter M, Schillinger W, Butter C, Hoffmann R, Corti R, Pedrazzini G, Swaans MJ, Neuss M, Rudolph V, Surder D, Grunenfelder J, Eulenburg C, Reichenspurner H, Meinertz T, Auricchio A. MitraClip(R) therapy in patients with end-stage systolic heart failure. Eur J Heart Fail. 2011;13(5): 569–76.
13. Pleger ST, Mereles D, Schulz-Schonhagen M, Krumsdorf U, Chorianopoulos E, Rottbauer W, Katus HA, Bekeredjian R. Acute safety and 30-day outcome after percutaneous edge-to-edge repair of mitral regurgitation in very high-risk patients. Am J Cardiol. 2011;108(10):1478–82.
14. Ussia GP, Cammalleri V, Sarkar K, Scandura S, Imme S, Pistritto AM, Caggegi A, Chiaranda M, Mangiafico S, Barbanti M, Scarabelli M, Mule M, Aruta P, Tamburino C. Quality of life following percutaneous mitral valve repair with the MitraClip system. Int J Cardiol. 2012;155(2):194–200.
15. Van den Branden BJ, Swaans MJ, Post MC, Rensing BJ, Eefting FD, Jaarsma W, Van der Heyden JA. Percutaneous edge-to-edge mitral valve repair in high-surgical-risk patients: do we hit the target? JACC Cardiovasc Interv. 2012;5(1):105–11.
16. Auricchio A, Schillinger W, Meyer S, Maisano F, Hoffmann R, Ussia GP, Pedrazzini GB, van der Heyden J, Fratini S, Klersy C, Komtebedde J, Franzen O. Correction of mitral regurgitation in nonresponders to cardiac resynchronization therapy by MitraClip improves symptoms and promotes reverse remodeling. J Am Coll Cardiol. 2011;58(21):2183–9.
17. Herrmann HC, Kar S, Siegel R, Fail P, Loghin C, Lim S, Hahn R, Rogers JH, Bommer WJ, Wang A, Berke A, Lerakis S, Kramer P, Wong SC, Foster E, Glower D, Feldman T. Effect of percutaneous mitral repair with the MitraClip device on mitral valve area and gradient. EuroIntervention. 2009;4(4):437–42.
18. Ladich E, Michaels MB, Jones RM, McDermott E, Coleman L, Komtebedde J, Glower D, Argenziano M, Feldman T, Nakano M, Virmani R. Pathological healing response of explanted MitraClip devices. Circulation. 2011;123(13):1418–27.
19. Argenziano M, Skipper E, Heimansohn D, Letsou GV, Woo YJ, Kron I, Alexander J, Cleveland J, Kong B, Davidson M, Vassiliades T, Krieger K, Sako E, Tibi P, Galloway A, Foster E, Feldman T, Glower D. Surgical revision after percutaneous mitral repair with the MitraClip device. Ann Thorac Surg. 2010;89(1):72–80; discussion 80.
20. Glower D, Young JN, Alexander J, Gangahar D, Skipper E, Cleveland J, Trento A, Feldman T. EVEREST II randomized clinical trial: a critical assessment of anatomical predictors of de novo mitral valve replacement or following the MitraClip procedure. J Am Coll Cardiol. 2010;56(13, Supplement 1):B25.
21. Geidel S, Ostermeyer J, Lass M, Schmoeckel M. Complex surgical valve repair after failed percutaneous mitral intervention using the MitraClip device. Ann Thorac Surg. 2010;90(1):277–9.
22. Rogers JH, Yeo KK, Carroll JD, Cleveland J, Reece TB, Gillinov AM, Rodriguez L, Whitlow P, Woo YJ, Herrmann HC, Young JN. Late surgical mitral valve repair after percutaneous repair with the MitraClip system. J Card Surg. 2009;24(6):677–81.
23. Magne J, Girerd N, Senechal M, Mathieu P, Dagenais F, Dumesnil JG, Charbonneau E, Voisine P, Pibarot P. Mitral repair versus replacement for ischemic mitral regurgitation: comparison of short-term and long-term survival. Circulation. 2009;120(11 Suppl): S104–11.
24. Johnston DR, Gillinov AM, Blackstone EH, Griffin B, Stewart W, Sabik 3rd JF, Mihaljevic T, Svensson LG, Houghtaling PL, Lytle BW. Surgical repair of posterior mitral valve prolapse: implications for guidelines and percutaneous repair. Ann Thorac Surg. 2010; 89(5):1385–94.
25. Seeburger J, Borger MA, Doll N, Walther T, Passage J, Falk V, Mohr FW. Comparison of outcomes of minimally invasive mitral valve surgery for posterior, anterior and bileaflet prolapse. Eur J Cardiothorac Surg. 2009;36(3):532–8.

26. Braun J, van de Veire NR, Klautz RJ, Versteegh MI, Holman ER, Westenberg JJ, Boersma E, van der Wall EE, Bax JJ, Dion RA. Restrictive mitral annuloplasty cures ischemic mitral regurgitation and heart failure. Ann Thorac Surg. 2008;85(2):430–6; discussion 436–7.
27. Calafiore AM, Gallina S, Di Mauro M, Gaeta F, Iaco AL, D'Alessandro S, Mazzei V, Di Giammarco G. Mitral valve procedure in dilated cardiomyopathy: repair or replacement? Ann Thorac Surg. 2001;71(4):1146–52; discussion 1152–53.
28. Magne J, Pibarot P, Dagenais F, Hachicha Z, Dumesnil JG, Senechal M. Preoperative posterior leaflet angle accurately predicts outcome after restrictive mitral valve annuloplasty for ischemic mitral regurgitation. Circulation. 2007;115(6):782–91.

Echocardiographic Evaluation of Patients Before and After MitraClip Mitral Valve Repair

5

Frank E. Silvestry

Abstract

Edge-to-edge mitral valve repair improves mitral leaflet coaptation and reduces mitral regurgitation (MR) by approximating the middle scallops of the mitral valve. The percutaneous transcatheter MitraClip™ system emulates edge-to-edge surgical repair. The MitraClip™ repair system has been shown to be effective in selected patients with either degenerative or functional MR. As with surgical mitral repair, the echocardiographic assessment of mitral valve anatomy and the determination of the mechanism and severity of MR are required to select appropriate patients who may benefit from percutaneous intervention and to tailor the repair strategy to the individual pathology. High quality transthoracic and transesophageal echocardiography as well as real-time 3D imaging is essential to evaluate the mitral valve for percutaneous repair, as well as to evaluate the efficacy of the repair after it has been performed. This chapter will cover the echocardiographic assessment of the mitral valve in patients who are being considered for percutaneous edge-to-edge repair, both with regard to assessing the severity of MR as well as anatomic inclusion and exclusion criteria that has been used in the US trials and outside the US clinically. It will also cover the echocardiographic assessment of patients following percutaneous edge-to-edge mitral repair.

Keywords

Echocardiography • Real time 3D TEE • Mitral regurgitation • Mitral regurgitation severity Mitraclip • Degenerative MR • Functional MR • Regurgitant orifice are • Regurgitant volume • Percutaneous mitral repair • Residual MR • Mitral stenosis

Introduction

Edge-to-edge mitral valve repair improves mitral leaflet coaptation and reduces or eliminates significant mitral regurgitation (MR) by approximating the middle scallops of the mitral valve, thus creating a double orifice for diastolic inflow to the left ventricle [1, 2]. The technique of surgical edge-to-edge repair is emulated by the Abbott percutaneous transcatheter MitraClip™ system, in which a clip is placed on the leaflets of the mitral valve via a steerable transseptally placed guiding system [3–5]. The MitraClip™ is a polyester fabric-covered cobalt–chromium implantable clip with two arms which can be opened and closed with a steerable-guiding mechanism. A steerable guide catheter as well as steerable clip delivery catheter that is inserted in the guide is used, allowing for precise and iterative placement of the clip in the desired location on the mitral valve.

The MitraClip™ repair system has been shown to be effective in selected patients with either degenerative (both prolapsed and flail leaflets) or functional MR due to ischemic

F.E. Silvestry, M.D., FACC, FASE
Cardiovascular Division,
University of Pennsylvania School of Medicine,
Philadelphia, PA, USA

Department of Medicine,
Hospital of the University of Pennsylvania,
3400 Spruce Street, 9007 E Gates,
Philadelphia, PA 19104, USA
e-mail: fsilvest@mail.med.upenn.edu

T. Feldman et al. (eds.), *Atlas of Percutaneous Edge-to-Edge Mitral Valve Repair*,
DOI 10.1007/978-1-4471-4294-2_5,

or dilated cardiomyopathy [5]. The presence of active endocarditis, rheumatic valve disease, and significant mitral stenosis is a contraindication to MitraClip™ therapy. The MitraClip™ has been used most extensively worldwide to successfully treat mitral regurgitation arising from the central aspect of the mitral valve, that is, MR that originates at the A2 and P2 scallops.

As the MitraClip™ is analogous to a surgical suture, it therefore can be used to approximate leaflets at many locations along the leaflet coaptation surface. Alternative uses, such as nonstandard medial or lateral commissural or zipper-like clip placement [6], have been reported, but the greatest experience is with the creation of a double-orifice mitral valve with approximation of the central portion of the valve at A2–P2 [5, 7]. Treating MR at the medial and lateral commissures requires caution, as the ability and clearance to maneuver the MitraClip™ within the left ventricle are more limited than with standard central application. Given the complex structure of the sub-commissural chordae, a higher risk of clip entanglement within the chords as well as the possibility of chordal rupture can be anticipated, and care should be taken to avoid this.

As with surgical mitral repair, the echocardiographic assessment of mitral valve anatomy and the determination of the mechanism and severity of MR are required to select appropriate patients who may benefit from percutaneous intervention and to tailor the repair strategy to the individual pathology. High-quality transthoracic and transesophageal echocardiography supplemented by a real-time 3-D imaging is essential to evaluate the mitral valve for percutaneous repair, as well as to evaluate the efficacy of the repair after it has been performed. This chapter will cover the echocardiographic assessment of the mitral valve in patients who are being considered for percutaneous edge-to-edge repair, both with regard to assessing the severity of MR as well as anatomic inclusion and exclusion criteria that have been used in the US trials and outside the USA clinically. It will also cover the echocardiographic assessment of patients following percutaneous edge-to-edge mitral repair.

The MitraClip™ has been evaluated in the USA as part of several important EVEREST (Endovascular Valve Edge-to-Edge Repair Study) clinical trials (EVEREST I and II, as well as the EVEREST high-risk registry) and a continued access registry following completion of the randomized trial. Outside the USA, there is extensive robust clinical experience in Europe reported in registries and other sites in high-risk patients as well. As the worldwide use of the device is increasing dramatically, further experience with novel applications of the device will no doubt expand its utility and expand the inclusion criteria.

General Imaging Considerations

Echocardiography is the diagnostic method of choice to assess patients with mitral valve disease. Identifying the etiology and underlying lesion that result in mitral valve dysfunction is important for therapeutic decision-making in general and particularly in a patient considered for percutaneous edge-to-edge mitral repair. A precise morphologic assessment is necessary to identify the most appropriate treatment approach, whether percutaneous or surgical.

In most cases, the etiology and localization of the involved leaflets and segments can be identified by high-quality transthoracic echocardiography (TTE). A systematic approach to evaluating the MV is recommended, since a combination of lesions may contribute to the valve dysfunction and produce MR. Transesophageal echocardiography (TEE) allows an even more precise assessment of mitral functional anatomy as well as MR severity, and should be performed when the information obtained by TTE is inadequate for delineation of MV disease or MR severity. TTE and TEE were required for the assessment of patients prior to EVEREST I and II enrollment. The availability of 3-D echocardiography (especially TEE) provides additional information to determine the exact localization of lesions. In particular real-time 3-D TEE has produced significant insights into mitral valve disease both in surgical planning and in percutaneous repair [8–12].

Mitral Regurgitation Severity

The echocardiographic quantification of mitral regurgitation severity should also comprise an integrative approach of both qualitative and quantitative signs. Guidelines from the American Society of Echocardiography [13] and European Association of Echocardiography [14] exist to assist in this assessment. Table 5.1 summarizes this assessment. MR parameters are measured and then integrated for the accurate quantification of mitral regurgitation severity. In addition to quantitative parameters, supportive signs of MR severity have been defined [13, 14]. Figures 5.1, 5.2, 5.3, 5.4, 5.5, 5.6, 5.7, 5.8, 5.9, 5.10, 5.11, 5.12, 5.13, 5.14, and 5.15 demonstrate the assessment of MR severity by both transthoracic and transesophageal echocardiography. Specific signs for the presence of a severe mitral regurgitation include a vena contracta width ≥0.7 cm (Fig. 5.4), a large central regurgitant jet (Figs. 5.1 and 5.2; with a jet area of greater than 40 % of left atrium) or a wall-impinging eccentric jet of any size (Figs. 5.3 and 5.6), a large proximal flow convergence (Figs. 5.12 and 5.13), systolic pulmonary vein flow reversal in multiple veins (Fig. 5.15), and a large prominent flail mitral valve leaflet (Figs. 5.10 and 5.12). Supportive signs of severe mitral regurgitation include a dense, triangular continuous-wave Doppler MR jet envelope on spectral display (Fig. 5.5), elevated velocity of mitral inflow during passive early diastolic filling (E wave velocity greater than 1.2 m/s), as well as an enlarged left ventricle (*LV*) and left atrium (*LA*). Among the quantitative parameters, an effective regurgitant orifice area ≥0.40 cm^2, a regurgitant volume ≥60 mL, and a regurgitant fraction ≥50 % characterize severe organic mitral regurgitation due to degenerative disease and are associated with a poor outcome without treatment [15]. PISA is typically used to calculate the EROA and MR regurgitant volume (Figs 5.13 and 5.14). Real-time 3-D TEE may also be used to calculate the anatomic regurgitant orifice area (Figs. 5.7 and 5.11). In patients with functional MR due to dilated or ischemic cardiomyopathy, an effective regurgitant orifice area of ≥0.20 cm^2 and regurgitant volume of ≥30 mL predict poor outcome and may define severe functional MR [16]. As such, the estimation of effective regurgitant orifice area and regurgitant volume requires interpretation in causal context to best predict outcome and determine MR management.

Since most of the above measurements have limitations, the data from each variable should be combined and integrated. In addition, echocardiography allows estimation of pulmonary arterial pressure, measurement of LV systolic and diastolic dimension, and estimation of LVEF, which are all potentially important in the timing of mitral valve therapy. The assessment of the severity of mitral regurgitation should be correlated with the clinical evaluation as well.

Table 5.1 ASE qualitative and quantitative parameters in grading MR severity [13]

	1+ Mild	2+Moderate	3+ Moderate-severe	4+ Severe
Color flow Jet	Central, small	Central, moderate	Central, large	Central, large
	<4 cm^2	4–6 cm^2	>6 cm^2 <8 cm^2	>8 cm^2
	<10 % of LAA	10–30 % of LAA	>30 % <40 % of LAA	>40 % of LAA
			Eccentric reaching 1st PV	Eccentric reaching 2nd PV
Pulmonary vein flow	Systolic dominant	Diastolic dominant	All disatolic	Systolic flow reversal
Regurgitant volume	<30	30–44	45–59	>60
(ml/b) fraction (%)	<30	30–39	40–49	>60

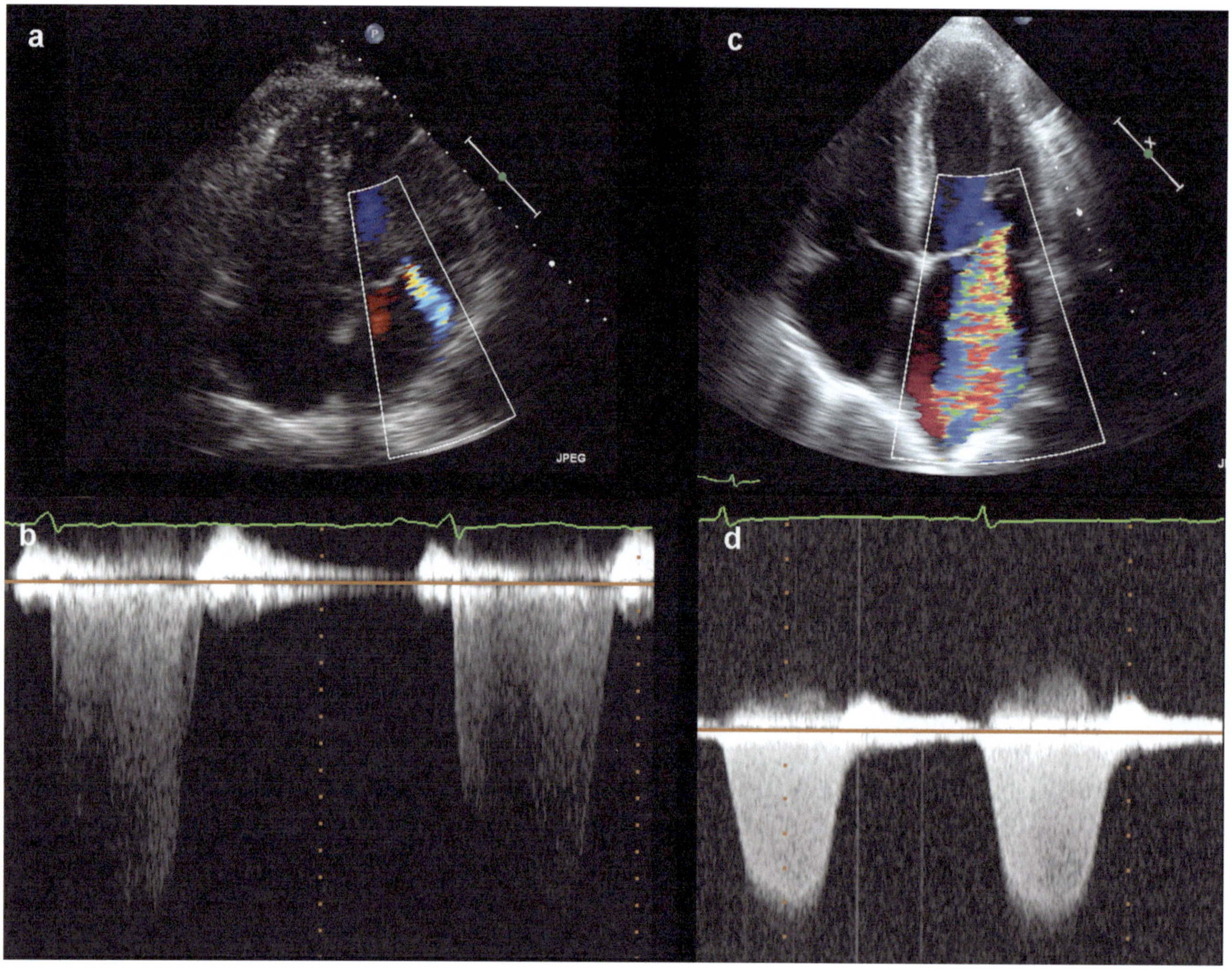

Fig. 5.1 Transthoracic echocardiography demonstrating (**a**) mild mitral regurgitation with a small regurgitant jet directed toward the lateral left atrial wall and (**b**) corresponding continuous-wave Doppler signal demonstrating a nondense jet. *Panel* **c** demonstrates moderately severe (3+) mitral regurgitation directed centrally with *panel* **d** demonstrating the corresponding dense signal on continuous-wave Doppler imaging

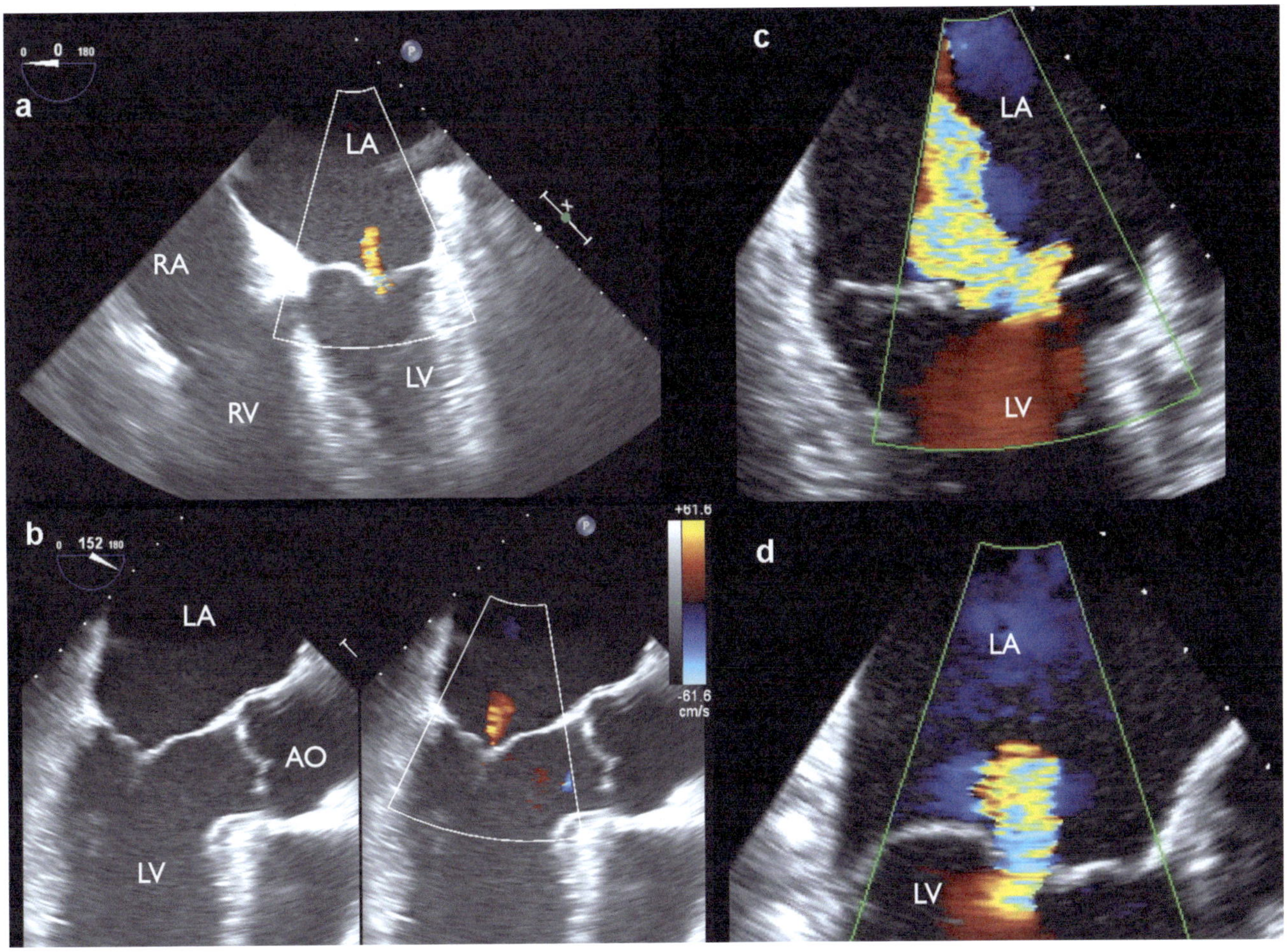

Fig. 5.2 Transesophageal echocardiography demonstrating (**a**) trivial mitral regurgitation with a small regurgitant jet directed centrally and (**b**) corresponding LV outflow tract view. *Panel* **c** demonstrates moderately severe (3+) mitral regurgitation directed slightly medially with *panel* **d** demonstrating the corresponding color Doppler jet in the LV outflow tract view. *LA* left atrium, *LV* left ventricle, *Ao* aorta

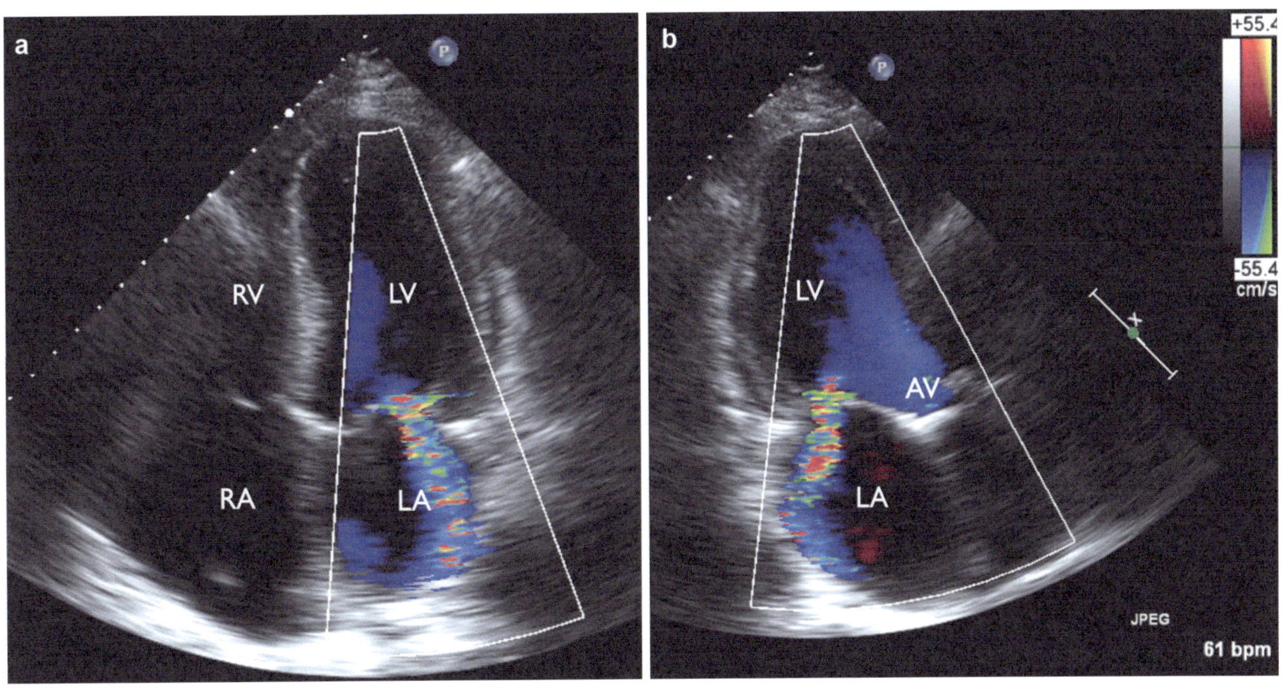

Fig. 5.3 Transthoracic echocardiography demonstrating (**a**) moderately severe (3+) mitral regurgitation with a large eccentric regurgitant jet directed toward the lateral left atrial wall in the four-chamber view and (**b**) corresponding three-chamber view of the highly eccentric jet directed posteriorly. *RV* right ventricle, *RA* right atrium, *LV* left ventricle, left atrium, *AV* aortic valve

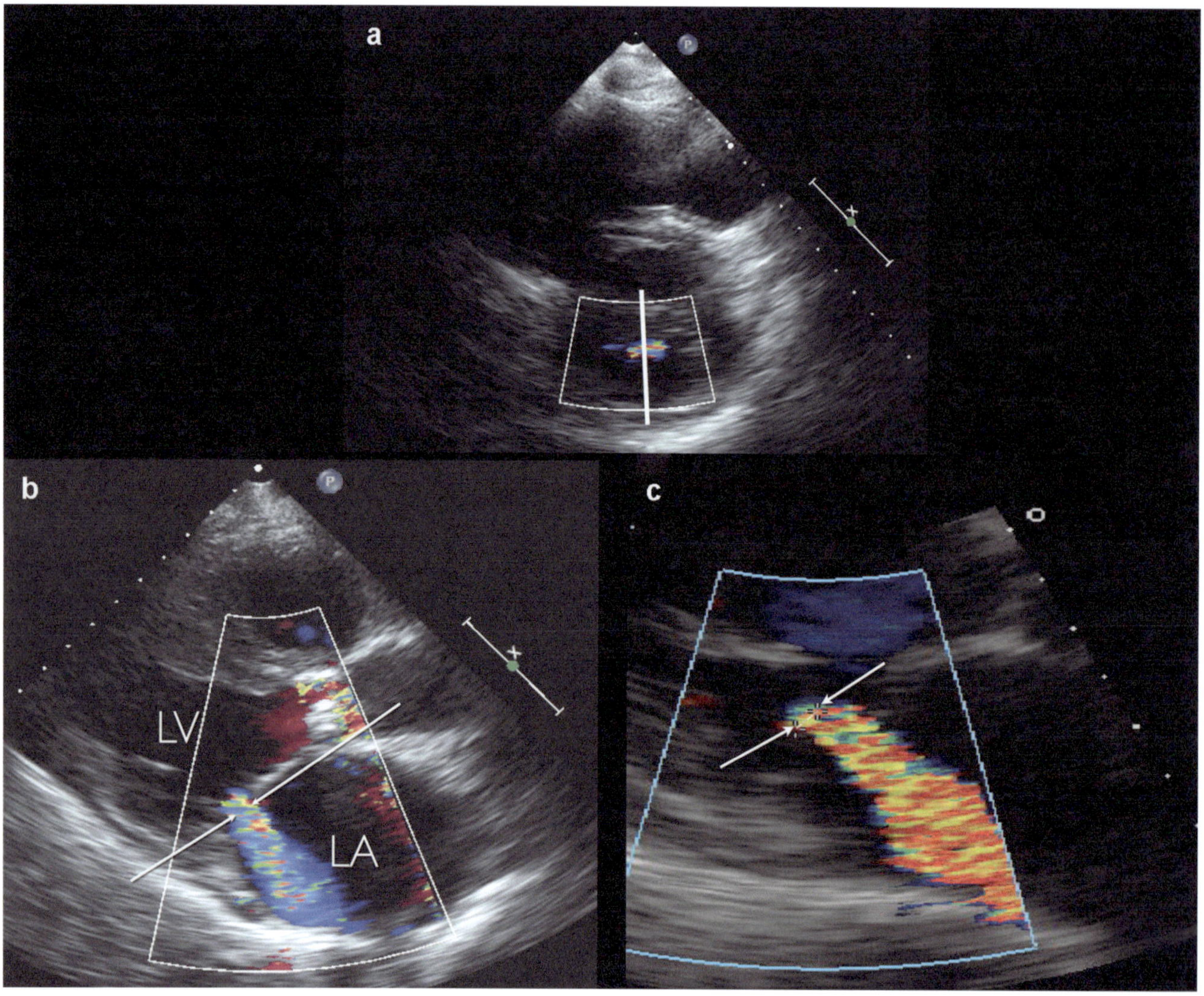

Fig. 5.4 Transthoracic echocardiography demonstrating (**a**) parasternal short-axis view of mitral regurgitation demonstrating the origin of the mitral regurgitation jet and the *white line* indicates the axis that the vena contracta is measured. *Panel* **b** demonstrates the parasternal long-axis view of a posteriorly directed jet with the vena contracta measurement (*arrows*). *Panel* **b** demonstrates a zoomed view of the vena contracta measurement. *LV* left ventricle, *LA* left atrium

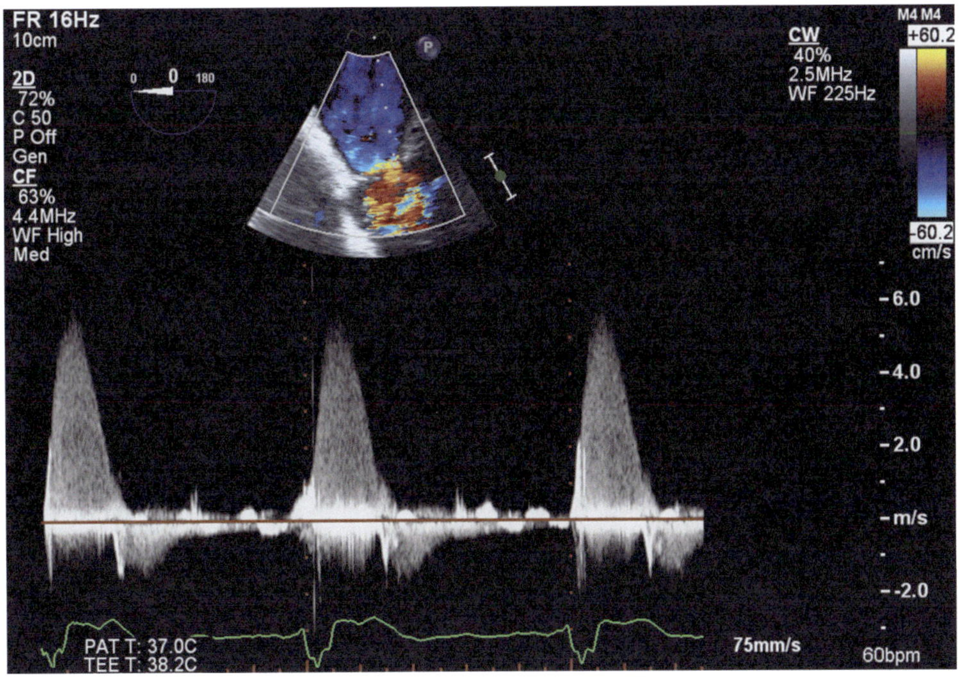

Fig. 5.5 The shape of a continuous-wave Doppler jet of severe (4+) mitral regurgitation is triangular and nonparabolic

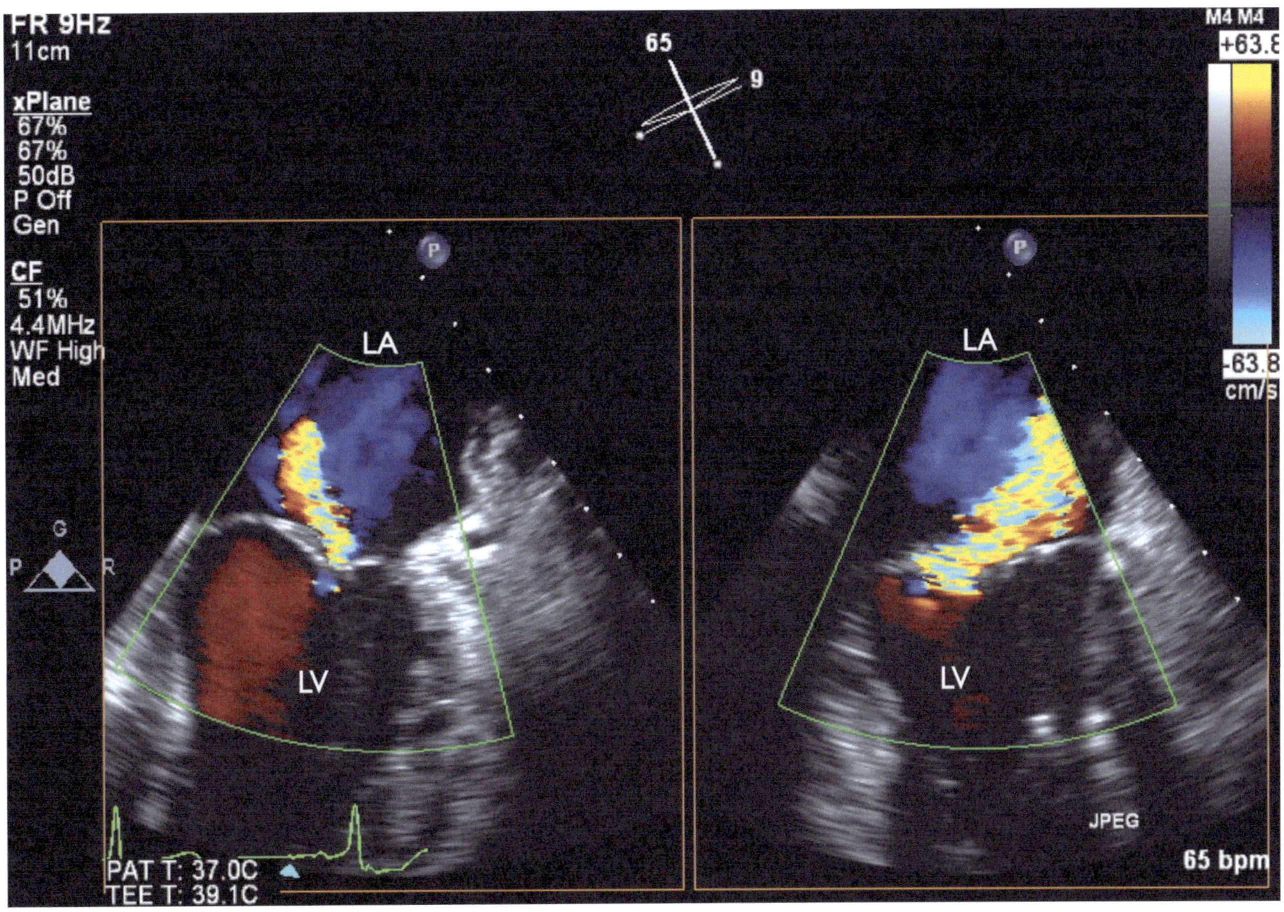

Fig. 5.6 Transesophageal echocardiography using simultaneous biplane (or X-plane imaging) demonstrating (*left*) moderate to severe mitral regurgitation in a zoomed four-chamber view with a regurgitant jet directed slightly laterally and (*right*) corresponding simultaneous two-chamber view demonstrating the same mitral regurgitation jet directed anteriorly. *LA* left atrium, *LV* left ventricle

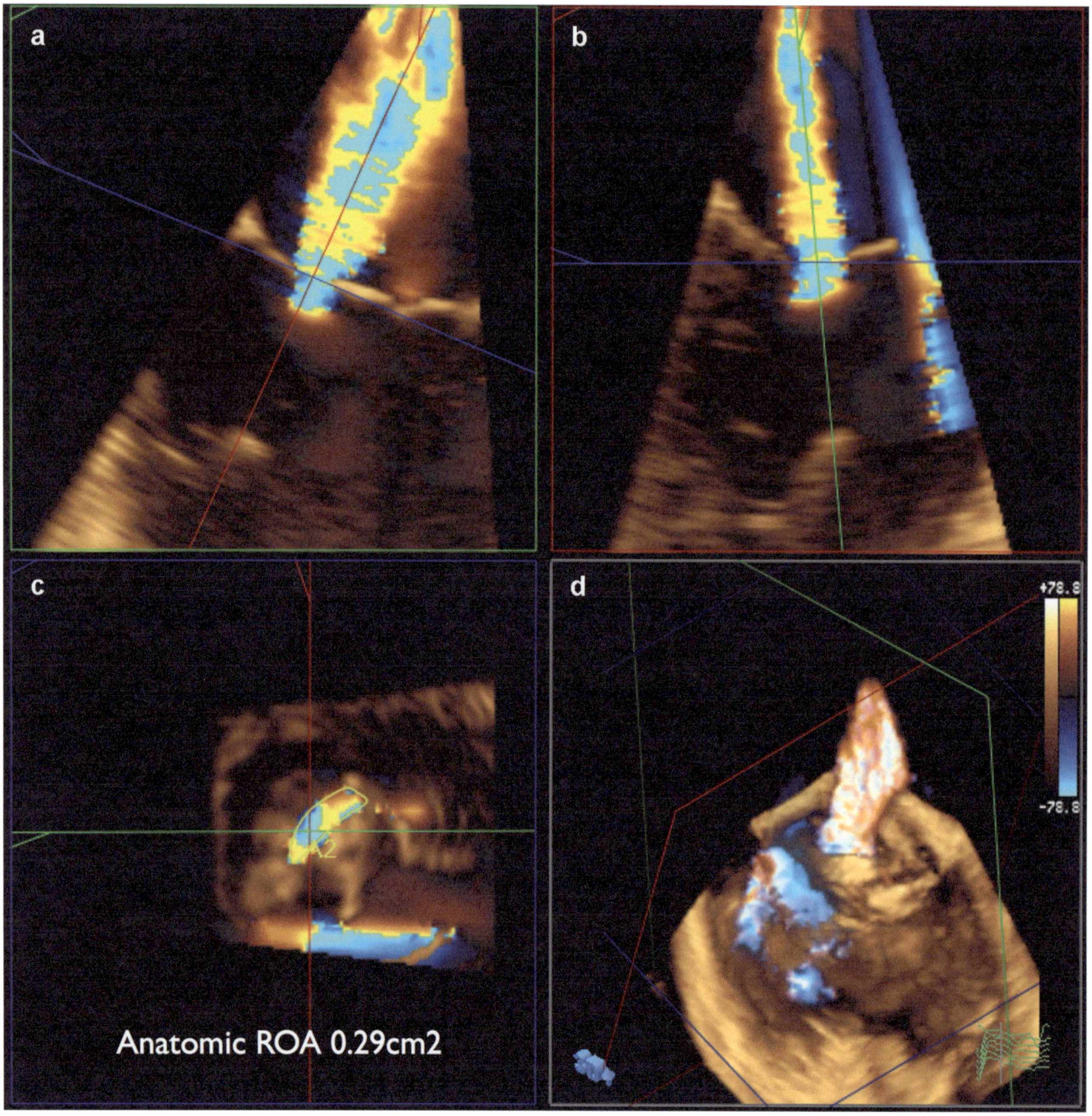

Fig. 5.7 Use of 3D software (MVQ) to align planes of mitral regurgitation on 3D TEE imaging. (**a**, **b**) Corresponding simultaneous four-chamber and two-chamber views of 2 to 3+ MR. Aligning the red, green, and blue cut planes at the origin of MR regurgitant orifice allows for planimetry of the anatomic regurgitant orifice from a true en face view (*panel* **c**). *Panel* **d** represents the corresponding rendered volume with color mapping

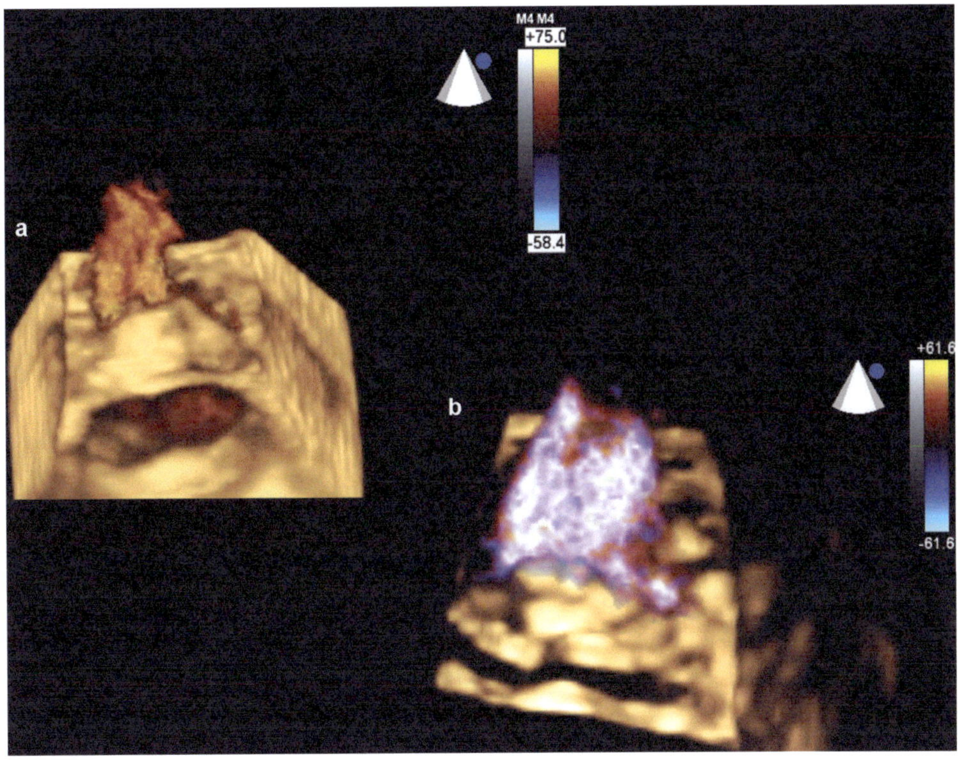

Fig. 5.8 Rendered 3D TEE color full volume imaging of (**a**) two discrete origins of MR and (**b**) a very wide-based jet of severe MR originating along the entire line of coaptation of the MV

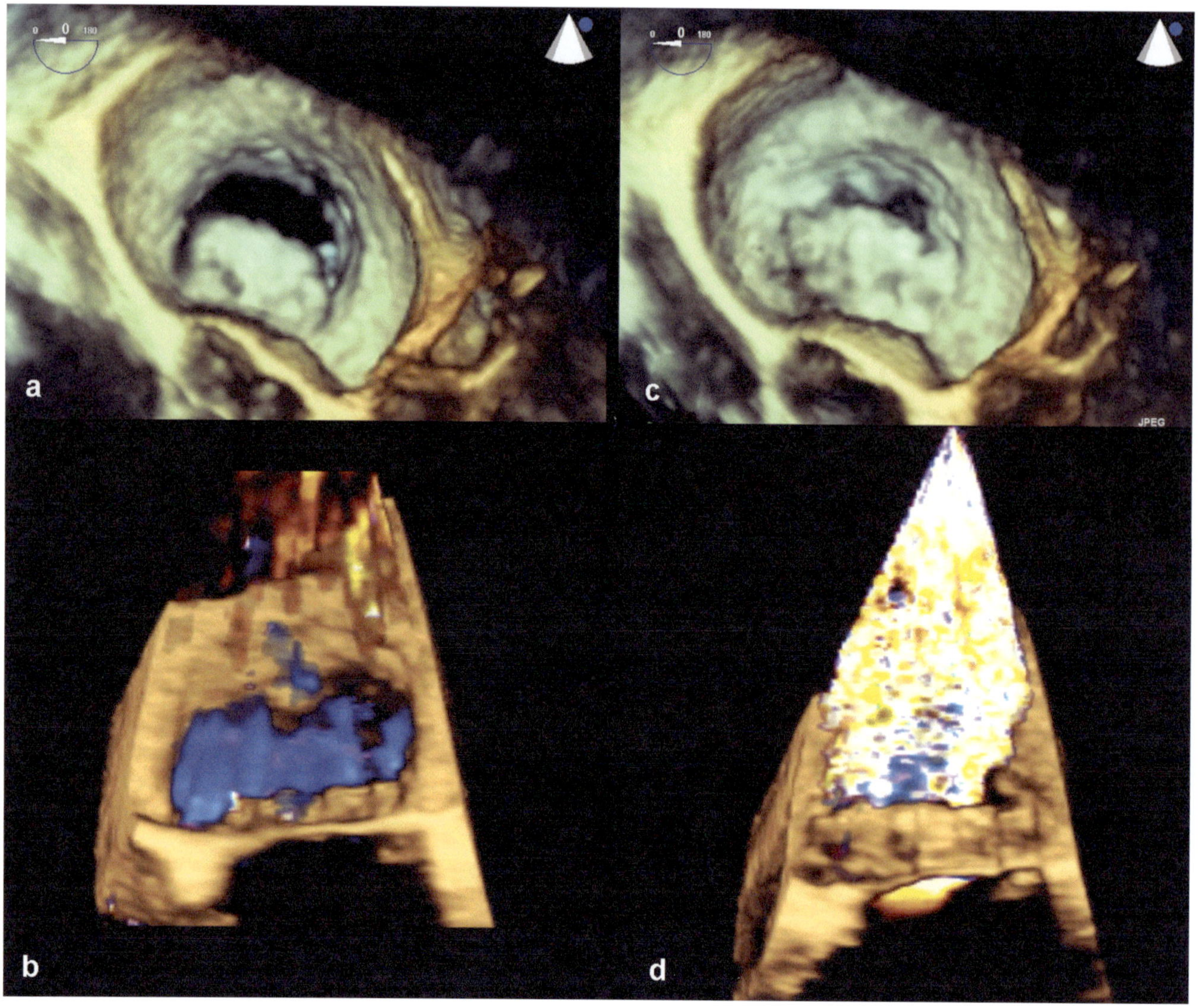

Fig. 5.9 RT3D TEE imaging of severe functional MR. *Panels* **a** and **b** are obtained during diastole, and *panels* **c** and **d** during systole. Marked restriction of posterior leaflet motion (Carpentier IIIb mitral dysfunction) is noted during systole due to ischemic LV remodeling, resulting in a wide jet of 4+ MR originating along the entire line of coaptation

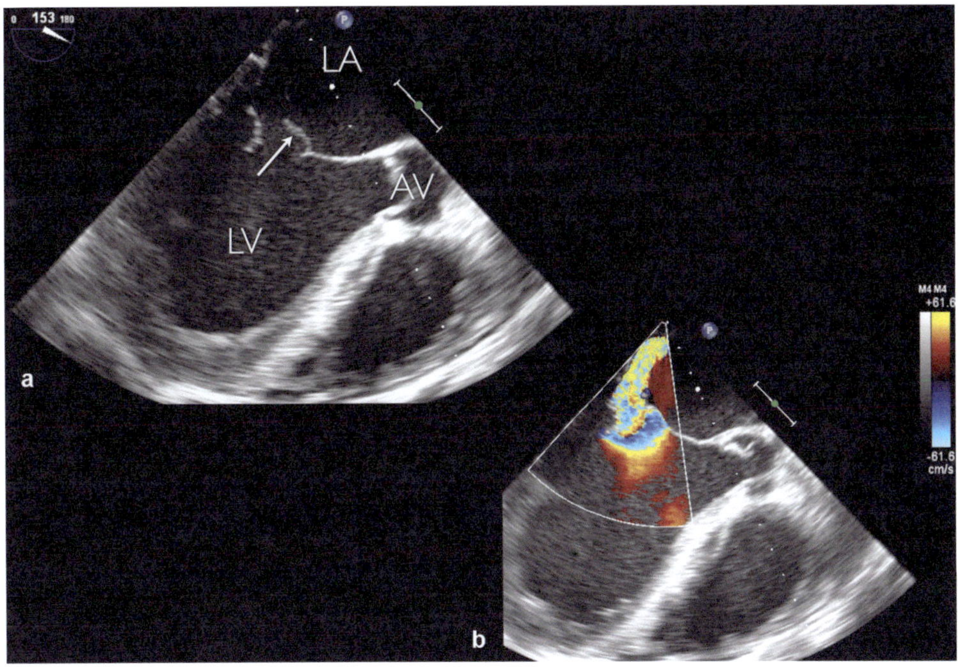

Fig. 5.10 Transesophageal echocardiography demonstrating (**a**) a flail anterior mitral valve leaflet and (**b**) corresponding color Doppler jet of severe (4+) MR in the LV outflow tract view. *LA* left atrium, *LV* left ventricle, *AV* aortic valve

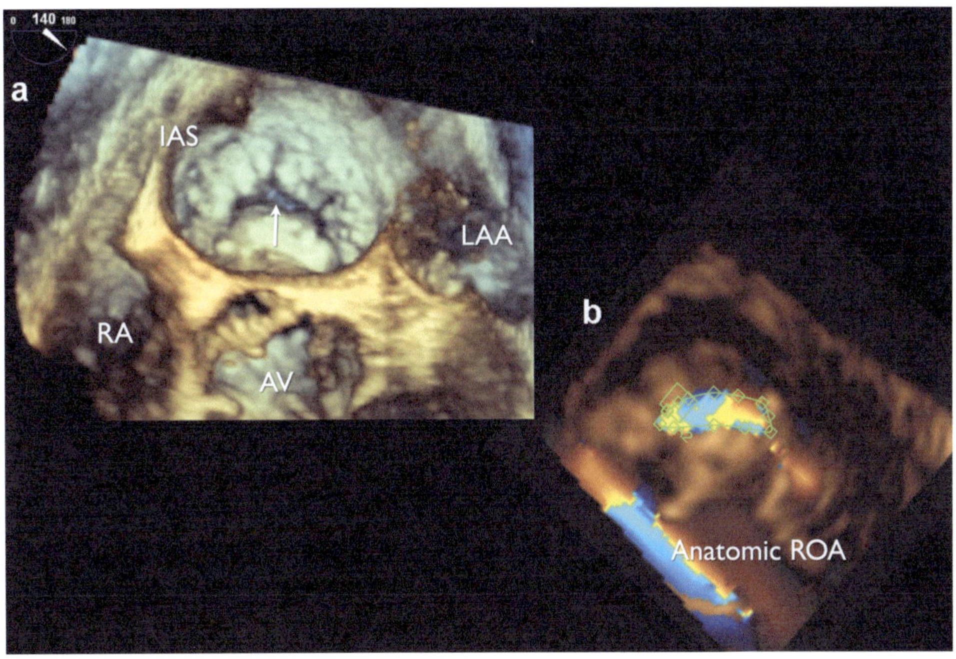

Fig. 5.11 (**a**) RT3D TEE image of myxomatous mitral valve (Barlow's) valve during systole with wide area of malcoaptation (*arrow*) and (**b**) corresponding anatomic regurgitant orifice area (*ROA*) derived from MVQ software 3D analysis. *LAA* left atrial appendage, *IAS* interatrial septum, *AV* aortic valve, *AR* right atrium

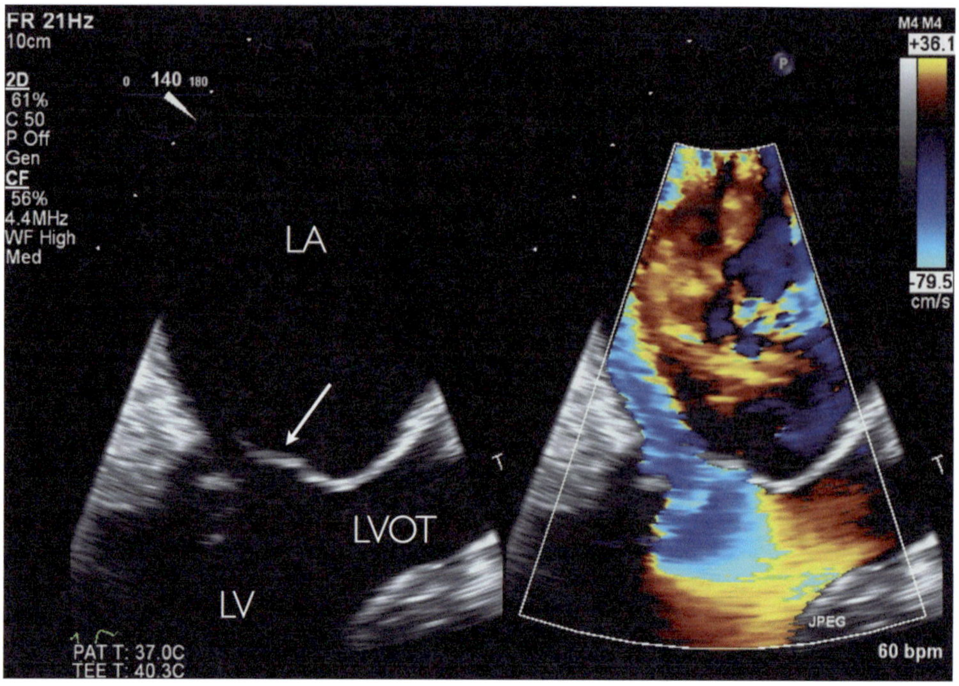

Fig. 5.12 TEE of severe MR. Note for large flail anterior leaflet (*arrow*) on the *left panel* and large proximal flow convergence (*right panel*). *LA* left atrium, *LV* left ventricle, *LVOT* left ventricular outflow tract

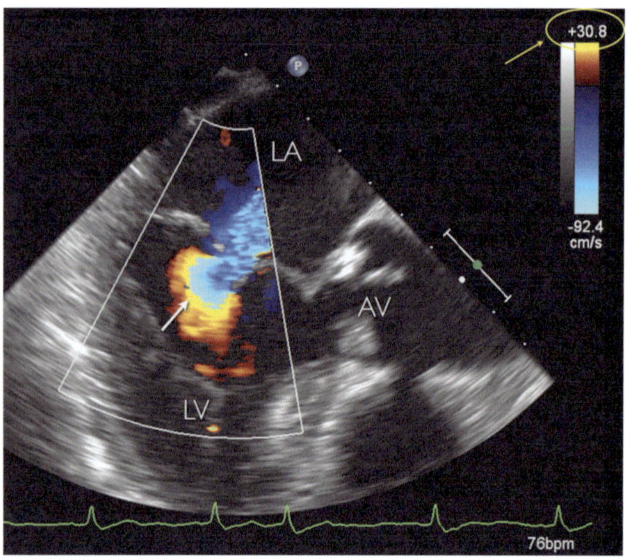

Fig. 5.13 Estimation of MR severity by the PISA technique. Note the large proximal flow convergence TEE imaging. *LA* left atrium, *LV* left ventricle, *AV* aortic valve. Note baseline shifted toward the direction of MR to allow for lower aliasing velocity (*arrow*, *circle*) to 30.8 cm/s, which facilitates accurate measurement of the radius of convergence. This information can be then used to calculate regurgitant orifice area and regurgitant volume

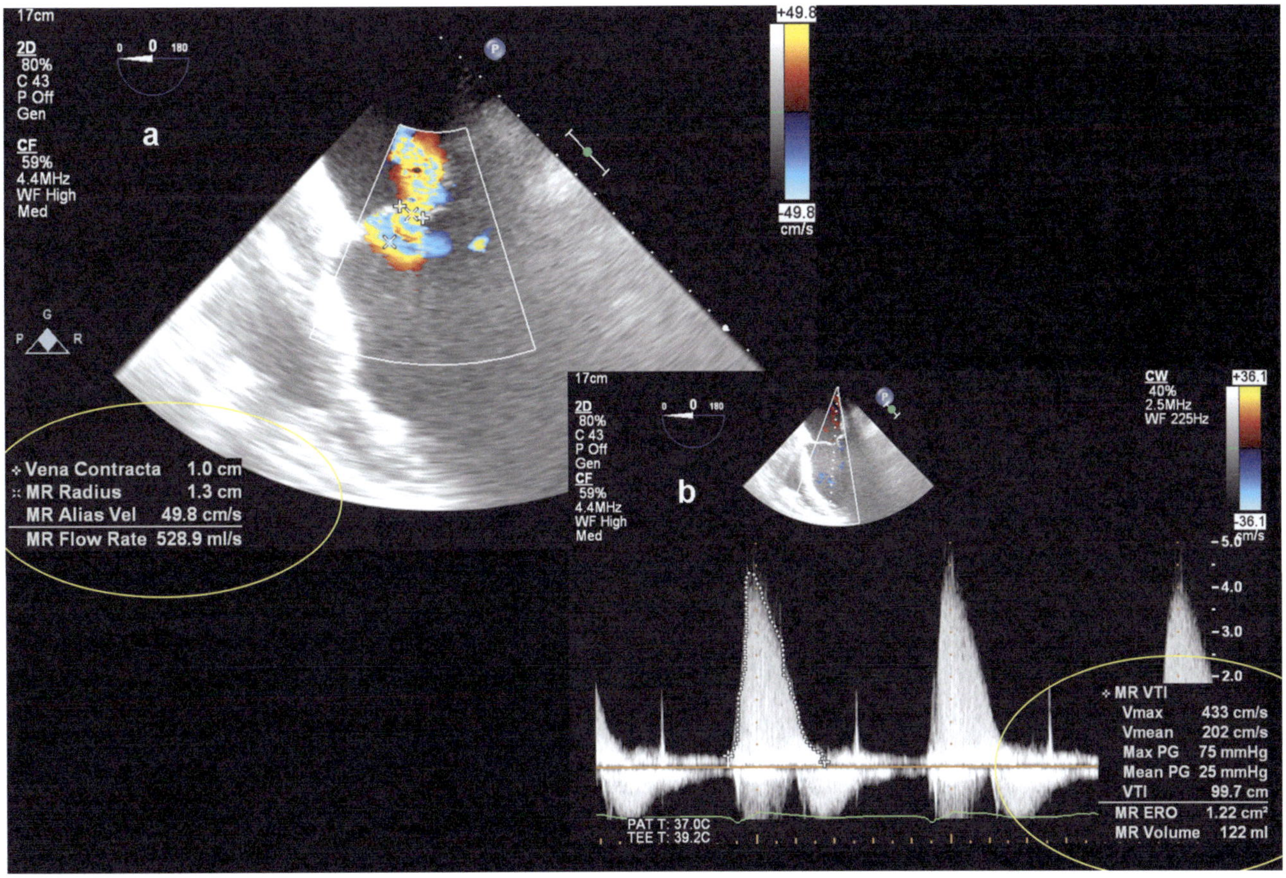

Fig. 5.14 Estimation of MR severity by the PISA technique. *Panel* **a** – note the large proximal flow convergence on TEE imaging. The radius of the MR convergence is measured and the aliasing velocity noted (*circled*). The vena contracta width can also be measured. This information can be then used to calculate regurgitant orifice area and regurgitant volume using the MR velocity and velocity time integral (*VTI*) of MR. A regurgitant orifice area (MRERO) of >0.4 cm^2, and regurgitant volume (MR volume) of >60 ml indicate severe MR. This information can be then used to calculate regurgitant orifice area and regurgitant volume using the MR velocity and velocity time integral (VTI) of MR (*panel* **b**)."

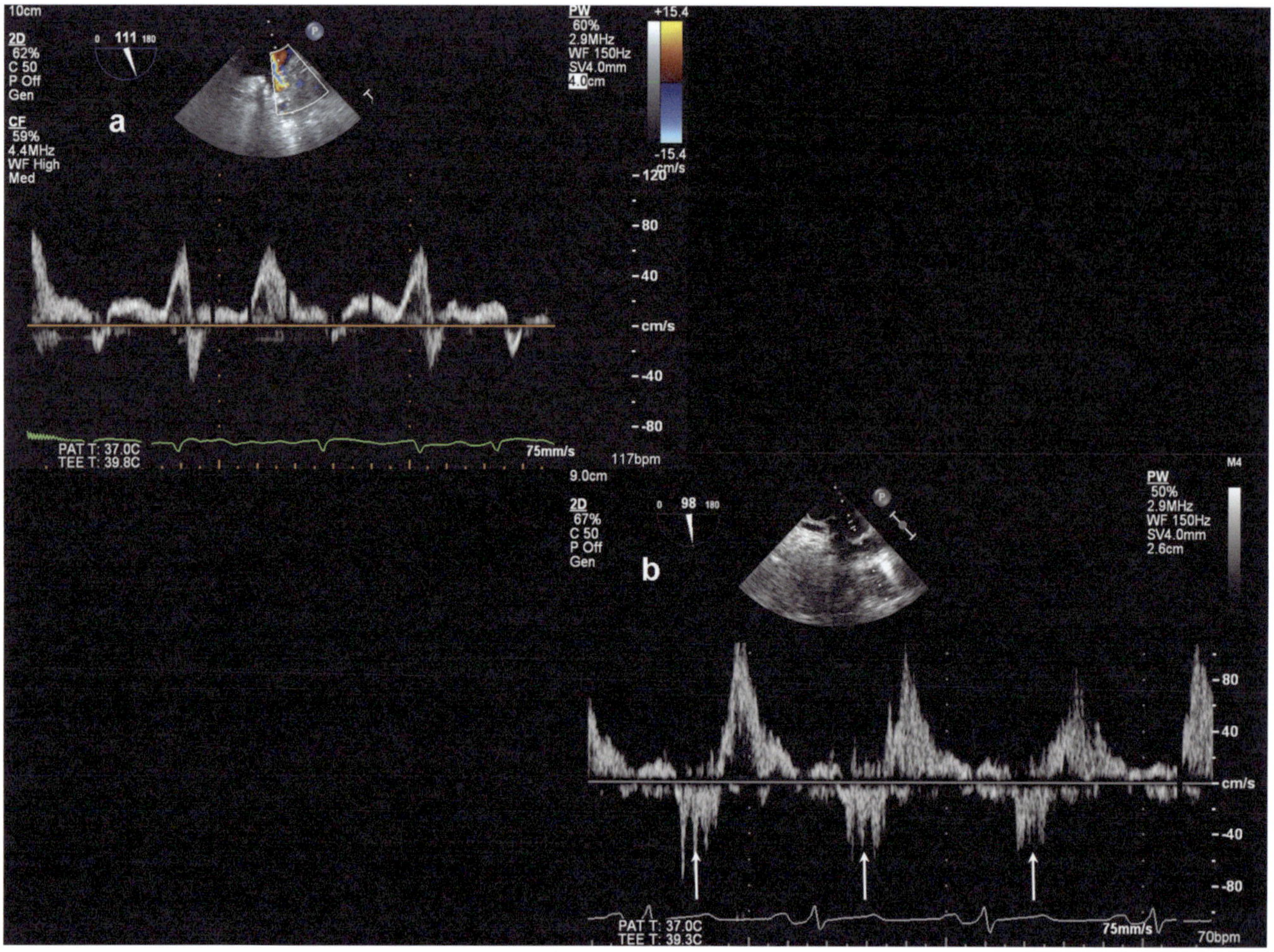

Fig. 5.15 (**a**) Systolic blunting of left superior pulmonary vein flow and (**b**) reversal of systolic flow (*arrows*) due to severe MR

Mitral Regurgitation Severity in EVEREST I and II

The MitraClip™ system is designed to treat patients with hemodynamically significant mitral regurgitation. In the EVEREST I and II cohorts, as well as in European registries [17–19], the MitraClip™ has been studied in patients with moderately severe (3+) or severe (4+) mitral regurgitation. In the EVEREST I and II trial, mitral regurgitation was rigorously graded before and after intervention by an echocardiography core laboratory according to the American Society of Echocardiography quantitation of native valve regurgitation guidelines [13], with the use of quantitative criteria (regurgitant volume, regurgitant fraction, and effective regurgitant orifice area) and qualitative criteria (color Doppler and pulmonary venous flow). Table 5.2 summarizes the inclusion criteria for moderate–severe (3+) and severe (4+) mitral regurgitation in the EVEREST I and II trials.

Screening transthoracic and transesophageal echocardiograms were reviewed by the principal investigator at the echocardiography core laboratory in EVEREST I and II using these criteria for assessing MR. Transthoracic echocardiography (TTE) was primarily used for the assessment of MR severity whereas transesophageal echocardiography (TEE) was used for mitral valve morphology and function. A minimum of three of the six criteria for moderate–severe (3+) or severe (4+) MR were required for entry; at least one of these three criteria had to be quantitative (Table 5.2). Key eligibility and exclusion criteria for the EVEREST cohort overall are listed in Table 5.3.

Table 5.2 Echocardiographic criteria for moderate–severe (3+) or severe (4+) MR in EVEREST I and II

Mitral regurgitant severity of moderate-to-severe or severe grade as defined by a minimum of three of the following criteria, one of which must be quantitative (i.e., 4, 5, or 6):
1. Color flow jet may be central and large (>6 cm^2 or >30 % of left atrial area) or smaller if eccentric, encircling the left atrium
2. Pulmonary vein flow may show systolic blunting or systolic flow reversal
3. Vena contracta width >0.3 cm measured in the parasternal long-axis view
4. Regurgitant volume of >45 ml/beat
5. Regurgitant fraction >40 %
6. Regurgitant orifice area >0.30 cm^2

Table 5.3 Key eligibility and exclusion criteria for the EVEREST cohort

Key eligibility criteria
Candidate for mitral valve repair or replacement surgery
Moderate-to-severe (3+) or severe (4+) chronic mitral regurgitation and symptomatic with LVEF > 25 % and LVIDs ≤ 55 mm
Asymptomatic moderate-to-severe (3+) or severe (4+) chronic mitral regurgitation with one of the following:
LVEF < 60 % (not less than 25 %)
LVIDs ≥ 40 mm (not wider than 55 mm)
New-onset atrial fibrillation
Pulmonary hypertension (pulmonary artery systolic pressure >50 mmHg at rest or >60 mmHg with exercise)
Key exclusion criteria[a]
Recent myocardial infarction
Any interventional or surgical procedure within 30 days of the index procedure
Mitral valve orifice area <4 cm^2
Renal insufficiency
Endocarditis
Rheumatic heart disease

[a]Previous mediastinal surgery was regarded as an exclusion criteria in the first 27 patients

Definitions: *EVEREST* Endovascular Valve Edge-to-Edge Repair Study, *LVEF* left ventricular ejection fraction, *LVIDs* left ventricular internal diameter, systole

Assessment of Mitral Valve Functional Morphology

The mitral valve apparatus is a complex three-dimensional anatomic structure comprised of two discrete leaflets (anterior and posterior), chordae with attachments to the two left ventricular papillary muscles, and the mitral annulus, and its geometry and function are in turn influenced by the geometry and function of the left atrium and left ventricle. The mitral valve leaflets (anterior and posterior) are each connected to two papillary muscles (anterolateral and posteromedial). The posterior mitral valve leaflet is further separated into three discrete sections with a cleft dividing it into three discrete segments named scallops P1 through P3 (from lateral to medial), and the anterior mitral leaflet is typically not anatomically divided per se, but its segments are named A1 to A3 according to the adjacent posterior scallop (Fig. 5.16).

The mitral annulus is a complex saddle-shaped structure with peaks anteriorly and posteriorly and nadirs medially and laterally. The anterior aspect of the mitral annulus is a rigid fibrous band that is shared with the aorta (aorto-mitral fibrosa or curtain), and the remaining medial, lateral, and posterior aspects are more vulnerable to remodeling and distortion of shape. The mitral valve is designed to provide unimpeded flow of blood into the LV during diastole and coapt or seal completely in systole, preventing backflow (or MR) against one of the highest naturally occurring pressure gradient produced within the body.

Mitral regurgitation (MR) may occur due to a variety of diverse clinical processes [20–22]. The pathophysiologic triad described by Carpentier separates the *disease* that produces a an *anatomic mitral valve lesion* and the subsequent *valve dysfunction* that produces MR. Carpentier classified MR into three distinct types of valve dysfunction [20]. Type I dysfunction is characterized by normal mitral leaflet motion and is typically seen in atrial fibrillation with atrial and mitral annular dilation [23, 24], as well as in endocarditis with leaflet perforation. Type II dysfunction is characterized by excessive systolic leaflet motion and is seen in degenerative mitral valve disease with either prolapse or flail of the mitral leaflets. Type IIIa dysfunction is characterized by reduced leaflet motion in both systole and diastole as is seen in rheumatic mitral disease, and type IIIb dysfunction is characterized by reduced systolic leaflet motion, as is typically seen in patients with dilated cardiomyopathy or MR due to ischemic LV remodeling. Type IIIb MR is often referred to as "functional MR." Please refer to the chapter on mitral valve anatomy for additional detail.

Patients with degenerative disease (type II dysfunction) as well as functional mitral regurgitation (type IIIb dysfunction) have been successfully treated with the MitraClip™ edge-to-edge mitral repair system. Successful percutaneous edge-to-edge repair depends upon, and *begins with*, appropriate patient selection.

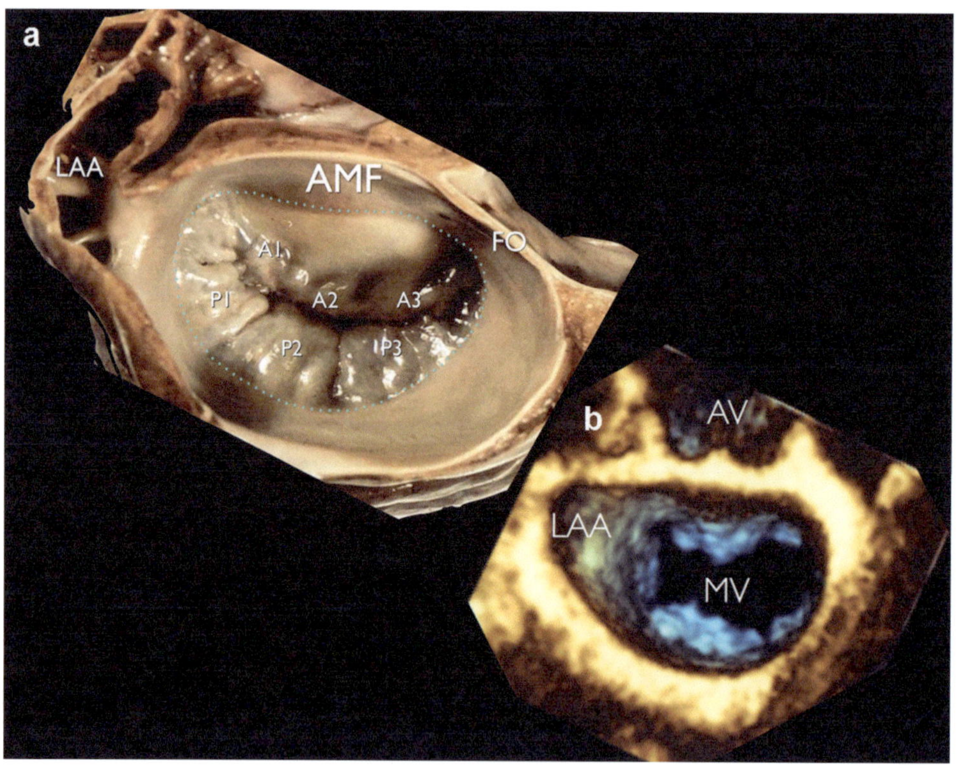

Fig. 5.16 (**a**) Anatomic specimen demonstrating mitral valve scalloping and (**b**) corresponding RT3D TEE image of the mitral valve in diastole *LAA* left atrial appendage, *AMF* aortic mitral fibrosa, *FO* fossa ovalis, *AV* aortic valve, *MV* mitral valve. A1–3 and P1–3 refer to the naming of the scallops of the anterior and posterior leaflets, respectively

Patient Selection: United States MitraClip™ Experience

In the US clinical trials EVEREST I and II, the mechanism of MR was required to originate from the central mitral scallops, either A2 or P2. Patients with degenerative MR with either prolapse or flail of the A2 and/or P2 scallops were most common, and this etiology represented 73 % of those patients enrolled in EVEREST II (Table 5.4) [5]. Similarly, patients with functional MR, either due to dilated cardiomyopathy or ischemic LV remodeling, were enrolled, provided the dominant MR jet arose from A2–P2. In EVEREST II, these patients represented 27 % of patients enrolled [5].

In the EVEREST trials, patients with significant MR originating the medial or lateral aspects of the valve were excluded per protocol, as were those with rheumatic mitral valve disease, history of endocarditis, and a baseline mitral valve area of less than 4.0 cm^2 by planimetry. Rheumatic disease represented exclusion due to concerns about (a) the ability to grasp a markedly thickened leaflet with the clip, (b) subvalvular apparatus involvement, as well as the (c) possibility of concurrent mitral stenosis. Endocarditis was a contraindication due to concern about infection of the implanted clip as well as interference with grasping due to damaged leaflets or healed vegetations. Obviously, leaflet perforation due to endocarditis cannot be addressed by edge-to-edge repair. A mitral valve area by planimetry of greater than 4.0 cm^2 was mandated prior to MitraClip™ placement to prevent the development of iatrogenic mitral stenosis, especially if two clips are placed. Additional exclusion criteria in EVEREST I and II also included abnormal thickness of the mitral leaflets or leaflet calcification if it would impede grasping with the MitraClip™ system.

Anatomic inclusion and exclusion for percutaneous edge-to-edge repair also depended in part upon the MR etiology. In patients with degenerative MR, those with a flail height of >10 mm and a flail width of >15 mm were excluded due to concerns of inability to grasp or hold the leaflet within the clip (Fig. 5.17). In patients with functional MR, adequate leaflet available for coaptation was required, and if it was less than 2 mm, the patients were excluded. Similarly, for FMR, a mitral coaptation depth of greater than 11 mm was also an anatomic basis for exclusion (Fig. 5.18) due to concerns about extensive leaflet distortion due to LV remodeling that the clip could potentially not address.

Table 5.4 Etiology of mitral regurgitation in EVEREST II [5]

Cause of MR—no. (%)	Percutaneous repair (N=184)	Surgery (N=95)
Functional	49 (27)	26 (27)
Degenerative		
With anterior or bileaflet flail or prolapse	58 (32)	25 (26)
With posterior flail or prolapse	72 (39)	42 (44)
With no flail and no prolapse	5 (3)	2 (2)

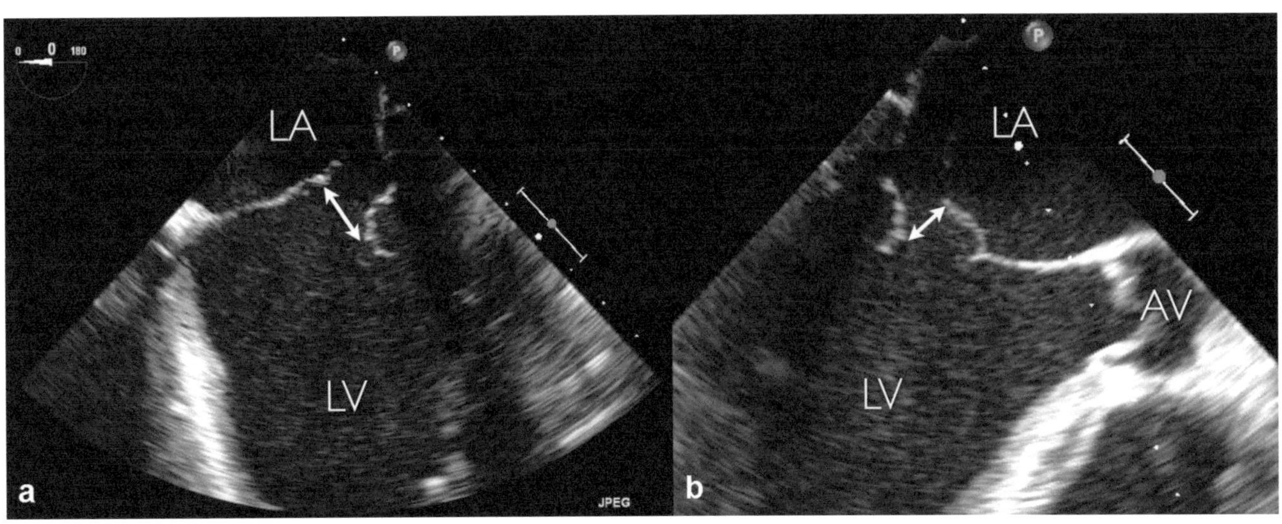

Fig. 5.17 Measurement of the flail gap in the (**a**) four-chamber view and (**b**) LVOT views. The *arrow* indicates the distance between the flail anterior leaflet and site of posterior leaflet coaptation. *LA* left atrium, *LV* left ventricle, *AV* aortic valve

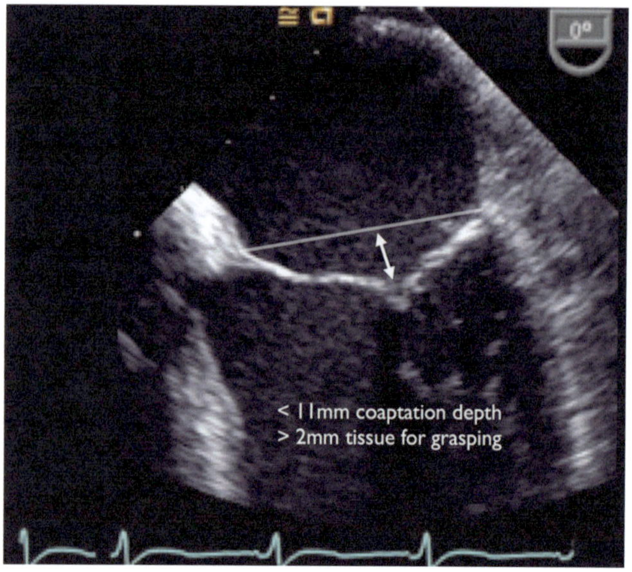

Fig. 5.18 Measurement of the depth of coaptation as well as leaflet available for coaptation for possible MitraClip therapy. *Gray line* indicates the mitral annular plane, *arrow* indicates distance from annulus to the point of coaptation in this TEE four-chamber view. At least 2 mm of tissue is required for grasping, and <11 mm of coaptation depth is consider ideal for MitraClip

Patient Selection: European MitraClip™ Experience

In 2008, the MitraClip™ received CE mark approval in Europe, and since then, the vast majority of worldwide MitraClip™ implants have been performed there. The European experience is still rapidly and dynamically evolving. In addition, the clinical and echocardiographic characteristics of European registry patients are significantly and fundamentally different than those enrolled in the EVEREST trials, as strict mitral leaflet anatomic inclusion and exclusion criteria are not required in Europe, and it is being applied to a typically high- or even prohibitive surgical-risk patient population. The two largest reports to date on the European MitraClip™ experience emanate from a single center in Germany and two centers in Italy.

Rudolph and Franzen et al. have reported their latest experience in Germany with the MitraClip™ system in patients who met current guideline criteria for treatment of MR but were not felt to be surgical candidates [18]. They have reported results in 104 patients with ≥3+MR who were deemed prohibitive for mitral valve surgical repair by their institutional interdisciplinary cardiac team. Inclusion criteria are summarized in Table 5.5. Their anatomic exclusion criteria were few and consisted of a mitral valve area (MVA) ≤ 2.0 cm², evidence for active endocarditis, or severely prolapsed or flail leaflets (prolapse width greater than 2.5 cm, flail gap greater than 2.0 cm). Patients in this series had significantly greater degree of left ventricular dysfunction and a greater degree of adverse valve morphology than those patients enrolled in the EVEREST trials. Specifically, there was no lower limit on LVEF or upper limit on LV size as was the case in EVEREST, and there was a broader spectrum of allowable leaflet anatomy and regurgitant jet location (even noncentral jet allowed). Patient and echocardiographic characteristics from this series are listed in Table 5.6.

In this series, the majority of patients had functional MR (66 %), with a smaller number with degenerative MR (27 %) or mixed disease (7 %). These authors have demonstrated the feasibility and midterm efficacy of the MitraClip™ in high surgical-risk patients, with a substantial proportion of patients treated that would have been excluded from the US EVEREST trials.

Tamburino et al. have reported results from the initial Italian clinical experience with the MitraClip™ at two centers [19]. Their multidisciplinary teams selected patients who met criteria for mitral intervention based on established guidelines and who were at high risk for surgery based on the consensus between cardiologist and cardiac surgeon, logistic EuroSCORE greater than 20, hepatic cirrhosis, autoimmune disease, severe renal failure requiring hemodialysis, or any contraindication to extracorporeal circulation.

Table 5.5 German experience [18]

Key mitral valve inclusion criteria
≥3+MR (central origin *not* required)
Prohibitive risk for mitral valve surgical repair by institutional interdisciplinary cardiac team
Mitral valve area (MVA) greater than 2.0 cm²
No evidence for active endocarditis
If degenerative MR:
Prolapse width less than 2.5 cm
Flail gap less than 2.0 cm
No lower limit on LVEF
No upper limit on LV dimension

Table 5.6 Baseline patient characteristics (*N*=104) in German registry [18]

Age (years)	74±9
Men	64 (62 %)
Logistic EuroSCORE (%)	36 (21–54)
Cardiomyopathy	
Ischemic	47 (45 %)
Dilated	34 (33 %)
Valvular	2 (2 %)
None	21 (20 %)
MR etiology	
Functional	69 (66 %)
Degenerative	28 (27 %)
Mixed	7 (7 %)
MR severity	
2+ (Mild to moderate)	1 (1 %)
3+ (Moderate to severe)	49 (47 %)
4+ (Severe)	54 (52 %)
LV ejection fraction (%)	43±16
LV end-diastolic diameter (mm)	65±12
LV end-systolic diameter (mm)	53±14
LV end-diastolic volume (ml)	212 (159–279)
LV end-systolic volume (ml)	123 (74–192)
Regurgitant volume (ml)	42 (28–56)
Regurgitant fraction (%)	48 (40–59)
Effective regurgitant orifice area (mm²)	35 (23–61)
Mitral valve orifice area (cm²)	4.1±1.0
Mean transmitral pressure gradient (mm Hg)	2.0 (1.0–3.0)

Values are mean±SD, *n* (%), or median (interquartile range)
EuroSCORE European System for Cardiac Operative Risk Evaluation, *LV* left ventricular, *MR* mitral regurgitation

Anatomic leaflet criteria, however, were similar to EVEREST criteria, with a requirement for primarily central regurgitation (at the A2/P2 interface) and sufficient leaflet tissue for mechanical coaptation. Key exclusion criteria were also similar to the EVEREST trials, including mitral valve orifice area >4.0 cm², flail width ≥15 mm, flail gap ≥10 mm, coaptation depth ≥11 mm, and coaptation length >2 mm. Importantly, unlike EVEREST, there was no exclusion for very low LV ejection fraction, nor was there an upper limit on LV size. Table 5.7 summarizes the inclusion criteria and Table 5.8 the exclusion criteria. As such, these patients also represent a high-risk cohort but one that is more closely anatomically related to the EVEREST cohort. This registry demonstrated the excellent acute safety and efficacy of MitraClip therapy in a population of patients similar to EVEREST patients but at higher surgical risk. Longer-term efficacy and durability in this initial cohort have not yet been reported.

The anatomic mitral leaflet criteria as well as clinical criteria for MitraClip patient selection were rigorously defined in the EVEREST trials, but the European experience has shown that the MitraClip can be used in cases of more complex (non-EVEREST) leaflet anatomy as well as in higher-risk patients. Although further investigation will undoubtedly refine our understanding of what constitutes "acceptable" leaflet anatomy, the main limitations still appear to be the ability to grasp both leaflets effectively, and the undesired development of mitral stenosis, especially when multiple clips are placed.

Table 5.7 Inclusion criteria Italian registry [19]

Echocardiographic and clinical inclusion criteria
Moderate-to-severe (3+) or severe (4+) chronic mitral valve regurgitation with symptoms or without symptoms but LVEF 60 % or left ventricle end-systolic diameter <45 mm
High-risk candidates for mitral valve surgery including cardiopulmonary bypass
Primary regurgitant jet originating from malcoaptation of the A2 and P2 scallops of the mitral valve; if a secondary jet exists, it must be considered clinically insignificant
Presence of sufficient leaflet tissue for a mechanical coaptation
Non-rheumatic/endocarditic valve morphology
Transseptal catheterization determined to be feasible by the treating physician

Table 5.8 Exclusion criteria Italian registry [19]

Exclusion criteria
Need for any other cardiac surgery including surgery for coronary artery disease, atrial fibrillation, pulmonic, aortic, or tricuspid valve disease
Mitral valve orifice area >4.0 cm^2
If leaflet *flail* is present (Degenerative MR):
Flail width <15 mm
Flail gap <10 mm
If leaflet *tethering* is present (Functional MR):
Coaptation depth <11 mm
Coaptation length >2 mm
Severe mitral annular calcification
Any leaflet anatomy which may preclude clip implantation, proper clip positioning on the leaflets, or sufficient reduction in MR
Systolic anterior motion of the mitral valve leaflet
Hypertrophic cardiomyopathy
Echocardiographic evidence of intracardiac mass, thrombus, or vegetation
History of, or active, endocarditis
History of, or active, rheumatic heart disease
History of atrial septal defect, whether repaired or not
History of patent foramen ovale associated with clinical symptoms (e.g., cerebral ischemia) or previously repaired or when, in the judgment of the investigator, an atrial septal aneurysm is present that may interfere with transseptal crossing
History of a stroke or documented TIA within the prior 6 months
Patients in whom TEE is contraindicated

Post-procedure Follow-up Echocardiography

The assessment of the efficacy of percutaneous mitral valve repair begins during the procedure and prior to the clip being released from the guiding system and continues for post-procedure follow-up to assess the integrity and durability of the repair. Results from the EVEREST randomized clinical trial as well as European registries and case series are discussed elsewhere in this book. Intraprocedural echocardiography is also covered separately, but what follows here is a *general overview* of the imaging issues in patients who have undergone percutaneous edge-to-edge mitral repair. TEE is used to guide the procedure and assess the post-procedure results in the catheterization laboratory, and either TTE or TEE can be used to perform serial long-term follow-up. In the EVEREST II randomized clinical trial cohort, TTE was used for regular follow-up intervals at 1 day post procedure, 1 month, 6 months, and annually thereafter post repair. TEE may be used to evaluate the mitral valve post MitraClip if TTE is technically inadequate or to evaluate for unlikely complications such as partial clip detachment as well as endocarditis.

During the case, TEE is used to evaluate MR prior to the release of the clip, and the follow-up assessment begins here. For serial outpatient follow-up echocardiography after the procedure has been completed when using either TTE or TEE, a careful search for any residual MR must also be undertaken, including standard and nonstandard views of the mitral valve to assess for residual MR. 3-D imaging with full-volume color Doppler analysis is also valuable in this setting. Figures 5.19, 5.20, 5.21, 5.22, 5.23, 5.24, 5.25, 5.26, 5.27, 5.28, 5.29, 5.30, 5.31, 5.32, 5.33, and 5.34 detail the post-procedure assessment.

A careful search for any MR jet origin, vena contracta, flow convergence, as well as associated hemodynamic findings is performed (Figs. 5.19, 5.20, 5.21, 5.22, 5.23, 5.24, 5.25, 5.26, 5.27, 5.28, 5.30, 5.31, and 5.32). It is imperative to carefully search for an eccentric regurgitant jet as MR can be *redirected* significantly after clip placement, and numerous additional nonstandard multiplane angles or TTE imaging angles should be used (Fig. 5.27). During the procedure, echo machine settings including color Doppler gain and Nyquist limit should be identical to those used for the pre-procedure assessment of mitral regurgitation during the case. Similarly, during the procedure, approximation of pre-procedure hemodynamic loading conditions is accomplished with saline and vasopressor agents such as phenylephrine if these parameters have changed significantly. This is particularly important in patients with functional MR, which is afterload dependent.

Quantitation of any residual MR is complicated by the creation of a double mitral orifice. The mitral inflow volume required for quantitative volumetric Doppler MR estimation cannot be obtained due to the creation of a double diastolic orifice. In the absence of significant aortic regurgitation, LV forward flow can be estimated as flow through the outflow tract using the continuity equation and LV stroke volume estimated from 3-D-derived estimates of end-diastolic and end-systolic volumes. The difference between the two (stroke volume – forward flow) represents the regurgitant volume, although this method is time-consuming and may be best suited to long-term follow-up as it is not easily performed in the lab during the case. Echocardiography may underestimate LV volume when compared to other modalities such as cardiac magnetic resonance imaging (CMR) [25], but experience with CMR in this population is also limited [26]. Serial post-procedure TTE follow-up may be better able to perform quantitation of MR using this technique.

During the procedure in the catheterization lab, color Doppler echocardiography using semiquantitative techniques based on regurgitant jet dimensions may be best suited for real-time intraprocedural assessment (Figs. 5.19, 5.20, 5.21, 5.22, 5.23, 5.24, 5.25, 5.26, 5.27, 5.28, 5.30, 5.31, and 5.32). If two or more jets are present (Figs. 5.22, 5.28, and 5.31), it is important to realize that color Doppler jet area mapping may overestimate the corresponding regurgitant volume [27].

Similarly, the PISA approach for calculating the effective regurgitant orifice area (EROA) has not been validated for multiple regurgitant jets that may exist post MitraClip with the double-orifice geometry created with this device. Accurate assessment of the EROA by PISA may not be possible or accurate due to clip shadowing artifact as well (see Fig. 5.34).

Included in the MR evaluation is a careful hemodynamic assessment that includes pulse-wave Doppler interrogation of the pulmonary veins (Figs. 5.19, 5.20, 5.21, 5.22, 5.23, 5.24, 5.25, 5.26, 5.27, 5.28, 5.30, 5.31, and 5.32). On follow-up TTE, an effort to interrogate both the right and left veins with pulse-wave Doppler should routinely be performed. As with native valve regurgitation prior to the procedure, an integrated approach is essential synthesizing all the available hemodynamic data to best assess the MR severity.

It is also important to measure the mitral diastolic transvalvular gradients and estimate the mitral valve area to exclude mitral stenosis—especially when two clips have been placed. This is accomplished by measuring the transvalvular gradient with continuous-wave Doppler (Fig. 5.32) and by performing planimetry the two orifices using en face 3-D or transgastric short-axis views. 3-D-assisted planimetry may be performed using included QLab software on the 3-D ultrasound machine. The pressure half-time method of MV assessment has not been validated for patients who have undergone percutaneous edge-to-edge mitral repair and is therefore not relied upon.

Clinically significant mitral stenosis has not been a significant limitation of the MitraClip™ procedure, largely as a result of careful pre-procedure screening of patients (pre-procedure mitral valve area by planimetry >4.0 cm²) and with careful Doppler and planimetered double-orifice MVA assessment during the procedure *prior* to clip release, especially when two clips are used [28, 29].

Using short-axis views from 2-D as well as 3-D echocardiography, it is possible to observe the mitral valve en face from both atrial (Fig. 5.29) and ventricular perspectives, documenting the dual orifices created by the clip(s). 3-D full volume with color mapping also provides delineation of the site(s) of origin of any residual regurgitation along with standard 2-D imaging (Fig. 5.26).

TTE is typically used for follow-up assessment of MitraClip patients, unless there is concern about significant residual MR, MS, partial clip detachment, or endocarditis. Figures 5.33 and 5.34 demonstrate representative TTE images in a patient with mild to moderate residual MR.

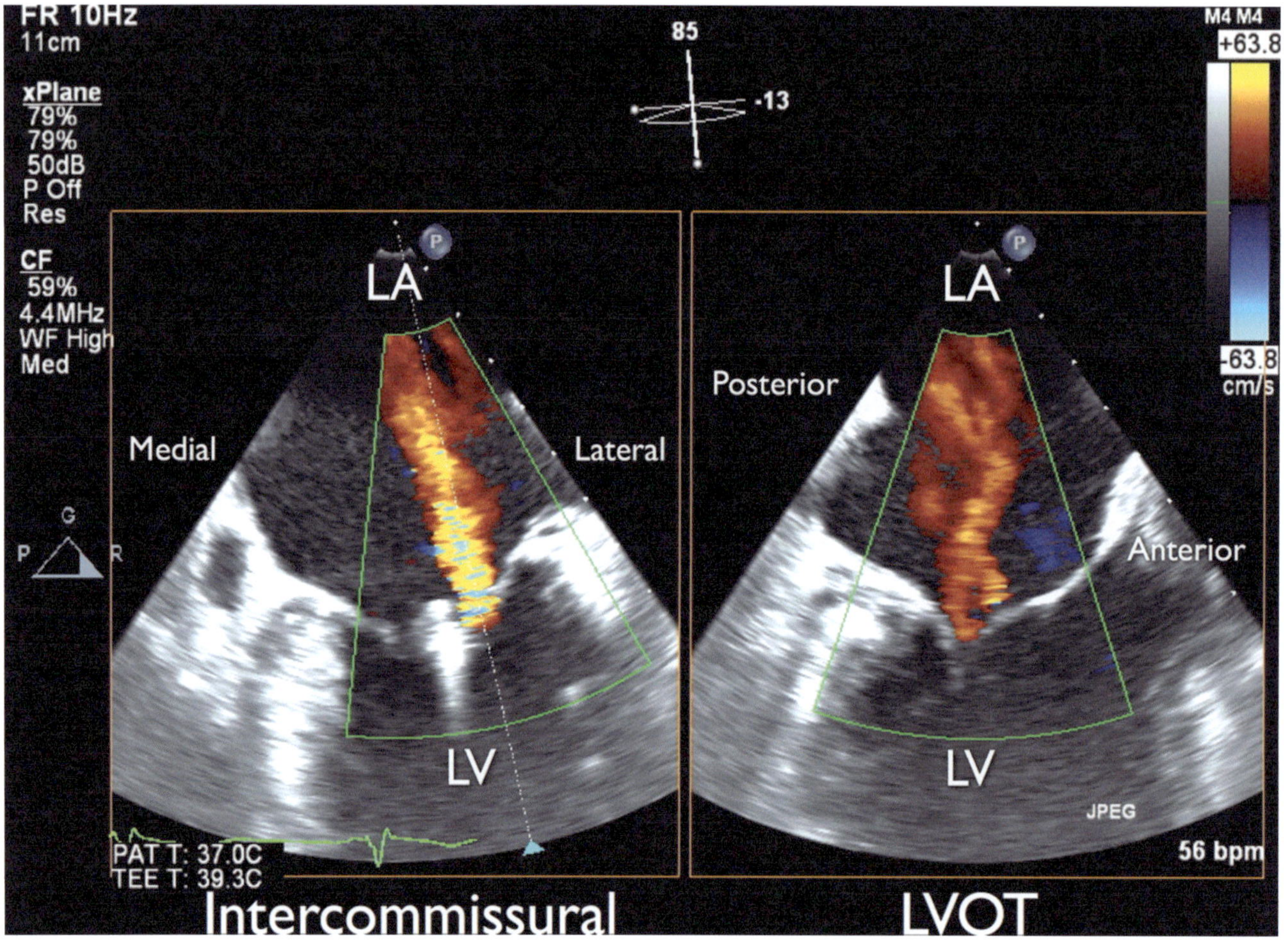

Fig. 5.19 Note a moderate degree of residual MR lateral to first clip placement in the intercommissural and LVOT views, prompting a decision to place second clip laterally. *LA* left atrium, *LV* left ventricle, *LVOT* left ventricular outflow tract

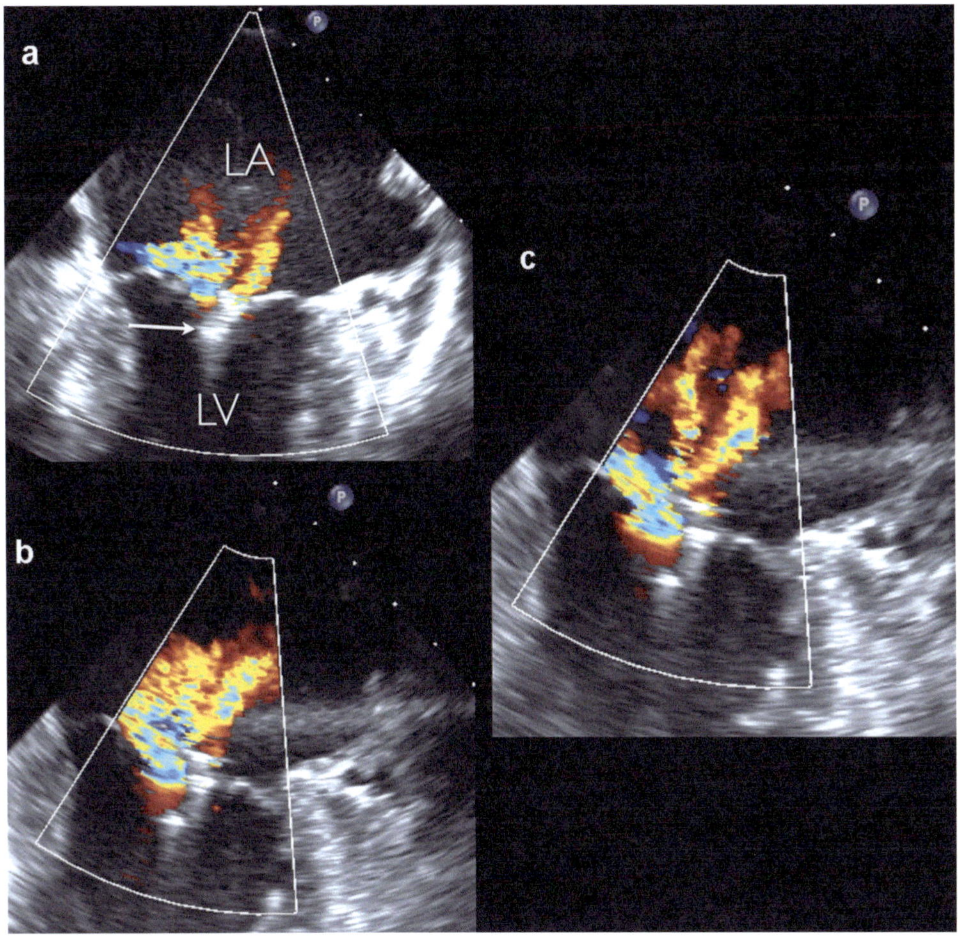

Fig. 5.20 Multiple larger residual MR jets seen serial systolic frames on TEE post placement of the MitraClip (*arrow*). Note the wider vena contracta at the origin of MR and larger proximal flow convergence. The decision between repositioning the clip vs. placing a second medial clip should be considered. This degree of MR reduction is unacceptable. *LA* left atrium, *LV* left ventricle

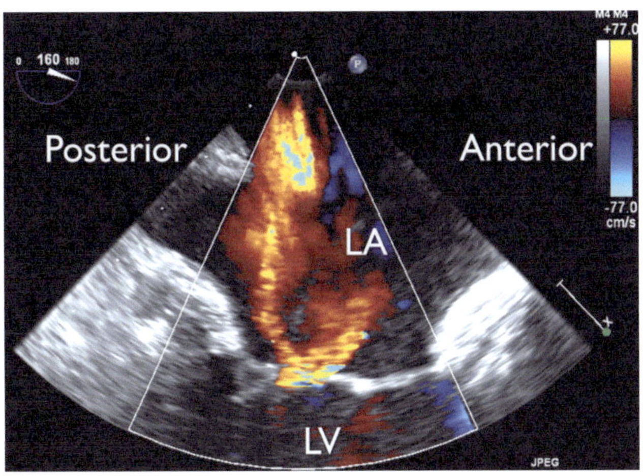

Fig. 5.21 Inadequate MR reduction after first clip placed in the zoomed LVOT view, prompting a repositioning of the MitraClip. *LA* left atrium, *LV* left ventricle

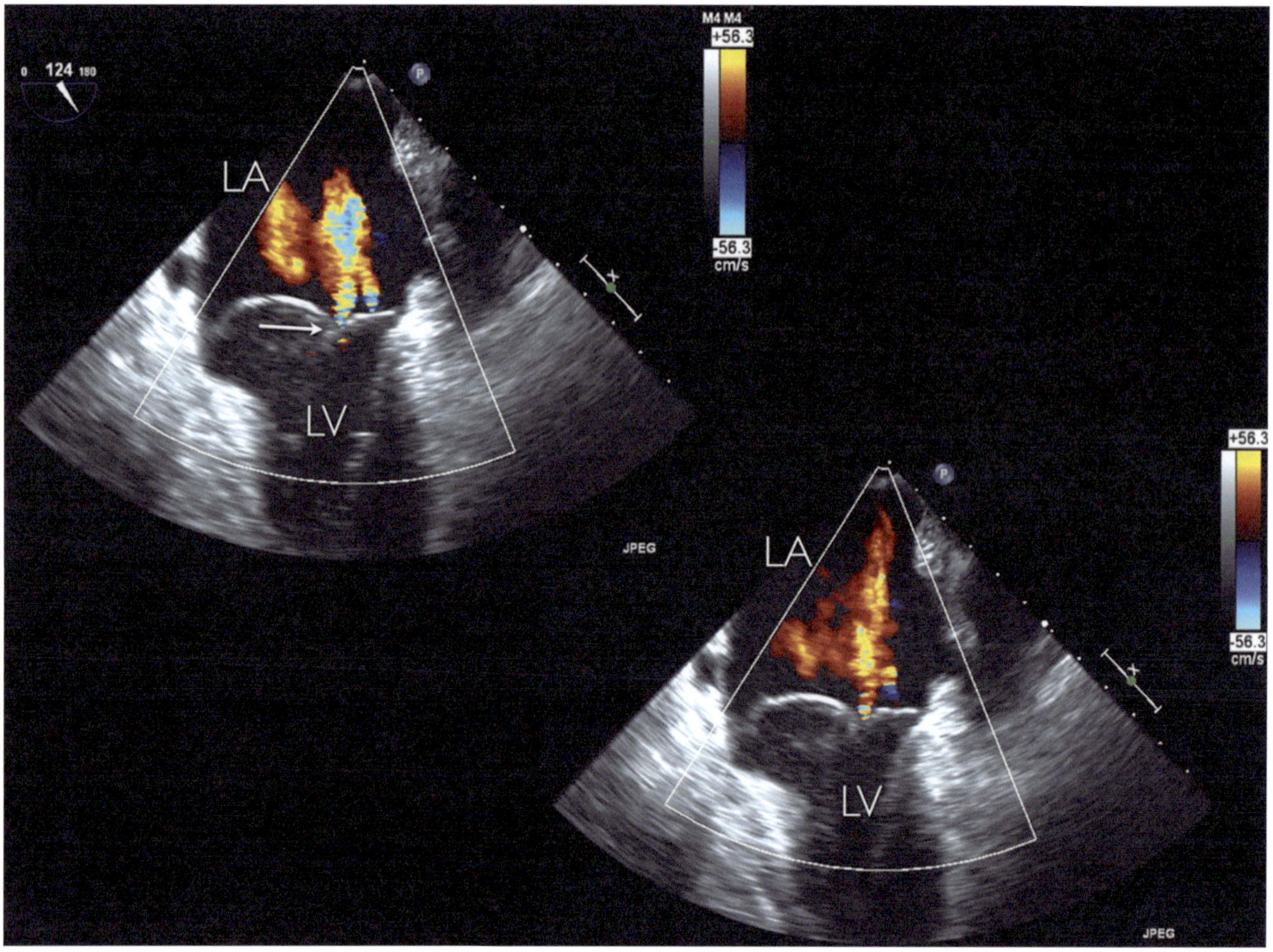

Fig. 5.22 Small residual MR jets are seen on multiple systolic frames from the same intercommissural views demonstrating complex significant MR post-placement of the MitraClip (*arrow*). *LA* left atrium, *LV* left ventricle

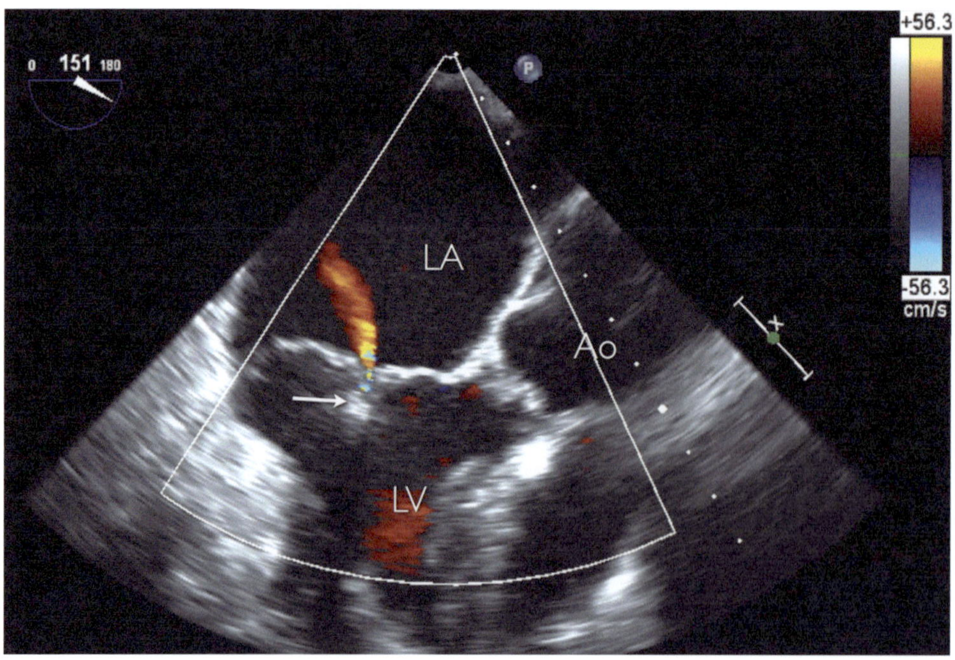

Fig. 5.23 Small residual MR jet seen in the LVOT view post-placement of the MitraClip (*arrow*). *LA* left atrium, *LV* left ventricle, *Ao* aorta

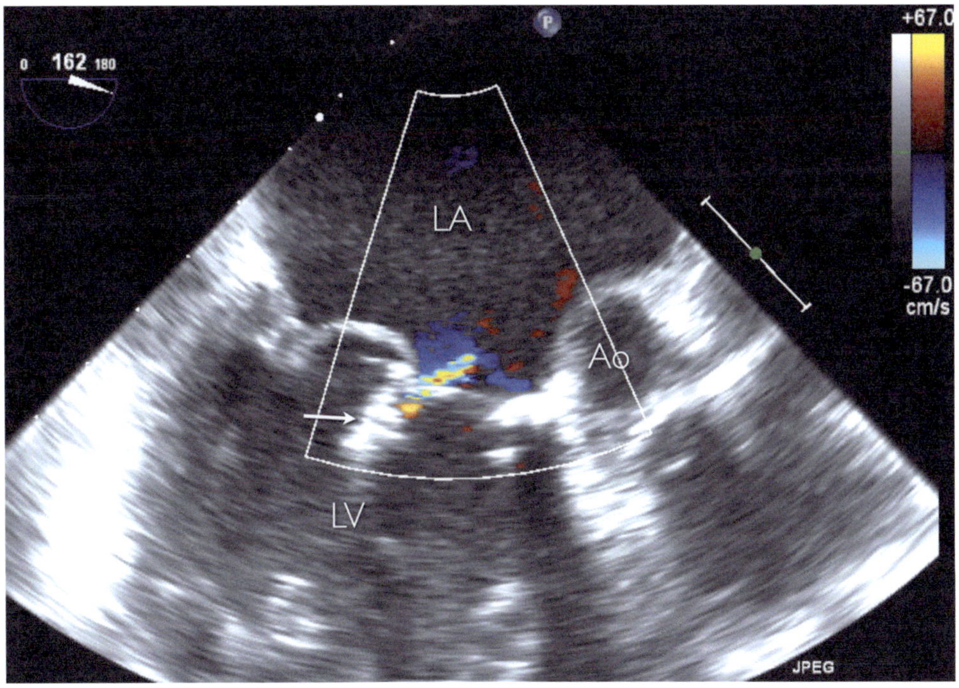

Fig. 5.24 Small residual MR jet seen in the LVOT view post-placement of the MitraClip (*arrow*). Note the narrow vena contracta at the origin of the MR anterior to the clip. *LA* left atrium, *LV* left ventricle, *Ao* aorta

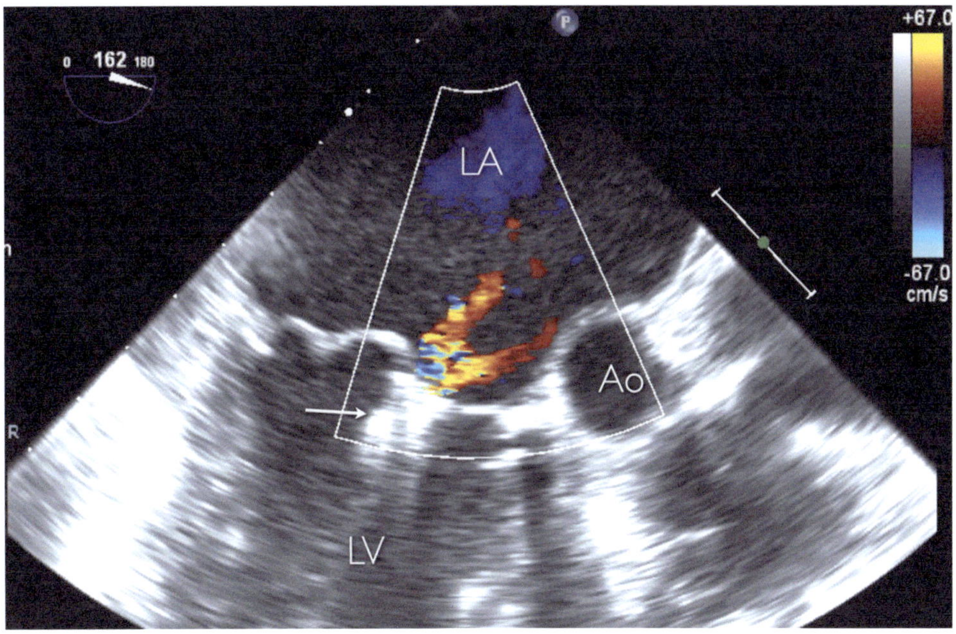

Fig. 5.25 Two small residual MR jet seen in the LVOT view post-placement of the MitraClip (*arrow*). Note the narrow vena contracta at the origin of the MR anterior to the clip. *LA* left atrium, *LV* left ventricle, *Ao* aorta

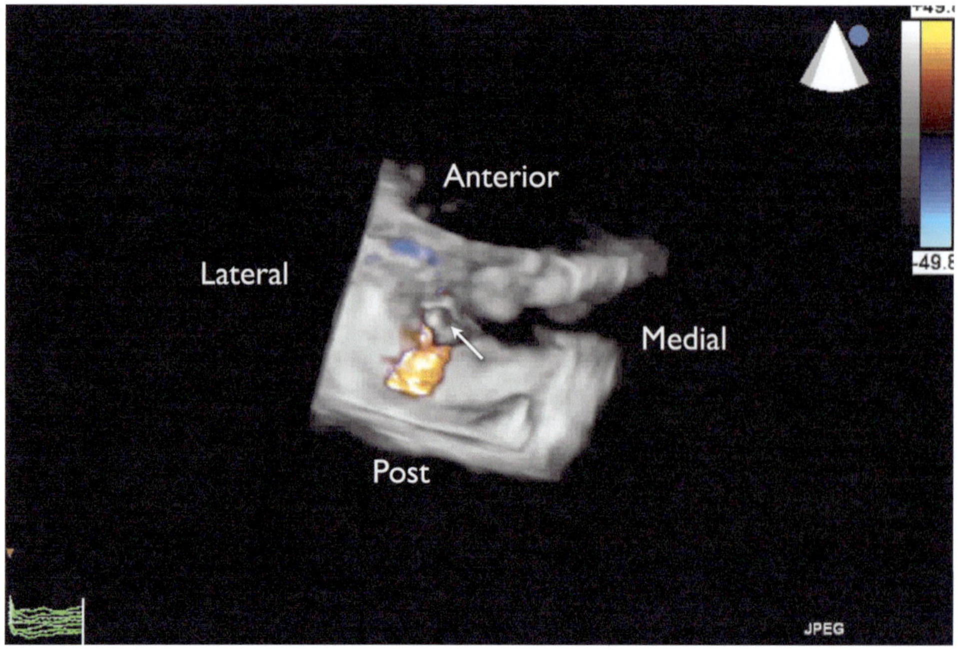

Fig. 5.26 Using color full volume on RT3D TEE imaging to identify a mild jet of eccentric MR post MitraClip (*arrow*)

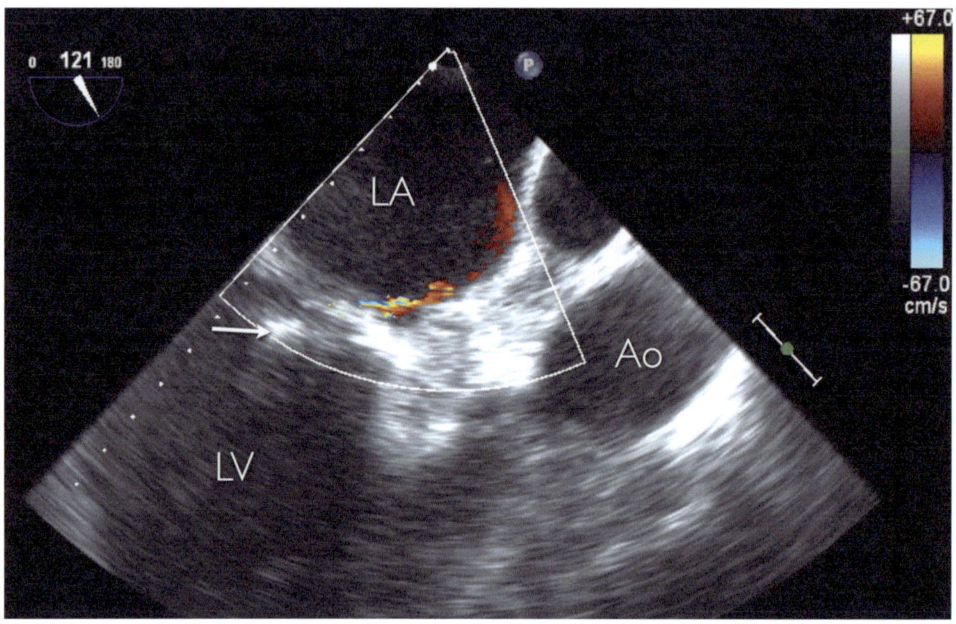

Fig. 5.27 A very small but highly eccentric residual MR jet seen in the LVOT view post-placement of the MitraClip (*arrow*). A careful search for eccentric MR is needed post-clip placement. *LA* left atrium, *LV* left ventricle, *Ao* aorta

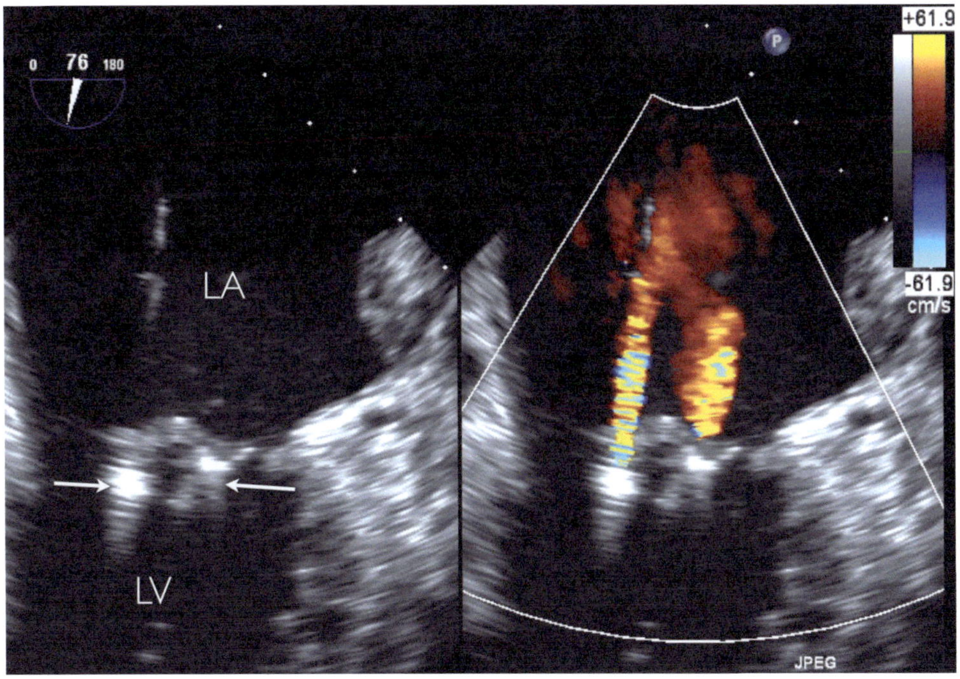

Fig. 5.28 Two small residual MR jet seen in the LVOT view post-placement of two central MitraClips (*arrows*). Note the narrow vena contracta at the origin of MR. *LA* left atrium, *LV* left ventricle

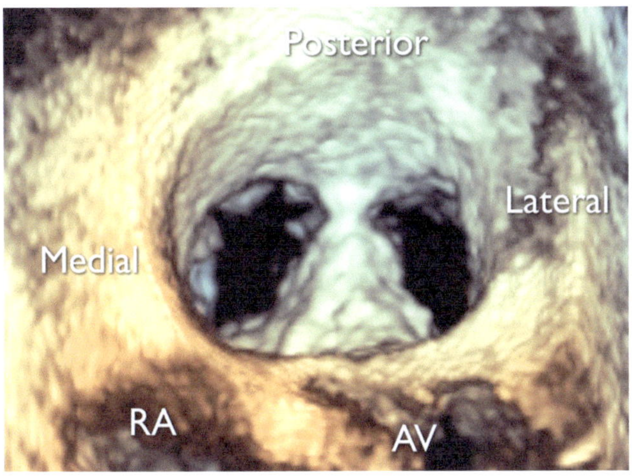

Fig. 5.29 3D zoom en face view post-MitraClip placement demonstrating double orifice MV. *RA* right atrium, *AV* aortic valve

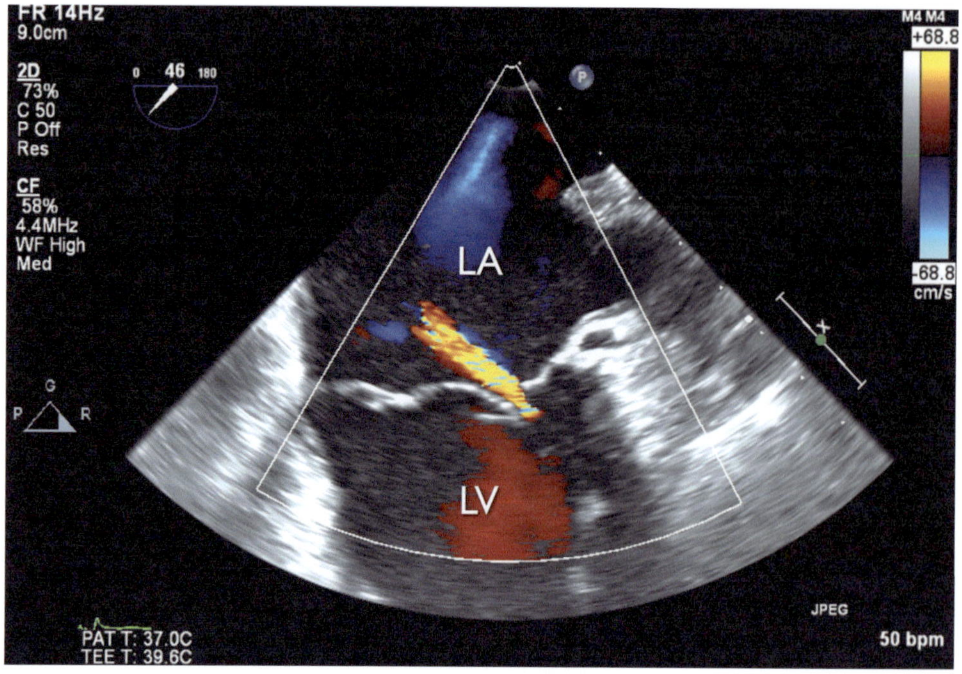

Fig. 5.30 Final residual MR shown in intercommissural view post-MitraClip placement. *LA* left atrium, *LV* left ventricle

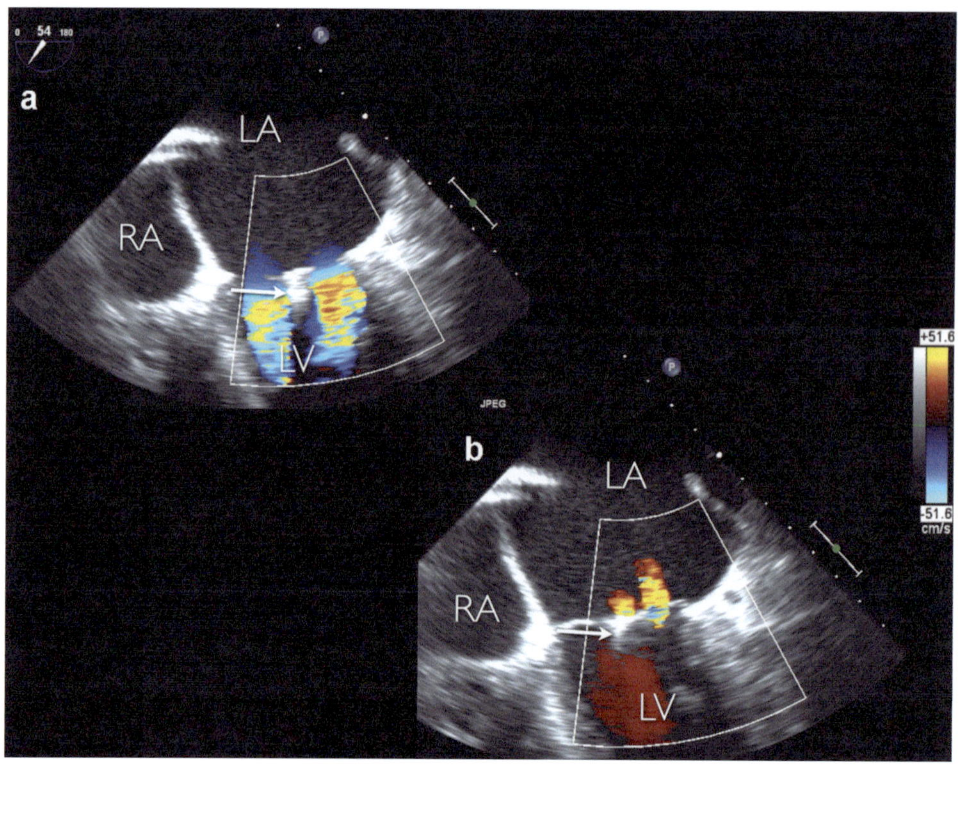

Fig. 5.31 (**a**) TEE four-chamber view post-MitraClip (*arrow*) placement demonstrating double orifice MV by color Doppler in diastole and (**b**) systolic frames demonstrating two jets of trivial residual MR. *RA* right atrium, *LA* left atrium, *LV* left ventricle

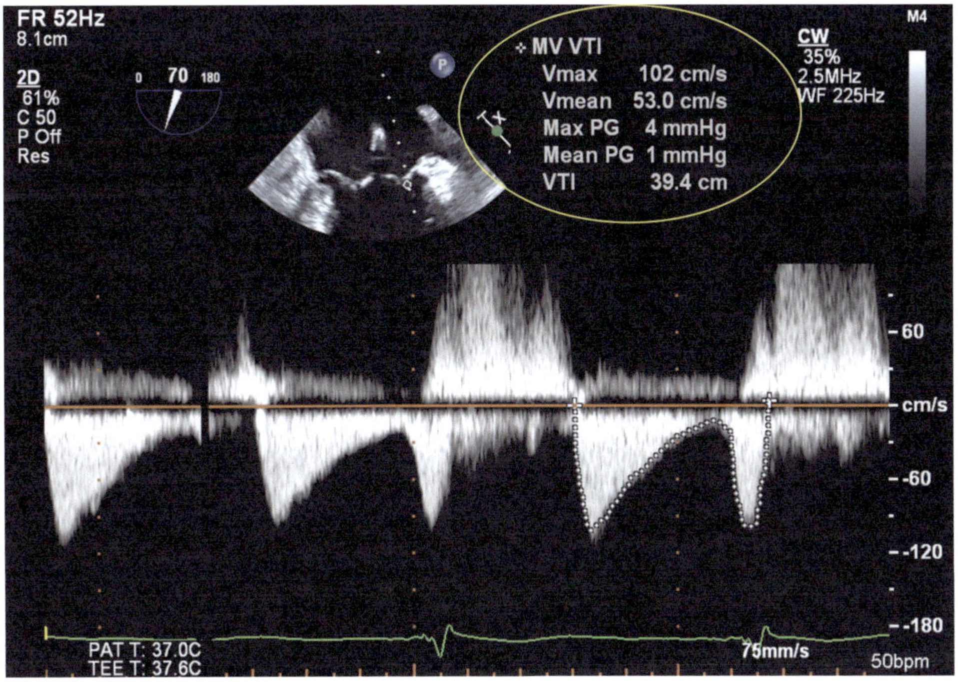

Fig. 5.32 Measurement of transmitral gradients with continuous-wave Doppler after MitraClip placement. The maximal gradient is 4 mmHg and the mean gradient 1 mmHg. A less than 4–5 mmHg mean gradient is desirable

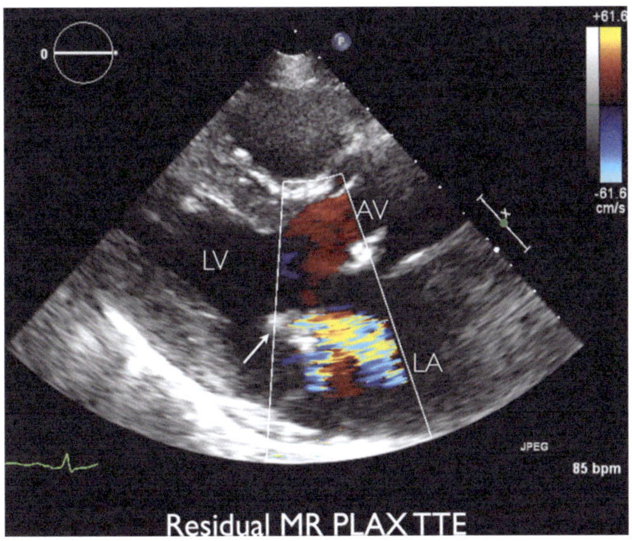

Fig. 5.33 Parasternal long-axis view post-MitraClip (*arrow*) placement mild residual MR. *LA* left atrium, *LV* left ventricle, *AV* aortic valve

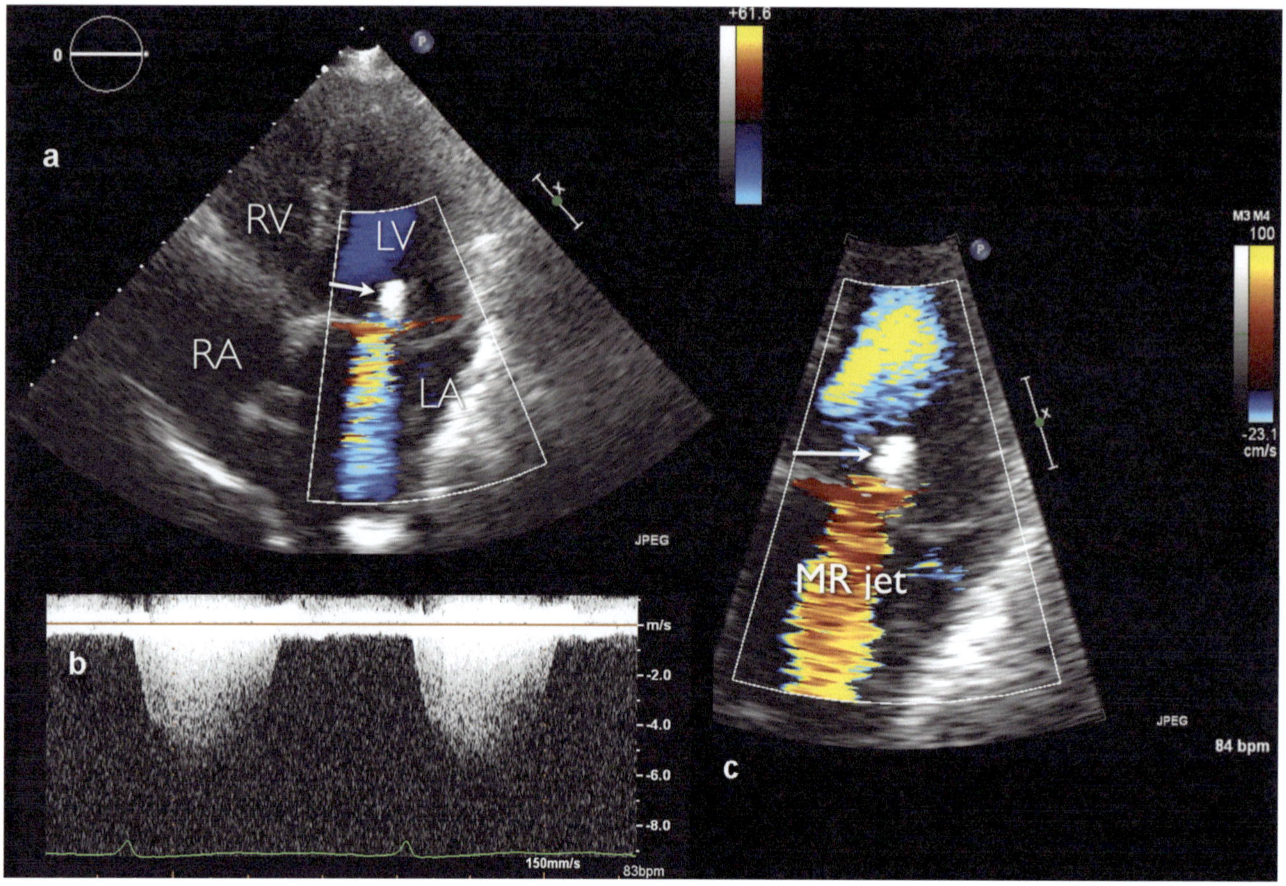

Fig. 5.34 Final MitraClip (*arrow*) result on TTE. (**a**) Four-chamber view of moderate 2+ residual MR and (**b**) corresponding nondense MR envelope on continuous wave Doppler imaging. (**c**) Difficulty in obtaining accurate PISA measurements post-MitraClip

Conclusion

Mitral valve repair with the MitraClip™ system is a safe and effective procedure that can be used to treat selected patients with significant mitral regurgitation. As with surgical mitral repair, the echocardiographic assessment of functional mitral valvular anatomy and the determination of the mechanism and severity of MR are required to select appropriate patients who may benefit from percutaneous intervention and to tailor the repair strategy to the individual pathology. High-quality transthoracic and transesophageal echocardiography supplemented by a real-time 3-D imaging is essential to evaluate the mitral valve for percutaneous repair as well as to evaluate the efficacy of the repair after it has been performed. Successful therapy with this system begins with appropriate patient selection.

References

1. Alfieri O, Maisano F, De Bonis M, Stefano PL, Torracca L, Oppizzi M, et al. The double-orifice technique in mitral valve repair: a simple solution for complex problems. J Thorac Cardiovasc Surg. 2001;122(4):674–81.
2. Maisano F, Vigano G, Blasio A, Colombo A, Calabrese C, Alfieri O. Surgical isolated edge-to-edge mitral valve repair without annuloplasty: clinical proof of the principle for an endovascular approach. EuroIntervention. 2006;2(2):181–6.
3. Goar FGS, Fann JI, Komtebedde J, Foster E, Oz MC, Fogarty TJ, et al. Endovascular edge-to-edge mitral valve repair: short-term results in a porcine model. Circulation. 2003;108(16):1990–3.
4. Feldman T, Wasserman HS, Herrmann HC, Gray W, Block PC, Whitlow P, et al. Percutaneous mitral valve repair using the edge-to-edge technique: six-month results of the EVEREST Phase I Clinical Trial. J Am Coll Cardiol. 2005;46(11):2134–40.
5. Feldman T, Foster E, Glower DD, Glower DG, Kar S, Rinaldi MJ, et al. Percutaneous repair or surgery for mitral regurgitation. N Engl J Med. 2011;364(15):1395–406.
6. Kische S, Nienaber C, Ince H. Use of four MitraClip devices in a patient with ischemic cardiomyopathy and mitral regurgitation: "Zipping by Clipping". Catheter Cardiovasc Interv. 2011. doi:10.1002/ccd.23431.
7. Rogers JH, Franzen O. Percutaneous edge-to-edge MitraClip therapy in the management of mitral regurgitation. Eur Heart J. 2011; 32(19):2350–7.
8. Ben Zekry S, Nagueh SF, Little SH, Quinones MA, McCulloch ML, Karanbir S, et al. Comparative accuracy of two- and three-dimensional transthoracic and transesophageal echocardiography in identifying mitral valve pathology in patients undergoing mitral valve repair: initial observations. J Am Soc Echocardiogr. 2011;24(10):1079–85.
9. Salcedo EE, Quaife RA, Seres T, Carroll JD. A framework for systematic characterization of the mitral valve by real-time three-dimensional transesophageal echocardiography. J Am Soc Echocardiogr. 2009; 22(10):1087–99.
10. Wei J, Hsiung MC, Tsai SK, Ou C-H, Chang C-Y, Chang YC, et al. The routine use of live three-dimensional transesophageal echocardiography in mitral valve surgery: clinical experience. Eur J Echocardiogr. 2010;11(1):14–8.
11. Silvestry FE, Kerber RE, Brook MM, Carroll JD, Eberman KM, Goldstein SA, et al. Echocardiography-guided interventions. J Am Soc Echocardiogr. 2009;22(3):213–31, quiz 316–7.
12. Zamorano JL, Badano LP, Bruce C, Chan K-L, Gonçalves A, Hahn RT, et al. EAE/ASE recommendations for the use of echocardiography in new transcatheter interventions for valvular heart disease. J Am Soc Echocardiogr. 2011;24(9):937–65.
13. Zoghbi W. Recommendations for evaluation of the severity of native valvular regurgitation with two-dimensional and Doppler echocardiography. J Am Soc Echocardiogr. 2003;16(7):777–802.
14. Lancellotti P, Moura L, Pierard LA, Agricola E, Popescu BA, Tribouilloy C, et al. European association of echocardiography recommendations for the assessment of valvular regurgitation. Part 2: mitral and tricuspid regurgitation (native valve disease). Eur J Echocardiogr. 2010;11(4):307–32.
15. Enriquez-Sarano M, Avierinos J-F, Messika-Zeitoun D, Detaint D, Capps M, Nkomo V, et al. Quantitative determinants of the outcome of asymptomatic mitral regurgitation. N Engl J Med. 2005;352(9): 875–83.
16. Topilsky Y, Grigioni F, Enriquez-Sarano M. Quantitation of mitral regurgitation. Semin Thorac Cardiovasc Surg. 2011;23(2):106–14.
17. Franzen O, Baldus S, Rudolph V, Meyer S, Knap M, Koschyk D, et al. Acute outcomes of MitraClip therapy for mitral regurgitation in high-surgical-risk patients: emphasis on adverse valve morphology and severe left ventricular dysfunction. Eur Heart J. 2010;31(11): 1373–81.
18. Rudolph V, Knap M, Franzen O, Schlüter M, de Vries T, Conradi L, et al. Echocardiographic and clinical outcomes of MitraClip therapy in patients not amenable to surgery. J Am Coll Cardiol. 2011;58(21):2190–5.
19. Tamburino C, Ussia GP, Maisano F, Capodanno D, La Canna G, Scandura S, et al. Percutaneous mitral valve repair with the MitraClip system: acute results from a real world setting. Eur Heart J. 2010;31(11):1382–9.
20. Carpentier A. Cardiac valve surgery – the "French correction". J Thorac Cardiovasc Surg. 1983;86(3):323–37.
21. Adams DH, Rosenhek R, Falk V. Degenerative mitral valve regurgitation: best practice revolution. Eur Heart J. 2010;31(16): 1958–66.
22. Barlow JB, Pocock WA. The significance of late systolic murmurs and mid-late systolic clicks. Md State Med J. 1963;12:76–7.
23. Gertz ZM, Raina A, Mountantonakis SE, Zado ES, Callans DJ, Marchlinski FE, et al. The impact of mitral regurgitation on patients undergoing catheter ablation of atrial fibrillation. Europace. 2011;13(8):1127–32.
24. Gertz ZM, Raina A, Saghy L, Zado ES, Callans DJ, Marchlinski FE, et al. Evidence of atrial functional mitral regurgitation due to atrial fibrillation: reversal with arrhythmia control. J Am Coll Cardiol. 2011;58(14):1474–81.
25. Shimada YJ, Shiota T. A meta-analysis and investigation for the source of bias of left ventricular volumes and function by three-dimensional echocardiography in comparison with magnetic resonance imaging. Am J Cardiol. 2011;107(1):126–38.
26. Radunski U, Lange M, Barmeyer A. Assessment of changes in cardiac volumes following MitraClip™ implantation using cardiac magnetic resonance imaging. J Cardiovasc Magn Reson. 2012; 14(1):101.
27. Lin BA, Forouhar AS, Pahlevan NM, Anastassiou CA, Grayburn PA, Thomas JD, et al. Color Doppler jet area overestimates regurgitant volume when multiple jets are present. J Am Soc Echocardiogr. 2010;23(9):993–1000.
28. Herrmann HC, Rohatgi S, Wasserman HS, Block P, Gray W, Hamilton A, et al. Mitral valve hemodynamic effects of percutaneous edge-to-edge repair with the MitraClip device for mitral regurgitation. Catheter Cardiovasc Interv. 2006;68(6):821–8.
29. Herrmann HC, Kar S, Siegel R, Fail P, Loghin C, Lim S, et al. Effect of percutaneous mitral repair with the MitraClip device on mitral valve area and gradient. EuroIntervention. 2009;4(4): 437–42.

MitraClip Procedural Echocardiography

6

Thomas W. Smith and William J. Bommer

Abstract
The MitraClip is a complex interventional procedure that is primarily guided by transesophageal echocardiography. A successful procedure is dependent on efficient and precise communication between the primary operator and the echocardiologist. In this chapter, key components of a safe and efficient procedural echocardiogram are described.

Keywords
Mitral regurgitation • MitraClip • Transesophageal echocardiography • Three-dimensional • Echocardiologist

In parallel with the rapid advancements in percutaneous structural heart disease intervention, echocardiography has made significant technological advancements. These advances in echocardiography have expanded the role of echocardiologists beyond identifying patients who would benefit from intervention to providing the necessary guidance during the procedure. Since the first MitraClip was placed, the use of three-dimensional (3-D) transesophageal echocardiography (TEE) has become widespread. 3-D systems allow the primary operators access to real-time images of the entire mitral valve and the clip. From this perspective, the operators can make device manipulations more effectively, enhancing the speed of the procedure by reducing the number of TEE manipulations necessary for clip delivery. Biplane ("xplane") imaging is also possible with 3-D probes, allowing the display of two separate two-dimensional images at the same time. This has the advantage of displaying high-resolution images in two different planes at the same time – an invaluable tool in transseptal puncture and clip alignment.

T.W. Smith, M.D. • W.J. Bommer, M.D.
Division of Cardiovascular Medicine,
Department of Internal Medicine, University of California, Davis,
4860 Y Street, Suite 2820, Sacramento, CA 95817, USA
e-mail: thomas.smith@ucdmc.ucdavis.edu;
william.bommer@ucdmc.ucdavis.edu

Equipment Checklist

In addition to an adequate display for the echocardiographer, the interventional operators need to have real-time access to the transesophageal echocardiogram images. This will involve a second monitor connected to the output from the TEE machine. Ideally, this should be placed on the monitor bank next to fluoroscopy and hemodynamics. Not all catheterization laboratories are capable of displaying multiple screens at once from machines of various vendors. A pre-procedure checklist is necessary prior to all procedures to verify proper function, cable and adapter availability, and equipment compatibility. The TEE probe should be carefully inspected before each procedure for any small cracks or defects which could result in esophageal trauma during more lengthy procedures.

Echocardiographer Positioning

The echocardiographer is usually positioned to the patient's left at the head of the table. Most cardiac catheterization tables do not have adequate radiation reduction mechanisms automatically in place for this location. In order to reduce the amount of radiation exposure to the echocardiographer, a portable shield should be placed between the patient and the echocardiographer. At times when fine manipulation is

T. Feldman et al. (eds.), *Atlas of Percutaneous Edge-to-Edge Mitral Valve Repair*,
DOI 10.1007/978-1-4471-4294-2_6, © Springer-Verlag London 2013

not necessary, the probe can be held in place with a clamp or tie affixed to the shield. Attention to adequate shielding and avoiding reaching into the fluoroscopic field will reduce the echocardiographer's radiation exposure. The interventional operator should be equally mindful of the risk to the echocardiographer and provide adequate warning when moving the image intensifier or when activating cine imaging.

Initial Imaging: Establish Working Views

Patients will have had comprehensive TEEs prior to the day of the procedure to establish eligibility for MitraClip placement. Following intubation and passage of the TEE probe, an abbreviated transesophageal echocardiogram is performed. The role of this procedure is to rule out direct contraindications to the procedure – such as a new left atrial appendage or left atrial thrombus, left ventricular thrombus, or new mitral valve lesion. Once the safety to proceed is established, then confirmation of the mitral anatomy, regurgitation severity, and jet orientation is required. Subsequently, it is necessary to establish working views and images that will be used during the procedure. These views include surgical three-dimensional view (Fig. 6.1), bicaval (80–110°, Fig. 6.2a), short axis at the base (10–40°, Fig. 6.2b), long axis (110–140°, Fig. 6.2c), and intercommissural (40–70°, Fig. 6.2d). Since diagnostic TEEs are usually performed with the patient in the left lateral position and the MitraClip procedure is in the supine position, heart orientation, angles, and probe manipulations may not always be standard.

Transseptal Puncture

The transseptal puncture establishes the critical sheath position relative to the mitral valve. This position is paramount to successful manipulation of the clip delivery system. Establishing the sheath too superior or inferior will complicate subtle manipulations at the valve level. Bicaval and short axis at the base views provide the operator with superior/inferior and anterior/posterior positioning. Biplane imaging displays both of these views simultaneously, thus allowing the operator to correct motion outside of the primary imaging plane (Fig. 6.3). Although the sector width in biplane is slightly reduced, the advantage of simultaneous orthogonal views is well worth it. Once the bicaval view is obtained, biplane is initiated with the complementary view rotated to produce a standard short axis at the base. Rotation of the complementary image is always required; by maintaining standard image orientation, any uncertainty of the orientation is eliminated. Once an appropriate location to cross the interatrial septum is established, then a modified four-chamber view is obtained to confirm the projected distance to the mitral valve leaflets (Fig. 6.4). The ideal height above the mitral annulus or valve coaptation plane (depending on the underlying valve disease) is 3.5–4.5 cm. Depending on the heart rotation and apical location, this may require either right lateral motion of the TEE probe or measurement in the 150–170° range in order to keep the tented portion of the septum and the mitral leaflets in plane.

After crossing the interatrial septum, the MitraClip guide-dilator assembly (with echogenic coils) is advanced over a 0.035 extra-stiff wire into the left atrium. The guide catheter is advanced until the radiopaque tip is approximately 3 cm into, and in the middle of, the left atrium (Figs. 6.5, 6.6, 6.7, and 6.8).

Steering Clip Delivery System Above Mitral Valve

After confirming sheath placement, the clip delivery system (CDS) is introduced and visualized exiting the sheath into the left atrium (Fig. 6.9). The delivery catheter with the clip attached is guided with the steerable sleeve down to the mitral valve with careful attention given to the lateral wall and the left atrial appendage as the clip is maneuvered into position approximately 1 cm above the mitral valve (Fig. 6.10). An iterative TEE approach is necessary starting with a four-chamber view and then modified to allow visualization of both the tip of the delivery system and the lateral wall as the clip is flexed and rotated into position above the valve. A similar protocol is necessary in reverse when removing the delivery system at the end of the case.

Orientation of Clip Over Mitral Valve

Once the CDS is positioned over the mitral valve, it is further oriented above the regurgitant jet. The primary views to establish appropriate position are the long-axis or left ventricular outflow tract (LVOT) and intercommissural views. These two views respectively provide anterior/posterior and lateral/medial orientation. As with crossing the transseptal, it is valuable to know how moving the device anteriorly affects the lateral/medial position. This can be accomplished either with live 3-D imaging or with biplane. Biplane has the advantage of providing real-time color along with higher frame rates and improved resolution when compared to real-time 3-D (Figs. 6.11 and 6.12). It is easiest to establish the intercommissural view first, then apply biplane and rotate the complementary plane to display the long-axis orientation.

Starting from the intercommissural view eliminates potential confusion regarding lateral and medial as the initial biplane image created when starting with the long-axis view is typically a reversed intercommissural view.

After positioning the CDS in line to split the regurgitant jet, the arms are opened in the left atrium. The clip arms need to be oriented perpendicular to the mitral valve scallop line of coaptation. While this can be confirmed by visualizing equal arm lengths in the long-axis view and lack of arms in the intercommissural view, ideally the valve and clip should be imaged in a short-axis plane. Prior to the widespread use of three-dimensional TEE imaging, this would be obtained with a transgastric short-axis view of the mitral valve (Figs. 6.13, 6.14, and 6.15). Three-dimensional TEE has essentially eliminated the need to obtain transgastric views since a projected short-axis view of the valve can be obtained from the esophagus in 3-D.

When orienting the clip arms, the mitral valve should be displayed with 3-D real-time echocardiography in the standard surgical view with the left atrial appendage on the left of the screen and the interatrial septum on the right. In this orientation, the operator can easily identify if a rotation of the device is necessary and visualize the subsequent correction in real time.

The device can then be advanced into the left ventricle (Fig. 6.16). This is best viewed in either the long axis or biplane with the complimentary intercommissural view. After advancing into the left ventricle, 3-D imaging can again verify clip arm orientation perpendicular to the scallops. If there is chordal interference, a zoomed view of the clip arms can reveal what subtle adjustments need to be made.

Leaflet Grasp

Adequate grasp of the leaflets is of paramount importance in ensuring a successful clip deployment. If there is inadequate grasp, there is at best a decrease in the MR reduction and at worst an increased risk of clip detachment. In order to increase frame rate and resolution, the sector width should be decreased to create a zoomed long-axis view of the clip and scallops. Gain and penetration must be optimized to visualize capture. The grasp maneuver requires specific coordination between the echocardiographer, anesthesiologist, and operator. In addition to a breath hold, we have developed an effective technique wherein a prolonged loop capture of 15–20 beats is acquired during the grasp. Following capture, the loop should be reviewed with the echocardiographer and operator to ensure visualization of adequate leaflet tissue capture. It is often helpful to review this loop frame by frame to allow precise visualization of the moment of leaflet capture (Fig. 6.17). Prior to assessing mitral regurgitation reduction, the quality of the grasp on the leaflets should be confirmed. This involves interrogation of the anterior and posterior scallops folding over the clip and under the arms (Figs. 6.18 and 6.19). Multiple views and probe manipulations are necessary – including rotation of the probe in the long-axis and intercommissural views. Once adequate grasp is confirmed, residual structural abnormalities and mitral regurgitation may be assessed.

Residual Mitral Valve Disease

With the clip arms closed, residual mitral regurgitation and structural abnormalities may be evaluated. Careful attention to the patient's blood pressure during this assessment is also important as ideally it should be the same as during the imaging in the beginning of the case. Since cardiac anesthesia can lower blood pressure, it should be restored with vasopressors prior to mitral regurgitation assessment. Imaging with and without color Doppler should be performed in the mid-esophageal view at 0° from the lateral to medial aspect of the valve, the long-axis with medial and lateral rotation, and the intercommissural view with anterior and posterior rotation. These views will allow assessment of any residual prolapse or flail segments. In order to establish a quantitative assessment of the residual MR, pulmonary vein pulsed-wave Doppler assessment in all veins should be compared to pre-procedure tracings (Fig. 6.20). The 2-D and color views along with the pulmonary vein Doppler will delineate the location and severity of any residual regurgitation. Mitral regurgitation severity is based on a composite estimate of jet width (vena contracta), jet area/left atrial area, and pulmonary vein tracings.

In addition to assessment of MR reduction, it is necessary to evaluate for iatrogenic mitral stenosis. This is most easily done by tracing the envelope from continuous or pulsed-wave Doppler through one of the mitral orifices and establishing a mean gradient. Pressure half-time provides additional information on valve area. Planimetry either in the transgastric short axis or with three-dimensional echocardiography can also be performed if there is a question of significant mitral stenosis.

If there is procedural success with significant reduction in MR and no significant MS, then the clip can be released (Figs. 6.21 and 6.22). If there is evidence of significant continued mitral regurgitation, then the etiology of that residual MR needs to be established. Based on the etiology of the residual MR, multiple options exist. Occasionally, tightening the MitraClip or releasing any stored tension on the delivery catheter can further reduce MR prior to release. If there is significant residual degenerative disease, then either the first clip can be removed and an alternate grasp can be performed or an additional clip can be placed on the residual prolapsed or flail scallop. In functional MR, residual MR may result from a very wide initial jet that was not adequately reduced with a single clip. In this setting, either another clip may be placed in addition to the current one or the current clip should be removed and placed more lateral or medial in the jet to allow placement of a second clip. When the second clip is oriented in the left atrium, the arms are opened; however, when advancing the clip into the left ventricle, the arms should be closed to avoid interfering with the first clip. Once in the left ventricle, the arms may once again be carefully opened.

After making the final decision to leave the clip in place, it can be released by the operator. The tension on the valve with the delivery system can alter the residual mitral regurgitation. Following release, a final assessment of the MR reduction should be performed using the same views as above to ensure adequate clip position and leaflet capture. Occasionally, if there is significant MR after release, another clip may reduce the residual regurgitation (Fig. 6.23).

Guidance for CDS Removal

During catheter withdrawal from the MV annulus into the LA, the CDS needs to be followed superiorly to the interatrial septum puncture site. Once again, simultaneous visualization of the tip of the catheter and the lateral wall is necessary to reduce the risk of left atrial injury. This is best visualized with either a modified 4C view or biplane.

Residual Atrial Septal Defect

Following guiding sheath removal, an atrial septal defect will be present (Fig. 6.24). With careful attention to the sheath placement and manipulations during the case, the defect should be relatively small. A biplane view of the bicaval and short-axis view at the base with color provides the most detailed image of this defect. 3-D imaging with color may also be valuable (Fig. 6.25). These septal defects tend to close in most patients over the next 6 months. If the defect is hemodynamically significant, then it can easily be closed with a septal occluder device.

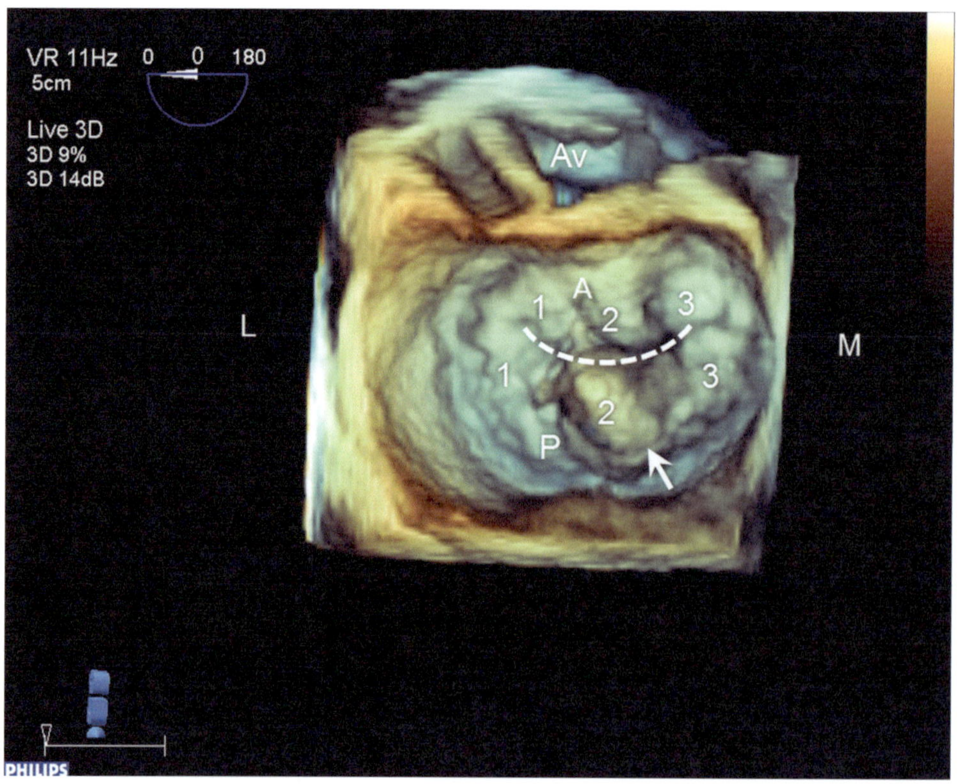

Fig. 6.1 Surgical view of mitral valve with 3-D transesophageal echocardiography demonstrating flail of the P2 scallop. *arrow Av* aortic valve, *L* lateral, *M* medial, *A* anterior mitral valve leaflet, *P* posterior mitral valve leaflet, *1–3* respective scallops of the anterior and posterior mitral valve leaflets, *Broken line* line of coaptation between anterior and posterior mitral valve leaflets

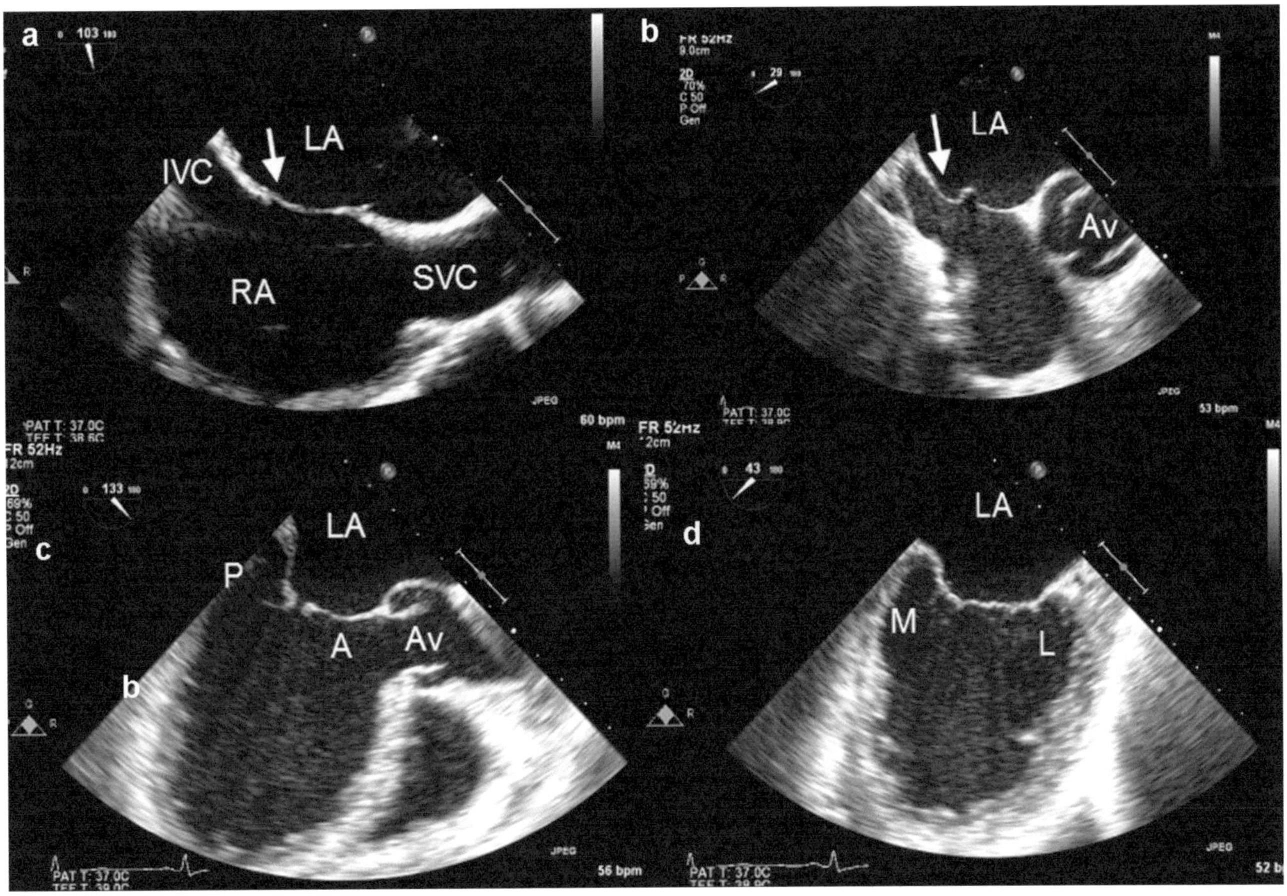

Fig. 6.2 Working views obtained at the beginning of the procedure. (**a**) Biplane image of interatrial septum. (**b**) Short-axis basal view with aortic valve in short axis. (**c**) Long-axis view. (**d**) Intercommissural view. *LA* left atrium, *RA* right atrium, *LV* left ventricle, *RV* right ventricle, *SVC* superior vena cava, *Av* aortic valve, *IVC* inferior vena cava, *P* posterior, *A* anterior, *M* medial, *L* lateral, *Arrow* interatrial septum

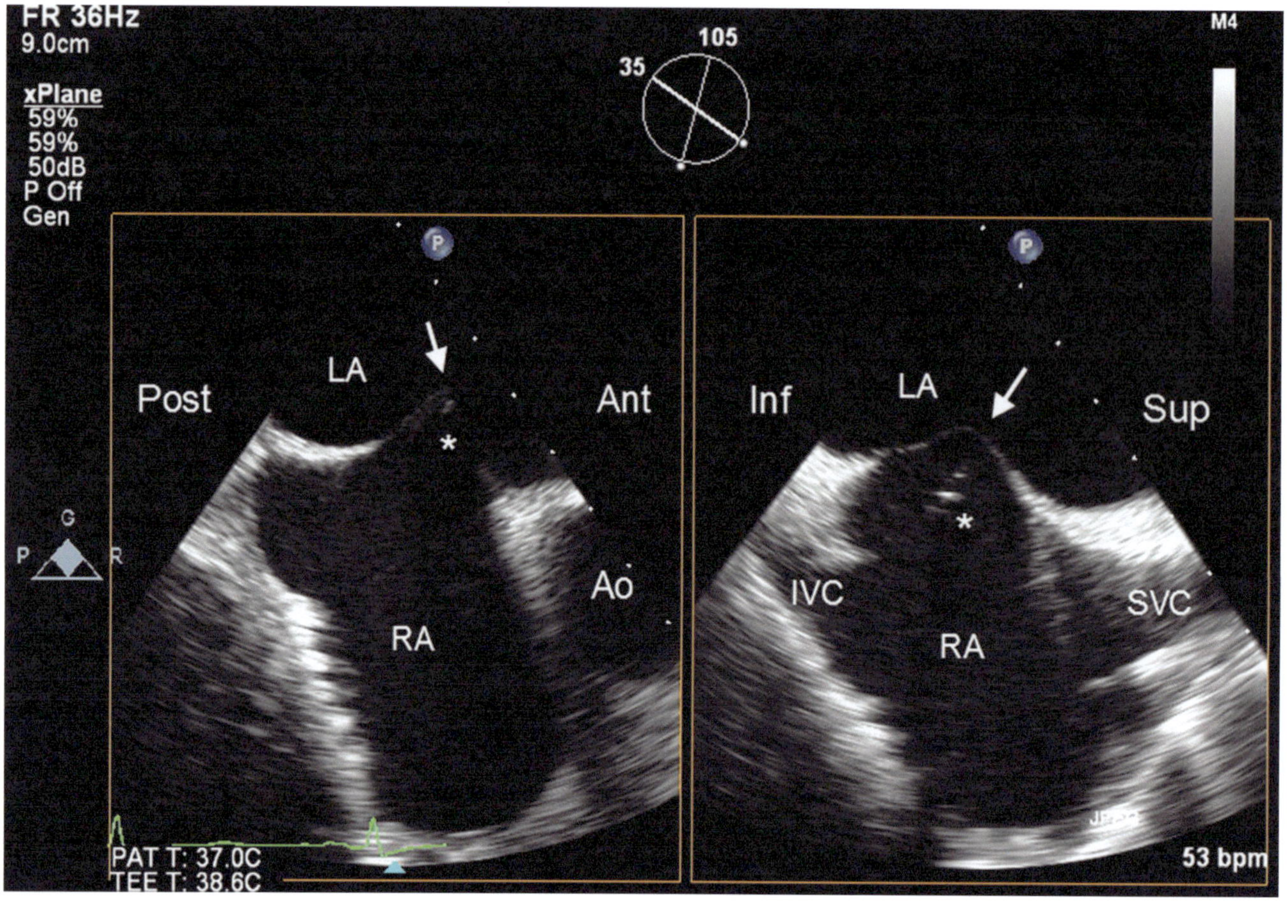

Fig. 6.3 Biplane image of interatrial septum during transseptal puncture. Tenting of the septum by the transseptal catheter (*) is visualized at the *arrow*. The biplane orientation allows real-time assessment of the catheter tip in the anterior/posterior and inferior/superior planes. *Post* posterior, *Ant* anterior, *Inf* inferior, *Sup* superior, *LA* left atrium, *RA* right atrium, *IVC* inferior vena cava, *SVC* superior vena cava, *Ao* aorta

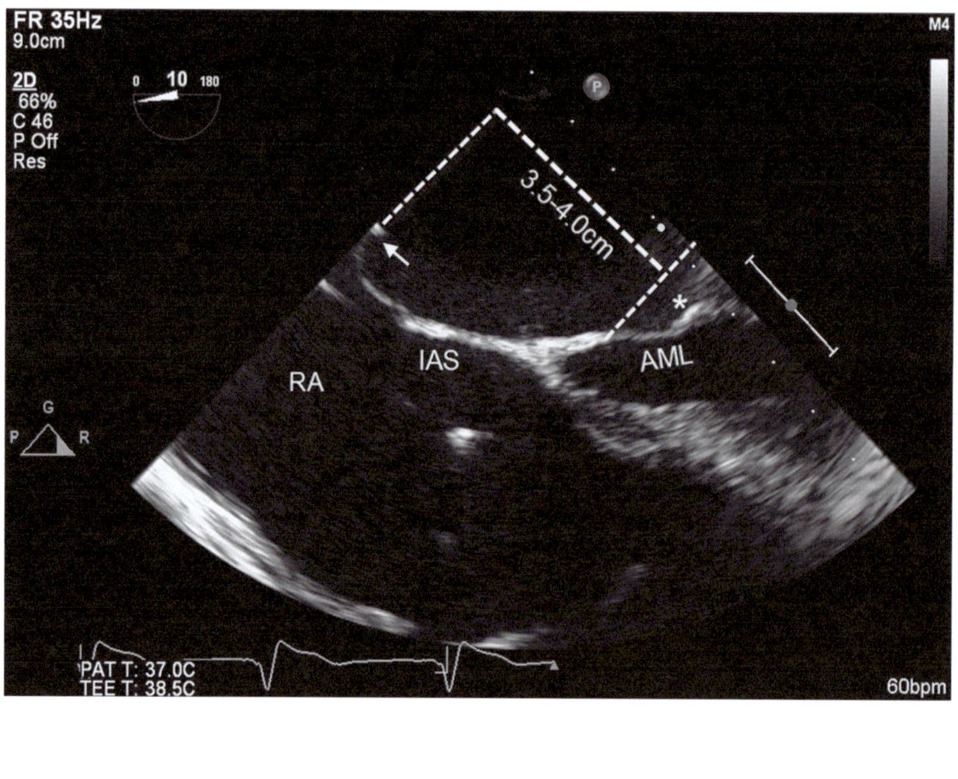

Fig. 6.4 Modified four-chamber view demonstrates the estimation of transseptal puncture to mitral valve annulus. *IAS* interatrial septum, *Arrow* tenting of IAS by transseptal needle/catheter, *RA* right atrium, *AML* anterior mitral valve leaflet, * coaptation point, *Vertical broken line* distance from mitral annuls to transseptal

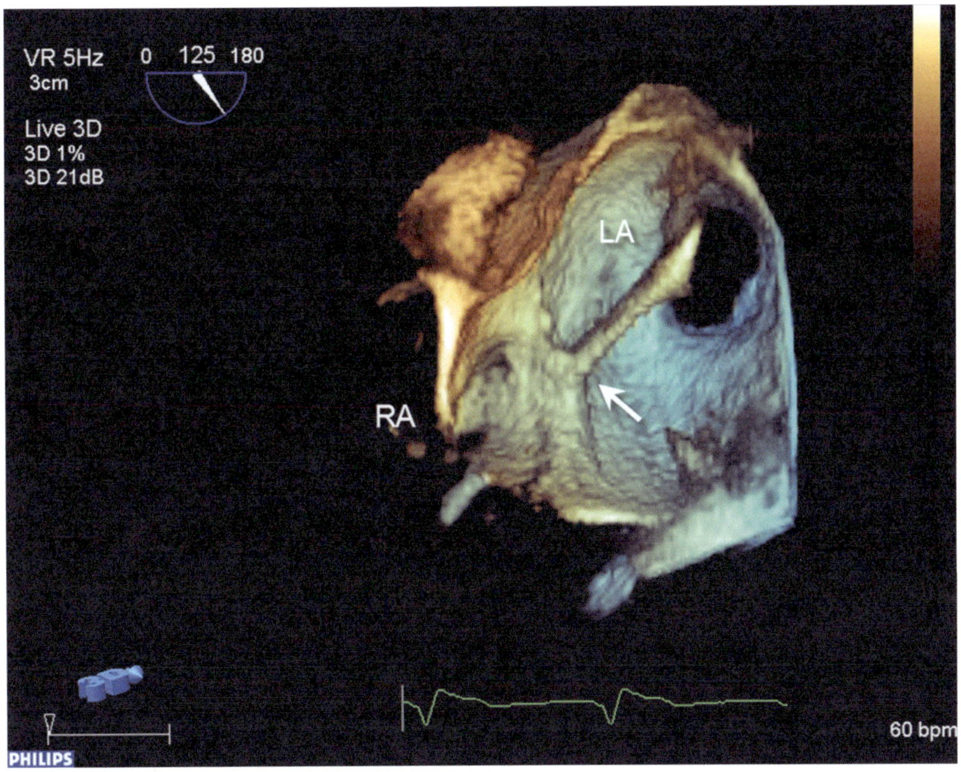

Fig. 6.5 3-D image of transseptal catheter crossing interatrial septum. Continued tenting is visible at the *arrow*. *LA* left atrium, *RA* right atrium

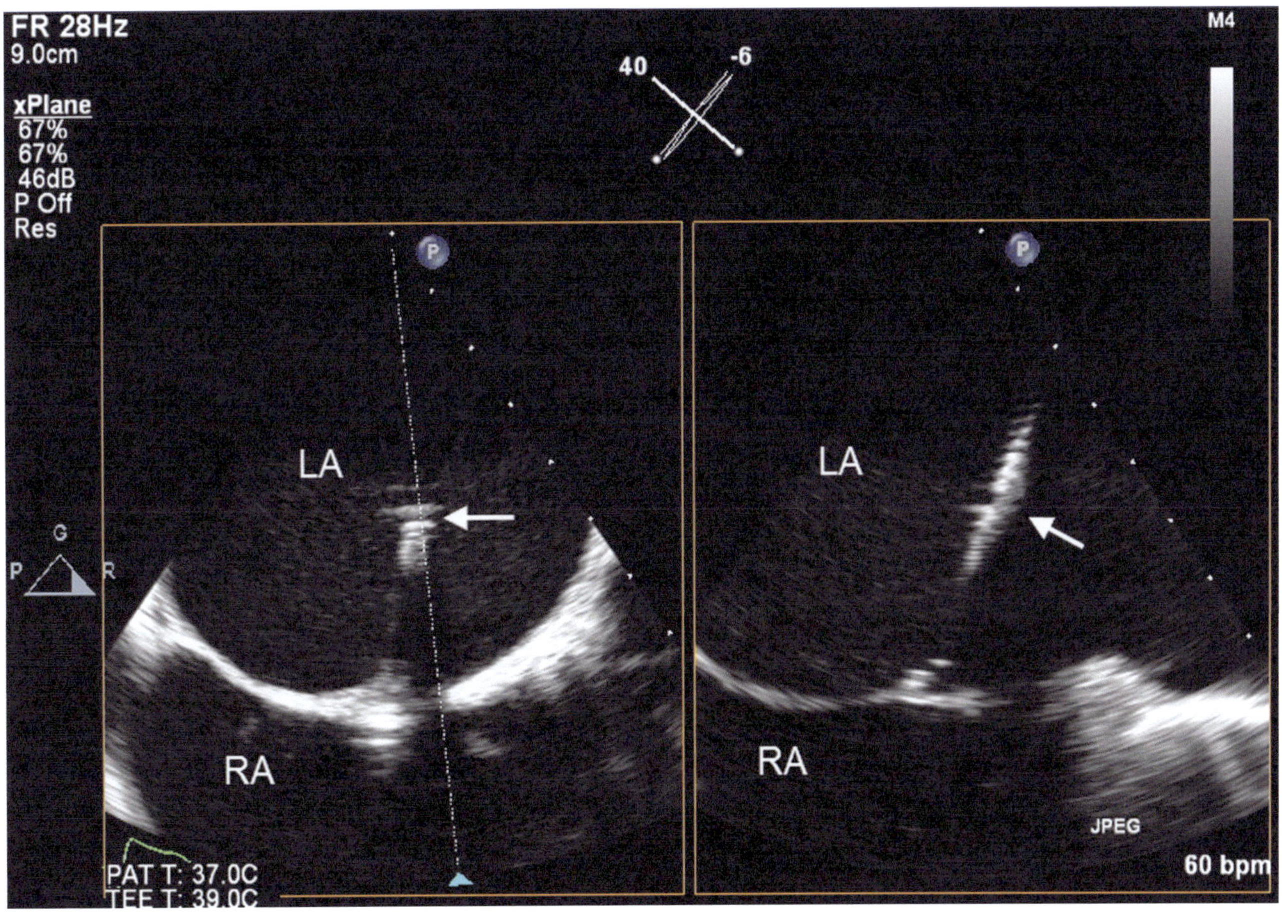

Fig. 6.6 Biplane orientation with placement of transseptal sheath across interatrial septum. *Arrow* delineates the transition between the sheath and dilator with echogenic coils. *LA* left atrium, *RA* right atrium

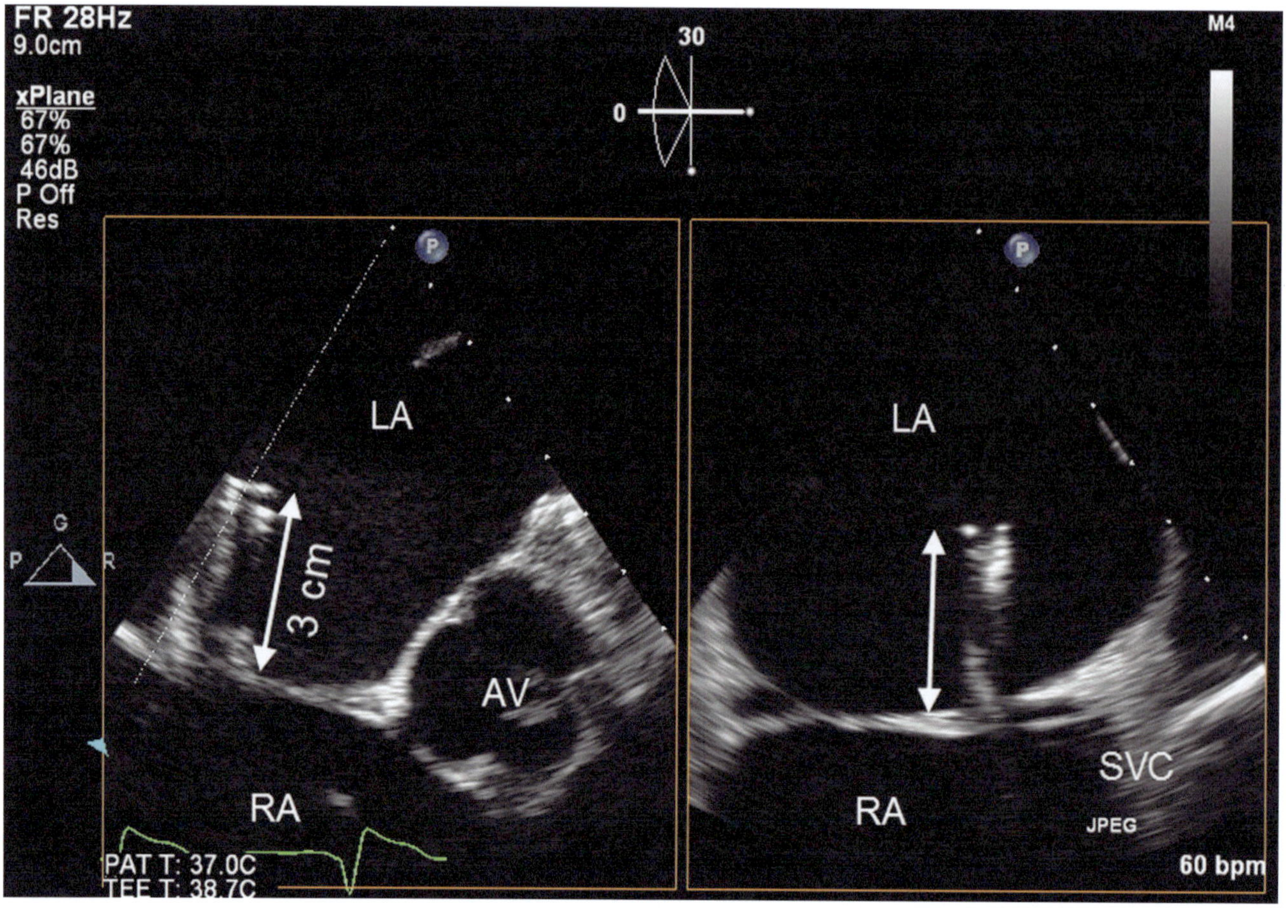

Fig. 6.7 Biplane orientation with sheath placed in working position approximately 3 cm across the interatrial septum. Dilator and wire have been removed compared with Fig. 6.6. *AV* aortic valve, *RA* right atrium, *LA* left atrium, *SVC* superior vena cava, *SVC* superior vena cava, *Two-sided arrow* sheath extending into left atrium

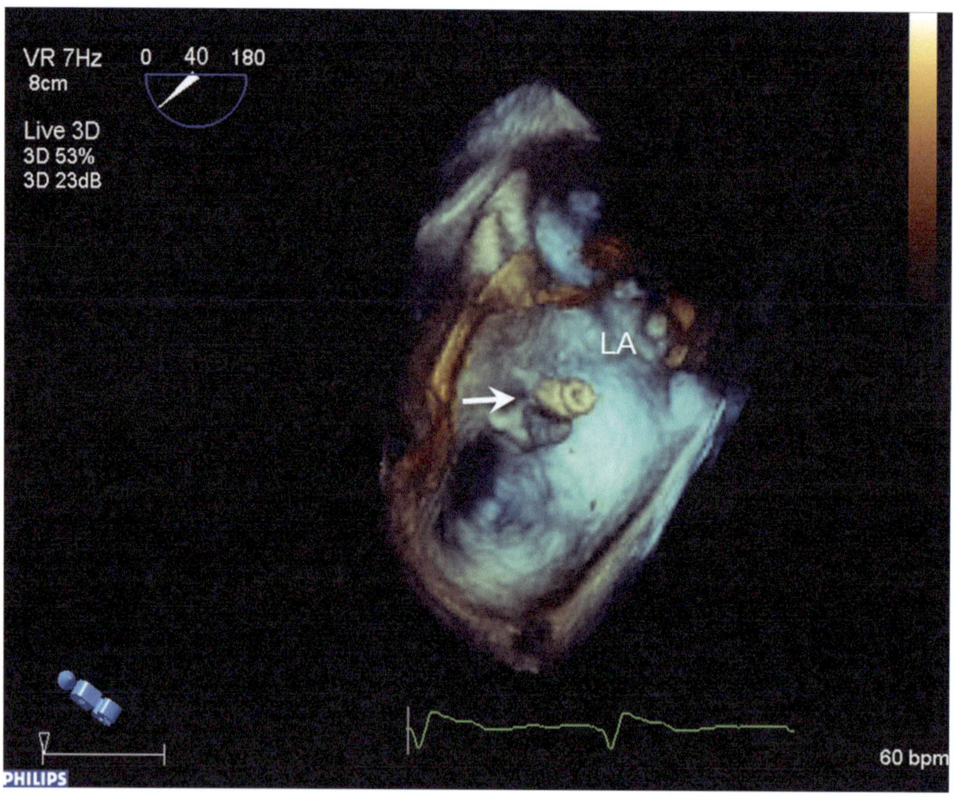

Fig. 6.8 3-D image with sheath extending into the left atrium. Wire has been removed. *Arrow* sheath, *LA* left atrium

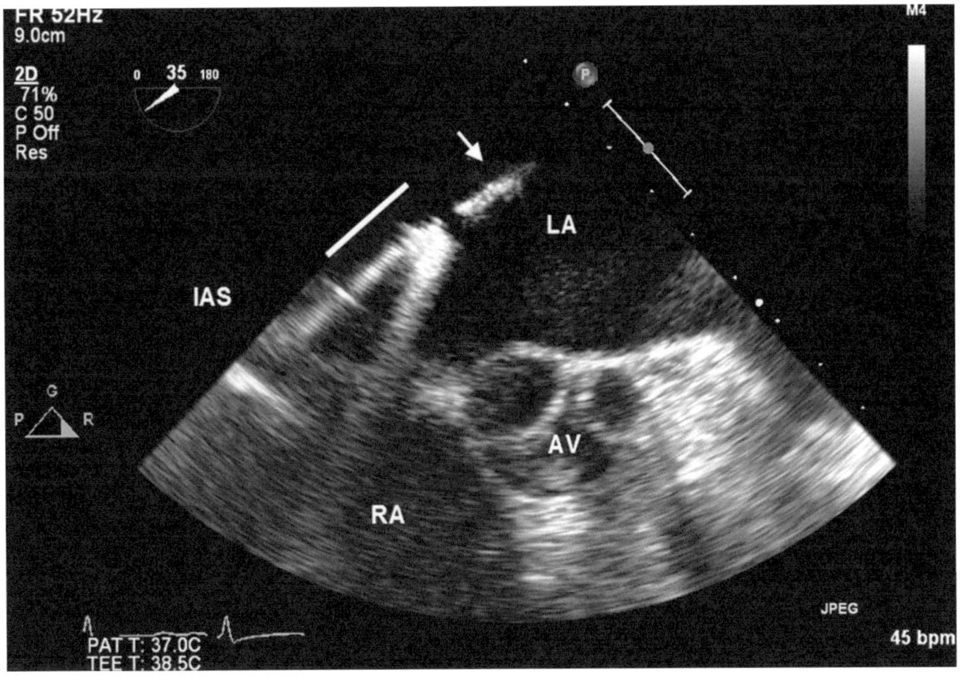

Fig. 6.9 Clip delivery system extending out of sheath and into left atrium. *Solid line*, delivery catheter and steerable sheath. The markers from the distal end of the guide catheter are visible just below the *white line*. *Arrow* clip implant, *LA* left atrium, *RA* right atrium, *IAS* interatrial septum, *AV* aortic valve

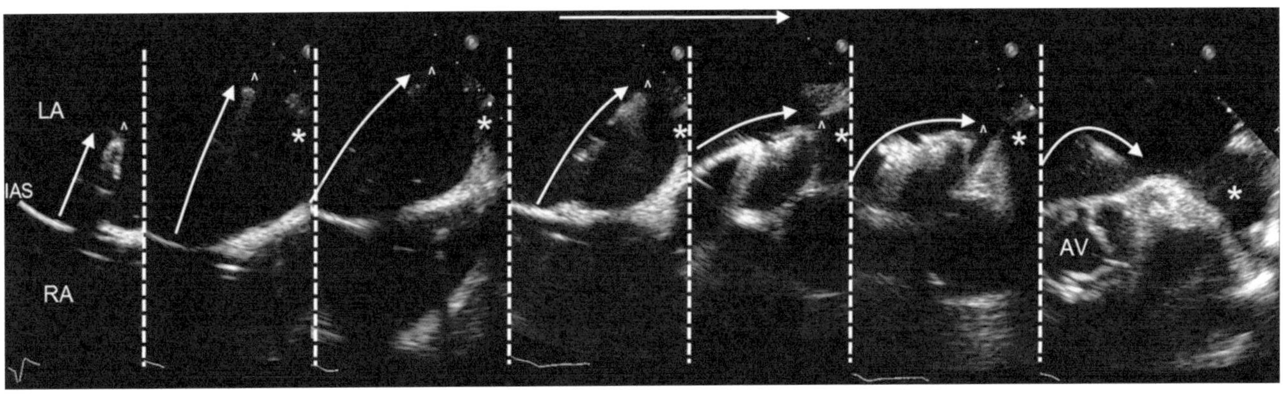

Fig. 6.10 Multiple 2-D images following the clip delivery system as it courses through the left atrium. This maneuver requires careful assessment of the proximity of the tip to the left atrial wall and left atrial appendage (*). *Solid arrow* clip delivery system, *RA* right atrium, *IAS* interatrial septum, *LA* left atrium, *AV* aortic valve, * medial aspect of left atrial appendage

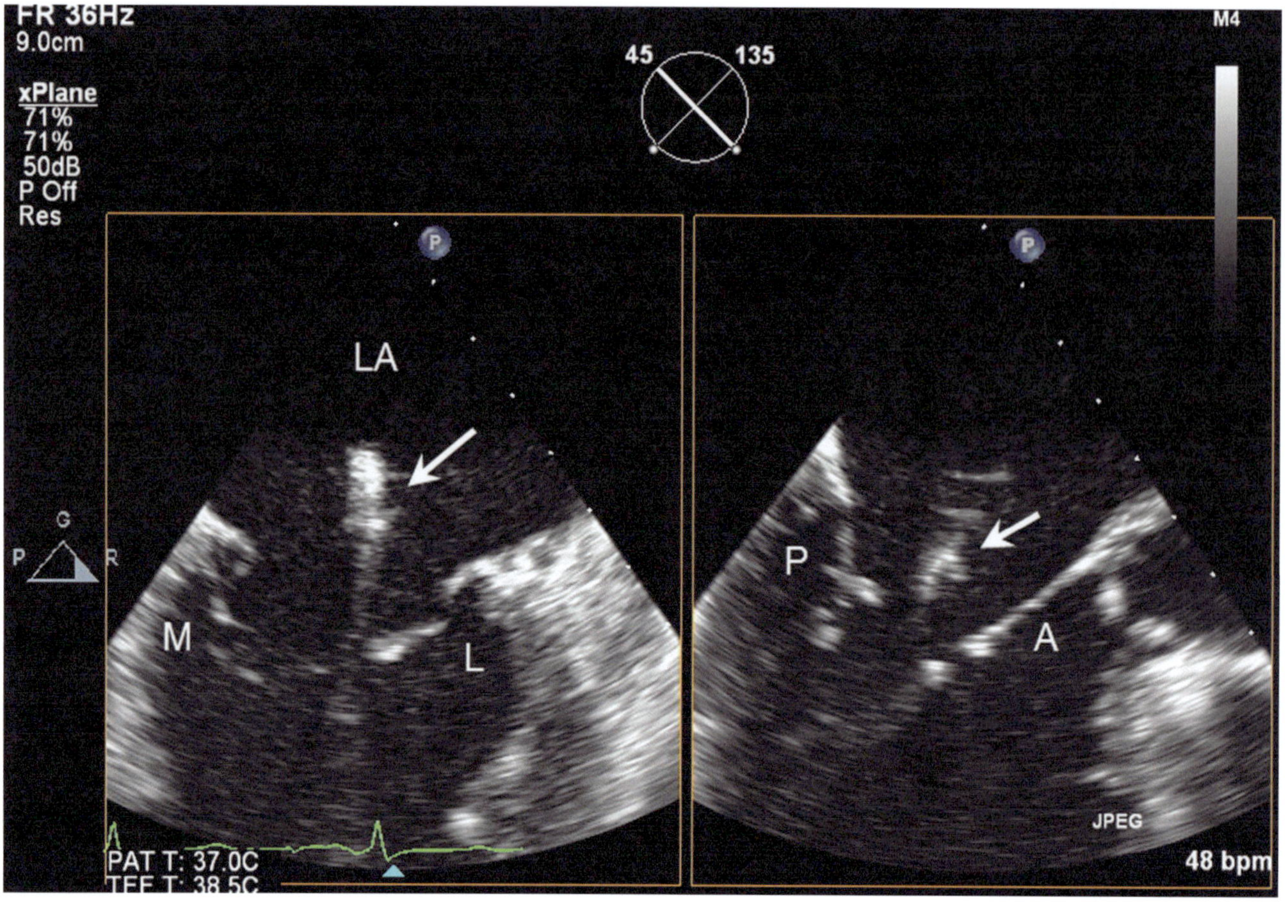

Fig. 6.11 Biplane imaging of clip positioning above the mitral valve. The *left panel* is an intercommissural view (45°), while the *right panel* is a long-axis view (135°). The clip is well positioned in the anterior/posterior plane although is located mildly lateral in the medial/lateral plane. *LA* left atrium, *M* medial *L* lateral, *P* posterior, *A* anterior, *Arrow* clip mechanism

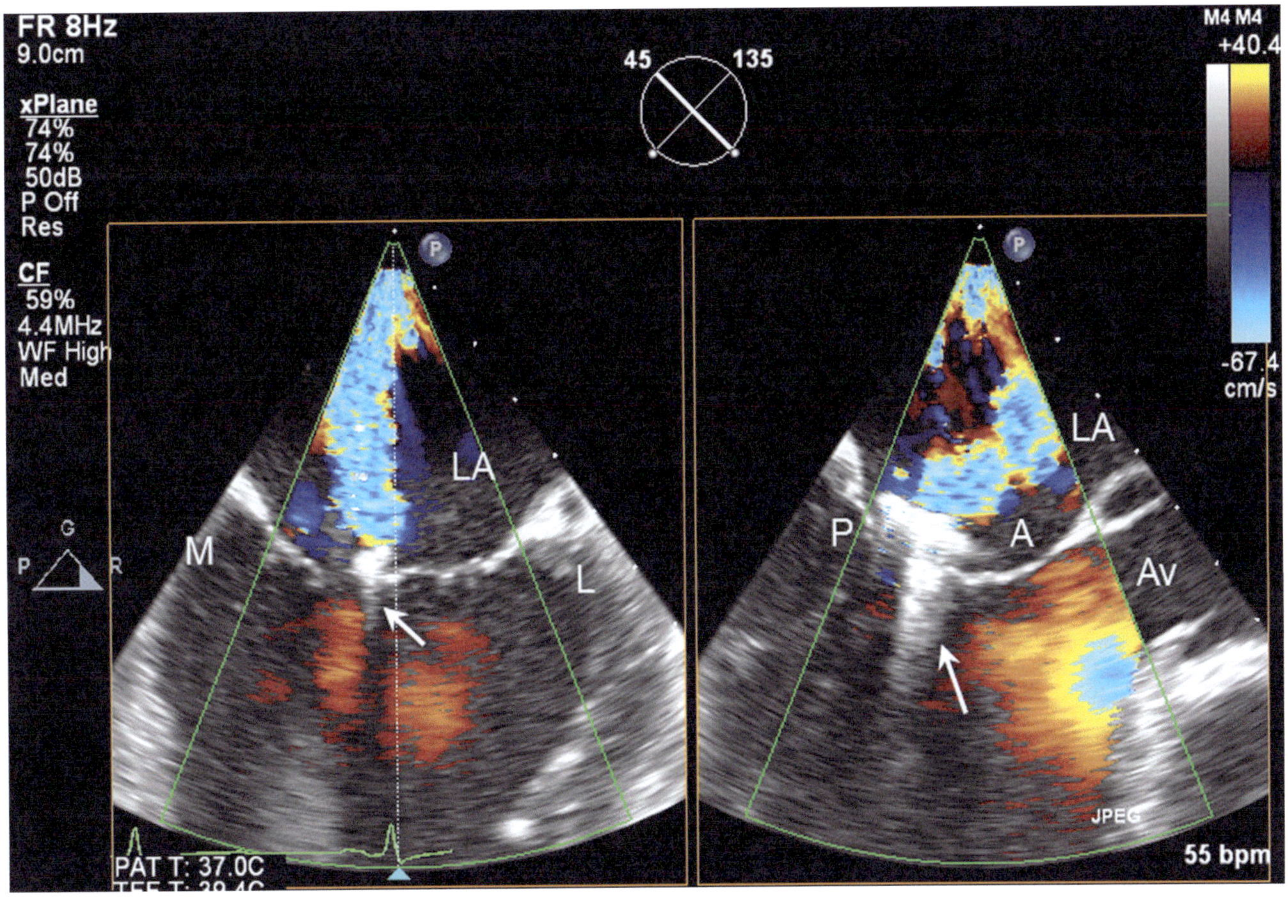

Fig. 6.12 Biplane imaging of clip positioning above the mitral valve with color Doppler demonstrating mitral regurgitation. The *left panel* is an inter-commissural view, while the *right panel* is a long-axis view. The mitral clip arms are open as demonstrated by the "T" shape of the clip in the *right panel*. The clip is splitting the color jet in both orientations. *LA* left atrium, *M* medial, *L* lateral, *P* posterior, *A* anterior, *AV* aortic valve *Arrow* clip mechanism

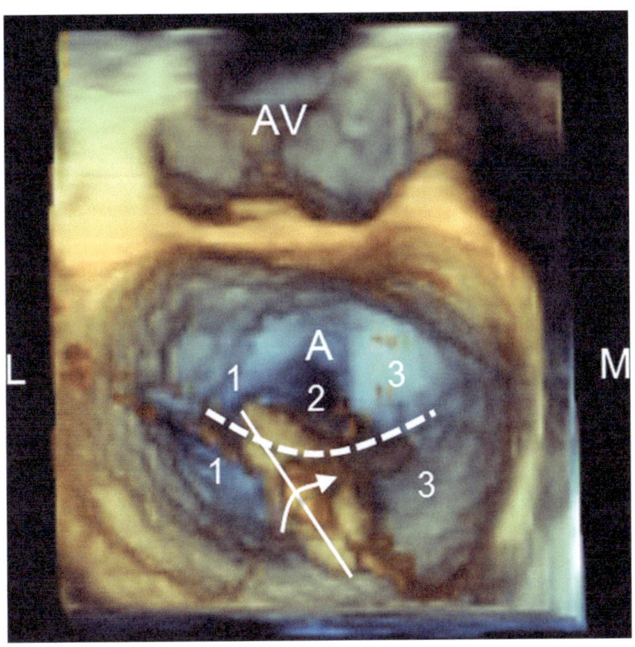

Fig. 6.13 Surgical view of mitral valve with 3-D transesophageal echocardiography demonstrating poor orientation of the clip with the anterior arm rotated laterally. *AV* Aortic valve, *L* lateral, *M* medial, *A* anterior mitral valve leaflet. *1–3* respective scallops of the anterior and posterior mitral valve leaflets, *Broken line* line of coaptation between anterior and posterior mitral valve leaflets, *Solid straight line* angle of clip, *Solid bent arrow* medial rotation that is necessary to align clip properly

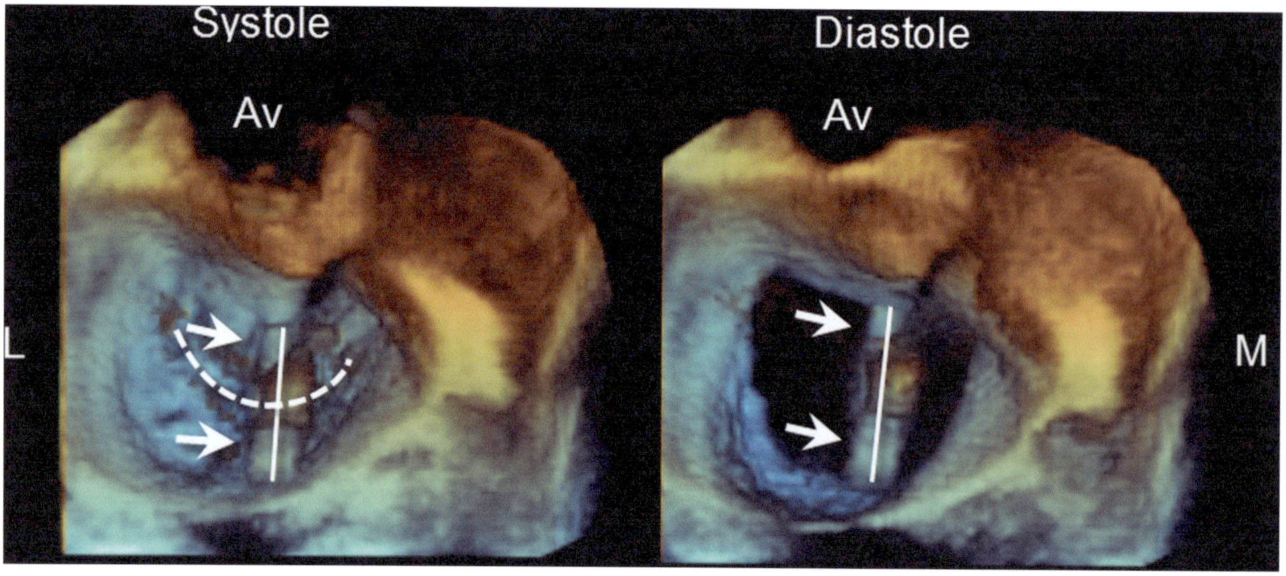

Fig. 6.14 Surgical view of the mitral valve with three-dimensional transesophageal echocardiography demonstrating appropriate angulation of clip arms in systole and diastole. The clip arms are perpendicular to the line of coaptation (*broken, curved line*), *Arrows* clip arms, *Av* aortic valve, *L* lateral, *M* medial

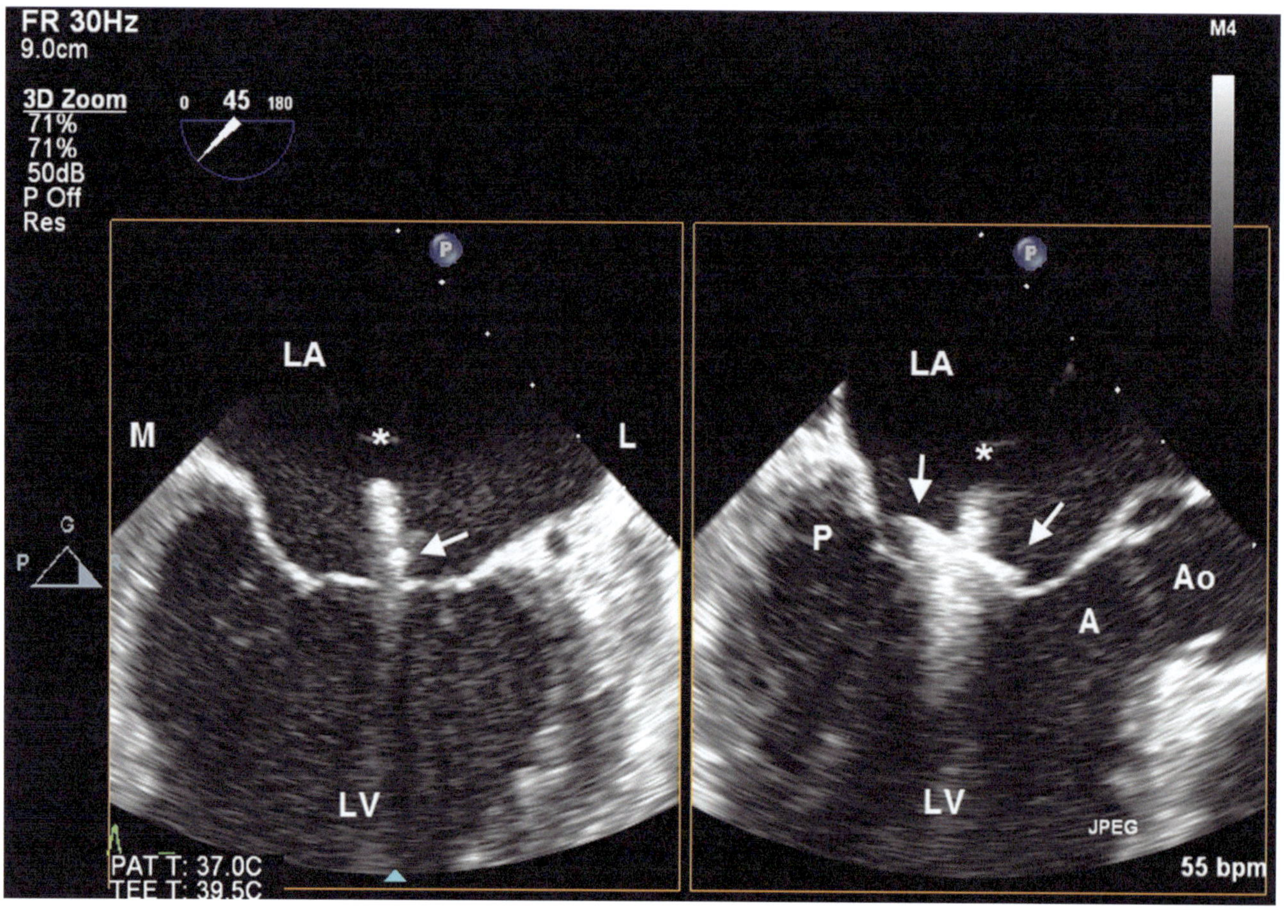

Fig. 6.15 Biplane commissural (*left panel*) and long-axis (*right panel*) view. The clip arms are extended (*arrows*). In the intercommissural view, one arm is oriented slightly laterally (*arrow*). * clip, *Arrow* clip arms, *A* anterior, *P* posterior, *M* medial, *L* lateral, *Ao* aorta, *LA* left atrium, *LV* left ventricle

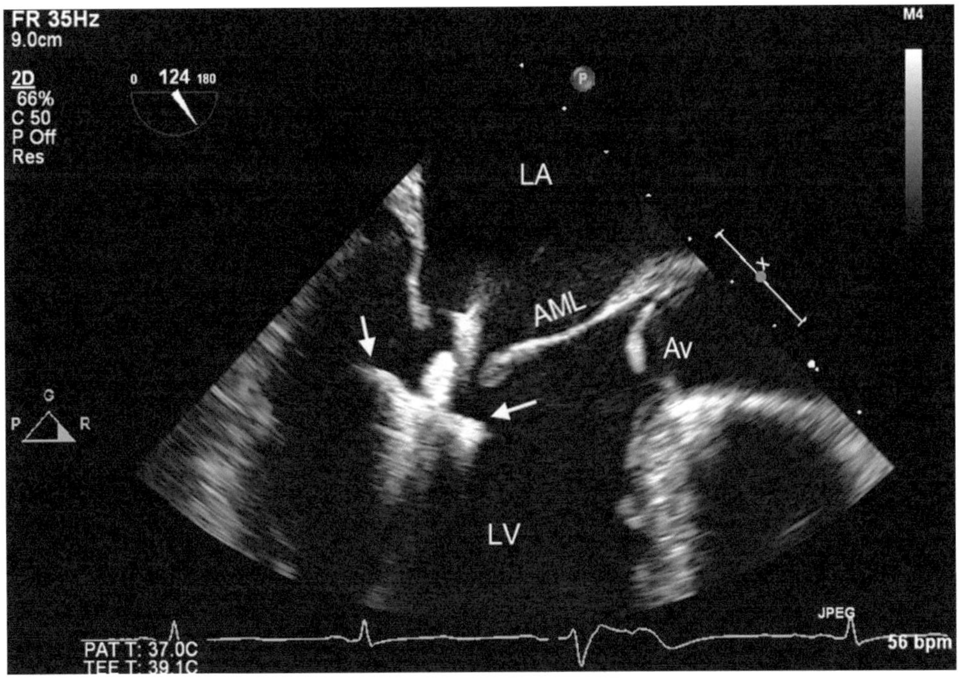

Fig. 6.16 Long-axis view with clip advanced into the left ventricle. Clip arms *Arrows* are oriented appropriately with equal lengths extending in the anterior and posterior directions. *LA* left atrium, *LV* left ventricle, *AML* anterior mitral valve leaflet, *Av* aortic valve

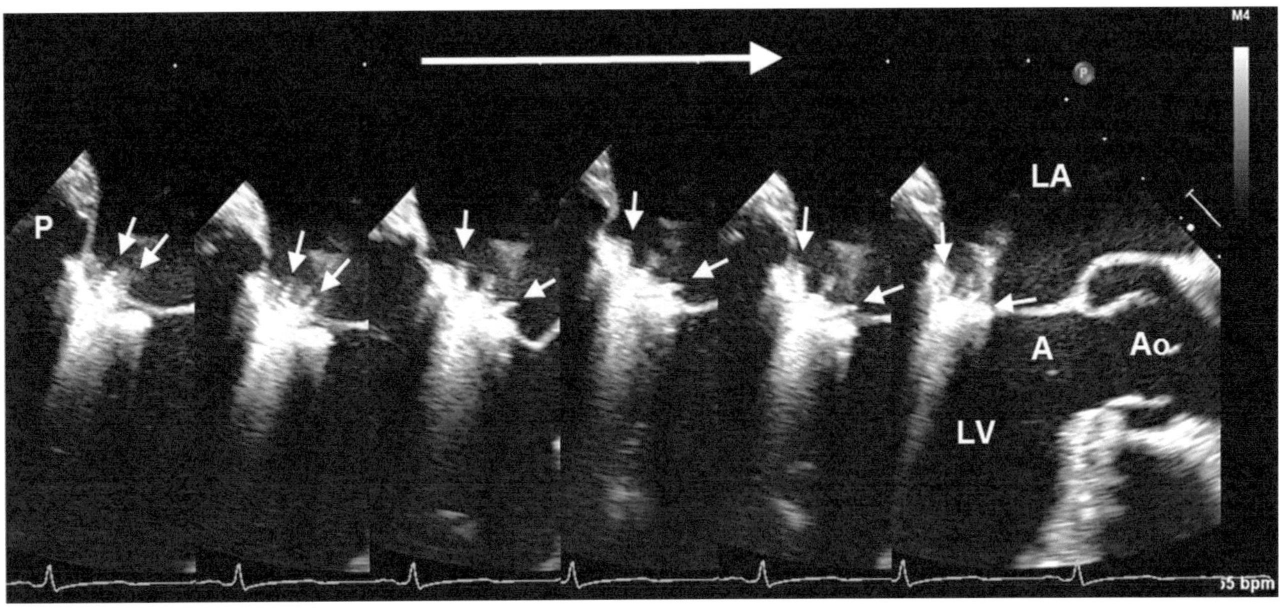

Fig. 6.17 Long axis, zoomed image of grasp. Images are taken from single echocardiographic loop. *Arrows* indicate the grippers coming down over the scallops and grasping the leaflets. *LA* left atrium, *LV* left ventricle, *A* anterior, *Ao* aorta, *P* posterior

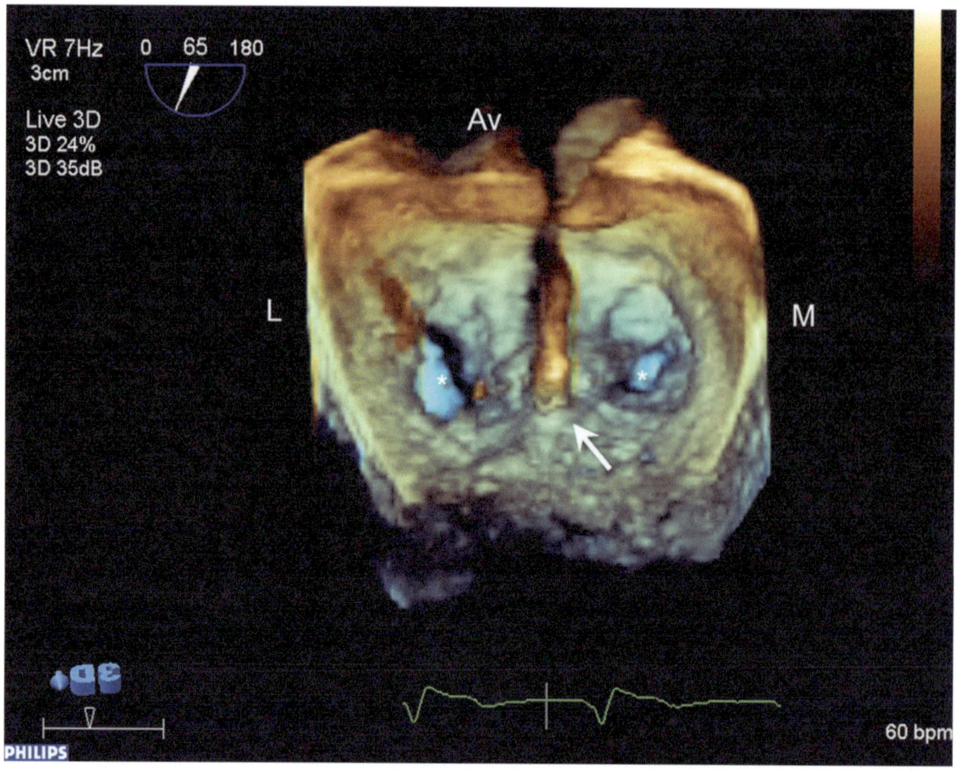

Fig. 6.18 3-D view of mitral valve from surgical view with clip closed on the second anterior and posterior scallops. The resolution of real-time 3-D echocardiography is not typically high enough to delineate the scallops between the clip arms and grippers. Confirmation of adequate capture requires higher-resolution images. * mitral valve orifices, *L* lateral, *M* medial, *Av* aortic valve, *Arrow* clip delivery system with scallops grasped

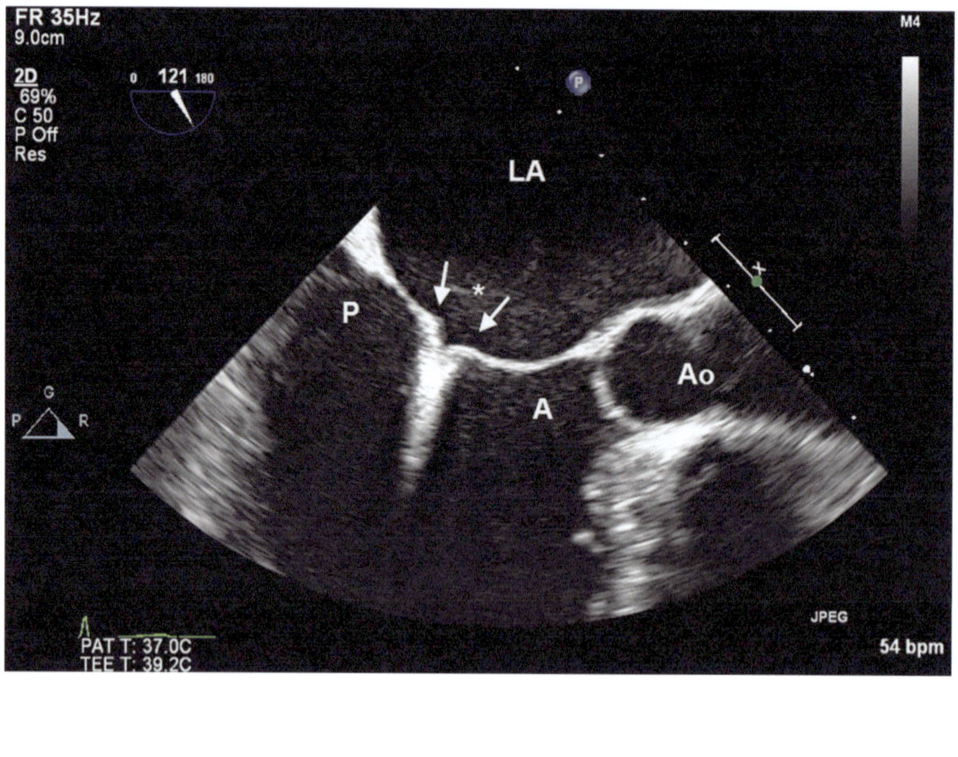

Fig. 6.19 Long-axis view after grasp maneuver. The clip delivery system is still attached to the clip (*). There is excellent draping of the scallops over the closed clip arms (*arrow*). *A* anterior, *P* posterior, *Ao* aorta, *LA* left atrium

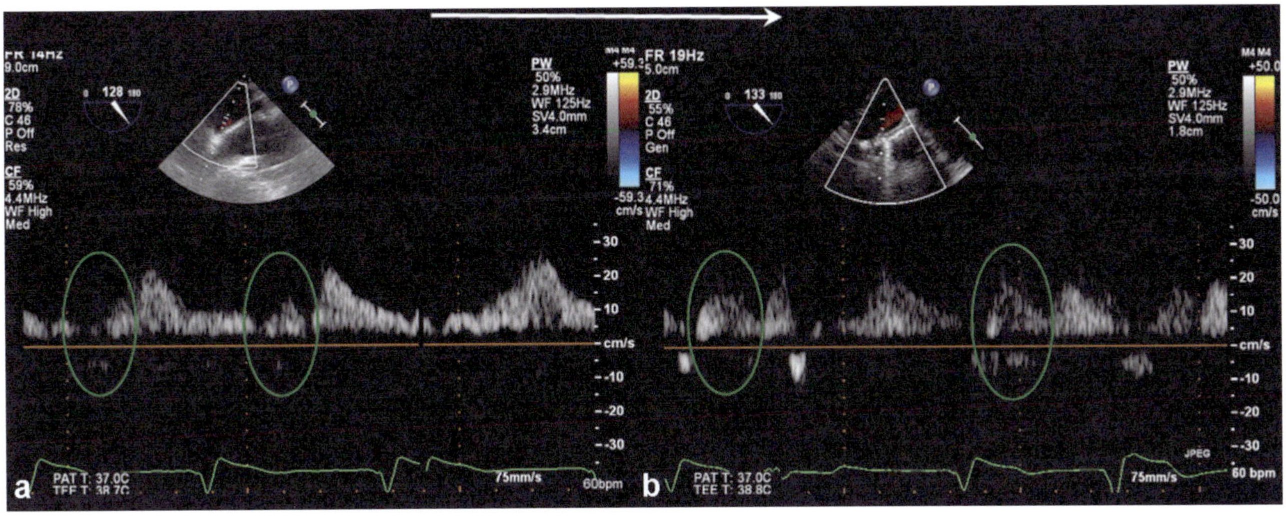

Fig. 6.20 Pulsed-wave Doppler of the left upper pulmonary vein. (**a**) Prior to clip deployment there is significant blunting of systolic flow (green circles) (**b**) After clip deployment the systolic flow has normalized (green circles). prior to and after clip placement. There is improved systolic forward flow in the pulmonary vein consistent with reduced mitral regurgitation

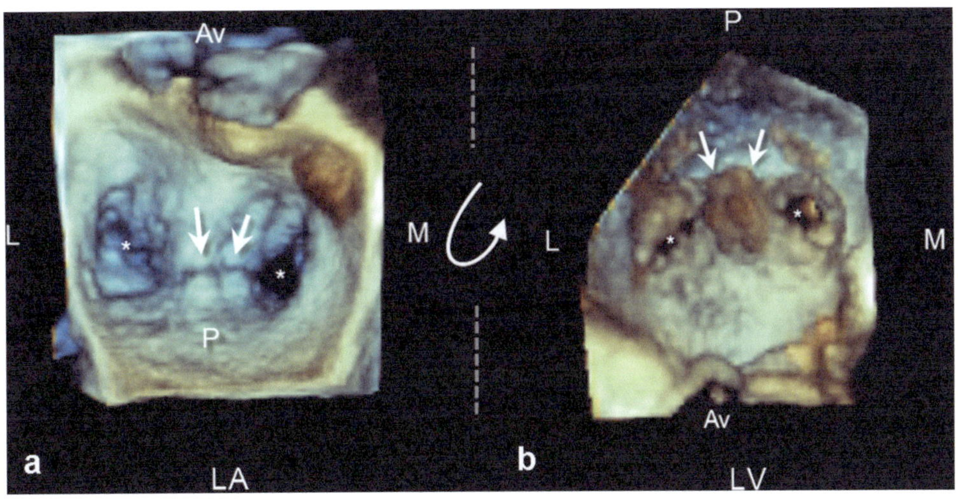

Fig. 6.21 3-D imaging of the mitral valve following two clips placed at the A2/P2 scallop interface (*arrows*). (**a**) Surgical view of the mitral valve. (**b**) Image rotated forward and viewed from the left ventricle looking at the inferior aspect of the mitral valve and clips. *Arrow* clips, * mitral valve orifice, *L* lateral, *M* medial, *Av* aortic valve, *P* posterior, *LA* left atrium, *LV* left ventricle

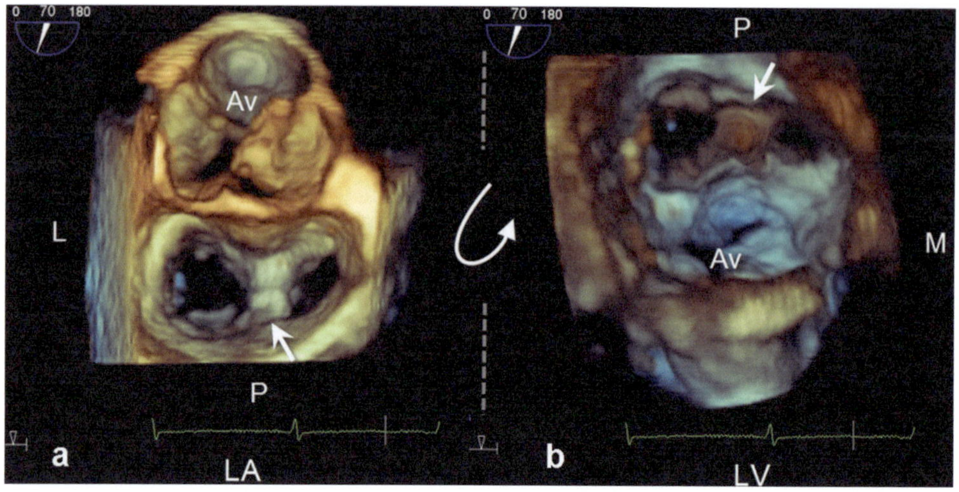

Fig. 6.22 3-D imaging of the mitral valve following single clip placed at the A2/P2 scallop interface (*arrow*). (**a**) Surgical view of the mitral valve. (**b**) Image rotated forward and viewed from the left ventricle looking at the inferior aspect of the mitral valve. *Arrow* clip, * mitral valve orifice, *L* lateral, *M* medial, *Av* aortic valve, *P* posterior, *LA* left atrium, *LV* left ventricle

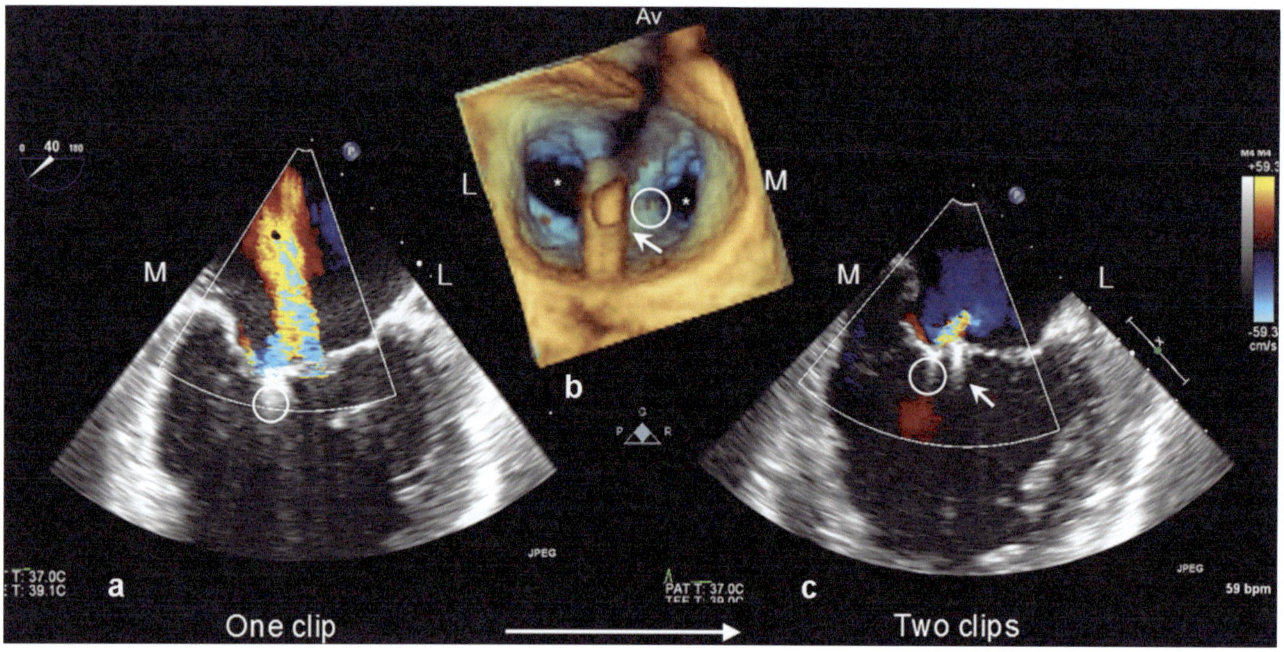

Fig. 6.23 Patient with moderate mitral regurgitation following single clip placement. (**a**) Intercommissural view demonstrating lateral residual mitral regurgitation. *Circle* delineates medial clip. (**b**) 3-D surgical view with clip positioned above mitral valve, lateral to the first clip. Of note, when this clip is advanced into the left ventricle, the arms will be closed to reduce disruption to first clip. (**c**) Commissural two-dimensional view with second clip placed (**l**) lateral, (**M**) medial, (**AV**) aortic valve, (*arrow*) and trace mitral regurgitation

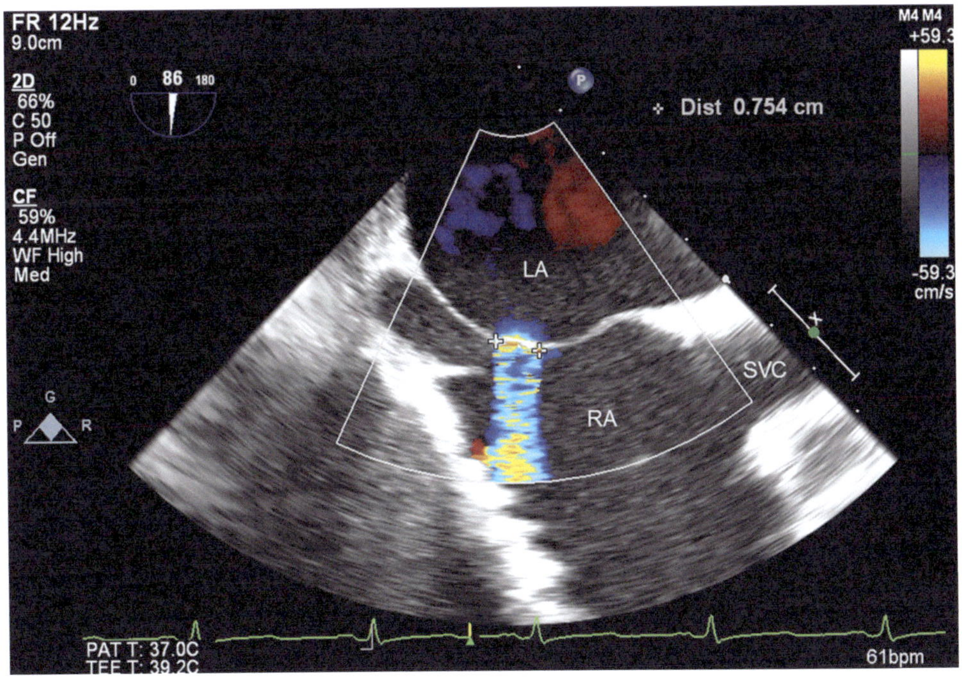

Fig. 6.24 Iatrogenic atrial septal defect measuring 0.75 cm in diameter with left to right shunting. *LA* left atrium, *RA* right atrium, *SVC* superior vena cava

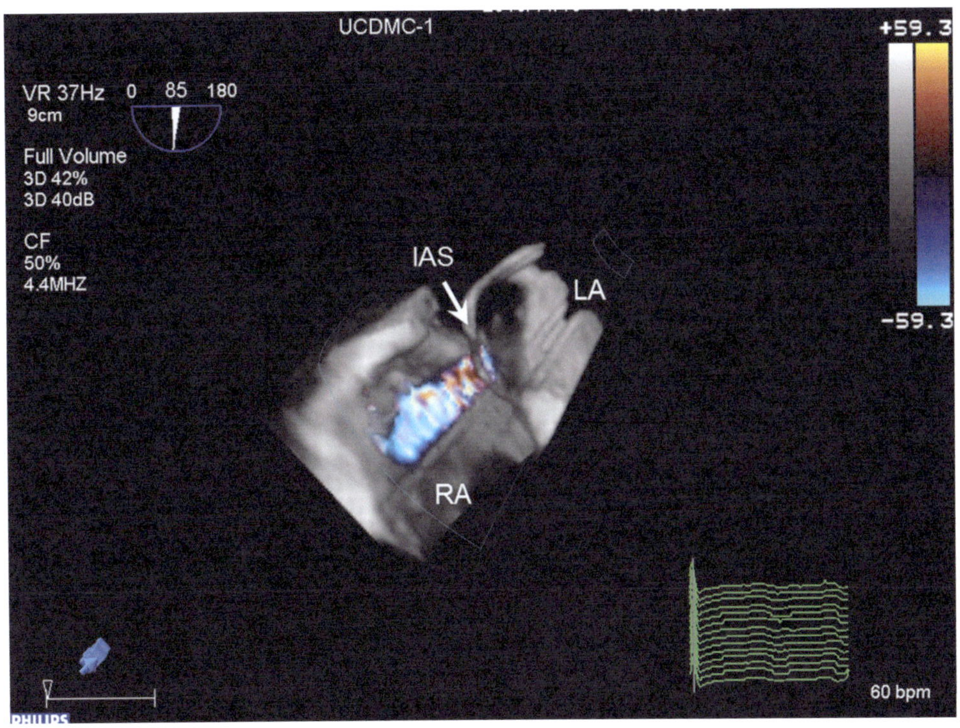

Fig. 6.25 3-D reconstruction of the interatrial septum with color Doppler demonstrating iatrogenic atrial septal defect. *IAS* interatrial septum, *RA* right atrium, *LA* left atrium

Transseptal Puncture

7

Khung Keong Yeo, Jason Rogers, and Reginald Low

Abstract

The transseptal puncture is a critical part of the MitraClip procedure. It is performed under transesophageal echocardiographic guidance because precise localization of the puncture site is crucial for the rest of the procedure. The location of the puncture determines the maneuverability of the MitraClip guide and the clip delivery system (CDS). A properly selected puncture site allows for a smooth and uncomplicated procedure, while a poorly selected location will result in difficulties in positioning the MitaClip and a prolonged procedure. In addition, transseptal puncture is also associated with risks of inadvertent puncture of the aorta, perforation of the atrium, and pericardial tamponade. This chapter reviews the key steps in the transseptal puncture for the MitraClip procedure.

Keywords

MitraClip • Transseptal • Transesophageal echocardiography • Intracardiac echocardiography • Patent foramen ovale • Atrial septal defect • Interatrial septal aneurysm

Importance of Transseptal Puncture

The transseptal puncture has been in use since its description in 1959 by Drs Ross, Braunwald and Morrow [1]. Through the years, its use has waxed and waned. In recent years, with the advent of complex structural heart interventions and complex electrophysiology ablation procedures, the transseptal puncture has seen a resurgence [2–4]. However, more so than any other procedure, it is a crucial part of the MitraClip procedure. It determines the height and position of the guiding catheter relative to the coaptation plane of the mitral leaflets and influences the degrees of freedom available for the clip delivery system (CDS) and guiding catheter to maneuver. Adequate range of movement of the CDS and guide is required to successfully deliver the MitraClip and grasp the leaflets.

A poorly positioned transseptal puncture will result in difficulty maneuvering the device in the left atrium. The guide may be too close to important structures such as the aorta by puncturing too anterior, or the guide may be directed toward the posterior wall of the left atrium by an inappropriately posterior puncture. The puncture may be too high above the valve coaptation plane, leaving insufficient height for the CDS and clip to reach and grasp the leaflets. Finally, the puncture may be too low, making it difficult to retract the CDS and grasp the leaflets.

A suboptimal transseptal puncture site may also limit the range of movement that is built into the MitraClip system. For example, an anterior puncture may result in an "aorta-hugger" scenario in which the CDS runs almost parallel to the aorta. In such a scenario, it is difficult for the CDS to orient perpendicular to the mitral valve.

K.K. Yeo, M.B.B.S., FACC, FSCAI (✉)
Department of Cardiovascular Medicine,
University of California, Davis Medical Center,
4860 Y Street, Suite 2820, Sacramento, CA 95817, USA

Department of Cardiology, National Heart Centre Singapore,
Mistri Wing, 17 Third Hospital Avenue, Singapore 168752, Singapore
e-mail: yeo_kk@yahoo.com, yeo.khung.keong@nhcs.com.sg

J. Rogers, M.D., FACC, FSCAI • R. Low, M.D., FACC
Department of Cardiovascular Medicine,
University of California, Davis Medical Center,
4860 Y Street, Suite 2820, Sacramento, CA 95817, USA
e-mail: jason.rogers@ucdmc.ucdavis.edu; ptcra@aol.com

T. Feldman et al. (eds.), *Atlas of Percutaneous Edge-to-Edge Mitral Valve Repair*,
DOI 10.1007/978-1-4471-4294-2_7, © Springer-Verlag London 2013

Equipment

The transseptal puncture can be performed safely using standard equipment and should be performed under transesophageal echocardiographic (TEE) guidance. This may include a Mullins sheath and dilator (Fig. 7.1) and a Brockenbrough needle. However, there are more options available currently, and operators may choose to use other commercially available needles and sheaths/dilators. These include the BRK series of transseptal needles and the SL series of transseptal sheaths (Figs. 7.2 and 7.3).

In general, we recommend using the SL-0 sheath and dilator with a BRK needle. The angle of the SL-0 sheath favors directing the subsequent Amplatz super-stiff wire toward the left upper pulmonary vein. However, the Mullins sheath is also commonly used and may be useful if extra curve is required. This may occur in situations where there is a patent foramen ovale (PFO) or when the left atrium (LA) is large. The Agilis NxT steerable introducers (St Jude Medical, St Paul, MN) are specialized catheters with adjustable curves that may be particularly suitable for complex anatomy. Depending on personal experience, preferences, and anatomy, operators may choose to utilize specific equipment. Regardless of the equipment chosen, the key to the transseptal procedure lies in clear visualization by TEE and careful selection of the puncture site.

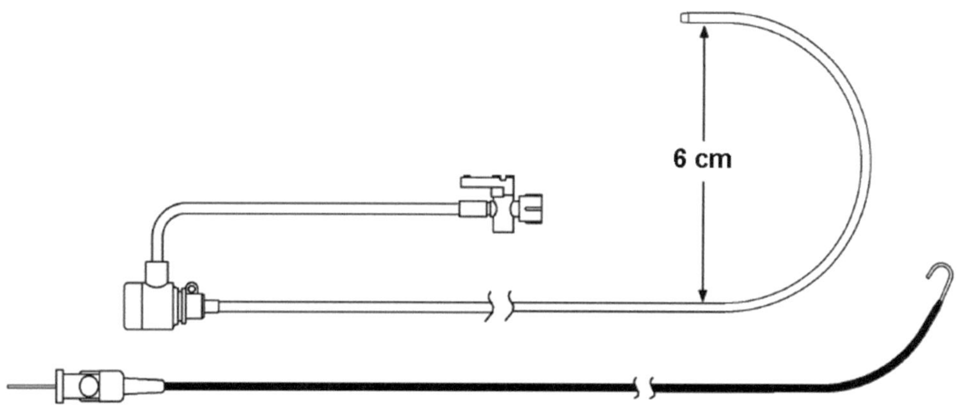

Fig. 7.1 Schematic of a Mullin's sheath (Image used courtesy of St. Jude Medical, Inc.)

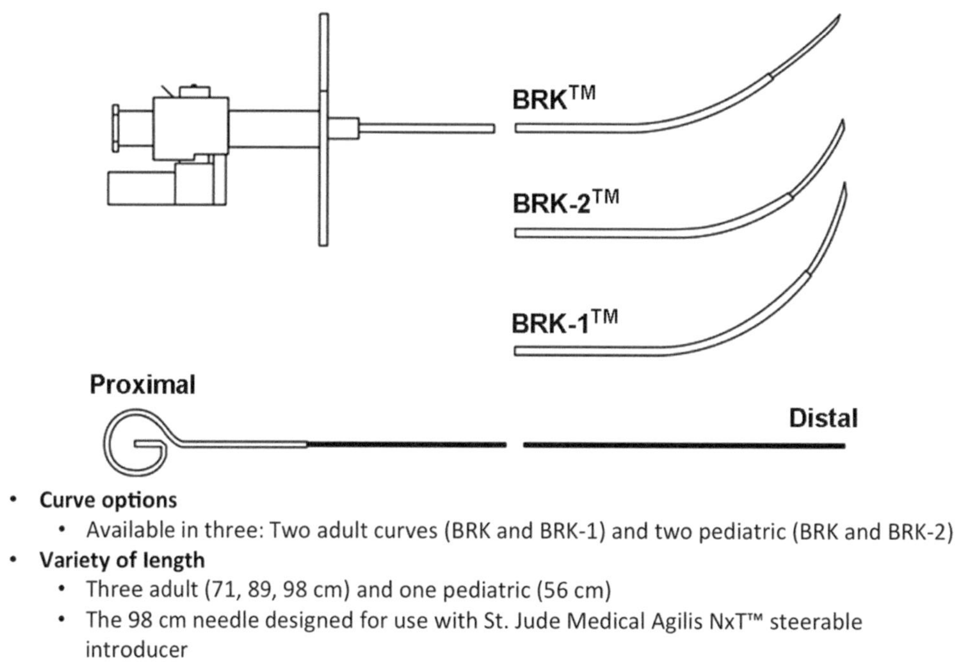

Fig. 7.2 Different curves and lengths for the transseptal needle

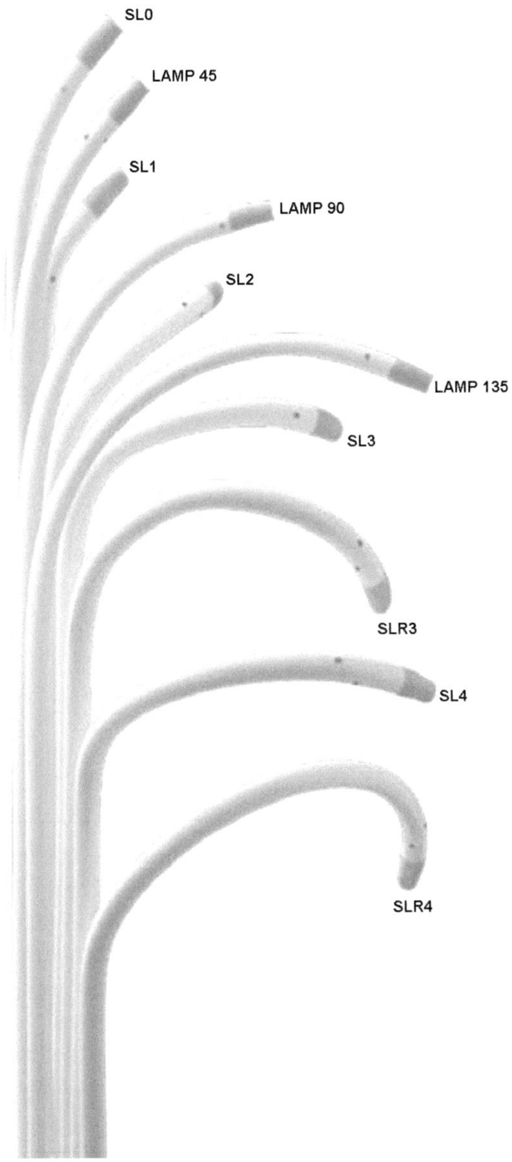

Fig. 7.3 Different transseptal catheters are available with different *curves* and *tip shapes*. These are generally available in both 8 and 8.5 F sizes (Image used courtesy of St. Jude Medical, Inc.)

Step-by-Step: Basic Transseptal Puncture

We review here step-by-step the basic transseptal puncture procedure. As discussed earlier, the transseptal puncture is critical, and it is worthwhile to invest time and attention to obtain an ideal puncture. After right femoral venous access is obtained, a 0.032 wire is advanced to the superior vena cava (SVC) under fluoroscopic guidance. The venous sheath is then exchanged out for a transseptal sheath and dilator such as the Mullins or SL-0 sheaths which are advanced into the SVC. The wire is then removed, and the transseptal needle is advanced to near the distal tip of the sheath and under fluoroscopic guidance (usually to ~1 cm from the tip of the dilator). The orientation of the needle and sheath must be maintained by matching the metal arrow on the needle's hub to the direction of sheath's sidearm. We find it is helpful to then move the needle and sheath together with one hand grasping both as a single unit. This technique also maintains a constant and safe needle distance from the tip of the dilator. Under fluoroscopic and TEE guidance, the sheath and needle are slowly and carefully pulled back to the junction of the SVC and right atrium (RA) (Fig. 7.4).

At this time, attention is focused almost completely on the TEE. The first view is the bicaval view in which the superior-inferior orientation of the puncture needed is determined (Fig. 7.4). The ideal position in a routine EVEREST II type patient would be just slightly superior from the midpoint in this view (Figs. 7.4, 7.5, and 7.6). The sheath dilator should be used to "tent" the septum (Fig. 7.7). Once this position is achieved, the TEE is used to display the short-axis view at the level of the aorta. This view provides an anterior-posterior perspective on the transseptal location. To manipulate the transseptal needle and sheath posteriorly, the entire system is torqued clockwise and counterclockwise for anterior orientation. The ideal position is slightly posterior of the midline (Fig. 7.8). It is important to recognize that if the dilator is tenting the septum too aggressively, clockwise or counterclockwise torque of the sheath may simply cause the tip of the sheath to "pivot" at the site of tenting. It may therefore be necessary to slightly disengage (pull back) the catheter from the septum to allow repositioning. The same principle applies when adjusting the sheath in an anterior-posterior direction by either advancing or withdrawing the catheter. Finally, since the fossa ovalis is an elliptical shape, movement of the sheath posterior may actually result in a more inferior position, so the operator should check orthogonal TEE views to ensure proper orientation in both planes before puncturing.

The next view is the four- or five-chamber view in which the perpendicular (vertical) height of the transseptal "tenting" from the mitral valve is measured. This distance should be between 3.5 and 4.5 cm (Fig. 7.9). The mitral valve reference point is either the mitral valve annular plane or the point of coaptation of the mitral valve leaflets. Usually, in patients who have mitral valve prolapse, the mitral annulus is a reasonable guide for height measurements. However, in functional mitral regurgitation (MR) patients, the point of coaptation is usually lower due to restricted leaflet mobility. Hence, we would recommend using the point of leaflet coaptation in patients with functional MR as a point of reference. Once the suitability of the proposed transseptal puncture site has been confirmed by the views described, puncture across the septum is performed. This is performed by advancing the needle just beyond the tip of the dilator and exerting a gentle forward pressure. The needle should be connected to a pressure transducer to confirm entry into the left atrium by appearance of a venous waveform. Generally, a small "pop" is felt as the needle traverses the interatrial septum. Once the tip of the needle enters the left atrium, the needle and sheath should be rotated slightly counterclockwise to avoid inadvertent puncture of the posterior wall of the left atrium. The dilator and sheath are then advanced over the needle into the left atrium, and the sheath is then advanced over the needle and dilator. The needle and dilator are then carefully removed, and the transseptal sheath is carefully aspirated and flushed to avoid any air entry or thrombus formation.

Once the transseptal puncture is done and the sheath or guide is across the interatrial septum, IV heparin to achieve an ACT > 250 s is given. A 0.035 Amplatz super-stiff guidewire is then advanced under fluoroscopic guidance to the left upper pulmonary vein (LUPV, Figs. 7.10 and 7.11). Sometimes, it is necessary to use a nested catheter such as a multipurpose catheter through the transseptal sheath to guide the wire into the LUPV. Usually, the echocardiographer will maintain real-time echo imaging of the left atrial appendage to warn the operator against advancing the wire into the appendage. This is a useful and important step to prevent complications.

The transseptal sheath is then removed carefully, maintaining wire access in the LUPV. A 16–18 F dilator is then used to dilate the femoral venous track. The MitraClip guide with its spiral dilator is then advanced slowly into the RA and against the interatrial septum. Gentle pressure is applied on the spiral dilator to cross the septum. It is important to do so cautiously though firmly. Overly aggressive pushing may tear the septum, resulting in significant interatrial shunting at the conclusion of the procedure.

Once the dilator and guide are across the septum, the dilator is withdrawn first into the guide and then the wire. The dilator and the wire are then both removed together from the guide while aspirating gently with the wire well within the dilator. This is important as the wire may compromise the hemostatic valve of the guide if it is pulled through the guide outside of the dilator.

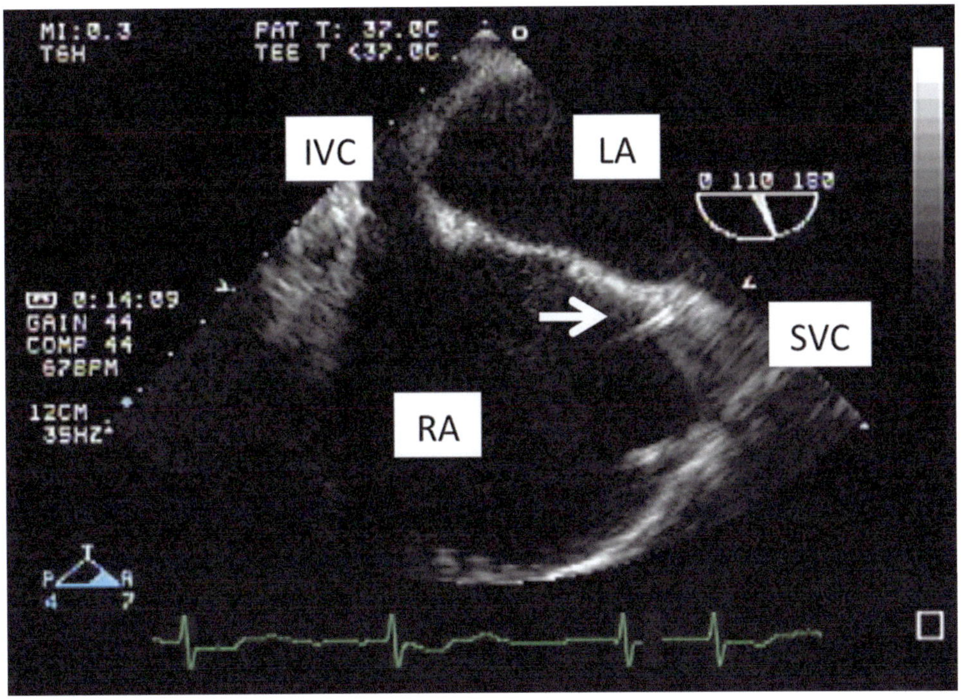

Fig. 7.4 TEE bicaval view showing the transseptal dilator (*arrow*) at the junction of the SVC and RA as it is slowly pulled down from the SVC. *LA* left atrium, *IVC* inferior vena cava, *SVC* superior vena cava, *RA* right atrium

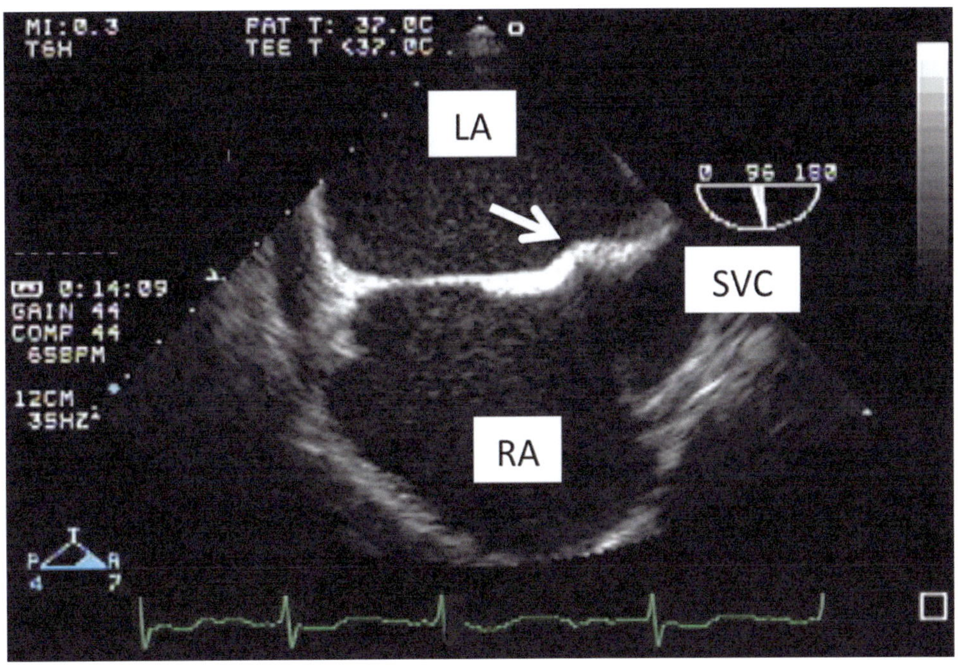

Fig. 7.5 Bicaval view showing the transseptal dilator (*arrow* at site of tenting) now at the septum secundum. *LA* left atrium, *SVC* superior vena cava, *RA* right atrium

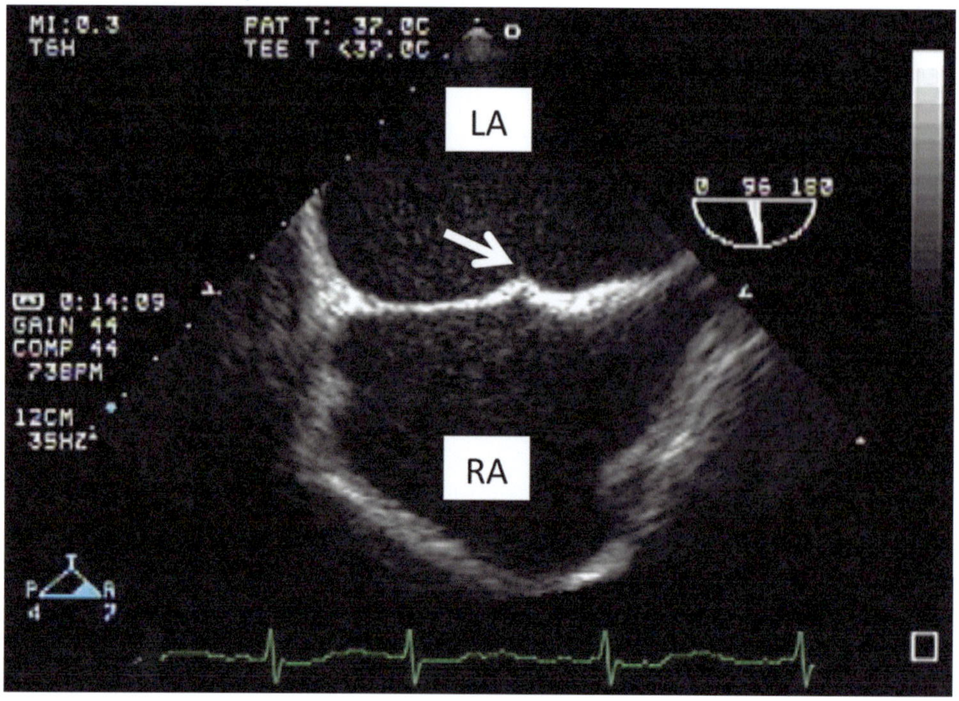

Fig. 7.6 Bicaval view showing the transseptal dilator (*arrow*) at the limbus of the fossa ovalis. *LA* left atrium, *RA* right atrium

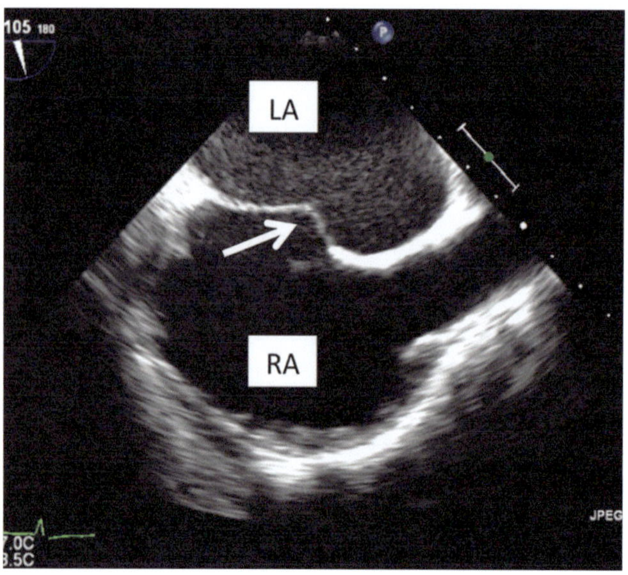

Fig. 7.7 Bicaval view showing the transseptal dilator (*arrow*) "tenting" the fossa ovalis (septum primum) at a location near the midpoint. *LA* left atrium, *RA* right atrium

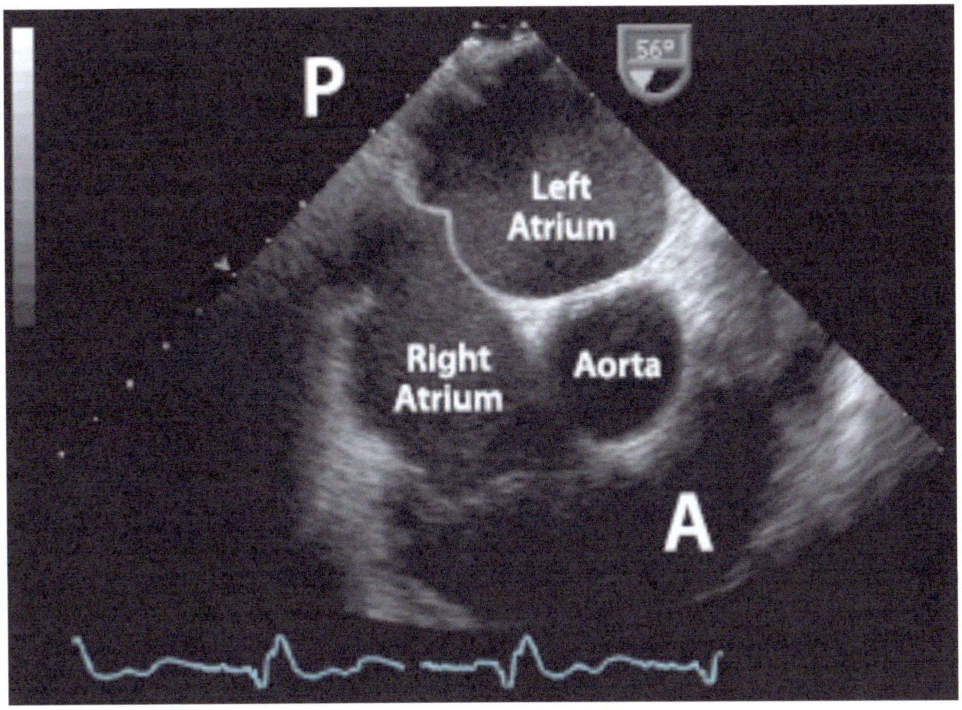

Fig. 7.8 Short-axis view at the level of the aorta. The transseptal dilator should avoid the aorta. In an ideal position, the needle should tent the interatrial septum slightly posterior to the midpoint of the septum as seen in this view. Tenting too anteriorly may risk puncture of the aorta. Also, an anterior puncture may result in an "aorta-hugger" situation during steering of the device. In such a situation, it becomes difficult for the MitraClip to approach the mitral valve plane perpendicularly. *A* Anterior *P* Posterior

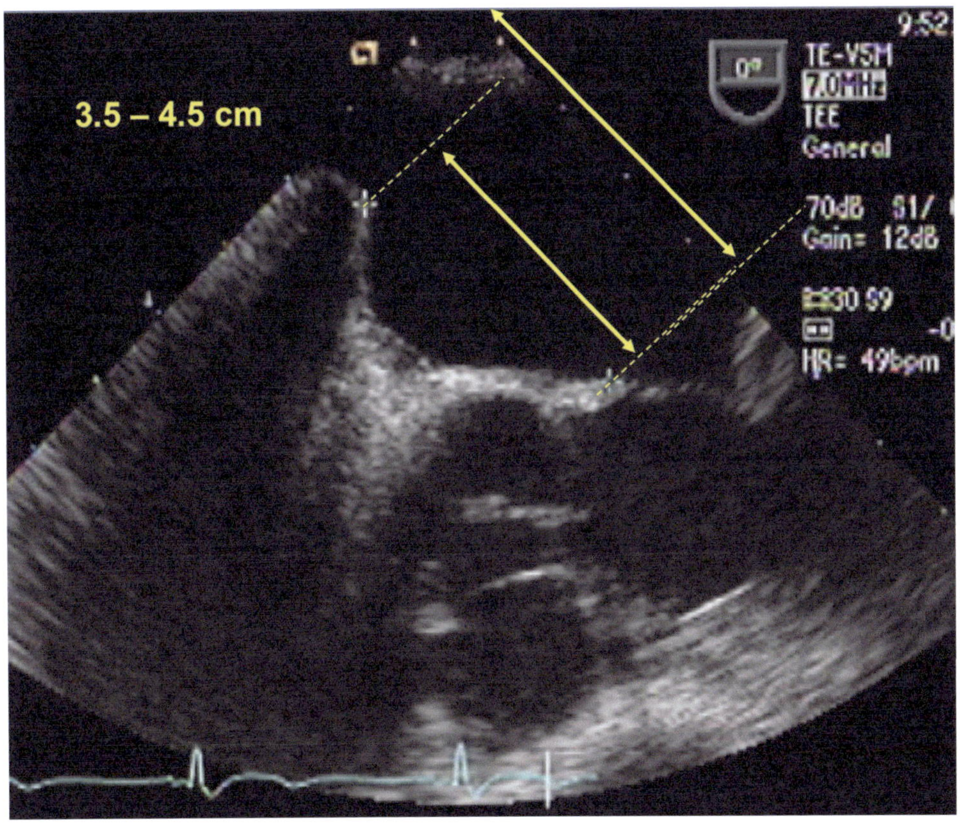

Fig. 7.9 Four-chamber or five-chamber view. This view is meant for assessment of "height" above the mitral valve. This is the perpendicular distance from the "tenting" point (*arrow*) to the mitral valve annulus. Some operators may choose to use the reference point as the point of mitral leaflet coaptation. Regardless, the generally accepted distance is 3.5–4.5 cm depending on the nature of the MR

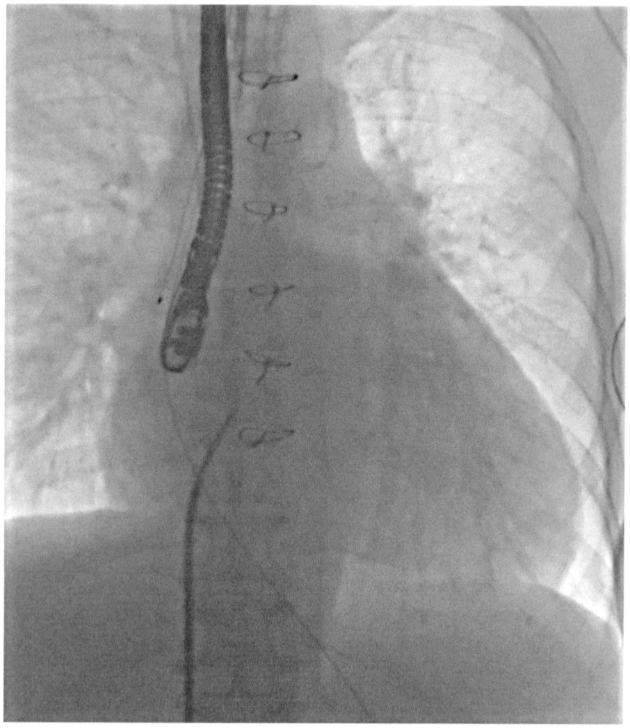

Fig. 7.10 This shows the transseptal needle and catheter at the interatrial septum before puncture

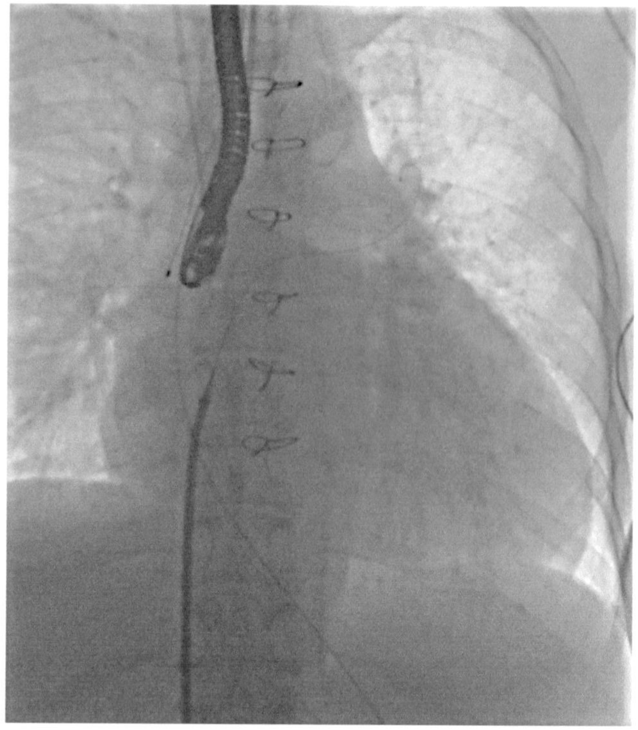

Fig. 7.11 This shows the transseptal needle and catheter with successful puncture across the interatrial septum and a wire advanced to the left upper pulmonary vein

Complications of Transseptal Puncture and Management

With proper technique and use of TEE imaging, complications related to transseptal puncture should be rare. However, familiarity with possible adverse events should increase procedural safety, awareness, and preparedness for managing complications.

The main category of transseptal complications is related to inadvertent puncture of cardiac structures besides the interatrial septum [5–11]. These structures might include the aorta, superior or inferior vena cava, right or left atria, pulmonary veins, and the left or right atrial appendages. Generally, if only the needle punctures a structure, retraction of the needle, reversal of anticoagulation, and observation will generally allow spontaneous sealing of the perforation. For larger perforations, emergent pericardiocentesis, volume resuscitation, and transfusion of blood products may be required. If the patient remains unstable, emergent cardiac surgical repair may be necessary.

Air embolism is always a risk when performing transseptal puncture, and meticulous attention must be paid to de-airing and properly flushing left atrial catheters. Cerebral and coronary air embolism (right coronary > left coronary) are the most frequent sites of involvement. Thrombus formation on the transseptal sheath and wire are also possible, which makes administration of heparin immediately after safe transseptal puncture mandatory. In general, wires tend to be more thrombogenic than catheters; therefore, wires should not be left in the left atrium for any extended period of time. An iatrogenic atrial septal defect is created universally after any transseptal procedure. These will usually close over time [12]. In rare cases due to clinically significant persistent interatrial shunting, transcatheter closure may be necessary.

Special Transseptal Situations

Transseptal Crossing in the Presence of a Patent Foramen Ovale (PFO)

A PFO may potentially make it more difficult to perform a transseptal puncture. In general, we do not recommend crossing the PFO to enter the LA. The PFO may bias the needle superiorly. If the needle or guide crosses at the PFO, it is often too "high" above the mitral valve plane and may limit steering of the device (Figs. 7.12, 7.13, and 7.14). Also, with a PFO or floppy interatrial septum, it may be difficult for a transseptal dilator or needle to find purchase on the interatrial septum. Even if the ideal position is identified, when the operator advances the needle, it may "slide" out of position due to difficulty in creating a "tent" (Fig. 7.14). In this case, the tiny wire dilator that is packaged within the transseptal needle may be helpful if advanced through the needle into the interatrial septum and may provide additional fixation to allow controlled puncture.

It is often necessary to puncture the interatrial septum separately from the PFO. To do so, a transseptal sheath with greater curvature may need to be used. For example, a Mullin's sheath instead of an SL-0 catheter may provide greater angulation to "catch" on the interatrial septum (Figs. 7.15 and 7.16). Similarly, a more curved transseptal needle may be required. For example, instead of the BRK needle, a BRK-1 needle may need to be used. The transseptal needles can also be reshaped by hand slightly before use. A gentle curve added near the IVC-RA junction may allow the top of the dilator to exert more of a horizontal vector against the septum. Figures 7.17 and 7.18 show the outcome in a case with a PFO.

In summary, it is important to identify the presence of a PFO prior to the MitraClip procedure. PFO location, tunnel length, diameter, and presence of a concomitant atrial septal aneurysm should be noted. If present, the MitraClip operator should anticipate using the techniques described to cross the septum at the chosen ideal location.

Transseptal Crossing in the Presence of an Atrial Septal Defect (ASD)

An atrial septal defect (ASD) severely limits the ability of the operator to determine the position of a transseptal puncture and, by extension, the ability to maneuver the device. The constraints of an ASD depend on its size, location, and whether it is single or fenestrated ASD. A very small ASD may not pose a significant problem. However, if a moderate-sized ASD is present and in a suboptimal location, a transseptal puncture in the preferred location may result in a tear of the interatrial septum causing massive left to right shunting.

If the ASD is in the ideal position, the MitraClip may theoretically be performed through the defect. However, operators should be cognizant of the inability to properly evaluate the position of the guide, as tenting with the transseptal needle is not possible.

If there is a moderate or large-sized ASD that precludes a separate puncture location, the operator may be obligated to cross the interatrial septum through the ASD. In some cases, this may result in issues such as insufficient height above the mitral valve (Figs. 7.19, 7.20, 7.21, and 7.22). Complex steering strategies will then be required to maneuver the device to the mitral valve. These techniques will be discussed in further detail in specific case samples and the chapter on complex and situational steering techniques.

Transseptal Crossing in the Presence of an Interatrial Septal Aneurysm

An interatrial septal aneurysm (IASA) can potentially complicate the transseptal puncture. The IAS is usually very floppy and may or may not be associated with a PFO. The floppy septum makes it difficult for a transseptal needle to cross into the LA as the needle often would create a very deep tent. In such situations, the operator has to be careful not to apply excessive pressure as the transseptal needle may puncture the wall of the LA when it finally crosses into the LA. Similarly, it may be difficult to advance the large 22 F guide across the IASA. In some cases, the septum may be tented all the way to the left upper pulmonary vein. In such situations, we recommend against the use of excessive force, instead; gentle pressure and patience is preferred. This will reduce the risk of in advertent perforation or tearing of the interatrial septum. In rare instance, it may be necessary to perform balloon dilatation of the septum. We recommend cautious stepwise inflations starting with a 6-mm balloon.

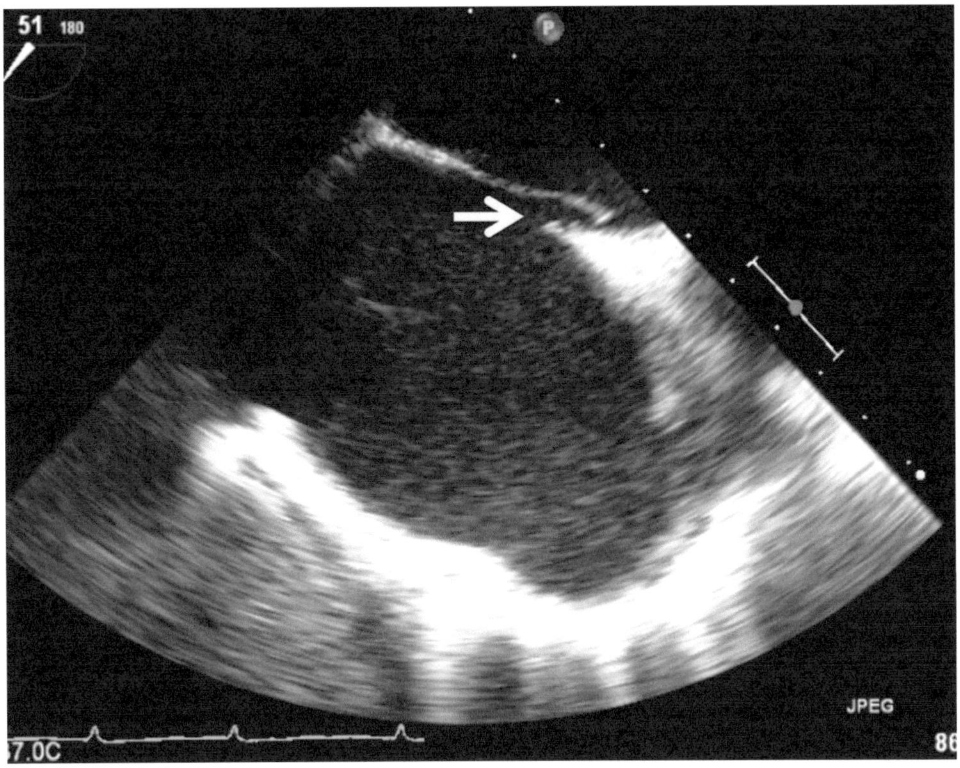

Fig. 7.12 Baseline echo shows the presence of a PFO (*arrow*)

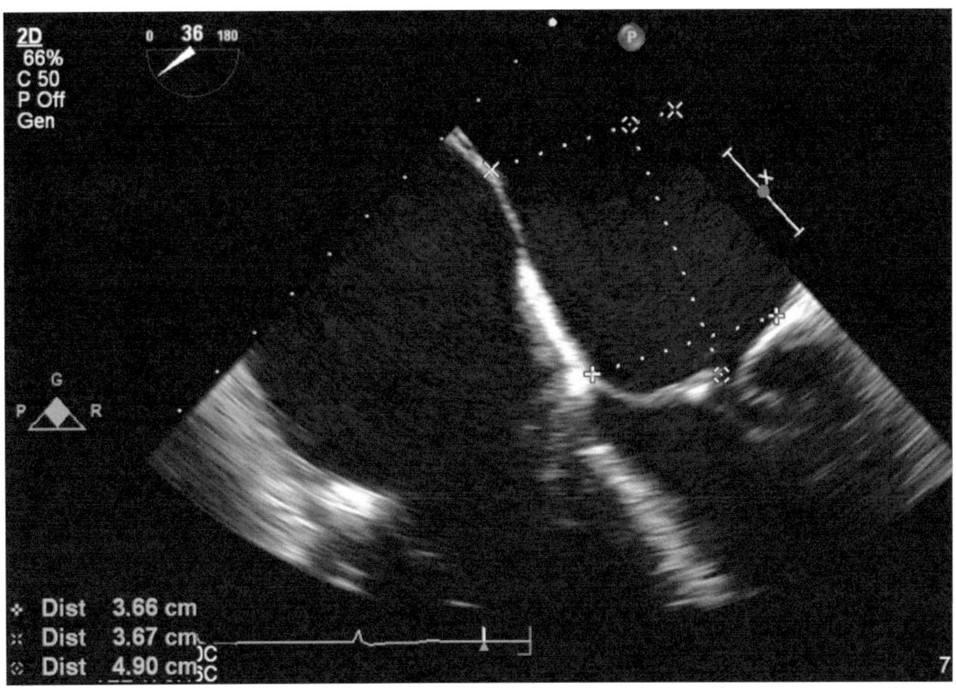

Fig. 7.13 The transseptal puncture height is too high with the PFO biasing the needle

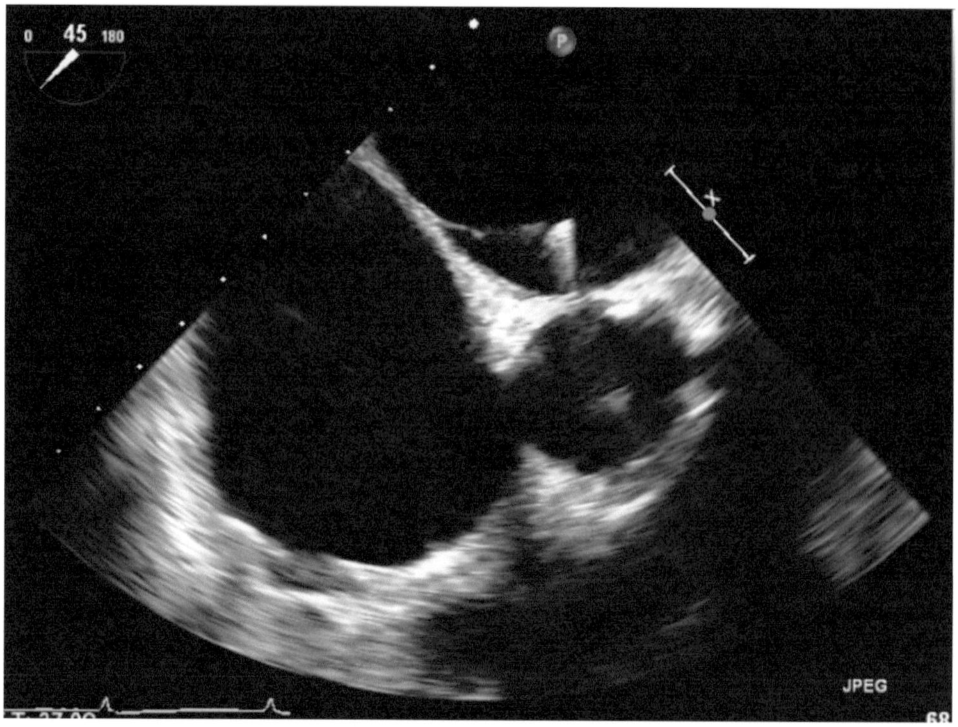

Fig. 7.14 The transseptal needle has entered the LA via the PFO

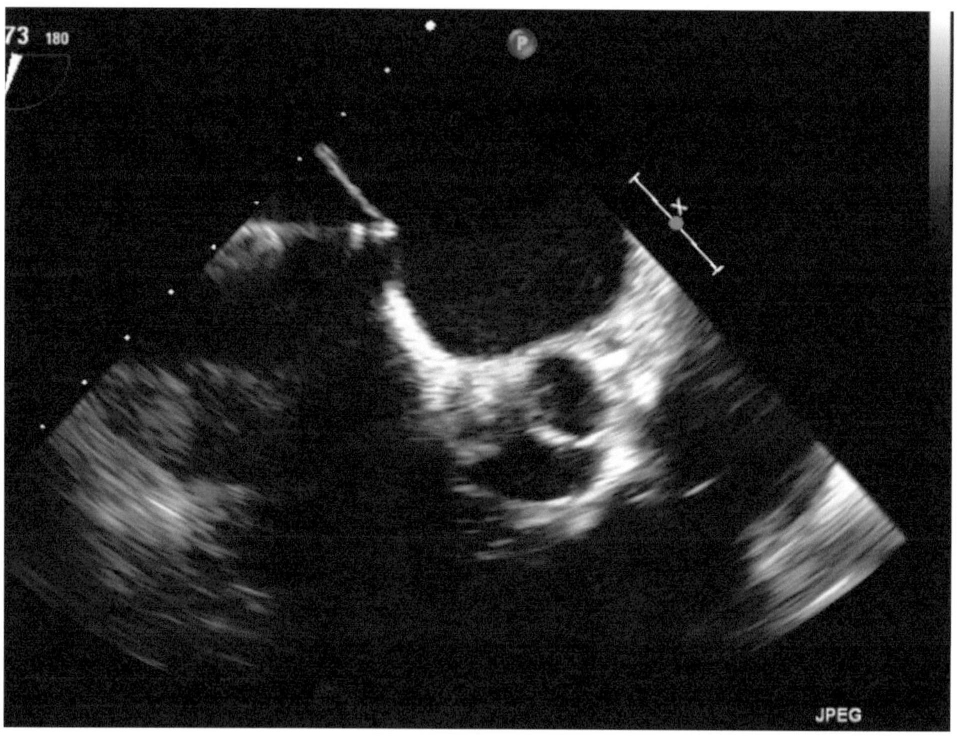

Fig. 7.15 An attempt is made to puncture the septum separate from the PFO. In this case, the operator has angled the puncture site more posteriorly

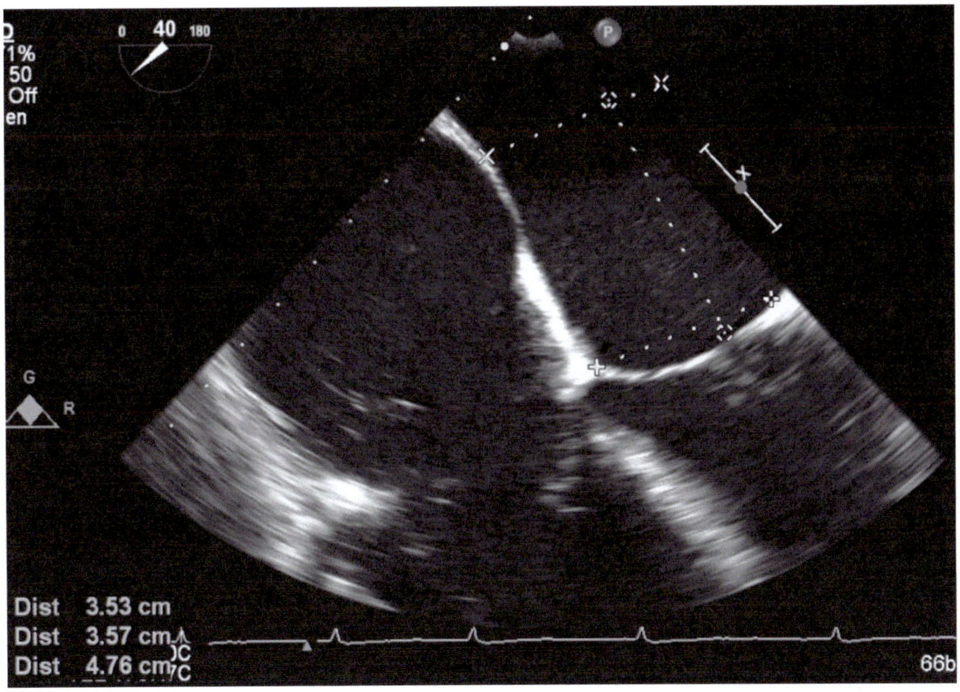

Fig. 7.16 The new transseptal puncture height at 4.76 cm is not as high as the initial position

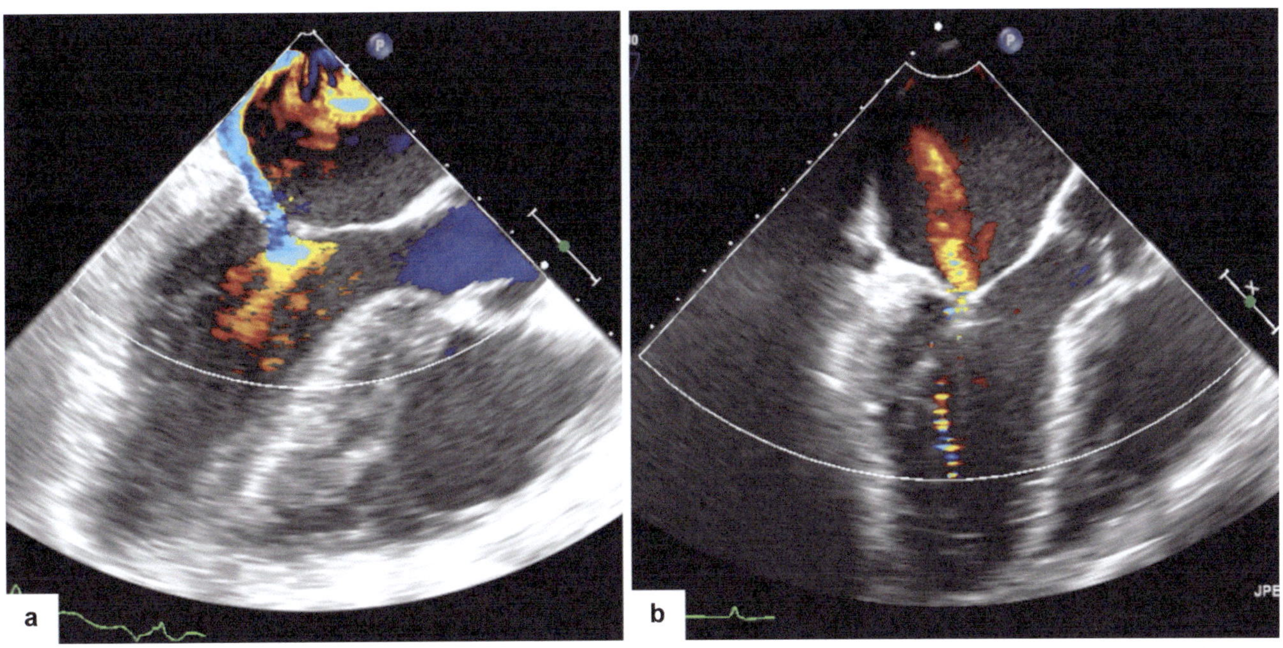

Fig. 7.17 Figure showing the MR before (**a**) and after (**b**) the MitraClip. The jet appears to have a smaller vena contracta and no longer hugs the atrial wall

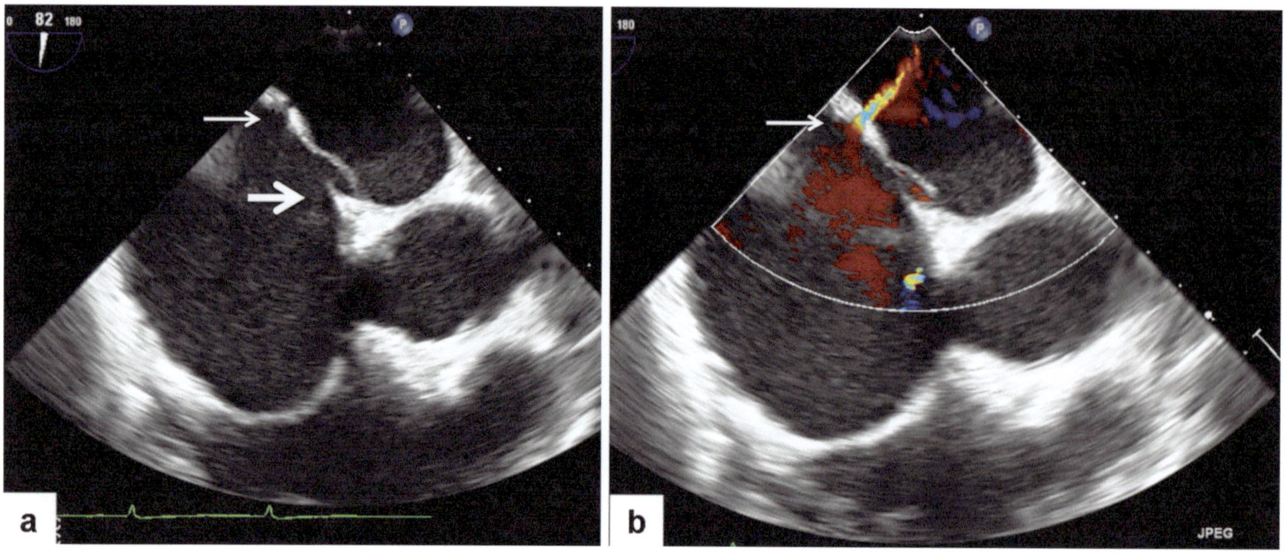

Fig. 7.18 This shows the preexisting PFO (**a**) (*fat arrow*) and the iatrogenic ASD (*thin arrows*) with some shunting seen on color Doppler (**b**) from right to left. This patient had high pulmonary pressures at baseline. Fortunately, this right to left shunt did not cause hypoxia

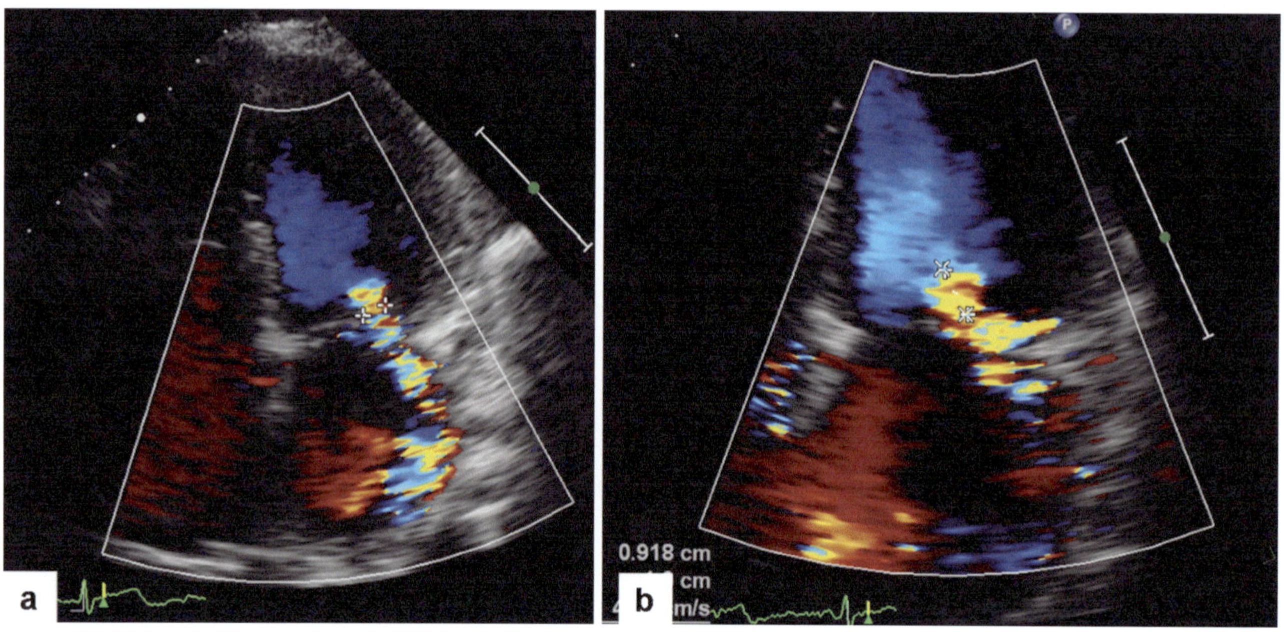

Fig. 7.19 Figures **a** and **b** show the baseline severe wall-hugging MR in a patient with an ASD

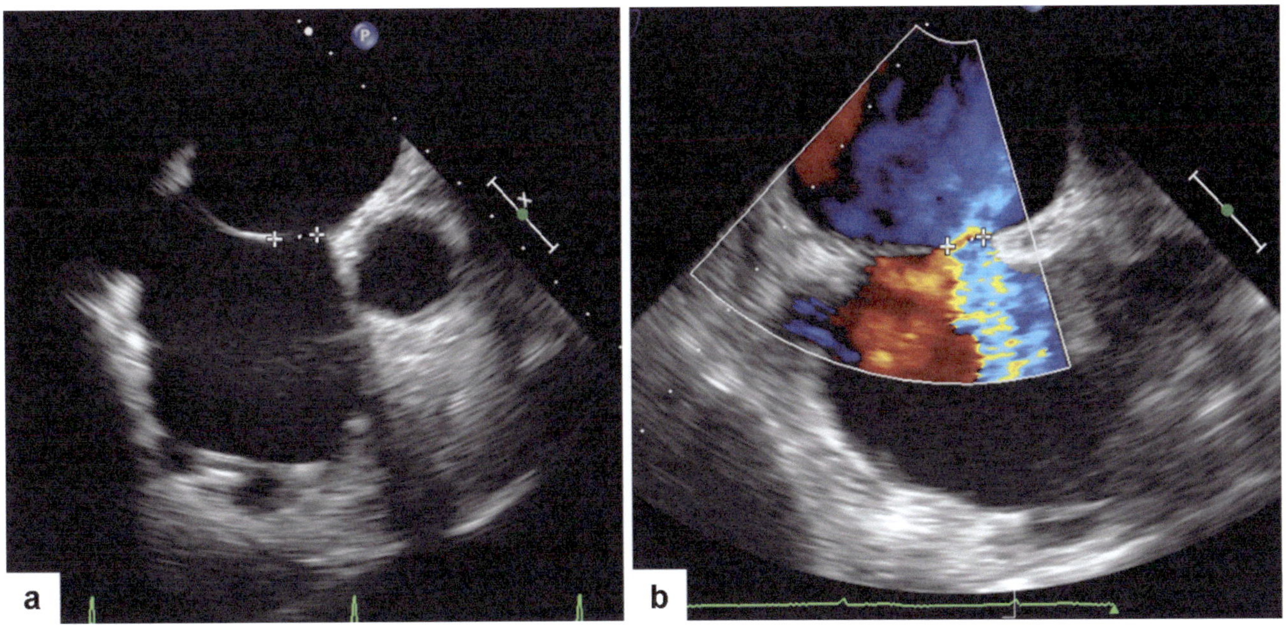

Fig. 7.20 Figure showing the moderate-sized ASD present at baseline (**a**) There is left to right shunting as seen on color Doppler (**b**)

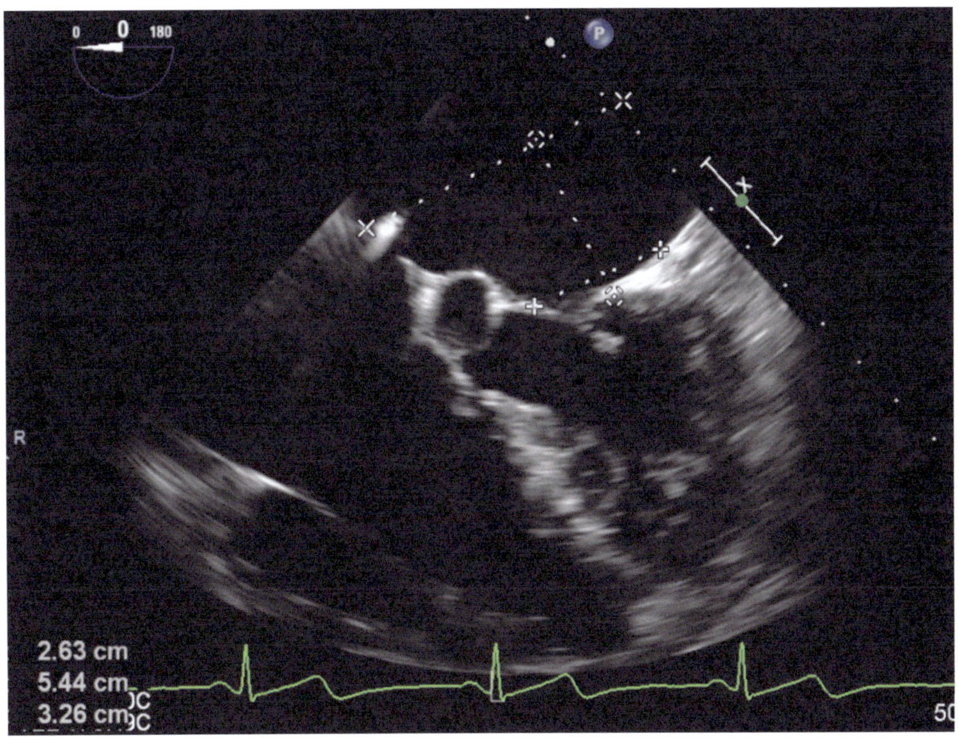

Fig. 7.21 The presence of the ASD made it difficult to puncture anywhere else on the septum. In this case, the transseptal sheath was located across the ASD. With the sheath across the ASD, the height above the mitral valve is low, making the procedure very complicated

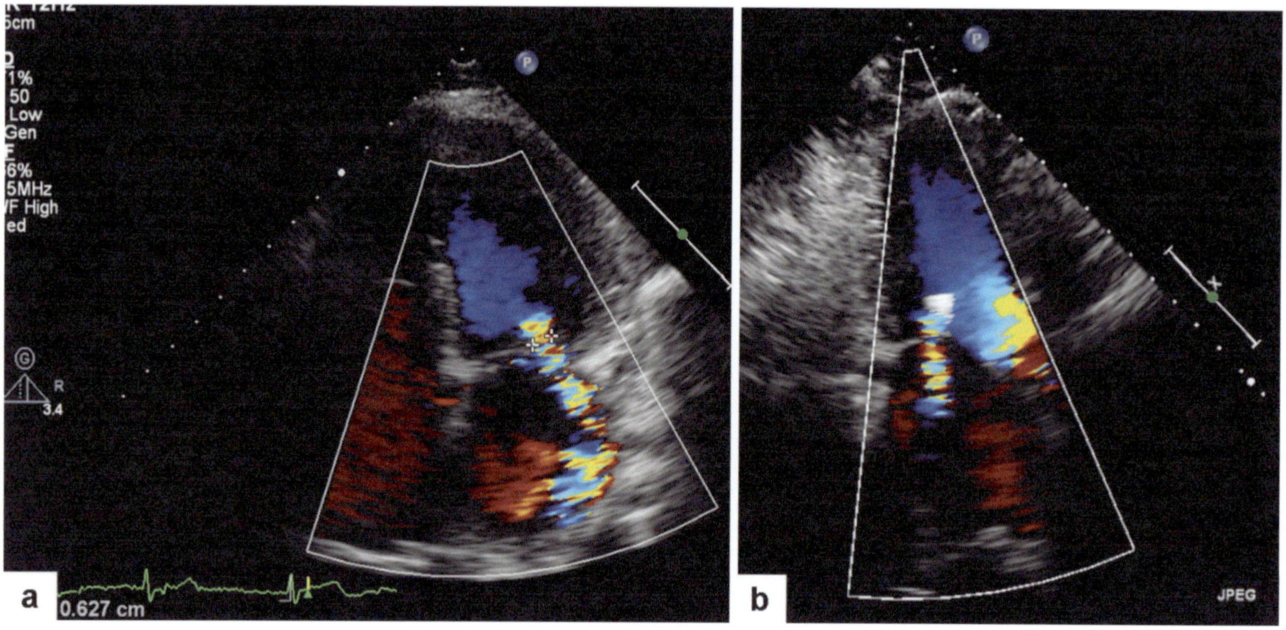

Fig. 7.22 Figure showing the MR before (**a**) and after (**b**) the MitraClip

Fig. 7.23 Step-by-step approach to the transseptal puncture for the MitraClip procedure

1. Advance the wire to the SVC
2. Exchange out the femoral venous sheath for the Mullins sheath or SL catheter
3. Remove guidewire and advance the transseptal needle into the catheter/sheath
4. Withdraw the catheter/sheath and needle to the desired position in the inter-atrial septum. This is the crucial step and is TEE guided
   - Superior/inferior orientation
     - Bicaval view. Tenting should be slightly superior
   - Anterior/posterior orientation
     - Short axis view at level of the aortic valve. Tenting should be slightly posterior
   - Height above the mitral valve
     - Four-chamber view. The tenting should be at a perpendicular height of 3.5 to 4.5cm above the point of coaptation. This height is different depending on MR etiologies
5. Puncture the IAS, and advance the SLO or Mullin's catheter in the LA. Full dose heparin given
6. Advance wire into the LUPV. Watch LAA on TEE to ensure wire does not encroach
7. Remove sheath or catheter, leaving wire in LUPV
8. Dilate the femoral vein track
9. Advance the MitraClip guide and dilator to the IAS
10. Cross into the LA under fluorscopic and TEE guidance
11. Dilator and wire removed

Role of Intracardiac echo

Although intracardiac echo (ICE) has been used in guiding a transseptal puncture in other procedures [13, 14], its use is limited by its 2-D functionality and absence of multiplane functionality (in commercial systems). It can be used to guide transseptal puncture in unusual situations where TEE may not offer adequate imaging of the septum (such as in a case of severe kyphoscoliosis or hiatal hernia). However, ICE cannot replace TEE for the rest of the MitraClip procedure, and it would not be generally recommended to use ICE for the entire MitraClip procedure at this time.

Conclusion

The transseptal puncture is a critical part of the MitraClip procedure. Care and attention are important for patient safety and in choosing the optimal puncture site. A step-by-step and methodical approach is recommended (Fig. 7.23). A properly selected puncture location reduces procedure time and improves the chances of procedural success.

References

1. Ross Jr J, Braunwald E, Morrow AG. Transseptal left atrial puncture; new technique for the measurement of left atrial pressure in man. Am J Cardiol. 1959;3:653–5.
2. Babaliaros VC, Green JT, Lerakis S, Lloyd M, Block PC. Emerging applications for transseptal left heart catheterization old techniques for new procedures. J Am Coll Cardiol. 2008;51:2116–22.
3. Schwagten B, Jordaens L, Rivero-Ayerza M, et al. A randomized comparison of transseptal and transaortic approaches for magnetically guided ablation of left-sided accessory pathways. Pacing Clin Electrophysiol. 2010;33:1298–303.
4. Linker NJ, Fitzpatrick AP. The transseptal approach for ablation of cardiac arrhythmias: experience of 104 procedures. Heart. 1998;79: 379–82.
5. Liu TJ, Lai HC, Lee WL, et al. Immediate and late outcomes of patients undergoing transseptal left-sided heart catheterization for symptomatic valvular and arrhythmic diseases. Am Heart J. 2006;151:235–41.
6. Gonzalez MD, Otomo K, Shah N, et al. Transseptal left heart catheterization for cardiac ablation procedures. J Interv Card Electrophysiol. 2001;5:89–95.
7. Tucker KJ, Curtis AB, Murphy J, et al. Transesophageal echocardiographic guidance of transseptal left heart catheterization during radiofrequency ablation of left-sided accessory pathways in humans. Pacing Clin Electrophysiol. 1996;19:272–81.
8. Roelke M, Smith AJ, Palacios IF. The technique and safety of transseptal left heart catheterization: the Massachusetts General Hospital experience with 1,279 procedures. Cathet Cardiovasc Diagn. 1994;32:332–9.
9. BL C, Olsson SB, Varnauskas E. Transseptal left heart catheterization: a review of 278 studies. Clin Cardiol. 1986;9:21–6.
10. Libanoff AJ, Silver AW. Complications of transseptal left heart catheterization. Am J Cardiol. 1965;16:390–3.
11. Adrouny ZA, Sutherland DW, Griswold HE, Ritzmann LW. Complications with transseptal left heart catheterization. Am Heart J. 1963;65:327–33.
12. McGinty PM, Smith TW, Rogers JH. Transseptal left heart catheterization and the incidence of persistent iatrogenic atrial septal defects. J Interv Cardiol. 2011;24:254–63.
13. Shalganov TN, Paprika D, Borbas S, Temesvari A, Szili-Torok T. Preventing complicated transseptal puncture with intracardiac echocardiography: case report. Cardiovasc Ultrasound. 2005;3:5.
14. Morton JB, Kalman JM. Intracardiac echocardiographic anatomy for the interventional electrophysiologist. J Interv Card Electrophysiol. 2005;13 Suppl 1:11–6.

Venous Access Management

8

Khung Keong Yeo and Jason Rogers

Abstract

Bleeding from the 24 F femoral venous access site in the MitraClip procedure is a potentially important complication. The access site is commonly managed using manual pressure, a figure-of-8 (or Z-tie), or using a preclose technique using two Proglide devices. This chapter reviews the steps of the latter two techniques.

Keywords

Venous access • Perclose • Preclose • Suture

Introduction

The MitraClip procedure utilizes a large guiding catheter that is 24 F in diameter at the femoral vein entry site and 22 F as it crosses the interatrial septum. The right femoral vein is the standard approach used for the procedure. Using the left femoral vein is technically possible but not recommended, as steering of the device may be unfavorably influenced by the reverse iliofemoral contours taken by the guide from the left side. While bleeding from a venous access site is generally less brisk and has fewer clinical consequences as compared to an arterial bleed, venous bleeding can nonetheless occur. Meticulous attention should be paid to proper access and postprocedure management of the MitraClip venous entry site, since this is the largest access required for the procedure. Hemodynamic monitoring and measurement of right-sided heart pressures are performed through much smaller sheaths, and bleeding complications at these sites are rare.

K.K. Yeo, M.B.B.S., FACC, FSCAI (✉)
Department of Cardiology, National Heart Centre Singapore,
Mistri Wing, 17 Third Hospital Avenue,
Singapore, 168752, Singapore

Department of Cardiovascular Medicine,
University of California, Davis Medical Center,
4860 Y Street, Suite 2820, Sacramento, CA 95817, USA
e-mail: yeo_kk@yahoo.com, yeo.khung.keong@nhcs.com.sg

J. Rogers, M.D., FACC, FSCAI
Department of Cardiovascular Medicine,
University of California, Davis Medical Center,
4860 Y Street, Suite 2820, Sacramento, CA 95817, USA
e-mail: jason.rogers@ucdmc.ucdavis.edu

Gaining Venous Access

When first accessing the femoral vein, a 7- or 8-F sidearm sheath is used. Access should be obtained over the femoral head to allow effective manual compression at the end of the procedure, and this location should be verified with fluoroscopic or ultrasound guidance. The angle of access into the vein should be approximately 45° from horizontal in anticipation of the angle that the guide will eventually enter the vein. The access angle may be particularly important in obese individuals where a long distance of soft tissue must be traversed before entering the vein. If the angle of entry does not approximate the final guide entry angle, it is possible to place excessive traction on the entry site which may increase the risk of intraprocedural hematoma formation. One should avoid inadvertent puncture of the right femoral artery during access as this increases the chances of hematoma or arteriovenous fistula formation.

After gaining access, a skin incision should be made sufficient to allow introduction of the 24-F guiding catheter. A wire is then advanced under fluoroscopic guidance into the

T. Feldman et al. (eds.), *Atlas of Percutaneous Edge-to-Edge Mitral Valve Repair*,
DOI 10.1007/978-1-4471-4294-2_8, © Springer-Verlag London 2013

inferior vena cava, and the access tract is predilated with a 16- or 18-F dilator. Predilation is important to achieve a controlled and gradual dilation of the entry site. The transseptal is then performed and a stiff Amplatz wire is placed in the left upper pulmonary vein as described separately in this atlas. The guiding catheter is then advanced over this wire slowly and carefully, first through the skin and then into the right common femoral vein.

After the procedure the guiding catheter is removed from the femoral vein. In general, hemostasis for the venous puncture site may be performed by one of three methods: manual compression, the Z-tie (also known as figure-of-8) suture technique, or by using the preclose technique using two 6-F Proglide devices (Abbott Vascular, Abbott Park, Menlo, CA). Manual compression can be performed in the standard manner per institutional protocols, although prolonged compression is often required.

Percutaneous Closure Techniques

Z-Tie or Figure-of-8 Suture Technique

The Z-tie or figure-of-8 is a simple technique utilizing a single 2-0 silk or prolene suture to create a soft tissue knot that puckers and compresses the venous access site. The concept is to mimic manual pressure by local placement of transcutaneous sutures. Intravenous protamine is often given to reverse anticoagulation from heparin. Frequently, additional manual compression for 5–10 min is required.

The Z-tie or figure-of-8 tie is shown step-by-step as follows:

Step 1: Using a 2.0 suture, the needle enters the skin on the side of the guide about 1 cm distal to the skin entry site of the guide. In this example, the needle enters on the medial side of guide. The operator makes a deep subcutaneous puncture under the guide to the opposite side. The needle exits the skin on the opposite (lateral) side of the guide (Figs. 8.1 and 8.2).

Step 2: The needle is then brought back to the medial side of the guide, this time approximately 1 cm proximal to the skin entry of the guide. This results in the suture crossing the guide (Fig. 8.3).

Step 3: A deep subcutaneous puncture from the medial side of the guide to the lateral side of the guide is then performed proximal to the skin entry site of the guide (Figs. 8.4 and 8.5).

Step 4: The two ends of the suture are then tied together into a slip knot onto the surface of the guide. The operator's assistant then prepares to pull the guide out (Figs. 8.6 and 8.7).

Step 5: As the guide is pulled out, the operator tightens the knot and holds manual pressure over the puncture site (Fig. 8.8).

Potential Complications of Z-Tie Technique

Success rates with hemostasis may be variable. Some operators have anecdotally reported success rates of only 60–80 % while others have had >90 % success. The success of this technique would appear to depend on several variables related to the patient's habitus, degree of anticoagulation, central venous pressure, and soft tissue compliance. This technique may not be ideal in thin patients as there is a less soft tissue present to serve as a "tissue knot." For thin patients, there is also the theoretical risk that an excessively deep needle bite may injure the neighboring artery. For obese patients, there is the risk of excessive soft tissue masking underlying failed hemostasis. Close observation is required after using this technique, and because of soft tissue distortion, the venous puncture site may also be more difficult to manually compress.

Preclose Technique Using Two Proglide Devices

The preclose technique is conceptually attractive as it employs direct suture-based closure of the vein at the entry site. The Proglide device was designed initially as a suture-based arteriotomy closure device (Fig. 8.9). It consists of two percutaneously delivered needles which allow a suture to be placed across the arteriotomy site. The device needles are spaced 6 mm apart and they deliver a prolene pretied suture. It has subsequently been used off-label for effective closure of venous access sites. In using the Proglide in a preclose fashion, we utilize a similar technique as preclosure of large-size arterial sheaths. Since veins are, in general, thin-walled and more delicate than arteries, care must be taken to avoid tearing the vein. Specifically, gentle movements are required while initially delivering the devices and when tensioning the sutures at the procedure conclusion. Note that the placement of the Proglide devices is performed during initial venous access before dilating the site with the guiding catheter.

Part 1: Preclose Steps

Step 1: An 0.035 wire is inserted via the right femoral venous sheath during initial venous access (Figs. 8.10 and 8.11). The sheath is then removed. The first Proglide is then advanced. The guidewire is removed when the white markers are at the surface of the skin.

Step 2: The first Proglide is then deployed at a 2–8 o'clock orientation and the 0.035 guidewire reinserted (Figs. 8.12, 8.13 and 8.14). The sutures are kept moist with a wet gauze and secured with a small clamp or sticker to the surrounding drape. These sutures should be labeled "1" as they are the first deployed and therefore the first to be tensioned at the end of the procedure.

Step 3: A second Proglide is then inserted (Fig. 8.15). Again, the guidewire is removed when the white markers of the device are at the level of the skin.

Step 4: The device is then deployed at 4–10 o'clock orientation and the 0.035 guidewire reinserted (Figs. 8.15 and 8.16).
Step 5: These second sutures are then harvested, secured away from the puncture site with a mosquito clamp, and placed under wet gauze. These sutures should be labeled "2" as they will be tensioned after the first set at the end of the procedure (Figs. 8.17 and 8.18).
Step 6: The 7 or 8 F sidearm sheath is then reinserted over the guidewire and the MitraClip procedure continues.

Part 2: Proglide Closure of Venotomy After the Procedure

Step 1: After the MitraClip procedure, with the guide still in the groin, preparations are made to close the venous puncture site.
Step 2: A long 0.035 wire is placed through the guide into the inferior vena cava. One assistant prepares to apply manual pressure at the groin during removal of the guide from the femoral vein. The main operator prepares to close the venous puncture site (Figs. 8.19 and 8.20).
Step 3: The main operator will use the initially deployed set of sutures (at 2–8 o'clock orientation) first (Figs. 8.21, 8.22, and 8.23). Failure to do so will result in tangling of the sutures in the access tract and inadequate closure. The sutures are tensioned and cut using the Proglide knot pusher and suture cutter.
Step 4: The second set of sutures is then tied, secured, and cut (Figs. 8.24 and 8.25). It is important during the entire process not to be too forceful in tying the knots as the veins are more delicate than arteries and may tear more easily.
Step 5: Manual pressure is held for ~5 min to secure hemostasis (Fig. 8.26). A cutaneous 2-0 or 3-0 suture or steri-strip may optionally be applied to appose the superficial cutaneous incision.

Potential Complications of Preclose Technique

Failure of hemostasis can occur but the exact rates are not known. Anecdotally, our success rate (as measured by acute success in the lab with no recurrent bleeding event during hospitalization) is very high. The main risk of this technique occurs with excessive pulling on the sutures resulting in tearing of the veins and bleeding. It should also be pointed out that the use of these two additional devices will add to the total cost of the procedure.

Conclusion

Successful hemostasis after withdrawal of the MitraClip guide is an important part of the entire MitraClip procedure. Lack of attention to this final step of the procedure may result in excessive bleeding and an unnecessary complication. This chapter reviews the key steps of two common techniques of securing hemostasis (other than manual compression). We recommend that operators become very familiar with one of the techniques.

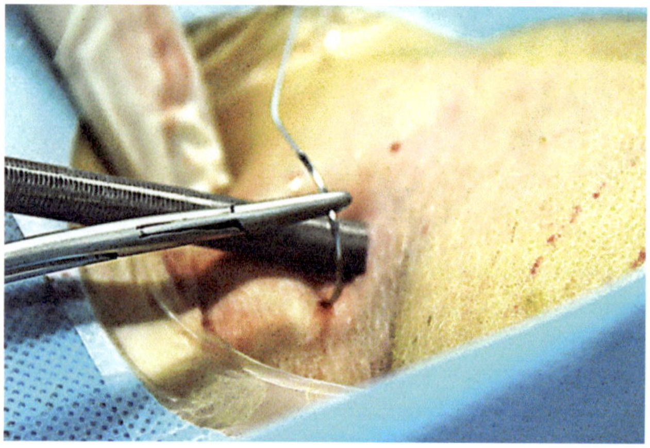

Fig. 8.1 Using a 2.0 suture, the needle enters the skin on the side of the guide about 1 cm distal to the skin entry site of the guide. (Courtesy of Dr Loh Poay Huan)

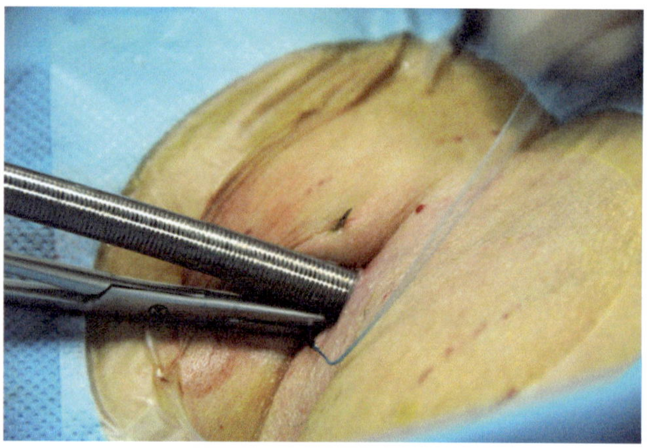

Fig. 8.2 The needle exits the skin on the opposite (lateral) side of the guide. (Courtesy of Dr Loh Poay Huan)

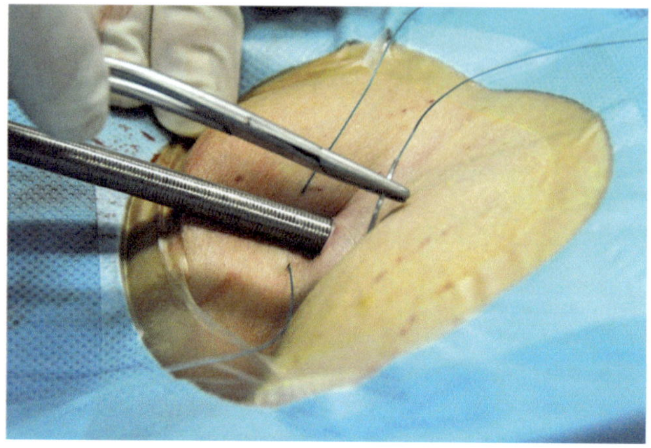

Fig. 8.3 The needle is then brought back to the medial side of the guide, this time approximately 1 cm proximal to the skin entry of the guide. This results in the suture crossing the guide. (Courtesy of Dr Loh Poay Huan)

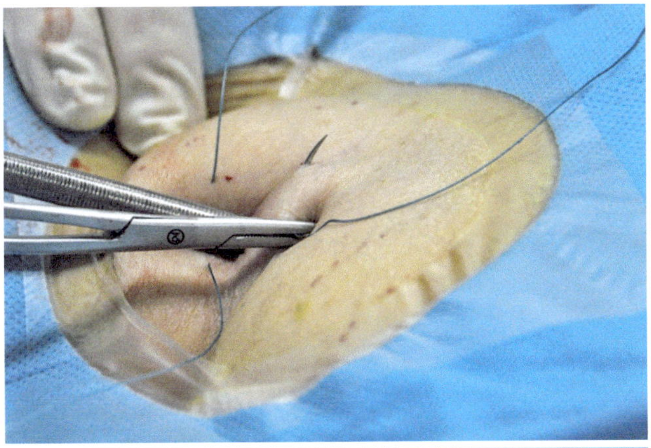

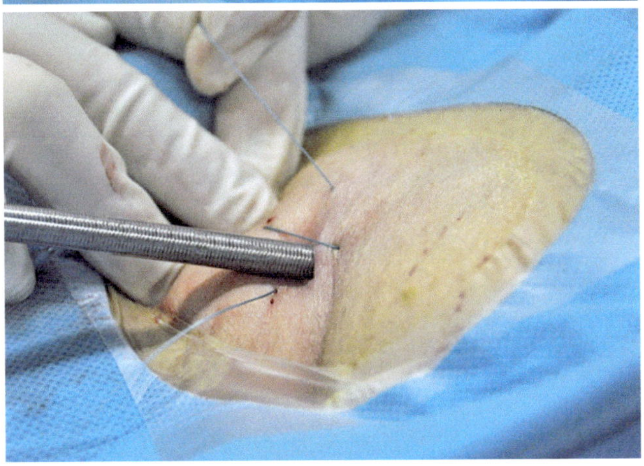

Figs. 8.4 and 8.5 A deep subcutaneous puncture from the medial side of the guide to the lateral side of the guide is then performed proximal to the skin entry site of the guide. (Courtesy of Dr Loh Poay Huan)

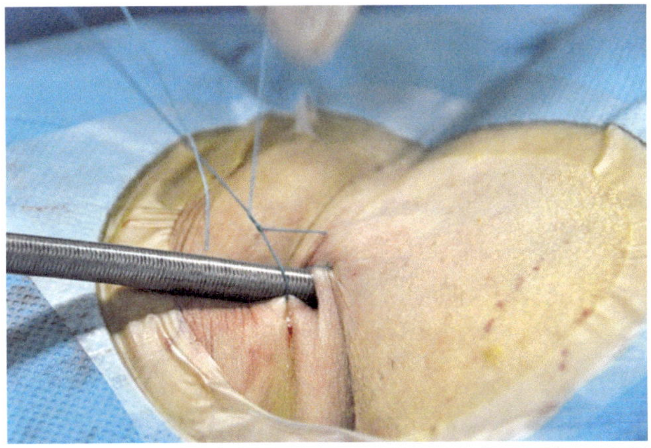

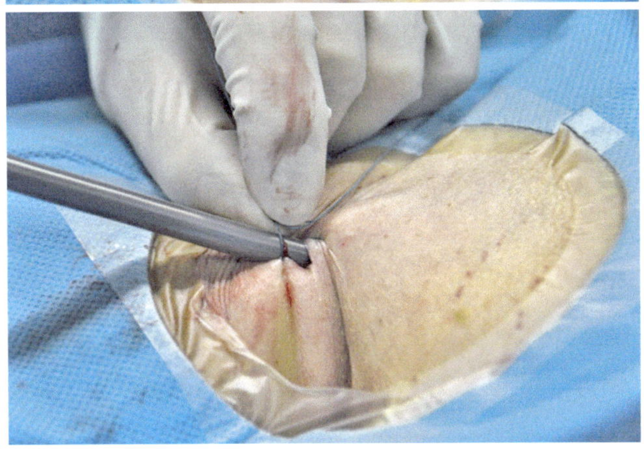

Figs. 8.6 and 8.7 The two ends of are then tied together into a slip knot onto the surface of the guide. The operator's assistant then prepares to pull the guide out. (Courtesy of Dr Loh Poay Huan)

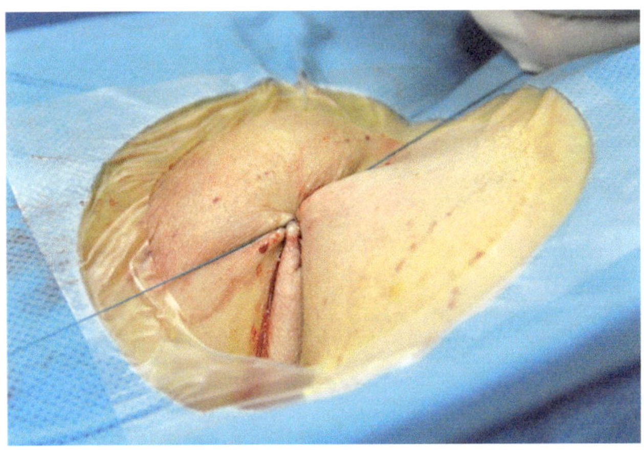

Fig. 8.8 As the guide is pulled out, the operator tightens the knot and holds manual pressure over the puncture site. (Courtesy of Dr Loh Poay Huan)

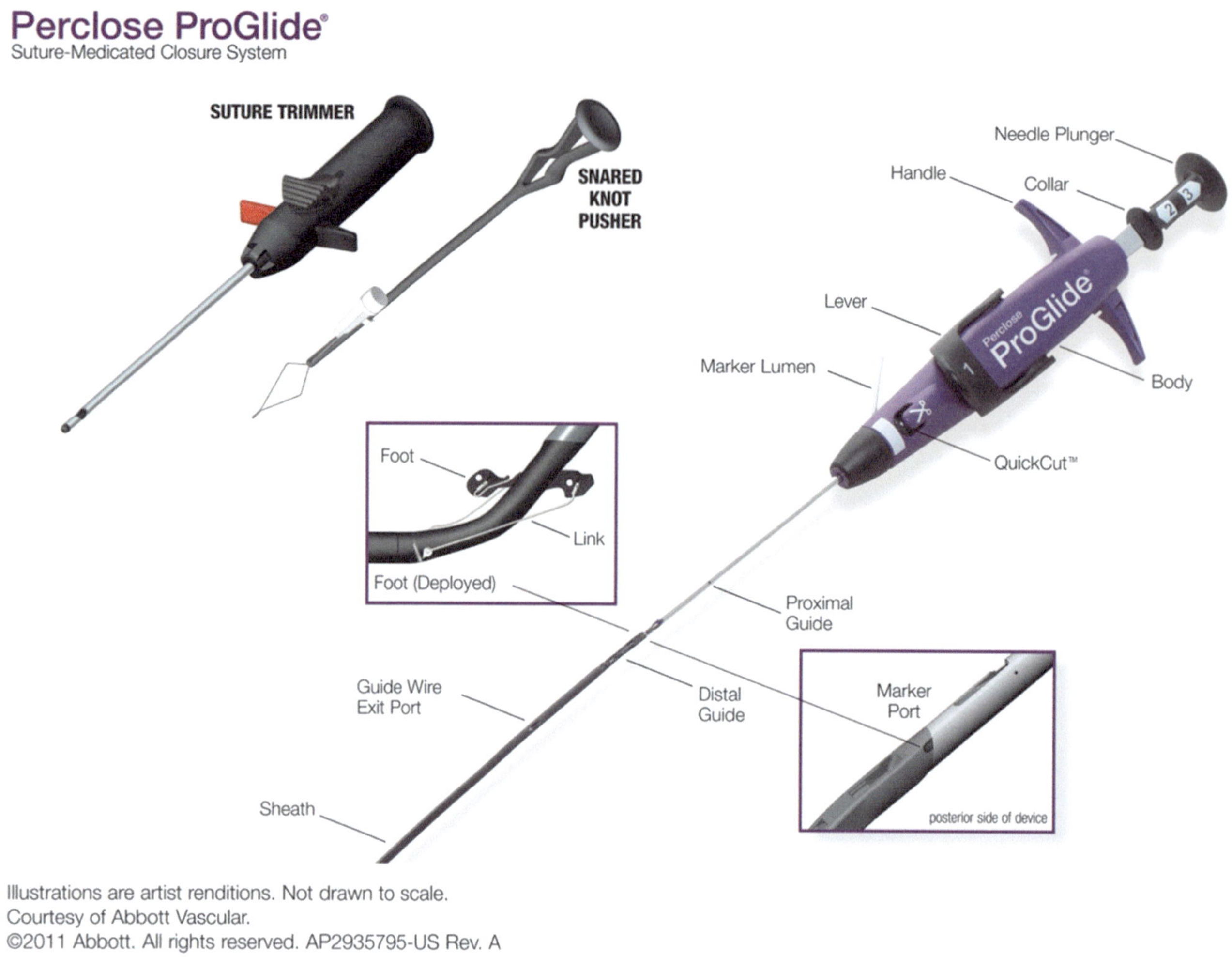

Fig. 8.9 The Perclose Proglide device with its components labeled

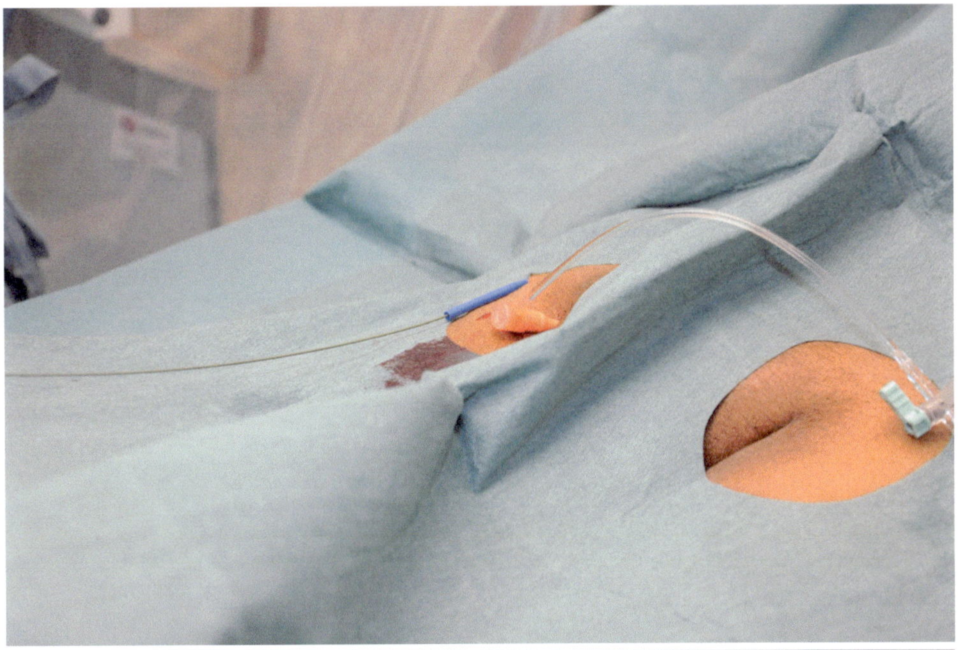

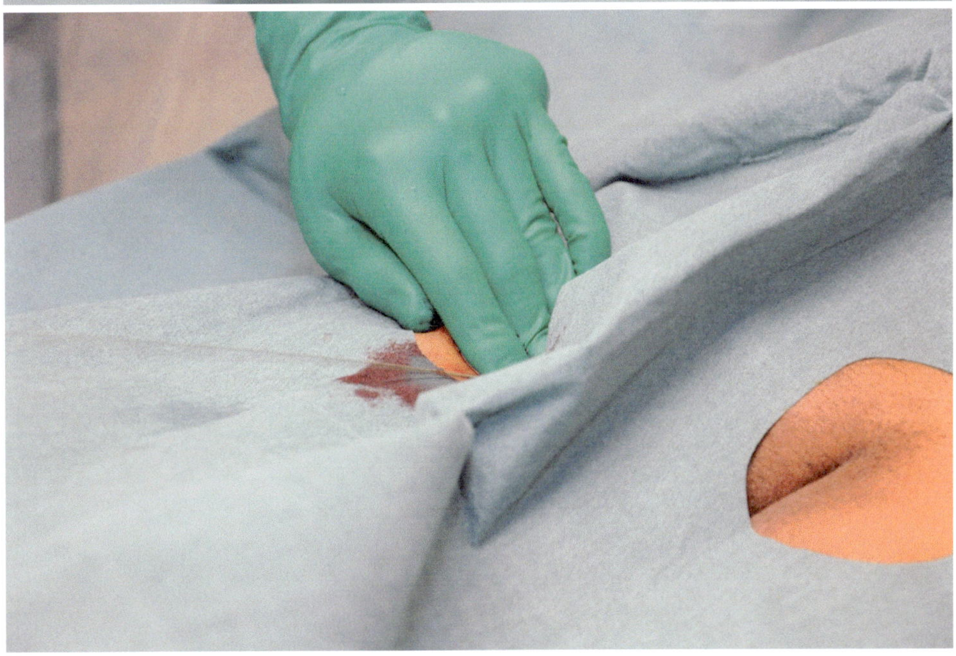

Figs. 8.10 and 8.11 An 0.035 wire is inserted via the right femoral venous sheath during initial venous access. The sheath is then removed

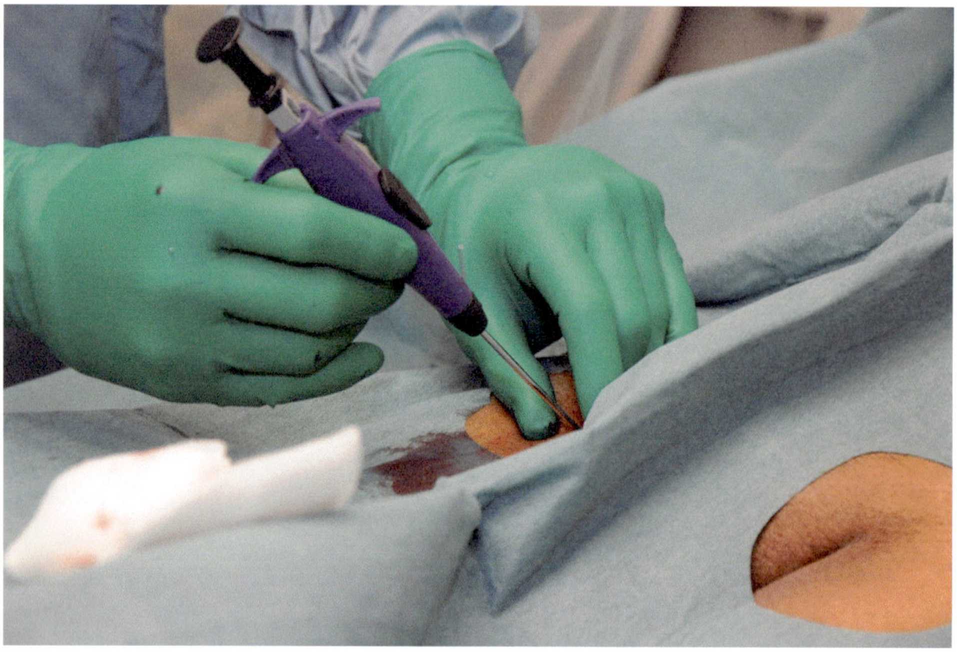

Figs. 8.12 The first Proglide is placed at a 2–8 o'clock orientation

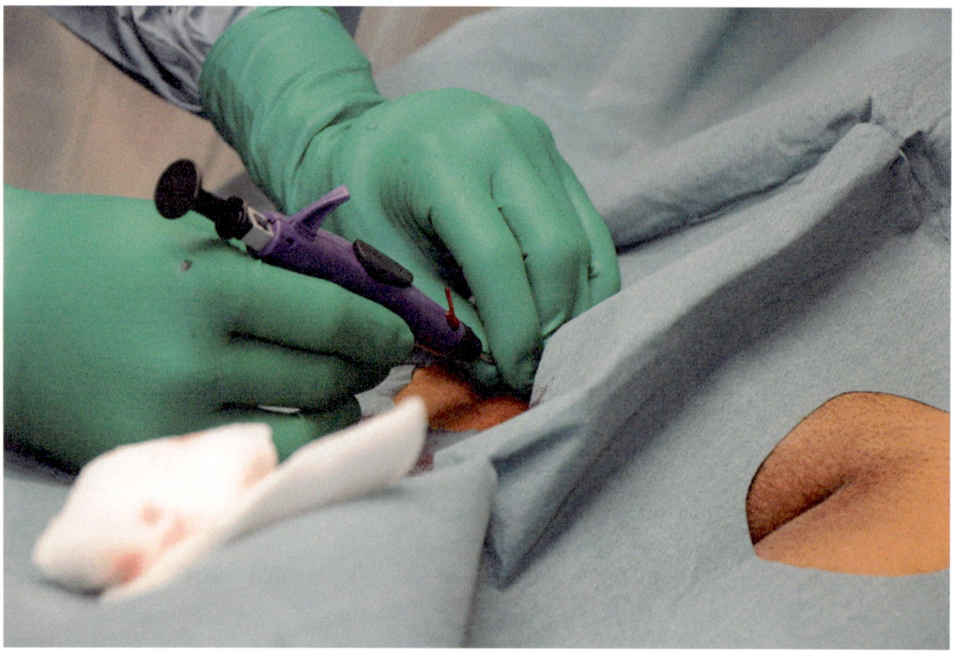

Fig. 8.13 Slow backflow of venous blood observed

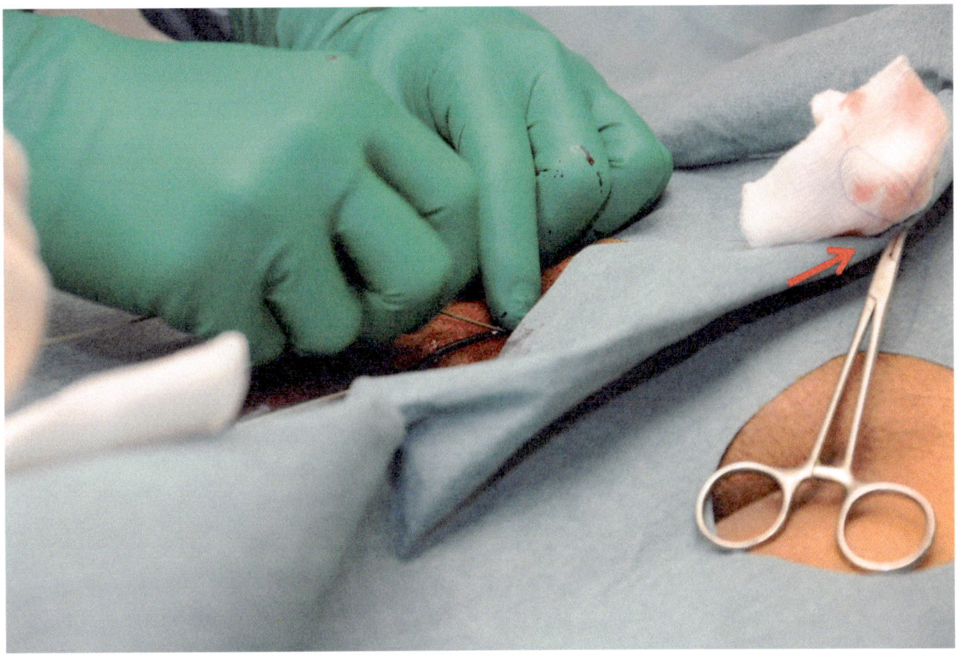

Fig. 8.14 Rewiring of the femoral vein via the Proglide after sutures harvested and clamped (*red arrow*)

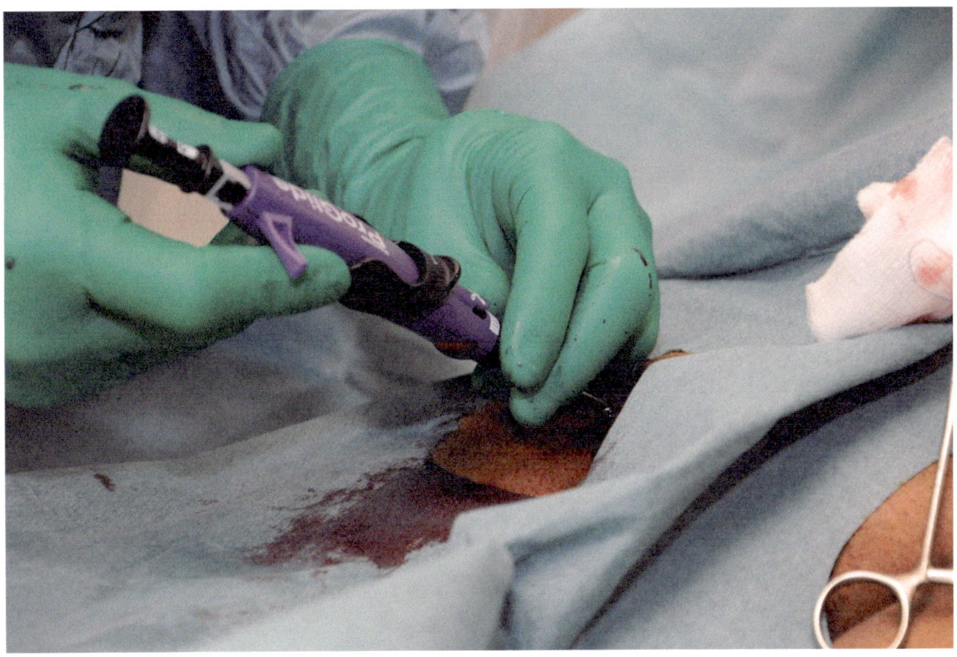

Fig. 8.15 The second Proglide is now placed via the guidewire and positioned at the 4–10 o'clock position, orthogonal to the first Proglide. Note the venous backflow

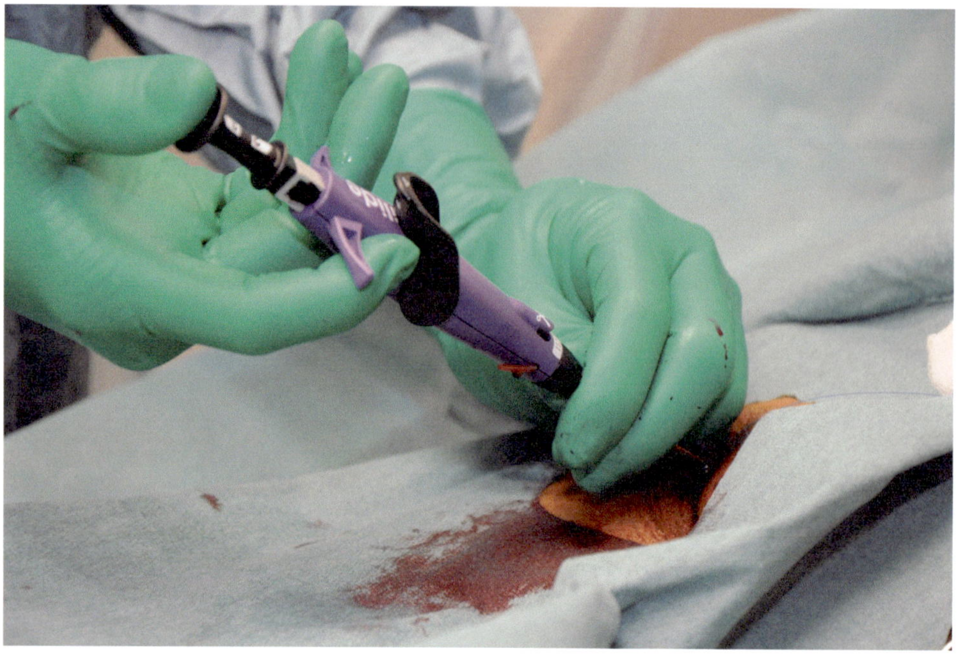

Fig. 8.16 The second Proglide is deployed

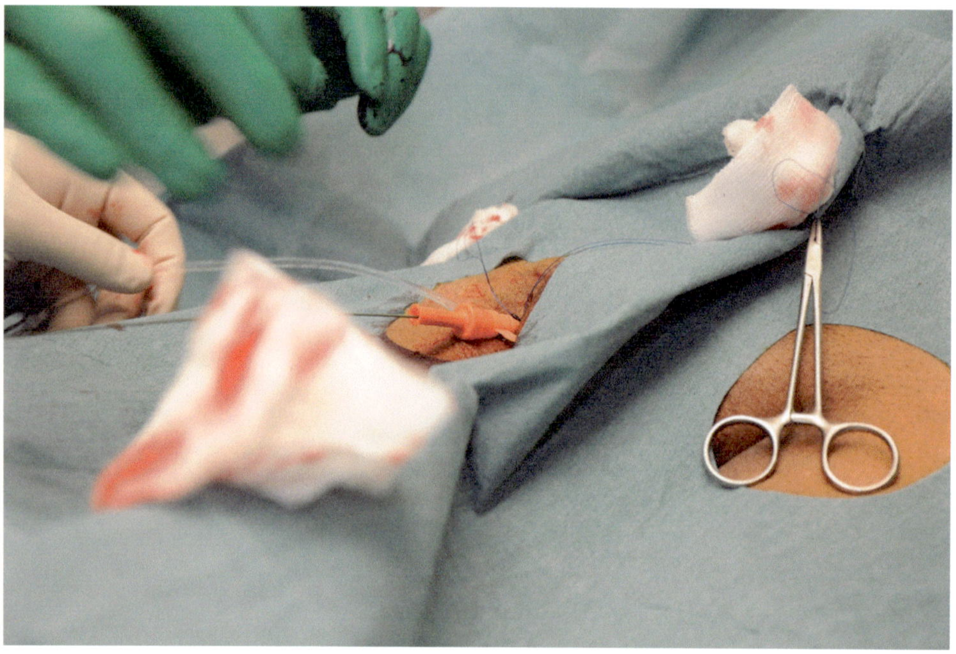

Fig. 8.17 The guidewire is replaced and the 7 F sheath is replaced

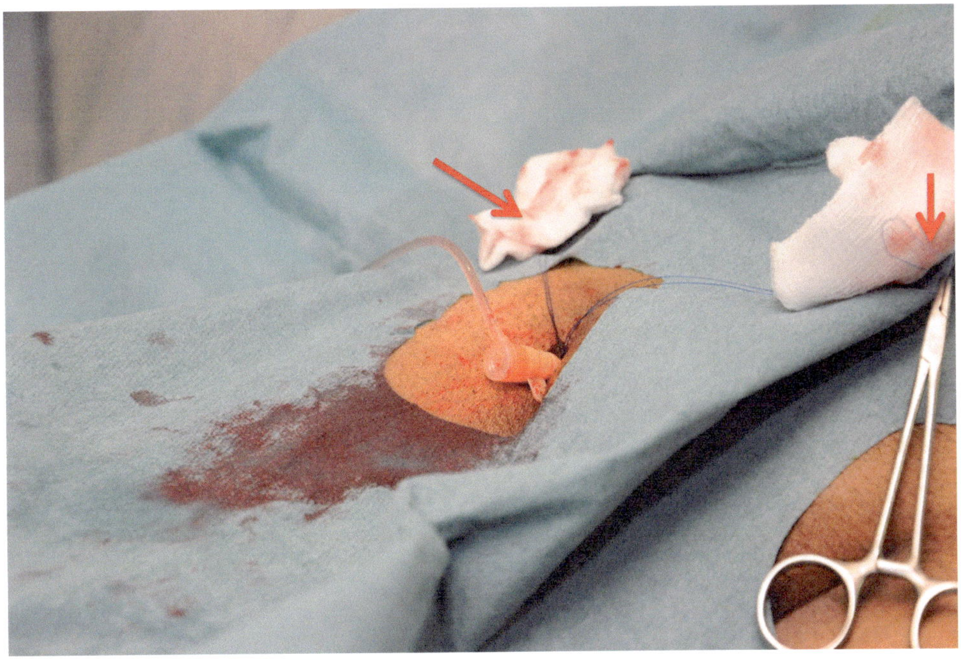

Fig. 8.18 The 7 F sheath is now in place. The two sets of sutures are placed by the side and clamped (*red arrows*), ready for use at the end of the procedure

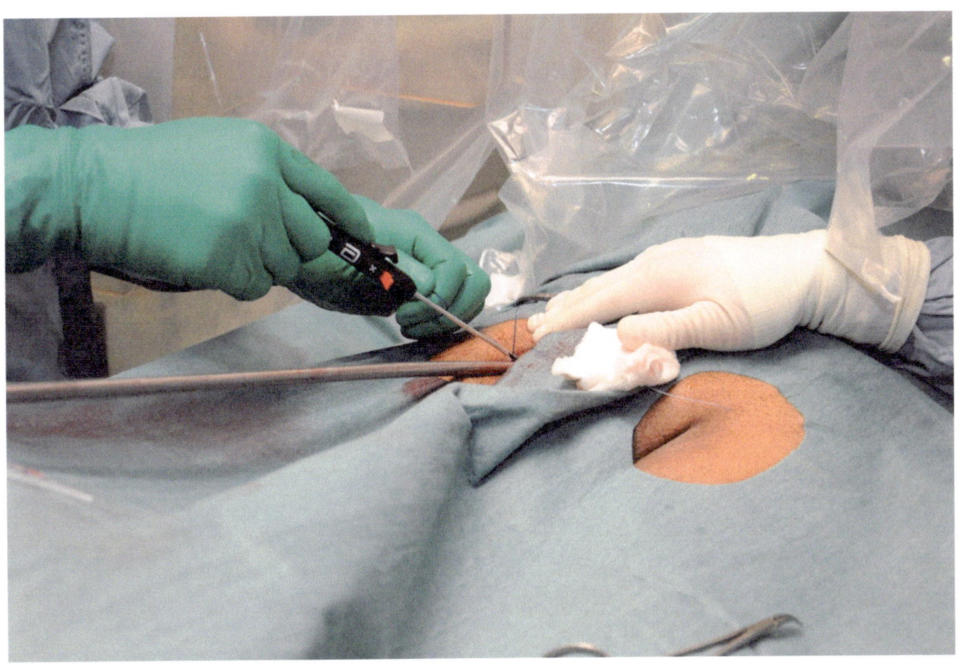

Fig. 8.19 The first Proglide suture is ready to be tied with the removal of the guide. An assistant makes ready to hold manual pressure

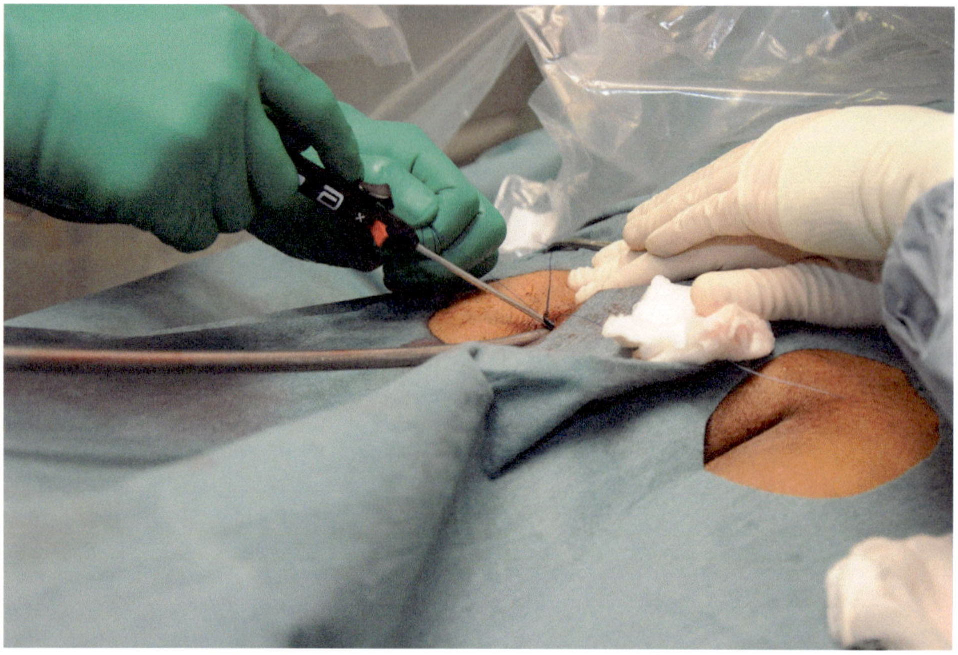

Fig. 8.20 The main operator prepares to close the venous puncture site

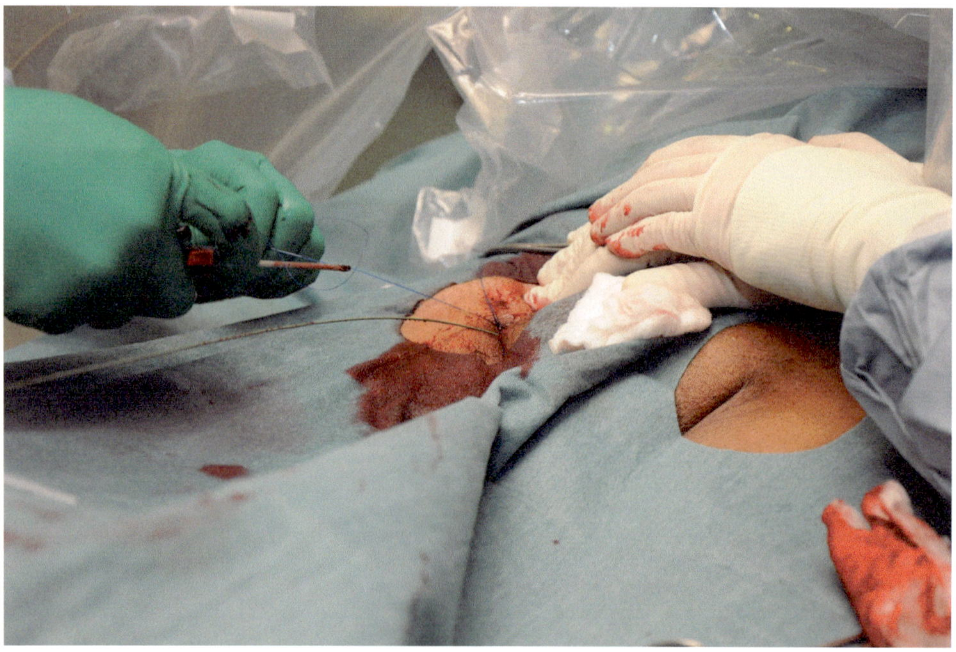

Figs. 8.21, 8.22, and 8.23 The knot is tied for the first Proglide suture

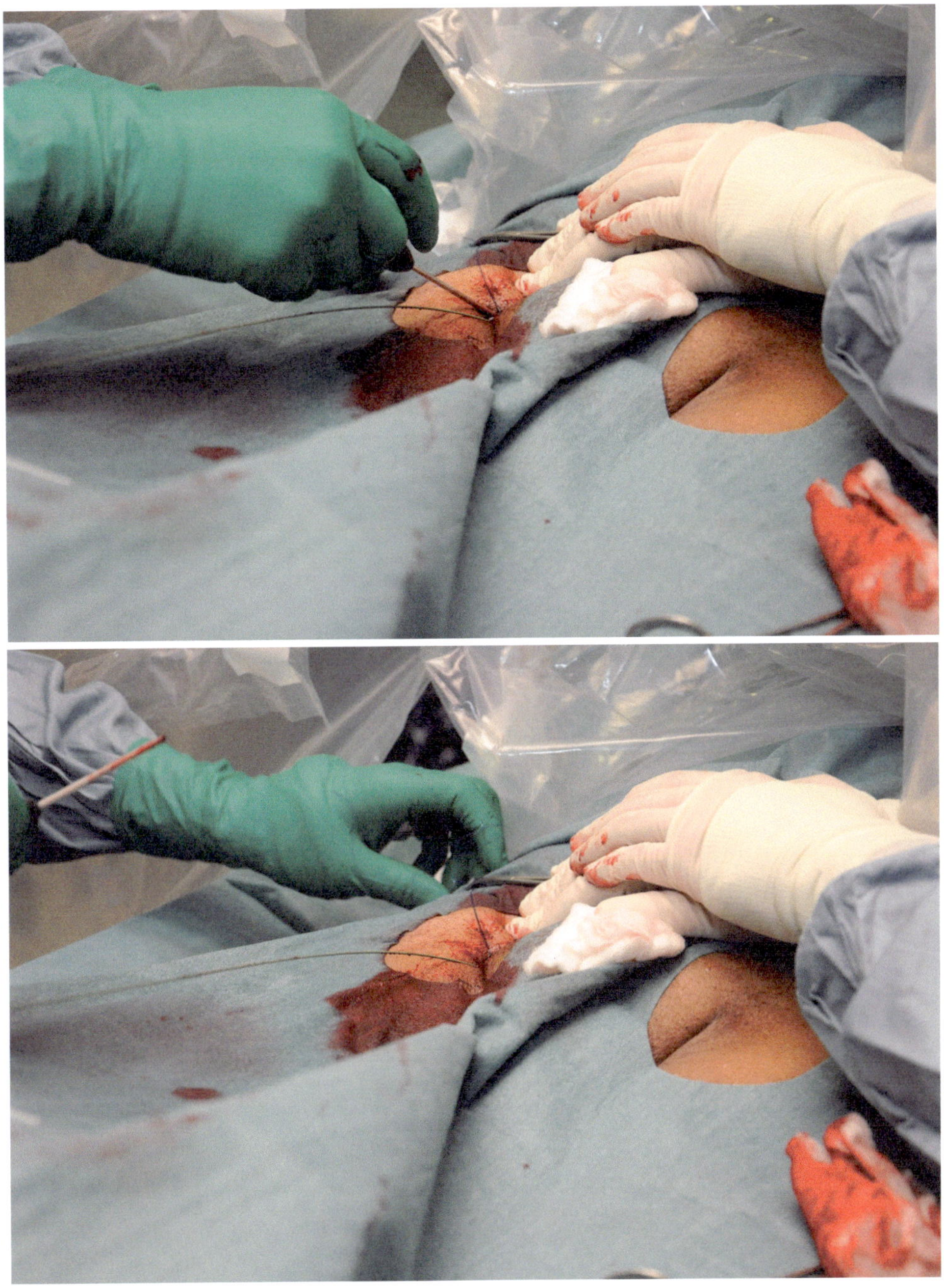

Figs. 8.21, 8.22, and 8.23 (continued)

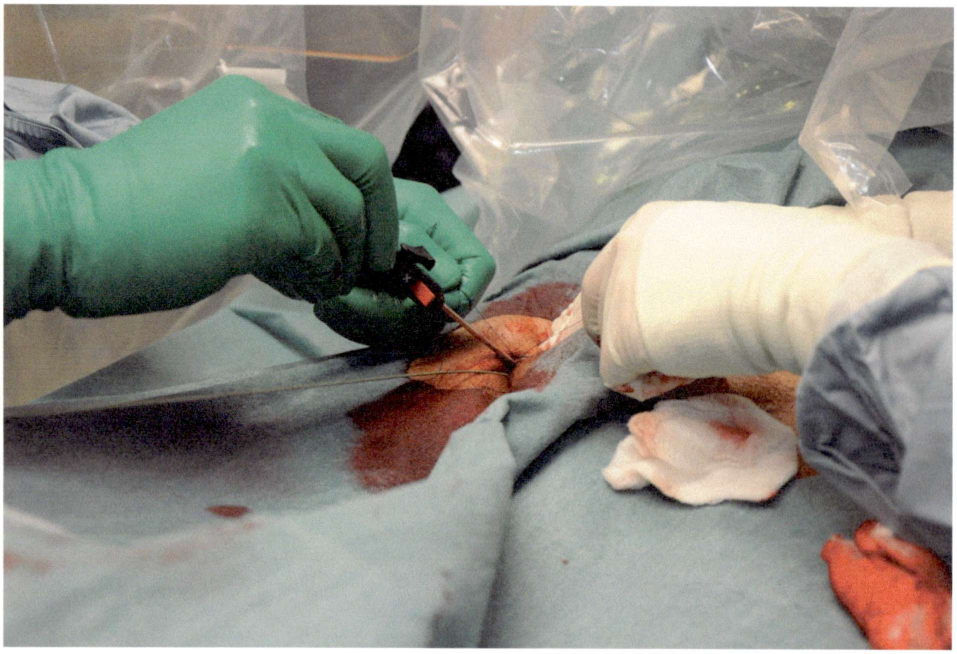

Fig. 8.24 The second Proglide knot is tied

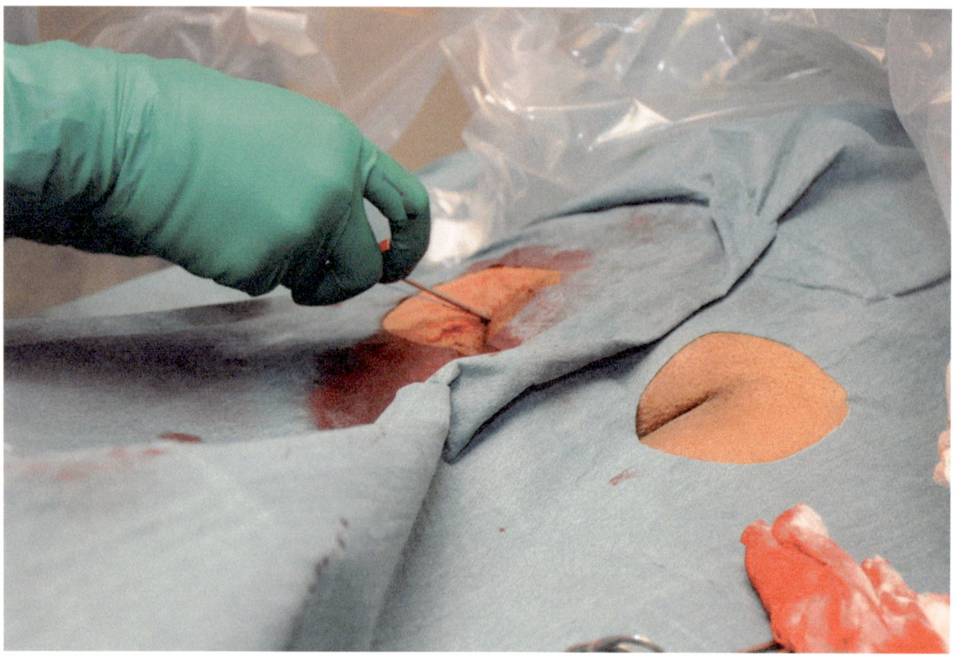

Fig. 8.25 The second Proglide knot is cut

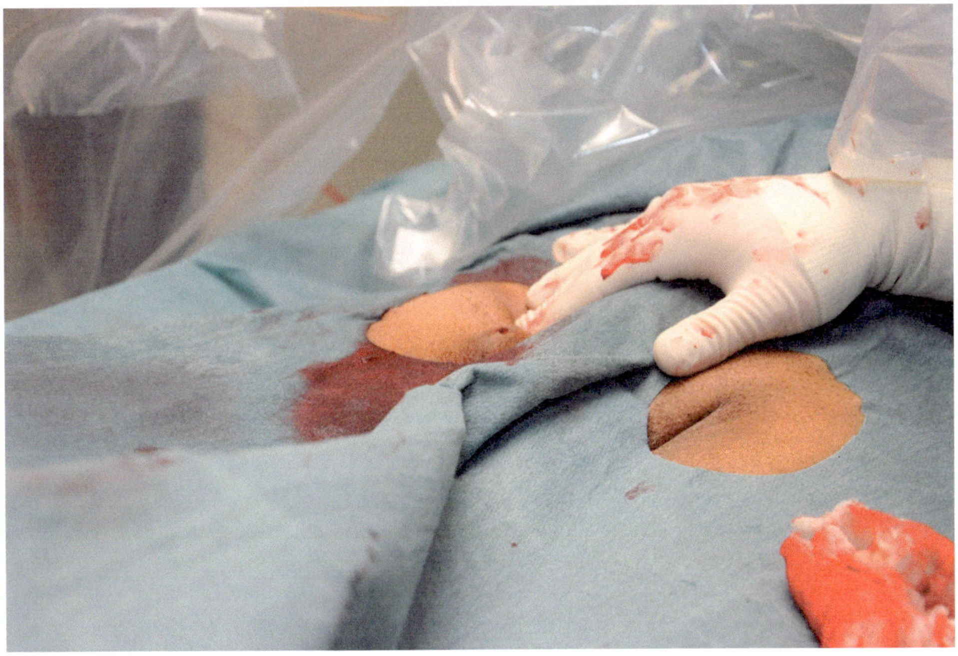

Fig. 8.26 Hemostasis is secured with light manual pressure

Hemodynamic Perspectives of Edge-to-Edge Mitral Valve Repair

9

Poay Huan Loh, Karsten Tange Veien, Oliver Gaemperli, and Roberto Corti

Abstract

Hemodynamic effects of mitral regurgitation (MR) are dependent on multiple factors including the chronicity of the regurgitation, orifice size, etiology, and loading conditions. Although the MitraClip procedure is very safe, significant hemodynamic changes can occur intraprocedurally, early and late postprocedure. Assessment and management of these hemodynamic changes can be complex, although most patients remain clinically stable throughout the procedure. This chapter reviews the hemodynamic effects of MR in the acute and chronic setting, the intra- and periprocedural effects of the MitraClip, as well as the role of various drugs used in anesthesia.

Keywords

Mitral regurgitation • MitraClip • Hemodynamics • Cardiac output • Atrial septal defect • General anesthesia

Introduction

The hemodynamic effects of mitral regurgitation (MR) are complex, and no single investigation can provide a thorough evaluation of the MR severity. This is mainly due to the fact that these hemodynamic variables can be affected by a variety of factors including the duration of mitral regurgitation, mitral regurgitant orifice, loading condition of the left ventricle, and left atrial compliance. In addition, many of the conventional measurements or methods of calculation for these variables are based on certain geometrical assumptions or physical models that are only rough approximations of the biological system. Many of these conventional theories remain the fundamental principles to the understanding of MR hemodynamics, based on which new methods have evolved. The progress in technology has also helped in the development of newer methods for assessing MR hemodynamics. Edge-to-edge mitral valve repair has posed further challenges to the assessment of hemodynamics especially in light of the fact that few published and validated data are available. This chapter gives an overview of the fundamental hemodynamic principles of MR, some relevant cardiac mechanics and mitral annular physiology, and the current understanding of double-orifice mitral valvular hemodynamics.

Adaptative Mechanisms to Mitral Regurgitation

Acute Mitral Regurgitation

The left ventricular response to MR is dependent on the time course of development and severity of the regurgitation. In

P.H. Loh, MB, BCh, BAO, MRCP(UK) (✉)
Department of Cardiology, Rigshospitalet University Hospital, Blegdamsvej 9, Copenhagen 2100, Denmark
e-mail: phloha@hotmail.com

K.T. Veien, M.D.
Department of Cardiology, Odense University Hospital, Sdr. Boulevard 29, Odense 5000, Denmark
e-mail: karsten.veien@ouh.regionsyddanmark.dk

O. Gaemperli, M.D. • R. Corti, M.D.
Department of Cardiology, University Hospital Zurich, Raemistrasse 100, Zurich CH-8091, Switzerland
e-mail: oliver.gaemperli@usz.ch; roberto.corti@usz.ch

T. Feldman et al. (eds.), *Atlas of Percutaneous Edge-to-Edge Mitral Valve Repair*, DOI 10.1007/978-1-4471-4294-2_9, © Springer-Verlag London 2013

acute and clinically relevant MR, there is an abrupt volume overload of the left ventricle (LV) leading to an increase in the left ventricular end-diastolic volume (LVEDV) and pressure (LVEDP), hence a rise in the left ventricular preload [1, 2]. More severe MR leads to a greater increase in LVEDV. However, with the constraint of a normal left ventricular compliance, the increase in LVEDV is only moderate. As there is no time for hypertrophy to develop, the increase in LVEDV is associated with LV wall thinning [1]. According to the law of Laplace, left ventricular wall tension is directly proportional to its pressure and radius but inversely proportional to its wall thickness. Therefore, the end-diastolic wall tension increases.

In acute MR, the left ventricular contractility is unchanged but the regurgitation augments the extent and rate of left ventricular emptying [3]. The LV and peak aortic systolic pressures also remain unchanged [1]. However, the LV pressure tends to reduce more rapidly during systole. As the rate of reduction in left ventricular volume and pressure increases [4] during the course of systole, the rate of decline of wall tension is accelerated. The average myocardial tension relative to an average left ventricular pressure is therefore reduced. Overall, the myocardial wall tension does not increase in acute MR [3]. This may partly explain the increase in myocardial energy requirement, or oxygen consumption is minimal despite a substantial increase in the stroke work of the left ventricle [3, 5, 6].

The Frank-Starling mechanism contributes to an increase in total stroke volume (TSV) with a reduction in left ventricular end-systolic volume (LVESV). In an experimental canine model, as the severity of acute MR increased from moderate to severe, left ventricular end-diastolic segmental length and the extent of systolic segmental shortening increased [7]. At the same time, the incompetent mitral valve allows the runoff of regurgitant stroke volume (RSV) into the lower-impedance left atrium (LA) leading to systolic unloading and lower left ventricular systolic pressure. The flow into the LA occurs throughout the systole, even during the preejection phase and after the forward flow into the aorta has stopped. These also contribute to the increase in TSV and a smaller LVESV [2]. However, much of the increase in TSV is attributed to the RSV, and the forward stroke volume (FSV) of the LV remains relatively unchanged [3].

The normal left atrium (LA) is not compliant [8, 9], and there is not enough time for the compensatory mechanisms of the left atrium to develop in acute MR. Corvisart was the first to recognize that LA does not enlarge in acute MR [10]. Hence, left atrium behaves as a poorly distensible reservoir for the regurgitant blood resulting in an abrupt increase in the left atrial pressure (LAP) [11]. This is generally reflected by a distinct *a* wave and prominent *v* wave on the LAP or pulmonary capillary wedge pressure (PCWP) tracing. In experimental canine model, LA chamber dilatation was accompanied by augmented LA muscle shortening via Frank-Starling mechanism in acute MR [7, 12]. The preload-dependent increase in LV stiffness also contributed to the increase in LAP [2]. The LA appendage began to balloon with each LV contraction [13]. As MR became severe, the LA continued to dilate to a certain extent, but the magnitude of muscle shortening was reduced markedly suggesting that the atrial myocardium was operating on the descending part of the Frank-Starling curve [7, 12]. In such setting, the use of vasodilators such as isoproterenol and nitroprusside decreased the LAP and LA diameter, restoring a more forceful atrial contraction [7].

Compared to chronic MR, the LA is smaller and less distensible in acute MR [11]. As the LA does not have time to enlarge to accommodate the regurgitant volume, it does not dampen the regurgitant pressure. Further, the pulmonary vascular resistance generally remains normal in acute MR [14, 15]. The increase in LAP is therefore transmitted retrogradely into the pulmonary artery (PA) leading to significant pulmonary hypertension [14, 15]. The systolic PA pressure waves typically have a triangular shape with a slow upslope and late peak due to the increase in right ventricular afterload [14]. In some cases, especially with severe acute MR, the *v* waves of LAP transmitted retrogradely into the PA are significantly elevated such that it is seen as a second peak in the descending part of the PA wave tracing. This gives a characteristic double-peak or "camel-back" appearance of the PA wave tracing which is not seen in chronic MR even if it was severe [14, 15] (Fig. 9.1).

The regurgitant volume across an incompetent mitral valve is related to the effective regurgitant orifice (ERO), ventricular-atrial systolic pressure gradient (VA-SPG) between the LV and LA, and the duration of ventricular systole [16, 17]. It is clear that the ERO is dynamic and the area varies under different hemodynamic conditions [18]. In experimental acute MR, volume expansion increased the RSV substantially while nitroprusside reduced the RSV without any significant change in the VA-SPG. Angiotensin increased aortic impedance and LVEDP, hence VA-SPG, leading to an increase in RSV that could only be partly explained by the raised VA-SPG. On the other hand, noradrenaline also increased aortic impedance and LVEDP with a substantial rise in LV contractility and VA-SPG but was associated with a drop in RSV [18]. These suggest that agents which increase the LV pressure or dimension can increase the ERO and hence the RSV, while agents that increase LV contractility can reduce the ERO and hence the severity of MR.

In a canine model with crushed sinoatrial nodes and a wide spectrum of MR severity, Yoran et al. elucidated the effects of heart rate on the hemodynamics of acute mitral regurgitation by LA pacing while maintaining a constant aortic pressure [19]. With increasing heart rate from 90 to

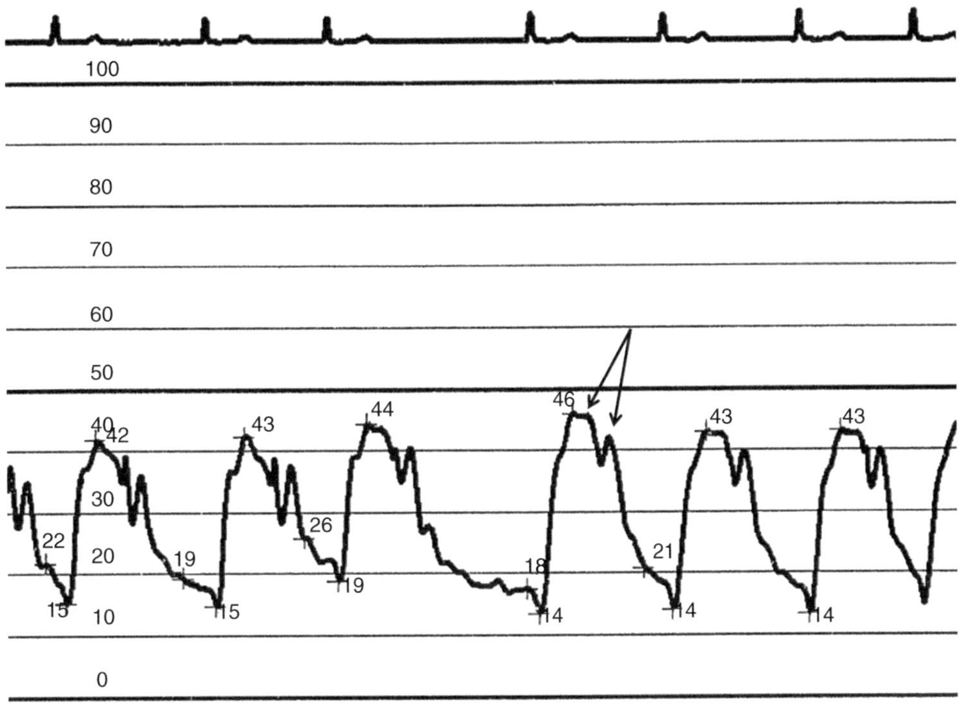

Fig. 9.1 The characteristic "double-peak" or "camel-hump" appearance of pulmonary arterial wave form in severe mitral regurgitation (*black arrow*)

180 beats/min, the LV filling volume, TSV, RSV, regurgitant time, and LVEDP decreased without any change in the total cardiac output (CO), forward CO, VA-SPG, mitral regurgitant fraction, and the regurgitant orifice. However, the LAP *v* wave amplitude was increased [19].

Acute severe MR is generally poorly tolerated. As pulmonary venous pressure becomes higher than oncotic pressure, pulmonary edema ensues. The FSV may also be significantly compromised as RSV constitutes higher proportion of the TSV. Hence, the effective cardiac output is reduced and patients will develop cardiogenic shock.

Chronic MR

Chronic MR is a progressive disease even in the absence of symptoms [20–22]. In patients with at least mild organic MR, the average rates of progression of the RSV, regurgitant fraction (RF), and ERO are 7.4 mL/year, 2.9 %/year, and 5.9 mm^2/year, respectively [23]. However, the same study found a wide variation in the progression of MR among the 74 patients with 51 % of them showing marked increase in the MR severity and 38 % remained stable, while regression in MR severity was observed in 11 % of these patients over the follow-up period of 561 ± 421 days [23]. In general, the progression of MR is characterized into three stages: compensated, transitional, and decompensated stages [2].

Compensated Stage

If acute MR can be managed medically or if the MR develops slowly over months to years, the patient will enter the chronic compensated stage of the disease. In this stage, the heart remodels in response to persistent volume overload in order to maintain adequate effective cardiac output while relieving pulmonary venous congestion.

During compensated stage of MR, the LV progressively enlarges with accompanied increases in LV wall thickness. This is achieved through LV hypertrophy and the remodeling of the extracellular matrix. The dissolution of extracellular fine collagen weave allows rearrangement and slippage of myocardial fibers such that these fibers align themselves side by side parallel to the surface of LV wall leading to chamber dilatation and eccentric hypertrophy [24, 25]. New sarcomeres are also added in series and this also contributes to LV dilatation [2]. This is in contrast to concentric hypertrophy that occurs during pressure overload where the myocardial fibers align themselves along the thickness of the LV wall leading to an increase in LV wall thickness rather than chamber dilatation [25]. The LVEDP that increases during acute MR remains the same or even decreases slightly during this stage of MR [1, 26]. In accordance to the Laplace principle, the development of eccentric hypertrophy leads to progressive reduction in the end-diastolic wall tension, but the level remains above the normal range [1].

The LV systolic pressure remains relatively stable throughout the acute and compensated phases of MR [1]. As

LV progressively enlarges so does the ESV; therefore, the systolic unloading that occurs during acute MR is also gradually replaced by normal or minimally increased systolic wall stress [27–29]. Using the recovery of LV function post-mitral valve replacement for patients with chronic severe MR to define compensated MR and failure of recovery or deterioration in LV function as decompensated MR, Zile et al. found that the LV peak systolic stress was similar in the patients with compensated and decompensated MR, but the end-systolic wall stress was higher in those with decompensated MR [30]. Corin et al. divided patients with chronic MR into those with LVEF ≥57 and <57 % and found that most of the measurements of systolic wall stress in those with LVEF ≥ 57 % were similar to or slightly higher than normal subjects with even higher measurements for the patients with LVEF < 57 % [31]. Hence, although MR seemingly provides systolic unloading through regurgitation into the lower-impedance LA, it is only in acute MR that the afterload in the LV becomes lower than normal. The afterload is normal or near normal in compensated chronic MR and increased in decompensated cases.

In experimental canine model, the percentage shortening and mean velocity of shortening of the mid-LV circumference (Vcf) corrected for a given end-diastolic dimension increased in acute MR and remained unchanged despite progressive LV dilatation during the compensated stage of MR [1]. As myocardial contractility is related to the Vcf and maximum systolic wall stress, it may be preserved throughout the compensated stage of MR in the presence of eccentric hypertrophy [29]. The length of individual sarcomere returns to normal during compensated stage of MR, and the loading conditions at each sarcomere also return to normal or near normal levels [32]. The presence of normal sarcomeric length despite progressive LV dilatation is suggestive that the enhanced myocardial function at this stage of MR is no longer depending on Frank-Starling mechanism [33]. Thus, LV dilatation is accomplished by an increase in the number of sarcomeres functioning at optimal length.

The LV also demonstrates significant regional differences in its response to chronic volume overload. The higher regional wall stress in the basal and mid-ventricular segments stimulates greater degree of hypertrophy in these regions resulting in a conical LV [34]. This is possibly an important compensatory mechanism to prevent excessive increase in diastolic LV wall stress [32]. As LV continues to dilate, its longitudinal segment length does not increase suggesting that the LV assumes a more globular geometry which may be an additional compensatory mechanism to prevent excessive wall stress [1].

Overall, the loading conditions seen in acute MR "normalize" in this compensated stage of chronic MR. Hence, the performance per unit of enlarged LV circumference is within the normal range [35]. In these patients the LVEF is often in the high normal range. As the left ventricular preload, afterload, and contractility are normal, the enhanced TSV is the result of increased LVEDV [35]. In this stage of chronic MR, the LV becomes a larger and compliant chamber that is better suited to deliver a larger stroke volume. The LA also dilates allowing the LAP to decrease. The patients may be asymptomatic and have normal exercise tolerance. Many patients with severe primary MR may remain in this stage for many years.

Transitional Stage

The transition from compensated to decompensated stage of chronic MR remains poorly understood. It has been postulated that the transition occurs as the result of an individual factor or combination of multiple factors including progressive increase in the regurgitant volume and/or chamber size, a reduction in LV contractile function, and an increase in afterload [2]. In addition, progressive remodeling of the extracellular matrix that provides structural support necessary for the maintenance of normal LV chamber geometry and for the translation of forces from individual cardiomyocytes to the LV chamber may also play a part [24]. Abnormal myocardial metabolism may also contribute to the progression into decompensated phase of chronic MR [36, 37]. Other factors implicated are loss of myofibrils [38], abnormal calcium metabolism and calcium overload in cardiomyocytes [39], and activation of the sympathetic nervous system [40].

Essentially the capacity of the compensatory mechanism is exceeded during this stage of MR and the cardiac output begins to decline. The myocardial contraction pattern remains normal but the forward cardiac output is reduced [41]. The LVEF reduces from 50 to 59 %. Most of the changes of LV in this transitional stage remain reversible following surgical treatment of the MR [2]. The decision to intervene is clear in symptomatic patients. However, some patients have little or no symptom and only become symptomatic when they have reached the decompensated stage of MR when LV dysfunction is irreversible.

Decompensated Stage

Decompensated stage of MR is characterized by substantial and progressive LV dilatation with impairment in LV contractility [2]. In a study comparing patients with isolated MR with LVEF ≥57 and <57 % to normal subjects, Corin et al. found that the LV EDP, EDV index (index to body surface area), and LV muscle mass index (index to body surface area) were elevated in patients with MR but these measurements were similar in the two groups of patient with MR [31]. Therefore, the end-diastolic stress was similar in both groups of patient with MR but higher than that in normal subjects. As discussed earlier, although the peak systolic stress may be similar in compensated and decompensated MR, the mean and end-systolic wall stress tend to be higher in those with decompensated MR [30, 31]. These suggest that although the preload may be similar, the afterload is higher in patients with decompensated than those with compensated MR.

As the impairment of LV contractility sets in, coupled with the increase in LV afterload, the LVEF, FSV, and CO are reduced [2]. As LV continues to dilate, the afterload increases and so do the impairment in LV contractility and severity of MR, perpetuating a vicious cycle that leads to the progression of the diseased state. The progression of volume overload in chronic MR was found to be mainly affected by the increase in ERO rather than the VA-SPG [23].

There are no definitive criteria to identify these three stages of MR, but rather, they are often defined according to the ability of LV function to recover after operation. However, there are relevant surrogate markers such as LV ESV and pulmonary arterial pressure which have been used in established guidelines to recommend mitral surgery [42, 43].

Assessment of LV Contractility in Chronic MR

Accurate evaluation of LV function is highly challenging as myocardial contractility is affected by the loading condition of the LV such that the contractility is inversely correlated with the afterload [27]. Therefore, the ejection or shortening phase indices of myocardial contractility such as LVEF, Vcf, and fractional shortening can be normal or elevated even in the presence of contractile abnormality [29–31, 44]. Hence, a low-normal range of ejection phase indices may reflect moderate contractile dysfunction, while moderately reduced levels are associated with more severe impairment of the LV contractility [45]. Satisfactory assessment of LV function is important in determining the timing of surgery, operative risk, and prognosis of the patients with chronic MR [28, 46]. In fact, surgical observations have raised the concern that removing the low-impedance regurgitant flow into the left atrium may abruptly increase the afterload and thereby affect LV performance resulting in an acute postoperative low-output state [4, 47–49].

The LV pressure-volume relation is one method whereby the LV function can be assessed independent of its loading condition [50]. The systolic and diastolic function indices can be derived from the end-systolic (ESPVR) and end-diastolic (EDPVR) pressure-volume relation, respectively. An established method to perform LV pressure-volume measurements is by using the conductance catheter which was first described by Baan and coworkers in the early 1980s [51]. This is based on the measurement of electrical conductance of blood within the LV cavity. The conductance method provides continuous LV volume tracings by applying a small amplitude electrical field to the LV cavity and measuring electrical conductance between a number of electrodes situated at regular intervals along a specially designed pigtail catheter (e.g., CDLeycom, Zoetermeer, the Netherlands, and Millar Instruments, Houston, USA). The segmental conductance of intracavitary blood between two electrodes reflects time-varying segmental LV volume, and total time-varying LV volume is calculated continuously by adding up all segmental signals. Using this method, the conductance catheter can be used to generate real-time pressure-volume (PV) loops and assess LV pump performance and its changes after clinical procedures that impose various hemodynamic challenges on the LV. Through the PV loop, indices of LV pump function (e.g., SV, CO, and stroke work), systolic function (ESV, ESP, EF, and peak ejection rate) and diastolic function (EDV, EDP, peak filling rate, and relaxation constant) can be determined directly. However, PV loops allow to calculate more sophisticated parameters of left ventricular contractility which are independent from LV loading conditions (Fig. 9.2). These include:

- End-systolic pressure-volume relationship (ESPVR): the ratio of end-systolic pressure over end-systolic volume
- End-systolic elastance (Ees): the slope of the ESPVR (which is extrapolated from ESPVR values by varying loading conditions, e.g., with balloon inflation in the inferior vena cava)
- Starling contractile state (SCI): +dP/dt during isovolumetric contraction phase divided by end-diastolic volume (EDV)
- Preload recruitable stroke work (PRSW): stroke work divided by EDV

Another way to characterize LV systolic function from these pressure-volume loops is by the ESV measurement at a predefined ESP [52]. Additionally, PV loops allow to calculate end-systolic and end-diastolic wall stress, a surrogate of afterload and preload, respectively. These calculations are based on the Laplace relationship which integrates simultaneous end-systolic or end-diastolic pressure and volume with LV wall thickness [53, 54].

In fact, percutaneous mitral valve repair (MVR) provides a unique pathophysiological model for assessing the hemodynamic effect of MR reduction on LV performance, eliminating any confounding effects from cardiopulmonary bypass or chordal ablation. Preliminary experiences in MitraClip cohorts with the conductance catheter suggest that despite an increase in end-systolic volume and decrease in LV ejection fraction, percutaneous edge-to-edge MVR does not negatively affect left ventricular contractility (Fig. 9.3) [55]. It is notable that, in contrast to surgical series, none of the patients

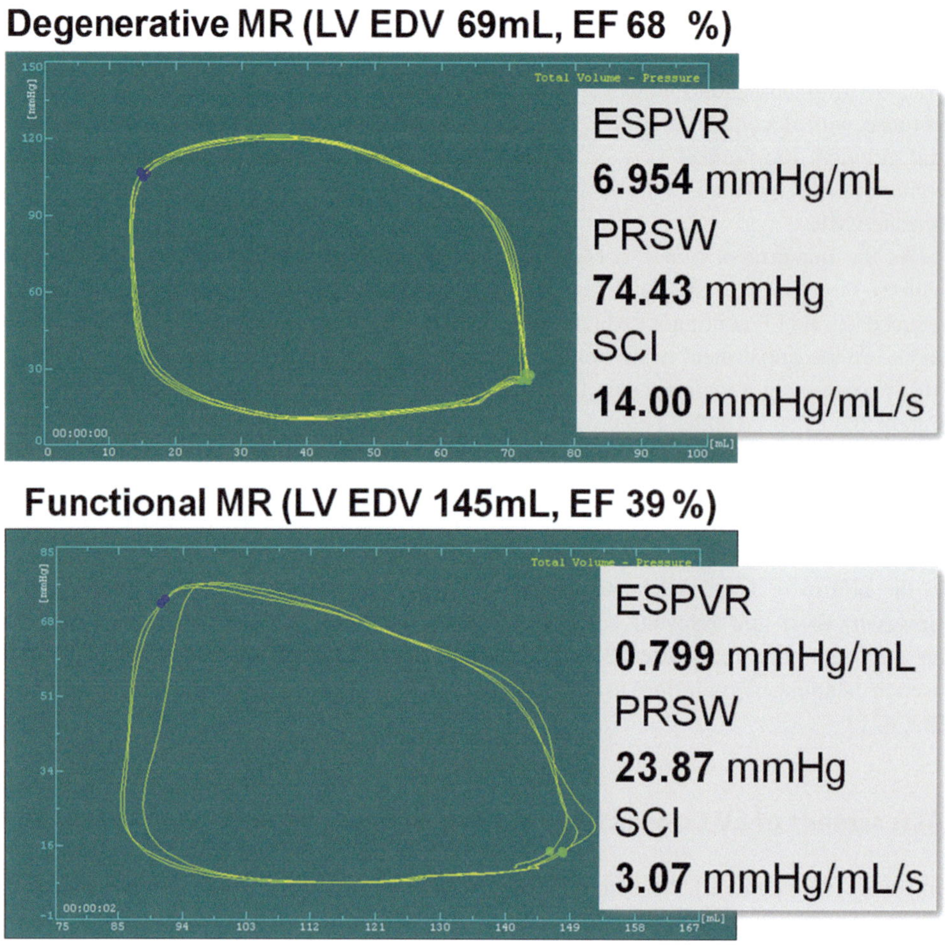

Fig. 9.2 Left ventricular pressure-volume loops in degenerative and ischemic mitral regurgitation (*MR*) using conductance catheter. (**a**) A 86-year-old lady with prolapse and flail posterior mitral leaflet and severe MR, left ventricular ejection fraction (*LVEF*) of 68 %, and an end-diastolic volume (*EDV*) of 69 mL. (**b**) A 61-year-old lady with ischemic cardiomyopathy, LVEF of 39 %, an EDV of 145 mL, and severe functional MR. A comparison of load-independent parameters of left ventricular contractility reveals higher values for end-systolic pressure volume relationship (*ESPVR*), preload-recruitable stroke work (*PRSW*), and Starling contractile index (*SCI*) in (**a**) compared to (**b**). End-systolic pressure volume point (*blue dot*); end-diastolic pressure volume point (*green dot*)

with successful MitraClip implantation experienced an acute low-output state after the procedure, which suggests that MitraClip implantation is safe even in patients with markedly compromised LV [55–57]. However, the mechanisms by which percutaneous edge-to-edge MVR may influence LV pump performance are yet to be explored and await larger investigations using PV loops.

LA Adaptation in Chronic Mitral Regurgitation

In patients with severe MR, the compliance of LA is a major determining factor of the hemodynamic and clinical picture. In general, there are three main groups of patients with severe MR and variable degree of LA compliance and pressure [9]. As mentioned earlier, there is a marked increase in LAP with relatively little LA enlargement (normal or reduced LA compliance) in acute MR leading to pulmonary congestion and/or edema. LA remodels with time leading to LA wall hypertrophy and reduced compliance. Although LA can contract more vigorously to enhance LV filling, the amplitude of *v* wave increases due to lower LA compliance. Over the next 6–12 months, significant changes occur in pulmonary vasculature leading to marked increase in pulmonary vascular resistance and pulmonary artery pressure. These changes include intimal proliferation and luminal narrowing of pulmonary veins, intimal proliferation of smaller muscular pulmonary arteries with obliteration of arteriolar branches, and intimal fibrosis and medial hypertrophy or larger muscular arteries [9].

At the other end of the spectrum is a group of patients with normal or mildly elevated LAP but grossly dilated LA due to long-standing severe MR, the syndrome of severe MR with normal LAP described by Braunwald and Awe (markedly increased LA compliance) [58]. The LA wall is thin with only small number of extremely elongated and thinned myocardial fibers surrounded by fibrous tissue [9]. Their resting pulmonary arterial pressure and vascular resistance may be normal or mildly raised. These patients almost invariably have atrial fibrillation and a low cardiac output [9]. However, the vast majority of patients will fall in between these two ends of the spectrum. They have variable degree of LA dilatation with elevated LAP (moderately increased LA compliance) [9].

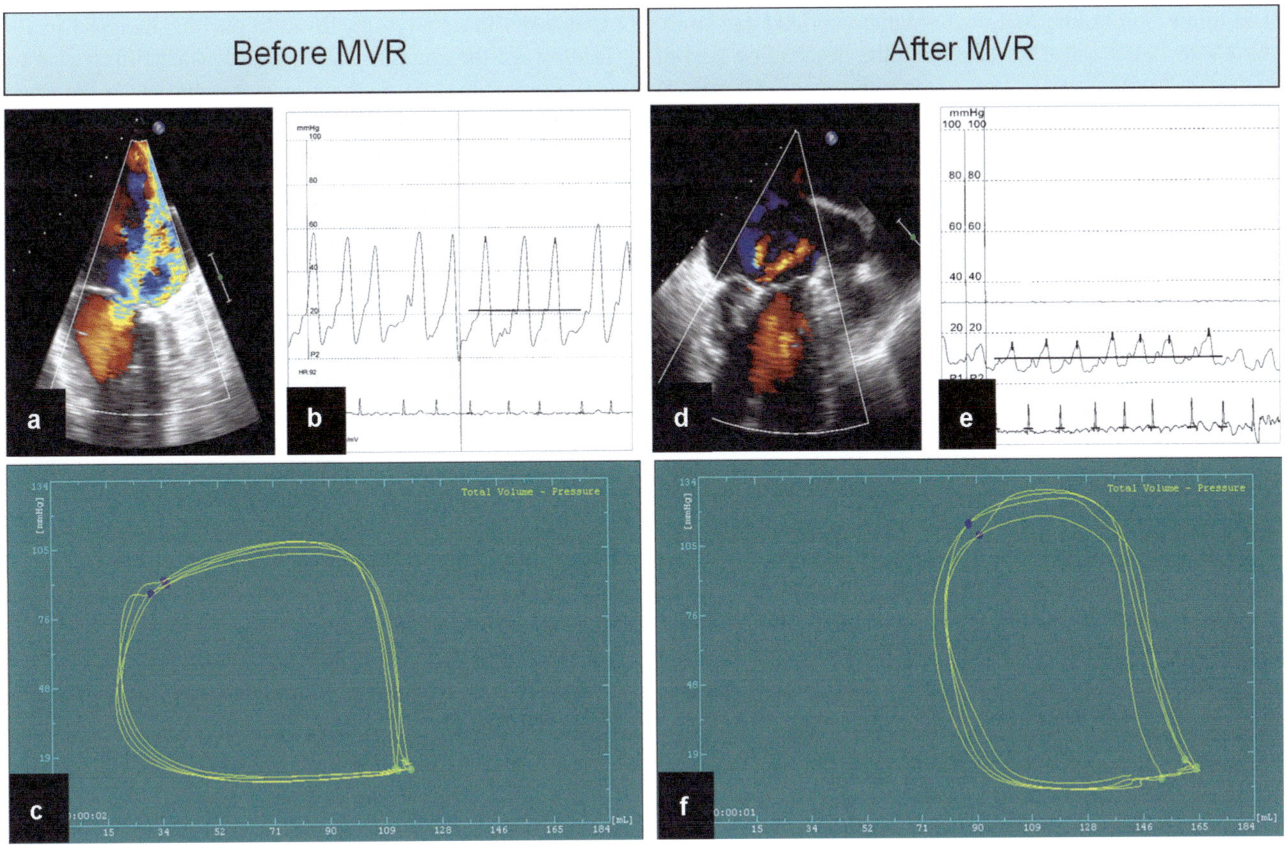

Fig. 9.3 Hemodynamic and left ventricular pump performance changes after percutaneous mitral valve repair (*MVR*) with three MitraClips in a 73-year-old man with prolapse of A3 and P3 segments of the mitral valve leaflets and severe (4+) mitral regurgitation (*MR*). Acute procedural success was documented by a reduction of MR from (4+) (**a**, *arrow*) to (1+) (**d**, *arrow*) on transesophageal echocardiography. Pressure tracings (**b**, **e**) show a reduction in mean pulmonary capillary wedge pressure (*PCWP*) from 22 to 10 mmHg. The *v* wave amplitude decreased from 54 to 17 mmHg. Similarly, the cardiac index increased from 3.6 to 4.8 L/min/m^2. Real-time pressure volume loops (**c**, **f**) (conductance catheter, CD Leycom, Zoetermeer, Netherlands) showed an upward and rightward displacement of the end-systolic pressure (*ESP*) volume point (*blue dot*) and a reduction in left ventricular ejection fraction (*LVEF*). Of note, end-diastolic pressures (*EDP*) are similar (*and at low level*) before and after MVR, indicating that the reduction in PCWP results from removal of the regurgitant burden on the pulmonary circulation rather than reduction in left ventricular filling pressure. End-diastolic pressure volume point in (*green dot*)

v Wave and Left Ventricular Pressure Curve

Hemodynamic parameters such as CO, PCWP, and *v* wave can be helpful in assessing the severity of MR. The *v* wave occurs during ventricular systole and indicates LA filling which can be antegrade filling from the pulmonary veins or regurgitant flow from the LV. In severe MR, the *v* wave amplitude is usually high but there are pitfalls. Mitral stenosis causes a high *v* wave because of antegrade flow into a LA with low compliance. In less severe MR, a high *v* wave may also be seen if the pressure in the LA is high because of ventricular septal rupture (increased flow) or congestive heart failure [59]. In heart failure patients, the LVEDP is high causing a high pressure in the LA and thus a higher *v* wave. The absolute value of the *v* wave alone cannot, therefore, be used to assess the severity of MR.

v wave and LA pressure are usually measured indirectly using PCWP. PCWP is a reliable estimation of the pressure in the LA, but there is a risk of inaccurate measurement due to artifact or inappropriately wedged catheter leading to dampened or inaccurately high curves [60].

Freihage et al. [60] compared different invasive hemodynamic factors in order to identify the factors that best corresponded to the severity of MR. In Freihage's study, 40 patients underwent transseptal cardiac catheterization under sedation while pressure in the LV and LA were measured. It was found that the ratio of the area under the *v* wave to the area under the LV systolic pressure (*v* wave/LV area) was best correlated to MR severity. With increasing MR, the area under the LA pressure–time curve increases, while the area under the LV pressure–time curve decreases. Thus, the forward or useful LV force gradually declines with prolonged duration and increasing severity of MR. In severe MR, the *v* wave occurs earlier during systole and can interfere with the *c* wave. Due to higher pressure in the LA, the LV loses more force to the LA. The LV must generate higher force causing it to dilate. In chronic MR, this volume overload can cause the LV to fail because LV works on the descending part of the Frank-Starling curve. In patients with severe MR, the LV generates a lower peak pressure and the curve under the LV decreases. As the LV gradually loses the useful forward flow, the backward flow into the LA increases. This pressure difference is taken into account by Freihage's new ratio *v* wave/LV area and is, therefore, a more useful indicator of MR severity than the *v* wave alone. In daily practice however, it is complicated to calculate this new indicator. Freihage found that PCWP did not correspond to LAP. Nevertheless, the LAP can easily be measured directly during percutaneous edge-to-edge MVR.

Although the *v* wave alone is not reliable for assessing the severity of MR, it can, in the same patient, be used together with the pressure curves in LA and LV to monitor the dynamic changes in MR during a procedure. Echocardiography is usually the standard examination used to evaluate the result of mitral repair. However, mitral valve has a double-orifice anatomy following MitraClip™ implantation and echocardiographic assessment with proximal isovelocity surface area, and vena contracta is probably invalid. In these cases, hemodynamics can be helpful in assessing the result of mitral repair [55, 61].

Double-Orifice Hemodynamics

Timely and competent mitral leaflet coaptation in the correct annular plane along their solitary zone of apposition and efficient opening to facilitate unimpeded left ventricular filling do not depend only on having a set of structurally normal mitral valvular complex. The dynamics of mitral annulus, geometrical orientation and function of subvalvular apparatus, and the left ventricular and atrial function are also essential [62].

Earlier animal studies and advance in imaging techniques have helped the understanding into mitral annular physiology. The mitral annulus is a saddle-shaped structure with two elevated segments ("peak") located at the septal and lateral aspects and two depressed segments ("trough") at the commissural ends [62, 63]. The mitral annulus is not a rigid structure. On the contrary, it maintains dynamic motion throughout the cardiac cycle [64]. In general, the mitral annular area (MAA) begins to reduce during presystolic phase, a result attributed to left LA contraction, reaching its smallest opening at end-systole before starting to increase at the onset of diastole to reach its maximum in the mid-to-end diastolic phase [63]. The reduction in MAA is mainly due to a reduction in the septolateral dimension of the annulus (reduction in interpeak distance and increase in eccentricity of the annulus) partly due to the inward movement of the septal portion of the annulus to accommodate aortic root expansion during systole. In addition, the increase in the "folding" of the annulus during systole (i.e., tilting of anterior annulus toward LA direction and reduction in the interpeak distance) also contributes to the reduction in MAA. The mitral annular plane is also displaced toward the apex by an average distance of around 1 cm during systole [63]. This conformational motion of mitral annulus ensures competent leaflet closure during systole and efficient LV filling during diastole. In normal human and based on 3D TEE and cardiac MRI studies, the maximum MAA is approximately 8–14 cm^2 and changes by 20–30 % during each cardiac cycle [65, 66].

The dynamic motion of mitral annulus can be affected by hemodynamic conditions and may be abolished by annuloplasty rings. During exercise, the increase in mitral inflow is accomplished mainly by an increase in the maximum diastolic mitral valve orifice without significant change in the velocity-time integral [67]. On the other hand, maximum diastolic MAA can be increased to a lesser extent or even reduced by inotropes when compared to exercise, but it is not altered by atrial pacing [68, 69]. Compared to normal subjects, patients with dilated cardiomyopathy and secondary MR have larger MAA and interpeak distance, more planar annular conformation, and lesser extent of MAA change (approximately 11–15 %) and basoapical displacement (approximately 0.5 cm) during each cardiac cycle [63, 65]. On the other hand, the presystolic MAA reduction is lost in atrial fibrillation and ischemia or abolished during ventricular pacing [70].

Percutaneous MVR using the MitraClip system is an effective treatment modality in selected patients with primary or secondary MR by cinching both mitral leaflets, creating a double-orifice mitral opening. How this affects the function of mitral valvular complex and its overall hemodynamic effects are not well understood. Current understanding is based on a few preliminary hemodynamic studies [55, 61], and much has to be extrapolated from experimental animal model, experience from surgical edge-to-edge mitral repair, and computer simulation model.

In a three-dimensional computational model, Maisano et al. has shown that the hemodynamic profile of a double-orifice mitral valve is similar to that of a physiological valve of the same total orifice area [71]. The transmitral velocity and pressure gradient are dependent on the total orifice area and not the configuration of the orifices. In addition, the velocities of the blood flowing through both orifices are similar regardless of the ratio of their areas [71]. Importantly, the velocity of transmitral inflow jet is at its lowest in the center of the jet and increases toward the periphery of the jet [71]. Consequently, the pressure gradient estimated using the transmitral flow velocity can differ up to 35 % depending on the position where the flow velocity is measured.

Acute Hemodynamic Effects After Percutaneous Mitral Valve Repair Using the MitraClip System

Immediately following acute MR reduction with the MitraClip system, some degree of reduction in the amplitude of *v* wave of the LAP or PCWP can often be seen on invasive hemodynamic measurement [55, 61]. The mean LAP, PCWP, pulmonary arterial pressure, and the LVEDP can decrease or remain unchanged [55, 56, 61]. Simultaneous measurement of the LV pressure allows the determination of the transmitral pressure gradient. This is particularly helpful when more than one clip is needed or in treating patients with sclerotic mitral leaflets and/or annulus. A significant rise in the transmitral gradient indicates hemodynamically important reduction in the effective mitral orifice [61]. However, in the presence of significant residual MR after clip deployment, a raised transmitral gradient may be observed without significant reduction in the effective mitral orifice. This phenomenon is due to the combination of the reduction in the effective mitral orifice and high transmitral blood flow leading to "relative mitral stenosis." On invasive hemodynamics, it is represented by a rapid upstroke of the LV pressure waveform [61]. In such cases, further reduction of MR using another clip may paradoxically ameliorate some of the transmitral gradient [61].

In the majority of patients, a reduction in MR is associated with an increase in the FSV and concomitant decrease in the systemic vascular resistance [56]. This results in an improvement in the forward cardiac output and cardiac index, in some cases, to near normal levels [55, 56, 61]. An increase in the systolic arterial pressure can also be observed, but the diastolic or mean arterial pressures remain unchanged [56].

However, anecdotal experience has suggested that in patients with severe left ventricular systolic dysfunction (LVSD), transient or persistent reduction in CO may occur following acute and substantial MR reduction (Fig. 9.4). The mechanism is unclear but likely that complex hemodynamic factors may be involved especially in those with very low LVEF [61]. The LV contractility is regulated by the Frank-Starling mechanism, force-frequency relationship, and neurohormonal control. The effectiveness of the later two mechanisms is impaired, but the Frank-Starling mechanism can be preserved even in end-stage heart failure [72]. Therefore, the maximum LV performance is achieved at much larger volumes in the failing LV than normal ones [73]. In experimental canine chronic heart failure model, a reduction of LVEDD to normal level by abrupt inferior vena cava occlusion led to further reduction in LV systolic function indicating the importance of LV preload to maintain LV systolic function in the failing hearts[74]. Therefore, an acute and significant reduction in MR may lead to a decrease in LVEDV (preload), compromising the Frank-Starling

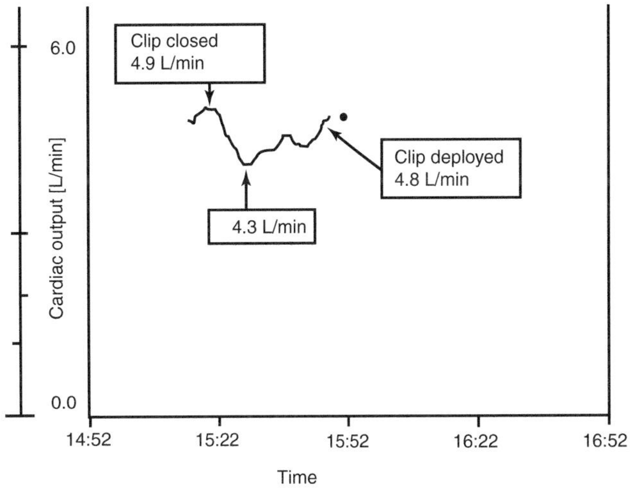

Fig. 9.4 Intraprocedural monitoring of cardiac output in a patient with poor left ventricular function. A patient with severe mitral regurgitation (*MR*) and poor left ventricular systolic function (left ventricular ejection fraction of 20 %) receiving cardiac resynchronization therapy underwent percutaneous MitraClip treatment. Upon grasping of both mitral leaflets, the MR was reduced to trace in severity (1+ or less). However, this was associated with an initial drop in the blood pressure and cardiac output measured using Swan-Ganz catheter. The patient was observed for a period of time, and the MitraClip was fully deployed only after the recovery of the blood pressure and cardiac output

compensatory mechanism and causes further deterioration in the LV systolic function. This is reminiscent of that observed in the Fontan circulation where preload is known to be the major determinant of CO especially in the presence of a dilated or impaired ventricle [75]. Another possible explanation is the poorly understood "pop-off valve" concept [76] which suggests that in patients with poor LV function, there is a need for the ventricle to off-load into the low-impedence LA. However, the improvement in the outcome of mitral valve surgery in patients with poor LV function and understanding about the importance of chordal preservation has disputed this concept [47, 77, 78]. In experimental canine model where an external LV-to-LA shunt was created to mimic the hemodynamic effects of MR, acute shunt closure led to an increase in the LV mean systolic pressure and wall stress (or afterload) [79, 80]. Closure of the shunt was associated with an improvement in the hemodynamic state with reduction in LVEDP and increased forward CO. However, in the presence of severe LVSD, LVEDP increased (or preload) despite a reduction in LV diastolic filling and the forward flow decreased [79]. The increase in LV systolic and diastolic wall stress leads to an increase in myocardial oxygen consumption, while increased LVEDP may reduce coronary blood flow leading to relative subendocardial ischemia [81]. Therefore, careful invasive hemodynamic monitoring in patients with significant LVSD during the procedure is warranted.

Longer-Term Hemodynamic Effects of MitraClip

To date, only acute hemodynamic effects of MitraClip are available as mentioned above, and all have been performed periprocedurally when the patients were under general anesthesia [55, 56]. Compared to the measurements taken in conscious nonsedated patients at a median of 19 days prior to their MitraClip procedure, most hemodynamic measurements taken during general anesthesia using propofol and remifentanil in the same patients were different. Under general anesthesia, these patients had lower mean arterial pressure, mean PAP, mean PCWP, systemic vascular resistance, and pulmonary vascular resistance but higher CO and CI [55]. Interestingly, the right atrial pressure and LVEDP were similar in conscious nonsedated state and under general anesthesia [55].

Although the longer-term hemodynamic effects of MitraClip is still unknown, reduction of MR with MitraClip leads to an early decrease in LV volumes and dimensions with associated minor decrease in LVEF which are sustained after 1 year [56, 82]. In addition, the acute changes in mean PCWP, the amplitude of the *v* wave of PCWP, and mean PAP measured intraprocedurally following clip deployment are associated with medium-term outcome including death, need for mitral surgery, and/or hospitalization for heart failure [55].

Without longer-term data, it is also unclear if the intraprocedural hemodynamic measurements correlate to longer-term hemodynamic effects of MitraClip. It is also unknown how the normal mitral annular mechanics are affected as the fibrous tissue bridge forms following the cinching of both mitral leaflets and reduction in septolateral annular dimension by MitraClip. In ovine model, the tension on the mitral leaflets exerted by Alfieri stitch during stress did not limit the annular motion in septolateral aspect and the dynamic changes in the MAA and dimensions throughout the cardiac cycle remained normal [64]. The data extrapolated from surgical edge-to-edge mitral repair are largely affected by concomitant mitral ring annuloplasty. In rare anecdotal cases where annuloplasty ring was not performed, increase in MAA associated with exercise could be observed after edge-to-edge mitral surgery although to a lesser extent when compared to a normal mitral valve [64, 83]. In the presence of concomitant ring annuloplasty, the MAA may or may not increase with exercise presumably depending on the surgical techniques and the type of ring used. There is also associated variable degree of increase in transmitral gradient and PAP during exercise [84–86]. This is a factor to be taken into consideration when treating patients using MitraClip especially in the presence of a sclerotic or calcified mitral annulus. It is reassuring that although MVA is reduced with an associated increase in transmitral gradient following MitraClip treatment, they remain stable over a period of 2 years without further reduction in the MVA or increase in the transmitral gradient [87].

Influence of Atrial Septal Puncture

Another aspect for consideration in transcatheter mitral valve intervention is whether atrial septal puncture affects the hemodynamic measurements and estimation of mitral valvular area. Based on studies of percutaneous mitral balloon valvotomy for mitral stenosis, left-to-right shunting of blood across the iatrogenic interatrial septal defect lead to an overestimation of the mitral valvular area by 12–29 % [88]. In 20 patients who had percutaneous mitral balloon valvotomy using 7F Inoue balloon catheter, Levin et al. found that balloon occlusion of the procedure-related atrial septal defect reduced cardiac output and hence the calculated mitral valvular area by 12 %. However, this difference was thought to be clinically insignificant, and all measurements, either with or without balloon occlusion of the atrial septal defect, correlated well to echocardiographic measurements [88]. The effect of a larger atrial septal defect created during MitraClip is unknown although anecdotal experience has suggested that the hemodynamic effect may also be clinically insignificant (Fig. 9.5). However, it may be reasonable to perform all postprocedural hemodynamic measurements with the MitraClip steerable guide in place.

General Anesthesia and Mitral Regurgitation

This part of the chapter will focus on how general anesthesia (GA) and blood pressure affect MR. Percutaneous mitral interventions are performed under GA partly due to the need for transesophageal echocardiogram. In such circumstances, it is important to know what and how the changes in hemodynamics will affect MR.

Anesthetic Agents

GA can alter the preload, afterload, and left ventricular contractility, all of which can affect the severity of MR. The commonly used anesthetic agents have varying influence on the hemodynamic factors. Generally, the blood pressure falls during GA thereby reducing the afterload of the LV. The agents most commonly used to induce anesthesia are sufentanil (an opioid) in combination with propofol or etomidate and fentanyl (an opioid). Sedation is often maintained by a combination of isoflurane/sevoflurane and nitrous oxide or a combination of isoflurane/sevoflurane and fentanyl.

Etomidate is often the drug of choice for anesthetizing hemodynamically compromised patient as it causes minimal

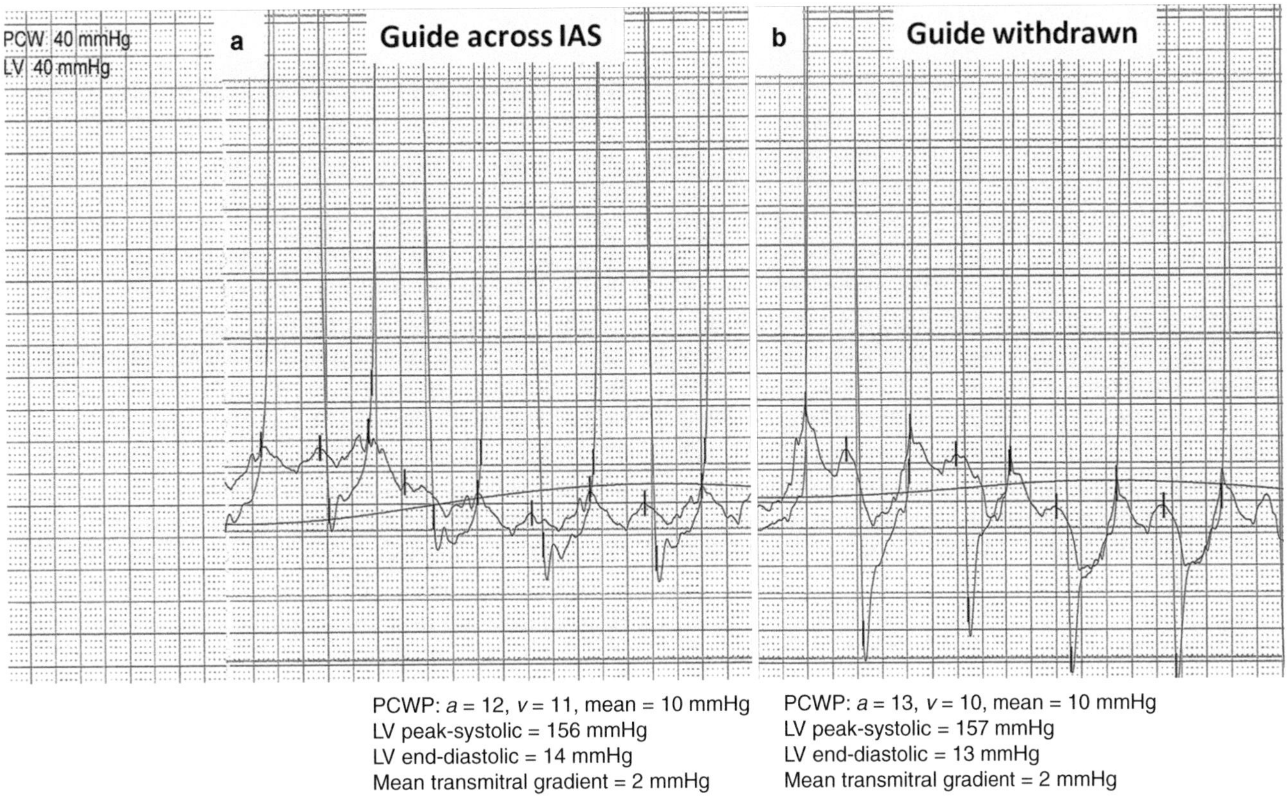

Fig. 9.5 Hemodynamic effect of interatrial septal (*IAS*) defect created for the steerable guide of MitraClip system. A 77-year-old patient with P2 prolapse and severe (4+) mitral regurgitation (*MR*) had an uncomplicated MitraClip procedure. The MR was successfully reduced to mild (1+) in severity. While the heat rate and systemic blood pressure were maintained relatively constant, the pulmonary capillary wedge pressure (*PCWP*) and mean transmitral gradient did not show any clinically relevant changes when measured (**a**) with the steerable guide kept across the IAS and (**b**) a minute after the guide was withdrawn from the IAS

cardiovascular depression. Similar to etomidate, ketamine is also a drug that can be used to induce anesthesia in high-risk patients as it maintains hemodynamic stability. Both etomidate and ketamine can only be used to induce anesthesia.

Opioids reduce sympathetic nervous system tone, respiratory depression, and analgesia. They induce a dose-dependent decrease in heart rate and arterial pressure leading to a reduction in afterload. Opioids have relatively few cardiovascular side effects and are especially valuable for patients with compromised ventricular function [89]. Due to decreased sympathetic outflow, high doses of fentanyl decrease heart rate, arterial pressure, and plasma concentrations of norepinephrine and epinephrine [90]. The combined administration of isoflurane and morphine enhances protection against myocardial infarction to a greater extent than that achieved by either drug alone [91].

Propofol is a common agent for inducing and maintaining anesthesia. It decreases sympathetic nervous tone, preload, vascular resistance (afterload), and myocardial contractility [92, 93]. The major hemodynamic consequences of propofol anesthesia in the setting of left ventricular dysfunction due to cardiomyopathy are venodilatation and LV preload reduction [94]. This results in a decrease in LVEDP and a reduction in chamber dimensions. These factors can explain why MR is reduced during anesthesia, especially with the use of propofol.

The inhaled agents, sevoflurane and isoflurane, can also be used to maintain anesthesia. Both agents are suitable for unstable patient, and they have more or less the same hemodynamic effects [95, 96]. Sevoflurane and isoflurane have a tendency to lower heart rate, blood pressure, and cardiac output without affecting LV filling pressures [95, 96].

Preload, Afterload, and Mitral Regurgitation Under General Anesthesia

Most of the agents used for anesthesia decrease preload and afterload thus reducing the severity of MR. This will increase the risk of underestimating, in particular, ischemic and functional MR if the preload and afterload are not corrected [97]. In ischemic MR, there is a tethering of the mitral leaflets secondary to papillary muscle displacement. Since GA reduces preload and afterload, there is a reduction in LV size and thereby a decrease in mitral valve tethering leading to lesser degree of MR [18, 68, 98]. The opposite can be brought on by exercise, volume overload, and severe hypertension [99]. Exercise increases functional MR because of increased preload, vascular resistance, and dilatation of the mitral annulus [100–102]. For heart failure patients, optimal medical therapy can lead to a reduction in functional MR because of lower filling pressures of the left and right heart and reduction in the dimensions of the LA, LV, and mitral annulus [103].

Under GA, the severity of MR is underestimated in approximately 50 % of the cases [98, 104]. Preload can be corrected by volume expansion. Byrne et al. [105] have suggested a provocative test with rapid transfusion of volume until the pulmonary capillary wedge pressure (PWCP) reaches 15–18 mmHg. If the MR is not reproduced, an afterload challenge can be carried out with intravenous phenylephrine until the mean arterial pressure reaches about 100 mmHg [105, 106].

Phenylephrine

Phenylephrine is a selective α_1-adrenergic receptor agonist commonly used in anesthesia or critical-care practices as a vasopressor to increase blood pressure in unstable patients with hypotension. It has the advantage of not being inotropic or chronotropic, thus elevating blood pressure without increasing heart rate or contractility. The elimination half-life of phenylephrine is about 2.5–3 h.

Following the induction of GA, systolic blood pressure often decreases by approximately 30 mmHg with associated reduction in the MR severity [99, 107]. Phenylephrine can restore the blood pressure but not the heart rate to the preanesthetic level. However, changes in heart rate have a limited effect on the degree of MR with heart rates below 150 beats/min [18, 68]. Mihalatos et al. [104] measured hemodynamic data for MR in 57 patients prior to, during, and after operation. Propofol and fentanyl were used to induce anesthesia, and isoflurane and nitrous oxide mixed with oxygen to maintain sedation. During GA, the MR severity was significantly underestimated in 47 % of the patients. The mean ERO fell from 0.59 to 0.39 cm^2 with associated reduction in the mean arterial pressure (MAP) and RSV. Phenylephrine could restore the MAP to preoperative level in 73 % of the patients. Although phenylephrine improved the accuracy of perioperative MR assessment in the majority of patients, MR was underestimated in six patients and overestimated in seven patients. The risk of overestimation of MR is higher when the blood pressure is raised above the preoperative level [99]. In patients with significant pulmonary hypertension, it may not be safe to increase afterload with phenylephrine due to the risk of pulmonary congestion [107].

Inotropes

While norepinephrine can also be used to increase blood pressure, there are fewer data on how it affects MR than on the effect of phenylephrine. In patients with chronic pulmonary hypertension, norepinephrine may be a better choice than phenylephrine as it causes less increase in pulmonary artery pressure thus preventing pulmonary edema [108]. However, inotropes such as norepinephrine and dobutamine increase LV contractility which can lead to a shrinking of the mitral annulus. In patients with dilated cardiomyopathy and functional MR, Keren et al. [109] found that dobutamine reduced MR even though the pressure gradient between the LV and LA increased. The reduction in MR was attributed to the reduction in the size of regurgitant orifice. Dobutamine reduces preload, systemic vascular resistance, and dilatation of the LV and leads to a reduction in the mitral annulus [100]. During dobutamine stress echocardiography in patients with ischemic or nonischemic cardiomyopathy, a low dose of dobutamine can improve myocardial contractility and attenuate mitral valvular tenting and functional MR [100, 110]. Dobutamine also causes an increase in the mean FSV, resulting in a decrease in MR and PCWP [109, 111].

Other inotropic agents such as adrenaline and dopamine also increase blood pressure and LV contractility, thus cause a reduction in MR [112, 113]. While milrinone, a phosphodiesterase inhibitor, has a similar cardiovascular profile to dobutamine, decreases pulmonary and systemic vascular resistance more than dobutamine [112]. The cardiovascular effects of levosimendan include increased heart rate, vasodilation, and prolonged LV contraction without any negative effect on the diastole. It can reduce secondary MR in patients with chronic heart failure [114].

When assessing MR under GA, it is recommended that phenylephrine to be used to increase the blood pressure (afterload) [18, 68, 98]. Phenylephrine does not increase the contractility of the LV and thus diminishes the risk of underestimating MR.

Hemodynamic Monitoring During Percutaneous MitraClip

Every laboratory should have an established protocol, experienced personnel, and the appropriate equipments to perform hemodynamic study and monitoring during the procedure. In addition to standard hemodynamic monitoring, other devices may help to provide instantaneous or rapid beat-to-beat hemodynamic indices. The knowledge on hemodynamic consequences of acute MR reduction by percutaneous MitraClip remains limited especially in patients with poor LV function or fragile hemodynamic state. Therefore, more robust hemodynamic monitoring may be prudent in these patients. Further, MitraClip also provides a unique setting which may help to improve understanding the effects of acute MR reduction.

As mentioned earlier, GA can affect the severity of MR making it difficult to be assessed. Awareness of patient's hemodynamic profile when assessing the severity of MR during periprocedural period is important in order to avoid inaccurate assessment. If necessary, agents such as phenylephrine may be helpful to increase the LV afterload and prevent underestimation of the severity of MR. However, care has to be taken to avoid increasing the afterload so much that the LV systolic function is compromised.

Further, the use of a pressure-conductance catheter allows a wide range of hemodynamic measurements and simultaneous assessment of LV contractility. The current commercially available Swan-Ganz catheter systems (e.g., Vigilance II and Advanced Technology Catheters, Edward Lifesciences, CA, USA) allow not only measurement of pulmonary arterial pressure and PCWP but also continuous measurement of CO, mixed venous oxygen saturation (SvO_2), EDV, systemic vascular resistance (SVR), SV, and right ventricular ejection fraction. One caveat is that the CO measurement is mainly based on thermodilution principle for practical reason. This technique may be unreliable in the presence of significant retrograde flow in the right heart (pulmonary or tricuspid regurgitation) or septal defect (atrial or ventricular). Therefore, CO measurement should be performed before the removal of the delivery guide system from the interatrial septum after the procedure. In addition, placing a pigtail catheter in the LV for simultaneous LV and LA or PCW pressure measurements will allow the assessment of transmitral gradient.

Conclusion

In transcatheter mitral valve intervention for MR, the complex interaction between various factors may affect the hemodynamic characteristics of MR and influence the assessment of its severity. Percutaneous MitraClip therapy offers a brilliant opportunity for studying the acute hemodynamic effect of MR reduction in a beating heart without confounding factors such as cardiopulmonary bypass. Further studies will help our understanding in these complex hemodynamic factors and may guide patient assessment and selection, periprocedural monitoring, and postprocedural follow-up. Current available data suggest that following the reduction in MR, percutaneous MitraClip can improve the hemodynamic profile in most of the patients, but caution should be given to those who have severe LVSD.

References

1. Lee JD, Sasayama S, Kihara Y, et al. Adaptations of the left ventricle to chronic volume overload induced by mitral regurgitation in conscious dogs. Heart Vessels. 1985;1:9–15.
2. Gaasch WH, Meyer TE. Left ventricular response to mitral regurgitation: implications for management. Circulation. 2008;118:2298–303.
3. Urschel CW, Covell JW, Sonnenblick EH, et al. Myocardial mechanics in aortic and mitral valvular regurgitation: the concept of instantaneous impedance as a determinant of the performance of the intact heart. J Clin Invest. 1968;47:867–83.
4. Leung DY, Griffin BP, Stewart WJ, et al. Left ventricular function after valve repair for chronic mitral regurgitation: predictive value of preoperative assessment of contractile reserve by exercise echocardiography. J Am Coll Cardiol. 1996;28:1198–205.
5. Evans CL, Matsuoka Y. The effect of various mechanical conditions on the gaseous metabolism and efficiency of the mammalian heart. J Physiol. 1915;49:378–405.
6. Urschel CW, Covell JW, Graham TP, et al. Effects of acute valvular regurgitation on the oxygen consumption of the canine heart. Circ Res. 1968;23:33–43.
7. Sasayama S, Takahashi M, Osakada G, et al. Dynamic geometry of the left atrium and left ventricle in acute mitral regurgitation. Circulation. 1979;60:177–86.
8. Stefanadis C, Dernellis J, Toutouzas P. A clinical appraisal of left atrial function. Eur Heart J. 2001;22:22–36.
9. Roberts WC, Braunwald E, Morrow AG. Acute severe mitral regurgitation secondary to ruptured chordae tendineae: clinical, hemodynamic, and pathologic considerations. Circulation. 1966;33:58–70.
10. Corvisart JN. An essay on the organic diseases of the heart and great vessels. Translated by Jacob Gates. Boston: Bradford & Read Co.; 1812.
11. Baxley WA, Kennedy JW, Feild B, Dodge HT. Hemodynamics in ruptured chordae tendineae and chronic rheumatic mitral regurgitation. Circulation. 1973;48:1288–94.
12. Sasayama S, Takahashi M, Kawai C. Left atrial function in acute mitral regurgitation. Factors which modify the regurgitant volume. Herz. 1981;6:156–65.
13. Haller JA, Morrow AG. Experimental mitral insufficiency. Surgery. 1955;38:518–26.
14. Friedman AW, Stein L. Pitfalls in bedside diagnosis of severe acute mitral regurgitation. Clinical and hemodynamic features. Chest. 1980;78:436–41.
15. Carley JE, Wong BY, Pugh DM, Dunn M. Clinical significance of the V wave in the main pulmonary artery. Am J Cardiol. 1977;39:982–5.
16. Gorlin R, Dexter L. Hydraulic formula for the calculation of the cross-sectional area of the mitral valve during regurgitation. Am Heart J. 1952;43:188–205.
17. Silverman ME, Hurst JW. The mitral complex. Interaction of the anatomy, physiology, and pathology of the mitral annulus, mitral valve leaflets, chordae tendineae, and papillary muscles. Am Heart J. 1968;76:399–418.
18. Yoran C, Yellin EL, Becker RM, et al. Dynamic aspects of acute mitral regurgitation: effects of ventricular volume, pressure and contractility on the effective regurgitant orifice area. Circulation. 1979;60:170–6.
19. Yoran C, Yellin EL, Hori M, et al. Effects of heart rate on experimentally produced mitral regurgitation in dogs. Am J Cardiol. 1983;52:1345–9.
20. Rosen SE, Borer JS, Hochreiter C, et al. Natural history of the asymptomatic/minimally symptomatic patient with severe mitral regurgitation secondary to mitral valve prolapse and normal

right and left ventricular performance. Am J Cardiol. 1994;74: 374–80.
21. Ling LH, Enriquez-Sarano M, Seward JB, et al. Clinical outcome of mitral regurgitation due to flail leaflet. N Engl J Med. 1996;335: 1417–23.
22. Enriquez-Sarano M, Tajik AJ. Natural history of mitral regurgitation due to flail leaflets. Eur Heart J. 1997;18:705–7.
23. Enriquez-Sarano M, Basmadjian AJ, Rossi A, et al. Progression of mitral regurgitation: a prospective Doppler echocardiographic study. J Am Coll Cardiol. 1999;34:1137–44.
24. Caulfield JB, Wolkowicz PE. Myocardial connective tissue alteration. Toxicol Pathol. 1990;18:488–96.
25. Tezuka F. Morphometric analysis of cardiac hypertrophy: left ventricular shape and number of muscle-fiber layers across left ventricular wall. Tohoku J Exp Med. 1982;138:1–6.
26. Zile MR, Tomita M, Nakano K, et al. Effects of left ventricular volume overload produced by mitral regurgitation on diastolic function. Am J Physiol. 1991;261:H1471–80.
27. Wisenbaugh T, Spann JF, Carabello BA. Differences in myocardial performance and load between patients with similar amounts of chronic aortic versus chronic mitral regurgitation. J Am Coll Cardiol. 1984;3:916–23.
28. Gaasch WH, Zile MR. Left ventricular function after surgical correction of chronic mitral regurgitation. Eur Heart J. 1991;12 (Suppl B):48–51.
29. Eckberg DL, Gault JH, Bouchard RL, et al. Mechanics of left ventricular contraction in chronic severe mitral regurgitation. Circulation. 1973;47:1252–9.
30. Zile MR, Gaasch WH, Levine HJ. Left ventricular stress-dimension-shortening relations before and after correction of chronic aortic and mitral regurgitation. Am J Cardiol. 1985;56:99–105.
31. Corin WJ, Monrad ES, Murakami T, et al. The relationship of afterload to ejection performance in chronic mitral regurgitation. Circulation. 1987;76:59–67.
32. Ross Jr J, Sonnenblick EH, Taylor RR, et al. Diastolic geometry and sarcomere lengths in the chronically dilated canine left ventricle. Circ Res. 1971;28:49–61.
33. Ross Jr J, McCullagh WH. Nature of enhanced performance of the dilated left ventricle in the dog during chronic volume overloading. Circ Res. 1972;30:549–56.
34. Badke FR, Covell JW. Early changes in left ventricular regional dimensions and function during chronic volume overloading in the conscious dog. Circ Res. 1979;45:420–8.
35. Ross Jr J. Adaptations of the left ventricle to chronic volume overload. Circ Res. 1974;35(suppl II):64–70.
36. Natarajan G, Nakhjavan FK, Kahn D, et al. Myocardial metabolic studies in prolapsing mitral leaflet syndrome. Circulation. 1975;52: 1105–10.
37. Conway MA, Bottomley PA, Ouwerkerk R, et al. Mitral regurgitation: impaired systolic function, eccentric hypertrophy, and increased severity are linked to lower phosphocreatine/ATP ratios in humans. Circulation. 1998;97:1716–23.
38. Urabe Y, Mann DL, Kent RL, et al. Cellular and ventricular contractile dysfunction in experimental canine mitral regurgitation. Circ Res. 1992;70:131–47.
39. Mulieri LA, Leavitt BJ, Martin BJ, et al. Myocardial force-frequency defect in mitral regurgitation heart failure is reversed by forskolin. Circulation. 1993;88:2700–4.
40. Mehta RH, Supiano MA, Oral H, et al. Relation of systemic sympathetic nervous system activation to echocardiographic left ventricular size and performance and its implications in patients with mitral regurgitation. Am J Cardiol. 2000;86:1193–7.
41. Rosenblatt A, Clark R, Burgess J, Cohn K. Echocardiographic assessment of the level of cardiac compensation in valvular heart disease. Circulation. 1976;54:509–18.
42. Bonow RO, Carabello BA, Chatterjee K, et al. 2008 Focused update incorporated into the ACC/AHA 2006 guidelines for the management of patients with valvular heart disease: a report of the American College of Cardiology/American Heart Association Task Force on Practice Guidelines (Writing committee to Revise the 1998 Guidelines for the Management of Patients With Valvular Heart Disease): Developed in collaboration with the Society of cardiovascular Anesthesiologists: endorsed by the Society for Cardiovascular Angiography and Interventions and the Society of Thoracic Surgeons. Circulation. 2008;118:e523–661.
43. Vahanian A, Baumgartner H, Bax J, et al. Guidelines on the management of valvular heart disease: The Task Force on the Management of Valvular Heart Disease of the European Society of Cardiology. Eur Heart J. 2007;28:230–68.
44. Berko B, Gaasch WH, Tanigawa N, et al. Disparity between ejection and end-systolic indexes of left ventricular contractility in mitral regurgitation. Circulation. 1987;75:1310–9.
45. Wisenbaugh T. Does normal pump function belie muscle dysfunction in patients with chronic severe mitral regurgitation? Circulation. 1988;77:515–25.
46. Enriquez-Sarano M, Tajik AJ, Schaff HV, et al. Echocardiographic prediction of survival after surgical correction of organic mitral regurgitation. Circulation. 1994;90:830–7.
47. Rozich JD, Carabello BA, Usher BW, et al. Mitral valve replacement with and without chordal preservation in patients with chronic mitral regurgitation. Mechanisms for differences in postoperative ejection performance. Circulation. 1992;86:1718–26.
48. Enriquez-Sarano M, Tajik AJ, Schaff HV, et al. Echocardiographic prediction of left ventricular function after correction of mitral regurgitation: results and clinical implications. J Am Coll Cardiol. 1994;24:1536–43.
49. Crawford MH, Souchek J, Oprian CA, et al. Determinants of survival and left ventricular performance after mitral valve replacement. Department of Veterans Affairs Cooperative Study on Valvular Heart Disease. Circulation. 1990;81:1173–81.
50. Sagawa K. The end-systolic pressure-volume relation of the ventricle: definition, modifications and clinical use. Circulation. 1981; 63:1223–7.
51. Baan J, van der Velde ET, de Bruin HG, et al. Continuous measurement of left ventricular volume in animals and humans by conductance catheter. Circulation. 1984;70:812–23.
52. van der Velde ET, Burkhoff D, Steendijk P, et al. Nonlinearity and load sensitivity of end-systolic pressure-volume relation of canine left ventricle in vivo. Circulation. 1991;83:315–27.
53. Schreuder JJ, Steendijk P, van der Veen FH, et al. Acute and short-term effects of partial left ventriculectomy in dilated cardiomyopathy: assessment by pressure-volume loops. J Am Coll Cardiol. 2000;36:2104–14.
54. Devereux RB, Alonso DR, Lutas EM, et al. Echocardiographic assessment of left ventricular hypertrophy: comparison to necropsy findings. Am J Cardiol. 1986;57:450–8.
55. Gaemperli O, Moccetti M, Surder D, et al. Acute haemodynamic changes after percutaneous mitral valve repair: relation to mid-term outcomes. Heart. 2012;98:126–32.
56. Siegel R, Biner S, Rafique AM, et al. The acute hemodynamic effects of MitraClip therapy. J Am Coll Cardiol. 2011;57:1658–65.
57. Franzen O, van der Heyden J, Baldus S, et al. MitraClip(R) therapy in patients with end-stage systolic heart failure. Eur J Heart Fail. 2011;13:569–76.
58. Braunwald E, Awe WC. The syndrome of severe mitral regurgitation with normal left atrial pressure. Circulation. 1963;27:29–35.
59. Kageji Y, Oki T, Iuchi A, et al. Relationship between pulmonary capillary wedge V wave and transmitral and pulmonary venous flow velocity patterns in various heart diseases. J Card Fail. 1996;2:215–22.

60. Freihage JH, Joyal D, Arab D, et al. Invasive assessment of mitral regurgitation: comparison of hemodynamic parameters. Catheter Cardiovasc Interv. 2007;69:303–12.
61. Jilaihawi H, Makkar R, Hussaini A, et al. Contemporary application of cardiovascular hemodynamics: transcatheter mitral valve interventions. Cardiol Clin. 2011;29:201–9.
62. Van Mieghem NM, Piazza N, Anderson RH, et al. Anatomy of the mitral valvular complex and its implications for transcatheter interventions for mitral regurgitation. J Am Coll Cardiol. 2010;56:617–26.
63. Kaplan SR, Bashein G, Sheehan FH, et al. Three-dimensional echocardiographic assessment of annular shape changes in the normal and regurgitant mitral valve. Am Heart J. 2000;139:378–87.
64. Timek TA, Miller DC. Experimental and clinical assessment of mitral annular area and dynamics: what are we actually measuring? Ann Thorac Surg. 2001;72:966–74.
65. Flachskampf FA, Chandra S, Gaddipatti A, et al. Analysis of shape and motion of the mitral annulus in subjects with and without cardiomyopathy by echocardiographic 3-dimensional reconstruction. J Am Soc Echocardiogr. 2000;13:277–87.
66. Komoda T, Hetzer R, Uyama C, et al. Mitral annular function assessed by 3D imaging for mitral valve surgery. J Heart Valve Dis. 1994;3:483–90.
67. Rassi Jr A, Crawford MH, Richards KL, Miller JF. Differing mechanisms of exercise flow augmentation at the mitral and aortic valves. Circulation. 1988;77:543–51.
68. Gorman 3rd JH, Jackson BM, Moainie SL, et al. Influence of inotropy and chronotropy on the mitral valve sphincter mechanism. Ann Thorac Surg. 2004;77:852–7; discussion 857–58.
69. Hecker SL, Zabalgoitia M, Ashline P, et al. Comparison of exercise and dobutamine stress echocardiography in assessing mitral stenosis. Am J Cardiol. 1997;80:1374–7.
70. Glasson JR, Komeda M, Daughters GT, et al. Most ovine mitral annular 3-D size reduction occurs before ventricular systole and is abolished with ventricular pacing. Circulation. 1997;96:II-115–23.
71. Maisano F, Vigano G, Blasio A, et al. Surgical isolated edge-to-edge mitral valve repair without annuloplasty: clinical proof of the principle for an endovascular approach. EuroIntervention. 2006; 2:181–6.
72. Weil J, Eschenhagen T, Hirt S, et al. Preserved Frank-Starling mechanism in human end stage heart failure. Cardiovasc Res. 1998;37:541–8.
73. Holubarsch C, Ruf T, Goldstein DJ, et al. Existence of the Frank-Starling mechanism in the failing human heart. Investigations on the organ, tissue, and sarcomere levels. Circulation. 1996;94:683–9.
74. Gill RM, Jones BD, Corbly AK, et al. Exhaustion of the Frank-Starling mechanism in conscious dogs with heart failure induced by chronic coronary microembolization. Life Sci. 2006;79:536–44.
75. Gewillig M, Brown SC, Eyskens B, et al. The Fontan circulation: who controls cardiac output? Interact Cardiovasc Thorac Surg. 2010;10:428–33.
76. Kirklin J. Replacement of mitral valve for mitral incompetence. Surgery. 1972;72:827–36.
77. Acker MA. Should moderate or greater mitral regurgitation be repaired in all patients with LVEF <30%? Mitral valve repair in patients with advanced heart failure and severe functional mitral insufficiency reverses left ventricular remodeling and improves symptoms. Circ Heart Fail. 2008;1:281–4.
78. Yun KL, Rayhill SC, Niczyporuk MA, et al. Mitral valve replacement in dilated canine hearts with chronic mitral regurgitation. Importance of the mitral subvalvular apparatus. Circulation. 1991;84:III112–24.
79. Rankin JS, Nicholas LM, Kouchoukos NT. Experimental mitral regurgitation: effects on left ventricular function before and after elimination of chronic regurgitation in the dog. J Thorac Cardiovasc Surg. 1975;70:478–88.
80. Spratt JA, Olsen CO, Tyson Jr GS, et al. Experimental mitral regurgitation. Physiological effects of correction on left ventricular dynamics. J Thorac Cardiovasc Surg. 1983;86:479–89.
81. Buckberg GD, Fixler DE, Archie JP, Hoffman JI. Experimental subendocardial ischemia in dogs with normal coronary arteries. Circ Res. 1972;30:67–81.
82. Feldman T, Foster E, Glower DG, et al. Percutaneous repair or surgery for mitral regurgitation. N Engl J Med. 2011;364: 1395–406.
83. Umana JP, Salehizadeh B, DeRose Jr JJ, et al. "Bow-tie" mitral valve repair: an adjuvant technique for ischemic mitral regurgitation. Ann Thorac Surg. 1998;66:1640–6.
84. Hori H, Fukunaga S, Arinaga K, et al. Edge-to-edge repair for mitral regurgitation: a clinical and exercise echocardiographic study. J Heart Valve Dis. 2008;17:476–84.
85. Agricola E, Maisano F, Oppizzi M, et al. Mitral valve reserve in double-orifice technique: an exercise echocardiographic study. J Heart Valve Dis. 2002;11:637–43.
86. Borghetti V, Campana M, Scotti C, et al. Preliminary observations on haemodynamics during physiological stress conditions following 'double-orifice' mitral valve repair. Eur J Cardiothorac Surg. 2001;20:262–8; discussion 268–9.
87. Herrmann HC, Kar S, Siegel R, et al. Effect of percutaneous mitral repair with the MitraClip device on mitral valve area and gradient. EuroIntervention. 2009;4:437–42.
88. Levin TN, Feldman T, Carroll JD. Effect of atrial septal occlusion on mitral area after Inoue balloon valvotomy. Cathet Cardiovasc Diagn. 1994;33:308–14.
89. Bovill JG. Intravenous anesthesia for the patient with left ventricular dysfunction. Semin Cardiothorac Vasc Anesth. 2006;10: 43–8.
90. Taneyama C, Goto H, Kohno N, et al. Effects of fentanyl, diazepam, and the combination of both on arterial baroreflex and sympathetic nerve activity in intact and baro-denervated dogs. Anesth Analg. 1993;77:44–8.
91. Ludwig LM, Patel HH, Gross GJ, et al. Morphine enhances pharmacological preconditioning by isoflurane: role of mitochondrial K(ATP) channels and opioid receptors. Anesthesiology. 2003;98:705–11.
92. Pagel PS, Hettrick DA, Kersten JR, et al. Cardiovascular effects of propofol in dogs with dilated cardiomyopathy. Anesthesiology. 1998;88:180–9.
93. Gelissen HP, Epema AH, Henning RH, et al. Inotropic effects of propofol, thiopental, midazolam, etomidate, and ketamine on isolated human atrial muscle. Anesthesiology. 1996;84: 397–403.
94. Lowe D, Hettrick DA, Pagel PS, Warltier DC. Propofol alters left ventricular afterload as evaluated by aortic input impedance in dogs. Anesthesiology. 1996;84:368–76.
95. Bennett SR, Griffin SC. Sevoflurane versus isoflurane in patients undergoing coronary artery bypass grafting: a hemodynamic and recovery study. J Cardiothorac Vasc Anesth. 1999;13:666–72.
96. Bennett SR, Griffin SC. Sevoflurane versus isoflurane in patients undergoing valvular cardiac surgery. J Cardiothorac Vasc Anesth. 2001;15:175–8.
97. Bach DS, Deeb GM, Bolling SF. Accuracy of intraoperative transesophageal echocardiography for estimating the severity of functional mitral regurgitation. Am J Cardiol. 1995;76: 508–12.
98. Grewal KS, Malkowski MJ, Piracha AR, et al. Effect of general anesthesia on the severity of mitral regurgitation by transesophageal echocardiography. Am J Cardiol. 2000;85: 199–203.
99. Shiran A, Merdler A, Ismir E, et al. Intraoperative transesophageal echocardiography using a quantitative dynamic loading test for

the evaluation of ischemic mitral regurgitation. J Am Soc Echocardiogr. 2007;20:690–7.
100. Tatsumi K, Kawai H, Sugiyama D, et al. Dobutamine-induced improvement in inferior myocardial contractile function predicts reduction in functional mitral regurgitation: a study using tissue Doppler strain rate imaging. Circ Cardiovasc Imaging. 2010;3: 638–46.
101. Lapu-Bula R, Robert A, Van Craeynest D, et al. Contribution of exercise-induced mitral regurgitation to exercise stroke volume and exercise capacity in patients with left ventricular systolic dysfunction. Circulation. 2002;106:1342–8.
102. Lancellotti P, Lebrun F, Pierard LA. Determinants of exercise-induced changes in mitral regurgitation in patients with coronary artery disease and left ventricular dysfunction. J Am Coll Cardiol. 2003;42:1921–8.
103. Rosario LB, Stevenson LW, Solomon SD, et al. The mechanism of decrease in dynamic mitral regurgitation during heart failure treatment: importance of reduction in the regurgitant orifice size. J Am Coll Cardiol. 1998;32:1819–24.
104. Mihalatos DG, Gopal AS, Kates R, et al. Intraoperative assessment of mitral regurgitation: role of phenylephrine challenge. J Am Soc Echocardiogr. 2006;19:1158–64.
105. Byrne JG, Aklog L, Adams DH. Assessment and management of functional or ischaemic mitral regurgitation. Lancet. 2000;355: 1743–4.
106. Dion R, Benetis R, Elias B, et al. Mitral valve procedures in ischemic regurgitation. J Heart Valve Dis. 1995;4 Suppl 2:S124–9; discussion S129-131.
107. Konstadt SN, Louie EK, Shore-Lesserson L, et al. The effects of loading changes on intraoperative Doppler assessment of mitral regurgitation. J Cardiothorac Vasc Anesth. 1994;8:19–23.
108. Kwak YL, Lee CS, Park YH, Hong YW. The effect of phenylephrine and norepinephrine in patients with chronic pulmonary hypertension. Anaesthesia. 2002;57:9–14.
109. Keren G, Laniado S, Sonnenblick EH, Lejemtel TH. Dynamics of functional mitral regurgitation during dobutamine therapy in patients with severe congestive heart failure: a Doppler echocardiographic study. Am Heart J. 1989;118:748–54.
110. Abe Y, Imai T, Ohue K, et al. Relation between reduction in ischaemic mitral regurgitation and improvement in regional left ventricular contractility during low dose dobutamine stress echocardiography. Heart. 2005;91:1092–3.
111. Keren G, Katz S, Strom J, et al. Dynamic mitral regurgitation. An important determinant of the hemodynamic response to load alterations and inotropic therapy in severe heart failure. Circulation. 1989;80:306–13.
112. El-Tahan MR. Preoperative ephedrine counters hypotension with propofol anesthesia during valve surgery: a dose dependent study. Ann Card Anaesth. 2011;14:30–40.
113. Bangash MN, Kong ML, Pearse RM. Use of inotropes and vasopressor agents in critically ill patients. Br J Pharmacol. 2012;165:2015–33.
114. Branzi G, Malfatto G, Villani A, et al. Acute effects of levosimendan on mitral regurgitation and diastolic function in patients with advanced chronic heart failure. J Cardiovasc Med (Hagerstown). 2010;11:662–8.

Situational Steering Techniques

10

Gretchen T. Gary and Olaf Franzen

Abstract

In situations where there is suboptimal positioning of the transseptal puncture or where anatomic factors complicate positioning of the MitraClip, advanced techniques may be required to successfully perform the procedure. These situational steering techniques rely on understanding how the various controls of the MitraClip Guide and Clip Delivery System work. In this chapter, the three most common and important situational steering scenarios are described. These include (1) inadequate height, (2) excessive height, and (3) aorta "hugger."

Keywords

Situational steering • Height • MitraClip

In order to successfully perform a MitraClip mitral valve repair, the MitraClip must first be delivered to the mitral valve at the area of greatest regurgitation. The initial MitraClip system positioning goals are (1) to position the MitraClip Device (Clip) centrally over the valve with respect to anterior-posterior and medial-lateral directions; (2) align the Clip so the Delivery Catheter shaft is perpendicular to the plane of the mitral valve; and (3) position the distal tip of the Clip at least 1 cm above the leaflets in order to achieve successful and adequate grasping of the mitral leaflets. Optimal steering and positioning of the Guide Catheter (Guide) and Clip Delivery System (CDS) can be influenced by the location of the transseptal puncture, the distance the guide tip is extended into the LA, and anatomical variations. A TEE-guided transseptal puncture should be performed relatively "high" and posterior in the fossa ovalis. Height above the mitral annulus (the ideal height from the annulus should be 3.5–4.0 cm) is necessary in order to achieve adequate working space for Delivery Catheter manipulations, Clip actuation, and Clip retraction during grasping.

The transseptal puncture should be optimally positioned more posterior from an anteroposterior perspective in the short axis at the base of the heart TEE view in order to enable Guide tip positioning near the line of leaflet coaptation (away from the aorta) and to allow torquing of the Guide Catheter both clockwise (posterior) and counterclockwise (anterior). If the transseptal puncture is placed too "low" in the fossa, the MitraClip Device may come to lie just above and too close to the mitral annular plane, and subsequent orientation of the CDS to position the clip appropriately and to grasp the leaflets may not be possible because of inadequate space in the LA above the annular plane. However, too much height above the valve may exceed the length of

G.T. Gary, B.A. (✉)
Department of Global Training,
Abbott Vascular Structural Heart,
4045 Campbell Avenue, Menlo Park, CA 94025, USA
e-mail: gretchen.gary@av.abbott.com

O. Franzen, M.D.
Department of Cardiology,
The Heart Center, Rigshospitalet, University of Copenhagen,
Blegdamsvej 9, Copenhagen 2100, Denmark

Royal Brompton Hospital, Royal Brompton
and Harefield NHS Foundation Trust, London, UK
e-mail: owfranzen@gmx.de

T. Feldman et al. (eds.), *Atlas of Percutaneous Edge-to-Edge Mitral Valve Repair*,
DOI 10.1007/978-1-4471-4294-2_10, © Springer-Verlag London 2013

Delivery Catheter available to advance the Clip into the LV far enough below the free edges of the leaflets to adequately grasp. An anterior transseptal position or an extreme medial Guide tip position in the LA may result in the base of the Delivery Catheter residing too anterior causing the Clip to approach the mitral valve plane with a posteriorly directed path that is adjacent and parallel to the aorta (an aorta "hugger").

These three scenarios, (1) insufficient height, (2) excessive height, and (3) aorta "hugger," are the most common and most important of the situational steering scenarios during a MitraClip procedure. If initial MitraClip system positioning maneuvers fail to align the Clip so the Delivery Catheter shaft is perpendicular to the plane of the mitral valve and fail to position the clip at the appropriate distance above the leaflets, then advanced situational steering techniques to increase height, decrease height, and/or optimize Delivery Catheter perpendicularity to the mitral valve plane will need to be employed. In the following sections, we review the steps employed to manage each of these scenarios.

How to Increase Height Above the Mitral Valve Plane

Fig. 10.1 Situation: Inadequate height above the mitral valve plane. The Clip has been steered down perpendicular to the mitral valve opening with respect to anterior-posterior and medial-lateral directions. However, the MitraClip Device has come to lie too close to the mitral annular plane and the Delivery Catheter radiopaque ring is fully retracted against the Sleeve radiopaque tip ring. Achieving additional height above the valve in order to adequately tension the leaflets during a grasp is not possible in this situation

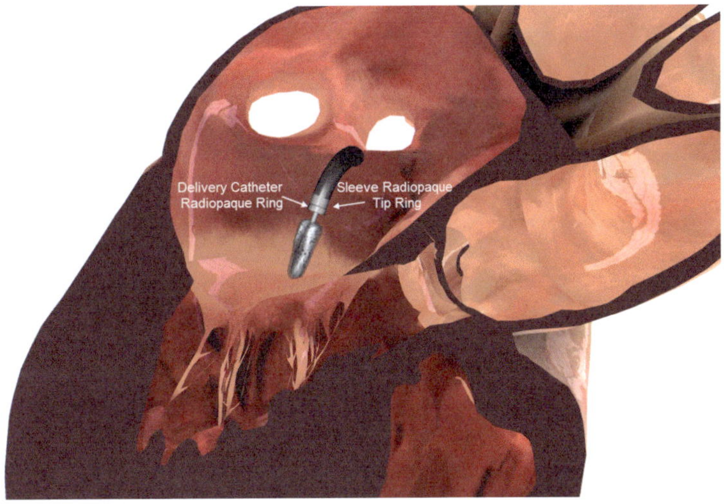

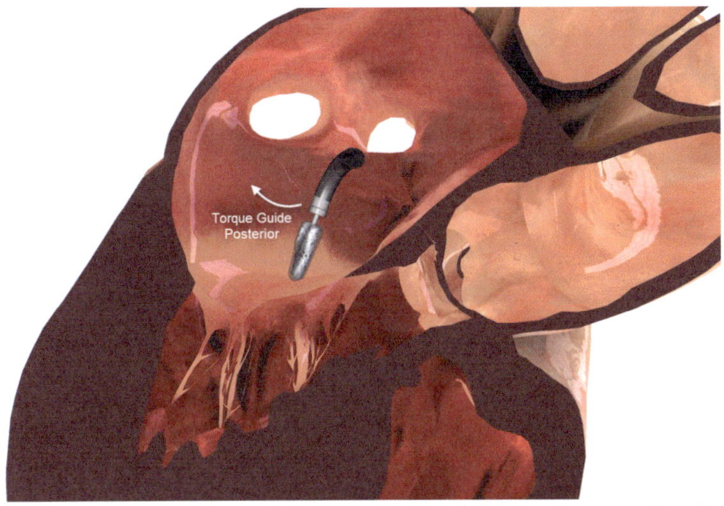

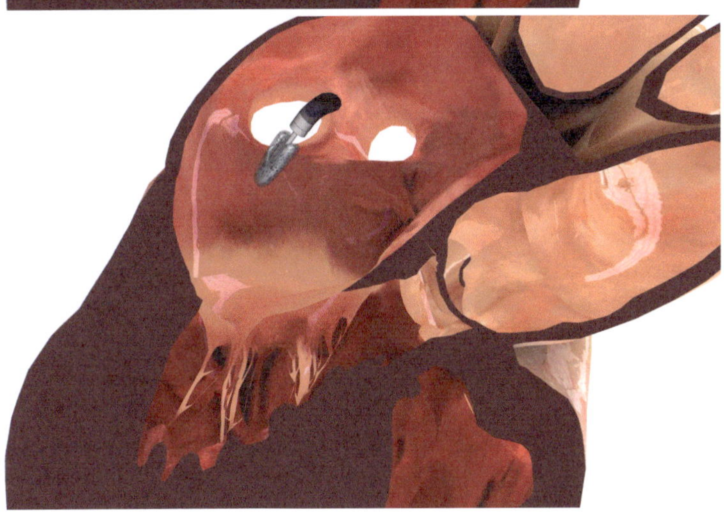

Fig. 10.2 To increase height. Torque the Guide handle posterior (clockwise) until the Clip is pointing at the posterior annulus. This will cause a change in height above the annulus but will affect the anterior-posterior position

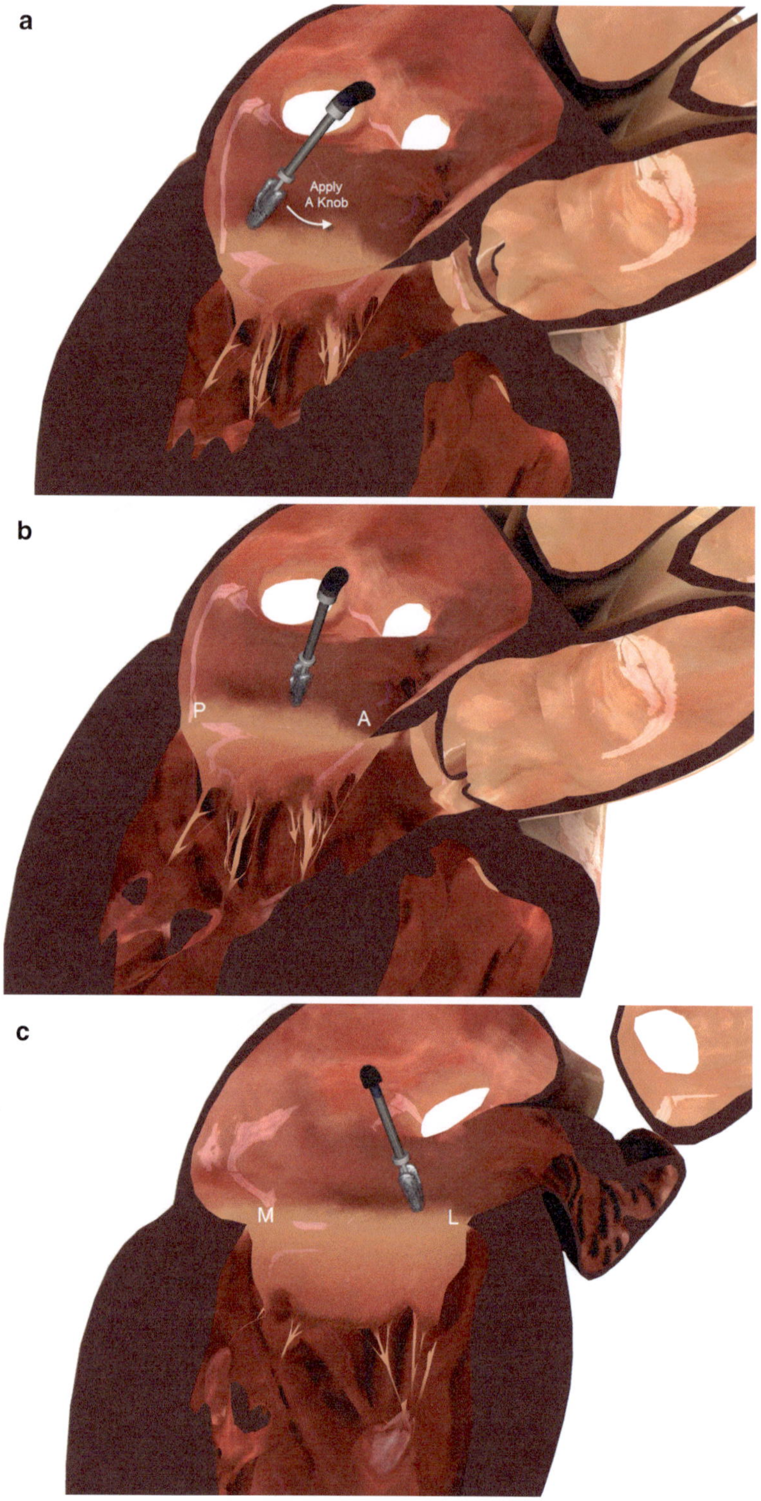

Fig. 10.3 Making an anterior adjustment. A knob is applied to compensate anterior while maintaining height (**a**). The Delivery Catheter moves toward the center of the valve from an anterior-posterior (A/P) perspective (**b**). However, applying A knob reduces the effect of M knob which releases some medial curvature thus resulting in the Delivery Catheter pointing lateral. It is necessary to verify alignment in the alternate long axis view (**c**)

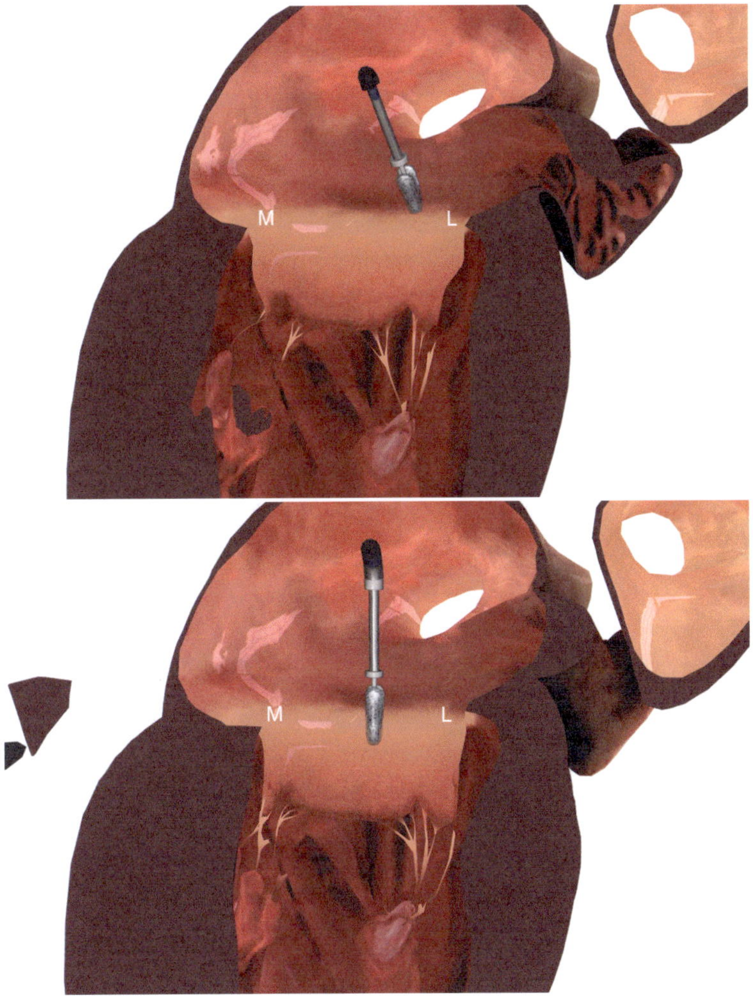

Fig. 10.4 Adjust medial-lateral position. M knob must be applied to realign the Clip in the medial-lateral plane

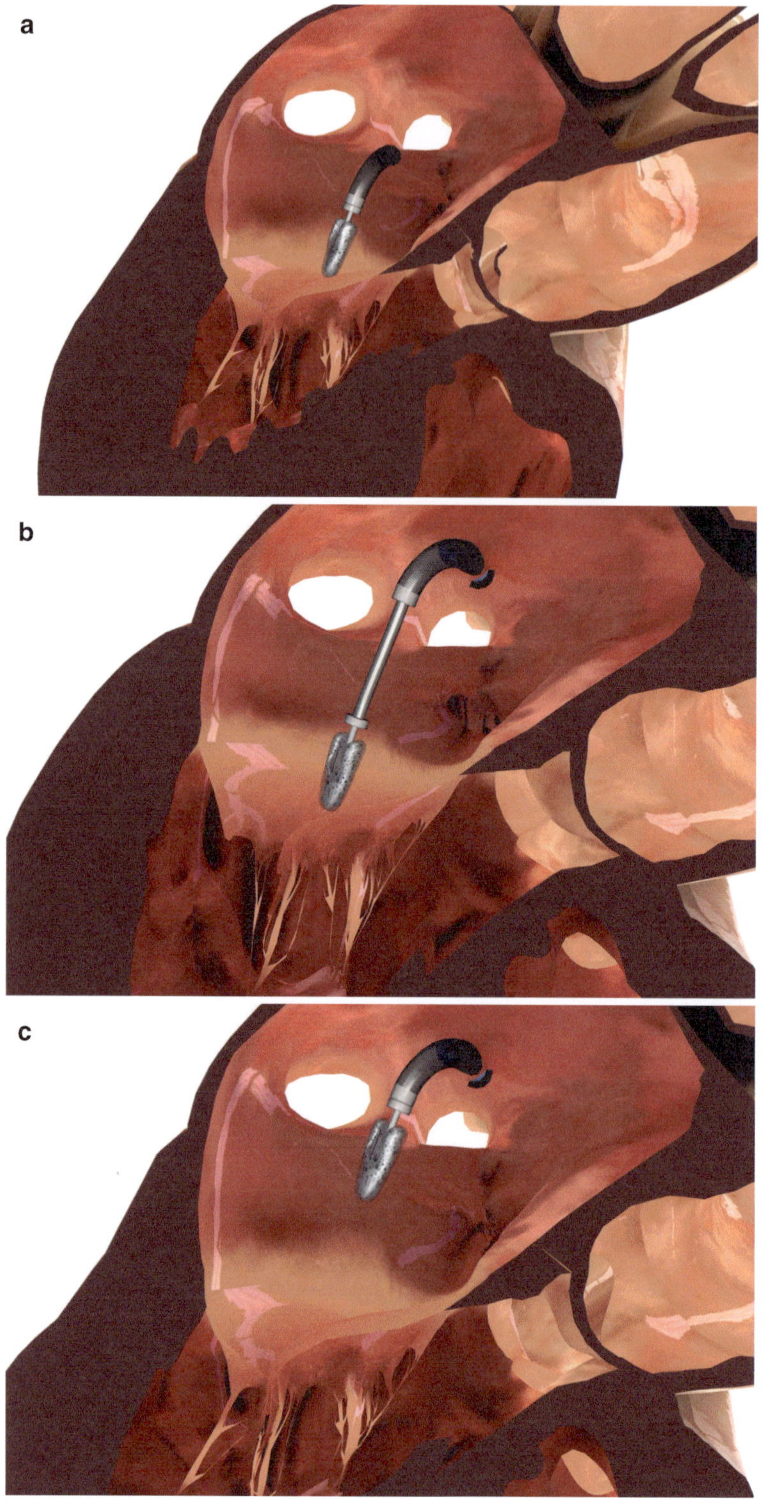

Fig. 10.5 Increasing height review: Inadequate height above the mitral valve plane is identified: the DC is fully retracted against the Sleeve and the tip of the clip is at or below the level of the annulus (**a**). After torquing the Guide catheter posterior, applying A knob, and adjusting the medial-lateral position, additional height above the valve is achieved to properly tension the leaflets in order to assure an adequate grasp (**b**, **c**)

How to Decrease Height Above the Mitral Valve Plane

Fig. 10.6 Situation: Excessive height above the mitral valve plane. The Clip has been steered down perpendicular to the mitral valve opening with respect to anterior-posterior and medial-lateral directions. However, the Delivery Catheter is fully extended, and therefore, it is not possible to adequately advance the Clip into the left ventricle far enough below the free edges to achieve a successful grasp in this situation (**a**, **b**)

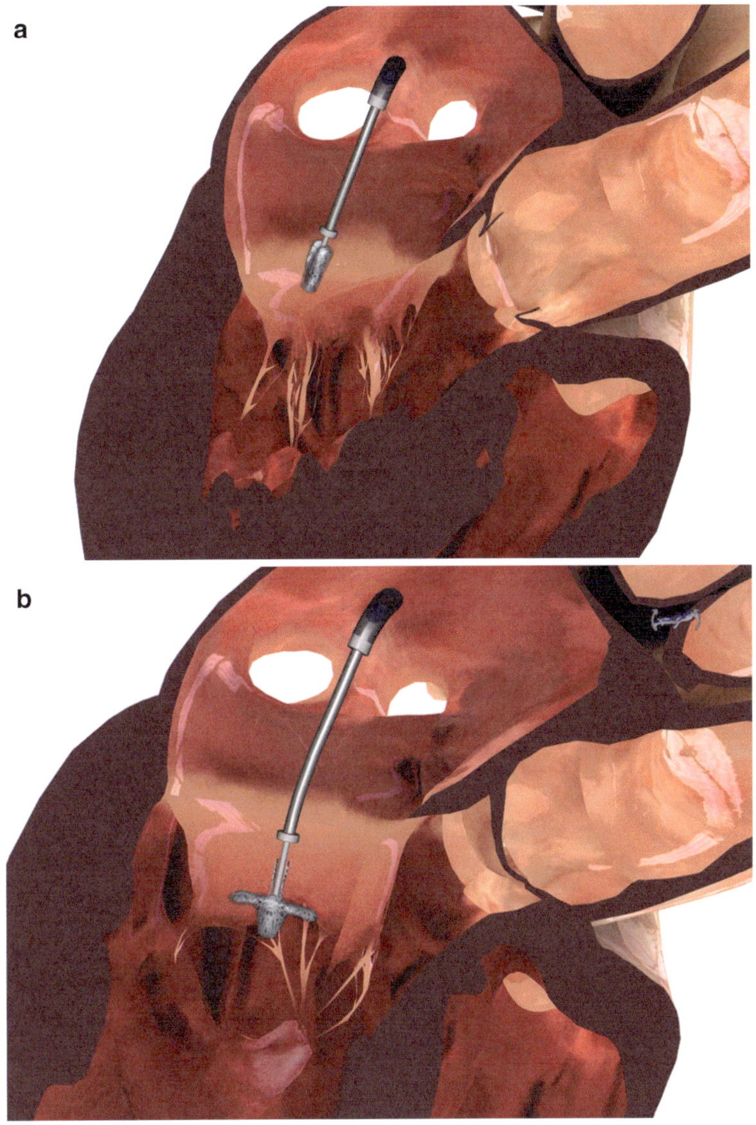

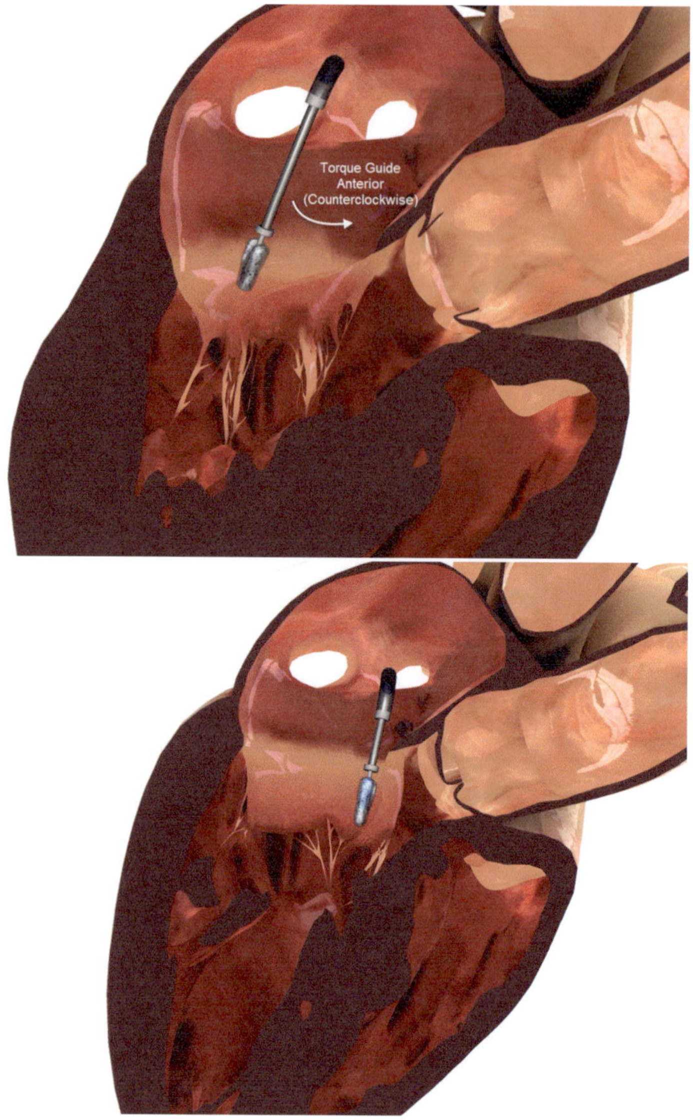

Fig. 10.7 To decrease height. Torque the Guide handle anterior (counterclockwise) until the Clip is pointing at the anterior annulus. This will cause a decrease in height above the annulus but will also affect the anterior-posterior position

Fig. 10.8 Making a posterior adjustment. P knob is applied to compensate posterior while maintaining the decrease in height (**a**). The Delivery Catheter moves toward the center of the valve from an anterior-posterior (A/P) perspective (**b**). However, applying P knob reinforces the effect of M knob which increases the medial curvature thus resulting in the Delivery Catheter pointing medial. It is necessary to verify alignment in the alternate long axis view (**c**)

a

b

c

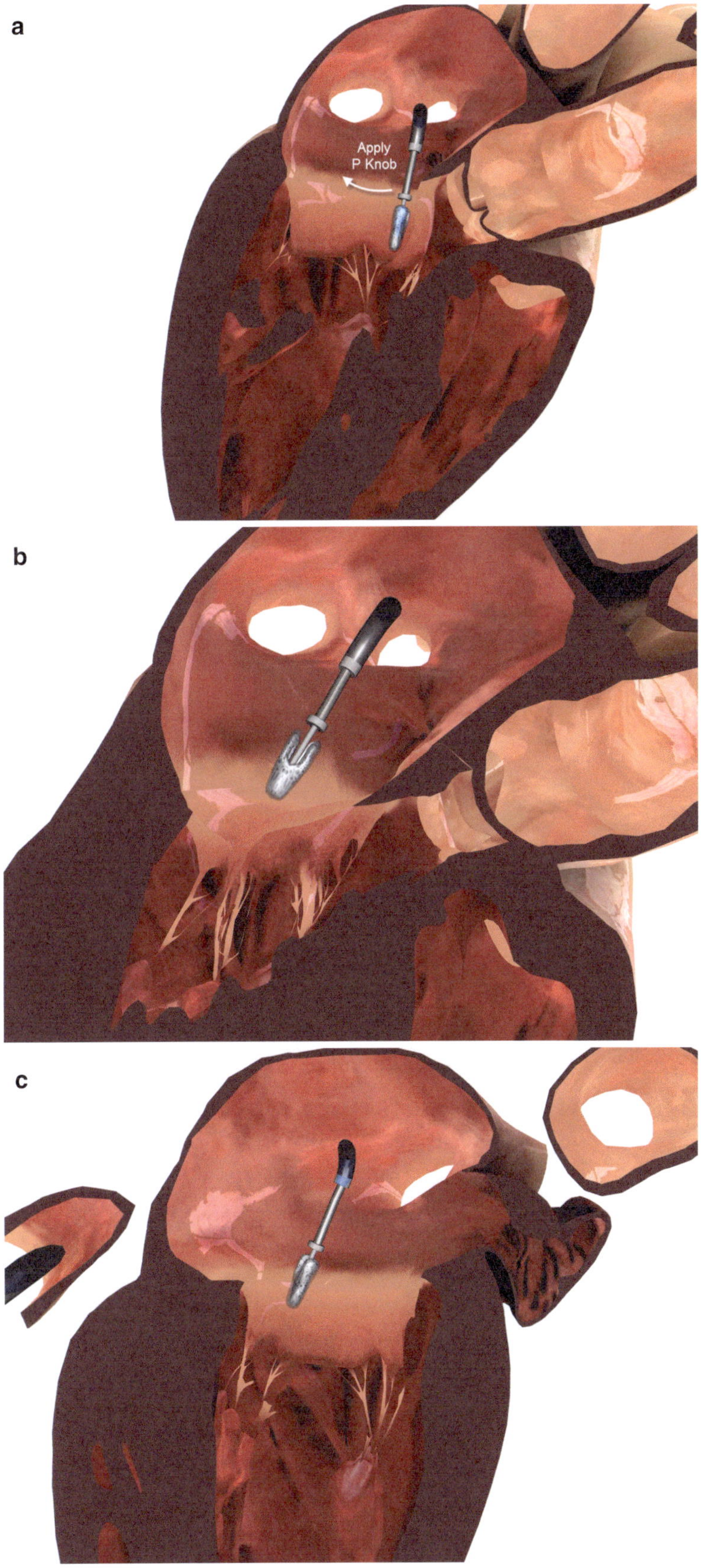

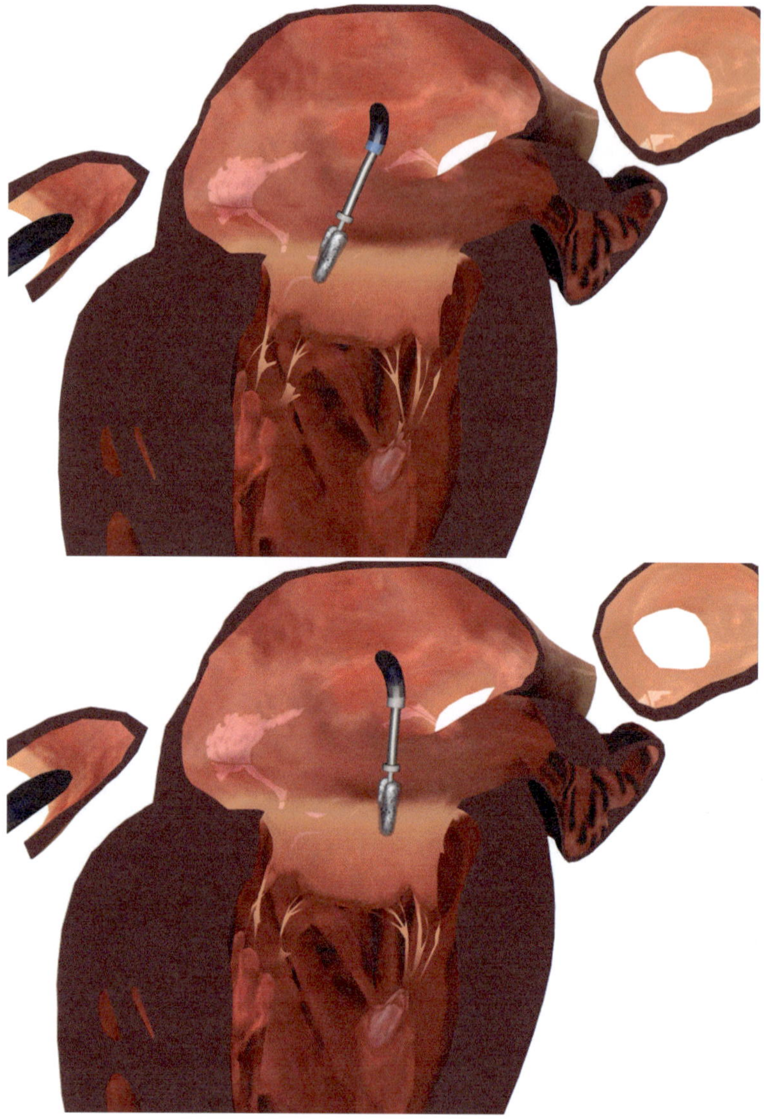

Fig. 10.9 Adjust medial-lateral position. M knob must be released in order to realign the clip in the medial-lateral plane

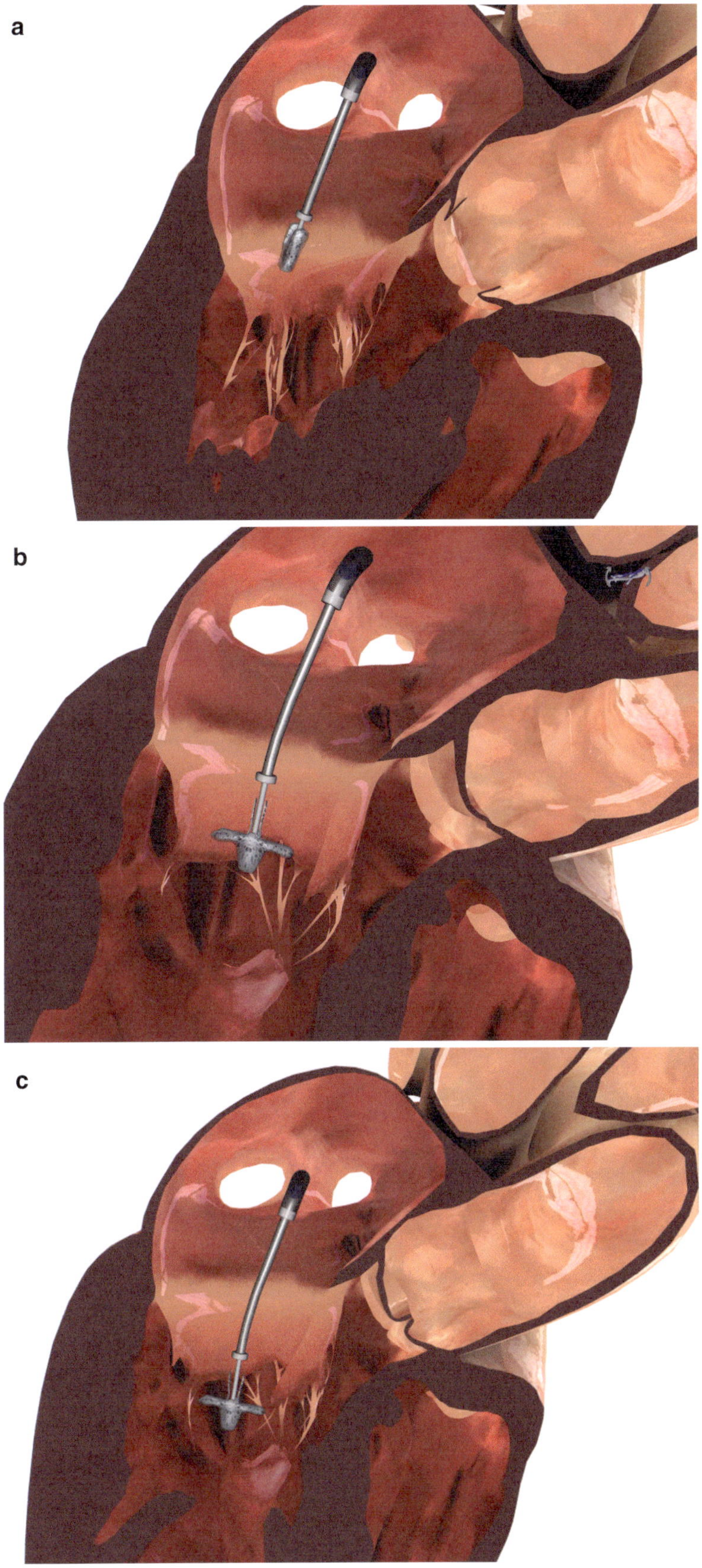

Fig. 10.10 Decreasing height review. Excessive height above the mitral valve plane is identified: The Delivery Catheter is fully extended and the tip of the clip is at or above the level of the annulus (**a**). Before decreasing height: the Clip is not able to be adequately advanced below the free edge of the leaflets (**b**). After torquing the Guide catheter handle anterior, applying P knob, and adjusting the medial-lateral position, a decrease in height above the valve is achieved to properly advance the Clip far enough into the left ventricle to permit free leaflet motion and ensure an adequate grasp (**c**)

How to Optimize Delivery Catheter Perpendicularity to the Mitral Valve Plane

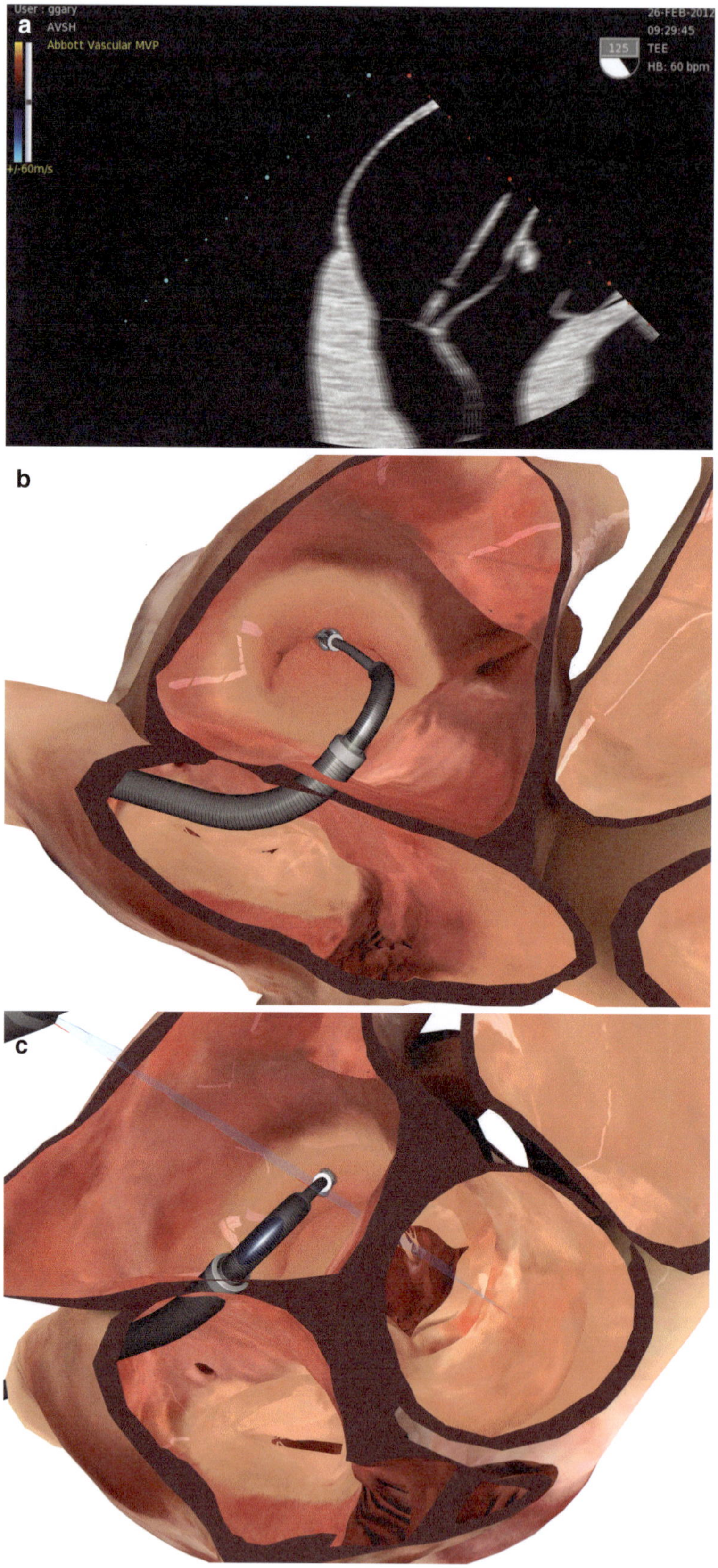

Fig. 10.11 Situation: The Clip has been steered down perpendicular to the mitral valve opening in the medial-lateral plane but has a significant posterior angle in the anterior-posterior plane (LVOT) (**a**). The base of the Delivery Catheter is too anterior due to an anterior transseptal location or an extreme medial Guide tip position in the LA causing the Clip to approach the mitral valve plane with a posteriorly directed path that is adjacent and parallel to the aorta (an aorta "hugger") (**b**, **c**). Grasping would not be effective in this situation as the anterior leaflet would not be well supported by the Clip

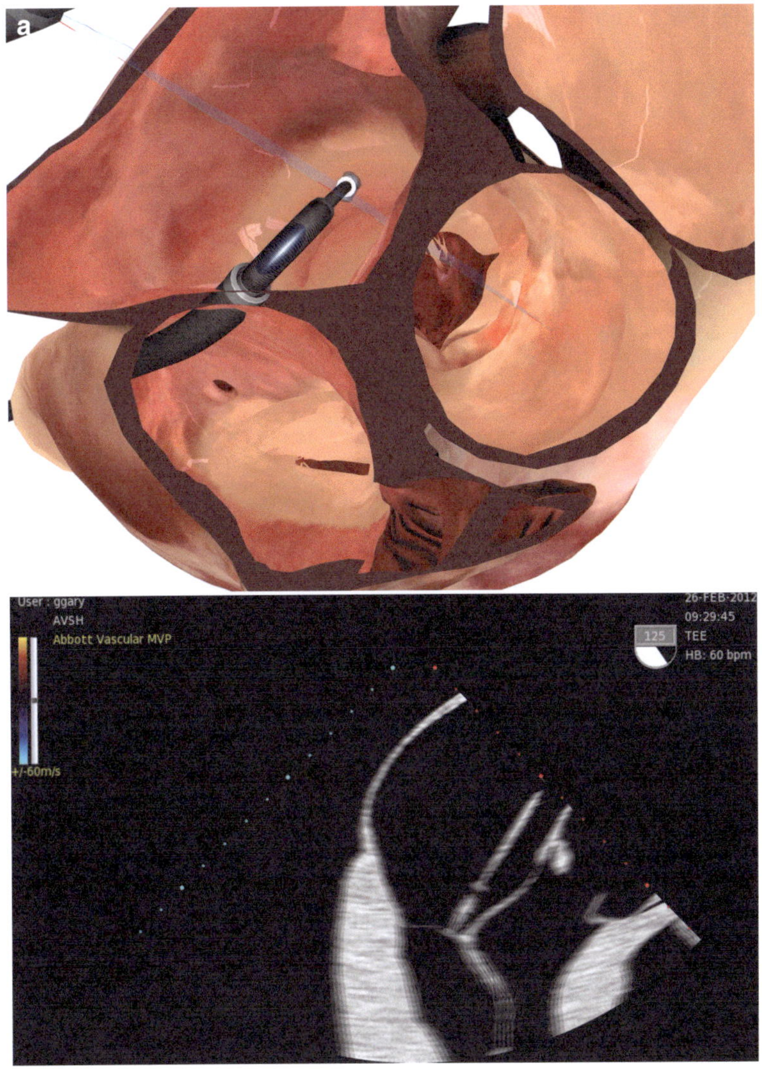

Fig. 10.12 To move the base of the catheter system posterior. To optimize the anterior-posterior path, add Guide positive (+) to reposition the base of the Guide and Delivery Catheter away from the aorta

Fig. 10.12 (continued)

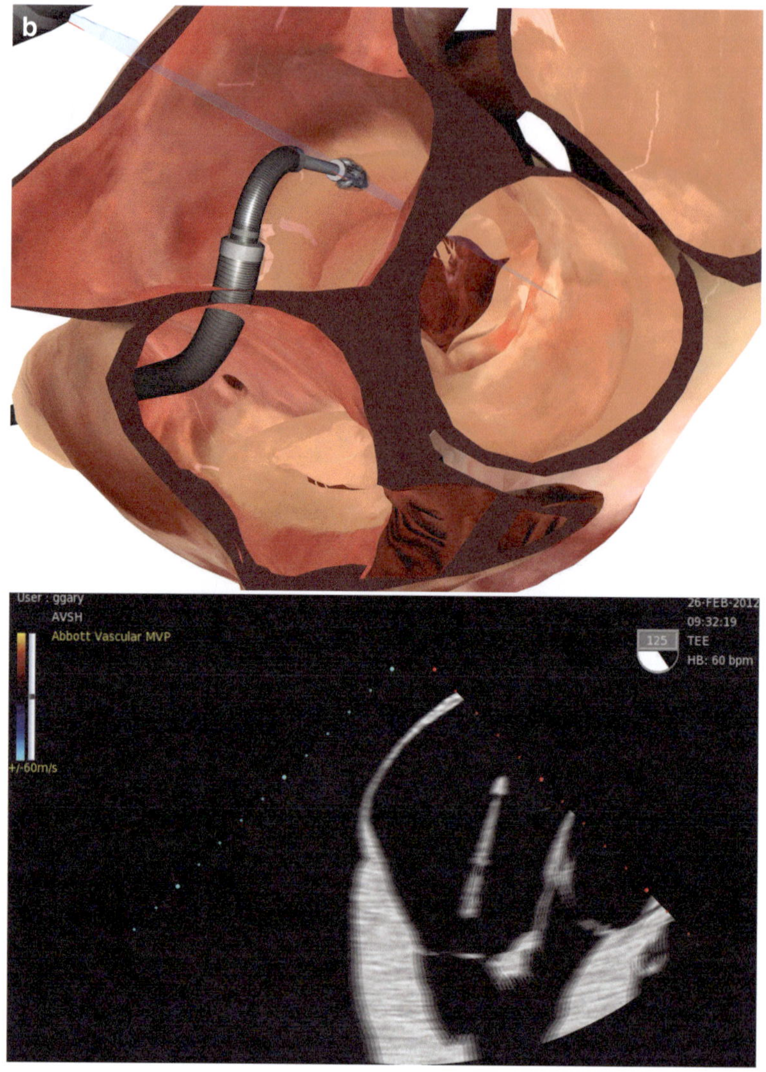

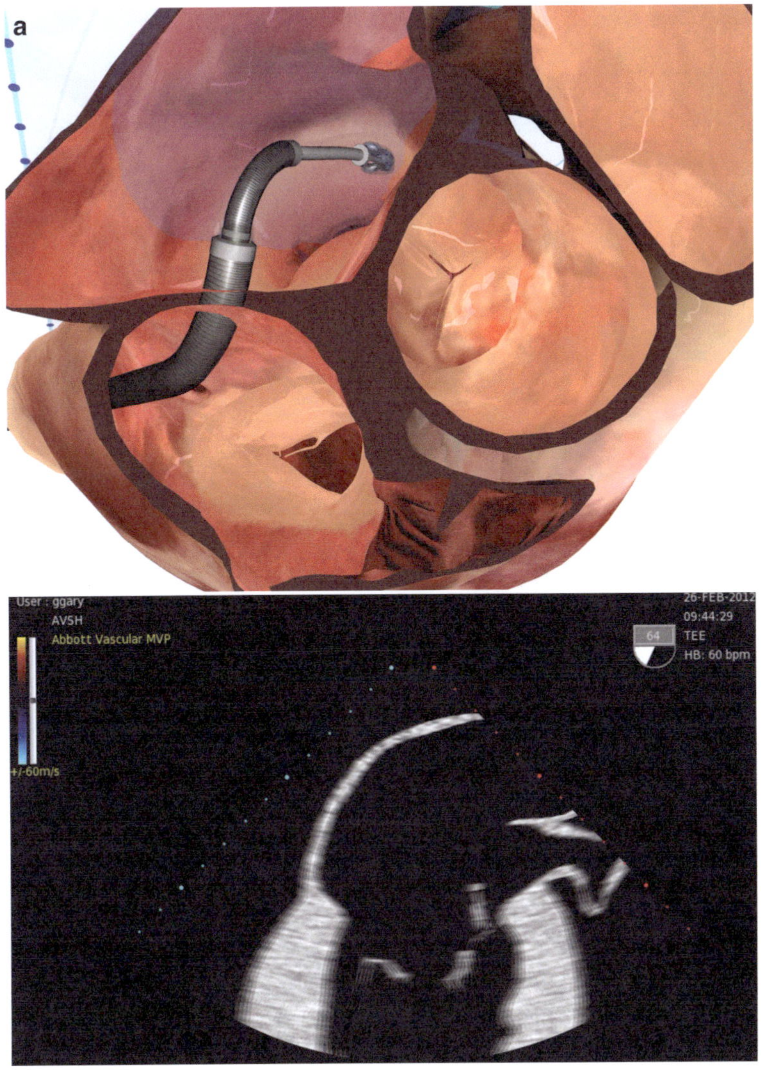

Fig. 10.13 Assess the medial-lateral position. After adding guide positive [+], it is necessary to verify alignment in the medial-lateral plane. Apply M knob as needed to realign the Clip. Advancing the entire system (stabilizer) may also be needed if the tip of the Guide is too close to the septum (**a**, **b**)

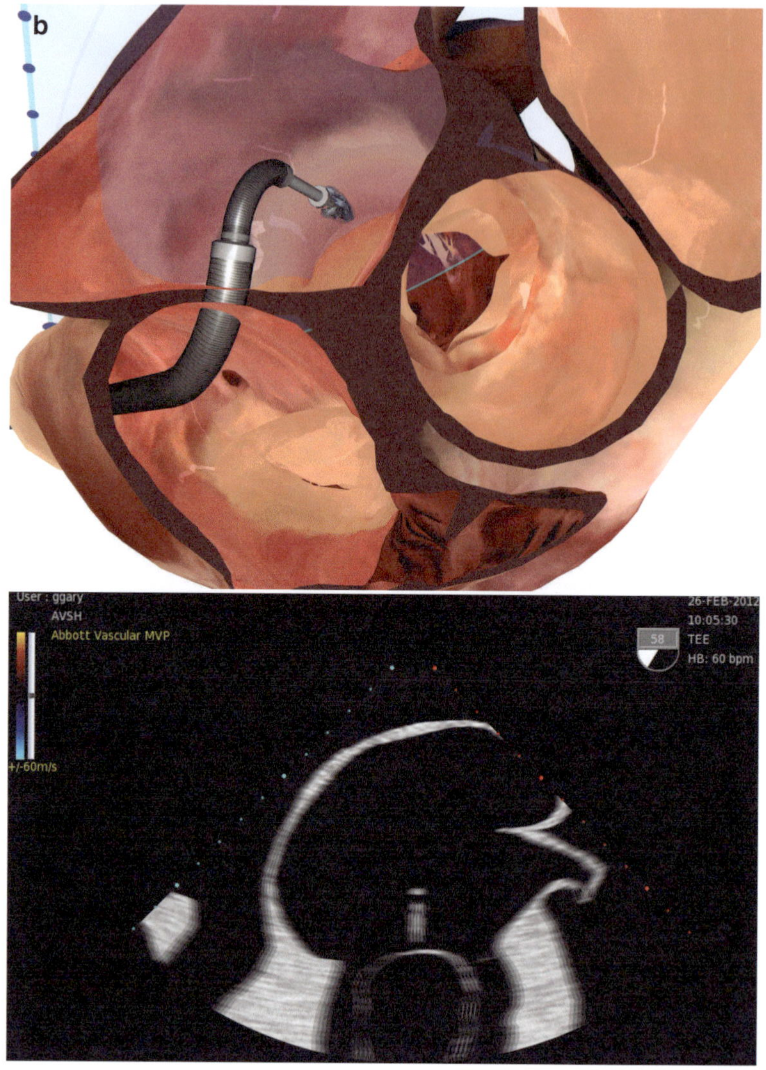

Fig. 10.13 (continued)

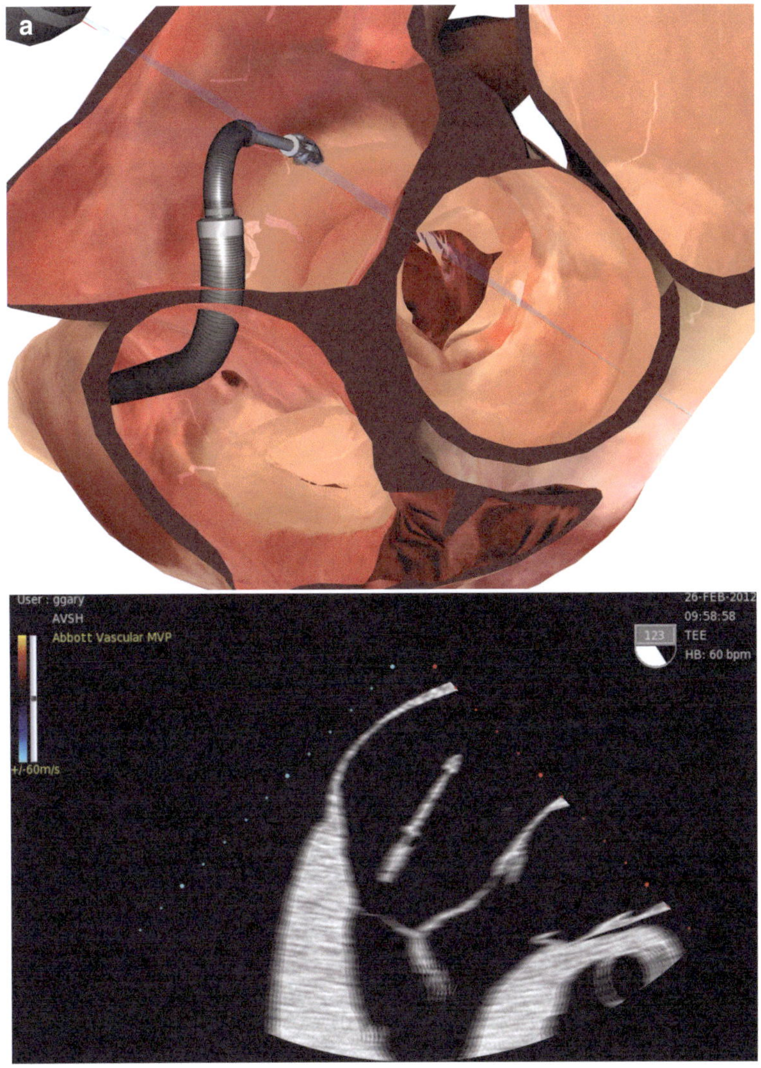

Fig. 10.14 Assess the anterior-posterior position. Adjust Guide torque as needed for axial alignment

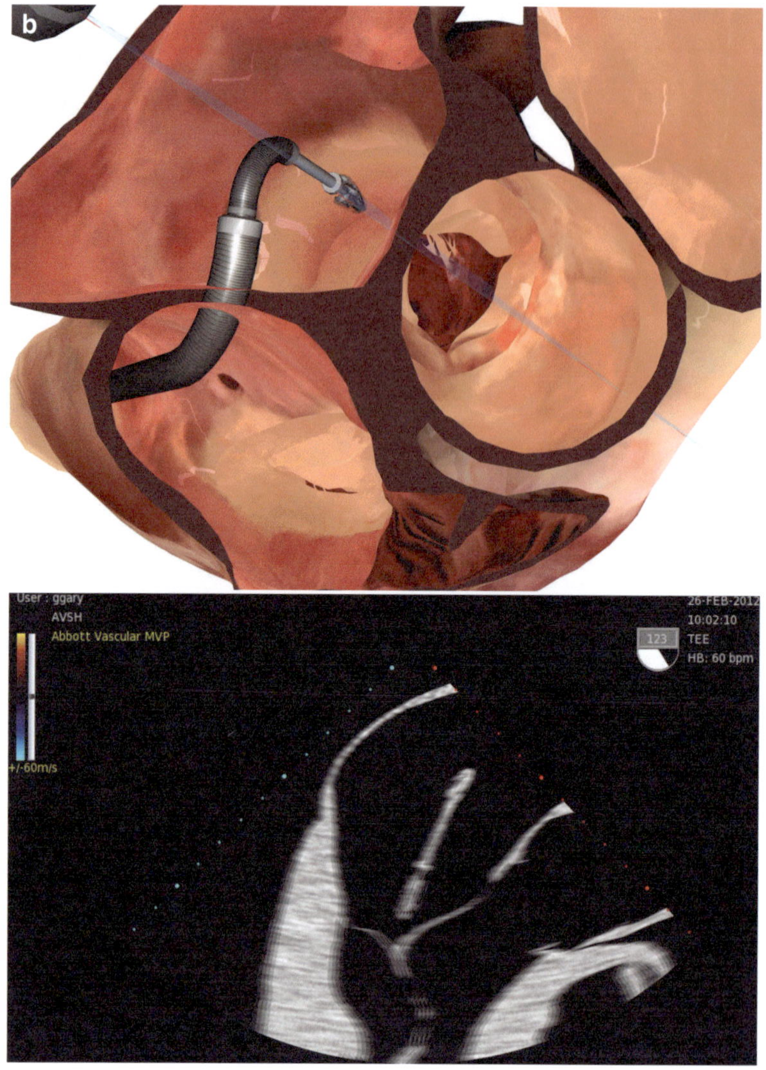

Fig. 10.14 (continued)

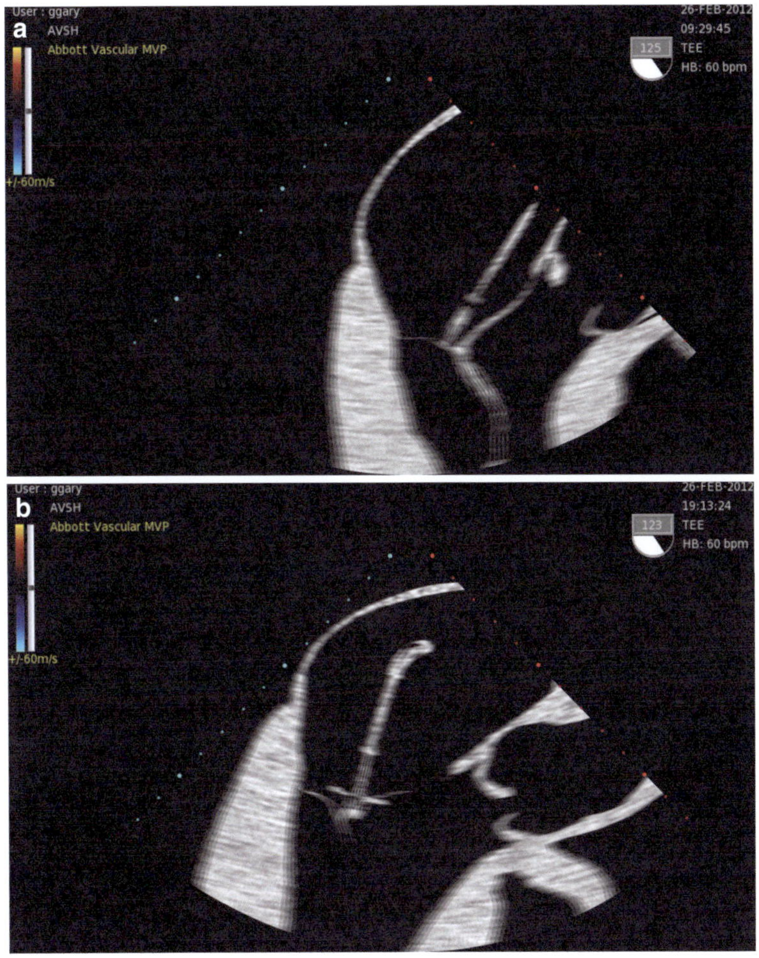

Fig. 10.15 Optimize Delivery Catheter perpendicularity to the mitral valve plane review. Apply Guide positive [+] to draw the base of the catheter system away from the aorta. Adjust M knob as needed for medial-lateral axial alignment. Adjust Guide torque as needed for anterior-posterior axial alignment. Advance system as needed to optimize the medial-lateral position

MitraClip: Basic Degenerative Case

11

Khung Keong Yeo, Eric Lim, Zee Pin Ding,
Soo Teik Lim, and Tian Hai Koh

Abstract

This is a case example of a patient with degenerative mitral regurgitation in Class II heart failure treated successfully with the MitraClip. This patient had declined surgery despite multiple hospital admissions and this case illustrates the step-by-step approach to such patients.

Keywords

Mitral regurgitation • Degenerative mitral regurgitation • MitraClip

Clinical History

A 73-year-old Chinese man with a known history of mitral valve prolapse presented with congestive heart failure requiring hospital admission on two separate occasions. He was NYHA Class II. He declined surgery. His transthoracic and transesophageal echo showed normal LV function (LVEF 55–60 %) and P2 prolapse. The mitral regurgitation (MR) was centrally directed. The estimated pulmonary systolic pressure was 54 mmHg. His only other significant comorbidity was atrial fibrillation and sick sinus syndrome requiring a permanent pacemaker.

Summary

In this case, the cause of the MR is a prolapsed P2 scallop. The procedural plan was to place one clip first with the expectation to use a second clip. The following Figs. 11.1, 11.2, 11.3, 11.4, 11.5, 11.6, 11.7, 11.8, 11.9, 11.10, 11.11, 11.12, 11.13, 11.14, 11.15, 11.16, and 11.17 demonstrate the key steps of this procedure.

K.K. Yeo, M.B.B.S., FACC, FSCAI (✉)
Department of Cardiology, National Heart Centre Singapore,
Mistri Wing, 17 Third Hospital Avenue,
Singapore 168752, Singapore

Department of Cardiovascular Medicine,
University of California, Davis Medical Center,
4860 Y Street, Suite 2820, Sacramento 95817, CA, USA
e-mail: yeo_kk@yahoo.com, yeo.khung.keong@nhcs.com.sg

E. Lim, M.B.B.S., M.A. (Cantab) • Z.P. Ding, M.B.B.S.
S.T. Lim, M.B.B.S. • T.H. Koh, M.B.B.S.
Department of Cardiology, National Heart Centre Singapore,
Mistri Wing, 17 Third Hospital Avenue, Singapore 168752, Singapore
e-mail: erictslim@gmail.com; ding.zee.pin@nhcs.com.sg;
lim.soo.teik@nhcs.com.sg; koh.tian.hai@nhcs.com.sg

T. Feldman et al. (eds.), *Atlas of Percutaneous Edge-to-Edge Mitral Valve Repair*,
DOI 10.1007/978-1-4471-4294-2_11, © Springer-Verlag London 2013

Learning Points

This case illustrates the basic steps in using the MitraClip to treat a patient with mitral valve prolapse involving the P2 scallop.

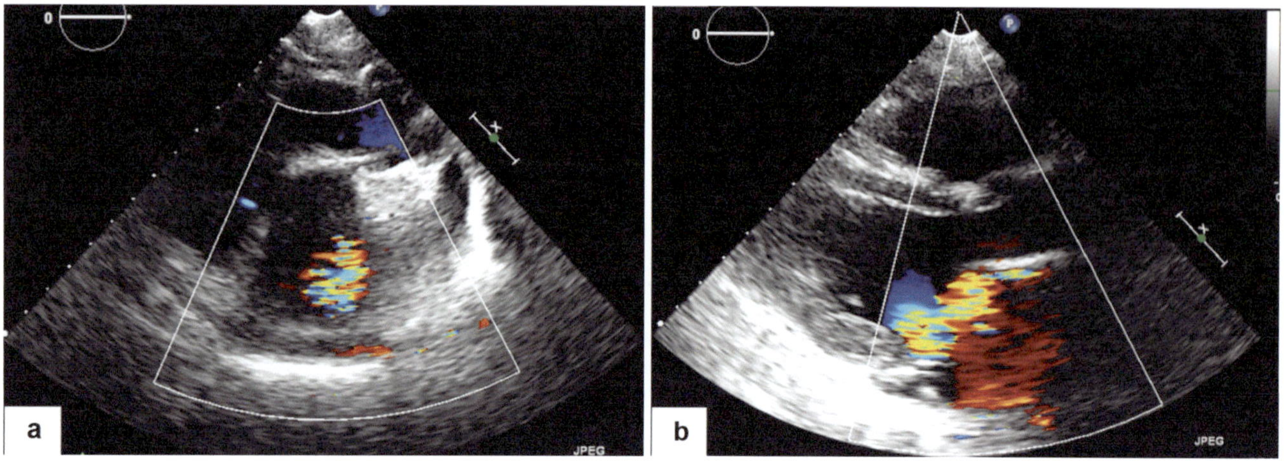

Fig. 11.1 Baseline transthoracic echo (*TTE*). (**a**) Short axis of the mitral valve with color showing a primarily central jet. (**b**) Parasternal long axis view showing an anteriorly directed mitral regurgitant jet

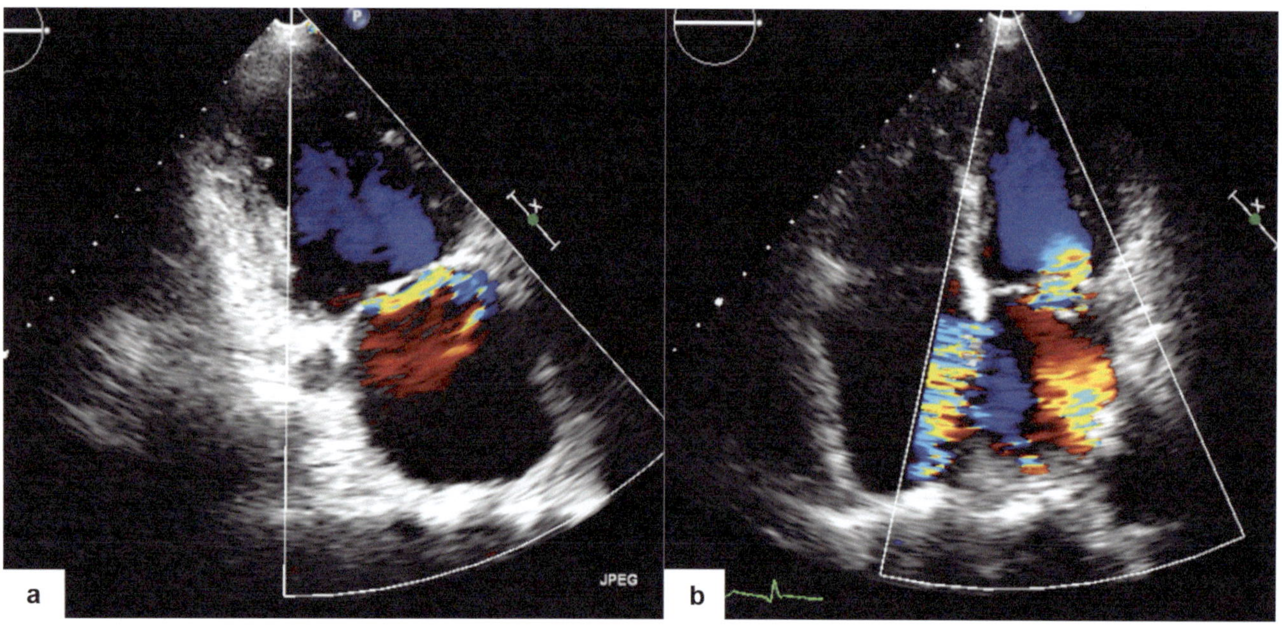

Fig. 11.2 Baseline TTE. (**a**) Transthoracic two-chamber view showing the eccentric MR jet. (**b**) Transthoracic four-chamber view showing the eccentric MR jet

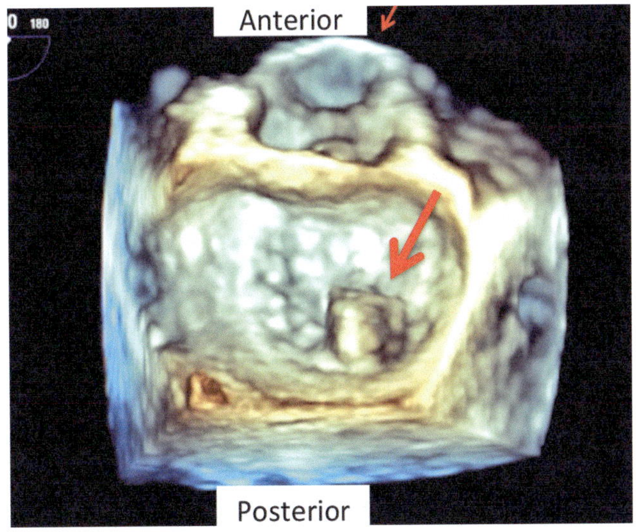

Fig. 11.3 TEE 3-D reconstruction as seen from the left atrium in the surgeon's view showing the P2 prolapse (*thick red arrow*). The aortic valve is seen anteriorly (*thin red arrow*)

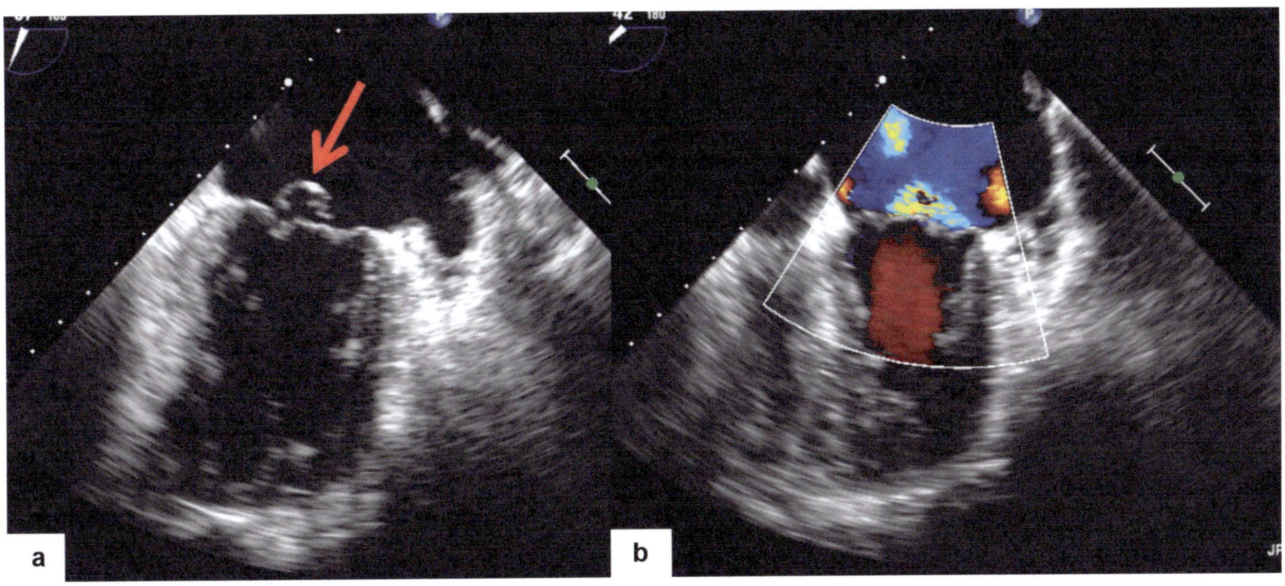

Fig. 11.4 Procedural TEE. (**a**) and (**b**) Final TEE LVOT view without and with color showing the MitraClips (*arrow*) with trace residual MR. (**b**) Final TEE intercommissural view without and with color showing the MitraClips (*arrow*) with trace residual MR"

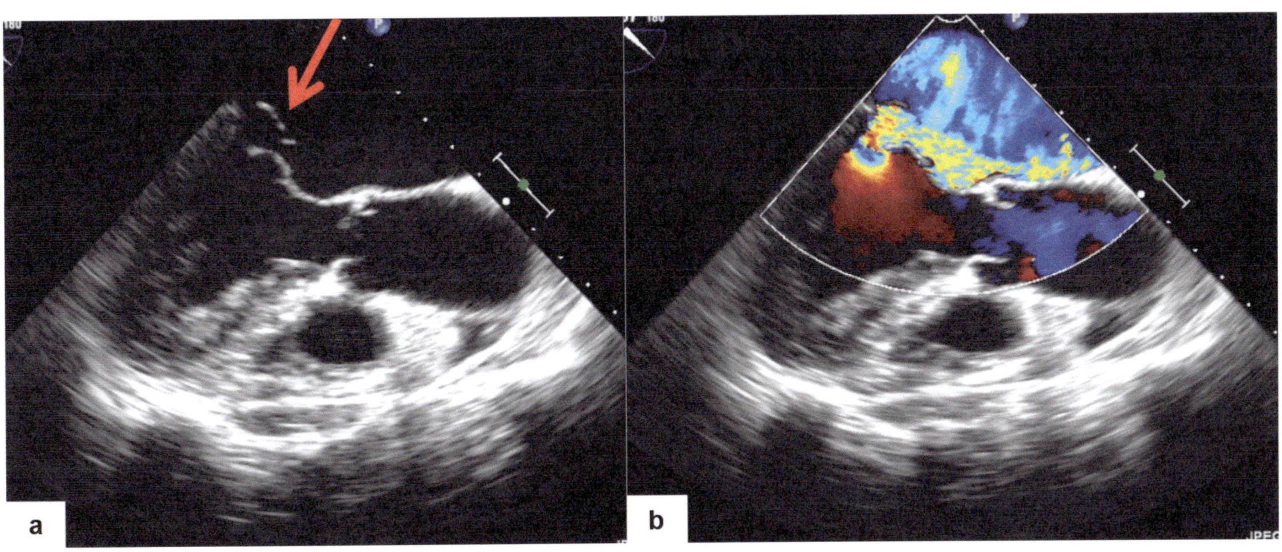

Fig. 11.5 Procedural TEE. (**a**) TEE 3-D reconstruction view from the left atrium showing the dual orifice mitral valve with the two MitraClips (*arrow*) attached. (**b**) Transgastric view of the two MitraClips (*arrow*) in a short axis view of the mitral valve"

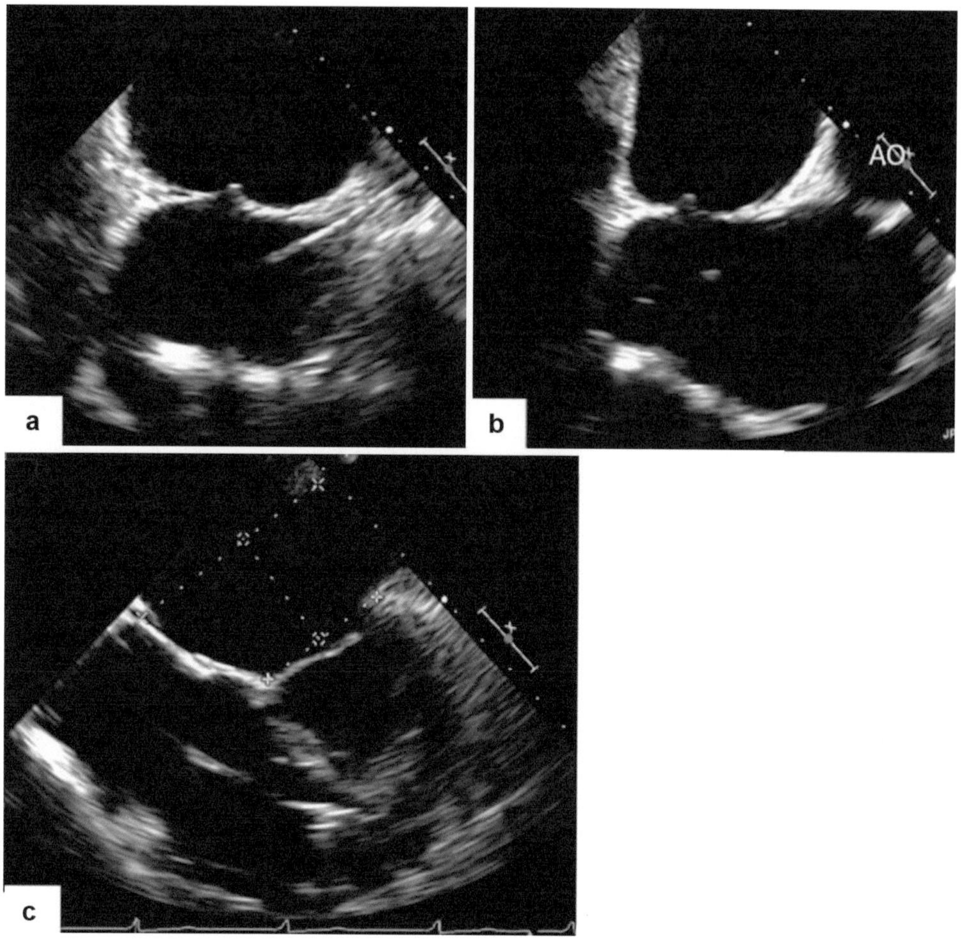

Fig. 11.6 Procedural TEE guiding the transseptal puncture. (**a**) TEE bicaval view showing tenting of the interatrial septum near the center. A pacemaker wire is seen entering from the SVC. (**b**) TEE short axis view showing tenting of the interatrial septum just posterior of the midpoint. The aorta is labeled "AO". (**c**) TEE four-chamber view showing the height of the tenting point from the valve plane. In this case, it was 3.5 cm

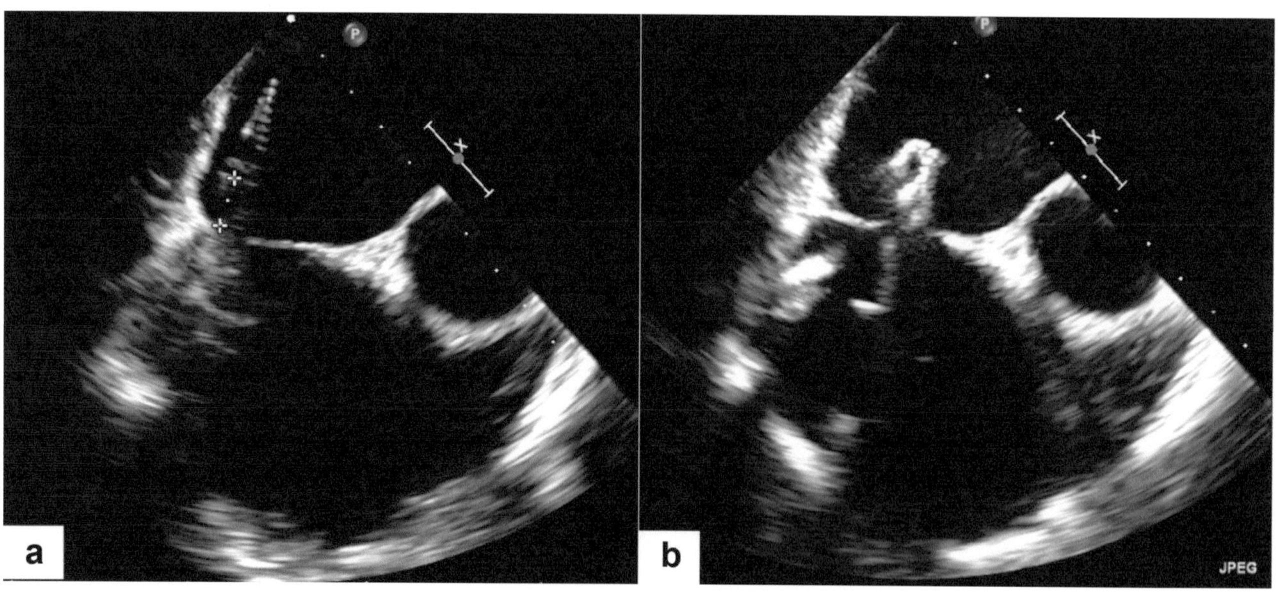

Fig. 11.7 Procedural TEE. (**a**) TEE short axis view showing the dilator and guide across the septum. The dilator is seen with spirals. (**b**) The guide is left in the left atrium after the dilator is removed

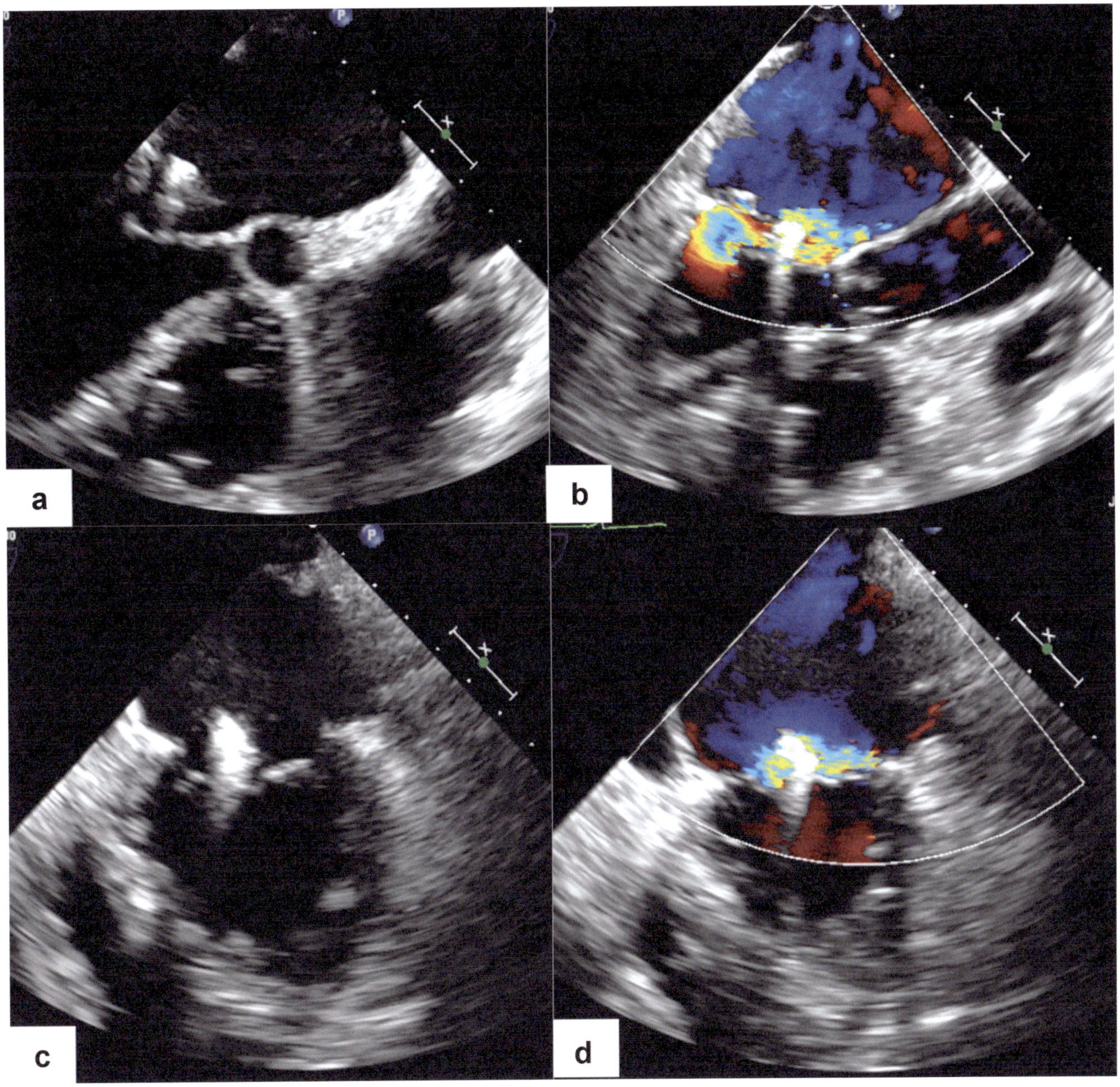

Fig. 11.8 Procedural TEE. (**a**, **b**) TEE LVOT view without and with color showing the tip of the clip as it is directed toward the regurgitant mitral valve. This view demonstrates the anterior-posterior orientation of the clip. (**c**, **d**) TEE intercommissural view without and with color showing the tip of the clip as it is directed toward the regurgitant mitral valve. This view demonstrates the medial-lateral orientation of the clip

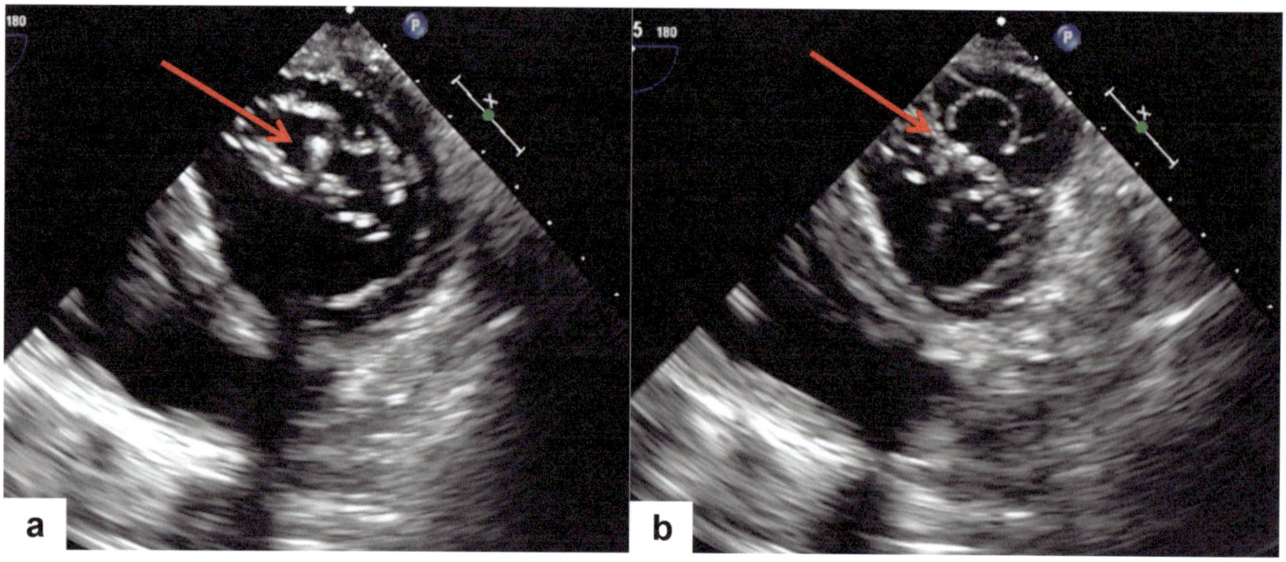

Fig. 11.9 Procedural TEE. (**a**, **b**) show TEE subgastric views of the tip of the clip (*red arrow*) as oriented perpendicular to the line of coaptation of the valve. In (**b**), the perpendicular arms are not seen as the view moves out the plane of the arms. However, they can be appreciated in (**a**)

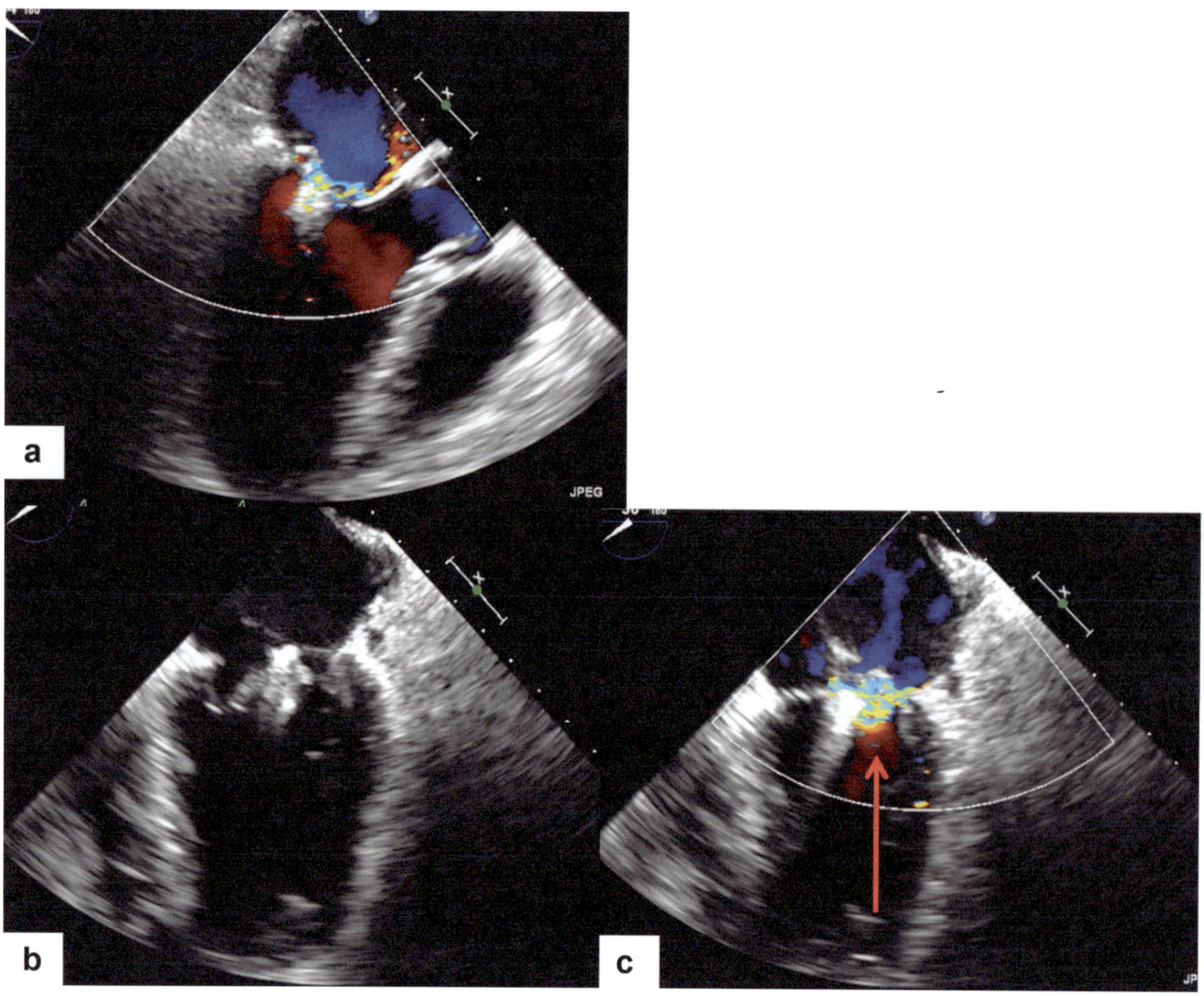

Fig. 11.10 Procedural TEE. (**a**) TEE LVOT view showing the residual moderate MR after the first MitraClip. (**b**, **c**) TEE intercommissural view showing the moderate MR arising lateral to the first MitraClip (*red arrow*)

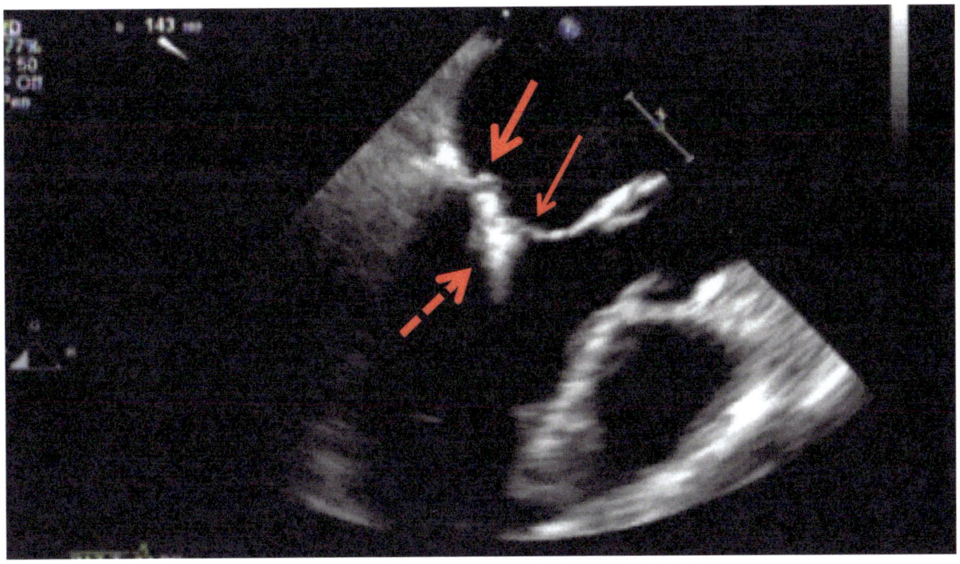

Fig. 11.11 Procedural TEE. Still frame showing verification of leaflet insertion in the LVOT view. The *thick arrow* shows the posterior leaflet riding over the top of the clip arm into the clip (*dotted arrow*). The *thin red arrow* shows the anterior leaflet entering the clip

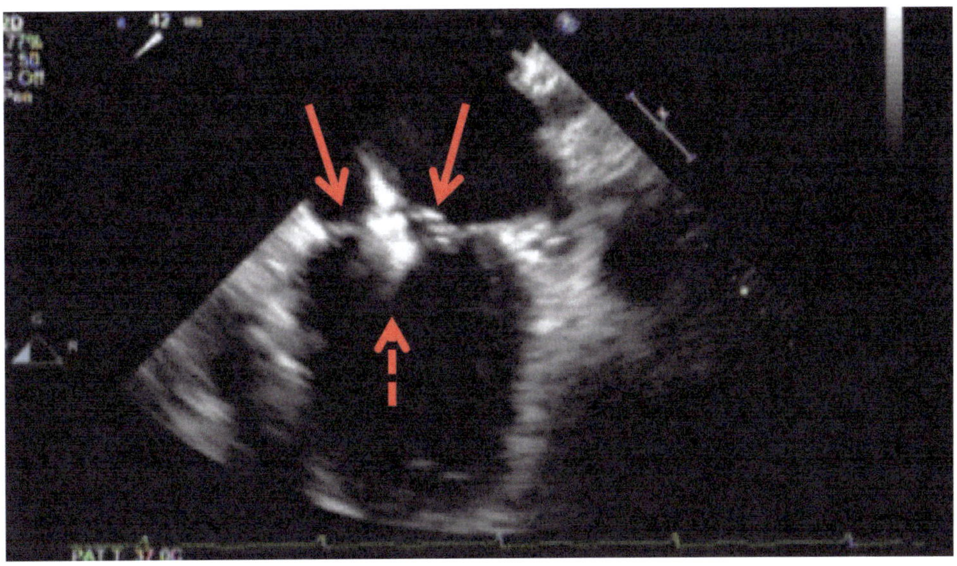

Fig. 11.12 Procedural TEE. Still frame in the intercommissural view showing the valve leaflets (*fill arrow*) bisecting the clip (*broken arrow*)

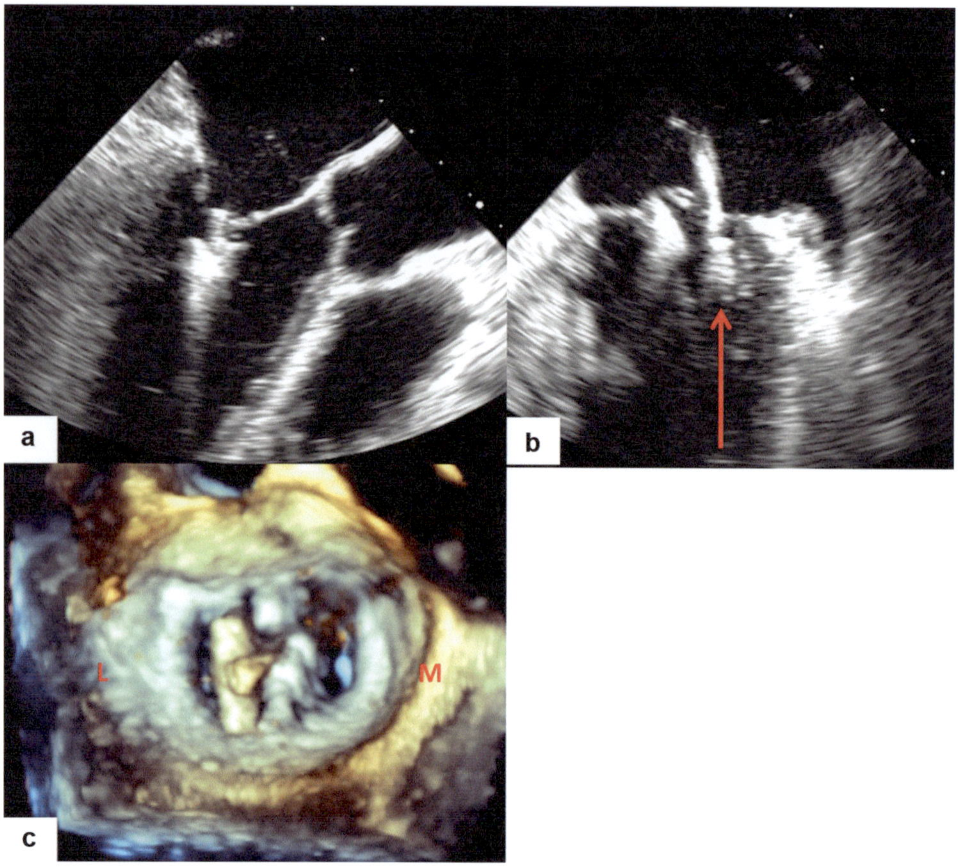

Fig. 11.13 Procedural TEE. (**a**) TEE LVOT view showing the second MitraClip being positioned. The first MitraClip is not well seen as it is off-plane. (**b**) TEE intercommissural view with the second MitraClip positioned lateral to the first MitraClip (*red arrow*). (**c**) TEE 3-D view as seen from the left atrium with the clip lateral to the first MitraClip. In this surgeon's view, note the medial (*M*) and lateral (*L*) orientation

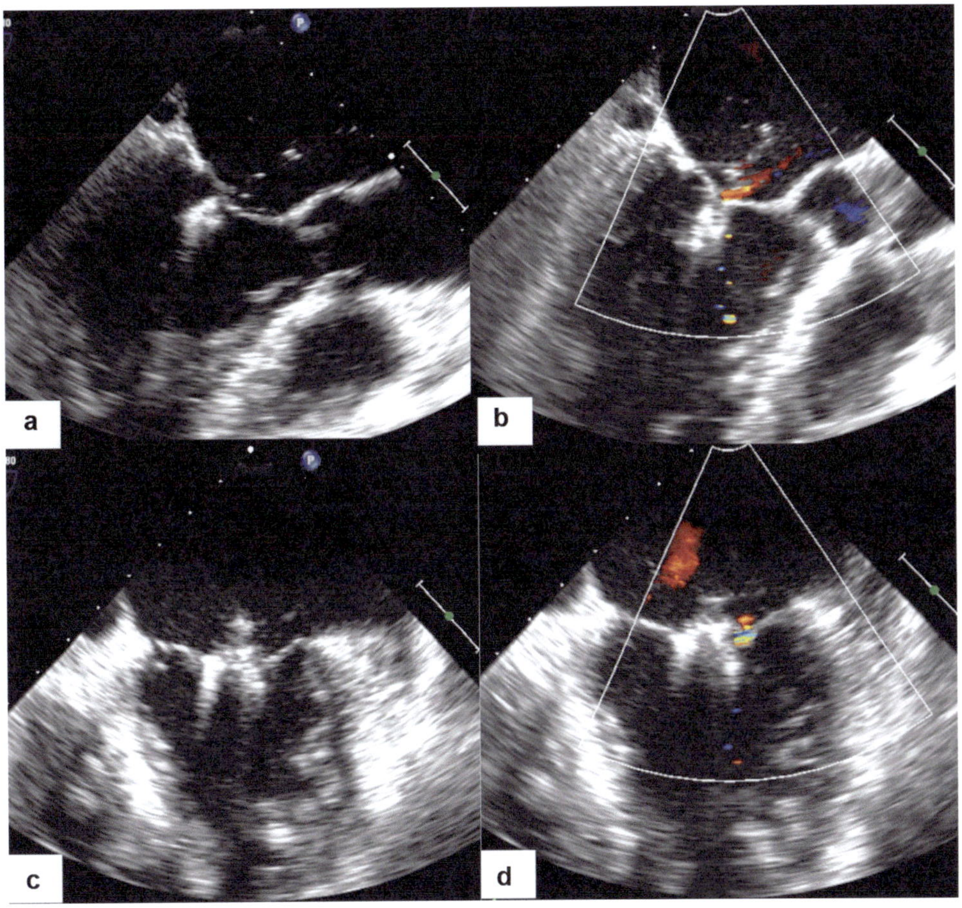

Fig. 11.14 Procedural TEE. (**a**) Final TEE LVOT view without and with color showing the MitraClips with trace residual MR. (**c**, **d**) Final TEE intercommissural view without and with color showing the MitraClips with trace residual MR

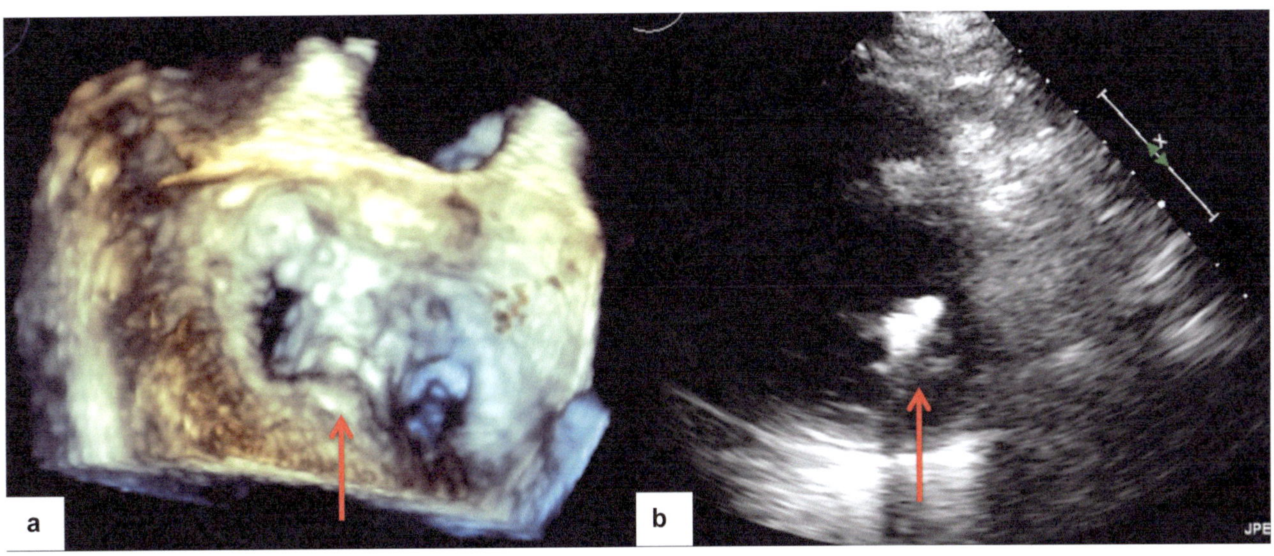

Fig. 11.15 Procedural TEE. (**a**) TEE 3-D reconstruction view from the left atrium showing the dual orifice mitral valve with the two MitraClips (*arrow*) attached. (**b**) Transgastric view of the two MitraClips (*arrow*) in a short axis view of the mitral valve

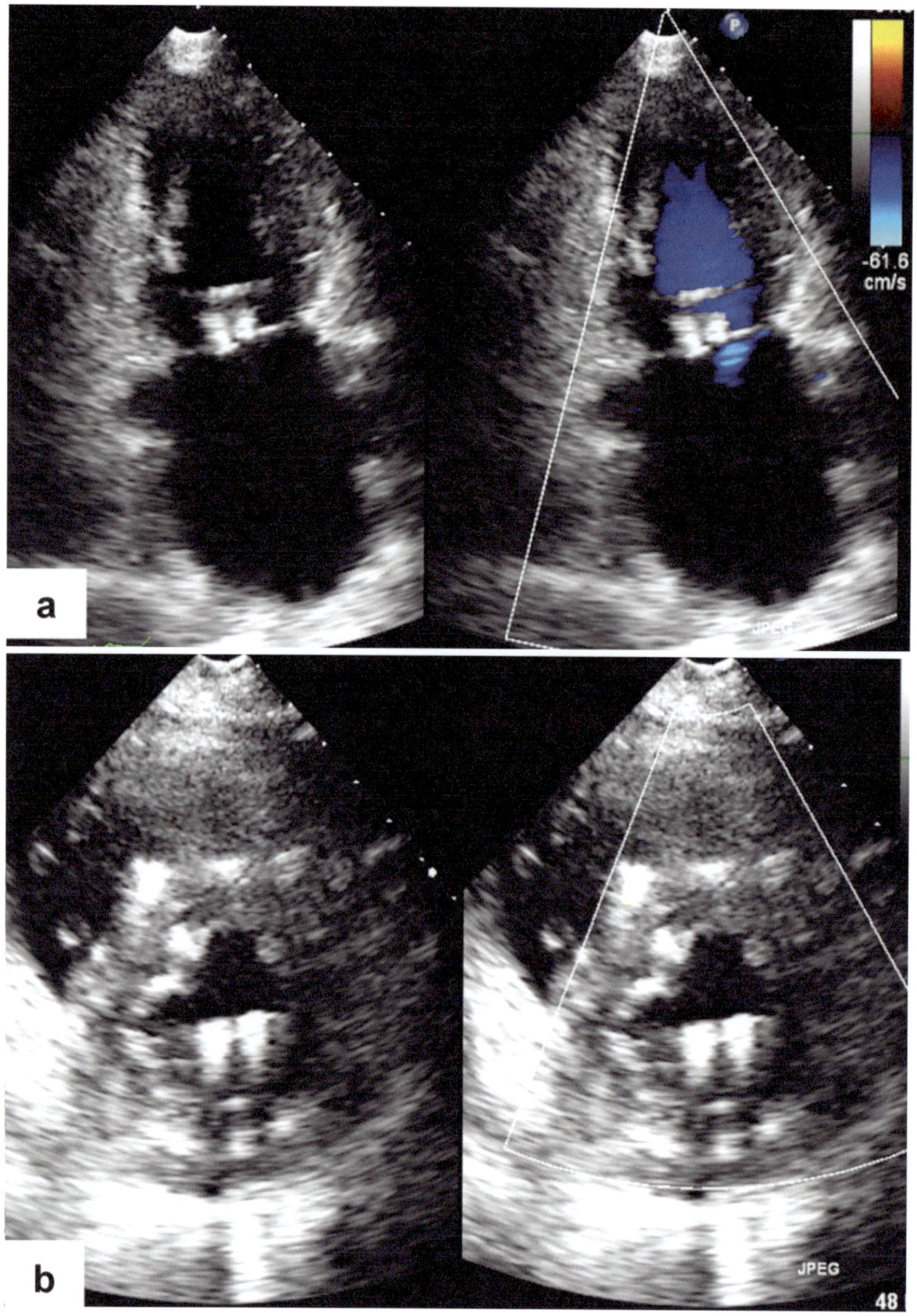

Fig. 11.16 One-month postprocedure TTE. (**a**) One-month postprocedure TTE two-chamber view showing the two MitraClips without and with color. (**b**) One-month postprocedure TTE parasternal short axis view showing the two MitraClips without and with color

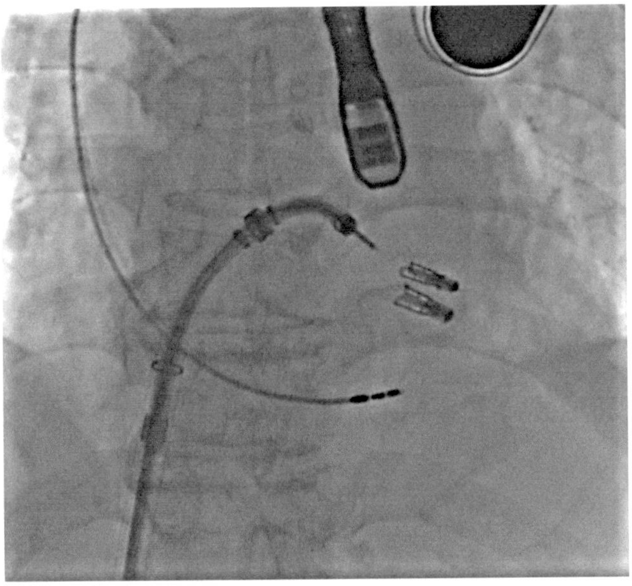

Fig. 11.17 Fluoroscopy showing the two MitraClips in place

12 EVEREST II Basic Functional Case Study

Ehrin J. Armstrong and Jason Rogers

Abstract

This is a case example of a patient with functional mitral regurgitation in Class III heart failure treated successfully with the MitraClip. This patient had significant surgical risk, and this case illustrates the step-by-step approach to such patients.

Keywords

Mitral regurgitation • Functional mitral regurgitation • MitraClip • High risk

Clinical History

An 84-year-old man with a history of prior myocardial infarction and coronary artery bypass grafting presented with dyspnea after mild to moderate exertion, consistent with NYHA Class III heart failure. Transthoracic echocardiography revealed functional MR and a depressed ejection fraction of 30 %. The patient was enrolled in the REALISM continued access registry.

E.J. Armstrong, M.D., M.Sc.
Division of Cardiovascular Medicine,
University of California, Davis Medical Center,
4860 Y Street, Suite 2820, Sacramento, CA 95817, USA
e-mail: ehrin.armstrong@ucdmc.ucdavis.edu

J. Rogers, M.D., FACC, FSCAI (✉)
Department of Cardiovascular Medicine,
University of California, Davis Medical Center,
4860 Y Street, Suite 2820, Sacramento, CA 95817, USA
e-mail: jason.rogers@ucdmc.ucdavis.edu

Summary

This patient represents a classic case of functional MR from ischemic cardiomyopathy who would be high risk for a surgical approach to mitral valve repair. The patient underwent implantation of two MitraClip devices in an uncomplicated procedure. Postprocedure, the patient's functional capacity improved dramatically, to the point where he was no longer limited in his level of activity. At 1 year postprocedure, he was asymptomatic with a dramatic improvement of his ejection fraction from 30 % preprocedure to 55 %. Patients such as this—with high or extreme risk for surgical intervention—represent a unique cohort who may derive significant clinical benefit from MitraClip implantation.

Learning Points

This case illustrates the step-by-step process of evaluating and treating a patient with functional MR.

Electronic supplementary material The online version of this chapter (doi:10.1007/978-1-4471-4294-2_12) contains supplementary material, which is available to authorized users.

T. Feldman et al. (eds.), *Atlas of Percutaneous Edge-to-Edge Mitral Valve Repair*,
DOI 10.1007/978-1-4471-4294-2_12, © Springer-Verlag London 2013

Screening Transthoracic Echo

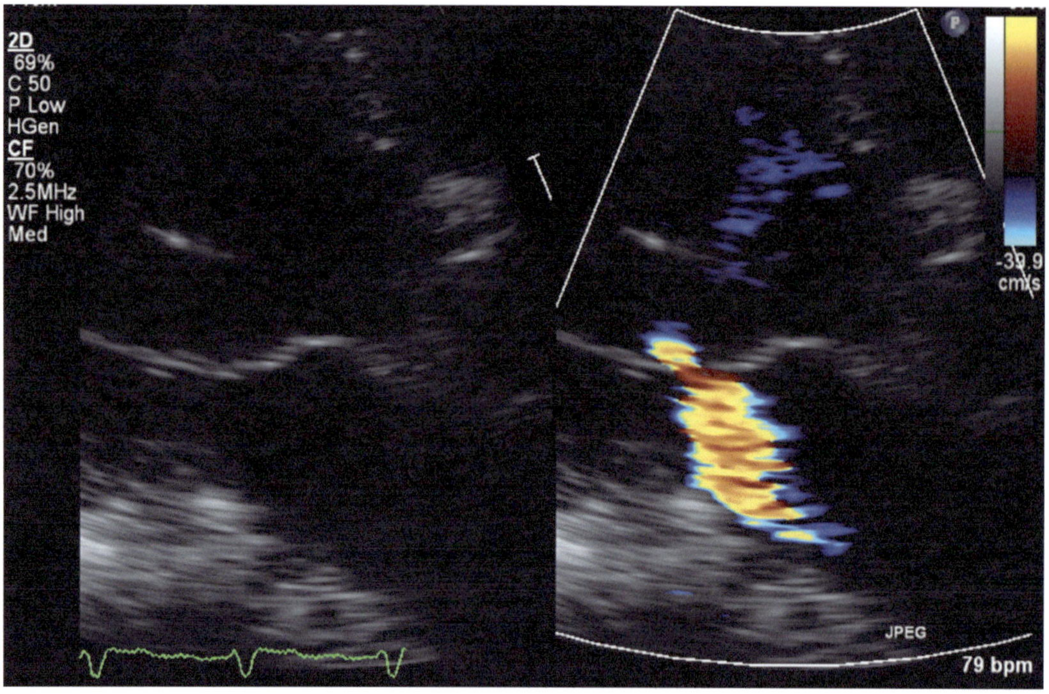

Fig. 12.1 TTE: parasternal LAX with and without color. There is significant tenting of the mitral leaflets and a posteriorly directed jet, consistent with a functional etiology and a restricted posterior leaflet secondary to the patient's ischemic cardiomyopathy and left ventricular remodeling

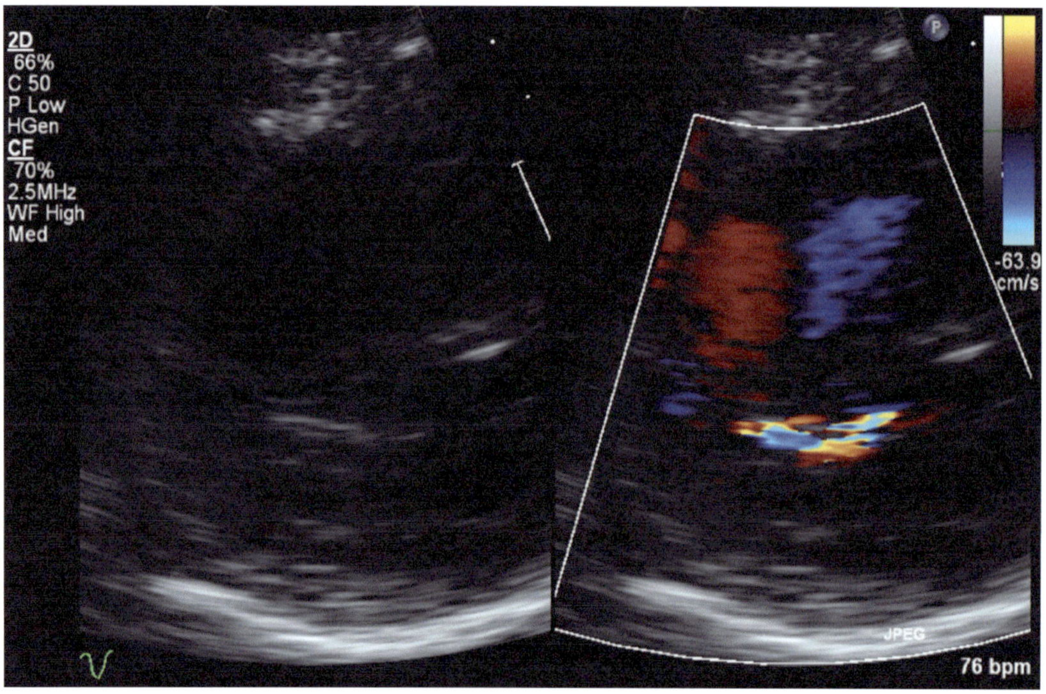

Fig. 12.2 TTE: parasternal SAX with and without color. The regurgitant jet has a central origin, primarily along the coaptation line of the A2 and P2 scallops

Screening Transthoracic Echo II

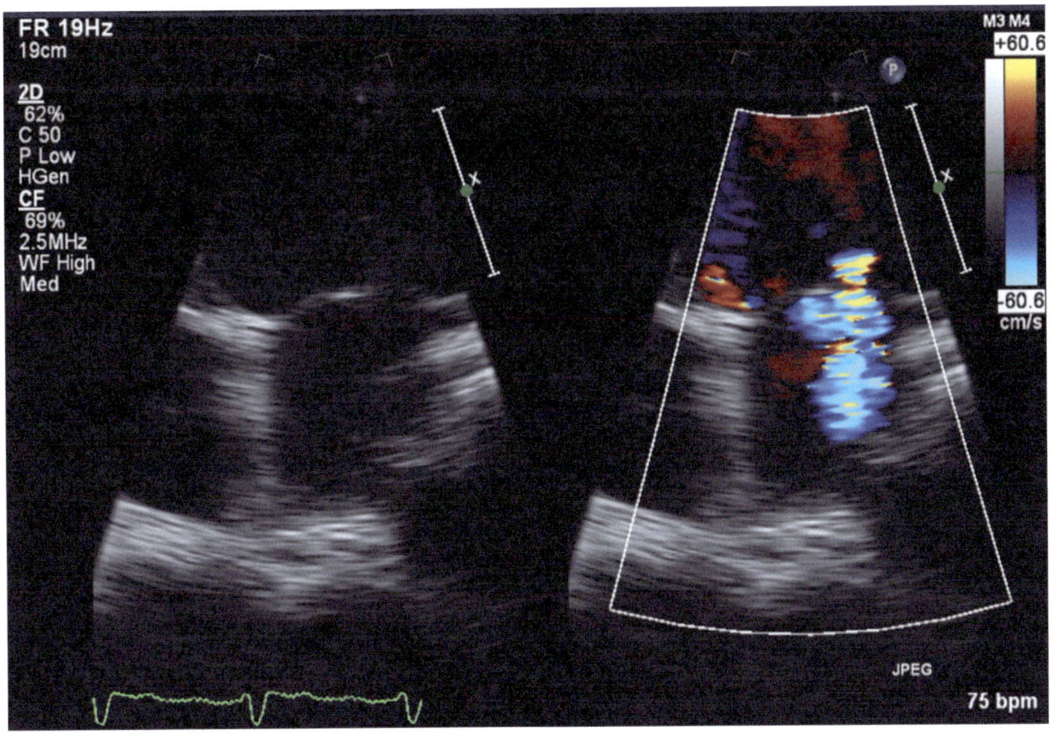

Fig. 12.3 TTE: apical 4C view with and without color. In the magnified 4C view, the leaflet tenting is again apparent. The lateral wall of the left atrium entrains the regurgitant jet and may therefore possibly decrease the apparent Doppler severity of the MR

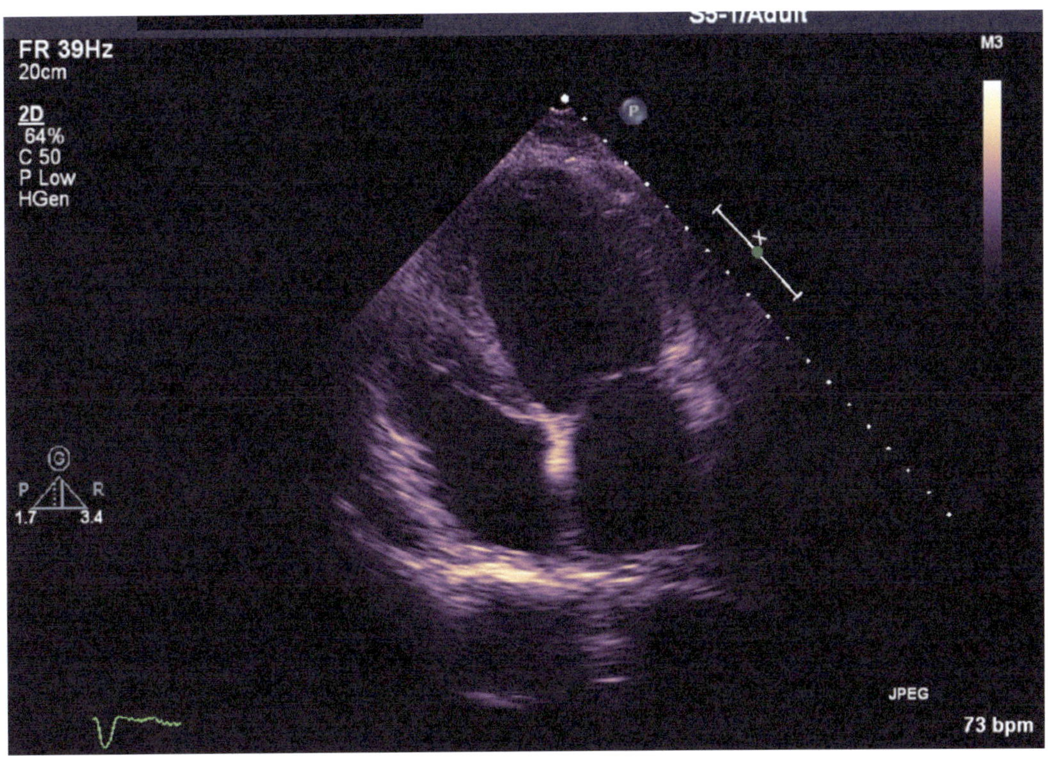

Fig. 12.4 TTE: apical 4C view. In this less magnified view, note the significant remodeling and spherical shape of the left ventricle

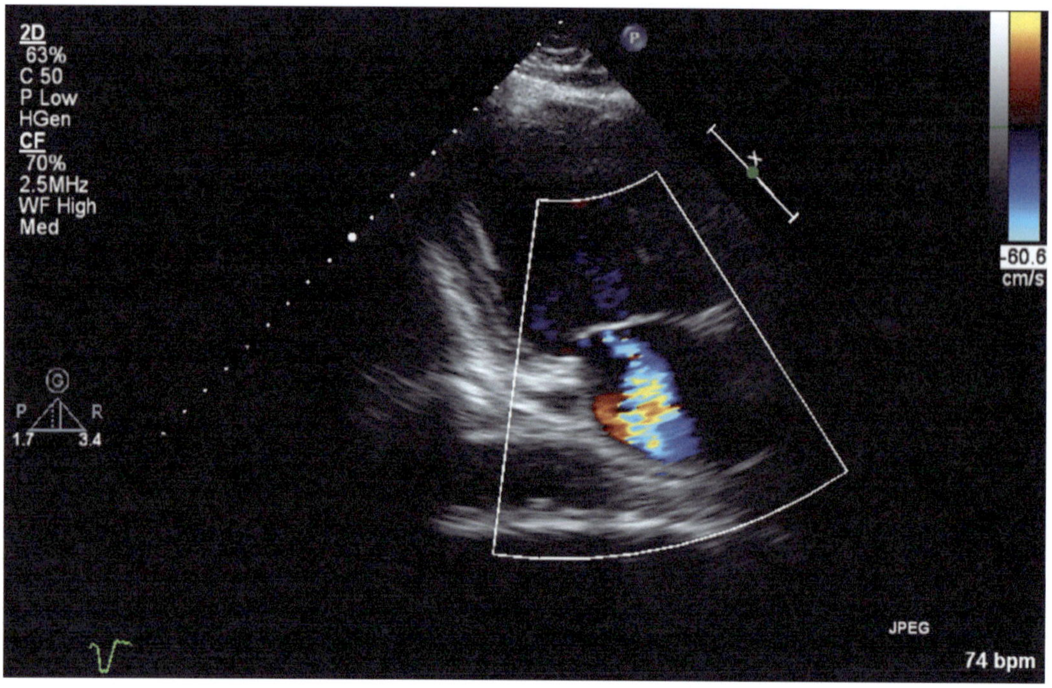

Fig. 12.5 TTE: apical 2C view. The regurgitant jet appears central in this view as well

Screening TEE

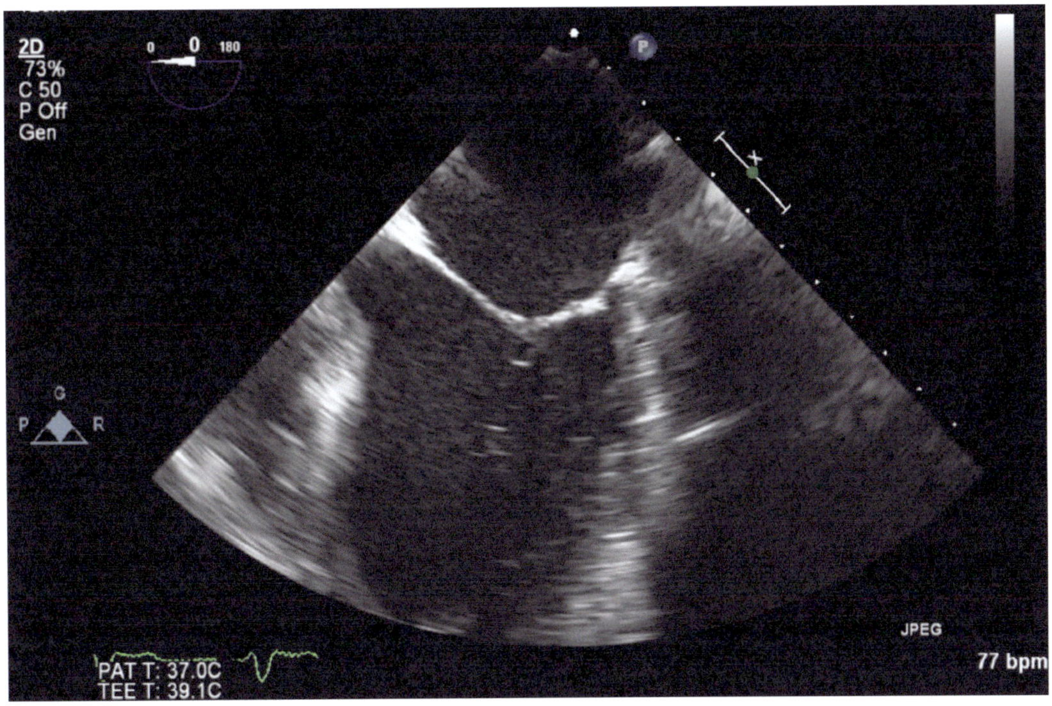

Fig. 12.6 TEE: 4C without color. The 4C views confirms significant tenting of the anterior and posterior leaflets

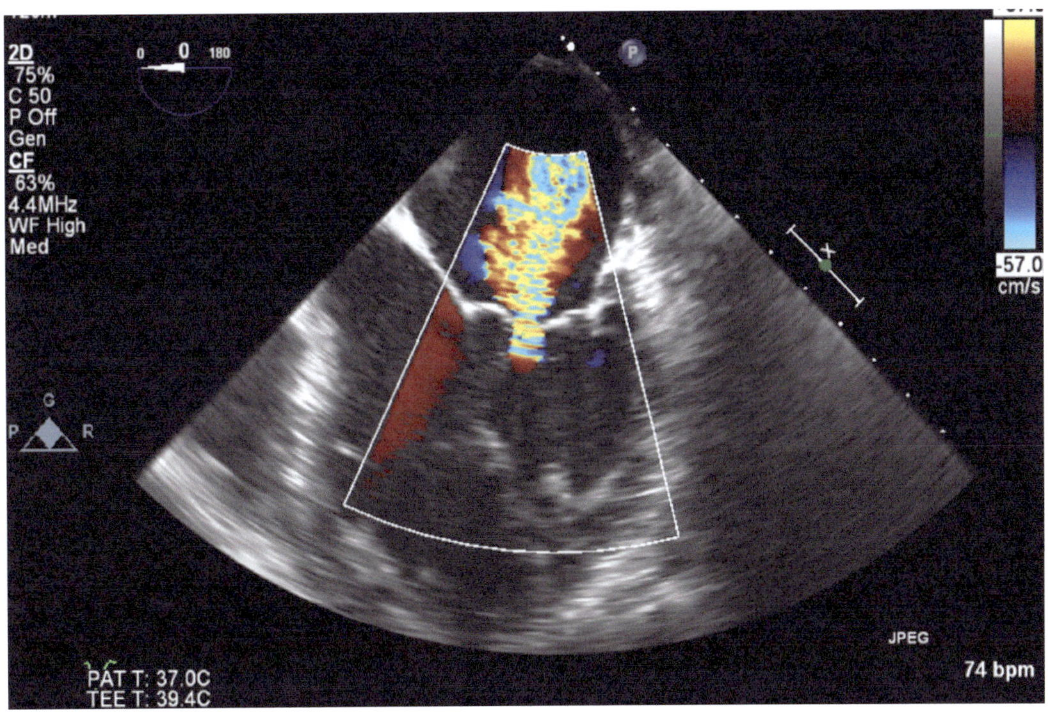

Fig. 12.7 TEE: 4C with color. There is a significant jet of posterior MR resulting from tethering of the leaflets

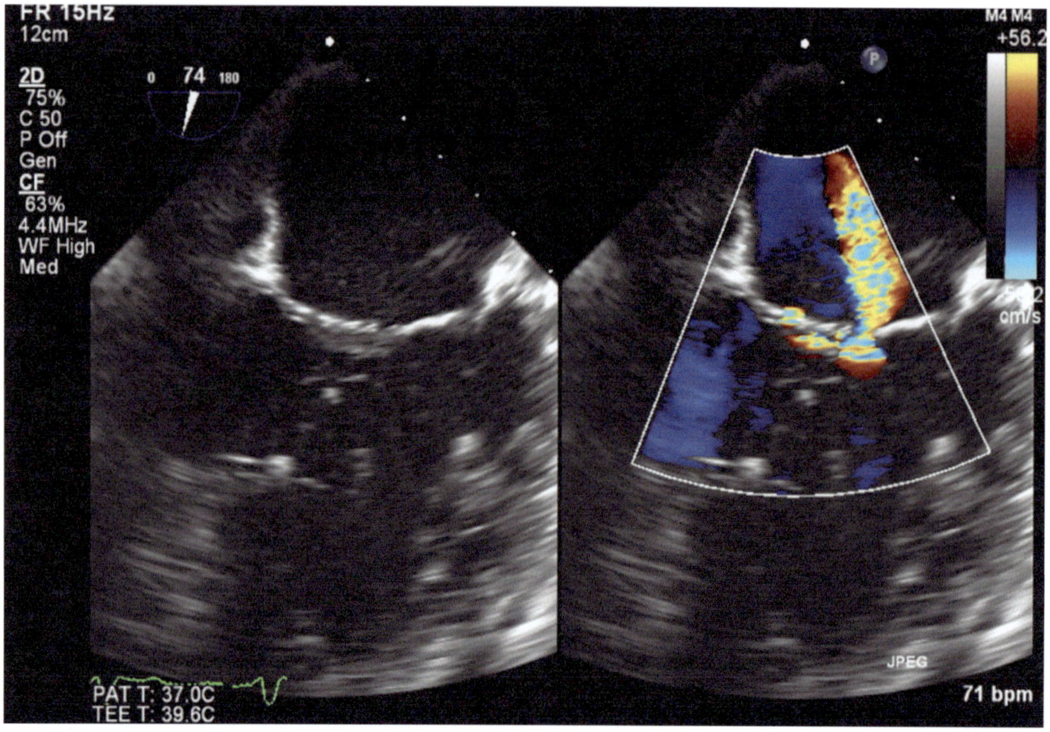

Fig. 12.8 TEE: bicom with and without color. The bicommissural view confirms a central location of the regurgitant jet

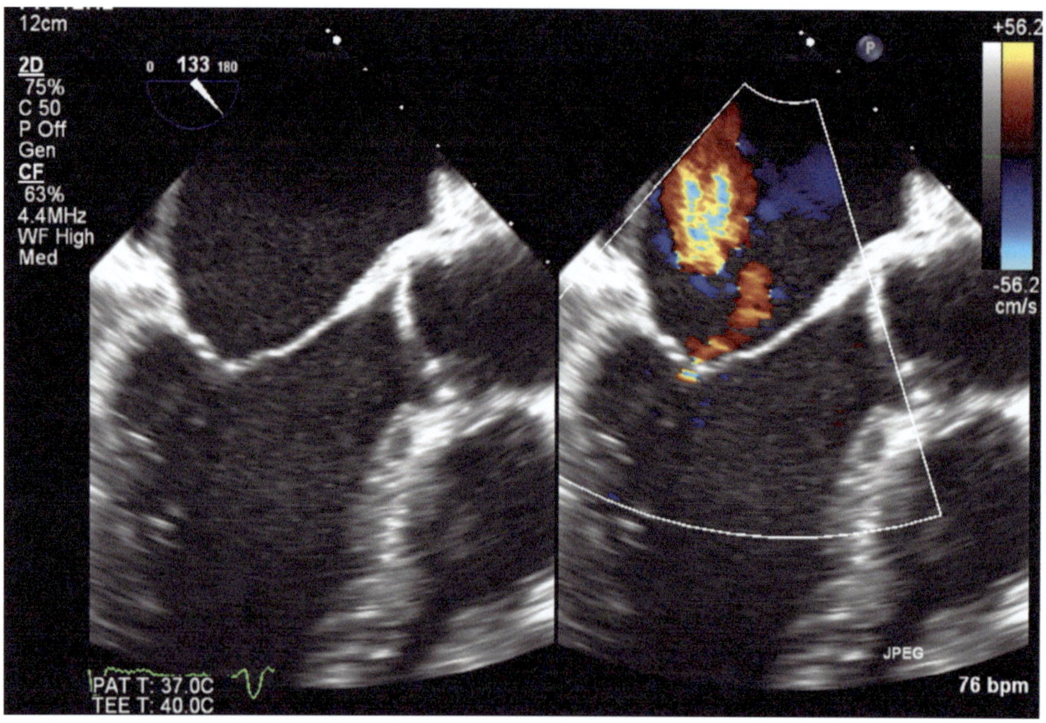

Fig. 12.9 TEE: 3C with and without color. The tenting is again apparent in the 3C view. The posterior leaflet appears somewhat shorter in this view, but there is not any significant leaflet calcification or thickening that might interfere with leaflet grasping

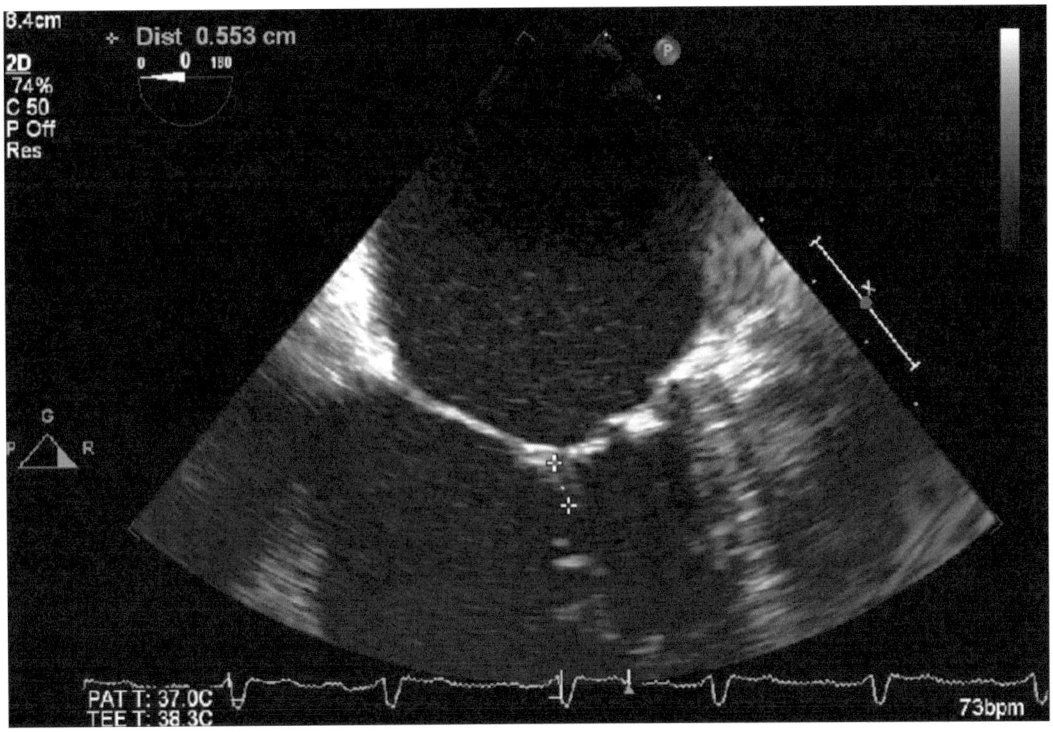

Fig. 12.10 TEE: 4C. The coaptation length is 5–6 mm, thereby providing enough leaflet tissue overlap to provide adequate grasping

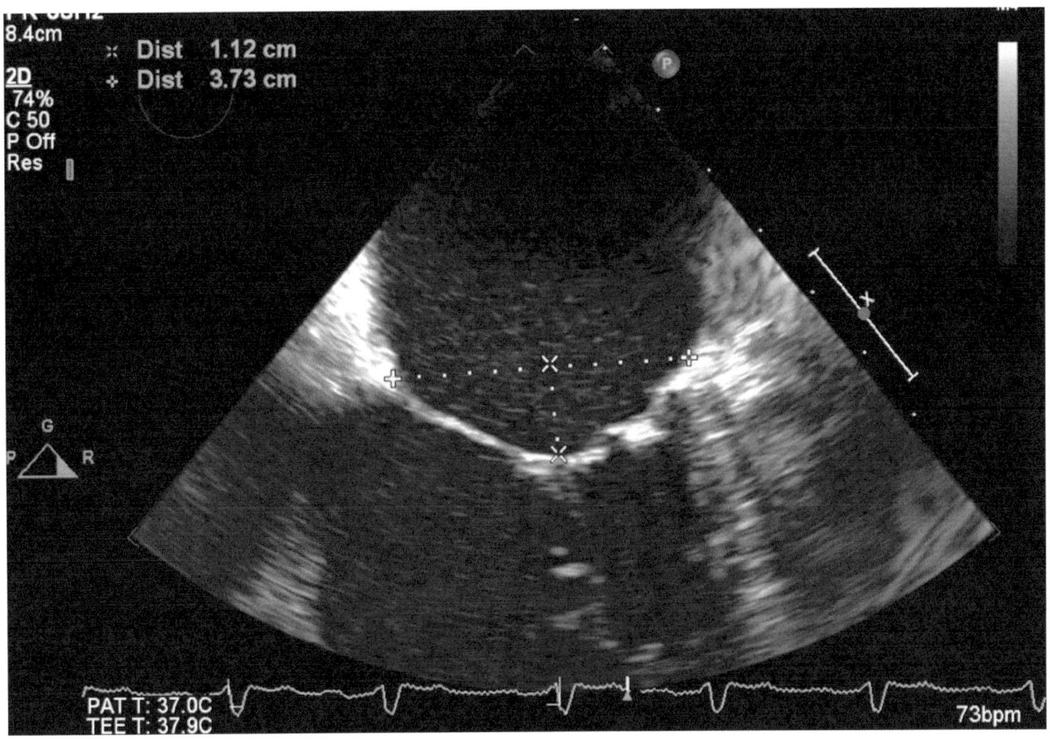

Fig. 12.11 TEE 4C. The coaptation depth is 11 mm, which is the approximate upper range of coaptation depth for inclusion in the EVEREST trials

Procedural TEE and Fluoro I

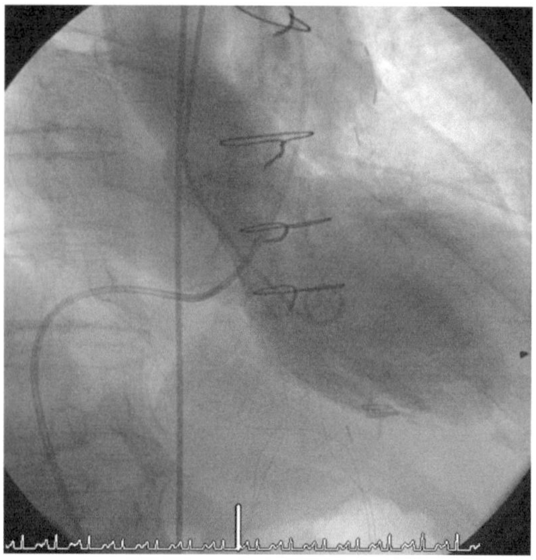

Fig. 12.12 Left ventricular cineangiography. Initial cineangiography is consistent with 3-4+ MR

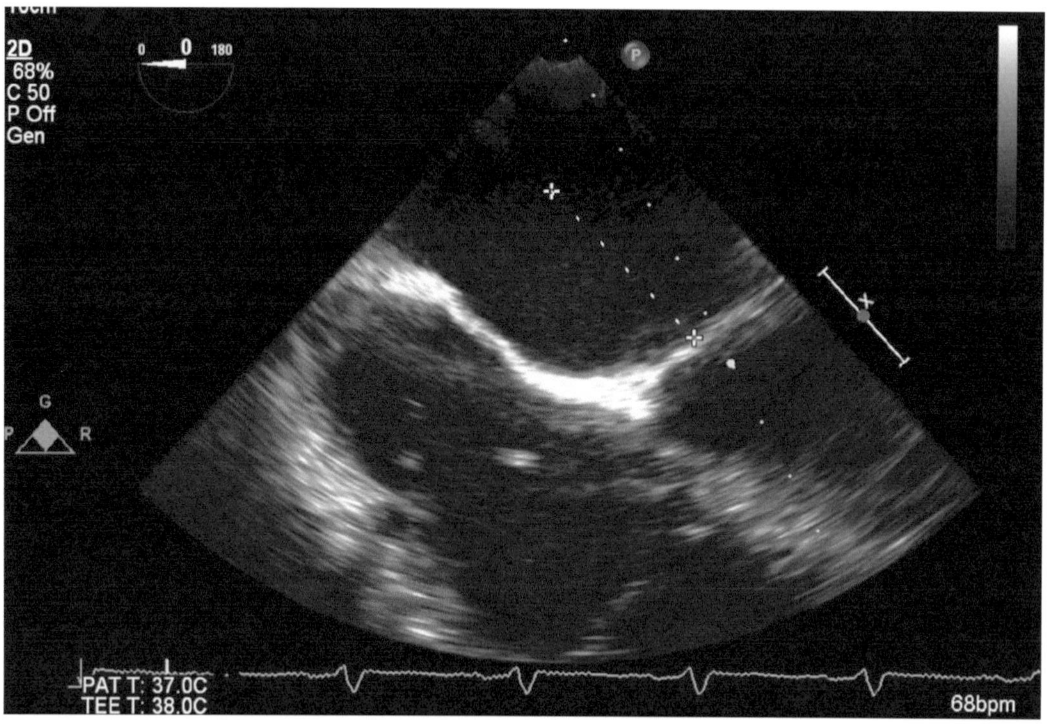

Fig. 12.13 TEE: 4C. The site of planned transseptal puncture is measured at approximately 4 cm above the annulus

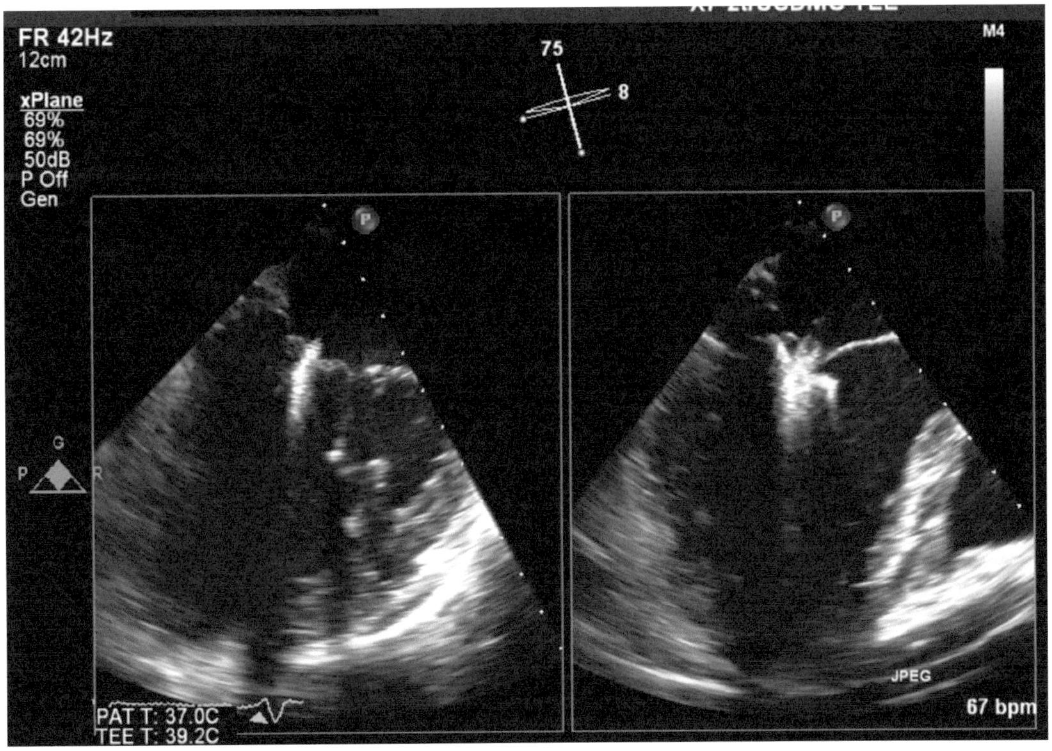

Fig. 12.14 TEE: biplane. Biplane echocardiography is used to align the device and confirm a central location prior to grasping the leaflets

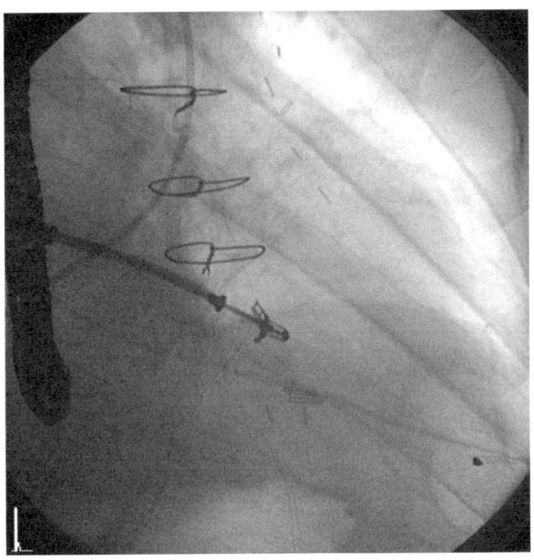

Fig. 12.15 Fluoroscopy. The first device is advanced across the mitral leaflets

Procedural TEE and Fluoro II

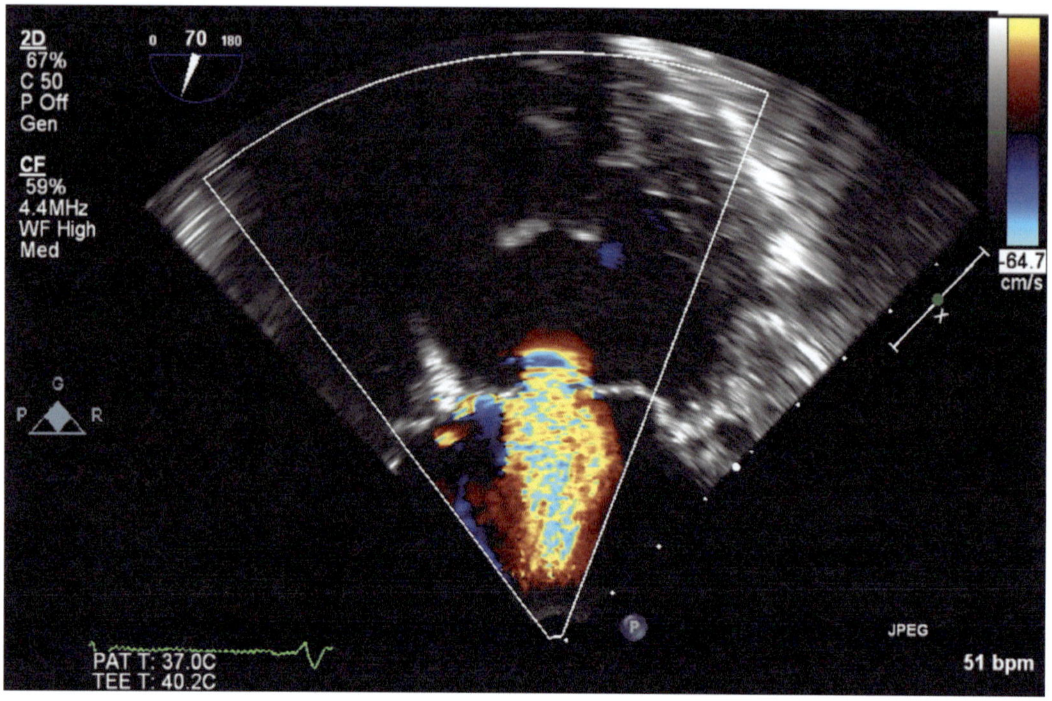

Fig. 12.16 TEE: bicom. After the first device is deployed, there is a persistent medial jet of MR

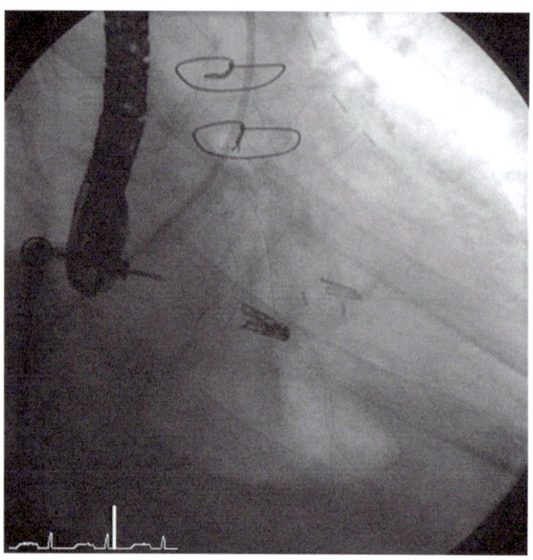

Fig. 12.17 Fluoroscopy. The first device appears well seated on fluoroscopy

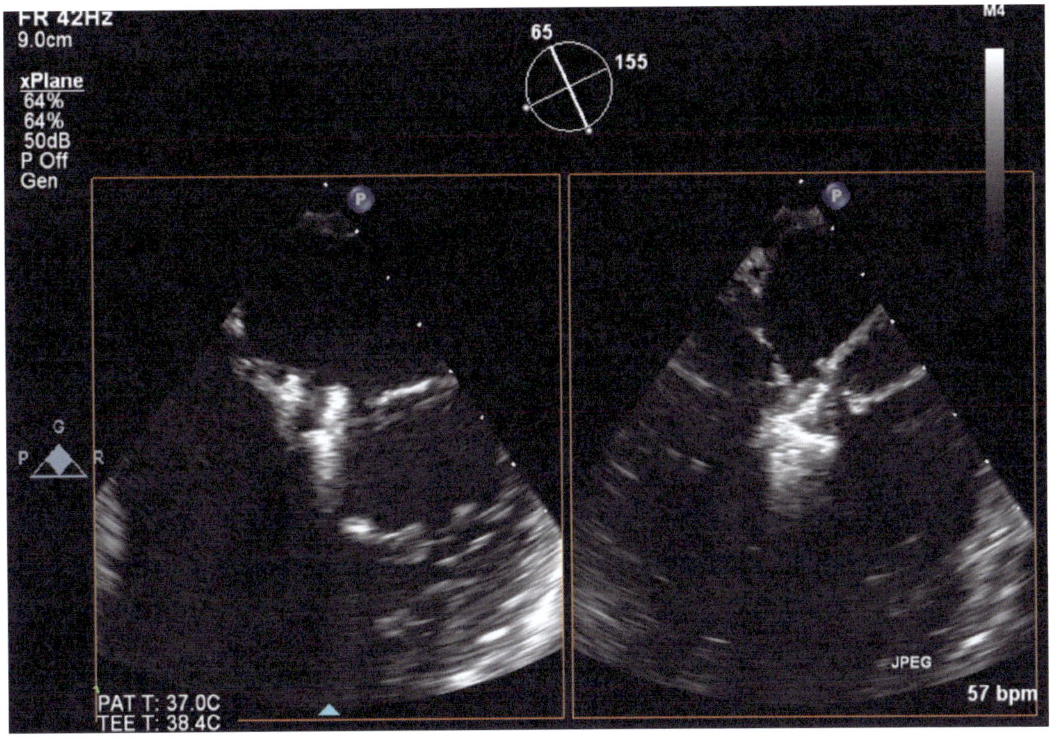

Fig. 12.18 TEE: biplane views. The second clip is deployed slightly medial to the first clip

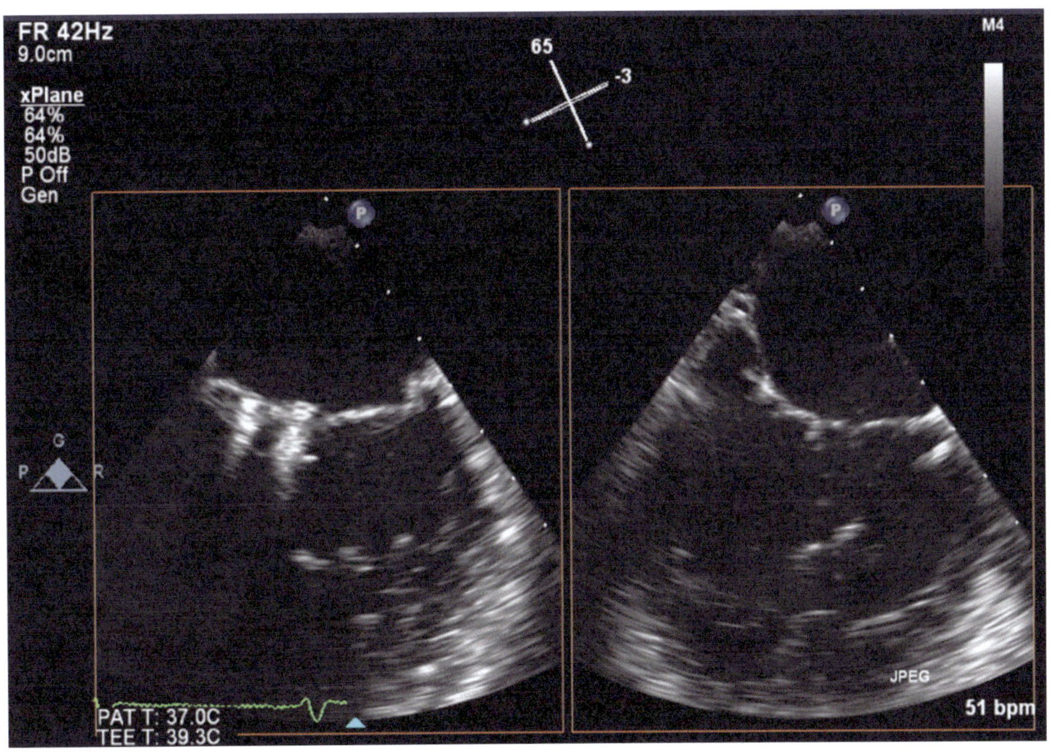

Fig. 12.19 TEE: biplane Doppler views after second clip. Postdeployment, the two devices appear well seated and parallel to one another

Procedural TEE and Fluoro III

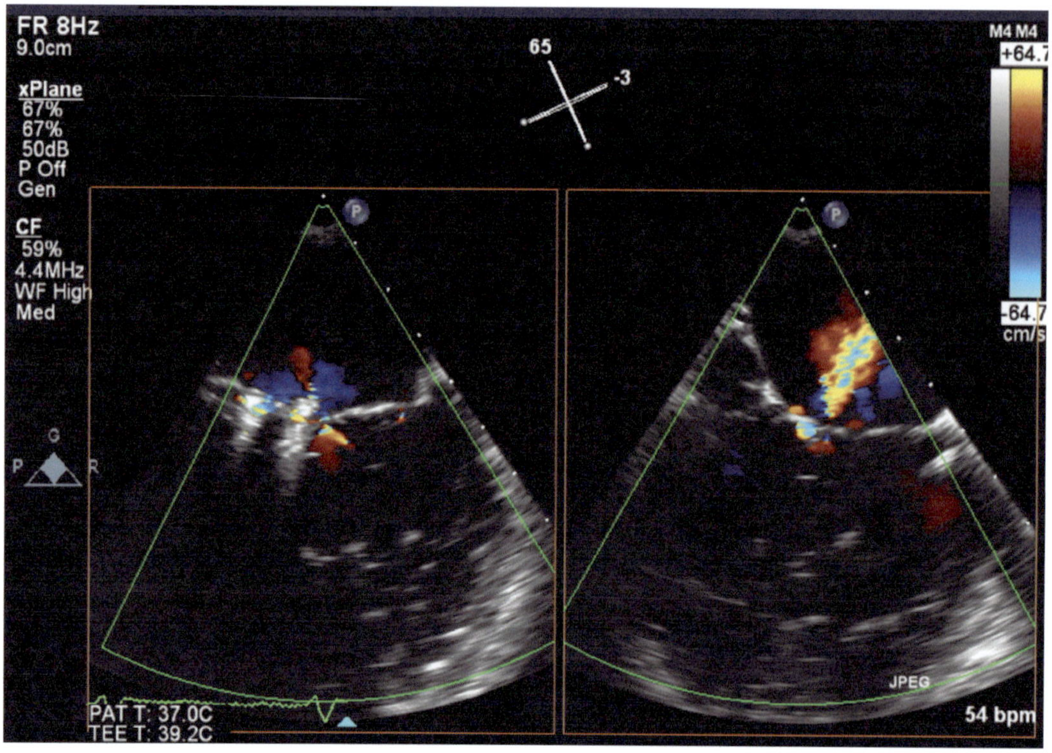

Fig. 12.20 TEE: biplane views. There is 1+ MR after deployment of two devices. The majority of the apparent MR originates from turbulence at the location of the leaflet grasping

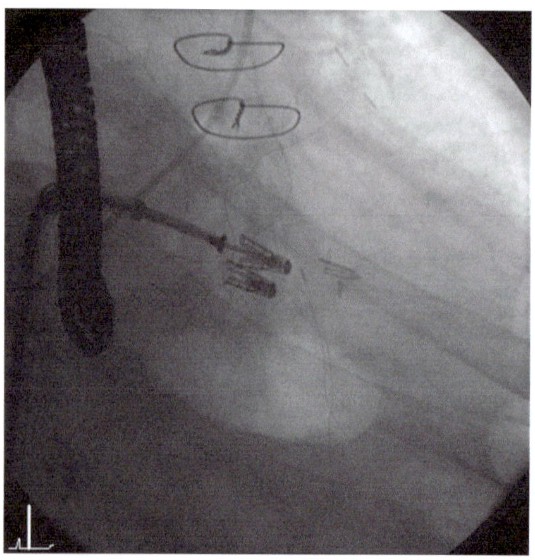

Fig. 12.21 Fluoroscopy. Correct positioning of the second device is also confirmed on fluoroscopy

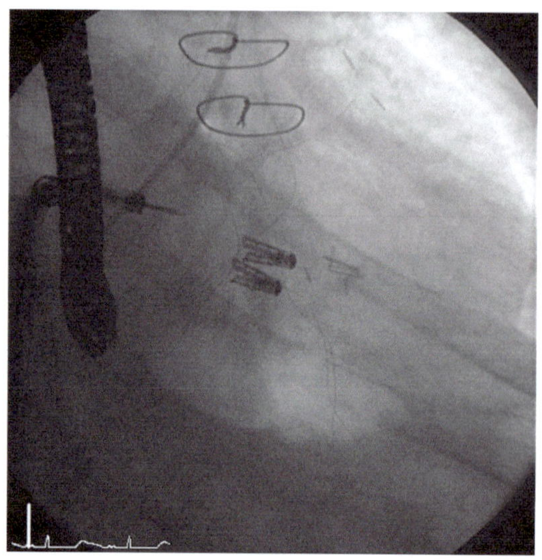

Fig. 12.22 Fluoroscopy. After deployment, the two devices are in a parallel position along the leaflet coaptation line

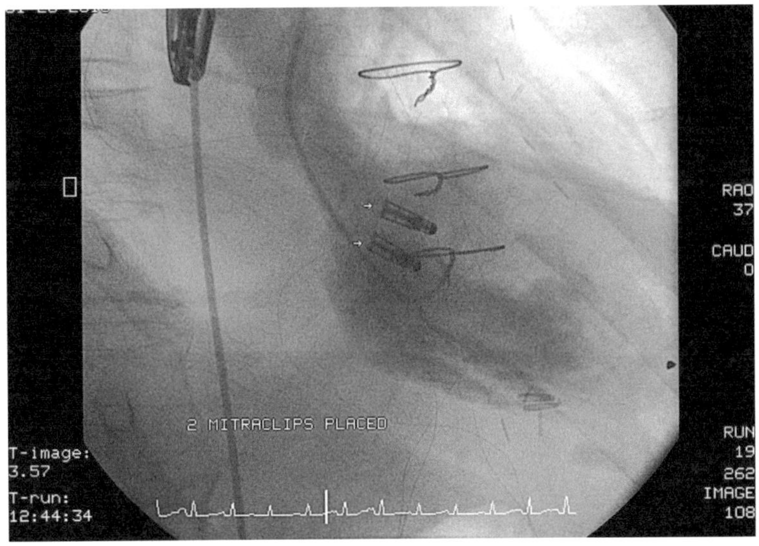

Fig. 12.23 Fluoroscopy. After deployment of both devices, there is only trace residual MR as assessed by left ventricular cineangiography. The arrows point to the atrial side of each MitraClip device

Postprocedure TTE

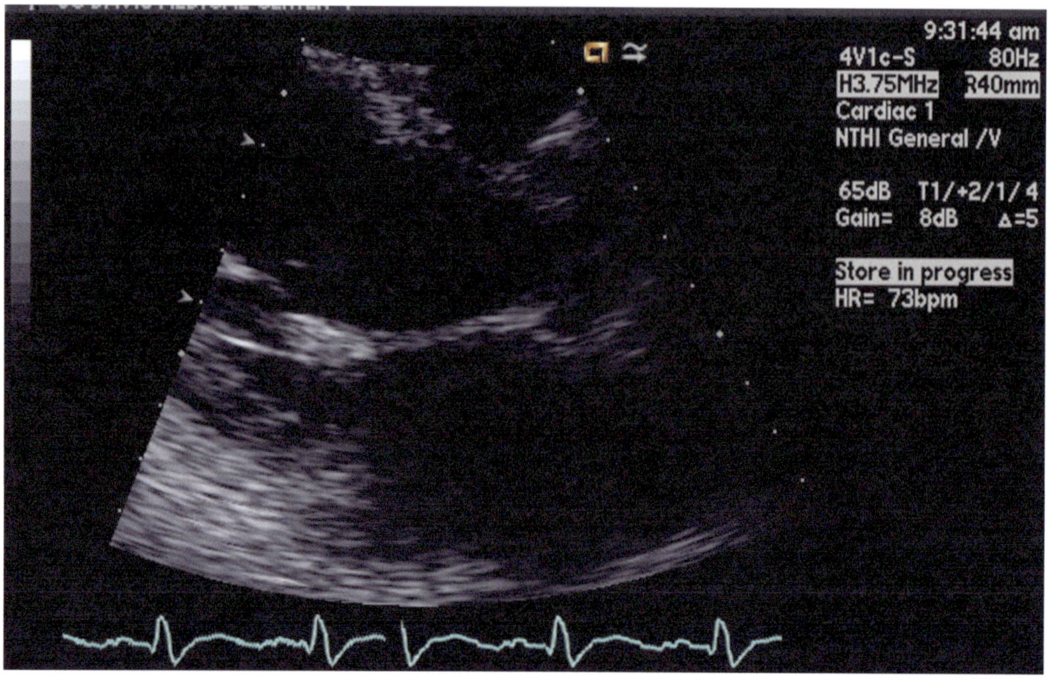

Fig. 12.24 TTE: parasternal LAX. The devices remain well oriented along the central portion of the mitral valve leaflets

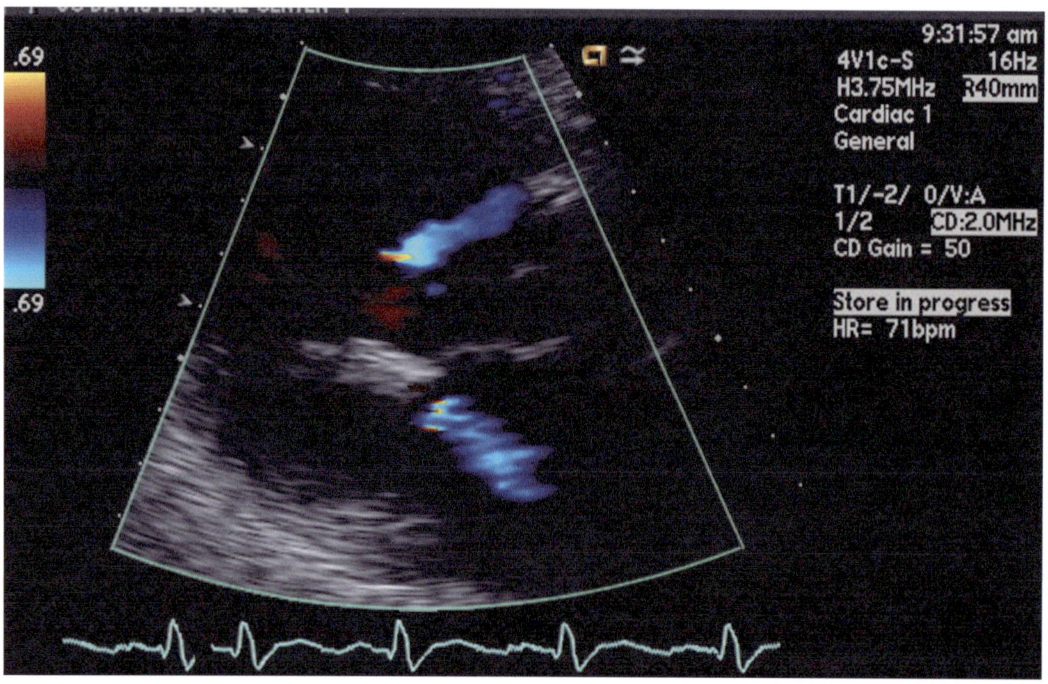

Fig. 12.25 TTE: parasternal LAX with color. Doppler shows only 1+ MR

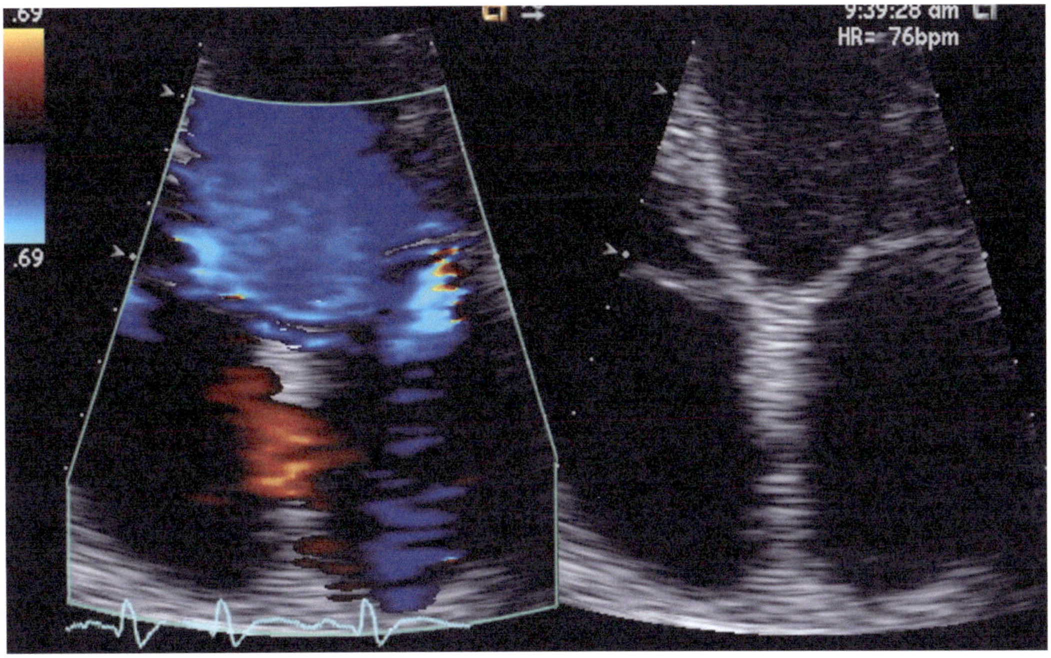

Fig. 12.26 TTE: 4C with and without color. In addition to the 1+ jet of MR on Doppler, note the persistent color flow across the interatrial septum, consistent with a small iatrogenic atrial septal defect

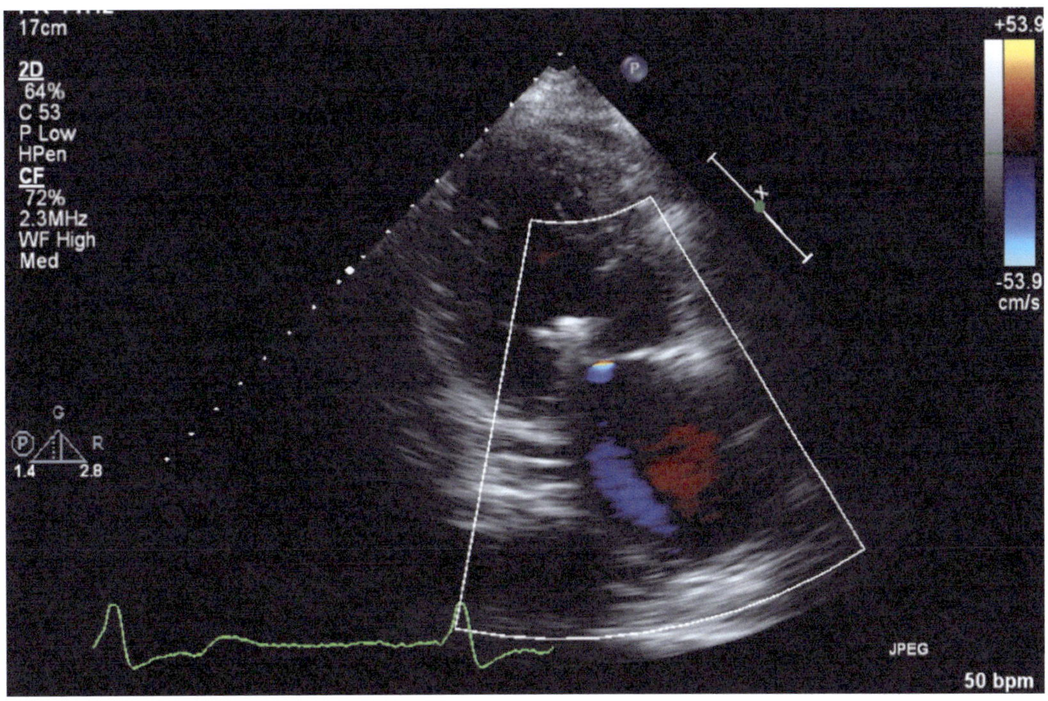

Fig. 12.27 TTE: 2C with color. In the 2C view, the 1+ jet of MR originates from a central location at the site of device coaptation

Barlow's Disease

13

Nikolaj Ihlemann, Lars Søndergaard, and Olaf Franzen

Abstract

Barlow's disease is an important cause of mitral valve prolapse and may result in mitral regurgitation. Repair of the valve using the MitraClip is more complex but technically possible. This chapter uses two case examples to illustrate some of the technical and procedural concerns and strategies when using the MitraClip to treat patients with Barlow's disease.

Keywords

Barlow's disease • Valve prolapse • Myxoid degeneration • Mitral regurgitation • MitraClip

Introduction

Barlow's disease is a disease entity characterized by excess of thickened mitral leaflets as a result of myxoid degeneration. It accounts for approximately 30 % of patients with degenerative mitral valve disease and mitral regurgitation, usually affecting the younger segment of patients below 60 years of age.

The microscopic changes include myxoid infiltration and replacement of elastic fibers with collagen fibers. Macroscopically, the annulus is dilated, the valves are thickened with excess tissue and billowing, and there is usually bileaflet prolapse or multiple sites of prolapse with multiple regurgitant jets [1, 2].

Surgical correction of Barlow's disease can be challenging. With progressive disease, results are usually poorer than in other patients with degenerative mitral valve disease. Surgical techniques include the "edge-to-edge" Alfieri repair, leaflet resection, sliding annuloplasty, and the use of neochordae [3].

Treating patients with Barlow's disease using the MitraClip is equally challenging, and a portion of patients are denied this treatment because of expected poor results [4]. It is of great importance to perform the diagnostic transesophageal echocardiography (TEE) thoroughly to identify the often multiple regurgitant jets to achieve the best outcome. Also, since the myxoid infiltration is heterogeneous, one should evaluate the tissue quality to choose leaflet areas most likely to endure the MitraClip grasp.

Case 1: Clinical History

A 90-year-old lady presented with New York Heart Association (NYHA) Class 3 heart failure but was otherwise in good health. Workup echocardiography revealed a floppy mitral valve with severe mitral regurgitation (Figs. 13.1 and 13.2), preserved left ventricular ejection fraction (LVEF), borderline pulmonary hypertension with estimated systolic pulmonary pressure of 40 mmHg, and no other valve disease.

N. Ihlemann, M.D., Ph.D. (✉)
Department of Cardiology,
Rigshospitalet, University Hospital of Copenhagen,
Blegdamsvej 9, Copenhagen 2100, Denmark
e-mail: nikolajihlemann@gmail.com

L. Søndergaard, M.D., Dm.Sc.
Department of Cardiology,
Rigshospitalet, University Hospital of Copenhagen,
Blegdamsvej 9, Copenhagen 2100, Denmark

Cardiology Invasive Laboratory, University Hospital of Copenhagen,
Blegdamsvej 9, Copenhagen 2100, Denmark
e-mail: lars.soendergaard@rh.regionh.dk

O. Franzen, M.D.
Department of Cardiology, The Heart Center, Rigshospitalet,
University of Copenhagen,
Blegdamsvej 9, Copenhagen 2100, Denmark

Royal Brompton Hospital, Royal Brompton
and Harefield NHS Foundation Trust, London, UK
e-mail: owfranzen@gmx.de

T. Feldman et al. (eds.), *Atlas of Percutaneous Edge-to-Edge Mitral Valve Repair*,
DOI 10.1007/978-1-4471-4294-2_13, © Springer-Verlag London 2013

Coronary angiography showed no significant stenosis. The patient was discussed at the hospital's multidisciplinary heart conference, and transcatheter treatment with the MitraClip was chosen because of advanced age and frailty.

Preprocedural TEE in two-chamber view, with and without color Doppler, showed thickened leaflets with bileaflet prolapse, yet most pronounced at the P1 scallop. Preprocedural two- and three-dimensional TEE showed thickened leaflets with bileaflet prolapse and several regurgitant jets. Integrating the two- and three-dimensional pictures helps to understand the valve anatomy and the placement of the regurgitant jets (see Figs. 13.1, 13.2, and 13.3). Since the patient had relatively small mitral annulus, with a mean gradient of 3.5 mmHg, a central clip strategy was planned (see Figs. 13.4 and 13.5).

After placement of the clip, one can appreciate the double orifice with prevalvular acceleration (see Fig. 13.6, left hand side). Figure 13.6, right-hand side, shows the two minor residual regurgitant jets, one small central and one lateral, the latter remains of the initial lateral jet. A second clip could not be placed taking care of the lateral jet, since the mean gradient was already increased from 3.5 to 6.5 mmHg (see Fig. 13.7). Due to the bileaflet prolapse, the clip moves vigorously throughout the heart cycle, which could possibly affect durability (see Fig. 13.8).

At 3 months follow-up, the patient experienced reduced symptoms of dyspnea as evaluated by changing from NYHA Class 3 to NYHA Class 2. Walking distance also increased as evaluated by a 6 min walk test increased from 170 to 330 m. Transthoracic echocardiography (TTE) showed minor mitral regurgitation, reduced left ventricular size (left ventricular diastole from 5.1 to 4.2 cm), but an increased transmitral VTI at 8 mmHg (see Fig. 13.9).

Case 2: Clinical History

Eighty-eight-year-old gentleman with severe dyspnea and NYHA Class 3 heart failure. TEE revealed a mitral valve with thickened leaflets and pronounced P2 to P3 prolapse (see Figs. 13.10 and 13.11). The mitral regurgitation was severe and LVEF was preserved. Coronary angiography showed no significant stenosis. The patient had a kyphotic thorax, with a slightly reduced pulmonary function. When discussed at the multidisciplinary heart team meeting, surgery was deemed unsuitable because of the advanced age and kyphotic thorax. Treatment with transcatheter mitral valve repair with the MitraClip system was planned (see Figs. 13.10, 13.11, and 13.12).

A strategy was chosen to start medially with the first clip rather than zippering from lateral to medial; again, three-dimensional pictures were helpful (see Fig. 13.13). After placing the first clip, a residual regurgitant jet called for placement of a second clip, after ensuring that the valve area was not reduced too much (see Figs. 13.14 and 13.15). After placement of the second clip, the final result was acceptable (see Figs. 13.16 and 13.17).

At 6-month follow-up, the patient symptoms improved from NYHA Class 3 to Class 1. His walking distance in a 6-min walk test improved from 185 to 360 m. LVEF was still normal and there was a mild residual mitral regurgitation (see Fig. 13.18). The systolic pulmonary pressure was improved from 53 to 23 mmHg.

Summary

Barlow's disease represents a challenging group of patients with mitral valve regurgitation. The special anatomy with excess thickened tissue and often bileaflet and severe prolapse makes grasping of the leaflets challenging. Tissue quality is heterogeneous and areas of weak tissue quality can be scattered in areas of more fibrous areas. Therefore, during the grasp, one has to choose the area for grasping not only after the regurgitant jet but also after the areas of good tissue quality. The extensive prolapse, and possible flail, can also limit or challenge the areas of possible grasping. Because the valve often presents with multiple jets, one should target the larger jet since it is not always possible to treat all the regurgitant jets. In Case 1, the mitral valve area limited our ability to place a second clip for further reduction of mitral regurgitation. A thorough baseline TEE is essential for planning which of the possible numerous jets to treat and in what order. Three-dimensional TEE can help to understand the anatomy and planning. During the procedure, assessment of the mitral valve opening area is essential to help choose the decision of when to stop reducing mitral regurgitation to avoid creating mitral stenosis.

Learning Points

1. In Barlow's disease, it is important to consider valve tissue quality when deciding on where to grasp the leaflets.
2. Plan a strategy that treats the area of the largest regurgitant jet in situations with multiple jets.

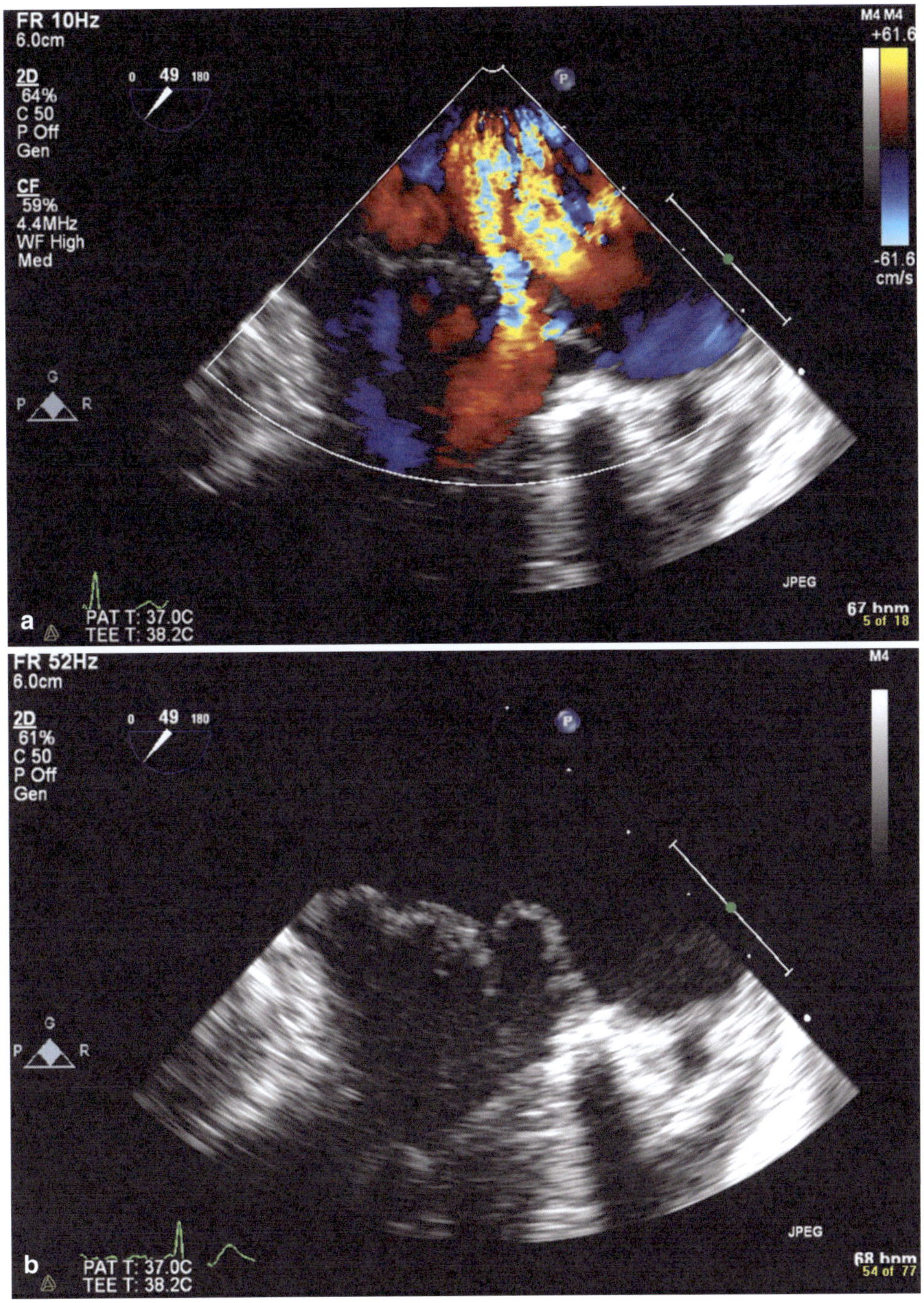

Fig. 13.1 Preprocedural TEE in two-chamber view, with (**a**) and without color Doppler (**b**), showing thickened leaflets with bileaflet prolapse, most pronounced at the P1 scallop

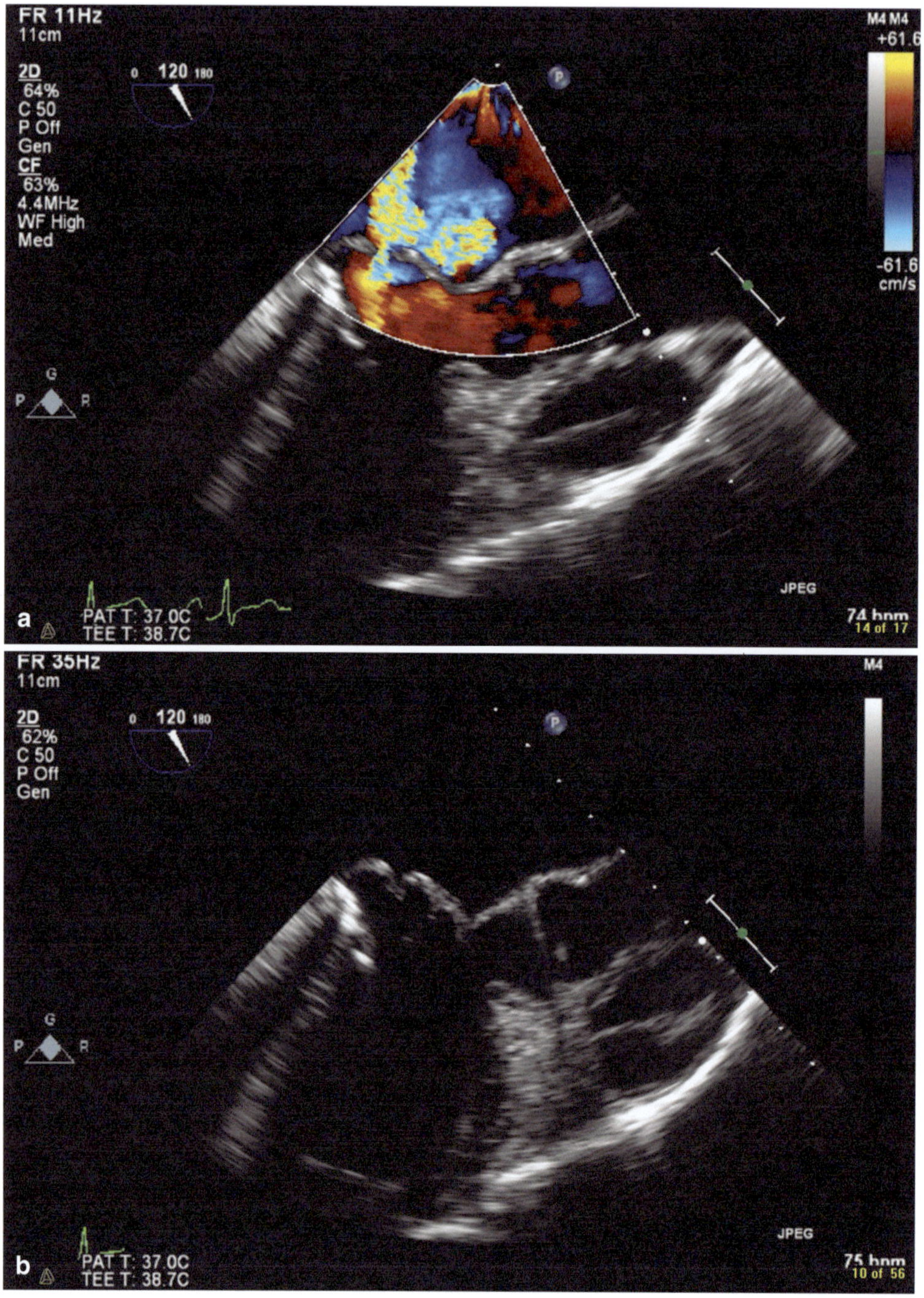

Fig. 13.2 Preprocedural TEE in three-chamber view, with (**a**) and without color Doppler (**b**), showing thickened leaflets with bileaflet prolapse. Note that there are several regurgitant jets

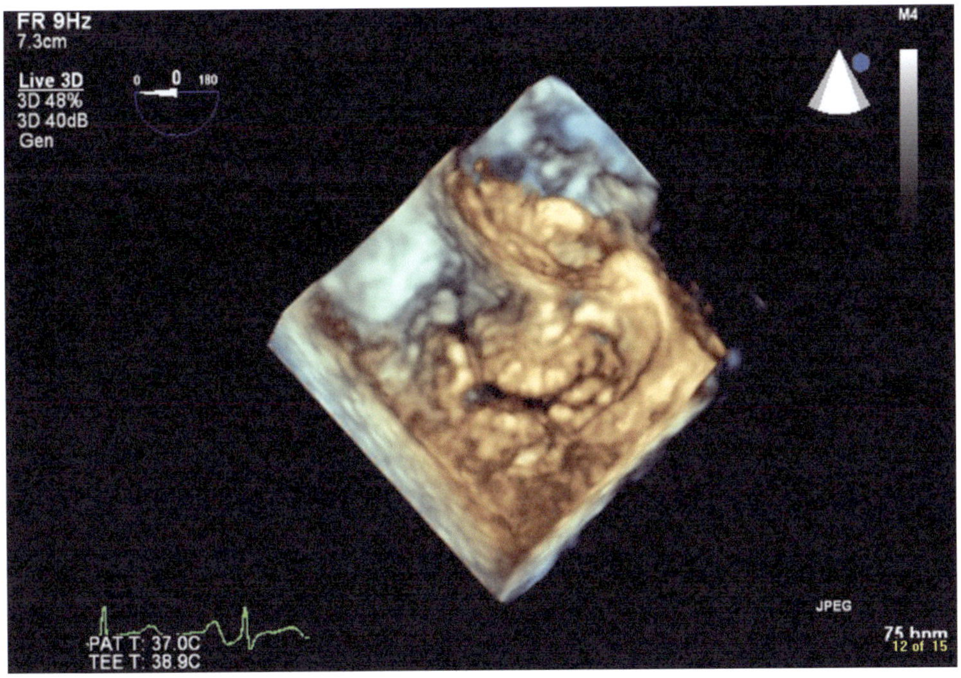

Fig. 13.3 Preprocedural three-dimensional TEE displayed in the "surgeon's view" with aorta in top of the picture. The picture shows the thickened leaflets and the bileaflet prolapse characteristic in Barlow's disease. Integrating this picture with the two-dimensional pictures helps the anatomic understanding. It is obvious there are two jets, one central and one lateral

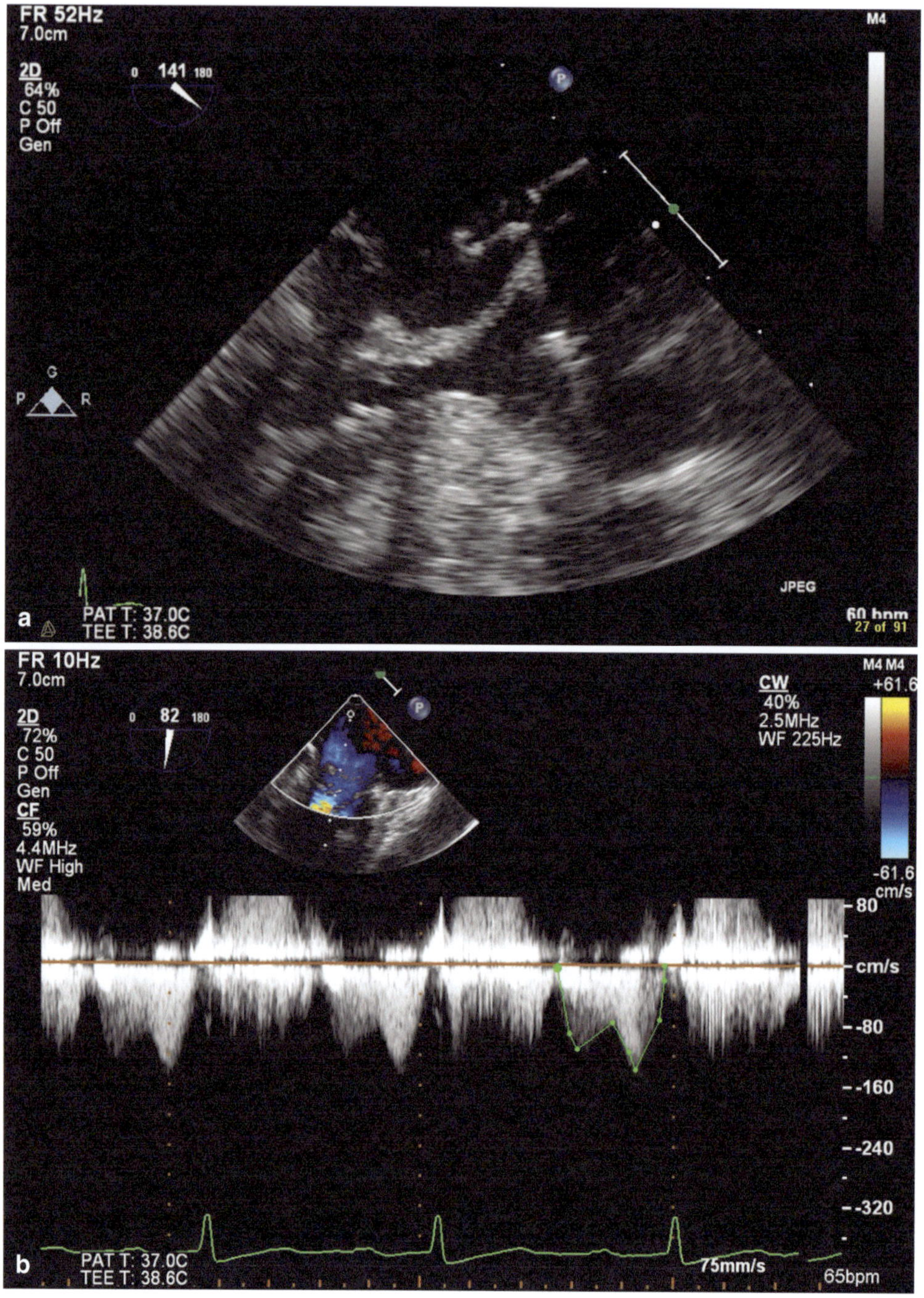

Fig. 13.4 Because of the relative small mitral annulus, in this patient, with a mean gradient of 3.5 mmHg, a central clip strategy was planned. The picture shows the clip approaching the mitral valve in a three-chamber view (**a**) and the mitral valve VTI (velocity time integral) (**b**)

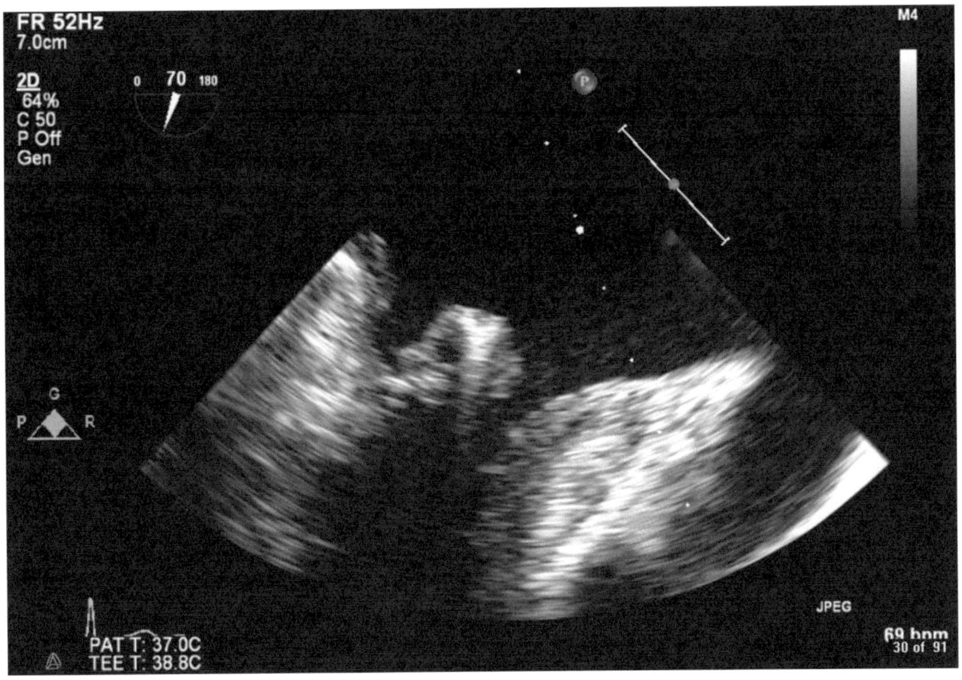

Fig. 13.5 TEE with a two-chamber view, in diastole, showing the central placement of the clip

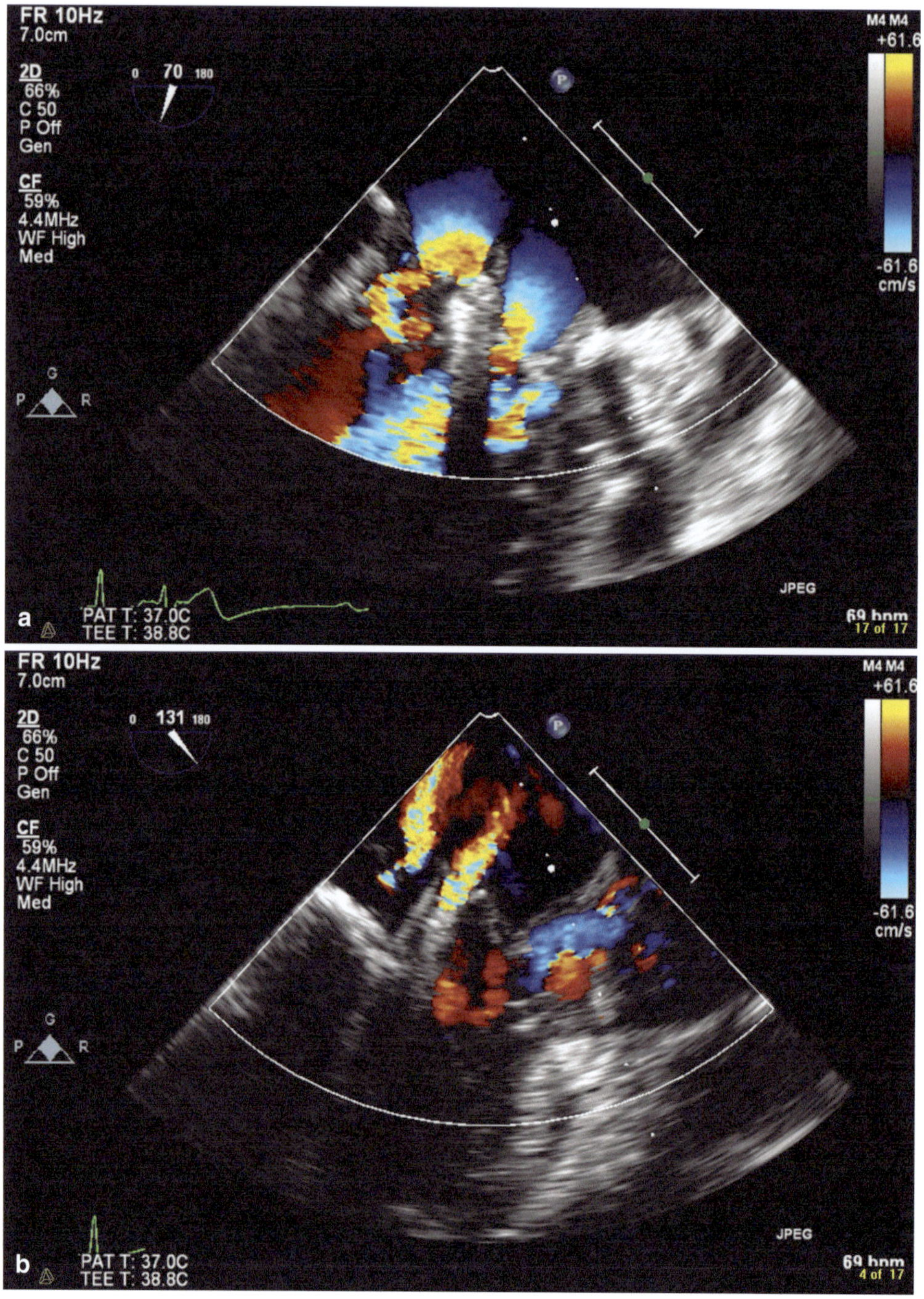

Fig. 13.6 After placement of the clip, one can appreciate the double orifice with prevalvular acceleration (**a**). TTE showing the two minor residual regurgitant jets, one small central and one lateral (**b**); the latter remains of the initial lateral jet. A second clip could not be placed, since the mean gradient had increased from 3.5 to 6.5 mmHg

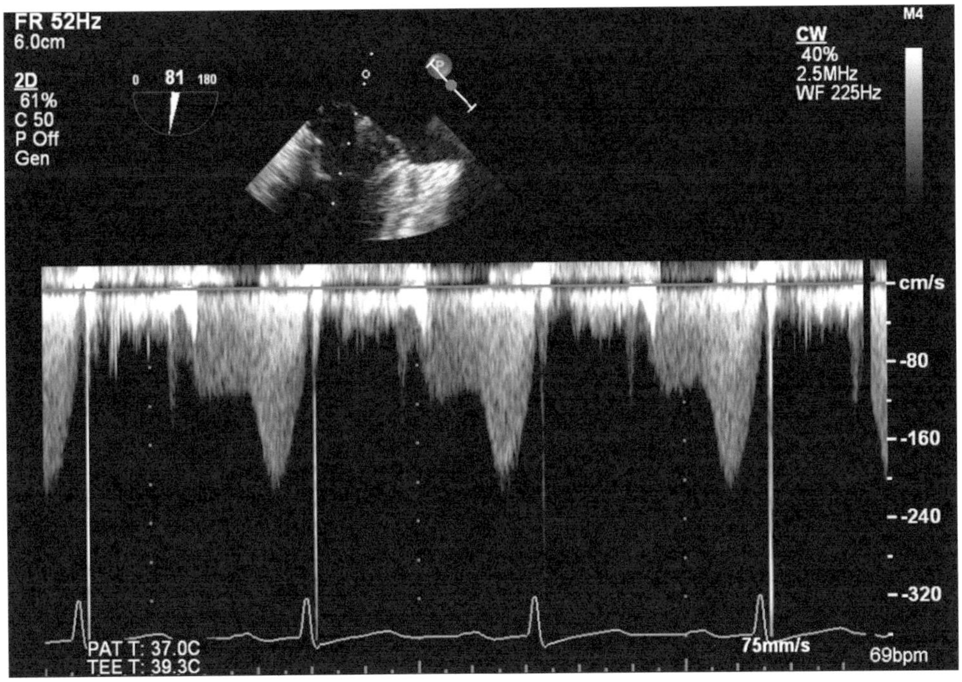

Fig. 13.7 Transmitral VTI after placement of the clip, the gradient rose from 3.5 to 6.5 mmHg after clip

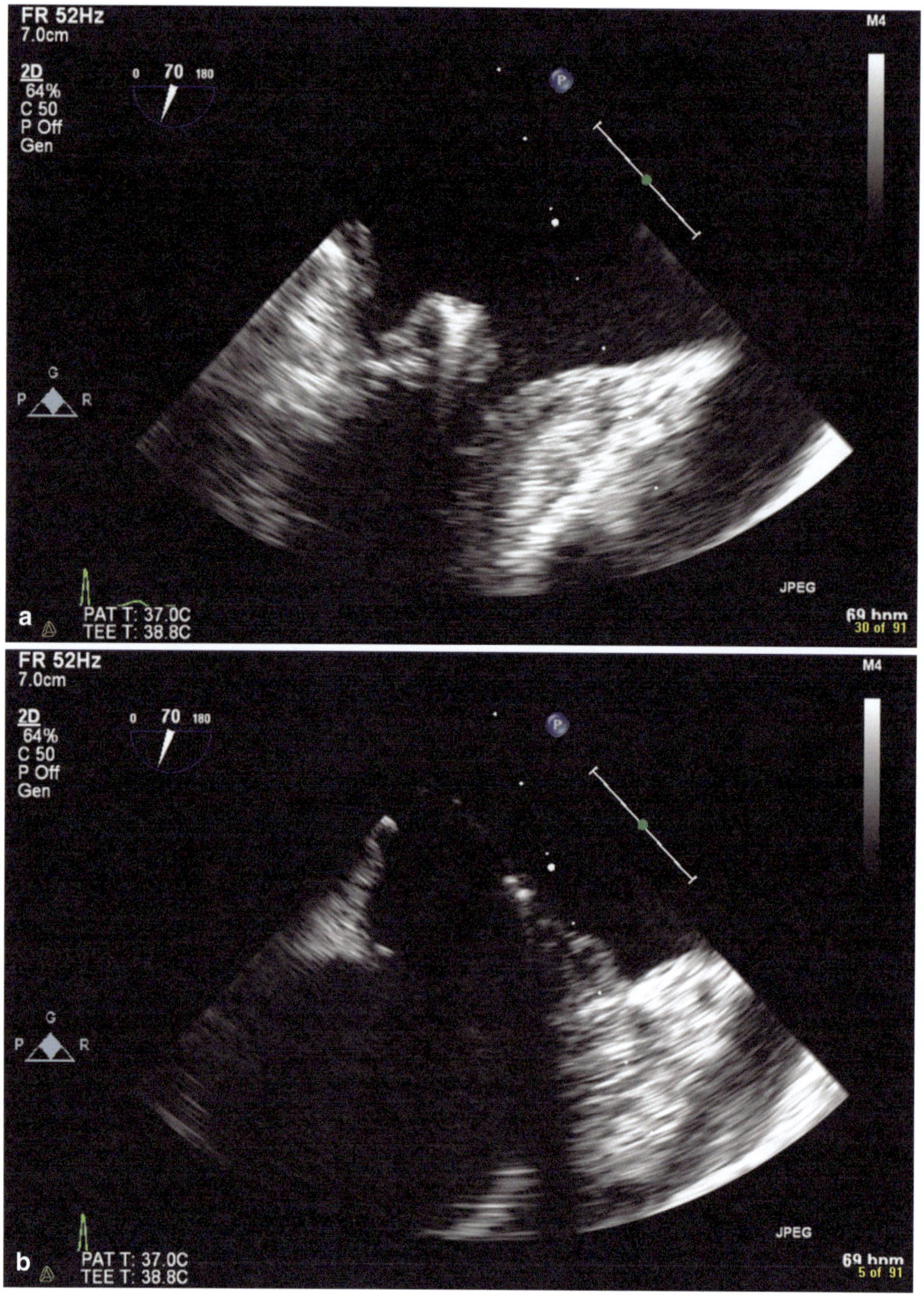

Fig. 13.8 This shows the mobility of the clip due to bileaflet prolapse. *Left panel* (**a**) shows the clip during diastole and the *right panel* (**b**) shows the billowing of the clip and leaflets during systole

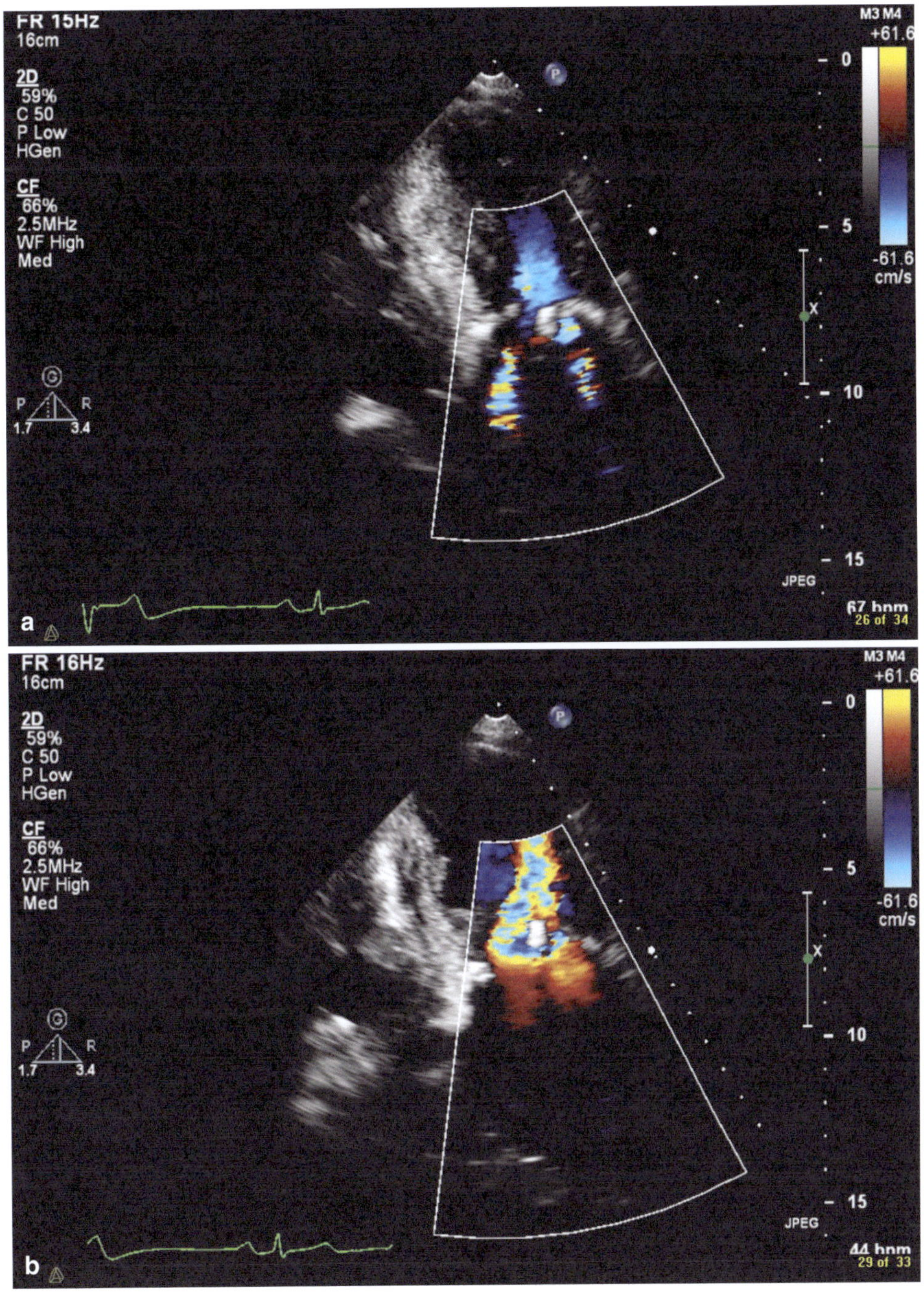

Fig. 13.9 TTE at 3-month follow-up. *Left panel* (**a**) shows the two residual regurgitant jets, and the *right panel* (**b**) shows the diastolic accelerated inflow giving no room for a multiple clip strategy

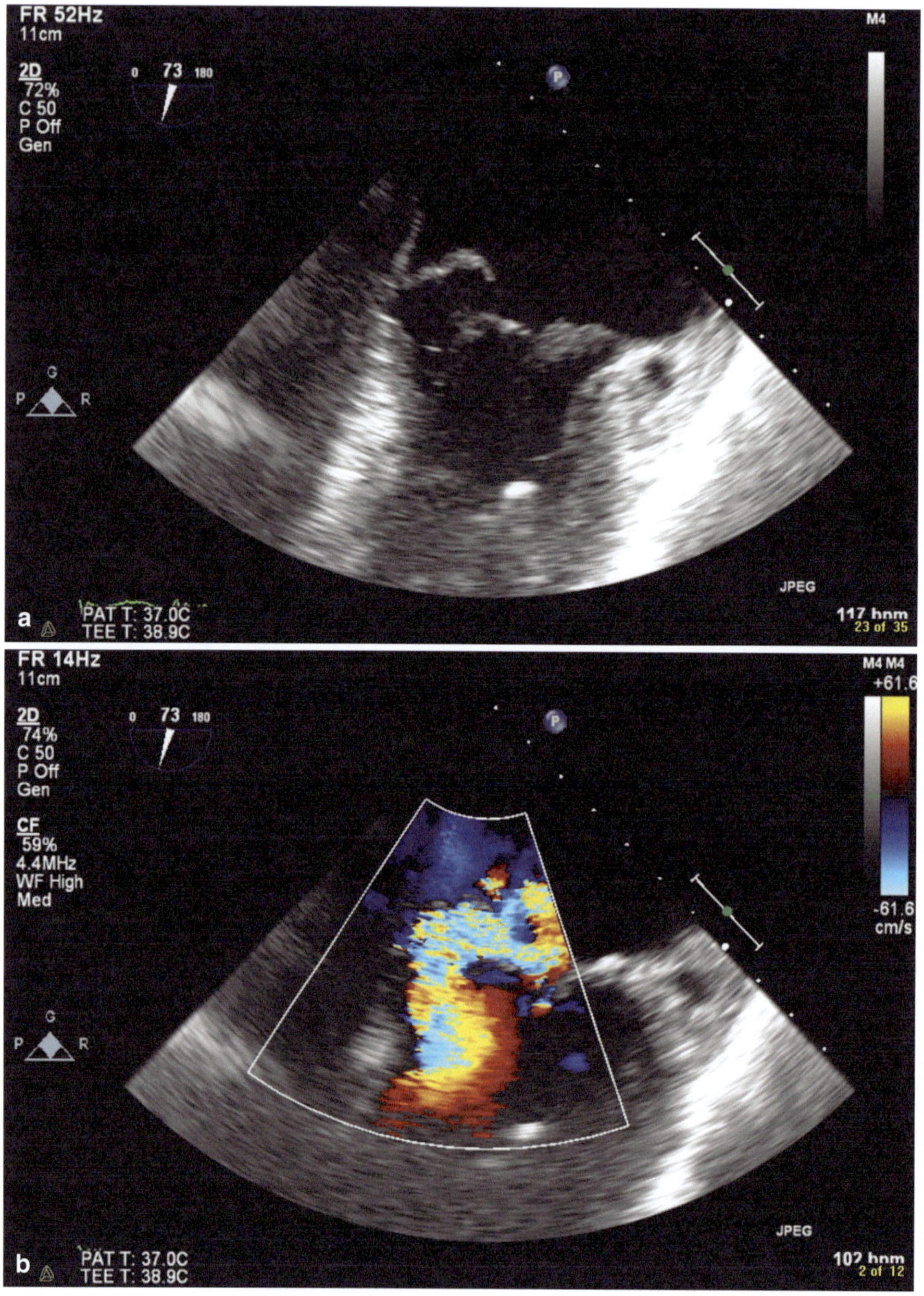

Fig. 13.10 TEE showing a two-chamber view. *Left panel* (**a**), the valve appears thickened and there is pronounced flail of the P3 segment. *Right panel* reveals severe regurgitation (**b**)

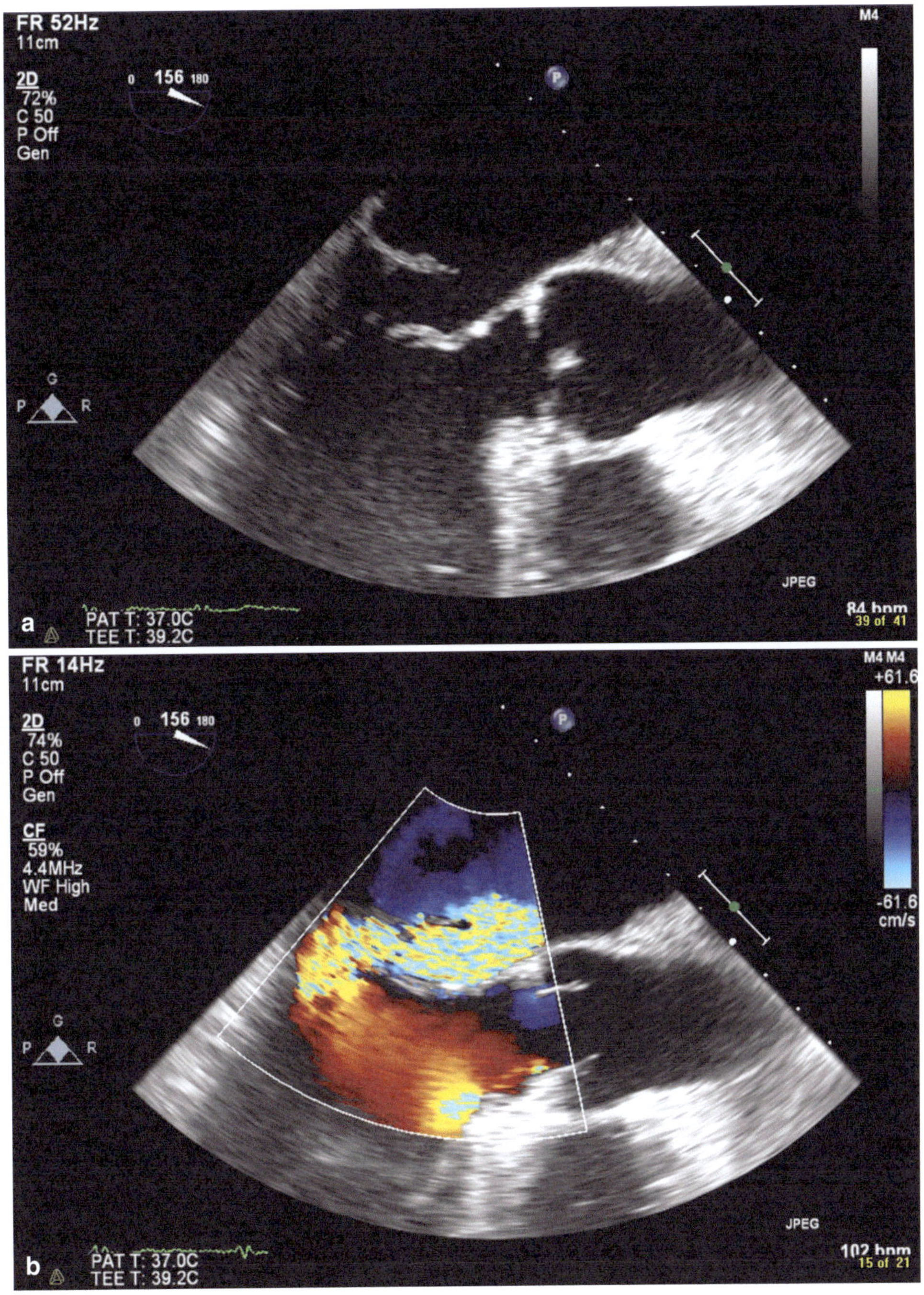

Fig. 13.11 TEE showing a three-chamber view. *Left panel* (**a**), the P2 segment is severe flail and the *right panel* reveals severe regurgitation (**b**)

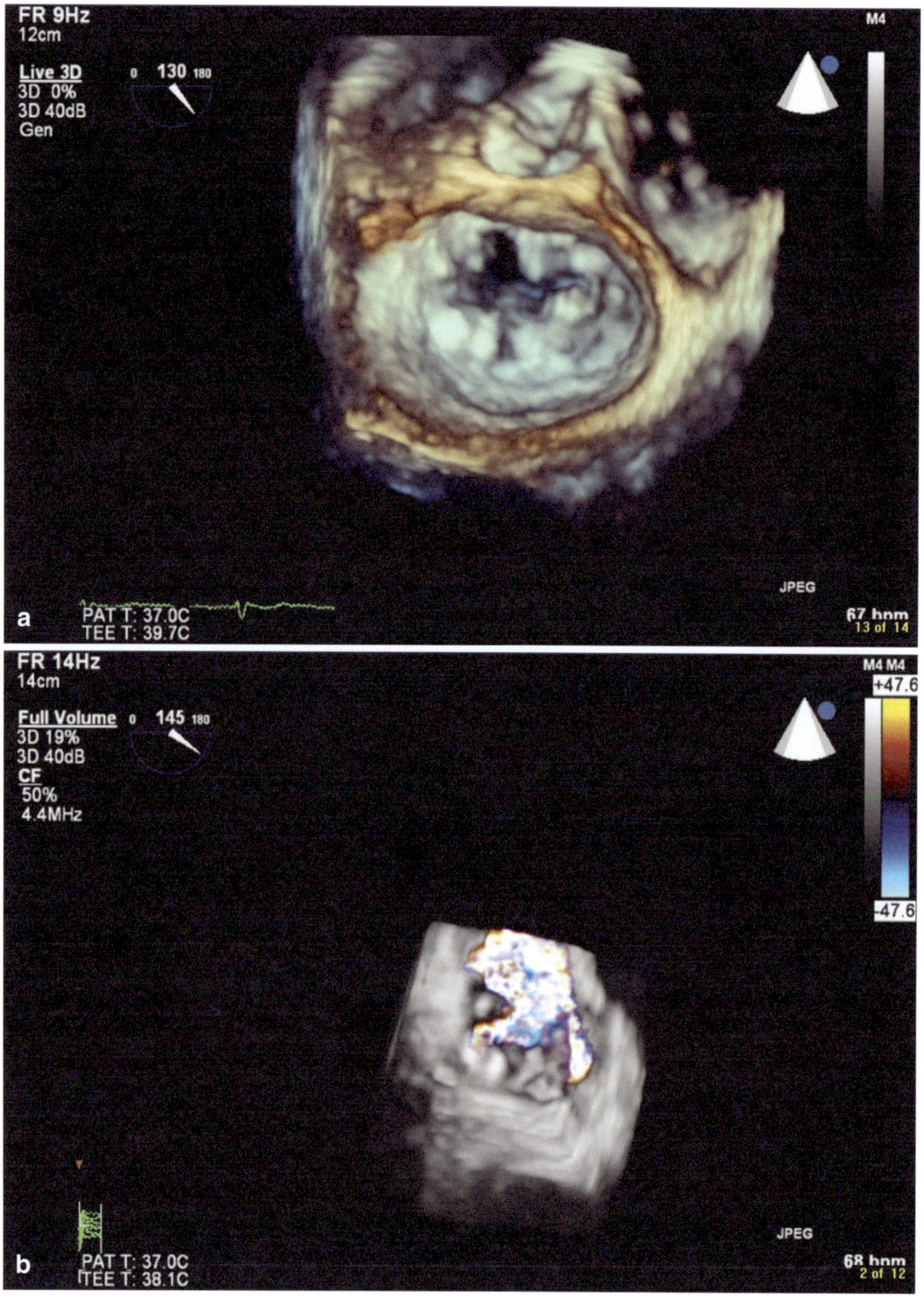

Fig. 13.12 Three-dimensional TEE, the mitral valve viewed from the atrium. *Left panel* (**a**) shows the thickened valve with the prolapsing P2 to P3 segment. The *right panel* (**b**) shows three-dimensional TEE with color showing that the major regurgitation originates from the P2 to P3 segment

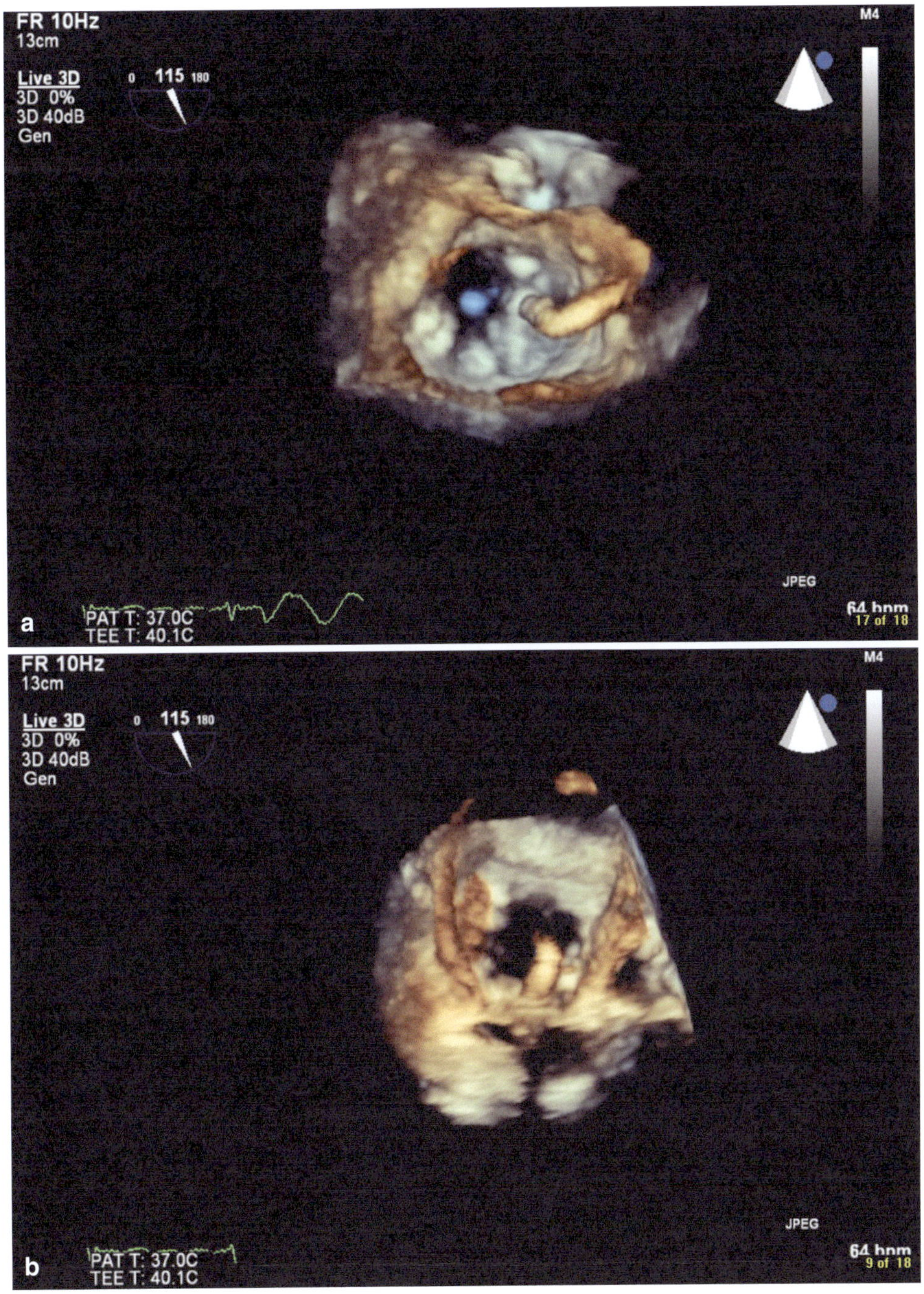

Fig. 13.13 Three-dimensional TEE pictures showing placement of the first clip. *Left panel* (**a**) shows the view from the atrium. A strategy was chosen to go start medial with the first clip rather than zippering from lateral to medial. *Right hand side* (**b**) shows the view turned and cropped. Now right is anterior, superior is lateral, and left is posterior

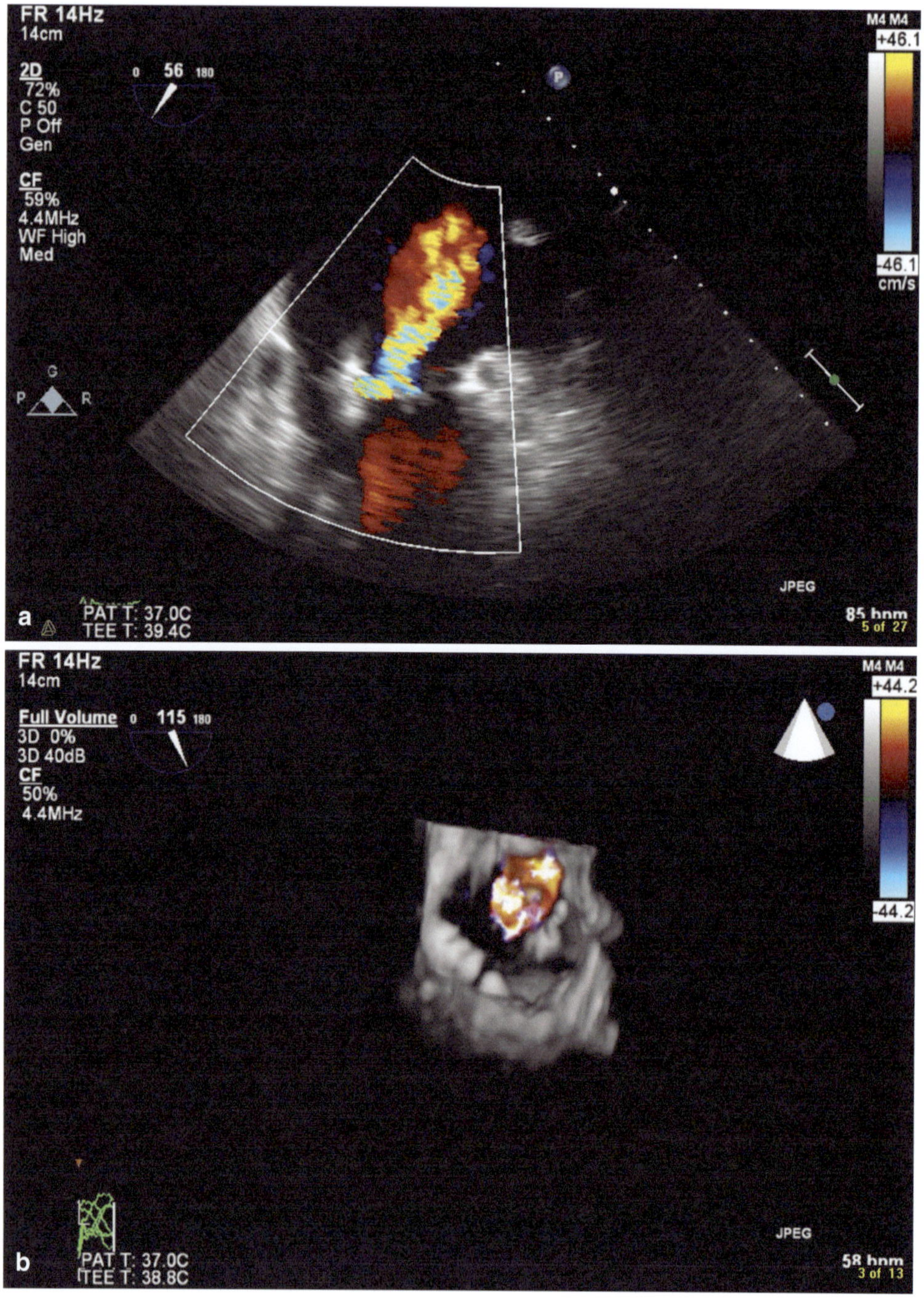

Fig. 13.14 After the first clip, the *left panel* (**a**) shows a two-chamber view with color Doppler, demonstrating a residual regurgitant jet medial to the first clip. This was as expected since the prolapse extends to the P2 segment. *Right panel* (**b**) shows a three-dimensional color view from the left atrium

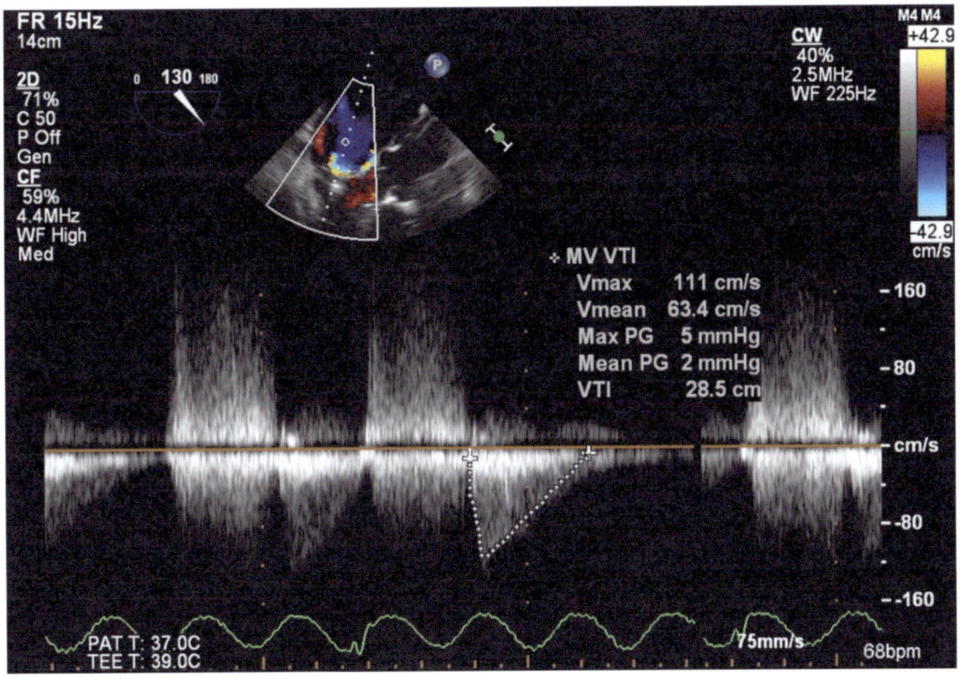

Fig. 13.15 Transmitral flow with continuous wave Doppler (*CW*) using velocity time integral (*VTI*) to estimate valve opening. A mean gradient of 2 mmHg allows for placement of a second clip to ensure a good reduction of the mitral regurgitation as well as stabilizing the first clip in the thickened and possible fragile leaflet tissue

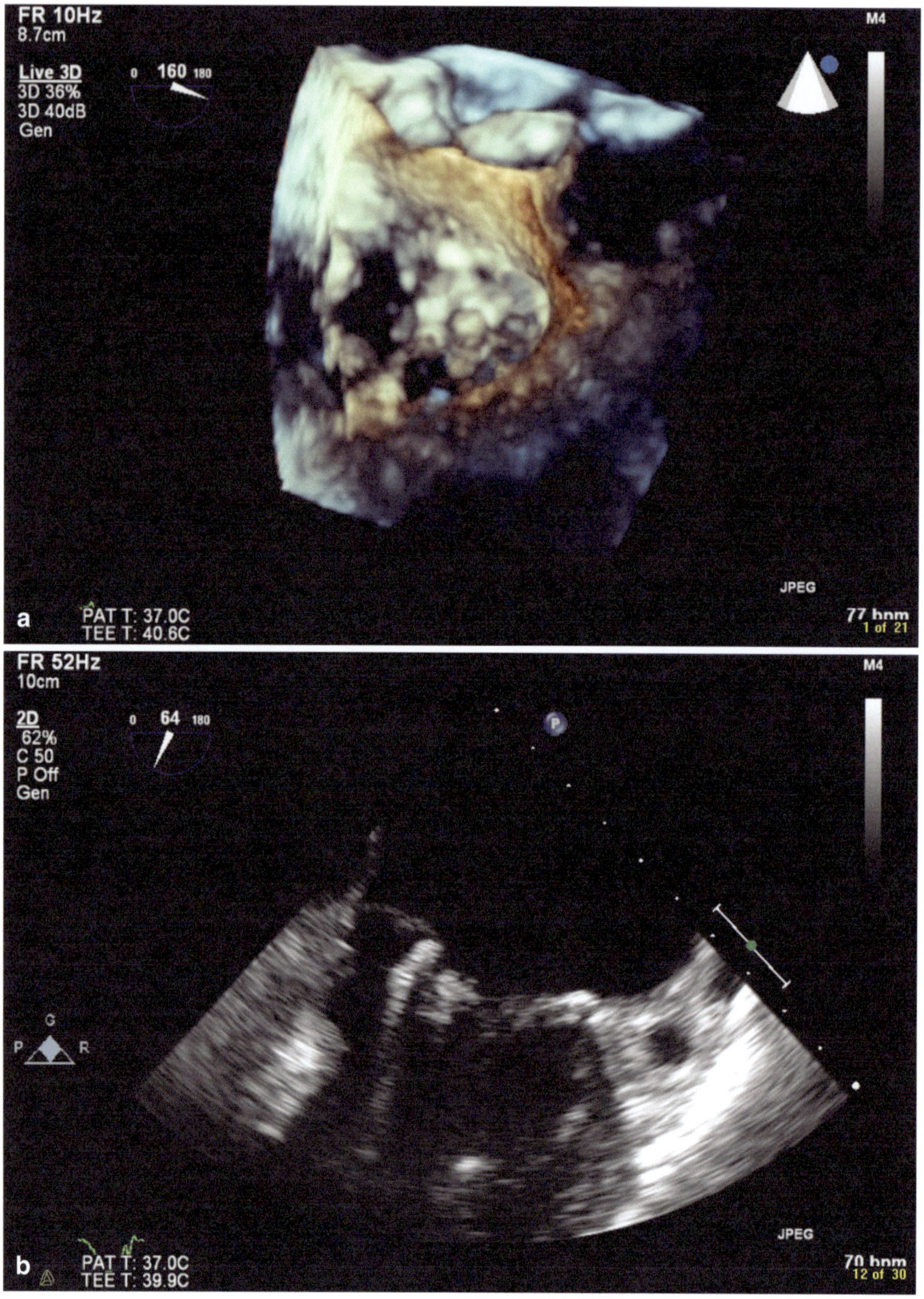

Fig. 13.16 Placement of the second clip. *Left panel* (**a**) shows three-dimensional TEE viewed from the atrium. The second clip is placed on the P2 segment. *Right hand side* (**b**) shows a two-chamber view with placement of the second clip lateral to the first. Note how the leaflets are thickened and billowing

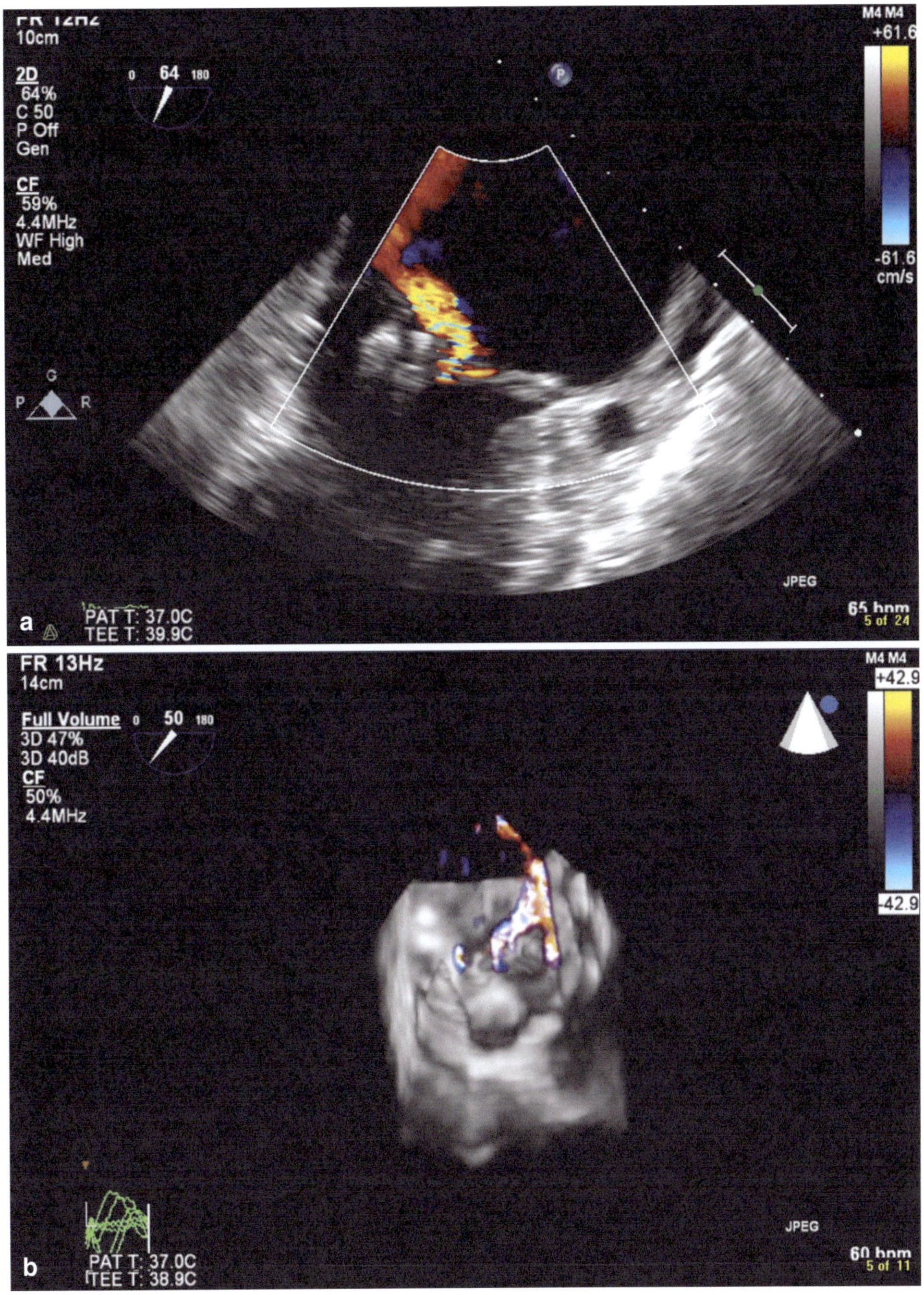

Fig. 13.17 Final result after placement of the second clip. *Left panel* (**a**) two-chamber view showing a residual jet placed lateral to the second clip. *Right panel* (**b**) shows a three-dimensional TEE viewed from the atrium showing that all residual jet is lateral to the second clip

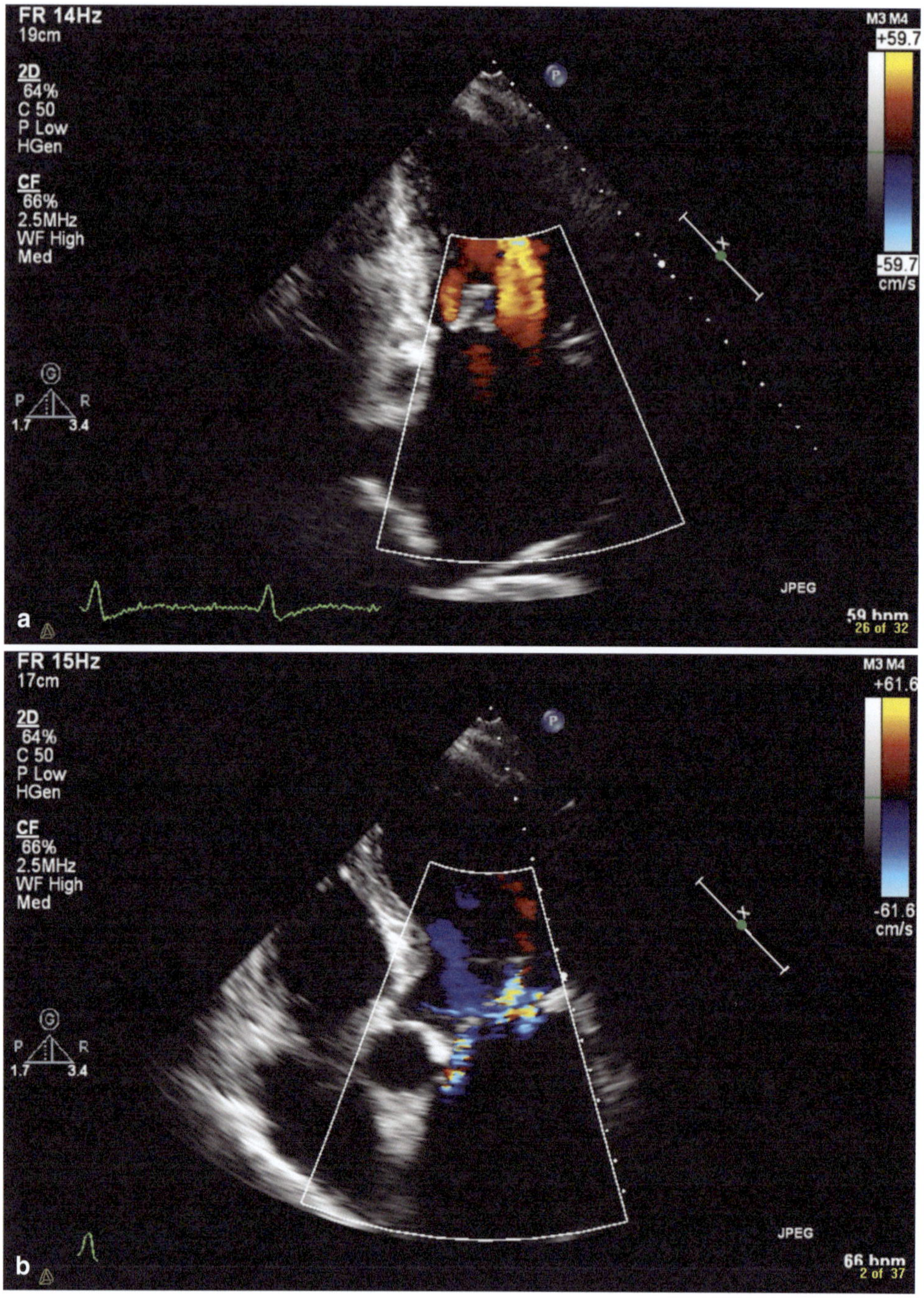

Fig. 13.18 TTE at 6 months follow-up. *Left panel* (**a**) shows two-chamber view in systole; there is no apparent inflow flow acceleration. *Right panel* (**b**) shows a three-chamber view visualizing a mild residual mitral regurgitation

References

1. Barlow JB, Bosman CK, Pocock WA, et al. Late systolic murmurs and non-ejection ("mid-late") systolic clicks. An analysis of 90 patients. Br Heart J. 1968;30:203.
2. Carpentier A, Chauvaud S, Fabini JN, et al. Reconstructive surgery of mitral valve incompetence: ten-year appraisal. J Thorac Cardiovasc Surg. 1980;79:338–48.
3. Jouan J, Berrebi A, Chauvaud S, et al. Mitral valve reconstruction in Barlow disease: long-term echographic results and implications for surgical management. J Thorac Cardiovasc Surg. 2012; 143(4):S17–20.
4. Grayburn PA, Roberts BJ, Aston S, et al. Mechanism and severity of mitral regurgitation by transesophageal echocardiography in patients referred for percutaneous valve repair. Am J Cardiol. 2011;108(6):882–7.

EVEREST II Case Study: Large Left Atrium

14

Satya S. Shreenivas and Howard C. Herrmann

Abstract

This case illustrates some of the challenges associated with performing the MitraClip procedure in a patient with a very large left atrium. These include modifying the usual landmarks used for selecting the ideal location for the transseptal puncture. In this case, the transseptal puncture was at the thick part of the septum, and required sequential balloon dilatations before the steerable guide would cross.

Keywords

Mitral stenosis • MitraClip • Balloon • Large left atrium

Clinical History

A 71-year-old male with past medical history significant for severe mitral regurgitation presented for percutaneous mitral valve repair utilizing the edge-to-edge MitralClip system. Due to his concomitant history of cirrhosis, he was deemed at high surgical risk for open repair.

Summary

This patient developed severe mitral regurgitation due to prolapse of the A2 segment likely secondary to ruptured chordae. Due to a large left atrial size of 8.6 cm, the transseptal puncture and subsequent delivery of the MitraClip was particularly challenging (Figs. 14.1, 14.2, 14.3, 14.4, 14.5 and Videos 14.1, 14.2, 14.3). We utilized 3-D transesophageal echocardiography to aid in both the transseptal puncture and in positioning the device.

The septum was crossed in a high posterior position through a thick part of the septum (Figs. 14.6, 14.7, 14.8 and Videos 14.4, 14.5). A 260 cm 0.032″ Amplatz wire was positioned in the left superior pulmonary vein. Despite serial dilations of the septum using 10, 12, 14, and 16 F dilators, we were not able to advance the sheath across the septum. A 6.0×30 mm Cordis PowerFlex balloon was used to dilate the transseptal puncture site twice (Figs. 14.9, 14.10 and Videos 14.6, 14.7). This allowed a 5-French MP catheter to cross the transseptal puncture site, and it was used to exchange the wire for a 300 cm 0.038″ Amplatz extra stiff wire. Next, the sheath was advanced into the left atrium over the wire (Figs. 14.11 and 14.12). The MitraClip delivery system was carefully positioned in the mitral valve orifice under both two-dimensional and three-dimensional transesophageal echocardiography and fluoroscopic guidance (Figs. 14.13, 14.14 and Video 14.8). Both the anterior and the posterior leaflets were grasped with the clip and the clip was then successfully released (Fig. 14.15). After the delivery of the first clip, transesophageal echocardiography revealed a moderate mitral regurgitant jet lateral to the MitraClip (Fig. 14.16 and Video 14.9). A second MitraClip was then placed lateral to the existing clip (Figs. 14.17, 14.18, 14.19 and Videos 14.10, 14.11). After delivery of both clips, there was only mild residual mitral regurgitation present (Fig. 14.20 and Video 14.12).

S.S. Shreenivas, M.D. • H.C. Herrmann, M.D. (✉)
Department of Medicine, University of Pennsylvania,
3400 Spruce Street, Philadelphia, PA 19010, USA
e-mail: satya.shreenivas@uphs.upenn.edu;
howard.herrmann@uphs.upenn.edu

Electronic supplementary material The online version of this chapter (doi:10.1007/978-1-4471-4294-2_14) contains supplementary material, which is available to authorized users.

T. Feldman et al. (eds.), *Atlas of Percutaneous Edge-to-Edge Mitral Valve Repair*,
DOI 10.1007/978-1-4471-4294-2_14, © Springer-Verlag London 2013

Learning Points

- In a patient with a large left atrium, the ideal transseptal puncture location may be in a location that is different from a usual case.
- In cases where the steerable guide catheter cannot cross the septum, balloon dilatation of the septum can be considered.

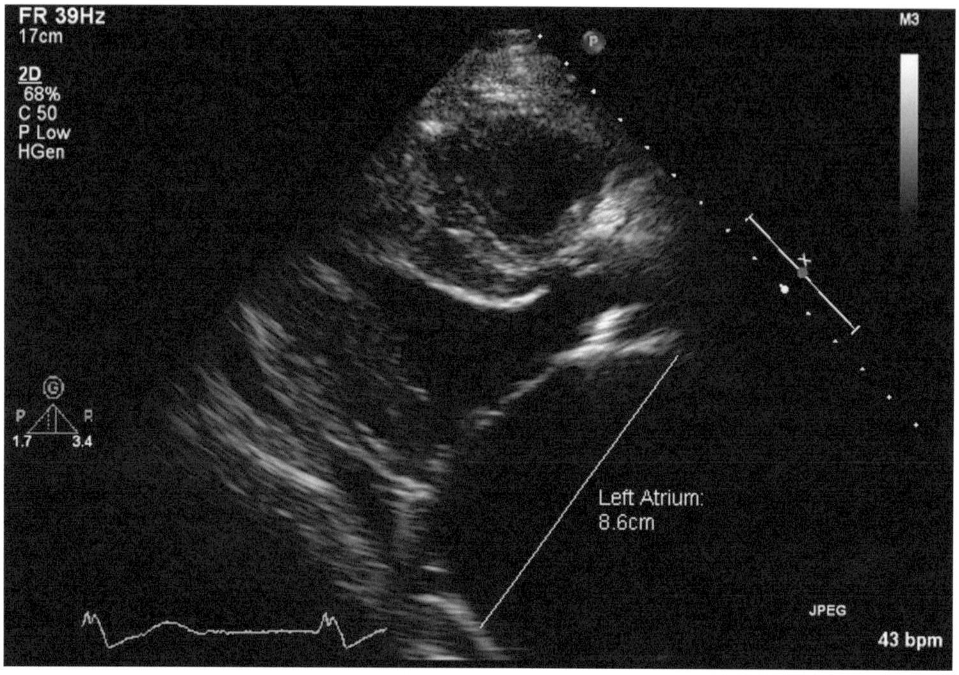

Fig. 14.1 Screening transthoracic echo. Parasternal long axis. The screening transthoracic echocardiogram shows a markedly dilated left atrium measuring 8.6 cm (Also see Video 14.1)

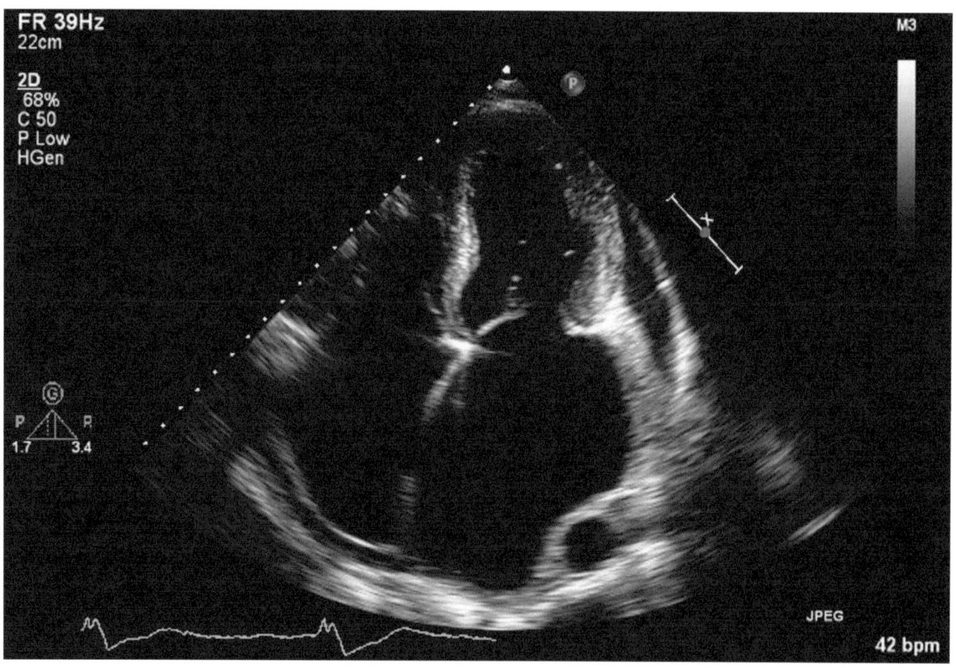

Fig. 14.2 Screening transthoracic echocardiogram. Apical four chamber. The apical four chamber confirms left atrial enlargement. Also seen are ruptured chordae attached to the anterior mitral valve leaflet

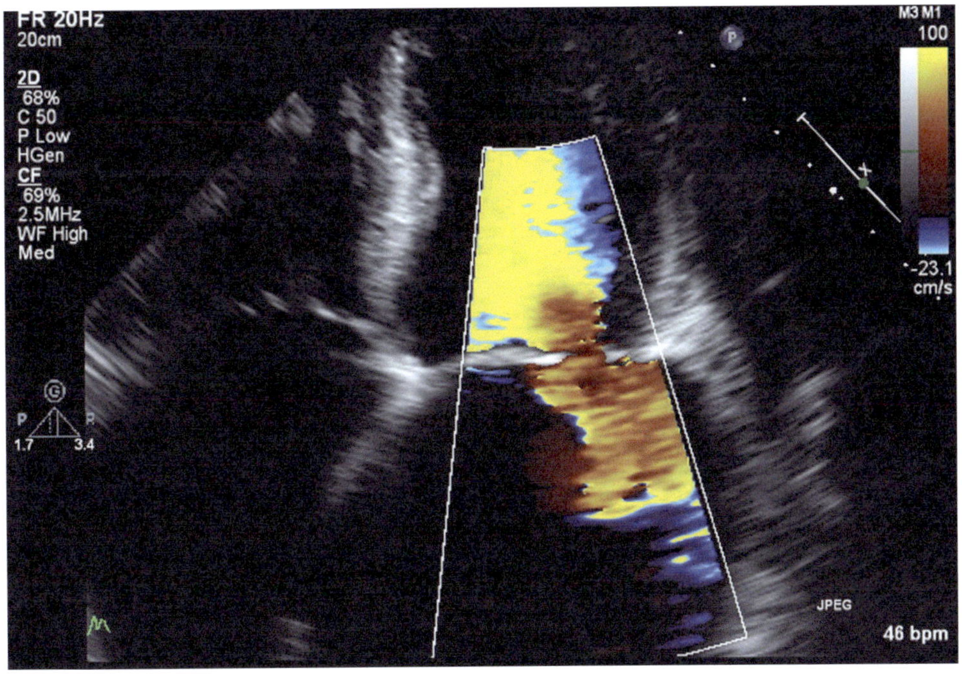

Fig. 14.3 Screening transthoracic echocardiogram. Apical four chamber with color. Adding color Doppler to the apical four chamber views shows severe mitral regurgitation with a laterally directed jet (Also see Video 14.2)

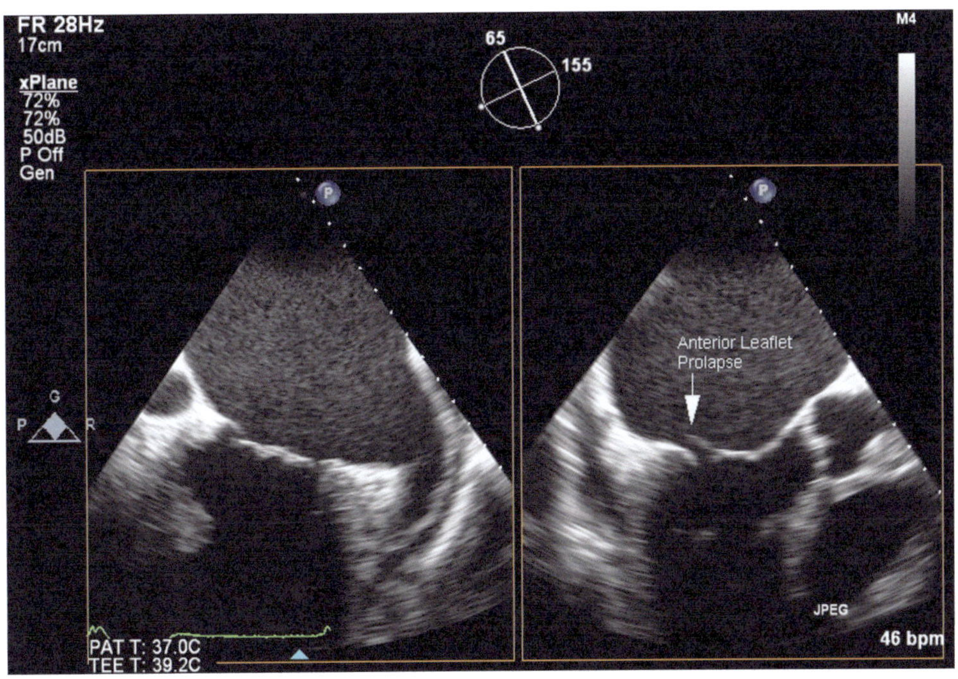

Fig. 14.4 Transesophageal echocardiogram. Two- and three-chamber views. The bicommissural and three-chamber views also confirm A2 prolapse

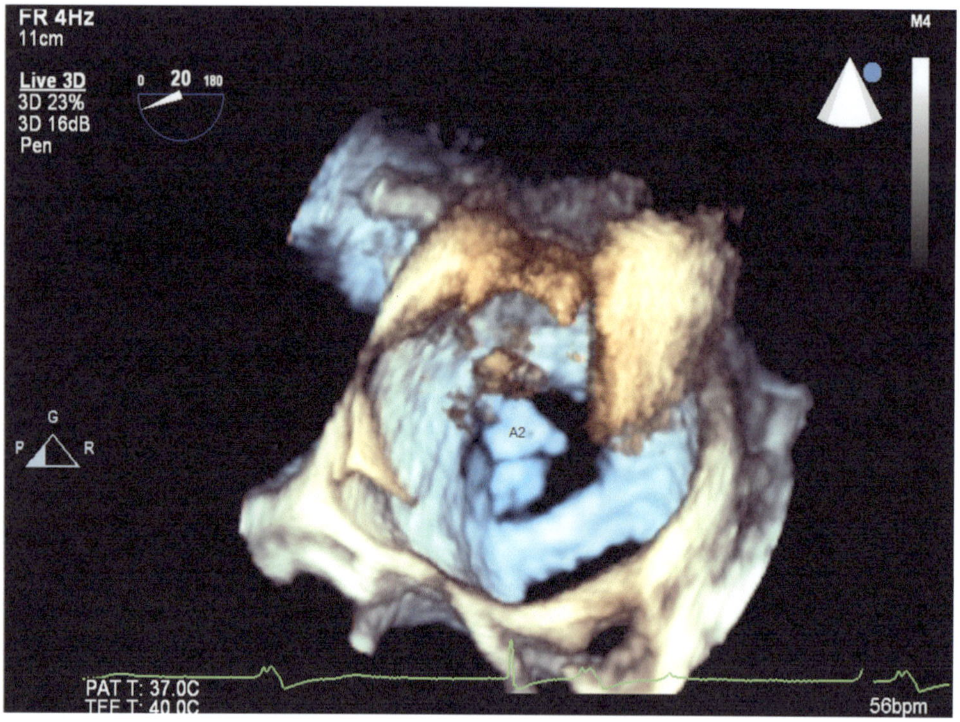

Fig. 14.5 3D transesophageal echocardiogram. 3D transesophageal view of the mitral valve also shows prolapse of the *A2* segment of the anterior leaflet (Also see Video 14.3)

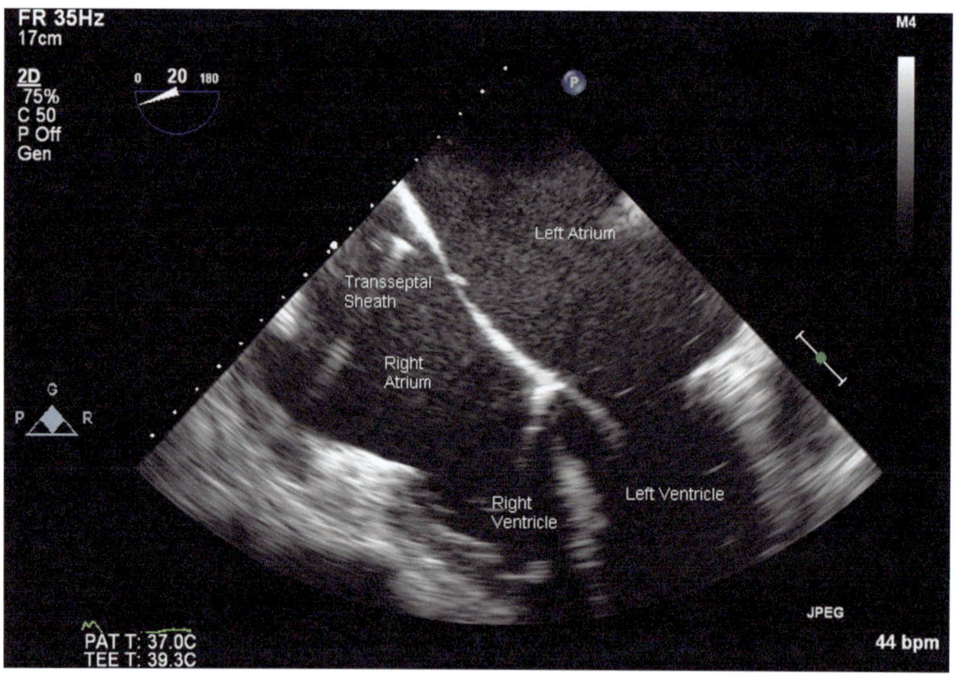

Fig. 14.6 Transesophageal four chamber. The transseptal needle can be seen in the right atrium abutting the septum in a fairly high location (Also see Video 14.4)

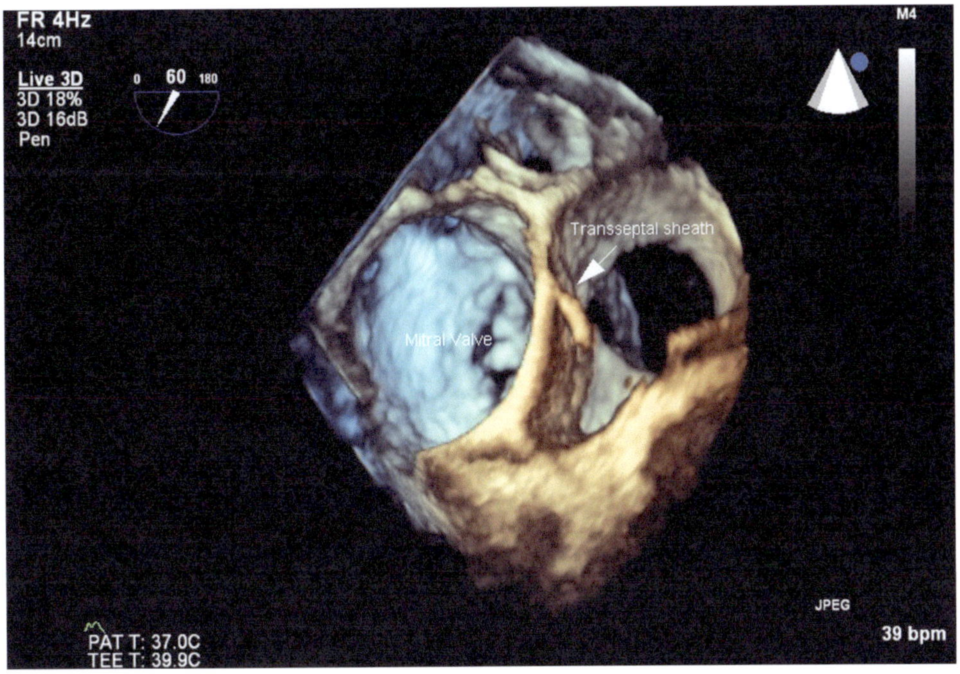

Fig. 14.7 3D transesophageal bicaval. 3D transesophageal echocardiogram confirms a high posterior location of transseptal puncture

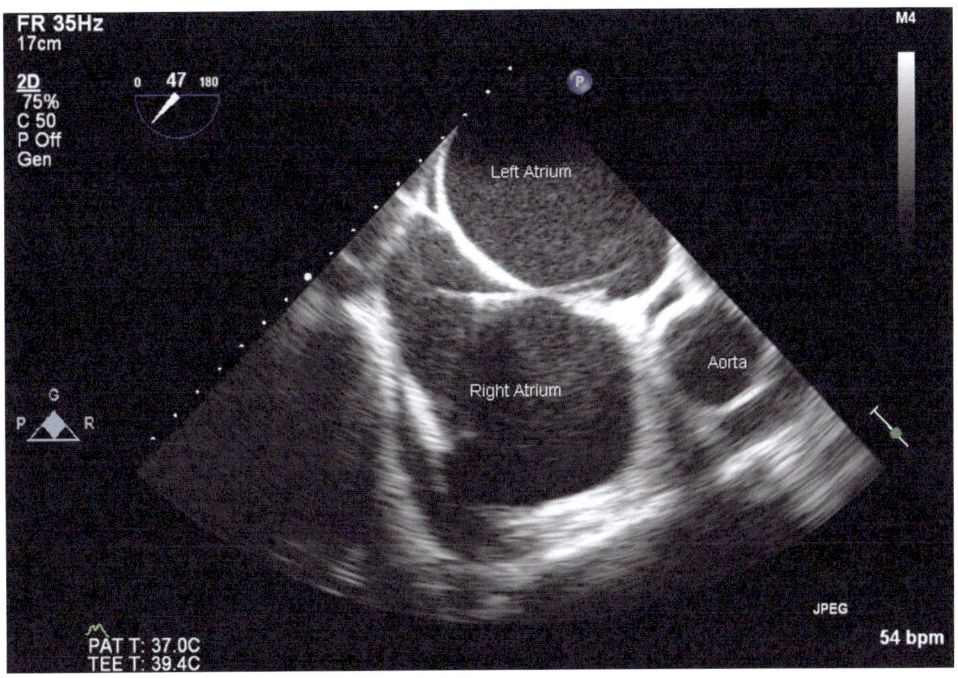

Fig. 14.8 Transesophageal bicaval off axis. A bicaval off-axis view shows the transseptal needle crossing into the left atrium. This view is also helpful to demonstrate the position of the aorta. Due to the very enlarged and bowed interatrial septum, the needle trajectory from the IVC across the septum forced a posterior to anterior angle resulting in a suboptimal anterior left atrial final position (Also see Video 14.5). Agitated saline injection confirms successful transseptal puncture

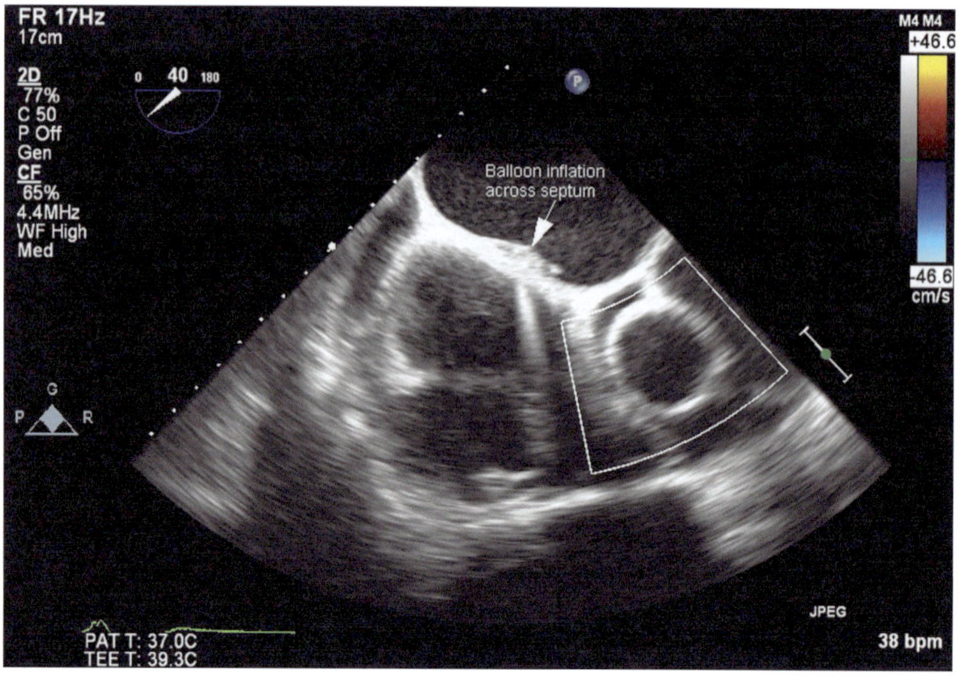

Fig. 14.9 Transesophageal bicaval off axis. After transseptal puncture, a Cordis PowerFlex Balloon is inflated across the septum to facilitate the insertion of a sheath into the left atrium (Also see Video 14.6)

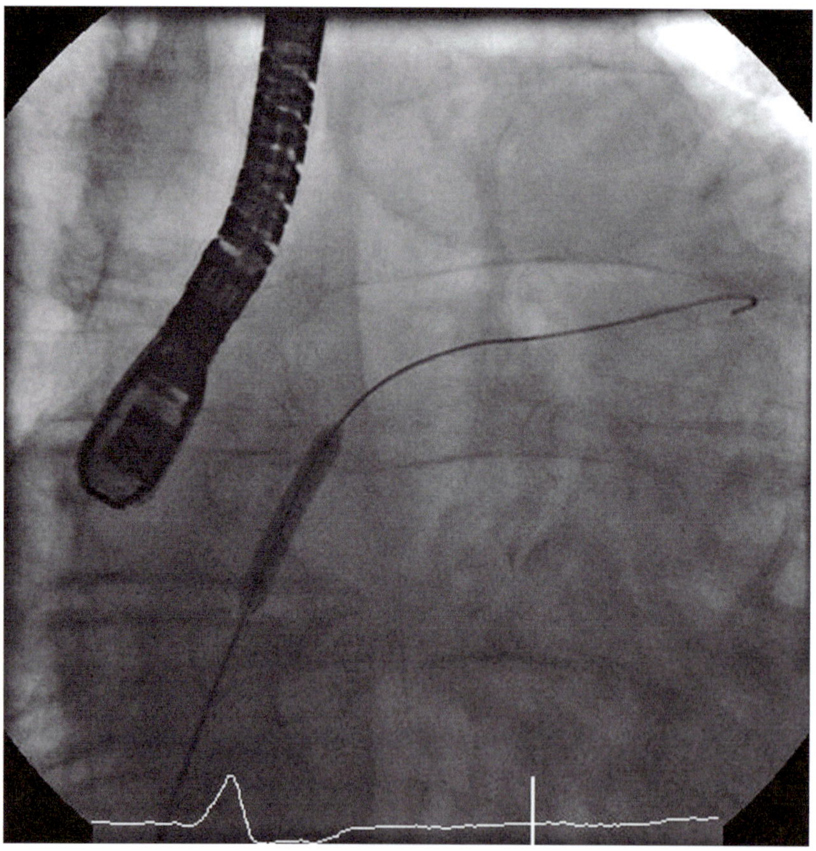

Fig. 14.10 Fluoroscopy. Balloon inflation across septum (Also see Video 14.7)

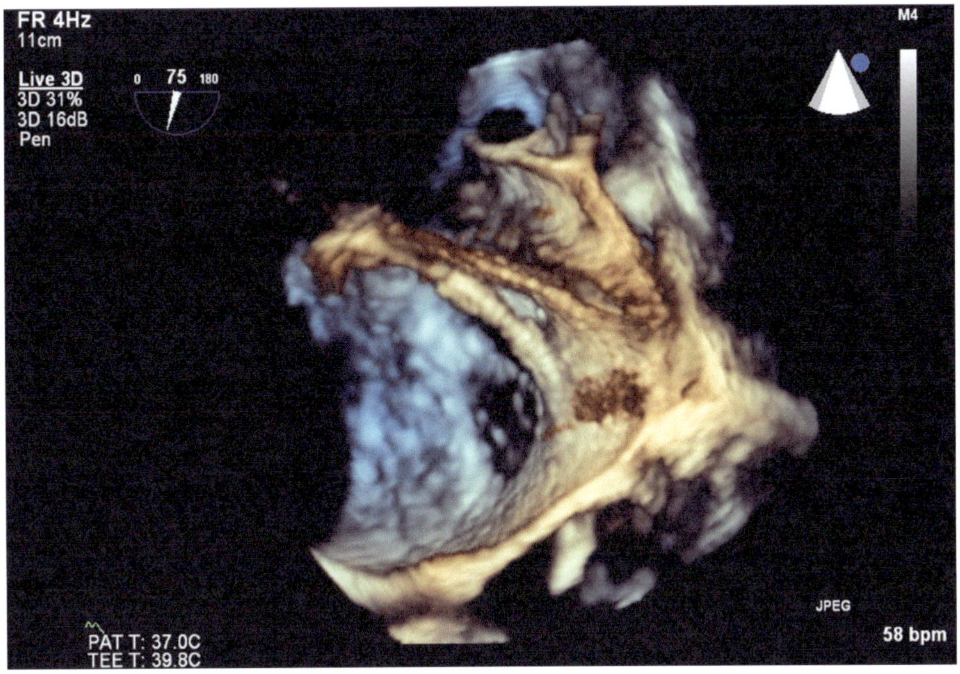

Fig. 14.11 3D transesophageal echocardiogram. The transseptal sheath is seen crossing from the right atrium into the left atrium and positioned close to the anterior and superior wall of the left atrium

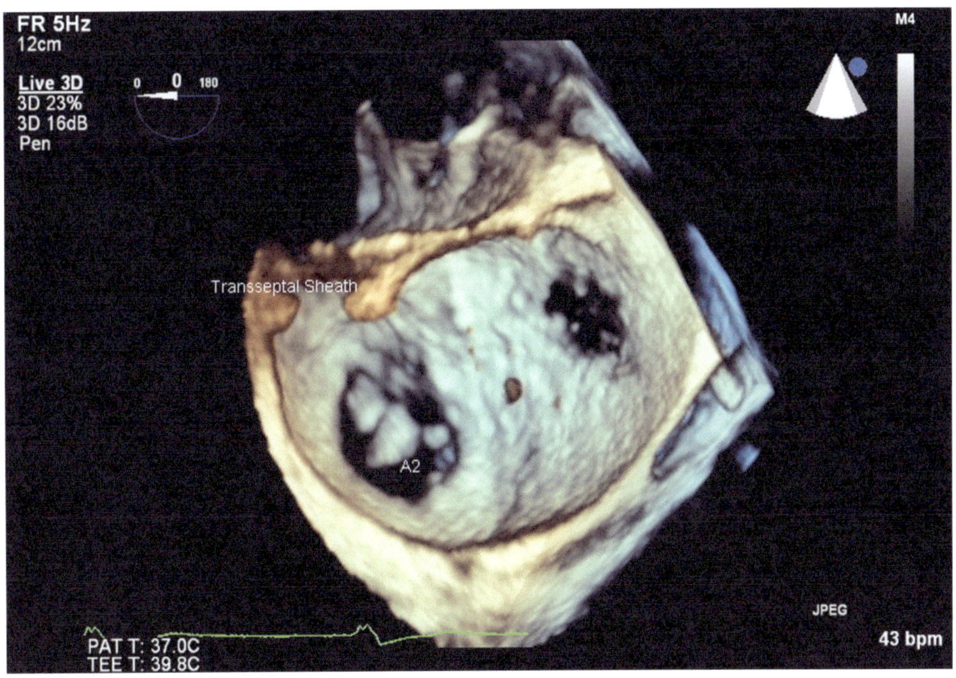

Fig. 14.12 3D transesophageal echocardiogram. Another view showing both the high location of the transseptal puncture and the mitral valve prolapse

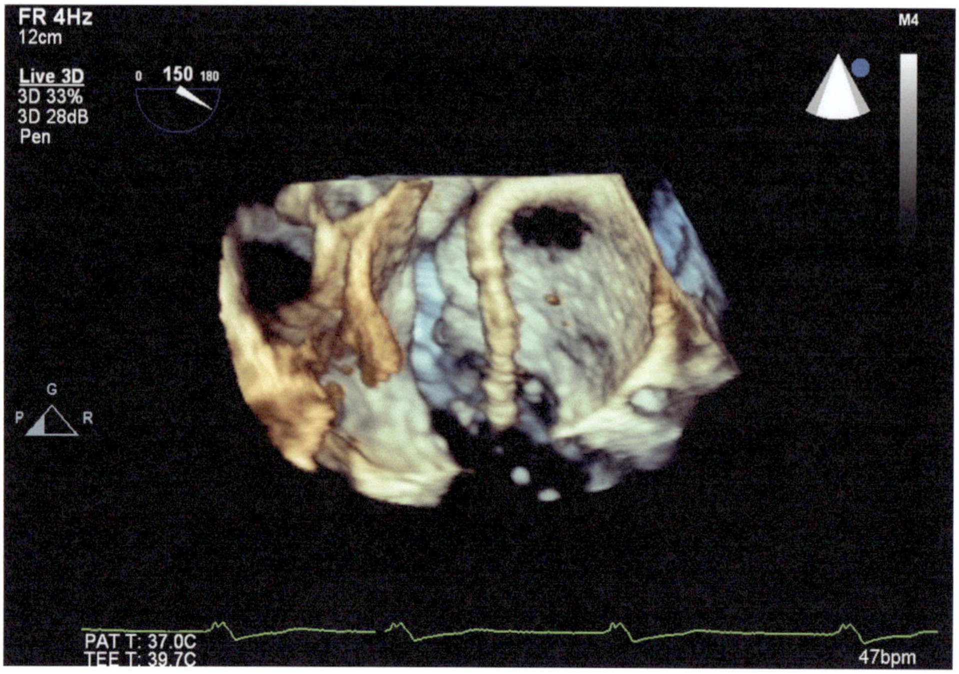

Fig. 14.13 3D transesophageal echocardiogram. Due to the high and posterior to anterior transseptal puncture, a large curve was needed to position the MitraClip more posteriorly in the left atrium over the mitral valve

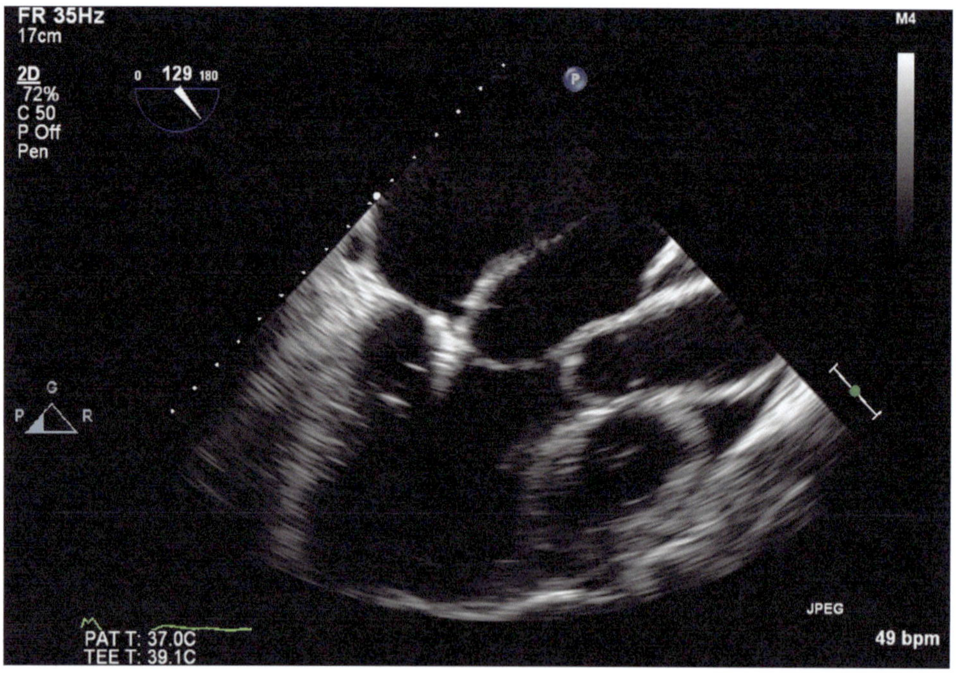

Fig. 14.14 Transesophageal echocardiogram left ventricular outflow tract view. The MitraClip is positioned across and holding both the anterior and posterior mitral valve leaflets (Also see Video 14.8)

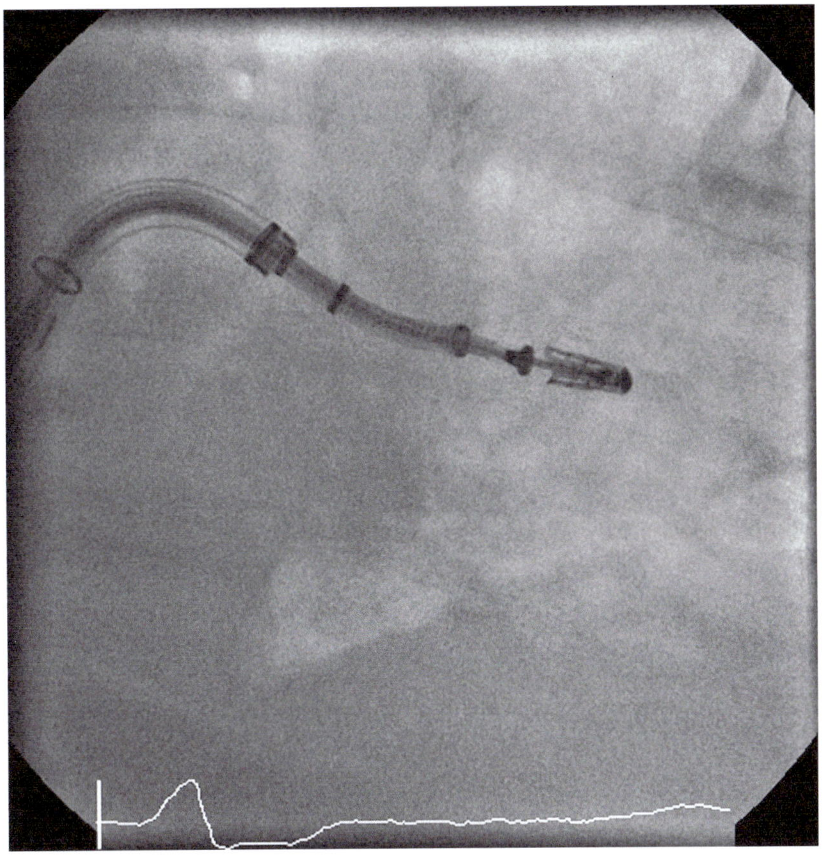

Fig. 14.15 Fluoroscopy. Deployment of clip 1

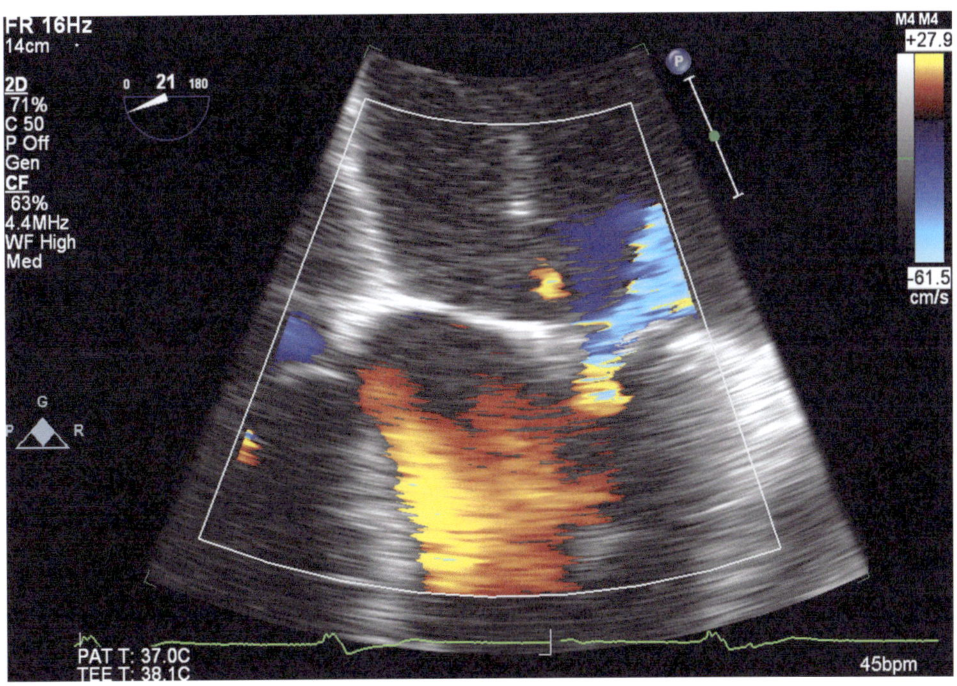

Fig. 14.16 Transesophageal echocardiogram four chamber with color. After deploying the first clip, there remained mild to moderate mitral regurgitation with the jet located laterally to the first clip (Also see Video 14.9)

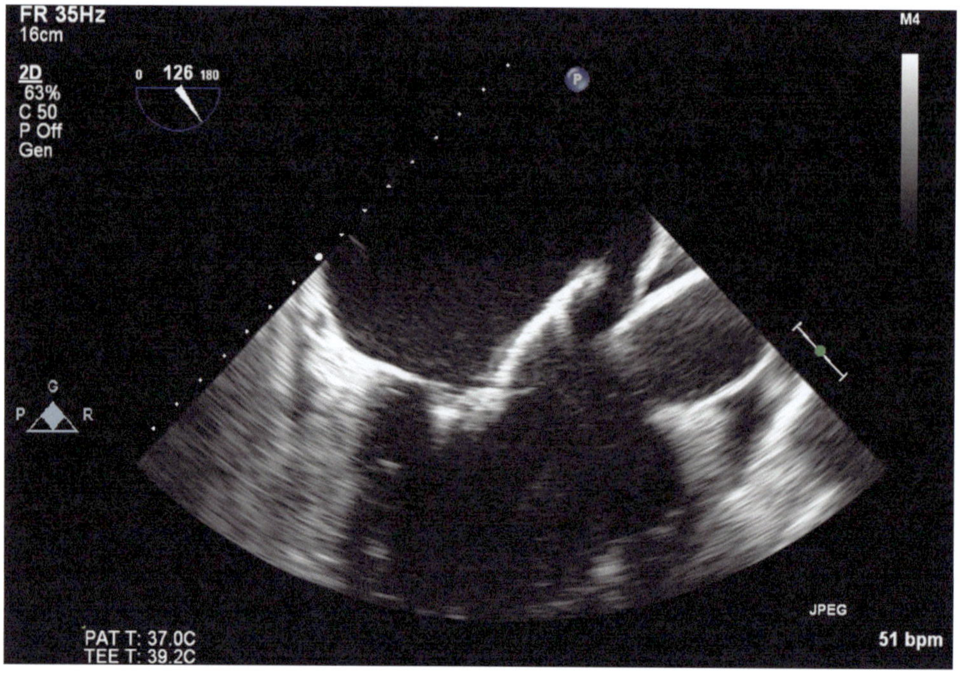

Fig. 14.17 Transesophageal echocardiogram three-chamber or LVOT view. The second MitraClip is positioned next to the first clip (Also see Video 14.10)

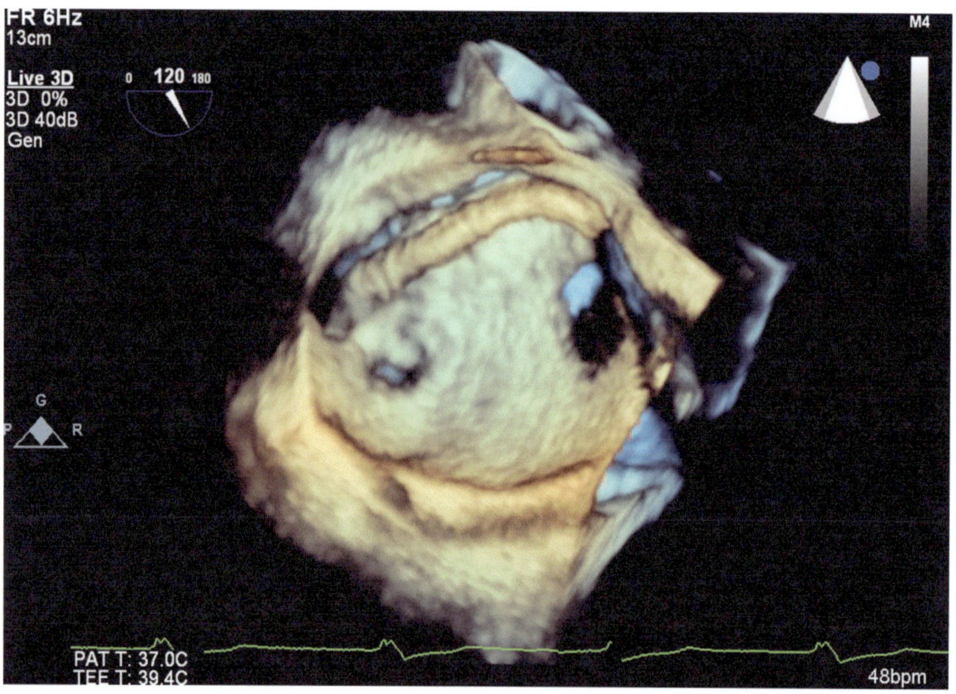

Fig. 14.18 3D transesophageal echocardiogram. 3D imaging is utilized to position and orient the opened second clip lateral to the first clip (Also see Video 14.11)

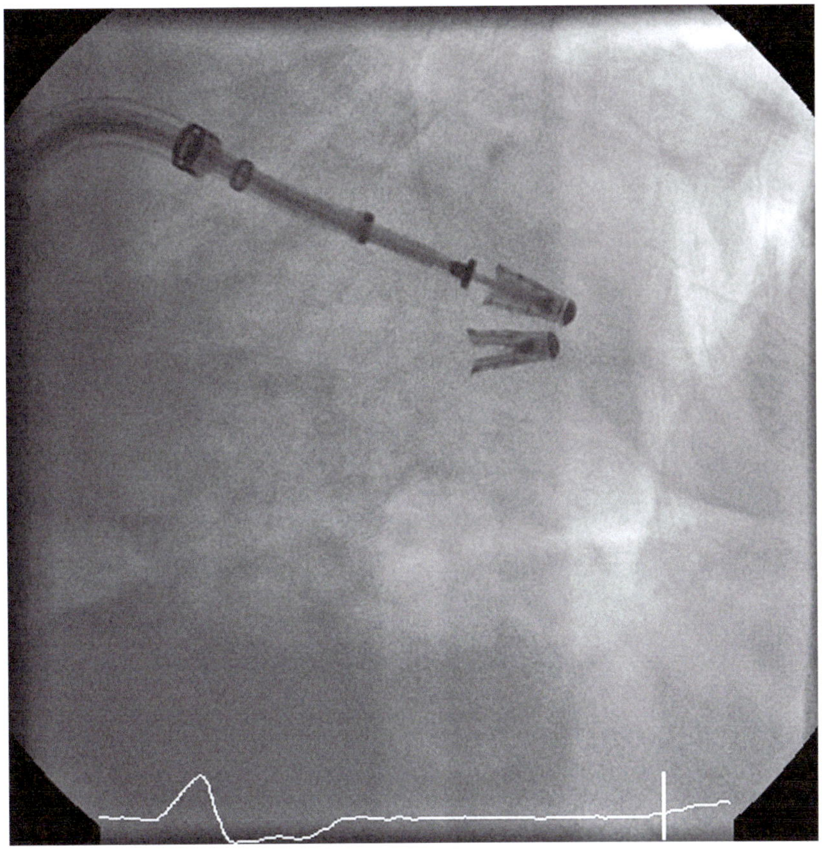

Fig. 14.19 Fluoroscopy. Deployment of clip 2

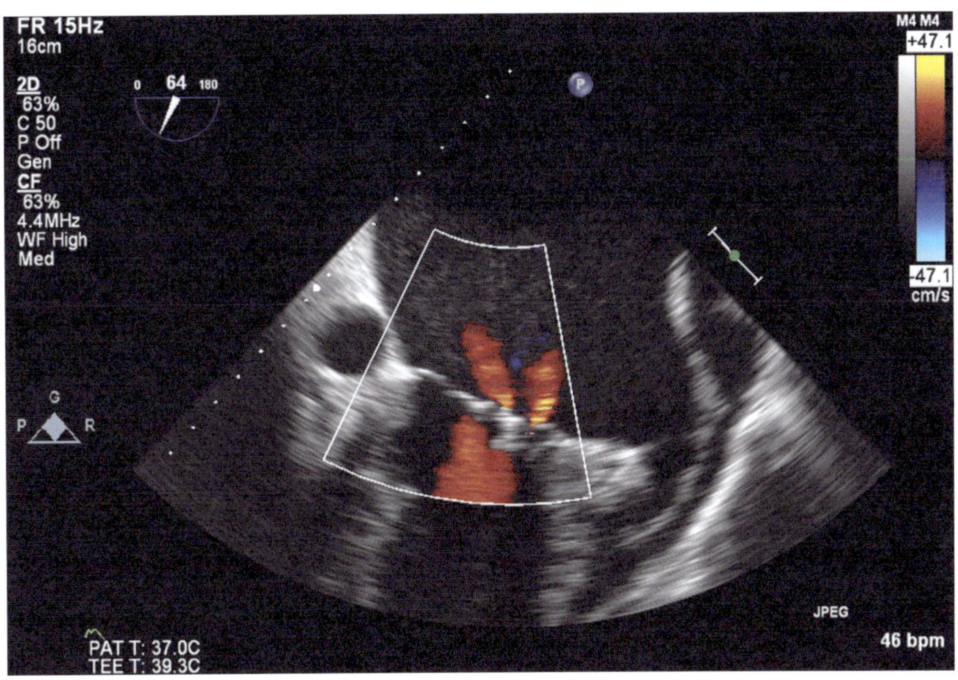

Fig. 14.20 Transesophageal echocardiogram bicommissural view. There is only mild mitral regurgitation after placement of both clips (Also see Video 14.12)

Approach to Mitral Regurgitation Requiring Multiple MitraClips

15

Hüseyin Ince, Liliya Paranskaya, Giuseppe D'Ancona, Stephan Kische, and Scott Lim

Abstract

The MitraClip is a percutaneous therapy for repairing severe MR in either degenerative or functional mitral regurgitation (MR). In the initial clinical experience with this therapy, one or two clips were used. However, with commercial use of the device, increasingly more complex anatomy has been treated with some cases requiring three or more clips. The use of multiple clips is highly dependent on valve anatomy, mechanism, and severity of MR. This chapter discusses the implantation strategy, technical considerations, and the potential pitfalls of using multiple clips in the use of the MitraClip therapy.

Keywords

Mitral regurgitation • MitraClip • Multiple clips

Introduction and Rationale for Using More Than One MitraClip

In this chapter, we will summarize our implantation strategy focusing particularly on the decision-making process for multiple clip implantation and its technical implications to create optimal correction of the MR and avoid iatrogenic mitral stenosis. The strategy of using more than one MitraClip to address MR can be classified into one of three intentions:

1. To address multiple sites of pathology on the mitral valve
2. To extend the width of tissue coaptation created by the MitraClip
3. To provide additional anchoring between anterior and posterior leaflets

With degenerative etiology of mitral pathology, multiple sites along the anterior or posterior leaflet may be affected, with prolapse or flail at one site and restriction at another. Figure 15.1a–c shows just such an example, in a patient with distinct pathologies along the different portions of the mitral apparatus. While a single MitraClip placed appropriately on a point of pathology may address that specific prolapsed or flail segment, this alone would leave significant residual mitral regurgitation at the other point of pathology. Therefore, a strategy of placing a second clip at the second point of pathology may be utilized, essentially creating a triple-orifice mitral valve. Clearly, for such a strategy to be successful, the native mitral valve orifice size must be adequate (at least > 5 cm^2). The other point worth noting is that frequently in patients with multiple locations of mitral pathology, at least one of those locations is into the commissures. Placing MitraClips onto commissural pathology incurs a risk of chordal entanglement, which can be managed, but should be noted.

Patients with both degenerative as well as functional etiologies of mitral regurgitation at times may benefit from extending the width of tissue coaptation created by the MitraClip, although for different reasons. For patients with

H. Ince, M.D., Ph.D. (✉) • L. Paranskaya, M.D.
G. D'Ancona, M.D., Ph.D. • S. Kische, M.D., Ph.D.
Department of Cardiology, Heart Center Rostock, University Hospital Rostock, Ernst-Heydemann-Str. 6, Rostock, MV 18057, Germany
e-mail: hueseyin.ince@med.uni-rostock.de; liliya.paranskaya@med.uni-rostock.de; rgea@hotmail.co; stephan.kische@uni-rostock.de

S. Lim, M.D.
Department of Cardiology, University of Virginia Medical Center, 1215 Lee Street, Hospital Expansion, Room 4038, Charlottesville, VA 22908, USA
e-mail: sl9pc@virginia.edu

T. Feldman et al. (eds.), *Atlas of Percutaneous Edge-to-Edge Mitral Valve Repair*,
DOI 10.1007/978-1-4471-4294-2_15, © Springer-Verlag London 2013

degenerative etiologies, in particular for those with a wide prolapse or flail width, a single MitraClip may not adequately capture all of the diseased mitral tissue within the MitraClip. Placing a second clip immediately adjacent to the first clip allows for extension of the width of tissue grabbed by the clip and thereby increasing the coaptation width between anterior and posterior leaflets. However, it is important to be careful when crossing into the ventricle immediately adjacent to a previously placed clip. It is advisable to set the appropriate trajectory and arm angles of the second clip while in the atria and then close the clip arms before crossing by the first clip, so as not to get hung up on the leaflet tissue going into the first clip. It also may be helpful to advance or withdraw the stabilizer system so the trajectory is maintained and the second clip is advanced through the largest portion of the residual orifice. Once into the ventricle, the clip arms may be opened and the clip delivery system moved close to the first clip (Fig. 15.2a, b).

One of the uncommon complications of the MitraClip procedure is partial leaflet detachment, also known as single leaflet clip insertion. When placed properly on the mitral valve, the mitral leaflet tissue is anchored within the MitraClip, between the arms of the MitraClip and the frictional gripper elements. However, inadequate leaflet insertion can occur when the leaflet is only grabbed to a small extent between the clip arm and the frictional gripper element. Unfortunately being able to determine the degree of leaflet tissue insertion is frequently difficult as there is a limitation resolution of echocardiography with the echo artifacts from the MitraClip materials. A single MitraClip may have a risk of inadequate leaflet insertion, but by placing a second clip, that risk is diminished ("two are better than one"). This benefit must be balanced against the risks of the procedure to place the second clip.

Whenever a second MitraClip is contemplated, certain hemodynamic considerations must be factored in. By placing a second MitraClip, the degree of leaflet apposition is increased but at the cost of decreasing mitral orifice area. Caution must be exercised to avoid hemodynamically significant mitral stenosis. In general, residual mitral regurgitation often can be adequately medically treated. However, if mitral stenosis is created, this is usually not amenable to further medical therapy and therefore should be avoided. Prior to a second clip being placed, the mean inflow gradient should be measured both by transesophageal echocardiography as well as by direct measurement off of the side arm of the steerable guide and with a catheter advanced retrograde to the left ventricle. An echocardiographic mean gradient of more than 5 mmHg or an invasively measured mean gradient of more than 2–3 mmHg unfortunately correlates with more severe stenosis if a second clip is placed. If a significant inflow gradient occurs only after the placement of a second clip, it also may be helpful to open up the arms of the second clip so that less tissue is pulled together, as long as the arm angle on the MitraClip is <60°. By doing so, the inflow gradient may be reduced, albeit with some increase in residual mitral regurgitation.

Patient Selection for Use of Two or More MitraClips

The indication to use multiple clips should be supported by hemodynamic evaluation and mitral anatomy. Different pathologic subtypes of MR require different approaches. We do not believe that a "one size fits all" strategy should be used to treat patients with different mechanisms of MR. The decision about the number of clips to implant should be rationalized preoperatively, confirmed intraoperatively, or eventually modified according to the intraprocedural real-time echocardiographic monitoring.

In our experience, patients with narrow jets involving a limited area of the mitral valve complex can frequently be addressed with a single clip. Patients with broader and more complex jets involving a more extended area of the MV should be considered for implantation of multiple clips.

It is important to emphasize that patients that are frequently referred for this novel procedure present, most often, with enlarged mitral annular dimensions and mitral inflow orifice areas. This is the result of global left ventricular dilatation from the increased volume load that in turn leads to stretching of the mitral subvalvular apparatus, consequent tethering of the MV leaflets, and deepening of the mitral coaptation depth. All these conditions will eventually lead to a wide regurgitant jet extending across the entire surface of the mitral valve.

Multiple MitraClips: Application of a Surgical Concept

The concept of multiple clipping is a surgical one. Multiple surgical sutures, either separate or by a running suture, apply a homogeneous distribution of the coaptation forces over the entire length of the suture line. In this way, the resistance to pulling forces is maximized and the risk of localized tissue tearing is minimized.

There are some surgical rules to keep into consideration when applying multiple MV clipping so to prevent tissue distortion and or excessive tissue restriction.

In surgical suturing, tissue distortion/restriction is prevented only when the consecutive sutures are placed in a parallel fashion and all have a similar angle in relationship to the wound's longitudinal plane. Furthermore, each stitch should theoretically incorporate the same amount (bite) of tissue at the two wound edges. When applying these rules to the mitral clipping with multiple clips, particular attention should be given to maintain a (1) *parallel* placement of the clips (almost linear along the new coaptation line) and to (2) *incorporate the same amount of MV tissue* within the corresponding opposite sections of the anterior and posterior leaflet (Fig. 15.3a, b).

Achievement of this goal is dependent on an in-depth intraoperative evaluation of the mitral pathologic anatomy and the MR jet shape.

Technical Approach to Use of Three or More MitraClips

There are some basic technical tips important to a multiple clipping procedure in order to minimize the time expenditure and risk of cardiac trauma. We have developed a stepwise strategy that has evolved since we first started using the MitraClip. The use of three or more MitraClips may be necessary to allow coaptation of a wide regurgitant jet, or may be used to treat mitral regurgitation which extends from the commissure into a more central portion of the valve.

After having evaluated the mitral pathologic anatomy and regurgitant jet shape, the determination of a single versus multiple mitral pathologies is made, which in turn helps to determine whether the procedure can be performed with one or more clips. The intraoperative echocardiography guides this decision. It should be emphasized that particularly with functional etiologies of MR, the intraoperative transesophageal echocardiography is affected by the patient's hemodynamic conditions during general anesthesia. Frequently, anesthesia induction leads to systemic vasodilatation and indirect decrease of the mitral regurgitant jet severity and morphology. For this reason we may utilize pharmacological measures to increase systemic arterial pressure and test the mitral valve function under more "physiologic" afterload conditions.

After having performed the transseptal puncture, entering the left atrium, and placing the MitraClip steerable guide, the first clip is placed. For wide jets that extend along the posteromedial aspect of the valve, the clipping is started at the posteromedial commissure (A3–P3), to create a percutaneous commissuroplasty and to initiate a progressive approximation of the two mitral leaflets along the new coaptation line. There are mechanical and technical reasons to use this strategy.

Mechanically, the commissural side of the MV can be compared to the hinges of a door. At this level the tissue is restrained to a greater degree, due to its proximity to the fibrous tissue of the commissure. Furthermore, the velocity of the movements of the two opposite quadrants of the MV leaflets (angular velocity) is reduced when compared to the middle portion of the MV leaflets, and the distance between the two edges is narrower. These conditions lead to an easier grasping and reduced tissue tearing.

From a technical standpoint, the decision where to place the first clip is governed by the transseptal puncture site and the design and maneuverability of the steerable guide. The transseptal puncture site is generally performed in the more superior part of the interatrial septum opposite to the anterolateral commissure. We prefer to move from the posteromedial commissure (A3–P3) toward the anterolateral one (A1–P1) (Fig. 15.4). Using this approach, there is less risk of accidentally making contact with a previously deployed clip since the initial approach of the clip toward the valve after exiting the guide is lateral to medial. As a general rule, we try to avoid placing a new clip between two previously implanted ones.

Intraoperative real-time 2D and 3D echocardiography guide the procedure in concert with fluoroscopy. The strategy of multiple clipping should be supported by real-time imaging that must document a progressive decrease in the severity of the MR and the necessity for additional clipping (Fig. 15.5a–c).

Conclusion

The hemodynamic and anatomical basis of MR may greatly differ from patient to patient, and for this reason, one cannot expect to treat all patients using the same operative strategy and in particular using the same number of clips. The common goal of every MitraClip procedure should be aimed at eliminating MR. This goal can be achieved minimizing the risk of iatrogenic MV stenosis only if the preoperative anatomy and the mechanism of MV regurgitation are adequately assessed. The use of multiple clips is feasible when performed carefully with special attention to technique and intraprocedural hemodynamic assessments to avoid mitral stenosis.

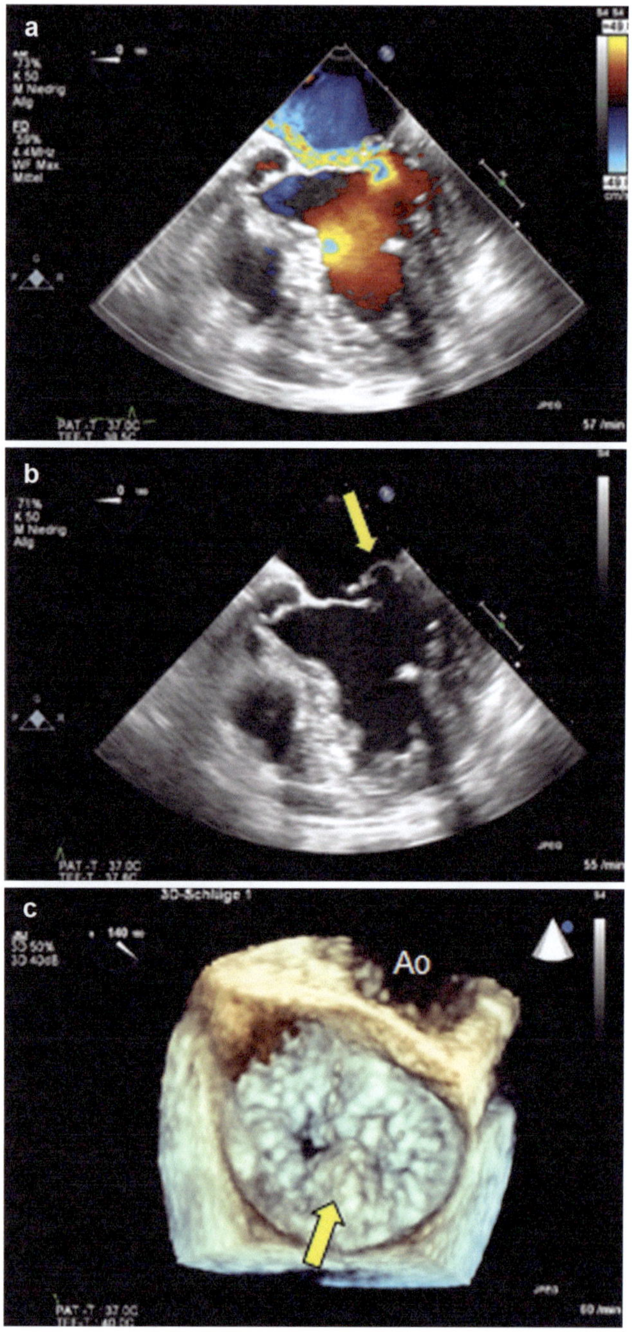

Fig. 15.1 2D color Doppler (four-chamber view) examination in similar orientation reveals severe eccentric mitral regurgitation (**a**). Transesophageal 2D (**b**) and 3D echocardiography (**c**) shows a prolapse of posterior mitral leaflet with flail (P2) scallops secondary to disruption of chordae (*yellow arrow*). *Ao* aorta

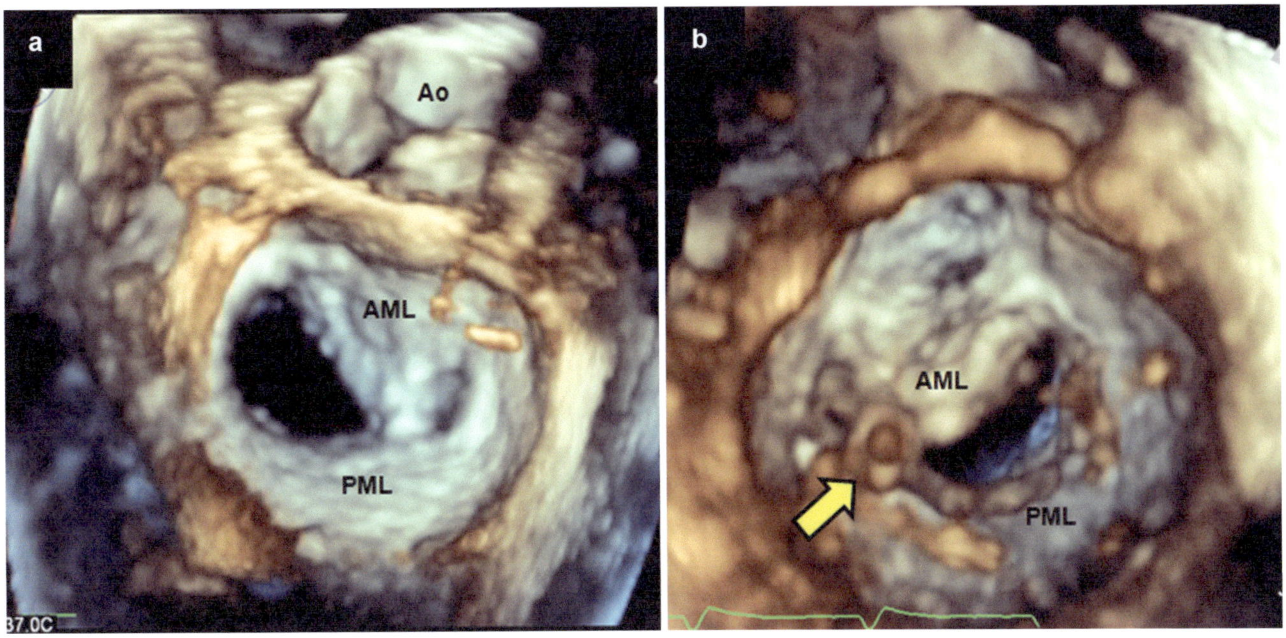

Fig. 15.2 Three-dimensional echocardiography showing the mitral valve from a left atrial (**a**) and a left ventricular view (**b**). The *yellow arrow* points to the first clip placed at the level of the posteromedial commissure. *AML* anterior mitral valve leaflet, *PML* posterior mitral valve leaflet, *Ao* aorta

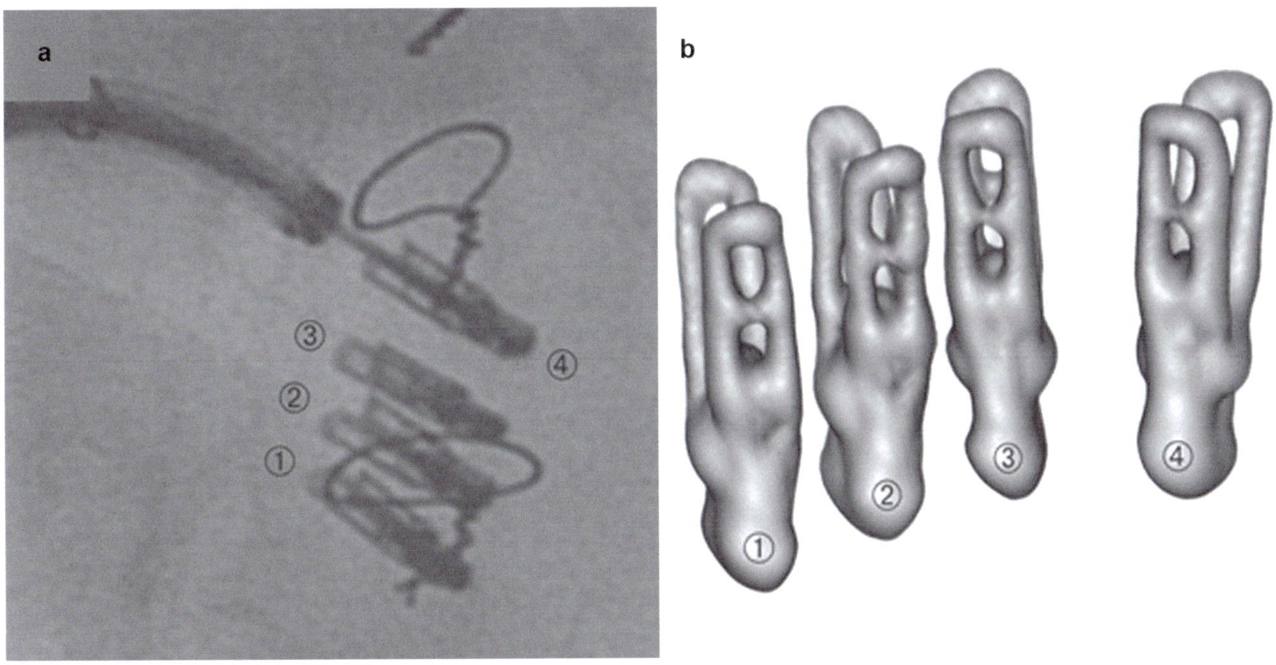

Fig. 15.3 Fluoroscopy (**a**) and 3D cardiac reconstruction (**b**) showing multiple clips (1, 2, 3, 4) implantation in a parallel fashion to reduce tissue retraction

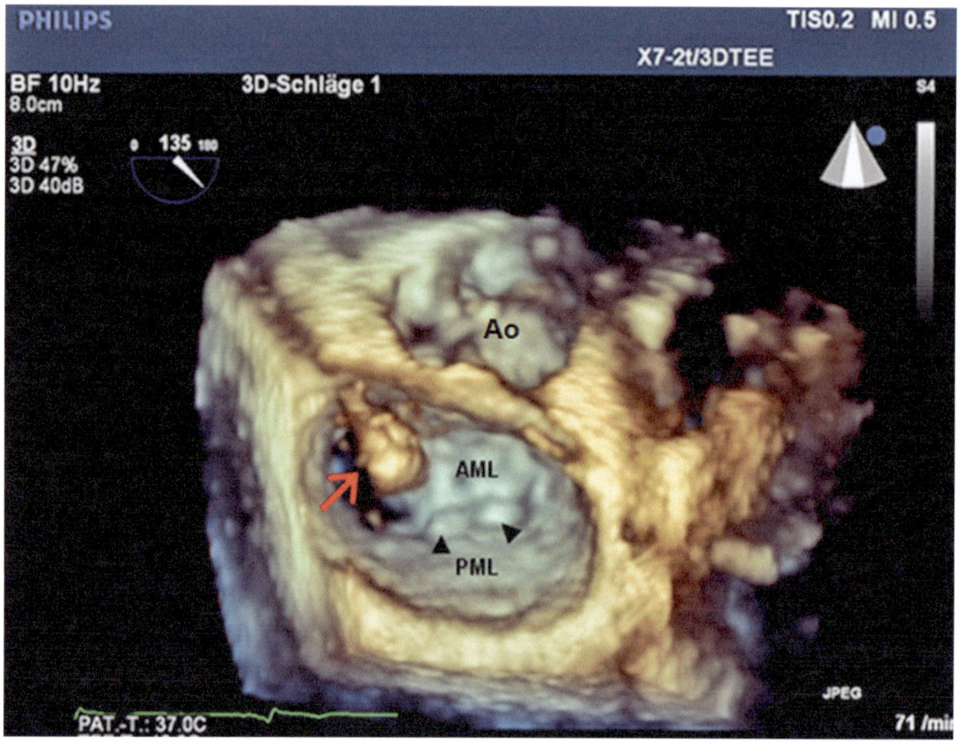

Fig. 15.4 Three-dimensional echocardiography showing the mitral valve from a left atrial view. *Black arrow heads* point to the two clips implanted consecutively starting at the level of the posteromedial commissure and moving toward the anterolateral commissure. Note that the MitraClip steerable guide and delivery catheter is being aimed at the level of the anterolateral commissure to release a third clip (*red arrow*). *AML* anterior mitral valve leaflet, *PML* posterior mitral valve leaflet, *Ao* aorta

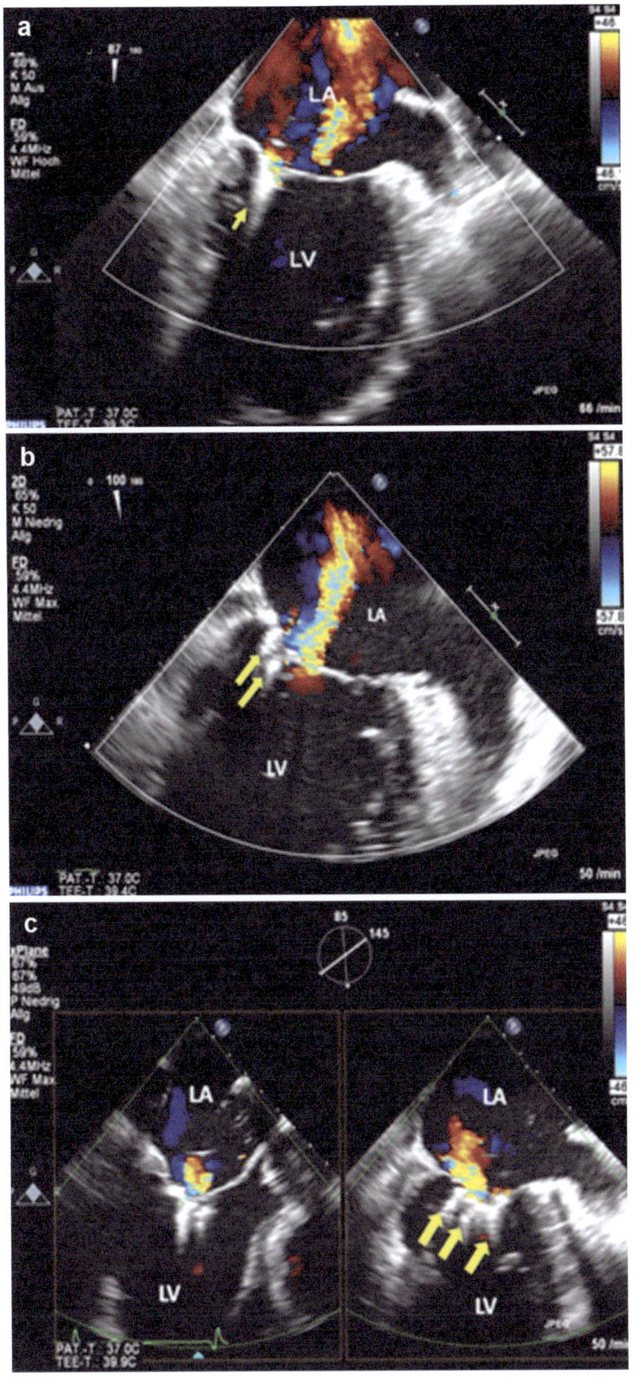

Fig. 15.5 (**a**–**c**) Standard transesophageal echocardiography with color Doppler (two chamber view) showing progressive mitral regurgitation jet reduction after consecutive clipping: (**a**) one clip, (**b**) two clips, (**c**) three clips. *Yellow arrows* point to the clips. *LA* left atrium, *LV* left ventricle

16 Case Example: Two Clips

Scott Lim

Abstract
This case sample demonstrates the steps in performing a two-Clip MitraClip procedure in a patient with severe functional mitral regurgitation (MR). The precise TEE localization of the residual MR after the first clip allowed for accurate placement of the second clip with excellent results.

Keywords
Mitral regurgitation • MitraClip • Functional mitral regurgitation • Multiple clips

Clinical History

An 84-year-old woman presented with NYHA Class III heart failure. She had a history of inferior myocardial infarction treated with coronary bypass grafting 10 years previously. Evaluation of her dyspnea demonstrated severe mitral regurgitation due to a restrictive posterior mitral leaflet with preserved ventricular function. Her coronary bypass grafts were patent, and her renal insufficiency was limiting (estimated glomerular filtration rate of 28 ml/min).

Summary

In this case, the patient developed an ischemic cardiomyopathy after her myocardial infarction, but with revascularization, she recovered her ventricular function. However, she remained with severe functional mitral regurgitation due to tethering of the posterior leaflet with incomplete coaptation. The origin of the mitral regurgitation was along the A2/P2 coaptation zone. Additionally, the moderate coaptation depth and adequate length of leaflet coaptation (>2 mm) made the mitral valve anatomy suitable for MitraClip implantation. After deployment of the first MitraClip, there was a lateral jet of residual mitral regurgitation. After deployment of the second MitraClip, there was only trace MR. Figures 16.1, 16.2, 16.3, 16.4, 16.5, 16.6, 16.7, 16.8, 16.9, 16.10, 16.11, 16.12, 16.13, 16.14, 16.15, 16.16, 16.17, 16.18, 16.19, 16.20, 16.21, 16.22, 16.23, and 16.24 show the step-by-step approach to evaluating a patient for and treating a patient with functional MR using the MitraClip. At follow-up, the patient reported greatly improved exercise tolerance, and follow-up TTE at 6 months showed 1+ MR.

Learning Points

This case demonstrates in a step-by-step fashion the steps taken for a two-Clip MitraClip procedure for functional MR.

S. Lim, M.D.
Department of Cardiology, University of Virginia Medical Center, 1215 Lee Street, Hospital Expansion, Room 4038, Charlottesville, VA 22908, USA
e-mail: sl9pc@virginia.edu

Electronic supplementary material The online version of this chapter (doi:10.1007/978-1-4471-4294-2_16) contains supplementary material, which is available to authorized users.

T. Feldman et al. (eds.), *Atlas of Percutaneous Edge-to-Edge Mitral Valve Repair*, DOI 10.1007/978-1-4471-4294-2_16, © Springer-Verlag London 2013

Screening Transthoracic Echo

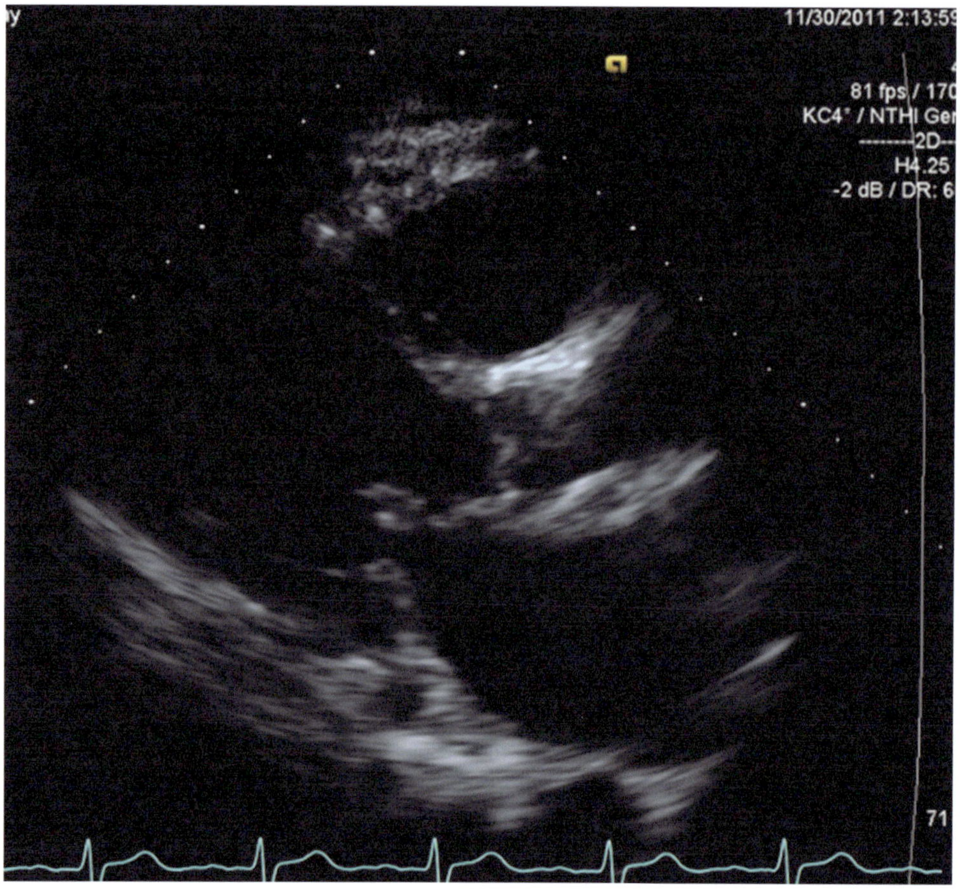

Fig. 16.1 TTE: parasternal LAX w/o color. The parasternal long axis demonstrates significant restriction of the posterior mitral leaflet, with a dilated left atrium and preserved ventricular function

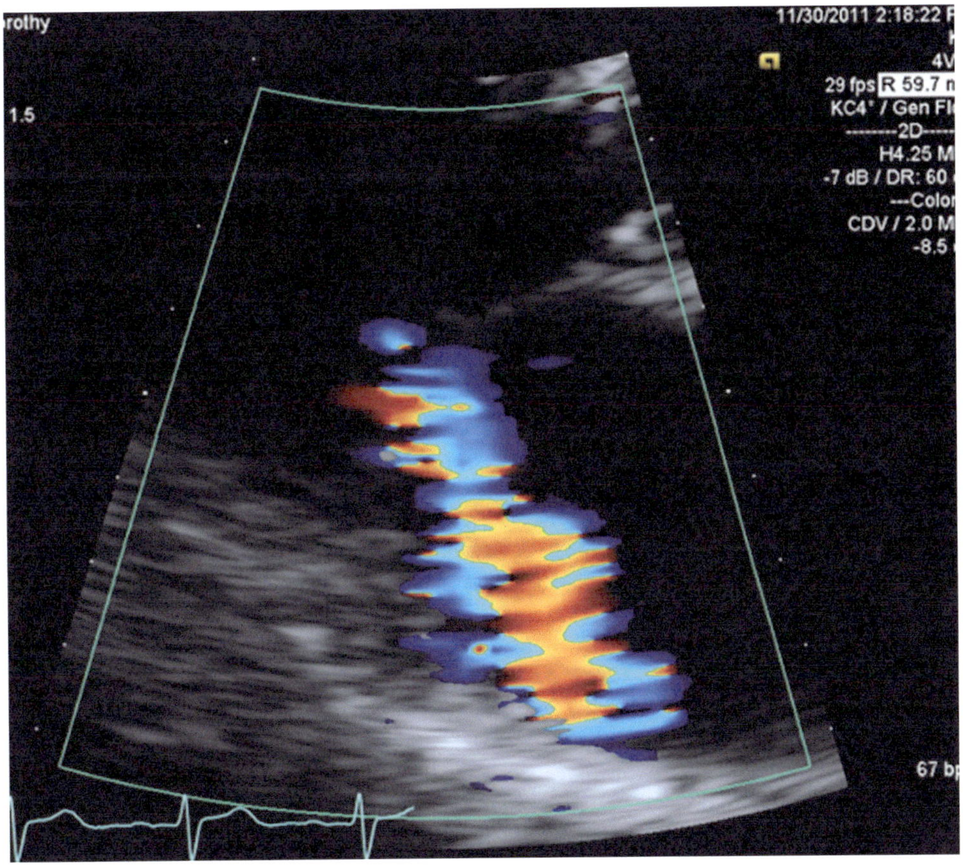

Fig. 16.2 TTE: parasternal LAX w/ color. This view zoomed in on the mitral valve with color Doppler demonstrates an eccentric, posteriorly directed jet, consistent with restriction of the anterior leaflet

Screening Transthoracic Echo

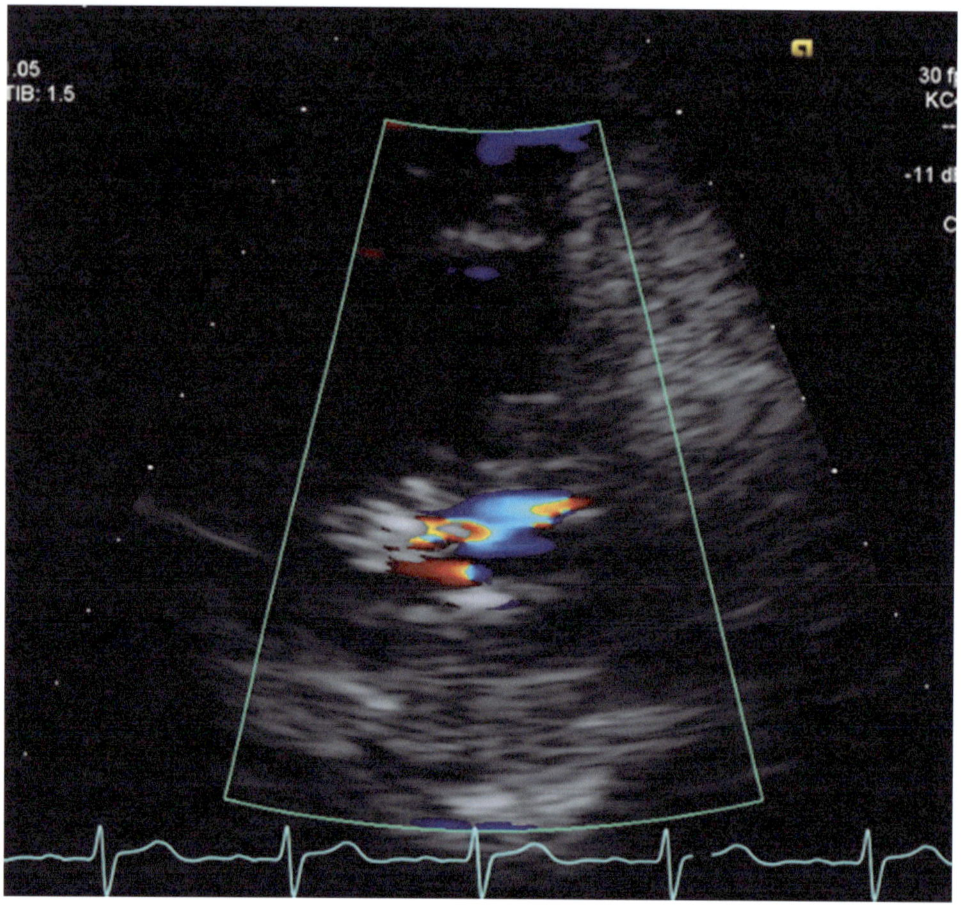

Fig. 16.3 TTE: parasternal SAX. Short axis view with color Doppler shows that the MR has a central origin along the A2/P2 interface

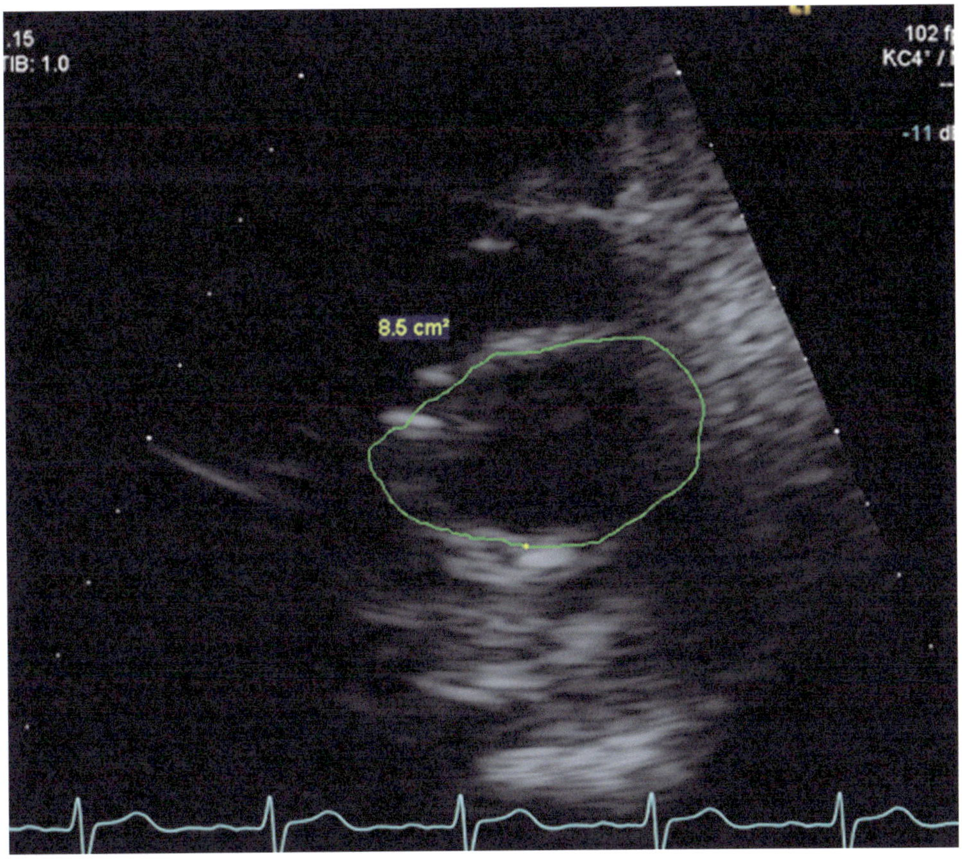

Fig. 16.4 TTE: apical 4C view. The Parasternal short axis view demonstrates a dilated mitral orifice area of 8.5 cm^2

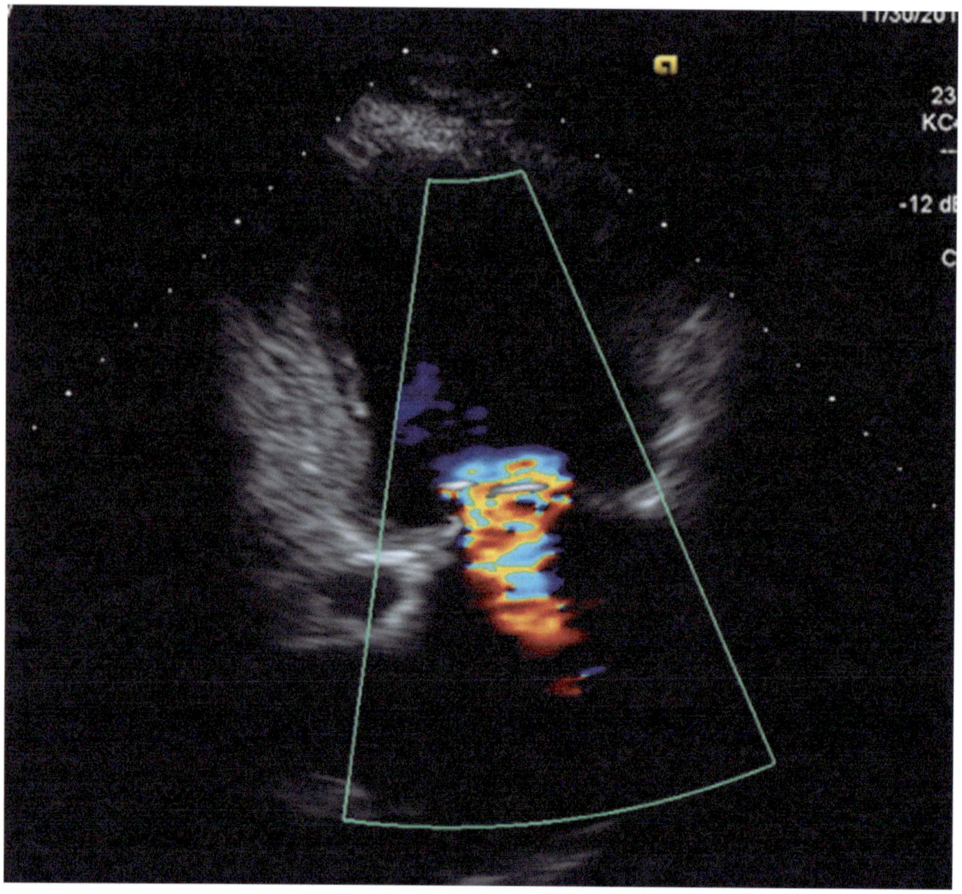

Fig. 16.5 TTE: 2C w color. In the apical two-chamber view, the very broad PISA of the eccentric MR jet is demonstrated, consistent with severe MR

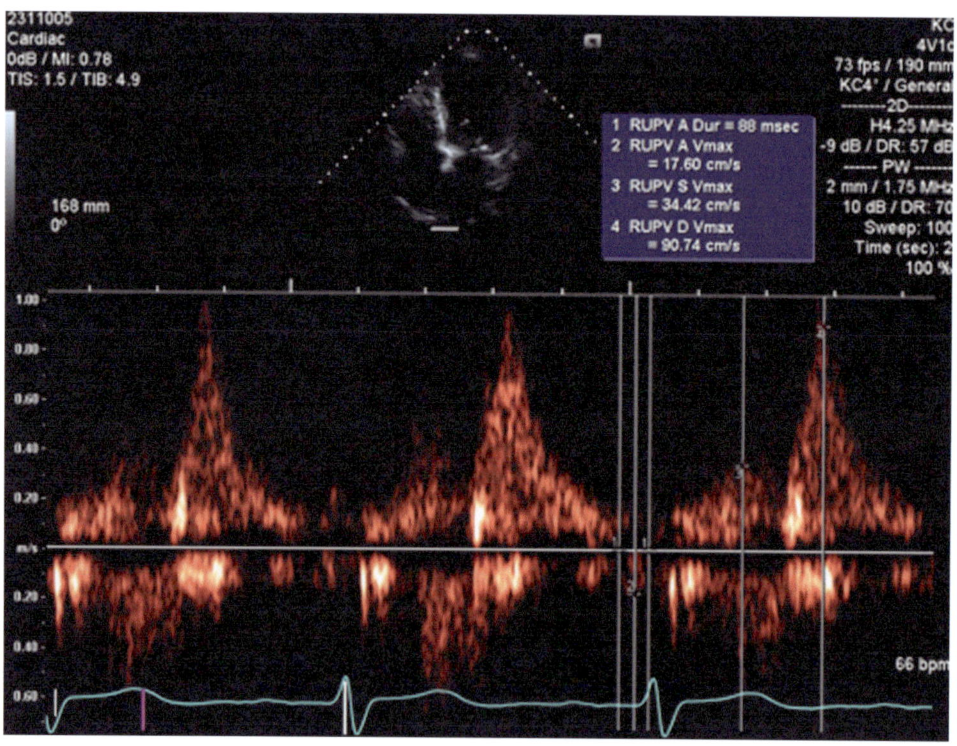

Fig. 16.6 TTE 4C. Pulmonary venous systolic flow reversal is demonstrated, consistent with severe MR

Screening TEE

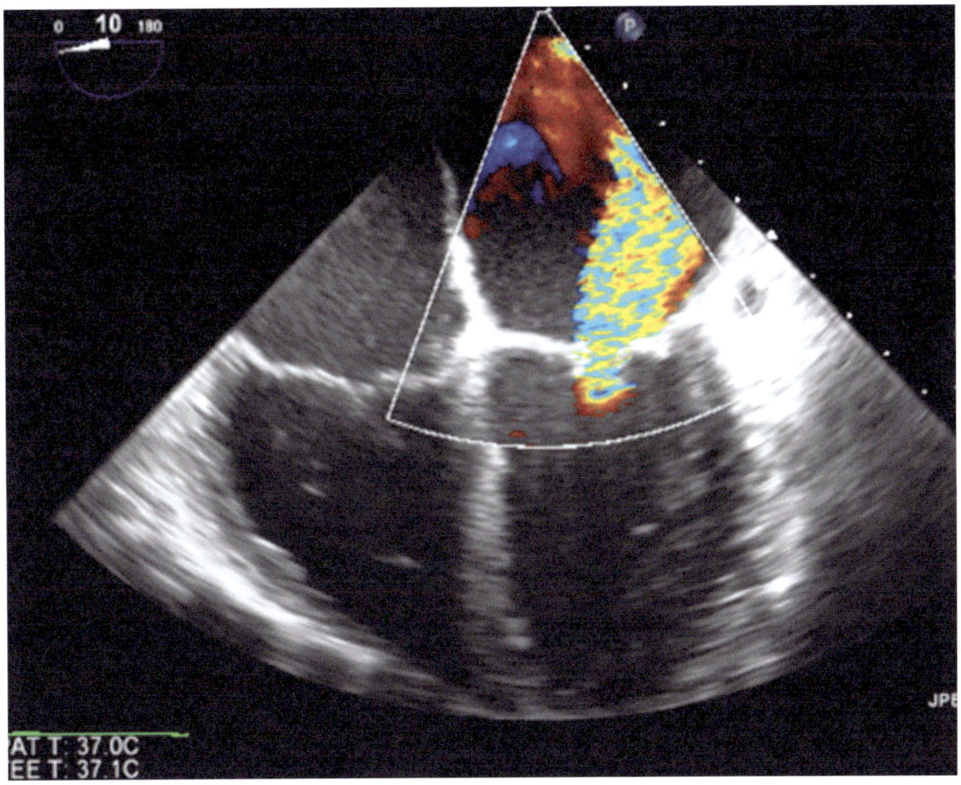

Fig. 16.7 TEE: 4C w color. The four chamber view at mid position demonstrates the broad jet originating from A2 to P2 with swirling in the dilated left atrium

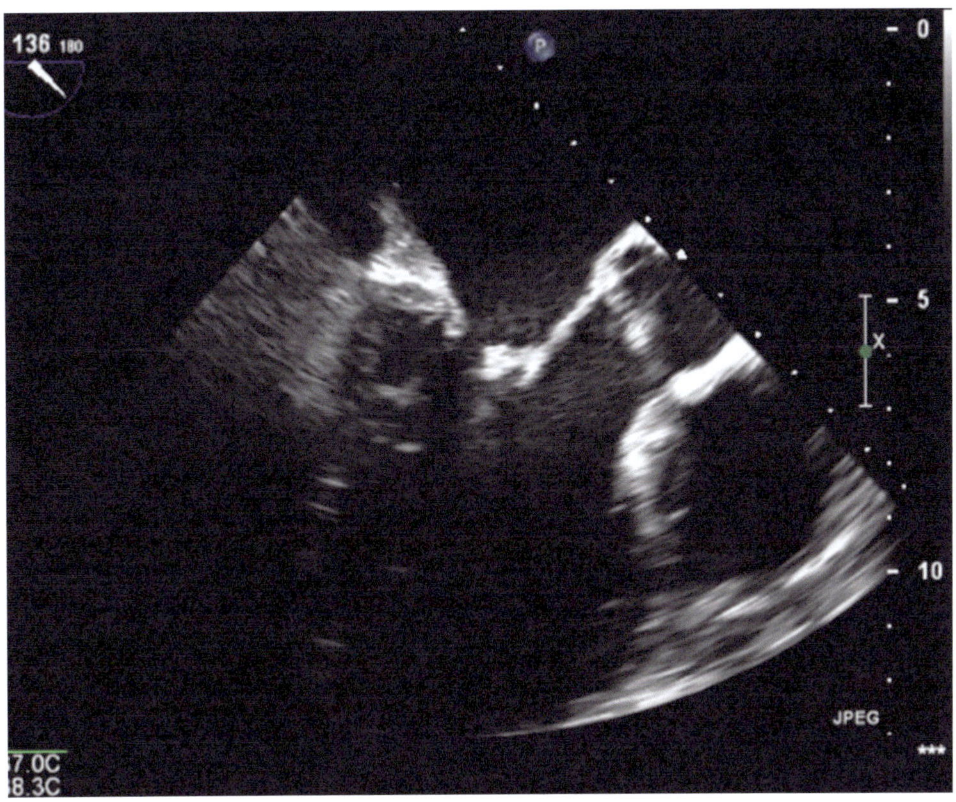

Fig. 16.8 TEE: LVOT w/o color. There is significant restriction of the P2 portion of the posterior leaflet

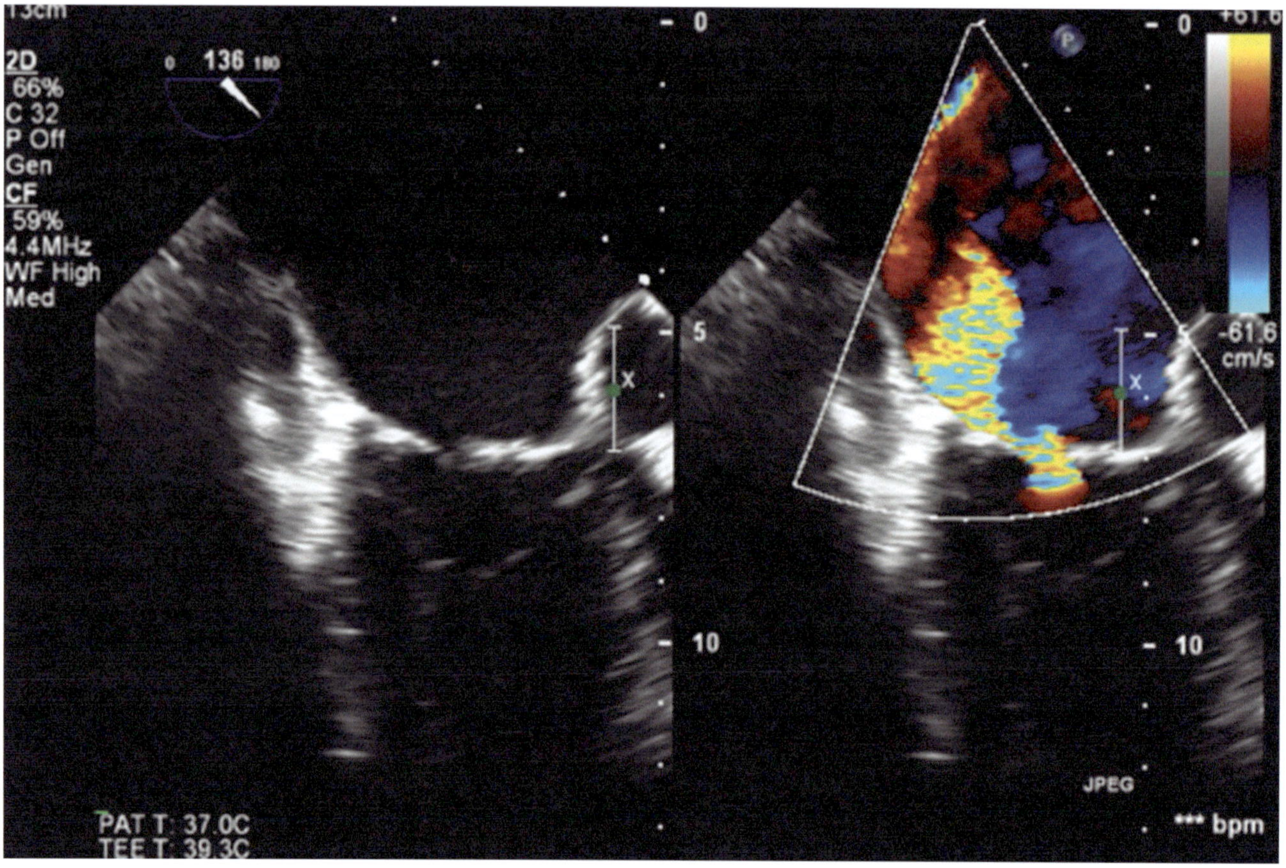

Fig. 16.9 TEE: LVOT w/ color. The LVOT view with color confirms a posteriorly directed jet originating at the A2/P2 interface due to restriction of P2

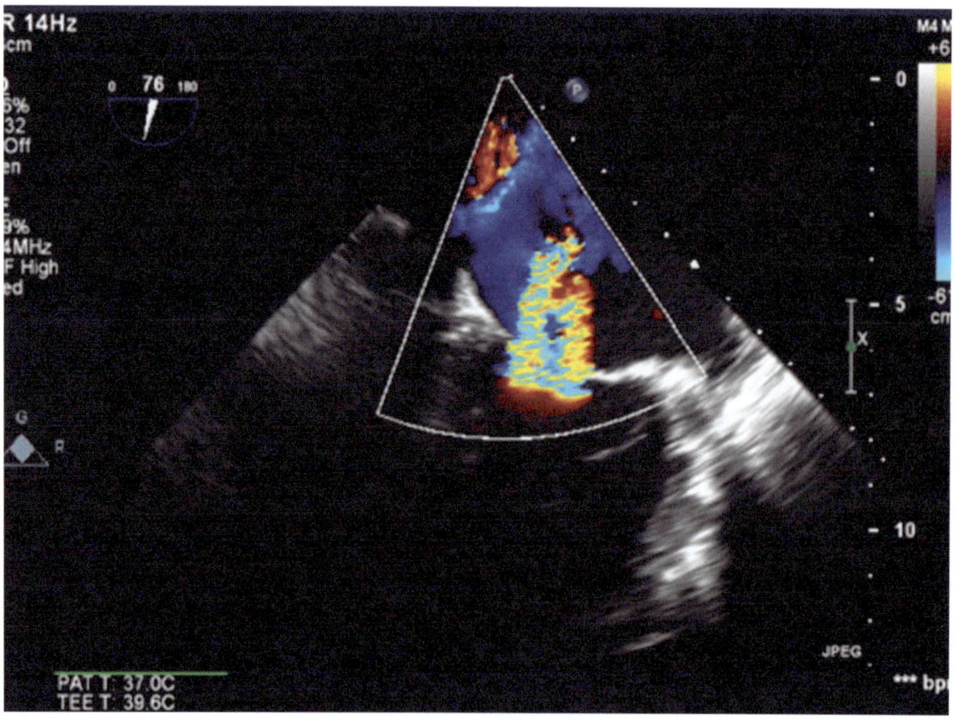

Fig. 16.10 TEE: 2C w/ color. There is a broad PISA from the A2-P2 zone consistent with severe MR

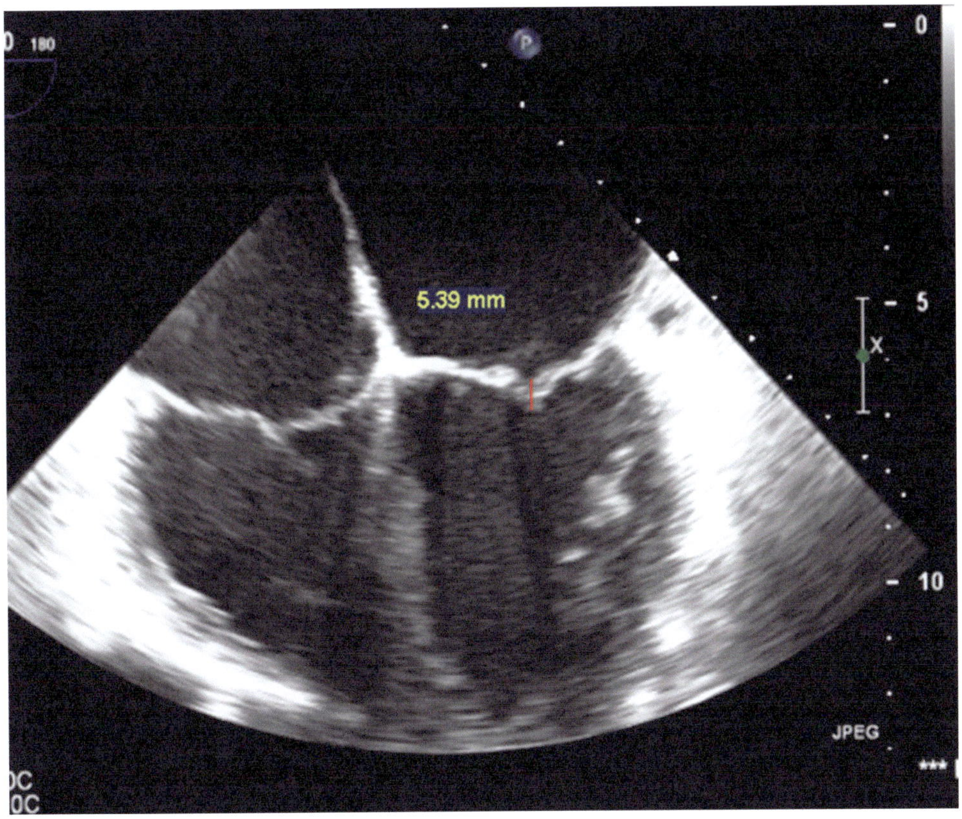

Fig. 16.11 TEE: 4C w/o color. The four chamber view shows a coaptation length of ~5 mm, suggesting favorable coaptation length for MitraClip

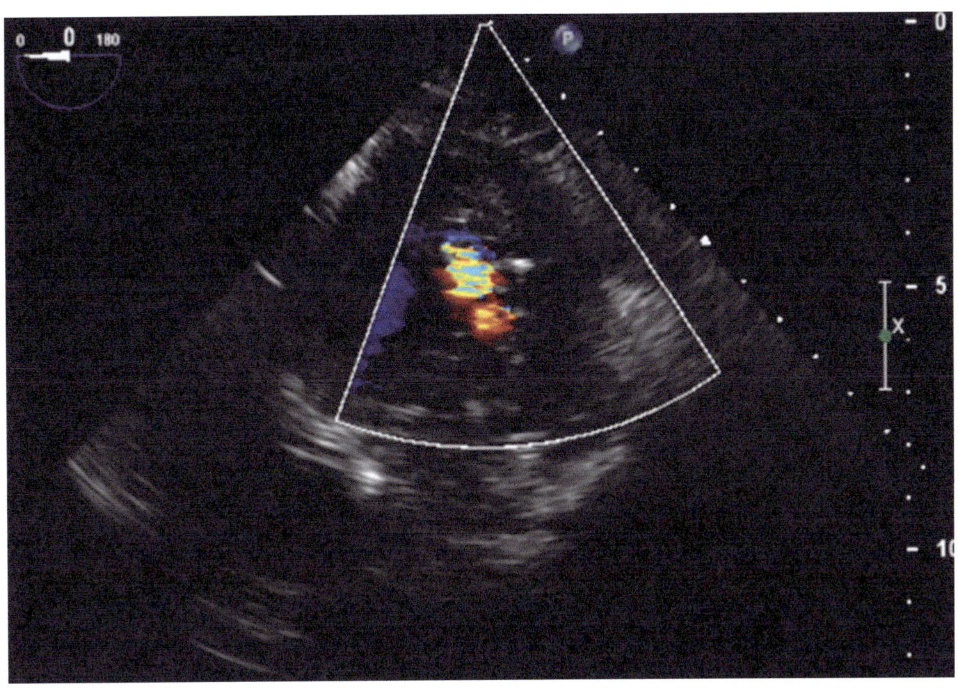

Fig. 16.12 TEE. Transgastric w/ color: the regurgitant jet has a central origin

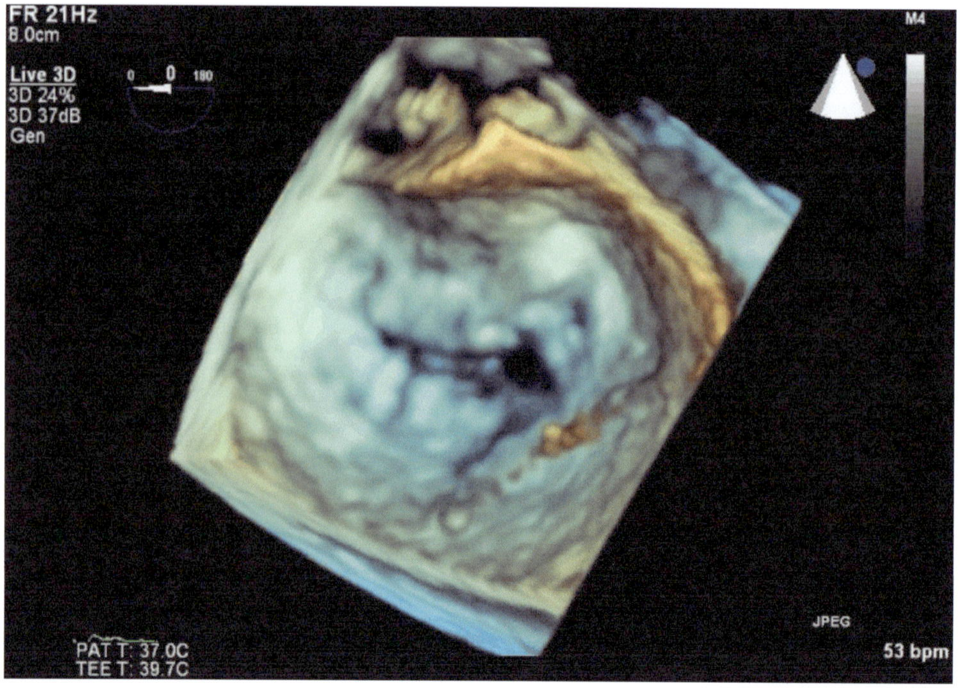

Fig. 16.13 TEE: 3D back of LA view. This real-time 3D view of the mitral valve from the LA demonstrates incomplete coaptation predominantly between the medial aspects of the A2–P2 zone

Transseptal Puncture

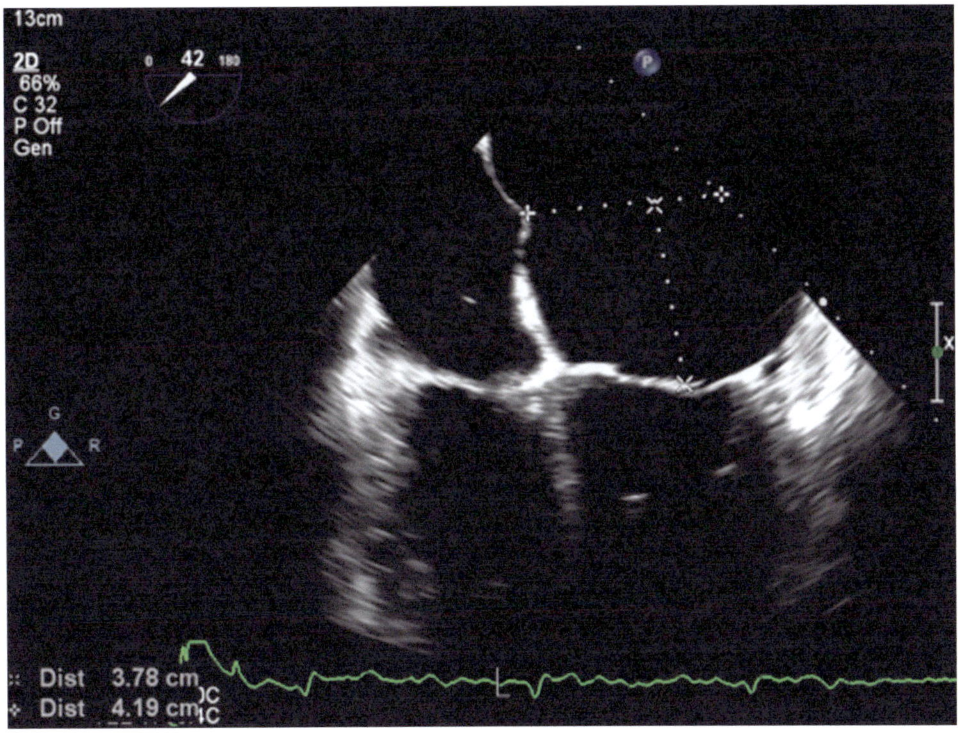

Fig. 16.14 TEE: 4C view. The transseptal dilator is tenting the interatrial septum at a height above the mitral annulus of 3.8 cm, appropriate for proper functioning of the MitraClip system

Procedural TEE and Fluoro I

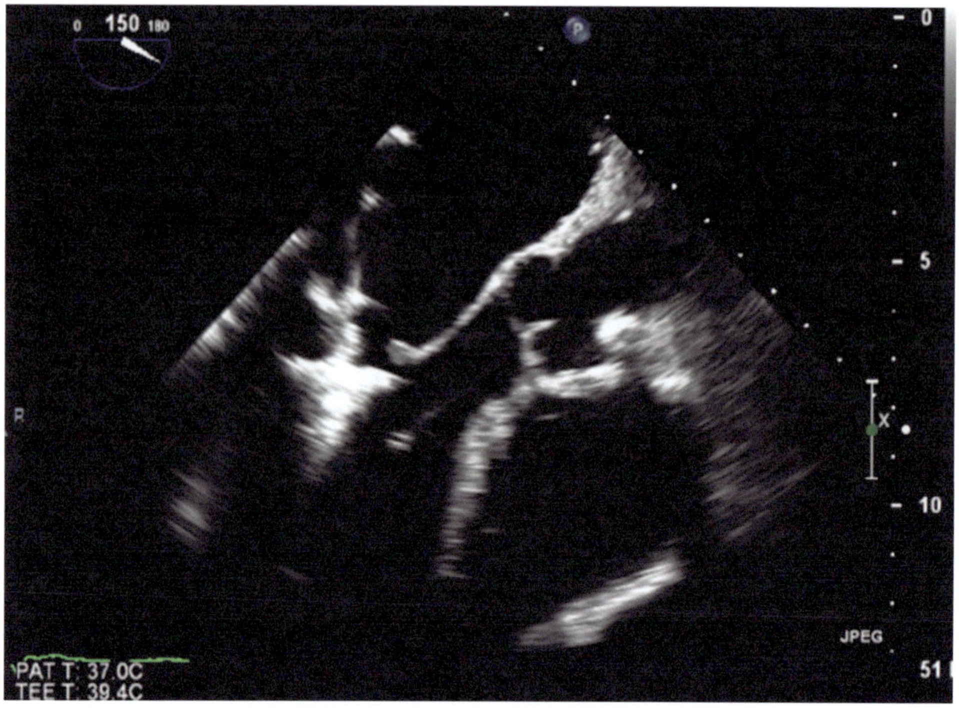

Fig. 16.15 TEE: LVOT. The MitraClip is advanced across the mitral valve, with arms perpendicular to the line of coaptation

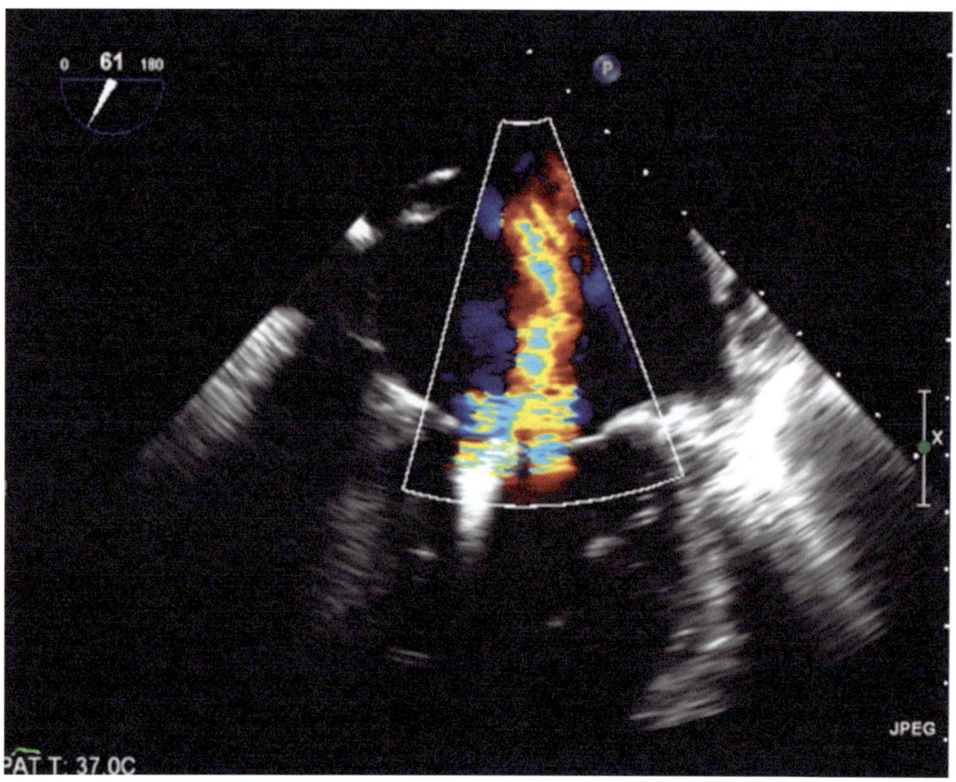

Fig. 16.16 TEE 2C. Following confirmation of adequate leaflet insertion, the MR severity is reduced with the clip arms tightened. The residual MR jet is isolated lateral to the first clip

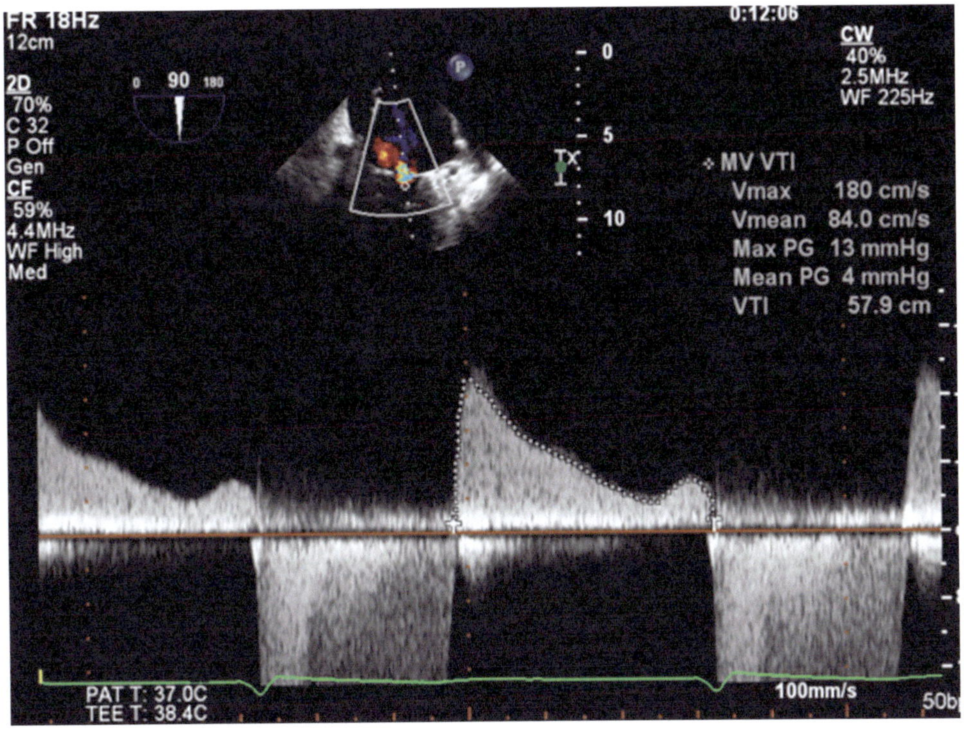

Fig. 16.17 Doppler. Following first clip deployment, minimal inflow gradient is demonstrated which was felt to be due to residual MR, and adequate for second clip placement

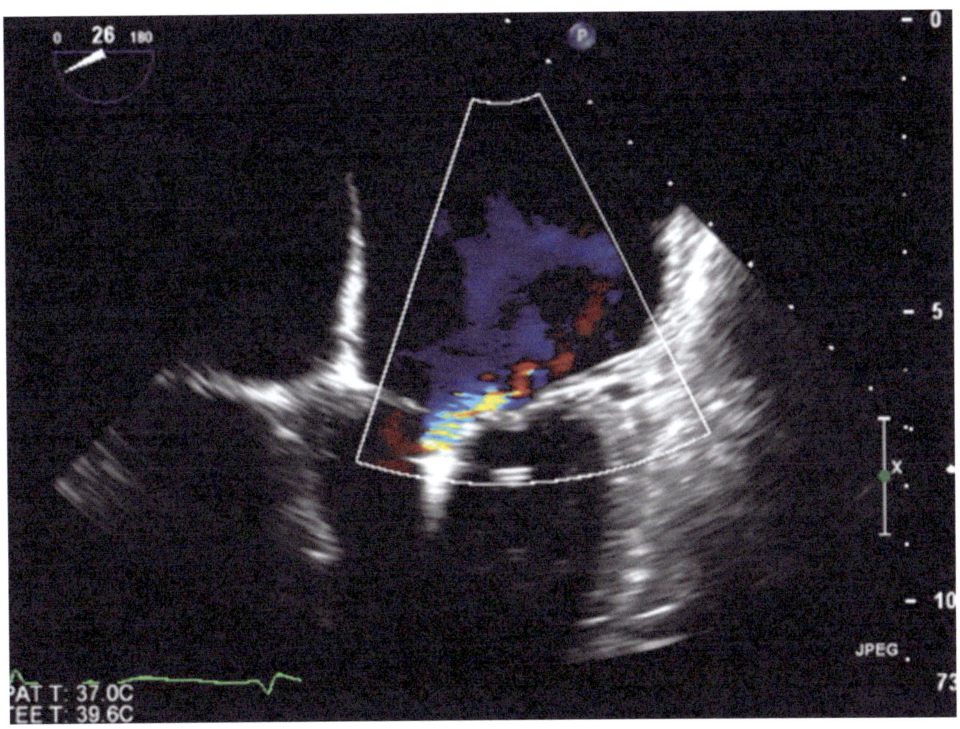

Fig. 16.18 TEE: after second clip deployment. Following second clip deployment, the larger lateral residual jet is abolished, leaving a small medial jet

Procedural TEE and Fluoro II

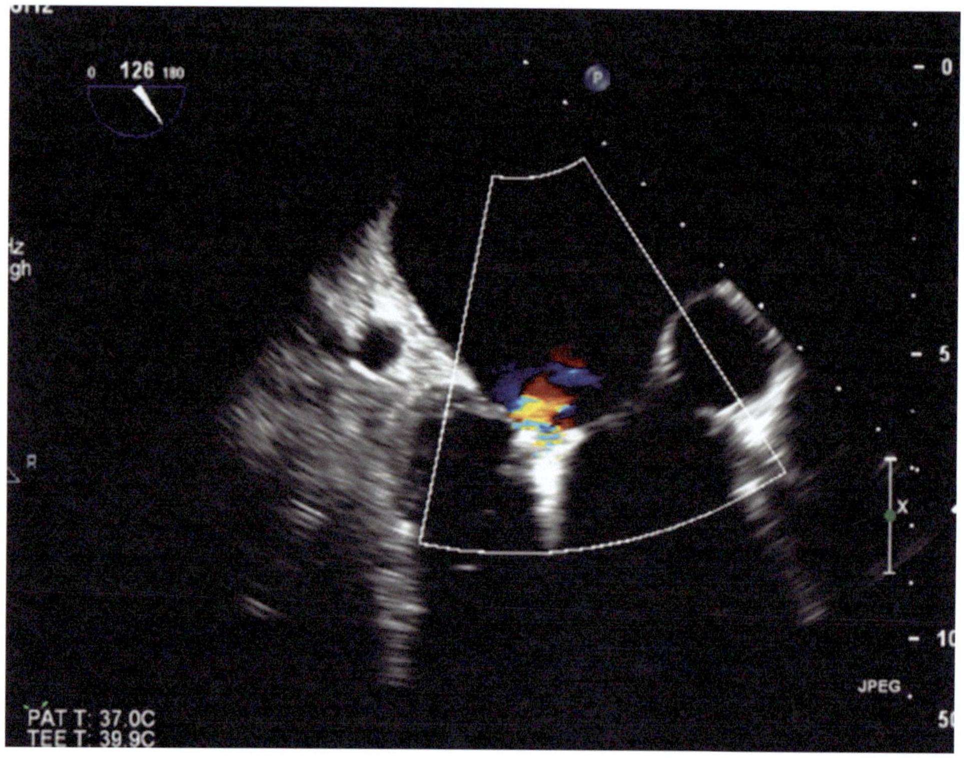

Fig. 16.19 TEE. The residual medial MR jet is judged to be mild

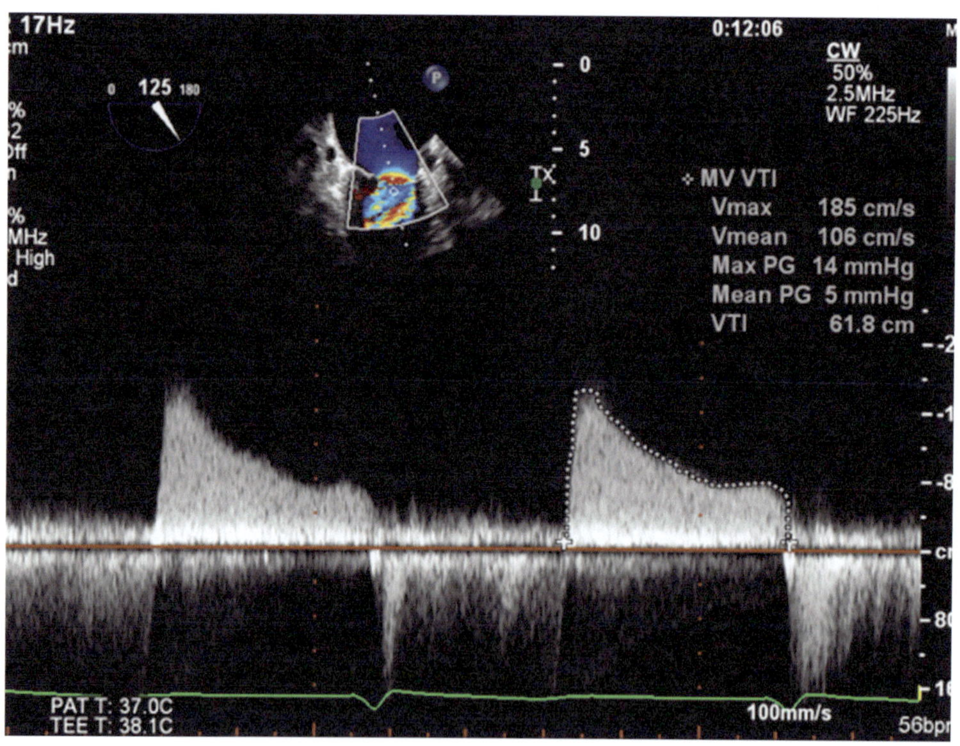

Fig. 16.20 Doppler. The final Doppler derived inflow gradient was judged to be negligible following two clips

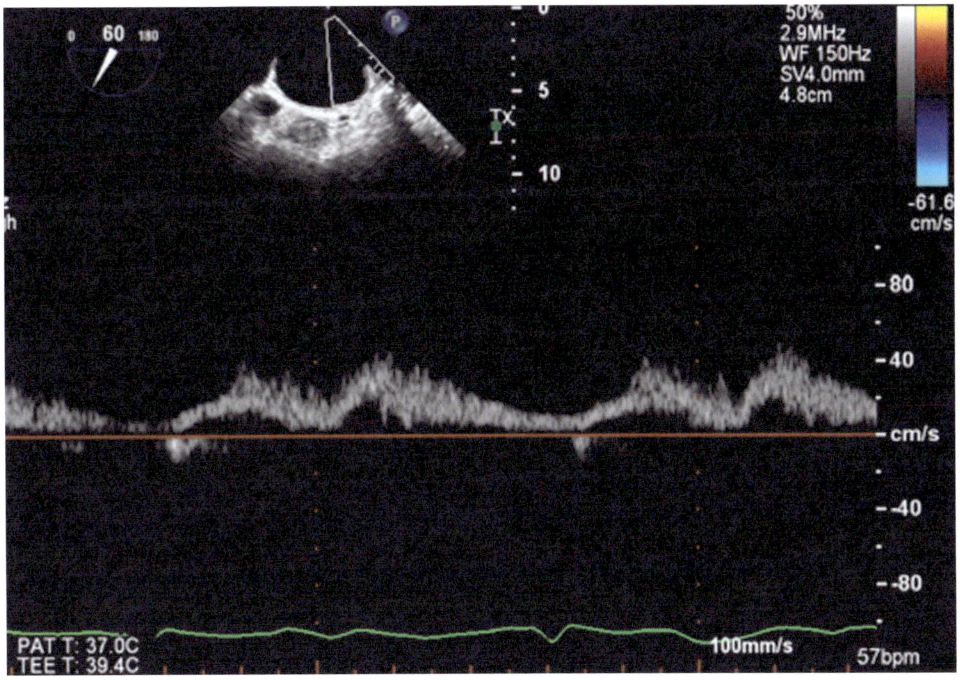

Fig. 16.21 TEE: pulmonary vein Doppler. The pulmonary venous flow pattern has normalized

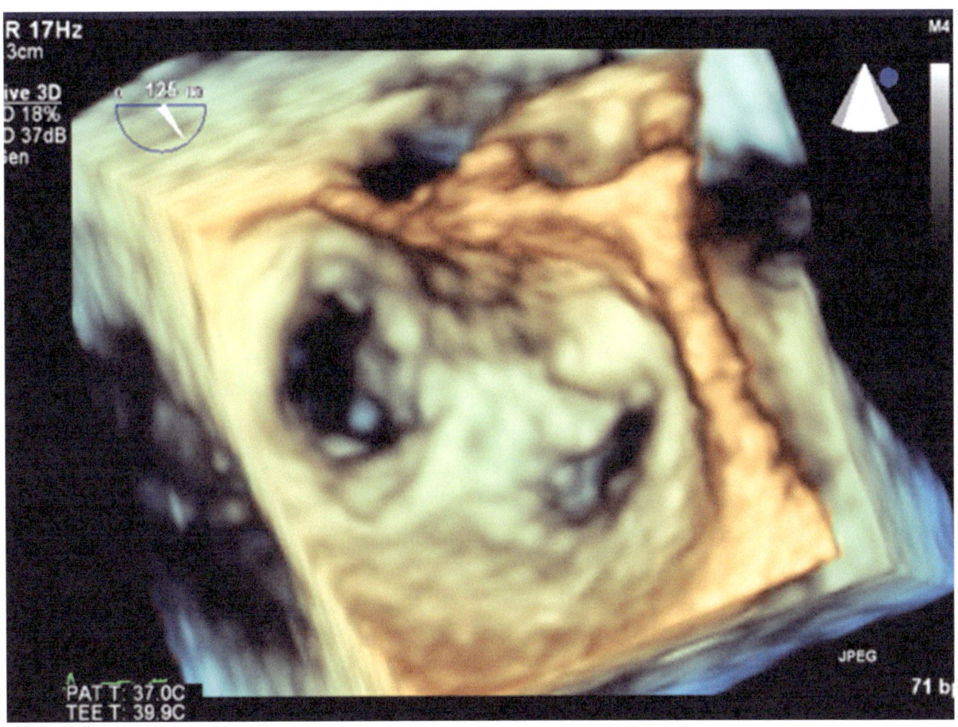

Fig. 16.22 TEE: 3D LA view of MV after second clip. Appropriate double orifice has been created

Procedural TEE and Fluoro III

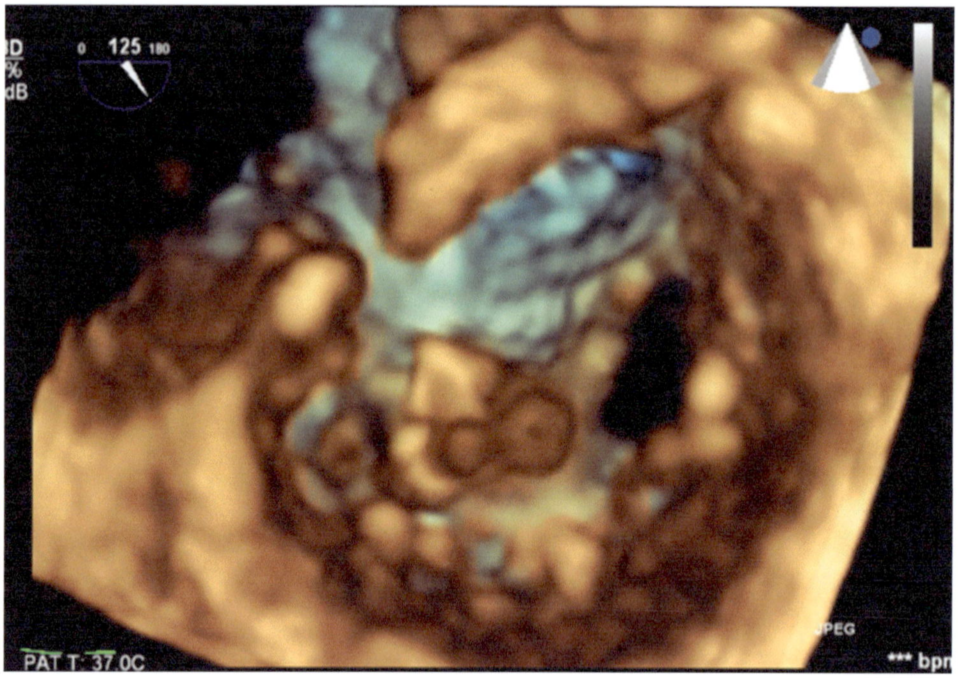

Fig. 16.23 TEE: 3D LV view of MV after second clip. Both clips are seen to have their arms perpendicular to the line of coaptation

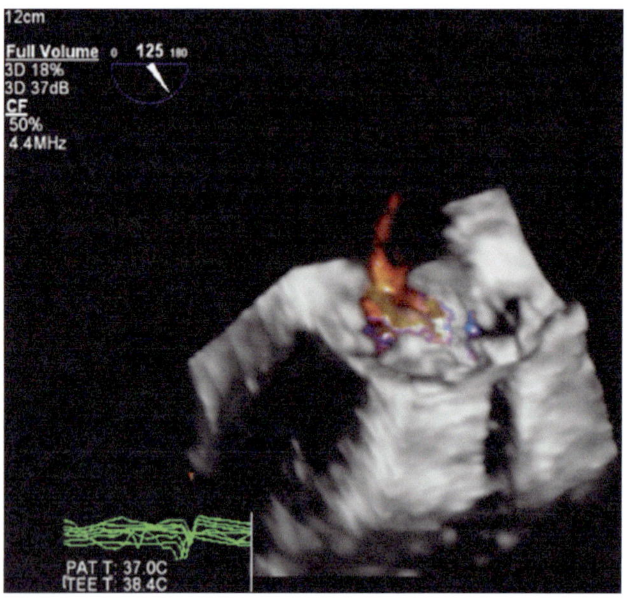

Fig. 16.24 TEE: 3D w/ color. Mild residual MR is demonstrated predominantly just medial to first clip

EVEREST II Delayed Second Clip for Early Recurrent MR

17

Ehrin J. Armstrong, Khung Keong Yeo, and Jason Rogers

Abstract

This case sample highlights the use of a second MitraClip in a patient who had developed early recurrent mitral regurgitation, likely secondary to partial clip detachment.

Keywords

Mitral regurgitation • Mitral valve prolapse • MitraClip • Partial clip detachment • Recurrent mitral regurgitation

Clinical History

A 68-year-old man with a history of severe MR and exertional dyspnea was enrolled in the REALISM continued access registry.

E.J. Armstrong, M.D., M.Sc.
Division of Cardiovascular Medicine,
University of California, Davis Medical Center,
4860 Y Street, Suite 2820, Sacramento, CA 95817, USA
e-mail: ehrin.armstrong@ucdmc.ucdavis.edu

K.K. Yeo, M.B.B.S., FACC, FSCAI
Department of Cardiology, National Heart Centre Singapore,
Mistri Wing, 17 Third Hospital Avenue,
Singapore 168752, Singapore

Department of Cardiovascular Medicine,
University of California, Davis Medical Center,
4860 Y Street, Suite 2820, Sacramento 95817, CA, USA
e-mail: yeo_kk@yahoo.com, yeo.khung.keong@nhcs.com.sg

J. Rogers, M.D., FACC, FSCAI (✉)
Department of Cardiovascular Medicine,
University of California, Davis Medical Center,
4860 Y Street, Suite 2820, Sacramento 95817, CA, USA
e-mail: jason.rogers@ucdmc.ucdavis.edu

Summary

Screening transthoracic and transesophageal echocardiograms revealed severe MR due to severe P2 prolapse and mild flail (Figs. 17.1, 17.2, 17.3, 17.4, 17.5, 17.6, 17.7, 17.8, 17.9, 17.10, 17.11 and Videos 17.1, 17.2, 17.3, 17.4, 17.5, 17.6, 17.7, 17.8, 17.9, 17.10, 17.11, 17.12, 17.13). The patient underwent uncomplicated single MitraClip device implantation with acute and postoperative day-one reduction in his MR from 4+ to 1+. On follow-up echocardiography 1 month later, a transthoracic echocardiogram revealed recurrent 4+ MR, possibly related to partial clip detachment and progressive P2 degenerative changes (Figs. 17.21, 17.22, 17.23, 17.24, 17.25, 17.26, 17.27, 17.28 and Videos 17.19, 17.20, 17.21, 17.22, 17.23, 17.24, 17.25, 17.26). He subsequently underwent a repeat procedure with implantation of a second device lateral to the first device with reduction of his MR from 4+ to 2+; the residual MR was mainly related to persistent regurgitation around the first device. This case illustrates early recurrent MR and ability to place a second device, but inability to completely reduce MR due to regurgitation around the partial clip detachment. Figures 17.12, 17.13, 17.14, 17.15, 17.16, 17.17, 17.18, 17.19, 17.20 and Videos

Electronic supplementary material The online version of this chapter (doi:10.1007/978-1-4471-4294-2_17) contains supplementary material, which is available to authorized users.

T. Feldman et al. (eds.), *Atlas of Percutaneous Edge-to-Edge Mitral Valve Repair*,
DOI 10.1007/978-1-4471-4294-2_17, © Springer-Verlag London 2013

17.14, 17.15, 17.16, 17.17, 17.18 show the steps in the initial procedure; Figs. 17.29, 17.30, 17.32, 17.33, 17.34, 17.35, 17.36, 17.37, 17.38, 17.39, 17.40 and Videos 17.27, 17.28, 17.29, 17.30, 17.31, 17.32, 17.33, 17.34 show the steps of the second procedure. At 6-month follow-up after the second device implantation, the patient was asymptomatic without any functional limitations (Figs. 17.41, 17.42, 17.43, 17.44 and Videos 17.35, 17.36, 17.37, 17.38).

Learning Points

- Partial clip detachment or single leaflet detachment can occur early after an initially successful MitraClip procedure.
- It is possible to re-intervene and place a second MitraClip in cases of early recurrent mitral regurgitation due to partial clip detachment.

Screening Transthoracic Echo

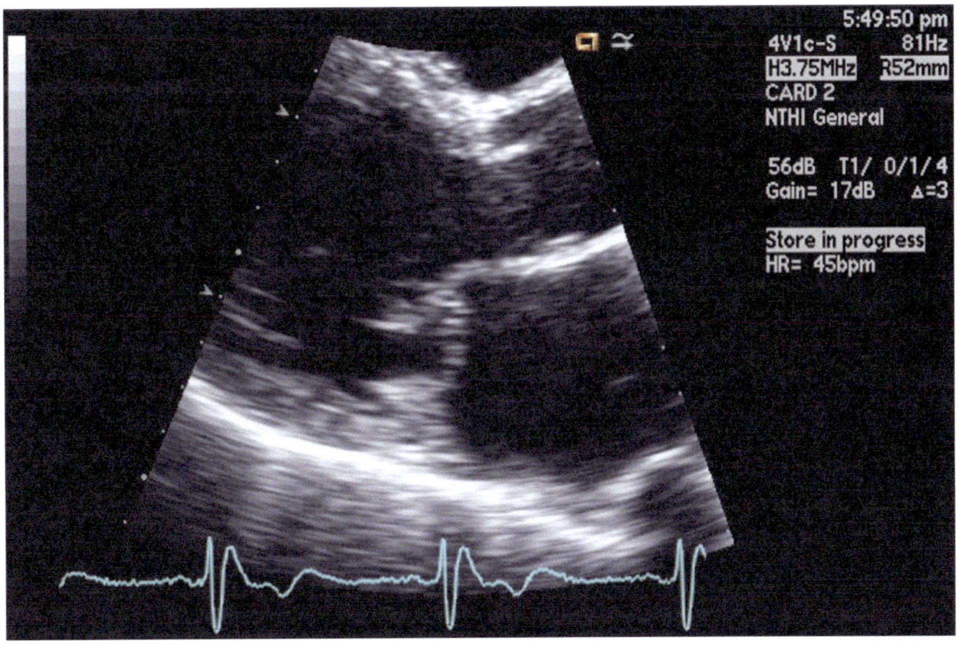

Fig. 17.1 TTE: parasternal LAX w/o color. The posterior leaflet has mild prolapse in systole

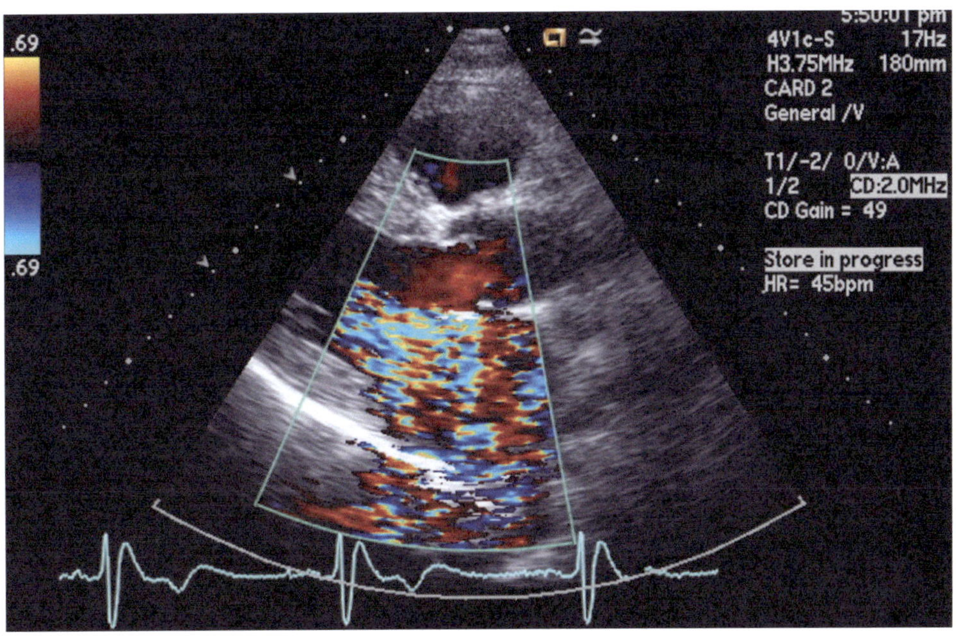

Fig. 17.2 TTE: parasternal LAX w/ color. Color flow Doppler suggests significant MR

Screening Transthoracic Echo

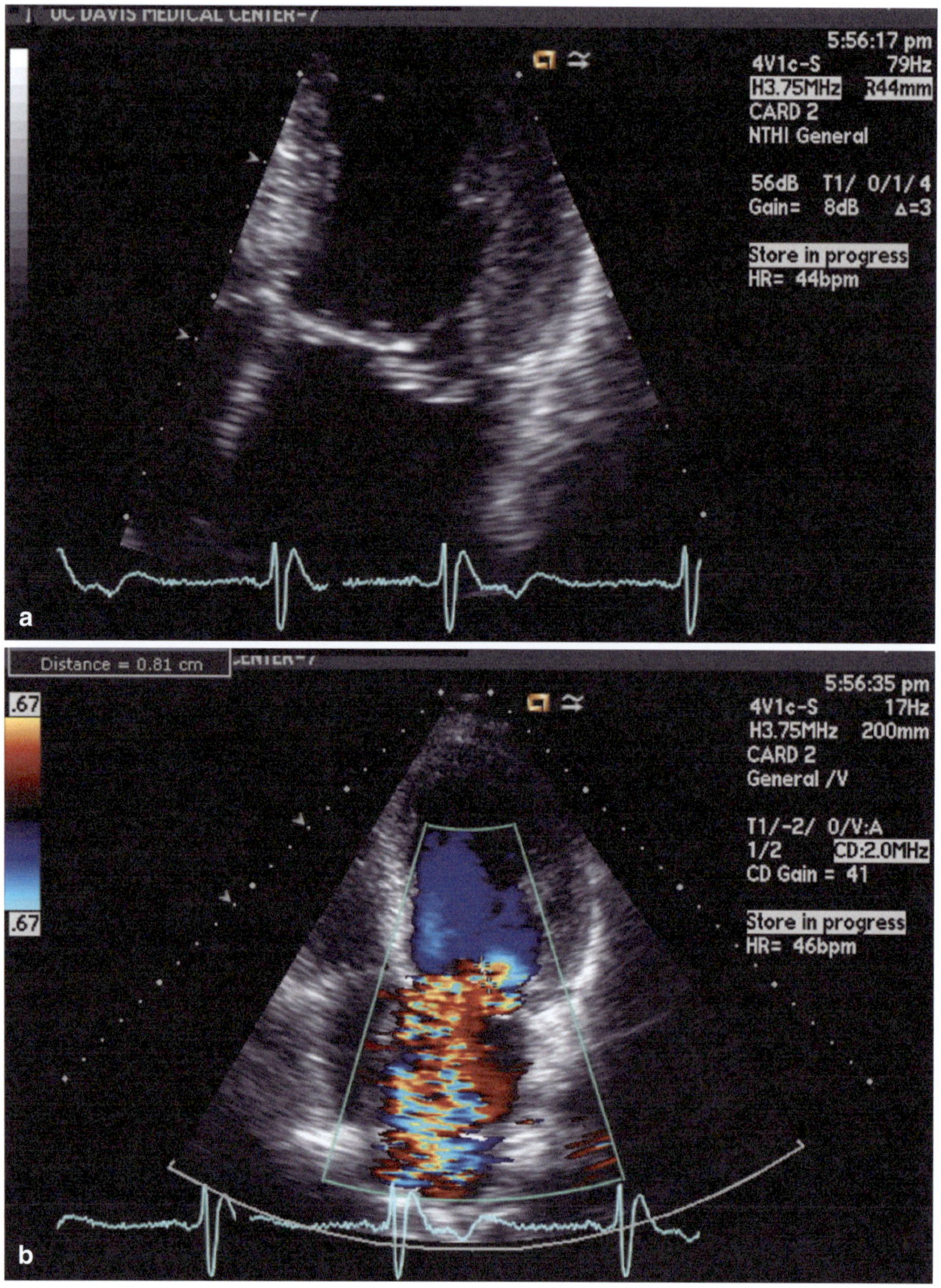

Fig. 17.3 TTE: apical 4C. The posterior leaflet can be seen prolapsing in systole (**a**), with an anteriorly directed jet of MR that reaches to the pulmonary veins (**b**)

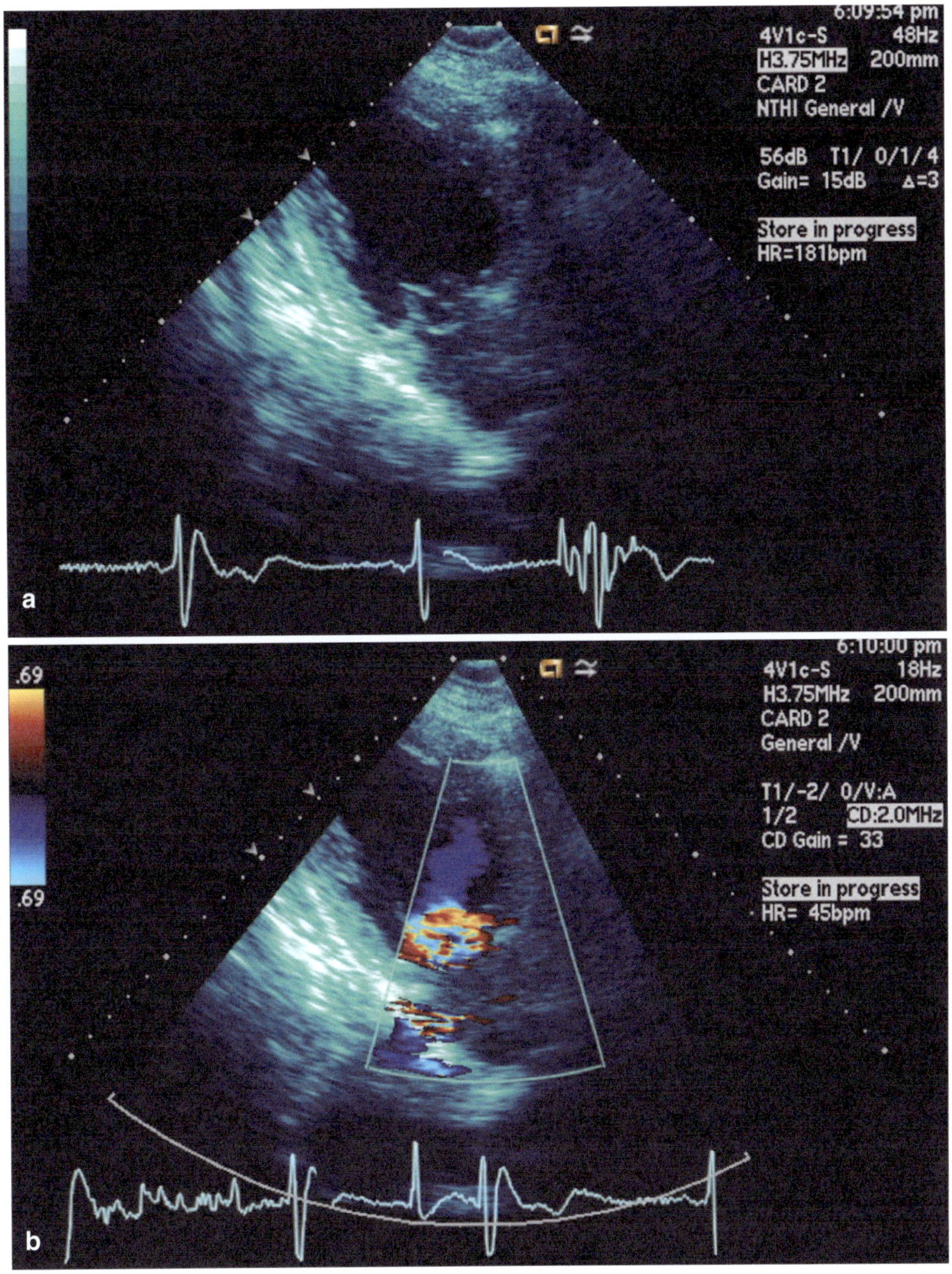

Fig. 17.4 TTE: apical 2C view. There is posterior leaflet prolapsed (**a**) with a central origin of the MR jet (**b**)

Screening TEE

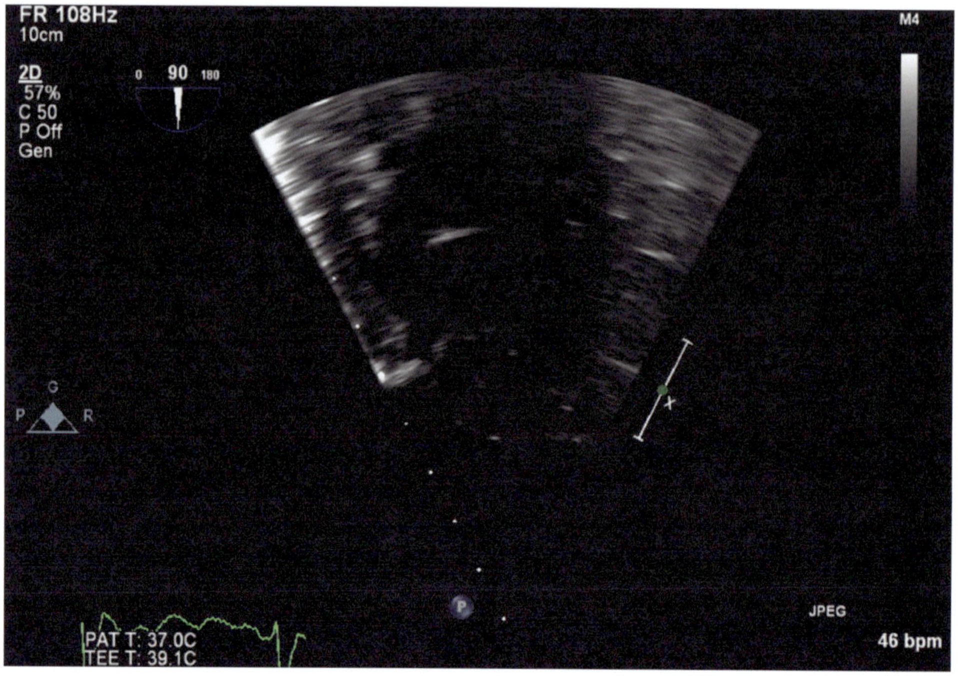

Fig. 17.5 TEE: bicommissural w/o color. The P2 segment can be seen prolapsing in the center of the valve

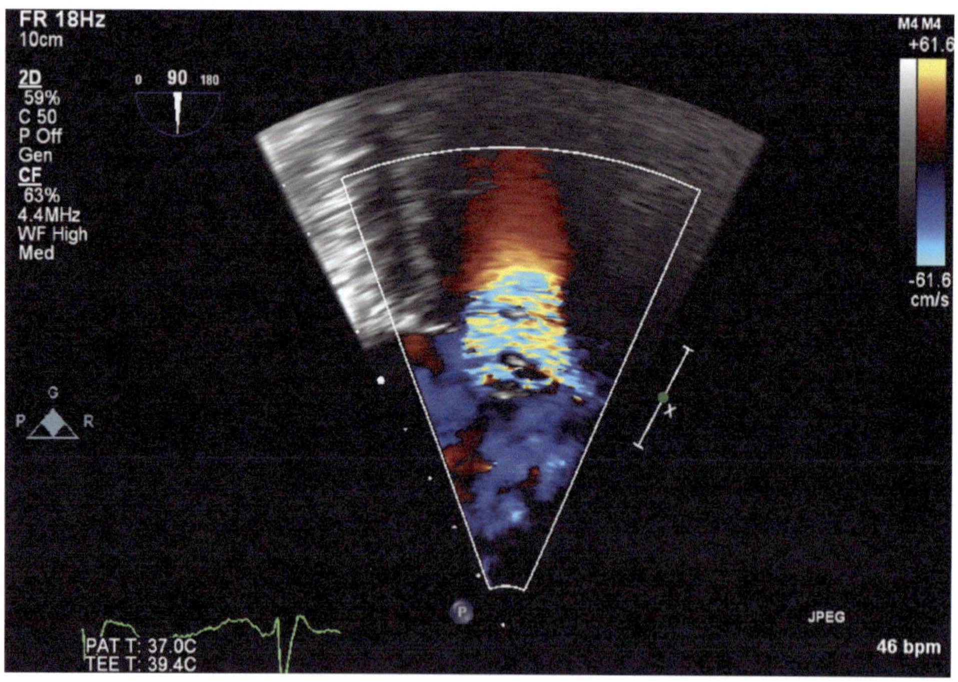

Fig. 17.6 TEE: bicommissural w color. There is significant MR with a central jet origin

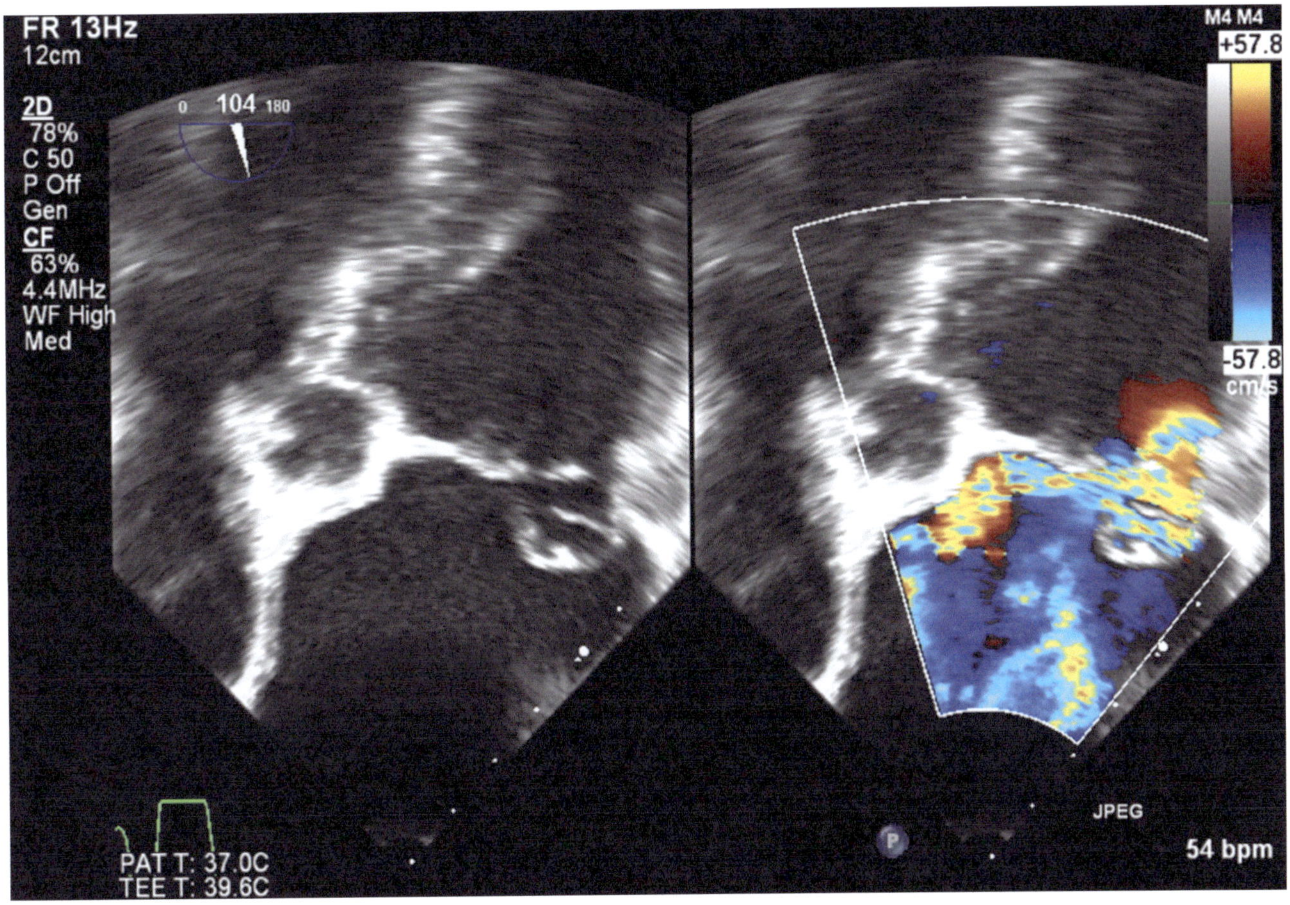

Fig. 17.7 TEE: 3C w/o color and w/ color. There is significant P2 prolapse with a small flail gap (*left*) and an anteriorly directed jet of MR (*right*)

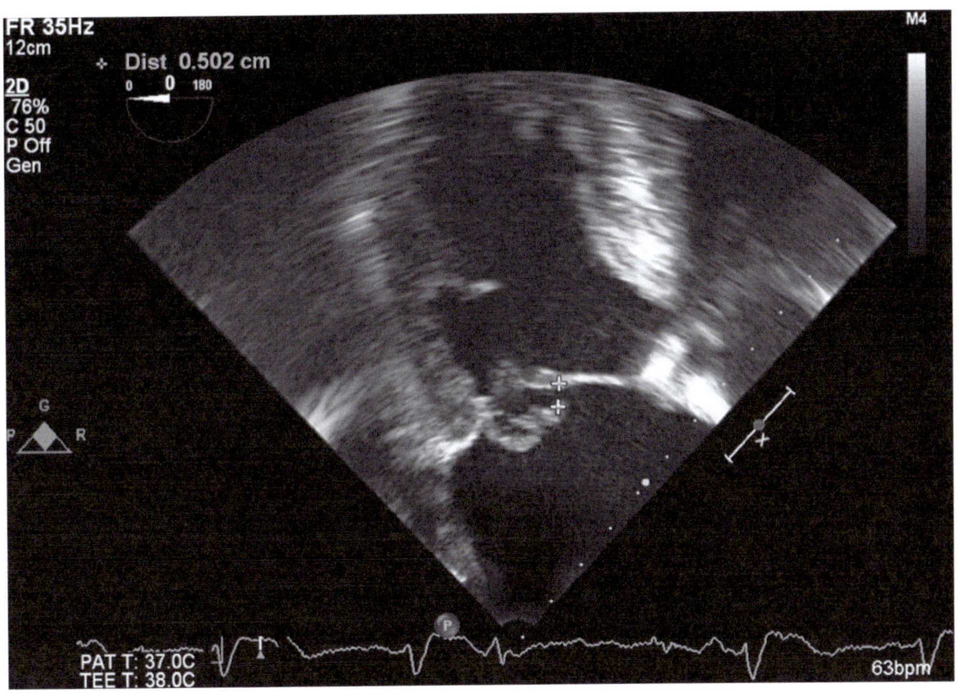

Fig. 17.8 TEE: 4C w/o color. There is P2 scallop prolapse with a small flail segment

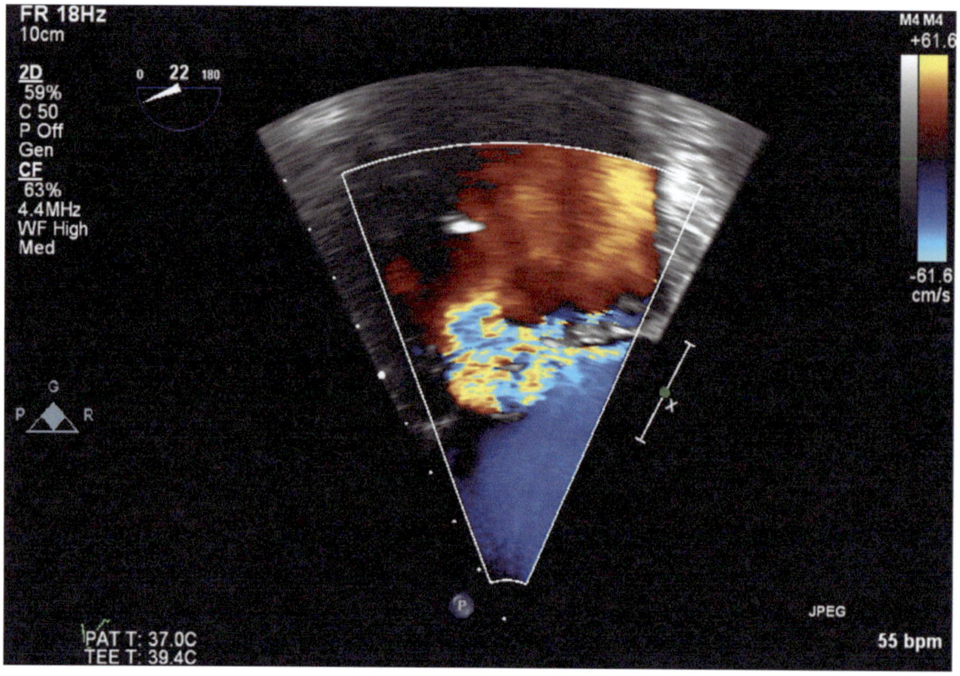

Fig. 17.9 TEE: 4C w/ color. The MR originates from the site of P2 prolapse

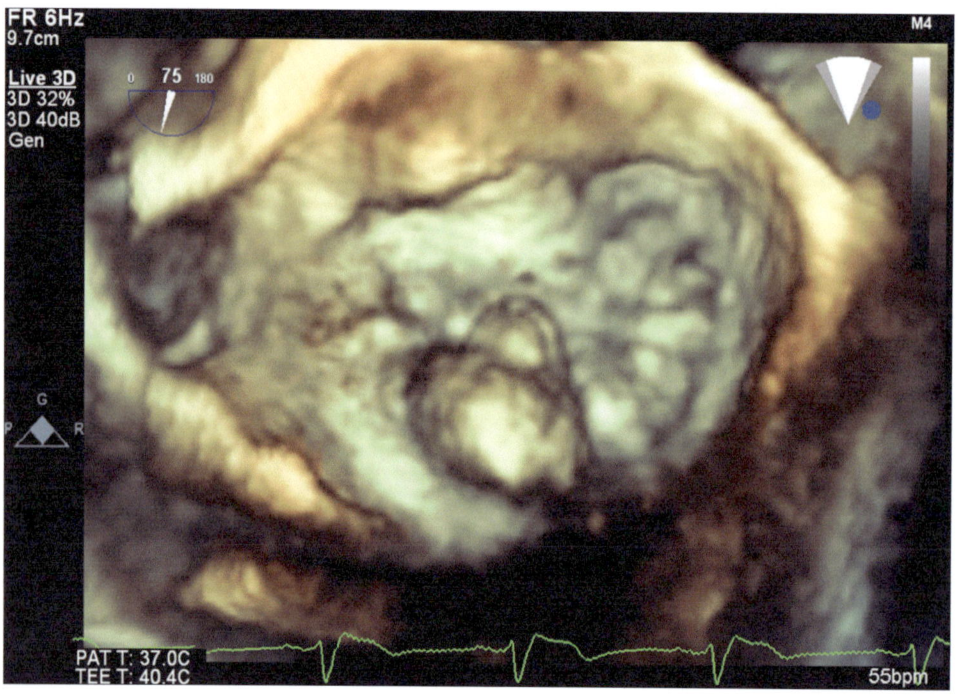

Fig. 17.10 TEE: 3D reconstruction. In systole, 3D reconstruction shows prolapse of the P2 scallop

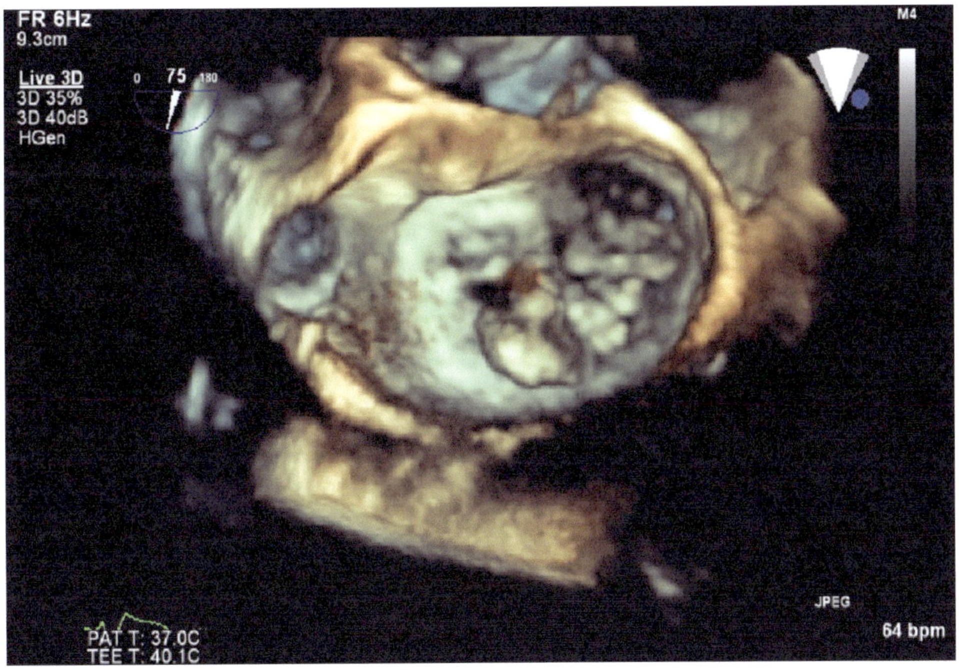

Fig. 17.11 TEE: 3D reconstruction. There is mild flail in mid systole

Procedural TEE and Fluoro 1

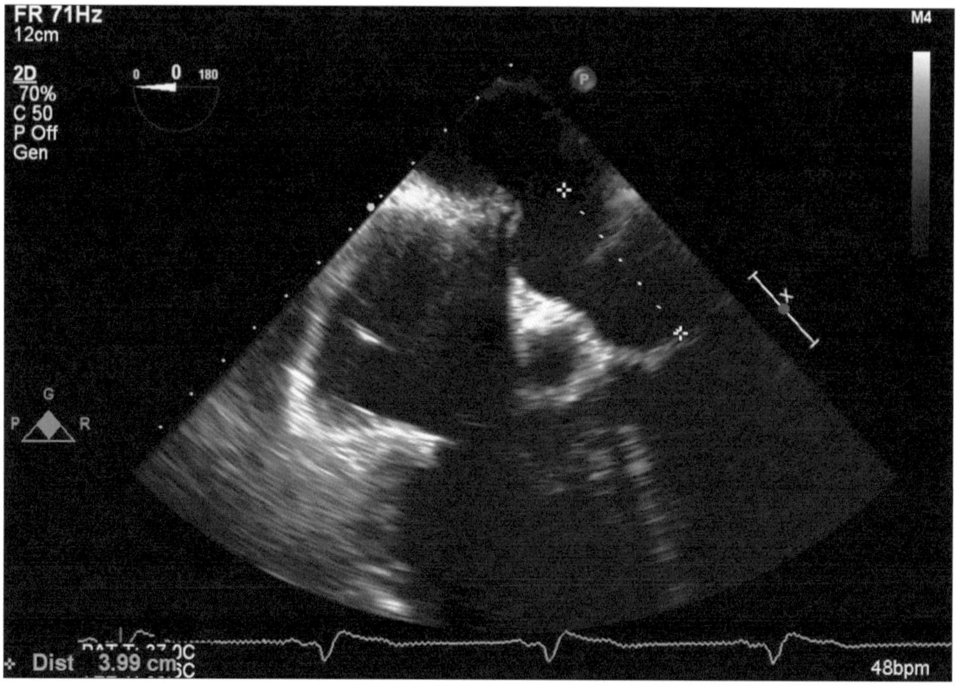

Fig. 17.12 TEE: 4C view. The transseptal puncture site is measured at 4 cm above the valve

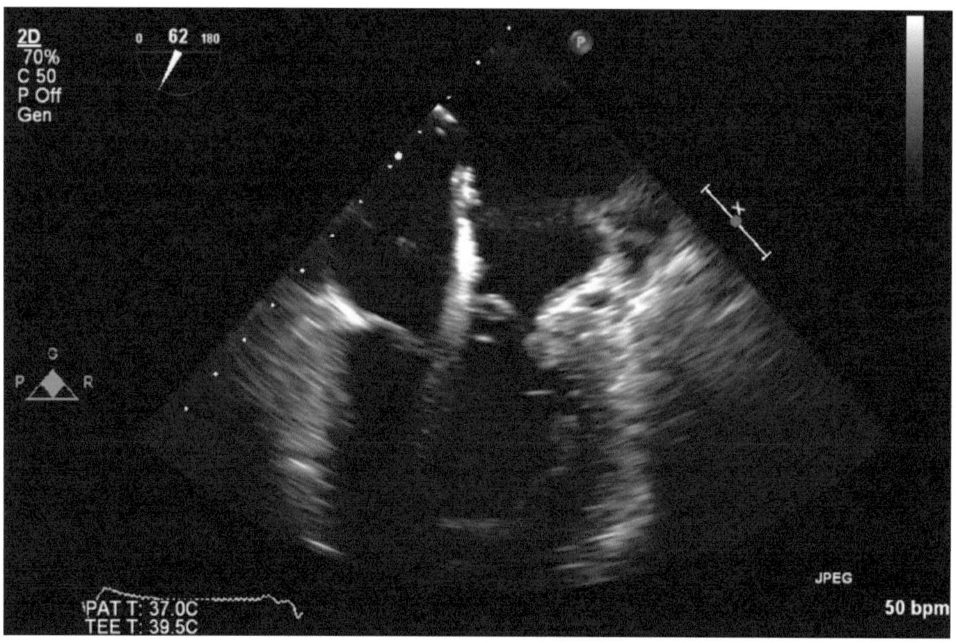

Fig. 17.13 TEE: Bicom view. The MitraClip device is oriented toward the center of the leaflets

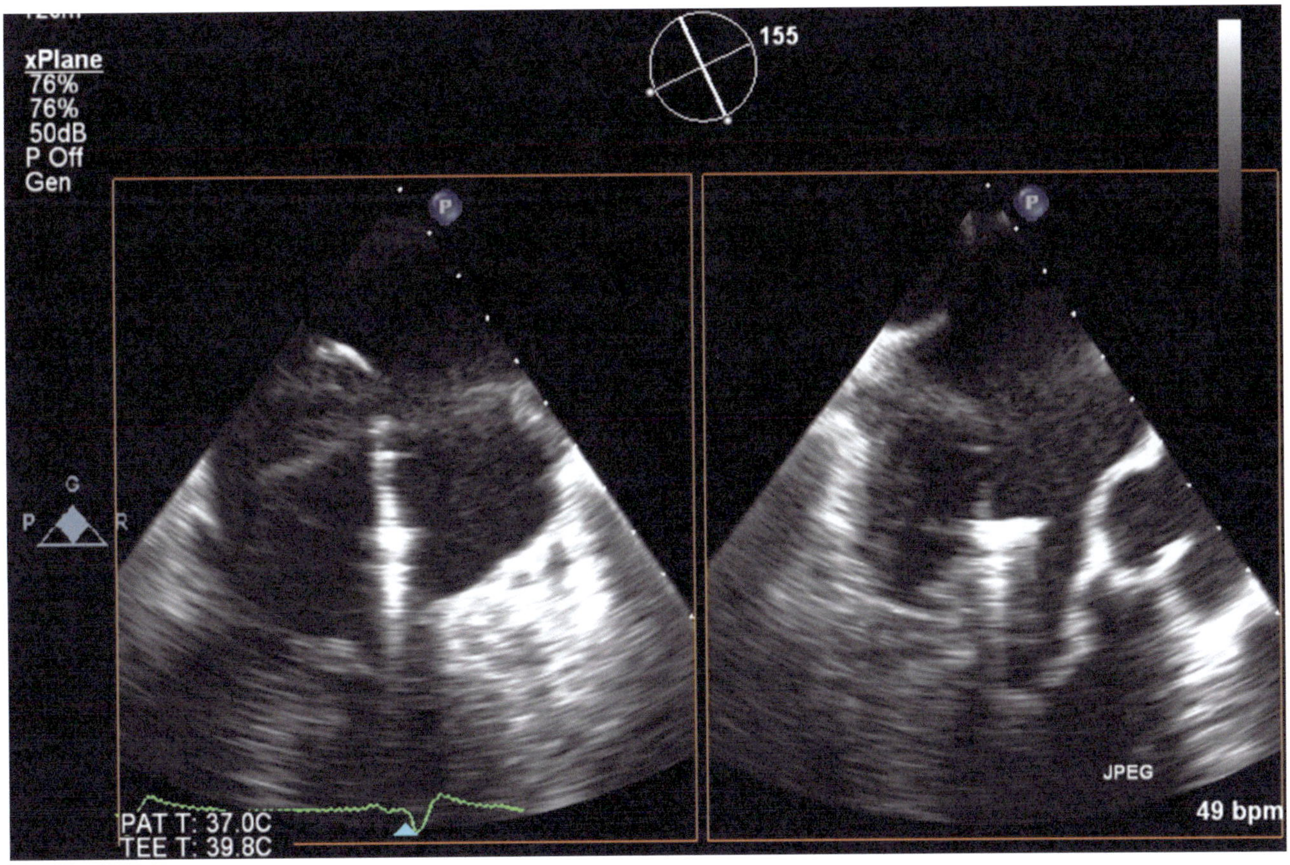

Fig. 17.14 TEE biplane views. The device is oriented to the center of the leaflets

Procedural TEE and Fluoro II

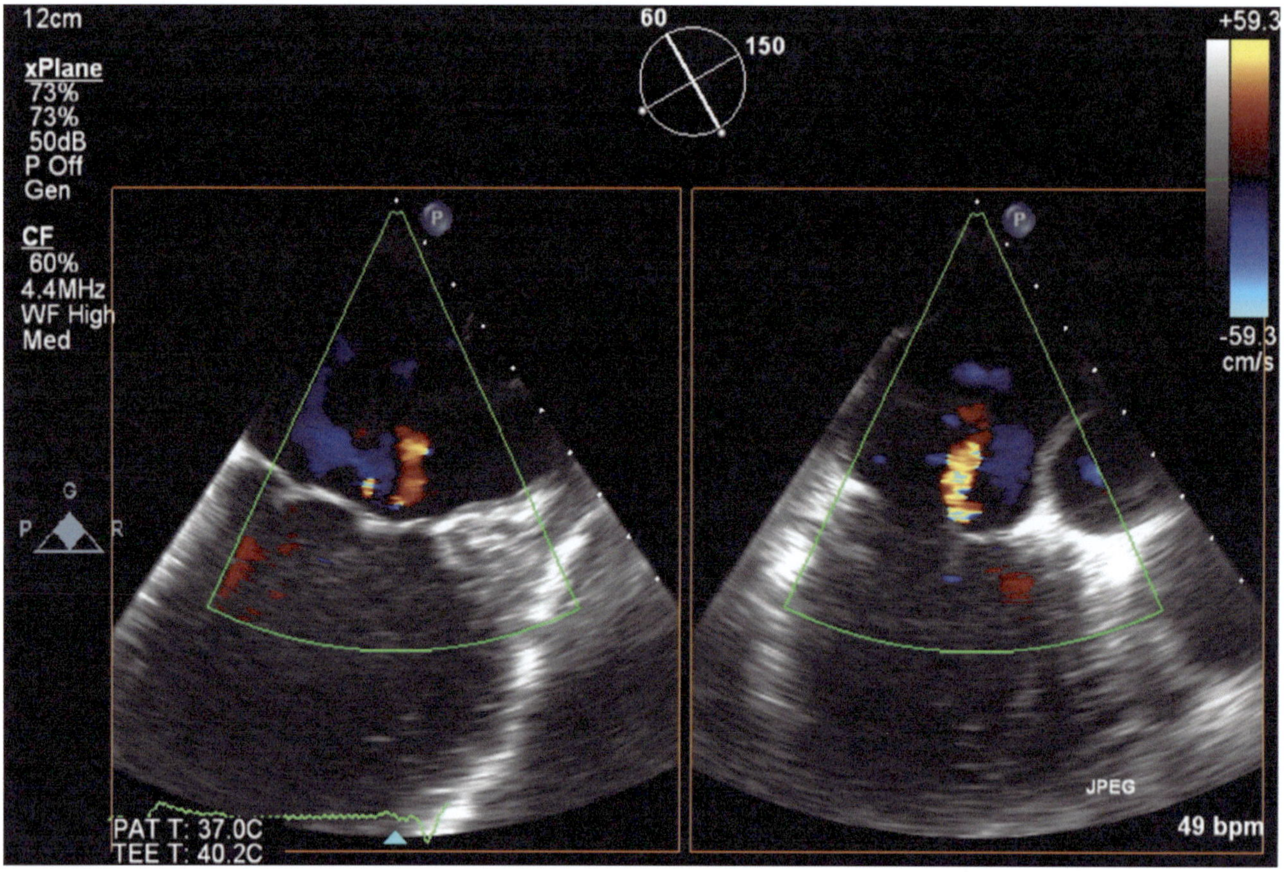

Fig. 17.15 Biplane TEE w/ Doppler. After deployment of one MitraClip, there is minimal Doppler MR on biplane views (*left* and *right*)

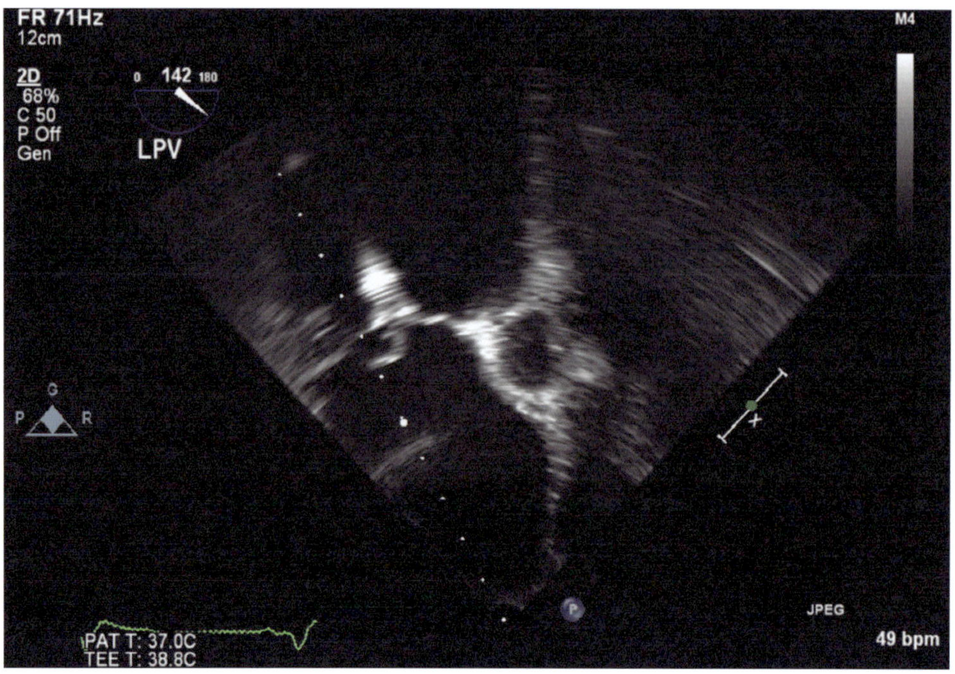

Fig. 17.16 TEE: 3C clip deployed. Once positioning is confirmed, the device is deployed

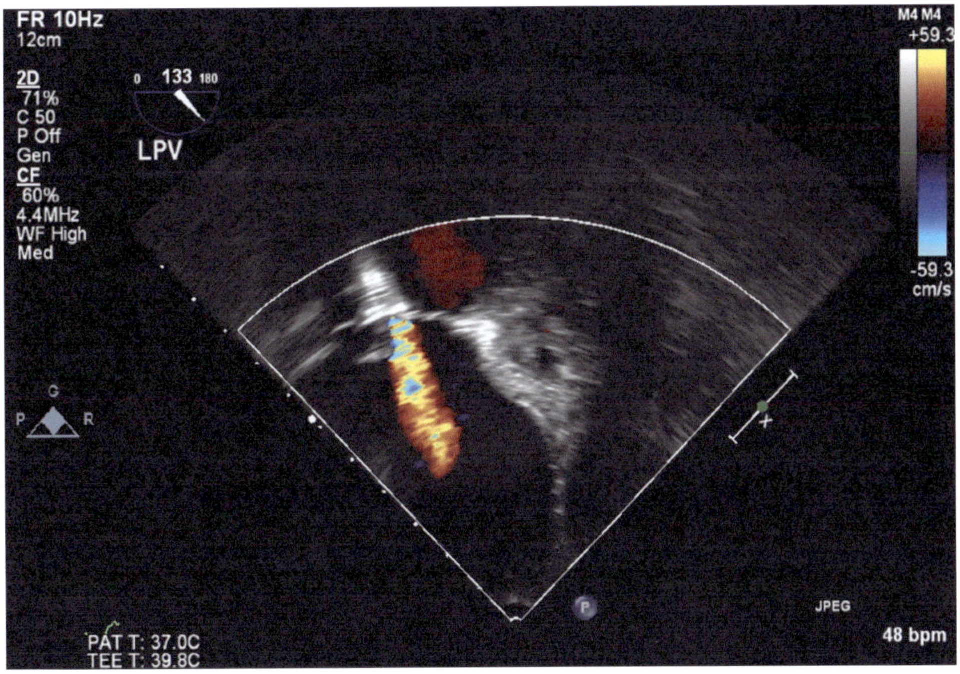

Fig. 17.17 TEE: 3C w/ Doppler. Post-deployment, there is a small jet of residual MR at the site of device deployment

Procedural TEE and Fluoro III

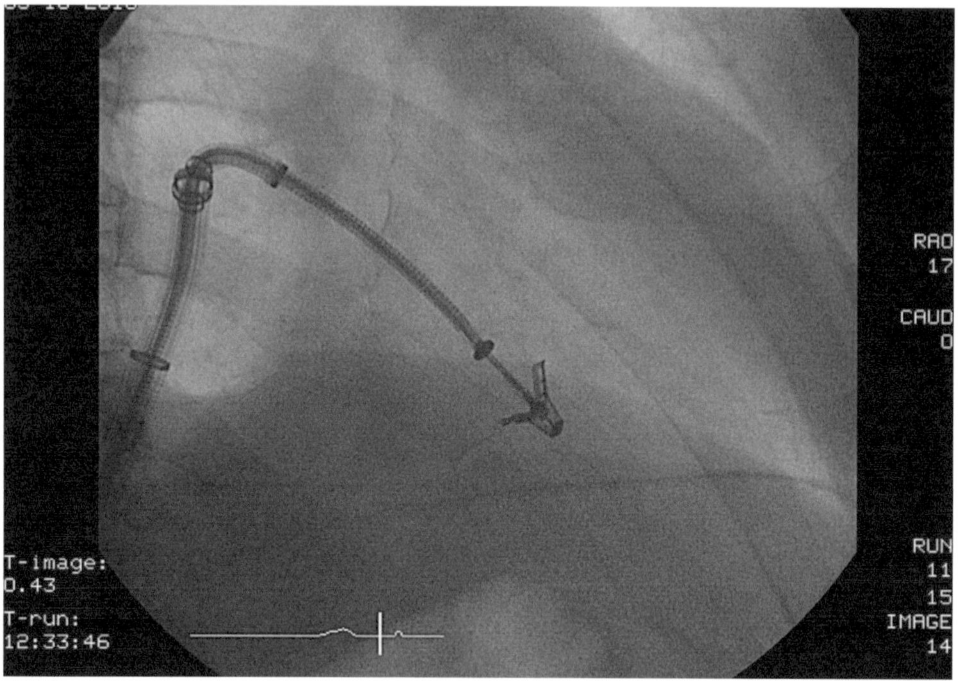

Fig. 17.18 Fluoroscopy. The first device is advanced across the mitral valve

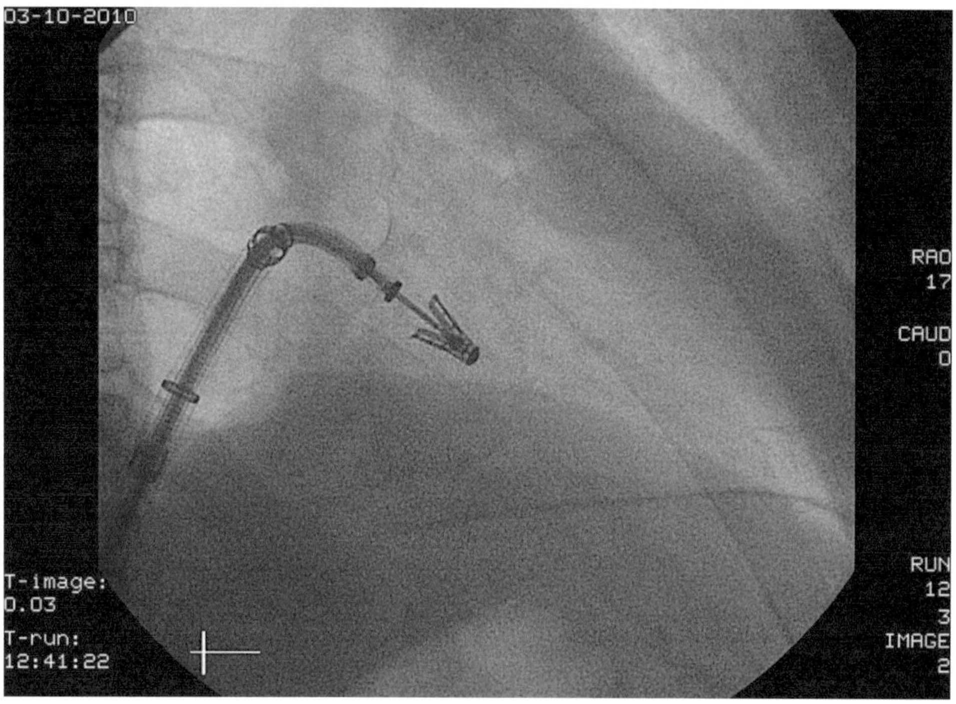

Fig. 17.19 Fluoroscopy. The device is pulled back and grasps the leaflet tissue

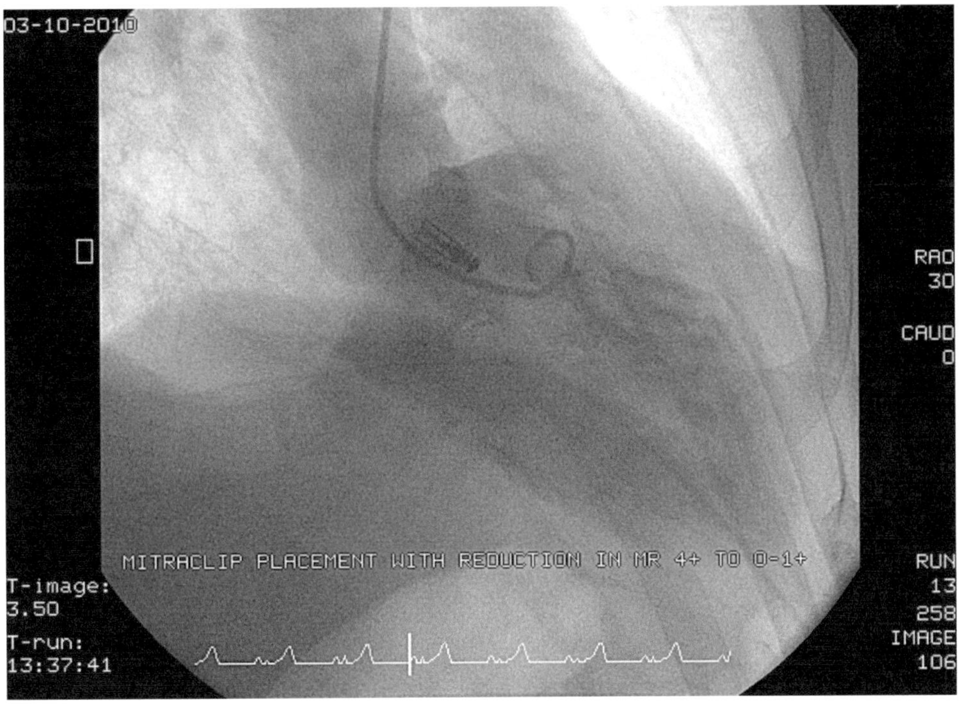

Fig. 17.20 Left ventricular cineangiography. Left ventriculogram at the conclusion of the procedure shows only trace MR and a well-positioned device

Follow-Up TTE I

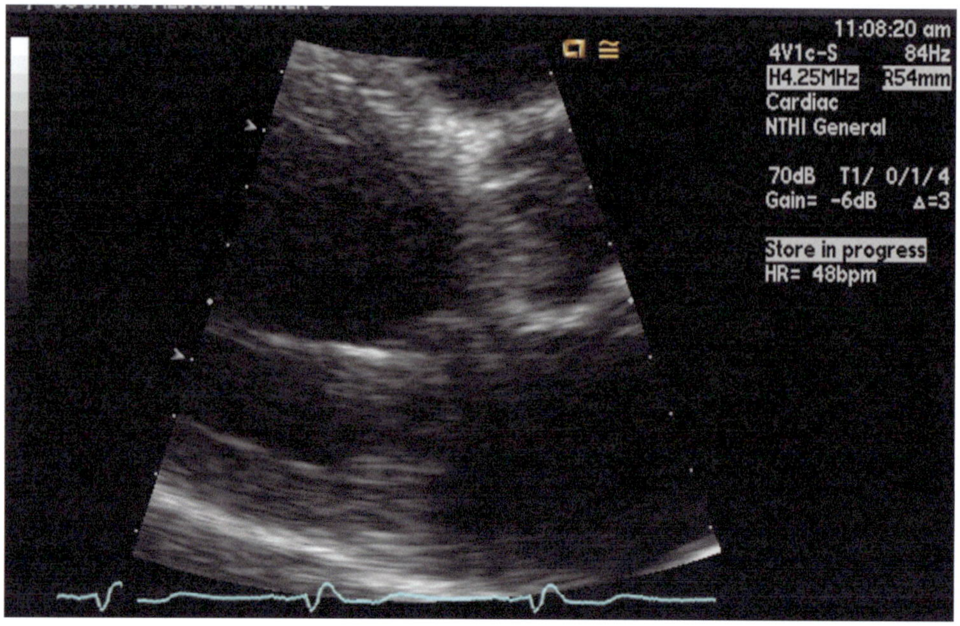

Fig. 17.21 TTE: parasternal LAX. At 1 month post-procedure, the device appears well seated along the midline of the mitral valve leaflets

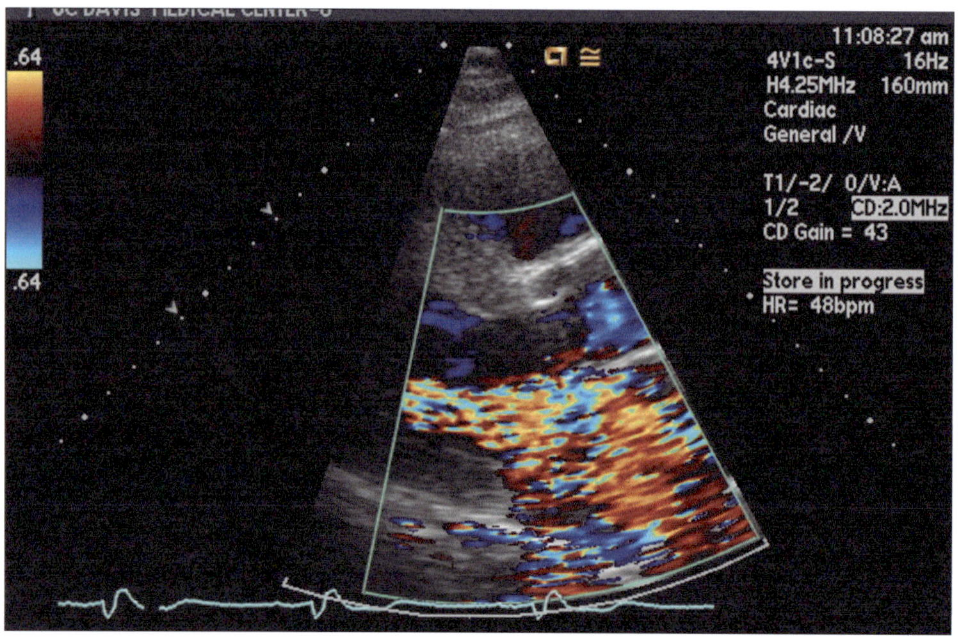

Fig. 17.22 TTE: parasternal LAX w/ color. In the intervening 1 month, severe MR has recurred, with a central jet origin

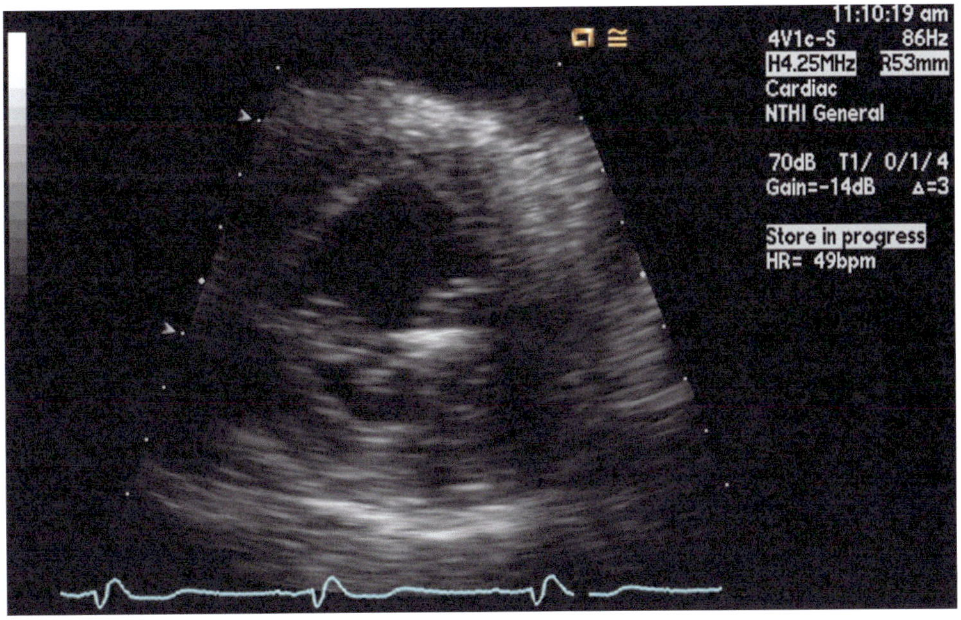

Fig. 17.23 TTE: short axis w/o color. On the short axis view, the MitraClip is apparent in the center of the leaflet coaptation line, with roughly similar size medial and lateral orifices

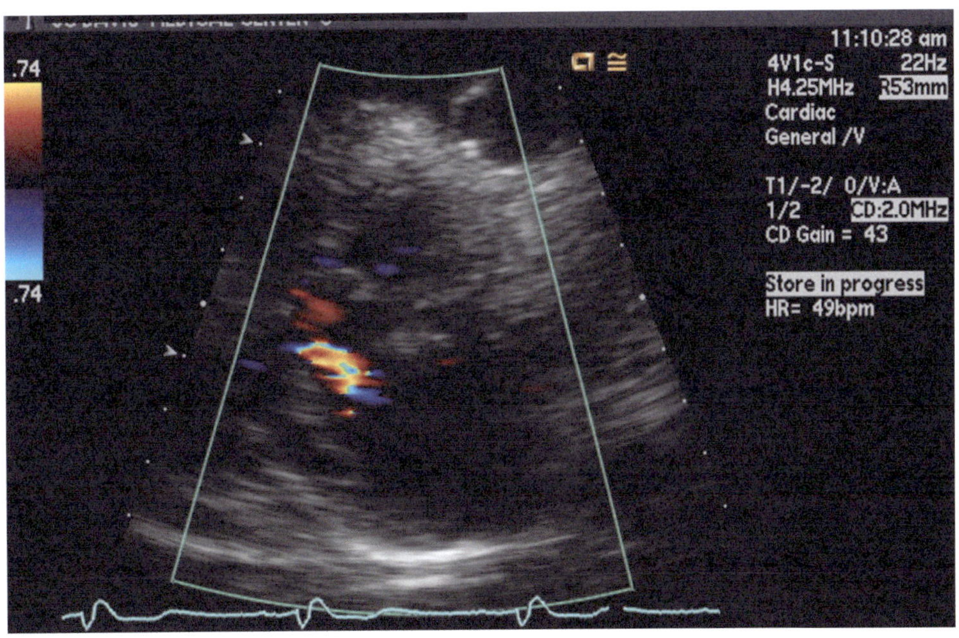

Fig. 17.24 TTE: short axis w/ color. The regurgitant jet appears to originate from the medial orifice

Follow-Up TTE II

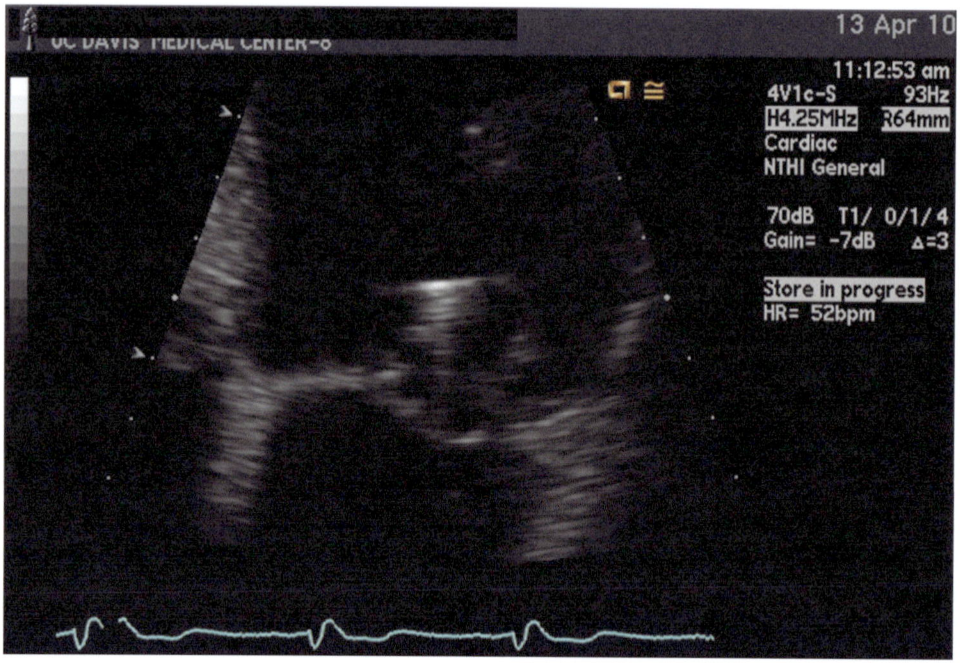

Fig. 17.25 TTE: apical 4C. The device appears well seated along the middle of the mitral valve leaflets

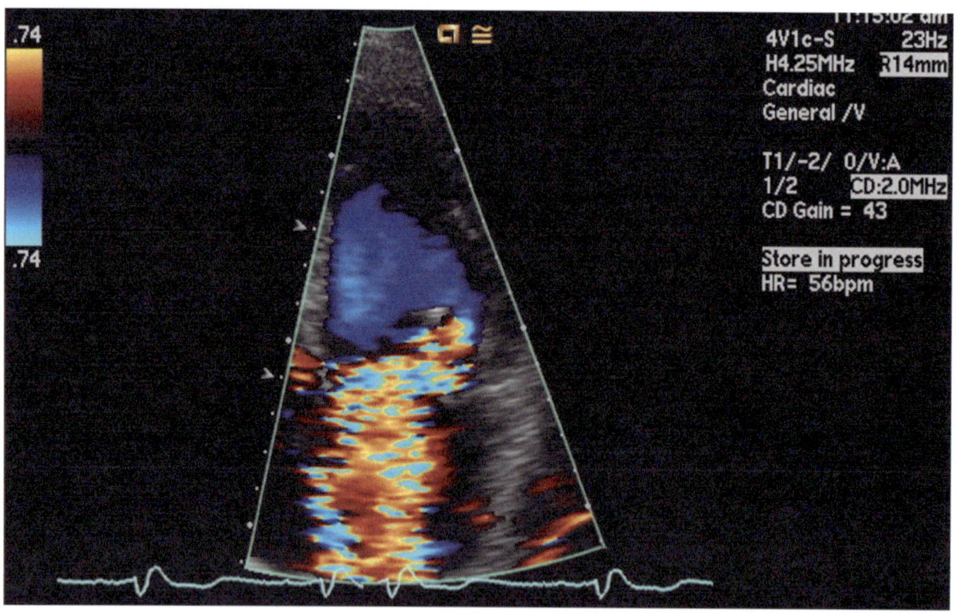

Fig. 17.26 TTE: apical 4C w/ color. The MR originated from near the device. The color flow Doppler is >2/3 of the left atrial area and reaches back to the pulmonary veins

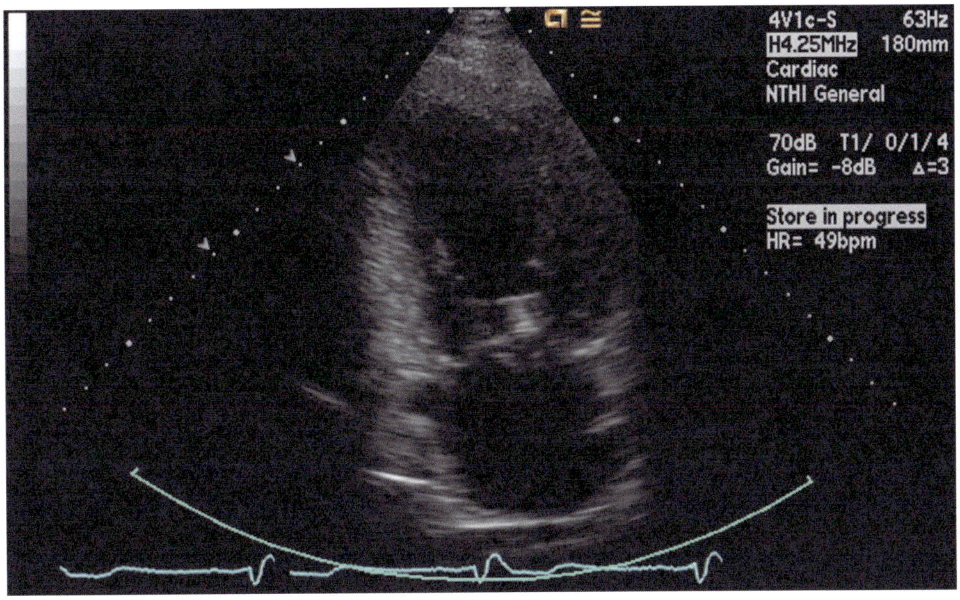

Fig. 17.27 TTE: apical 2C. In the two-chamber view, the device is central in location as well

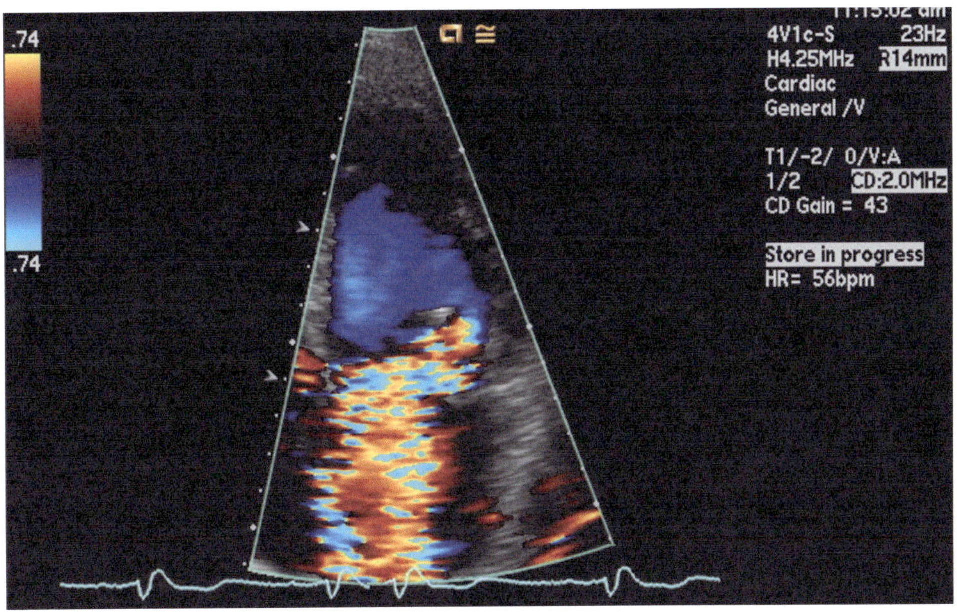

Fig. 17.28 TTE: apical 2C w/ color. Color Doppler again confirms a significant jet of MR

Second MitraClip Implantation Procedure I

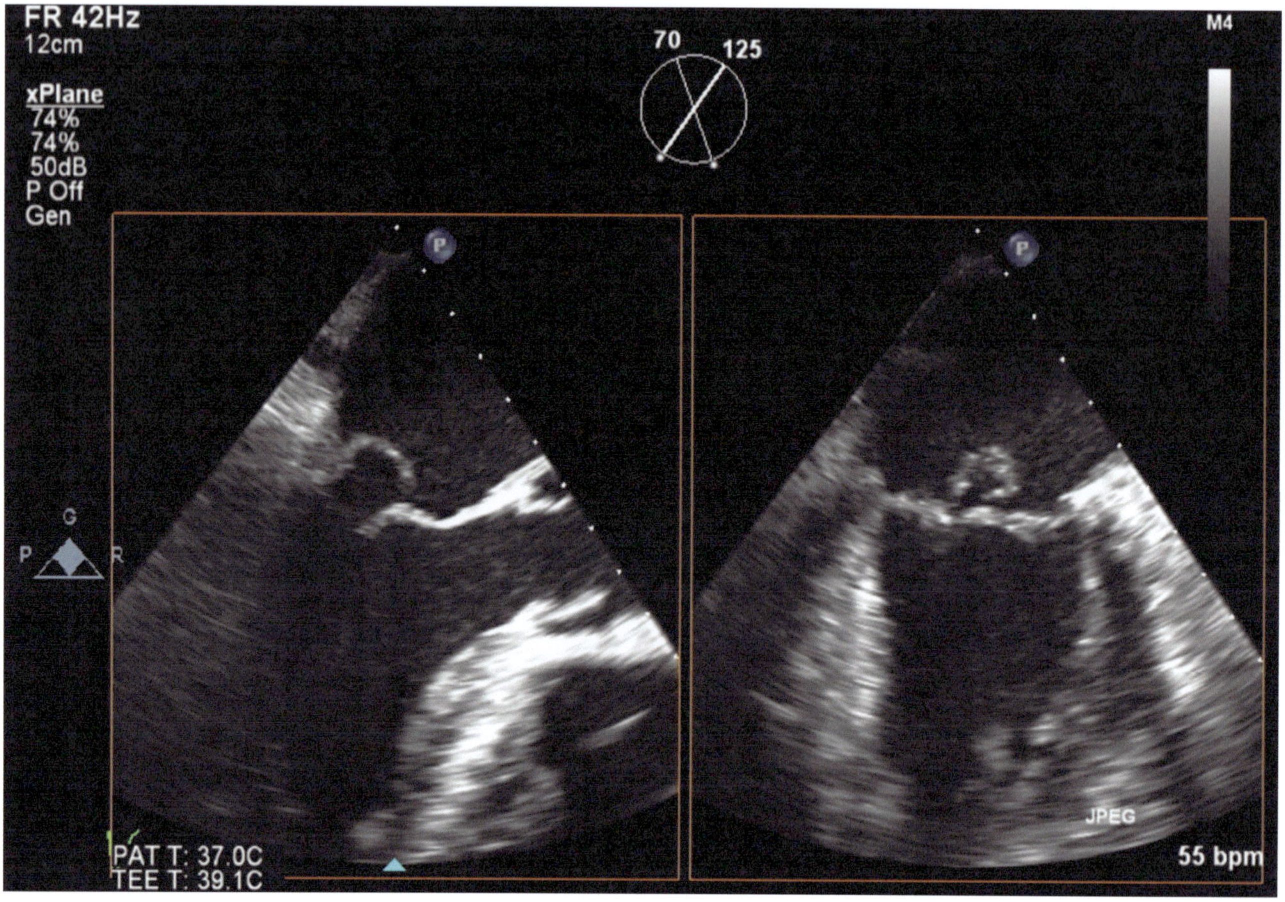

Fig. 17.29 TEE: biplane views. In the three-chamber and bicommissural views, there is significant prolapse of the P2 scallop

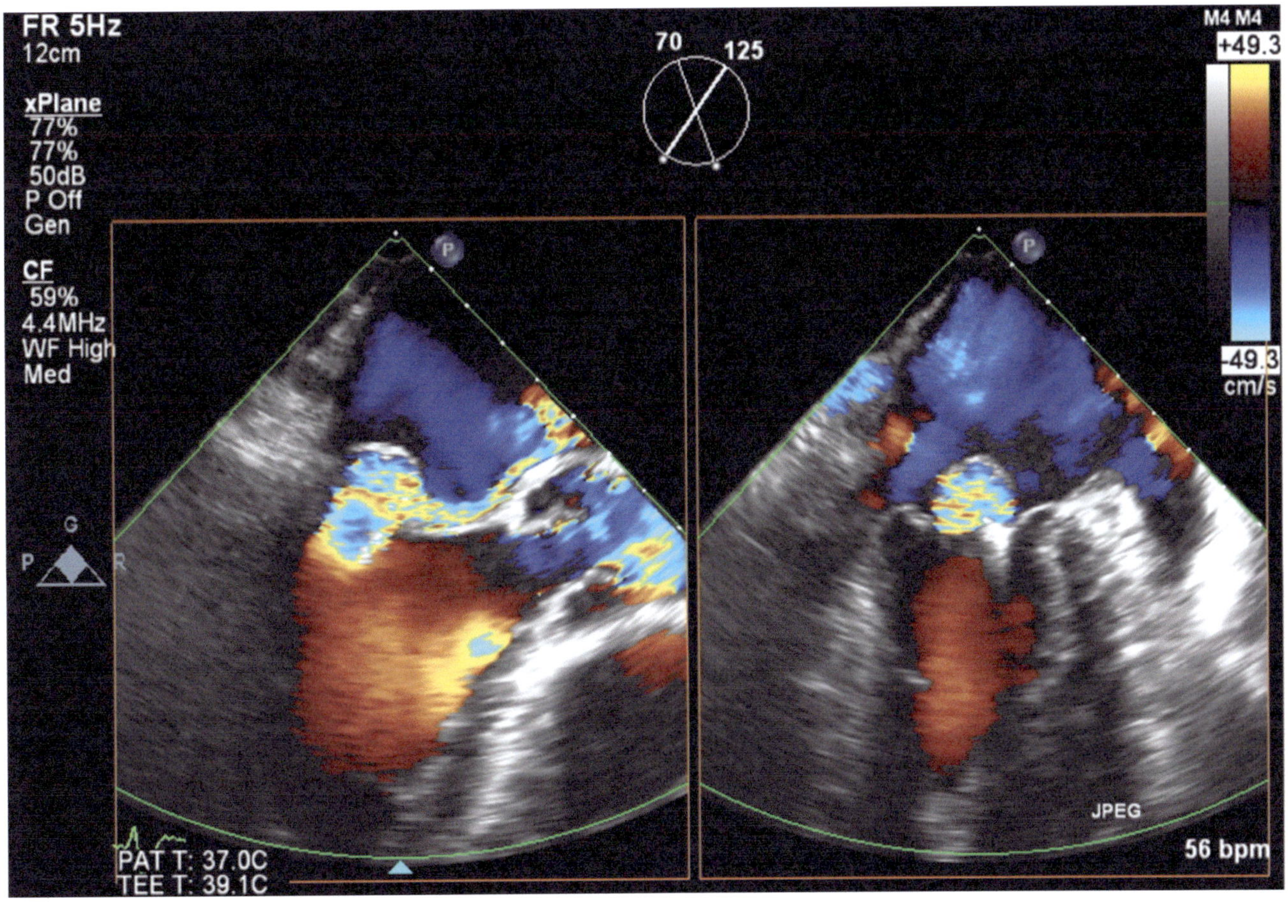

Fig. 17.30 TEE: biplane views w/ color. The regurgitant jet originates from the area of continued P2 prolapse and is directed anteriorly

Second MitraClip Implantation Procedure II

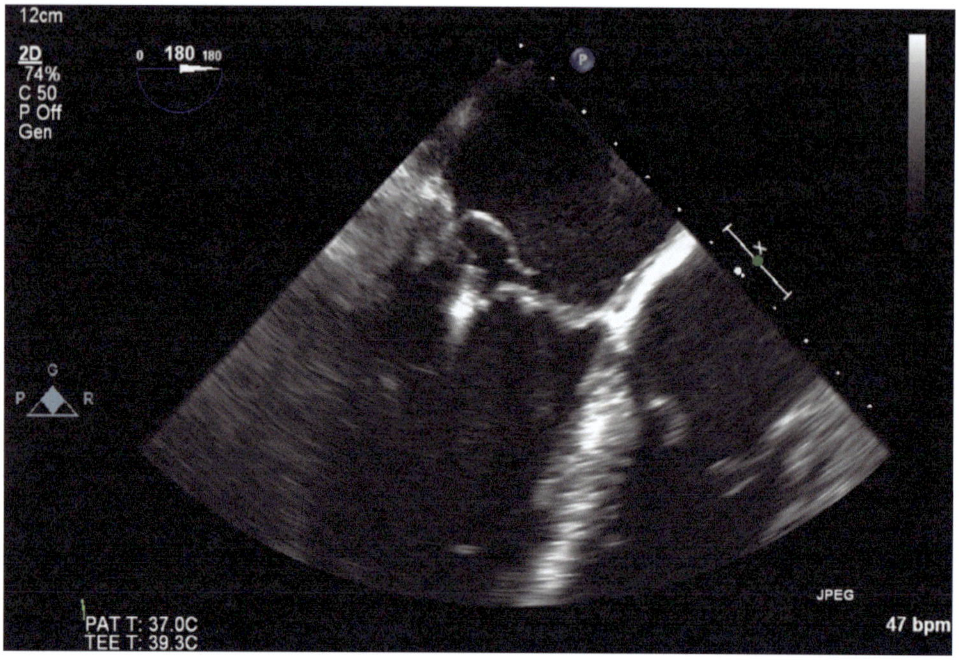

Fig. 17.31 TEE: 4C. In the four-chamber view, there is also some persistent flail of P2. Note that the image is left-right reversed

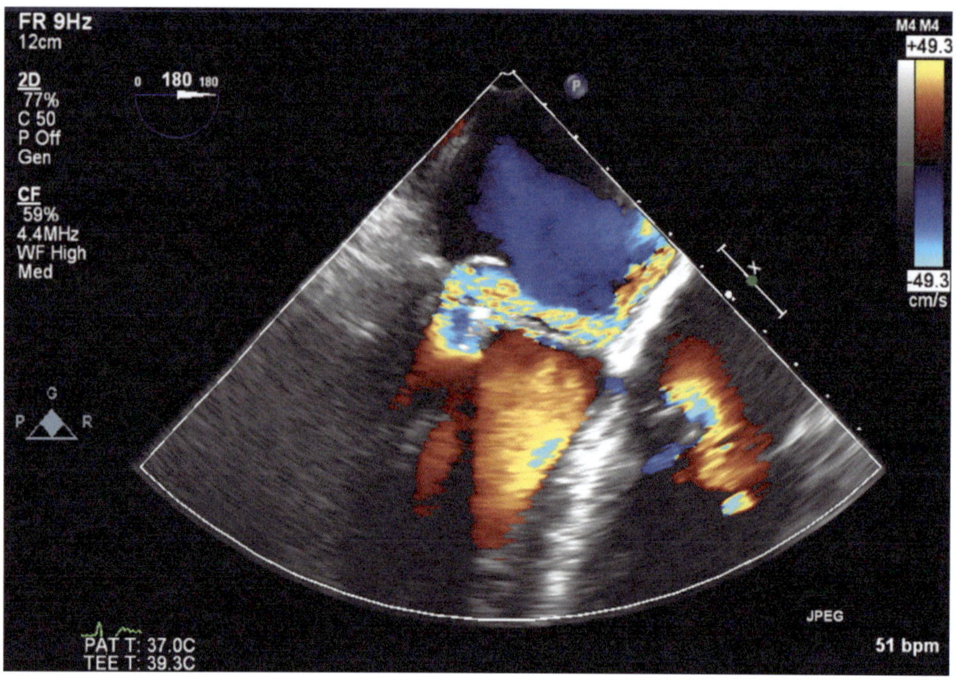

Fig. 17.32 TEE: 4C w/ color. The jet of MR is directed anteriorly

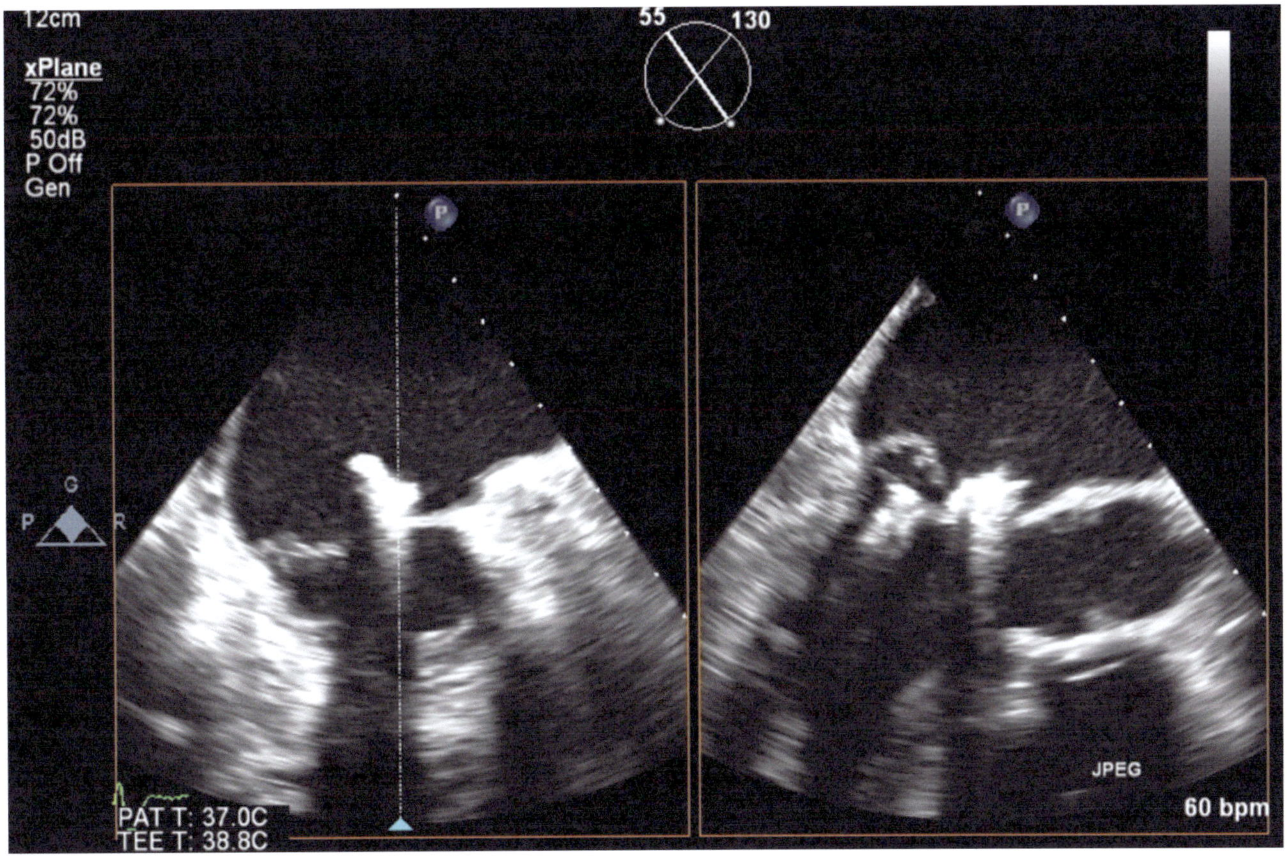

Fig. 17.33 TEE: biplane views. A second MitraClip device is directed at the A2-P2 interface in a central location (**a**, **b**)

Second MitraClip Implantation Procedure III

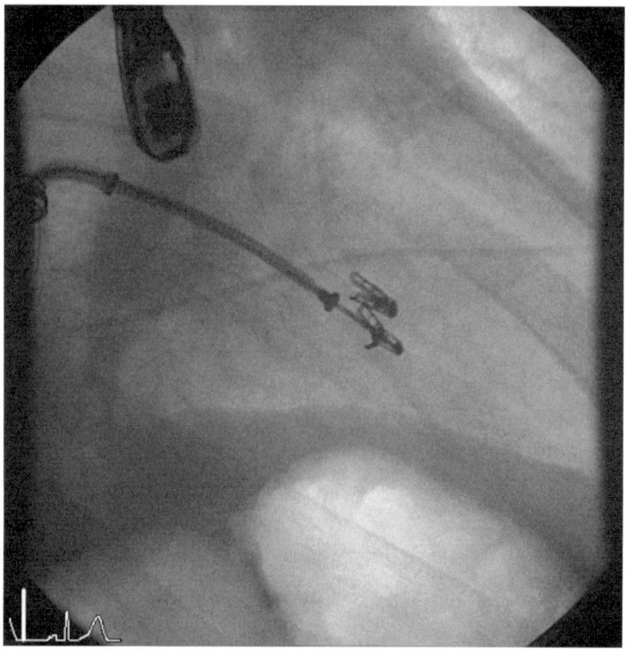

Fig. 17.34 Fluoroscopy. The second device is advanced parallel to previously deployed device

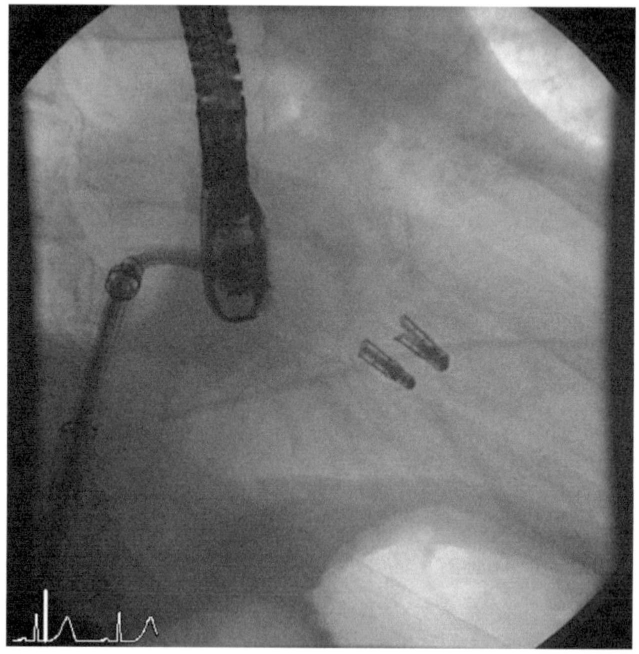

Fig. 17.35 Fluoroscopy. The devices have a parallel position

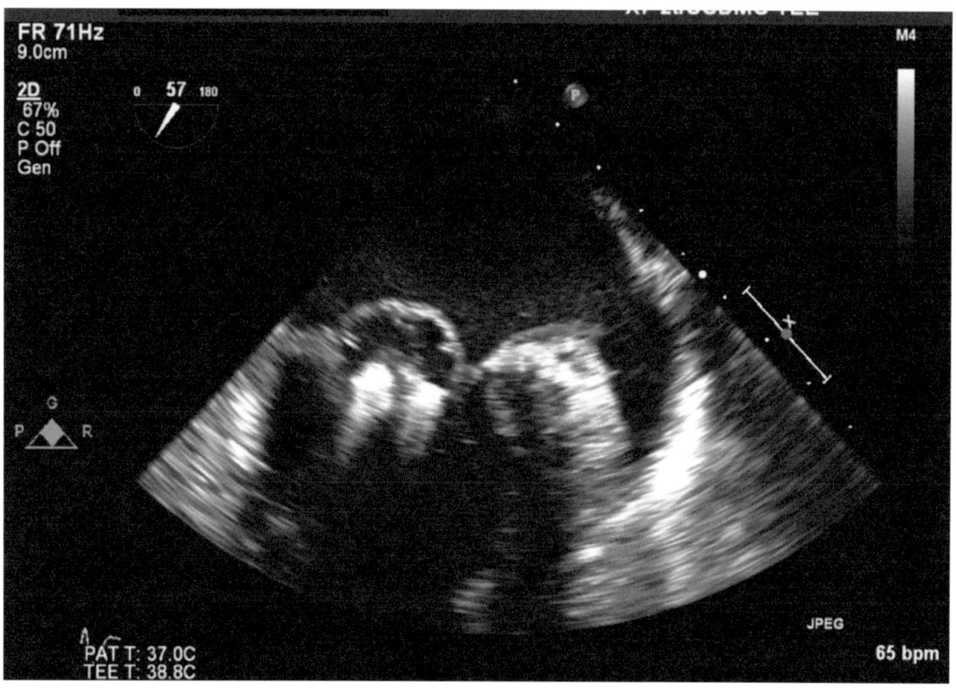

Fig. 17.36 TEE: Bicom view. Both devices can be seen in the bicommissural view

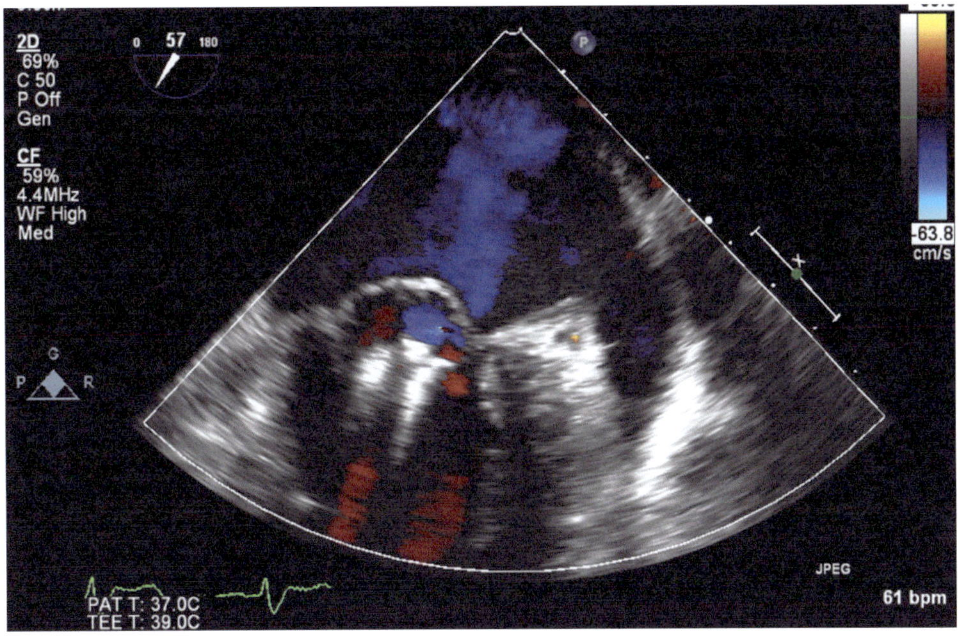

Fig. 17.37 TEE: Bicom view with Doppler. Although there is some mild prolapse of P2, there is only minimal MR

Second MitraClip Implantation Procedure IV

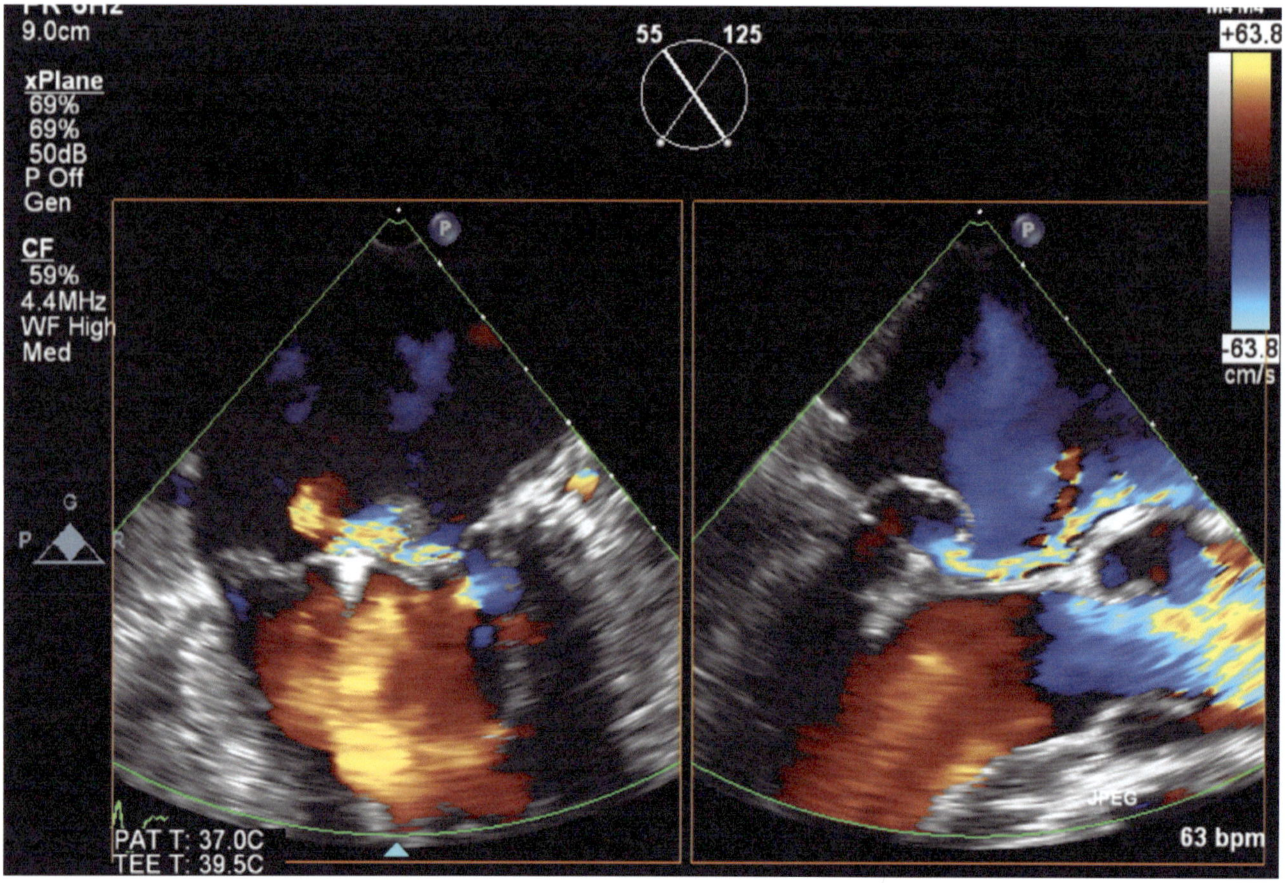

Fig. 17.38 TEE: biplane with Doppler. The residual MR is 1–2+

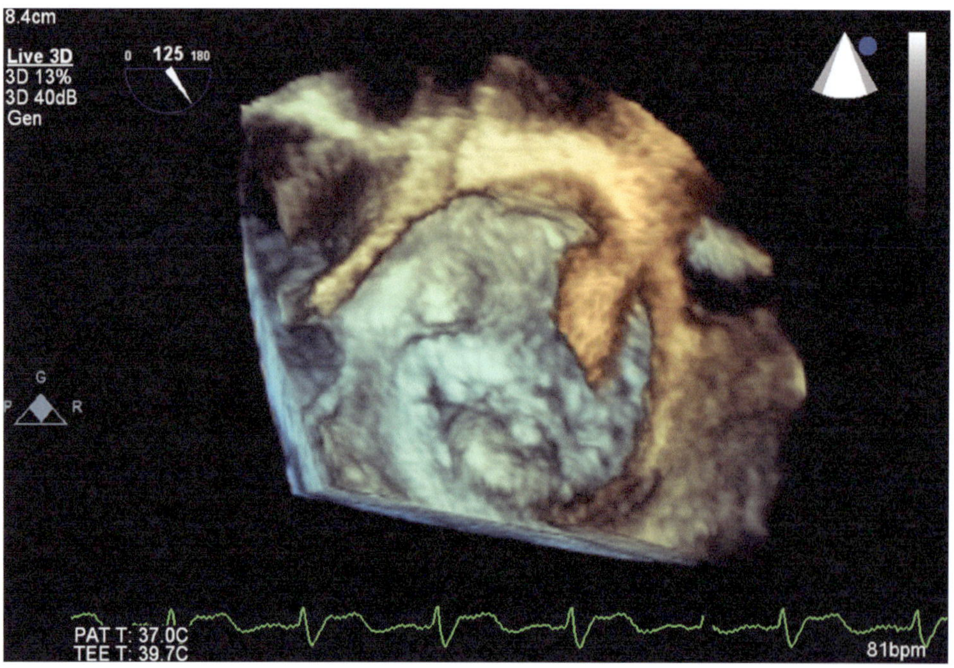

Fig. 17.39 TEE: 3D reconstruction. In systole, the leaflets appear to coapt well with some mild continued prolapse of P2

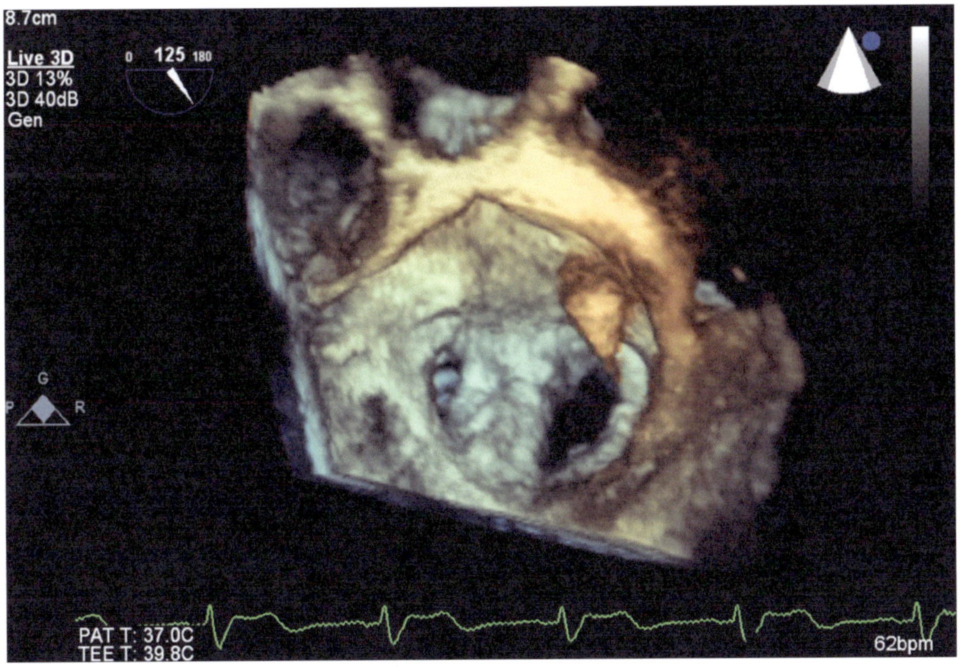

Fig. 17.40 TEE: 3D reconstruction. In diastole, the double orifice valve is apparent. The medial (right) orifice looks slightly larger than the lateral orifice, but this may also result from dropout of lateral structures on 3D reconstruction

Follow-Up Transthoracic Echocardiogram

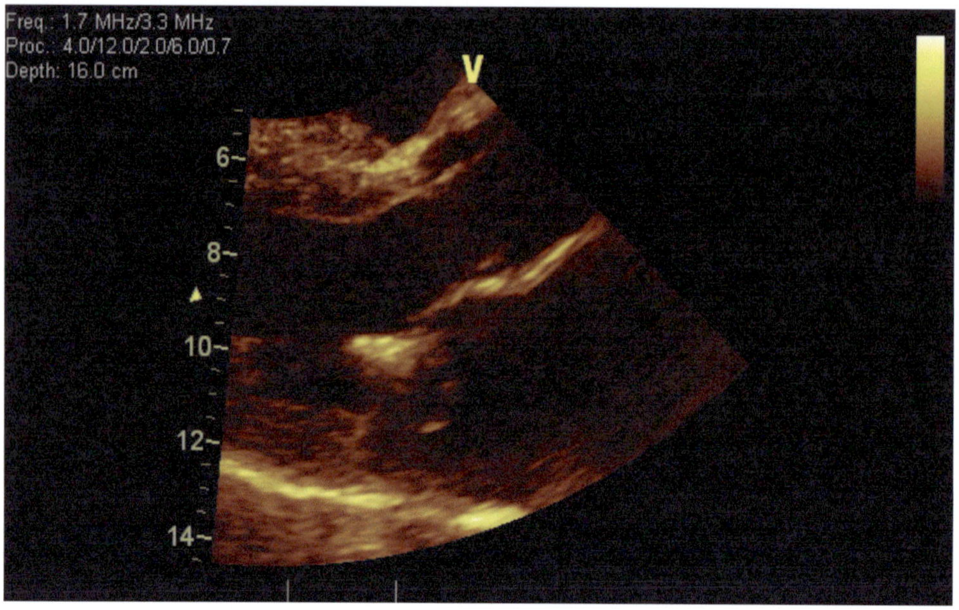

Fig. 17.41 TTE: parasternal long axis. The MitraClip devices can be oriented in the middle of the valve. Only one device can be seen in this parasternal long axis view

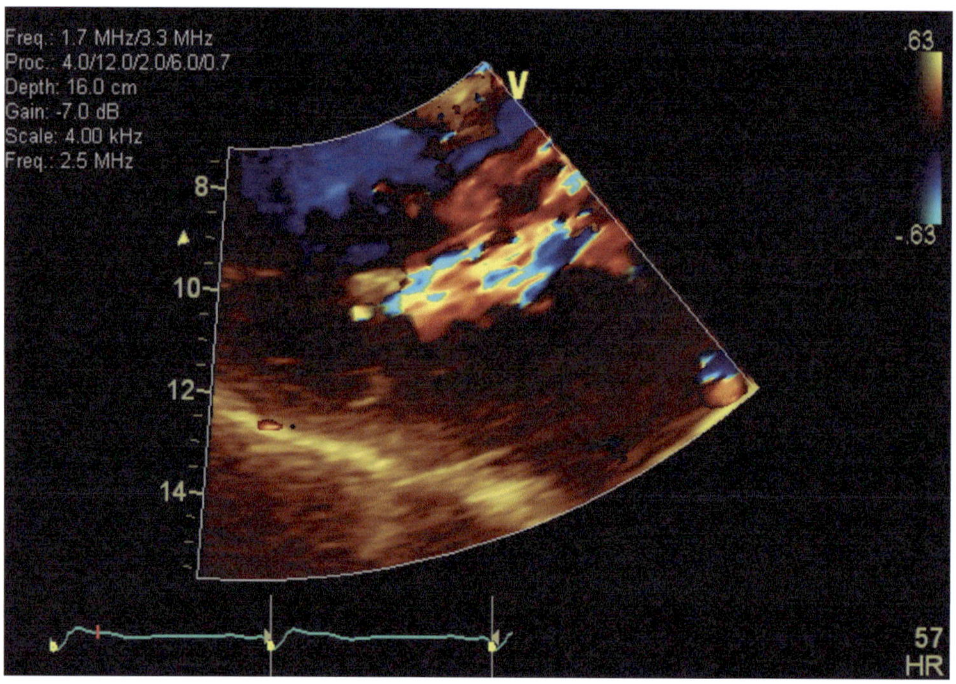

Fig. 17.42 TTE: parasternal long axis w/ Doppler. On Doppler imaging, there is 1–2+ persistent MR

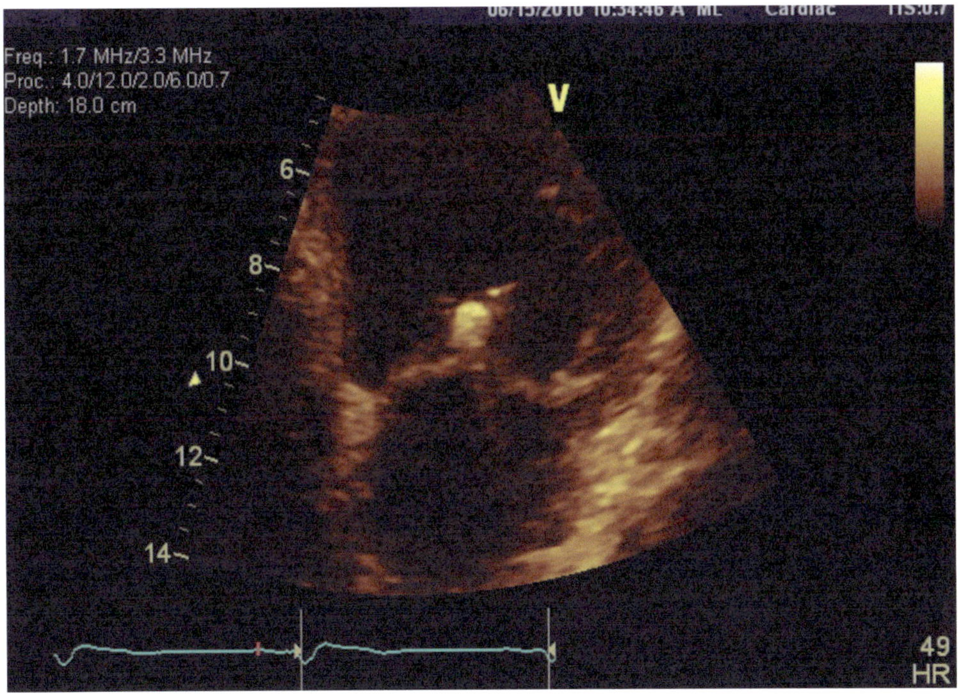

Fig. 17.43 TTE: apical 4C. The devices are oriented centrally

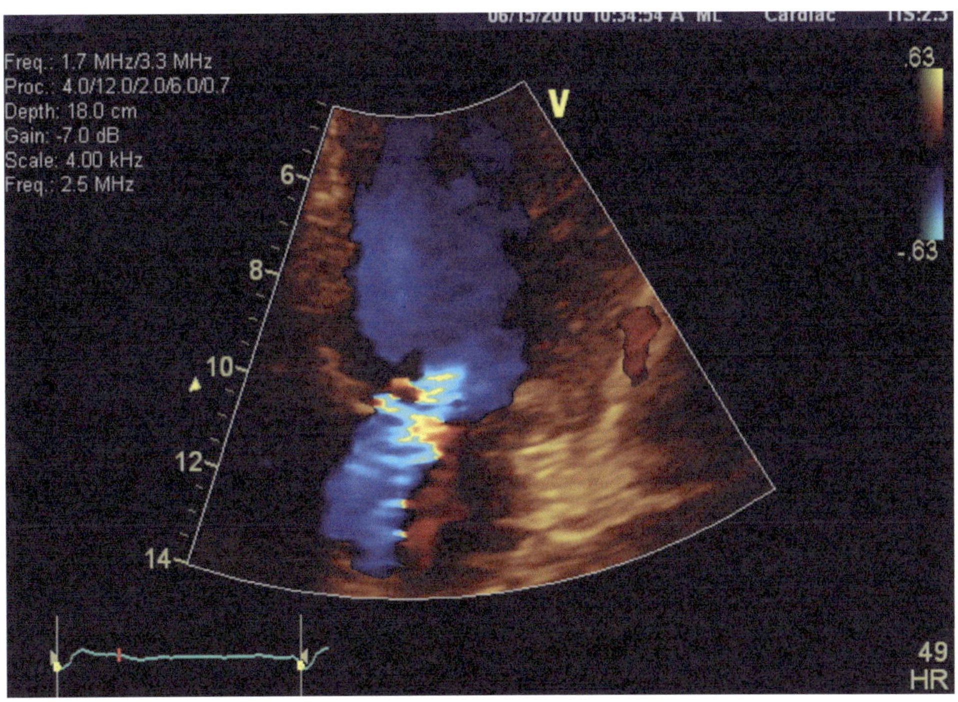

Fig. 17.44 TTE: apical 4C w/ Doppler. The Doppler MR again appears 1–2+

Secondary Mitral Regurgitation Due to Ischemic Mitral Valve Disease and Mild Rheumatic Mitral Valve Disease

18

Ali Vazir, Olaf Franzen, Neil Eric Moat, and Susanna Price

Abstract

A 72-year-old woman presenting with several episodes of decompensated heart failure was proven to have features of severe mitral regurgitation due to a combination of ischemic cardiomyopathy resulting in adverse LV remodeling and mild rheumatic heart disease. She underwent successful edge-to-edge repair with the MitraClip system.

Keywords

Mitral regurgitation • MitraClip • Mitral stenosis • Rheumatic heart disease

Clinical History

A 72-year-old female with previous history of coronary artery bypass surgery presented with NYHA III symptoms and several admissions with decompensated heart failure. Her comorbidities included renal dysfunction and type II diabetes mellitus. She had no history suggestive of rheumatic fever.

2D and Doppler echocardiography confirmed the presence of a dilated left ventricle (LVEDD of 5.8 cm, LVESD 3.8 cm, and LVEF by biplane Simpsons of 40 %), infarcted and scarred infero-posterior wall, and ischemic cardiomyopathy. There was severe mitral regurgitation (grade 4+) secondary to a combination of annular dilatation, left ventricular dilatation, and changes to LV geometry resulting in tenting of the mitral valve, bileaflet restriction with thickening and rolling of anterior and posterior leaflet edges, and thickening and calcification of the subvalvular apparatus. There was a minor degree of posterior commissural fusion, but no diastolic flow acceleration across the mitral valve, and no mitral stenosis (Figs. 18.1, 18.2, 18.3, 18.4, 18.5, 18.6, and 18.7).

She underwent the edge-to-edge mitral valve repair with the MitraClip system, reducing the severity of mitral regurgitation from 4+ to 1+. The patient was symptomatically significantly improved (NYHA II, with no further hospital admissions) following the procedure (Figs. 18.8, 18.9, and 18.10).

A. Vazir, MBBS, MRCP, CCDS, Ph.D. (✉)
Department of Cardiology, Royal Brompton Hospital, Royal Brompton and Harefield NHS Foundation Trust, Sydney Street, London SW3 6NP, UK

Department of Cardiology, Royal Brompton Hospital, National Heart and Lung Institute, Imperial College, London, UK
e-mail: a.vazir@rbht.nhs.uk, ali.vazir@btinternet.com

O. Franzen, M.D.
Department of Cardiology, The Heart Center, Rigshospitalet, University of Copenhagen, Blegdamsvej 9, Copenhagen 2100, Denmark

Royal Brompton Hospital, Royal Brompton and Harefield NHS Foundation Trust, London, UK
e-mail: owfranzen@gmx.de

N.E. Moat, MBBS, MS., FRCS
Department of Cardiac Surgery, Head of Trans-catheter valve programme, Royal Brompton Hospital, Sydney Street, London SW3 6NP, UK
e-mail: n.moat@rbht.nhs.uk

S. Price, MBBS, BSc, MRCP, EDICM, Ph.D., FFICM, FESC
Department of Cardiology, Royal Brompton Hospital, Sydney Street, London SW3 6NP, UK
e-mail: s.price@rbht.nhs.uk

T. Feldman et al. (eds.), *Atlas of Percutaneous Edge-to-Edge Mitral Valve Repair*, DOI 10.1007/978-1-4471-4294-2_18, © Springer-Verlag London 2013

Learning Points

1. The minor degree of rheumatic involvement did not impede the procedure and appeared to promote better apposition of the leaflet edges, possibly providing better tissue quality for gripping by the MitraClip arms.
2. The absence of anterior commissural fusion and deployment of only one clip meant the procedure did not result in any significant mitral stenosis.

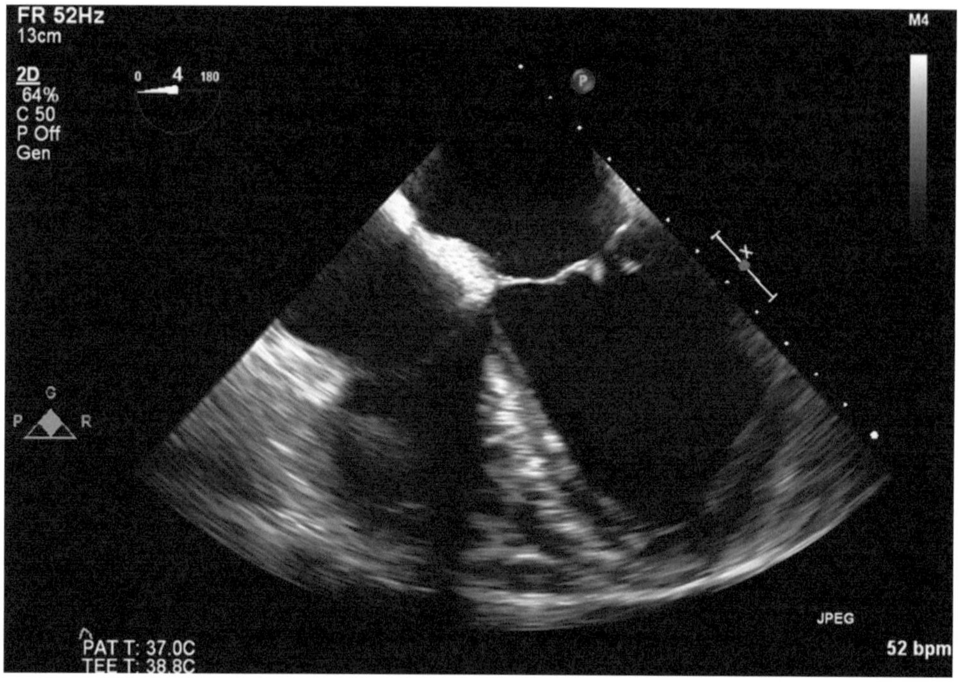

Fig. 18.1 Transesophageal four-chamber view shows rolled tips of the anterior and posterior mitral valve leaflets typical of rheumatic mitral valve disease

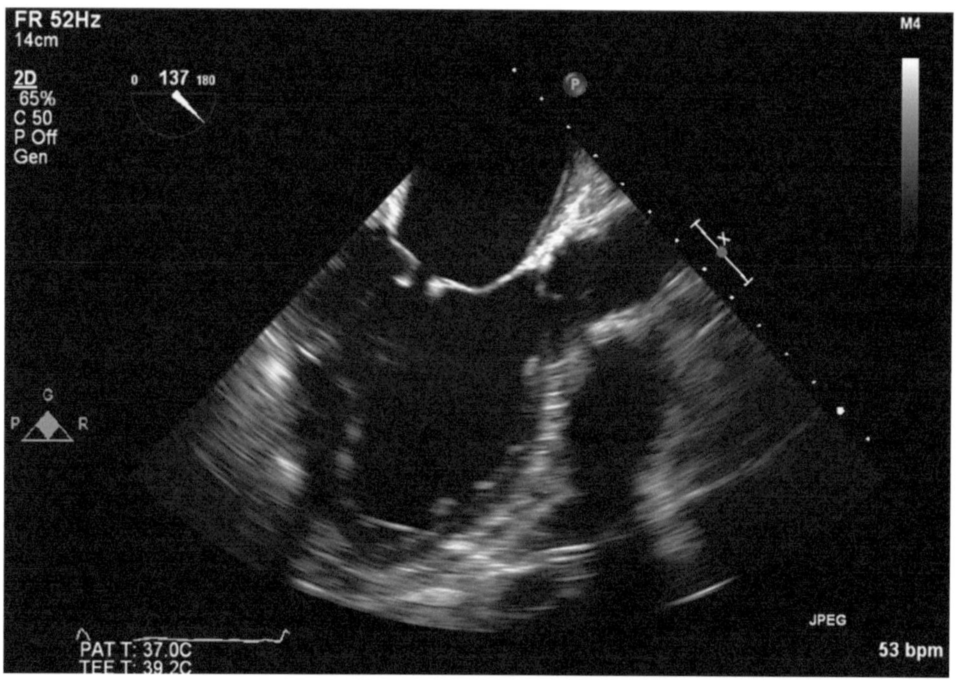

Fig. 18.2 Transesophageal long axis view shows rolled tips of the anterior and posterior mitral valve leaflets typical of rheumatic mitral valve disease

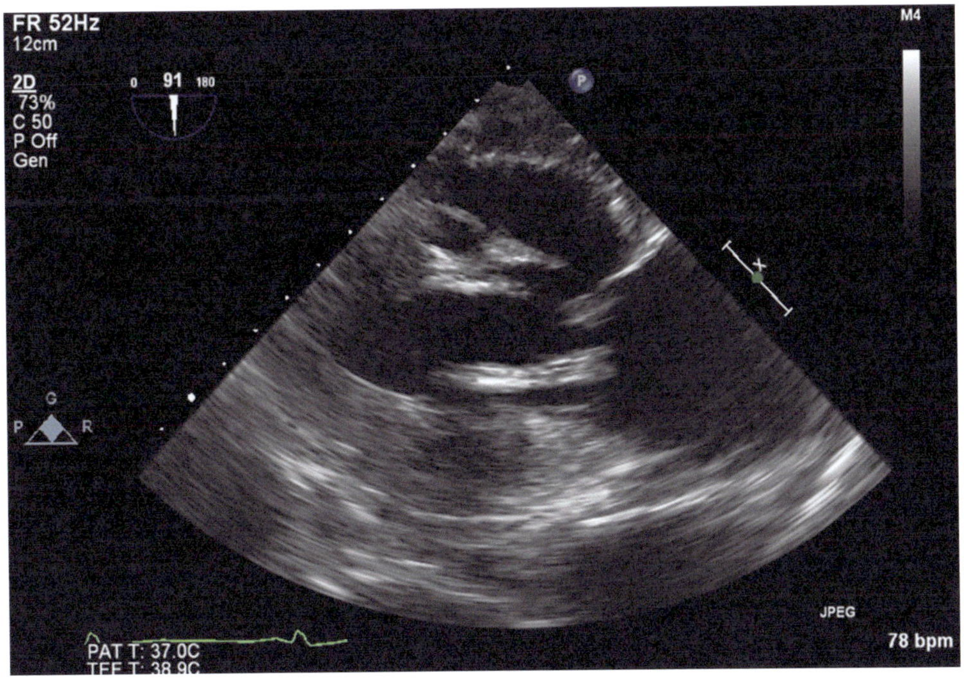

Fig. 18.3 Trans-gastric long axis view showing thickened and calcified subvalvular apparatus of the mitral valve typical of rheumatic mitral valve disease. Furthermore, the thin and scarred basal inferior wall is also evident

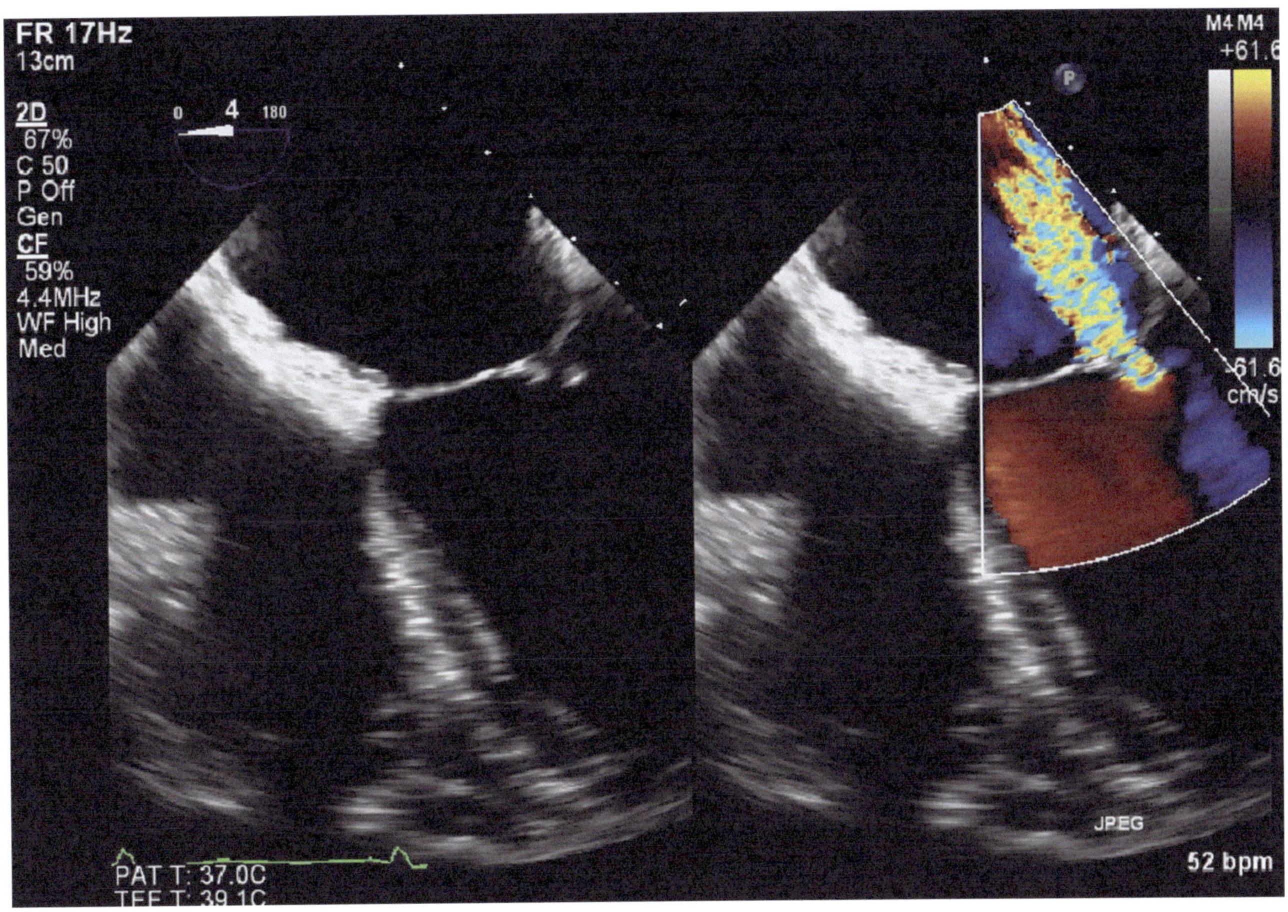

Fig. 18.4 Transesophageal four-chamber view shows severe mitral regurgitation during systole

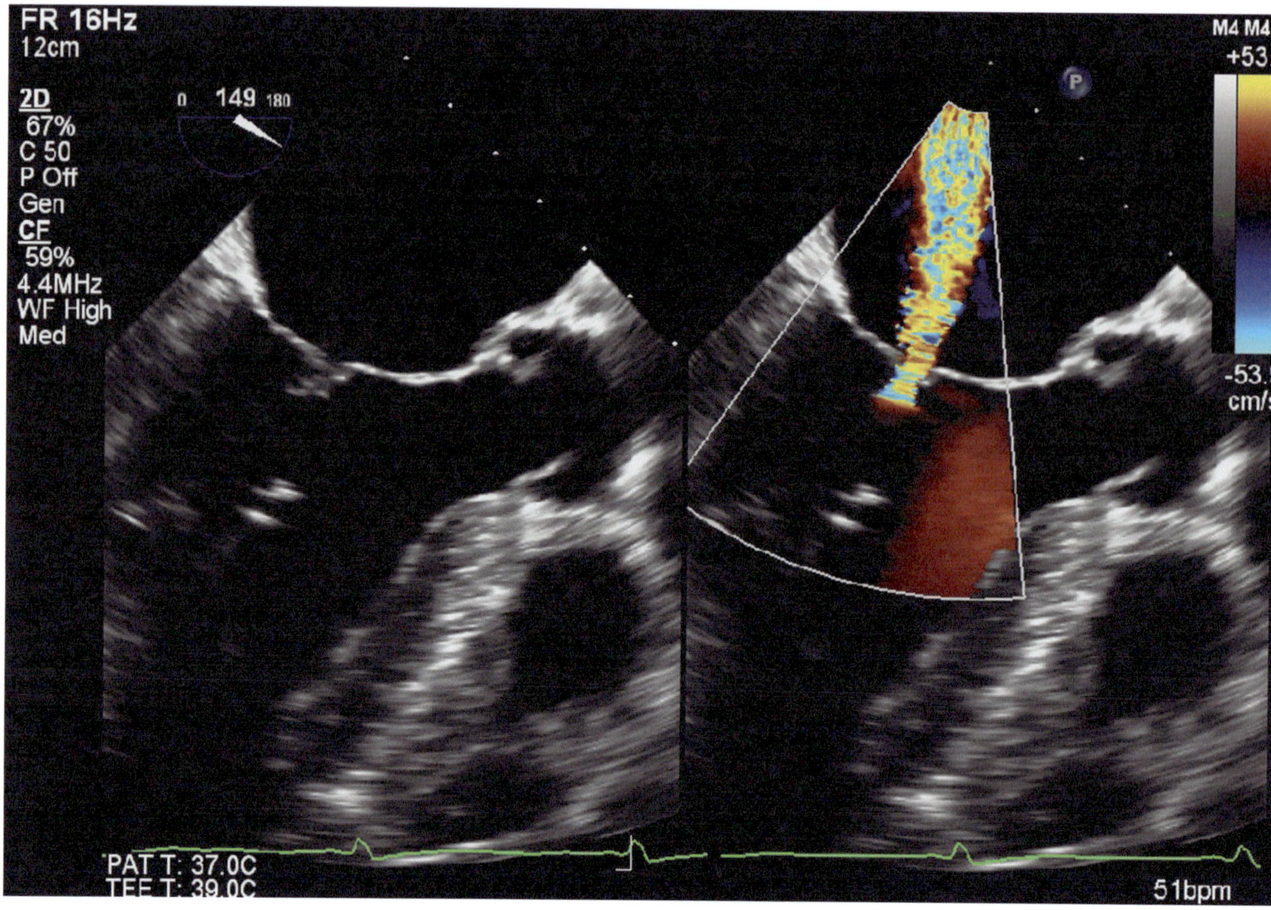

Fig. 18.5 Transesophageal long axis view shows severe mitral regurgitation during systole

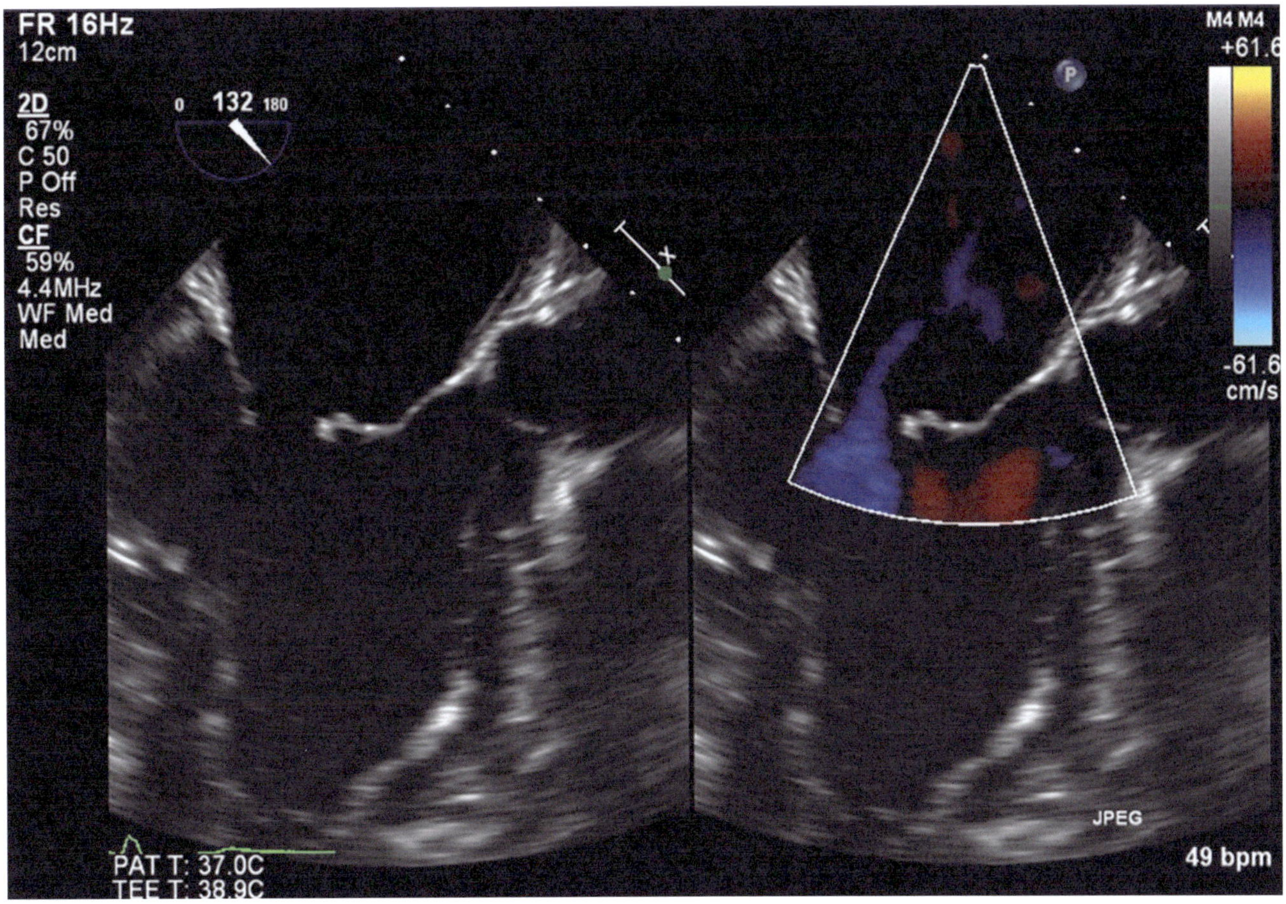

Fig. 18.6 Transesophageal long axis view during ventricular diastole with open mitral valve showing no turbulent flow to suggest mitral stenosis

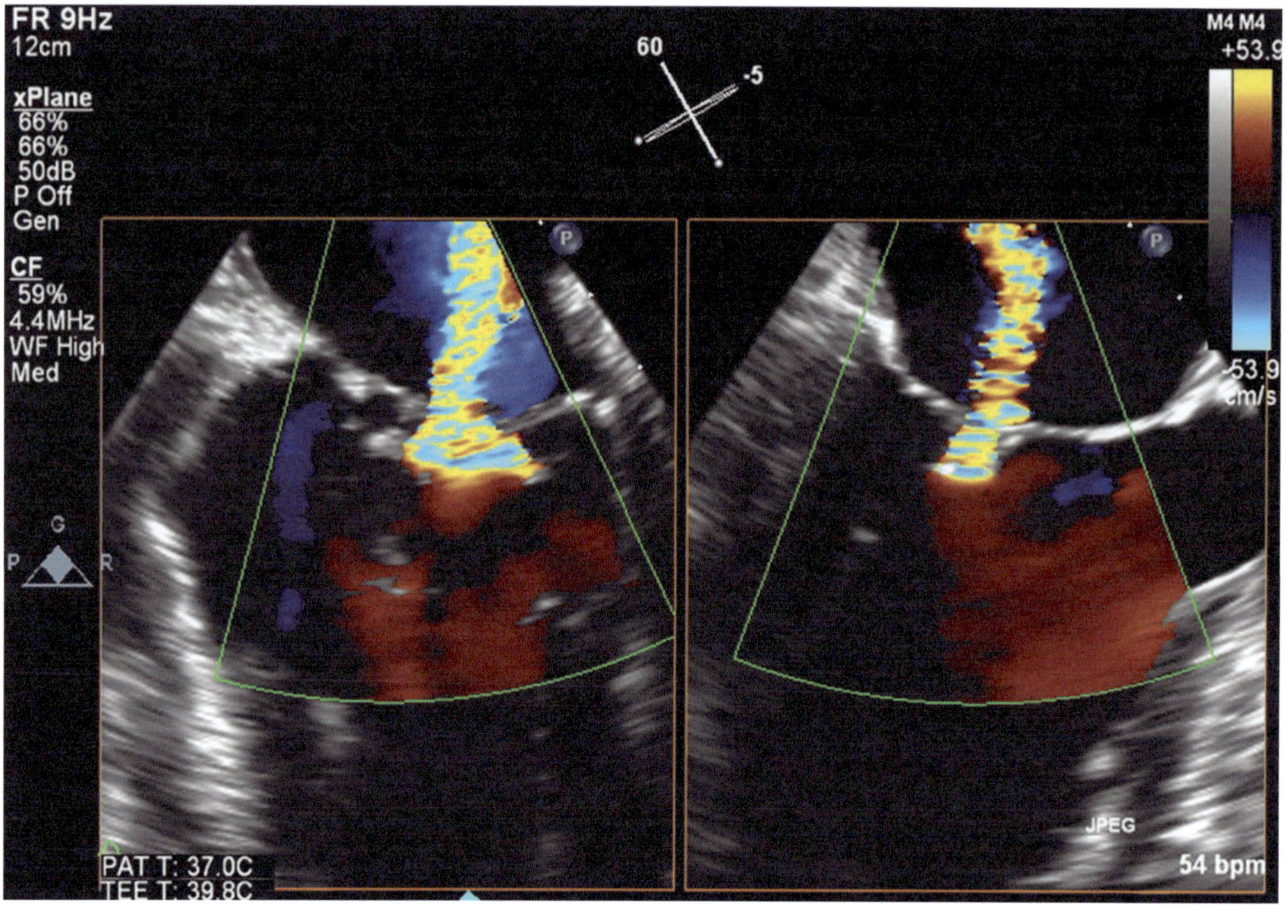

Fig. 18.7 Simultaneous transesophageal biplane of the bi-commissural view (*left*) and the long axis views (*right*) demonstrating severe mitral regurgitation at A2/P2 segments of the mitral valve

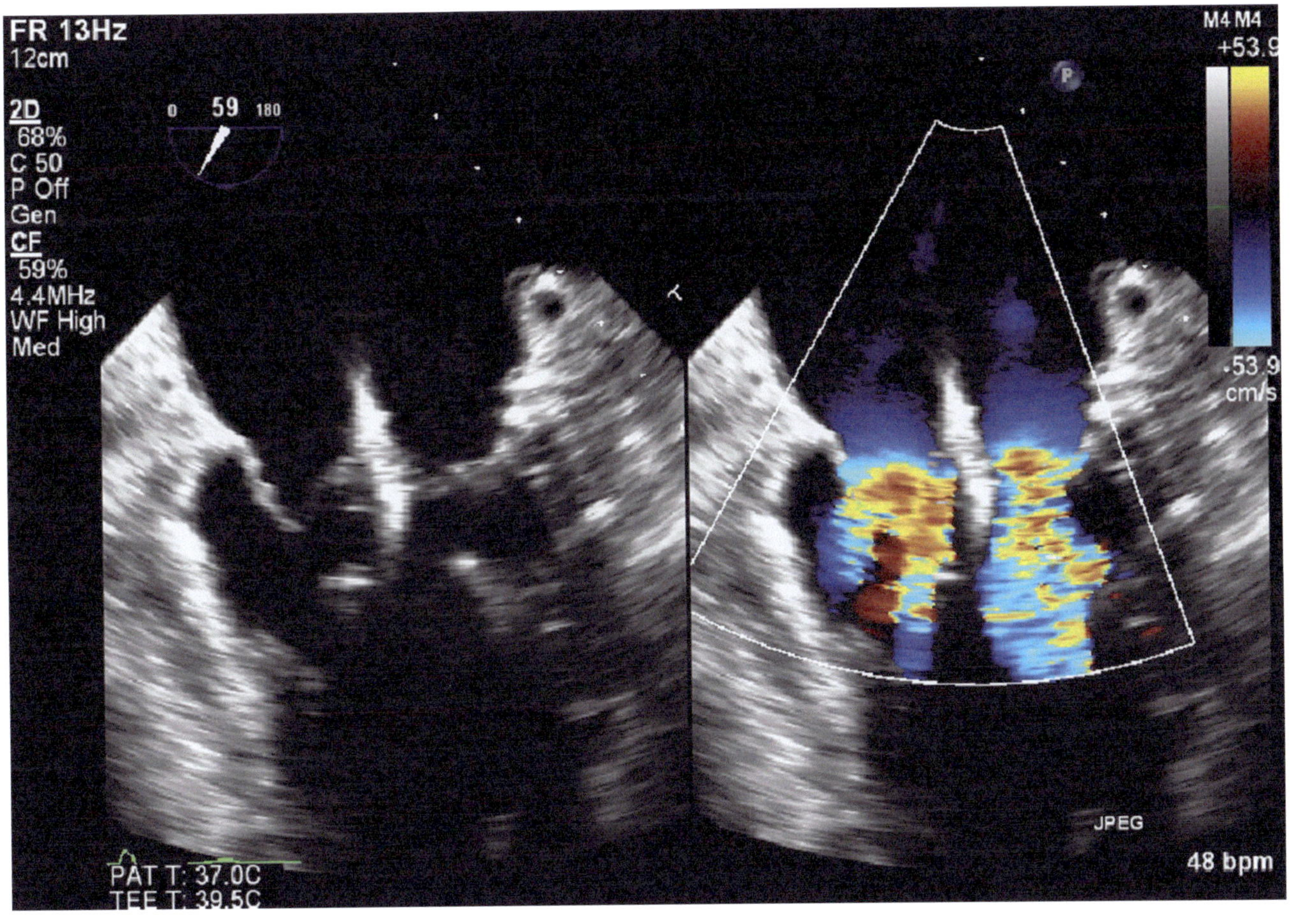

Fig. 18.8 Mid-esophageal bi-commissural view showing the presence of the MitraClip with closed arms at A2/P2 segments of the mitral valve during ventricular diastole with the resultant double orifice mitral valve

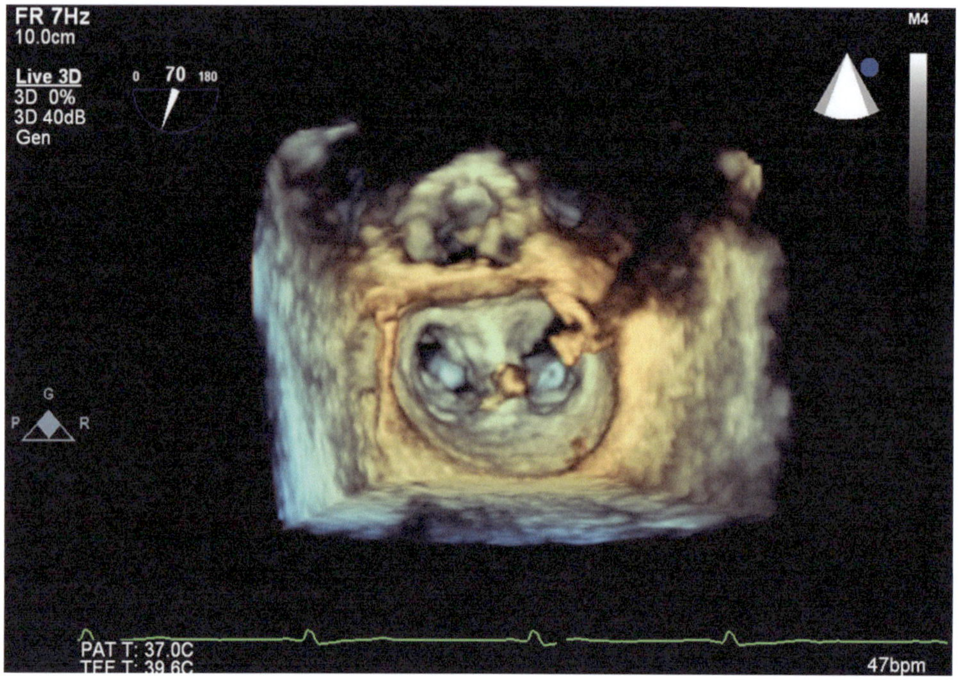

Fig. 18.9 3D image of the mitral valve showing the presence of the MitraClip with closed arms at A2/P2 segments of the mitral valve during ventricular diastole with the resultant double orifice mitral valve

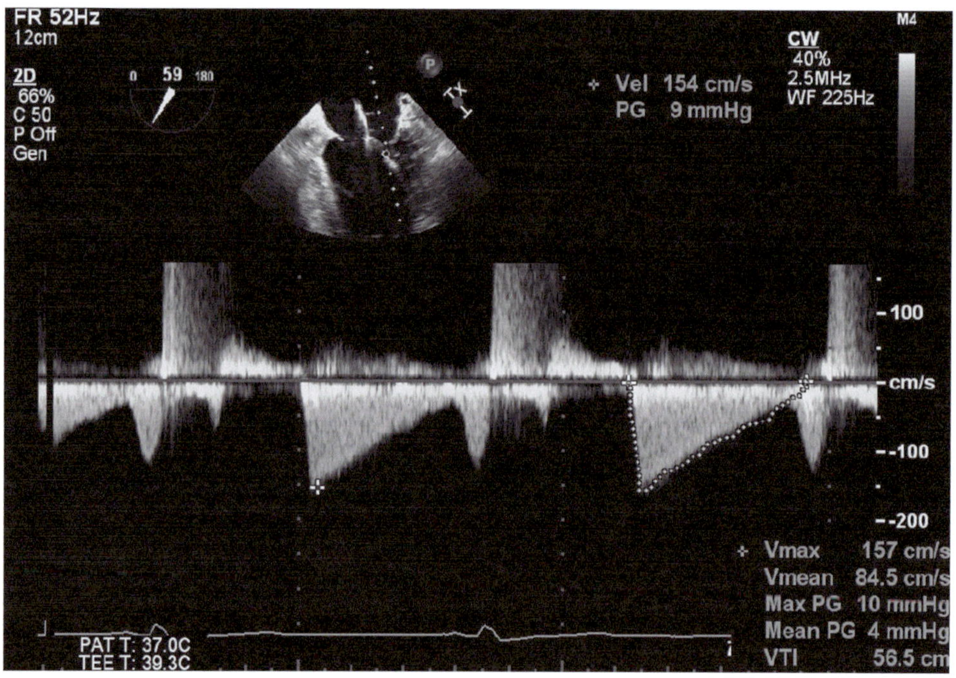

Fig. 18.10 Continuous wave Doppler across the lateral orifice of the double orifice mitral valve showing a mean pressure gradient of 4 mmHg

19 The Dilemma of Reducing Functional Mitral Regurgitation Versus Development of Mitral Stenosis

Ali Vazir, Olaf Franzen, Neil Eric Moat, and Susanna Price

Abstract

A 58-year-old man with a background history of ischemic heart disease and previous coronary bypass grafting presented with several episodes of heart failure. His echocardiogram showed severe mitral regurgitation with a broad jet secondary bileaflet restriction. He underwent edge-to-edge repair with the MitraClip system. An initial MitraClip was inserted, but the patient required a second clip, to further reduce the severity of the regurgitation, and the optimal position of the second clip was determined by balancing risk of reducing mitral regurgitation at the cost of producing mitral stenosis.

Keywords

Mitral stenosis • Mitral regurgitation • MitraClip

Clinical History

A 58-year-old man with history of heart failure secondary to ischemic heart disease, inferior myocardial infarction 1999, coronary artery bypass surgery 2001, hypertension and coexisting type II diabetes mellitus, renal dysfunction presented with NYHA III symptoms, and several episodes of pulmonary edema requiring intravenous diuretics. He was found to have a severe mitral regurgitation and evidence of severe tricuspid regurgitation with elevated pulmonary systolic pressure (PASP 60 mmHg).

His echocardiogram showed a non-dilated left ventricle (LVEDD 5.5 cm, LVESD 3.5 cm, biplane EF 66 %). The left atrium was significantly dilated. The mitral valve annulus was calcified with extension of a ridge of calcium onto the left ventricular surface of the posterior mitral valve leaflet. There was thickening of the mitral valve leaflets with rolled edges, and severe mitral regurgitation secondary to a combination of bileaflet restriction (both systolic and diastolic) and significant mitral annular dilatation. The maximum degree of regurgitation was present at A2/P2 and at A3/P3. See Figs. 19.1, 19.2, 19.3, and 19.4.

In view of his comorbidities, he was referred for percutaneous edge-to-edge repair of his mitral valve using the MitraClip system. It was recognized that given his mitral valve anatomy,

A. Vazir, MBBS, MRCP, CCDS, Ph.D. (✉)
Department of Cardiology, Royal Brompton Hospital, Royal Brompton and Harefield NHS Foundation Trust, Sydney Street, London SW3 6NP, UK

Department of Cardiology, Royal Brompton Hospital, National Heart and Lung Institute, Imperial College, London, UK
e-mail: a.vazir@rbht.nhs.uk, ali.vazir@btinternet.com

O. Franzen, M.D.
Department of Cardiology, The Heart Center, Rigshospitalet, University of Copenhagen, Blegdamsvej 9, Copenhagen 2100, Denmark

Royal Brompton Hospital, Royal Brompton and Harefield NHS Foundation Trust, London, UK
e-mail: owfranzen@gmx.de

N.E. Moat, MBBS, MS., FRCS
Department of Cardiac Surgery, Head of Trans-catheter Valve programme, Royal Brompton Hospital, Sydney Street, London SW3 6NP, UK
e-mail: n.moat@rbht.nhs.uk

S. Price, MBBS, BSc, MRCP, EDICM, Ph.D., FFICM, FESC
Department of Cardiology, Royal Brompton Hospital, Sydney Street, London SW3 6NP, UK
e-mail: s.price@rbht.nhs.uk

T. Feldman et al. (eds.), *Atlas of Percutaneous Edge-to-Edge Mitral Valve Repair*,
DOI 10.1007/978-1-4471-4294-2_19,

the procedure would be unlikely to completely resolve his mitral regurgitation, but the aim was to reduce its severity.

Figures 19.5, 19.6, 19.7, 19.8, 19.9, 19.10, 19.11, 19.12, 19.13, and 19.14 demonstrate successful deployment of the first MitraClip toward the posteromedial commissure, resulting in significant reduction in mitral regurgitation in the medial aspect of the valve, and no forward flow at this position. The central and lateral mitral regurgitation remained unchanged. A series of attempts were then made to determine the optimal position of the second clip: initially centrally (A2:P2), then moving more anterolaterally (Figs. 19.15, 19.16, 19.17, 19.18, 19.19, 19.20, 19.21, and 19.22). The more lateral the clip position, the more effective the reduction in mitral regurgitation, but at the expense of increased mitral stenosis with a reduced valve area. Finally, the second clip was deployed at the lateral aspect of A2/P2 with significant reduction of mitral regurgitation from 4+ to 1+, with some increase in forward velocities across the valve, and a degree of mitral stenosis, mitral valve area of 1.6–1.8 cm^2, mean forward mitral valve gradient of 9 mmHg (across the central orifice, between the two clips); see Figs. 19.23, 19.24, 19.25, 19.26, and 19.27.

Twelve months later, the patient presented with congestive cardiac failure with pulmonary edema and peripheral edema. He was found to be in atrial flutter, which was thought to be the possible cause of his decompensation. His echocardiogram showed 2+ mitral regurgitation and a degree of mitral stenosis, as suggested forward mean gradient of 9 mmHg across the mitral valve (Figs. 19.28 and 19.29). In his decompensated state, his tricuspid regurgitation appeared more significant with further elevation in pulmonary artery systolic pressure to 60–70 mmHg (Figs. 19.30 and 19.31).

He was treated initially with diuretics and ACE inhibitor. Once he was off loaded, he underwent a successful right-sided flutter ablation. He also had a right-sided heart catheterization that measured pulmonary artery systolic, diastolic, and mean pressures to be 68, 20, and 44 mmHg, respectively, and his mean wedge pressure to be 40 mmHg, with no evidence of systolic waves. Left ventricular end diastolic measurements were not taken.

Six months after the ablation, he remains in sinus rhythm with significant improvement in exercise capacity and no further episodes of heart failure since the ablation.

Learning Points

1. It is important to recognize the aims of the procedure: in some patients, it may not be possible to completely abolish the mitral regurgitation, but a significant reduction may be sufficient.
2. In positioning a number of clips, there has to be a balance between reduction of mitral regurgitation and causing mitral stenosis.

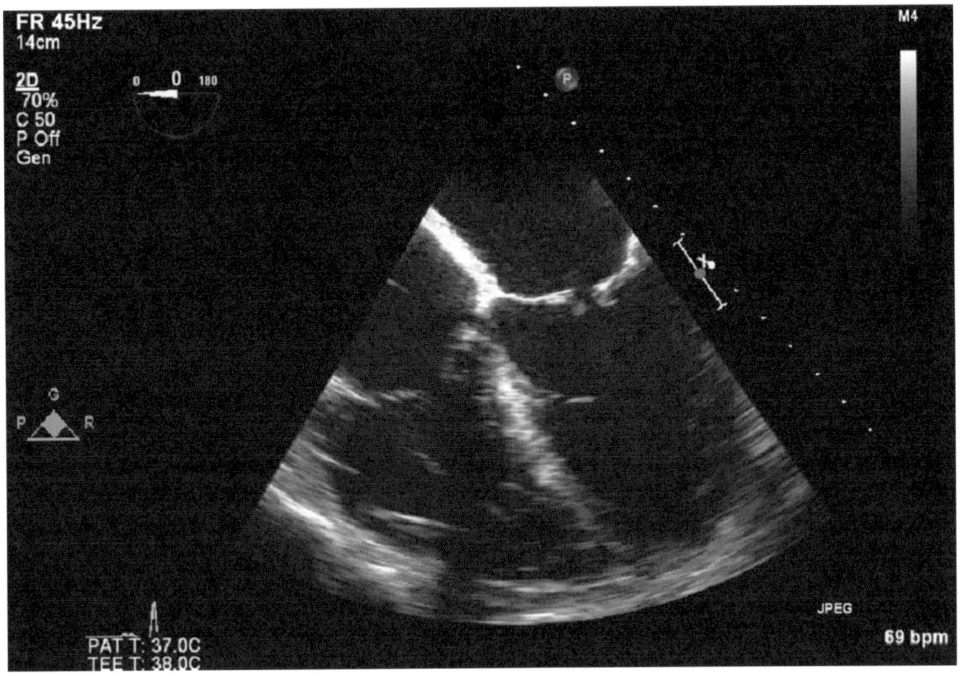

Fig. 19.1 Transesophageal four-chamber view showing calcified mitral valve annulus and thickening of the mitral valve leaflets with rolled edges

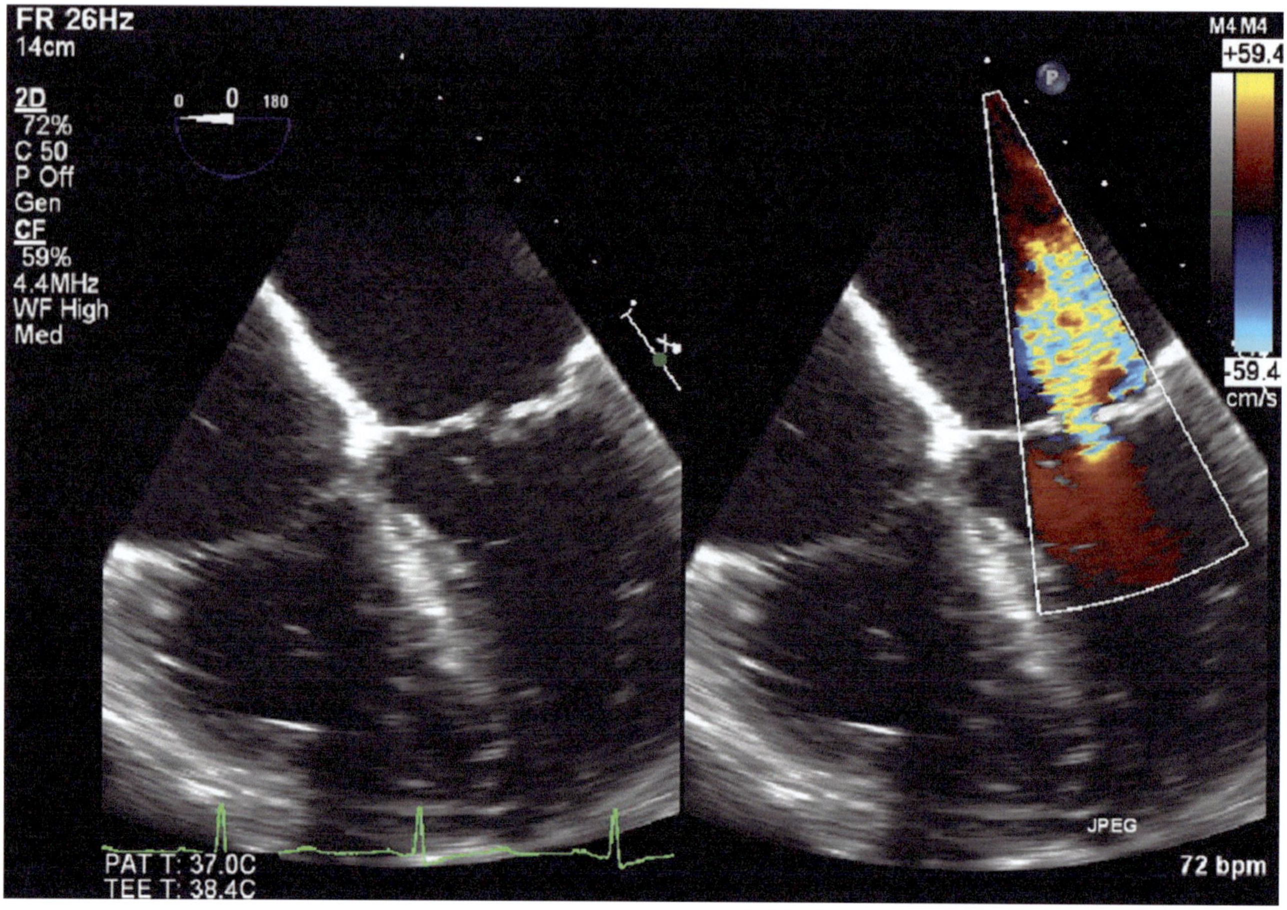

Fig. 19.2 Transesophageal four-chamber view showing severe mitral regurgitation with central jet

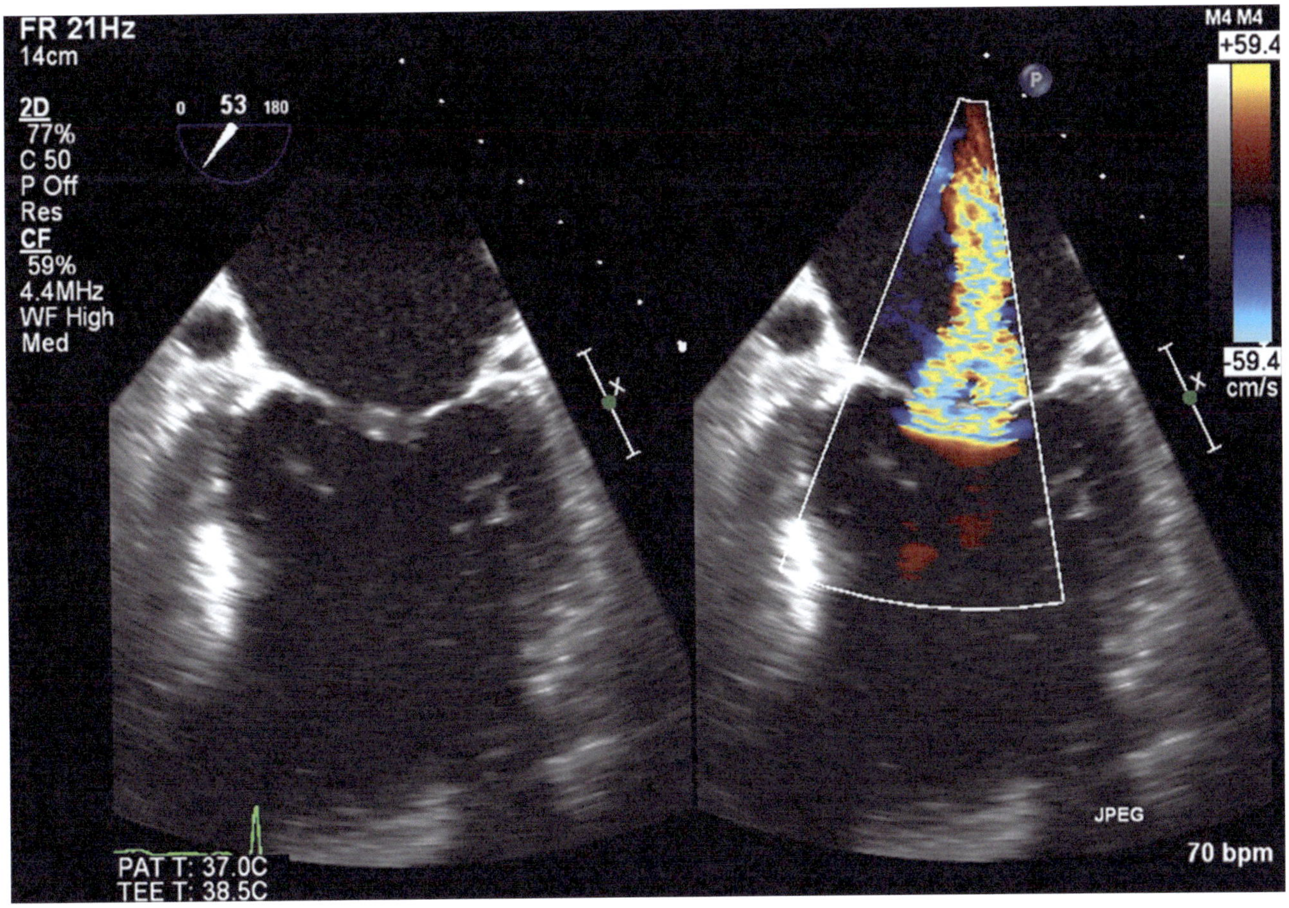

Fig. 19.3 Transesophageal bi-commissural view showing severe mitral regurgitation with a broad central jet across lateral aspect of A3/P3, A2/P2, and medial aspect of A1/P2

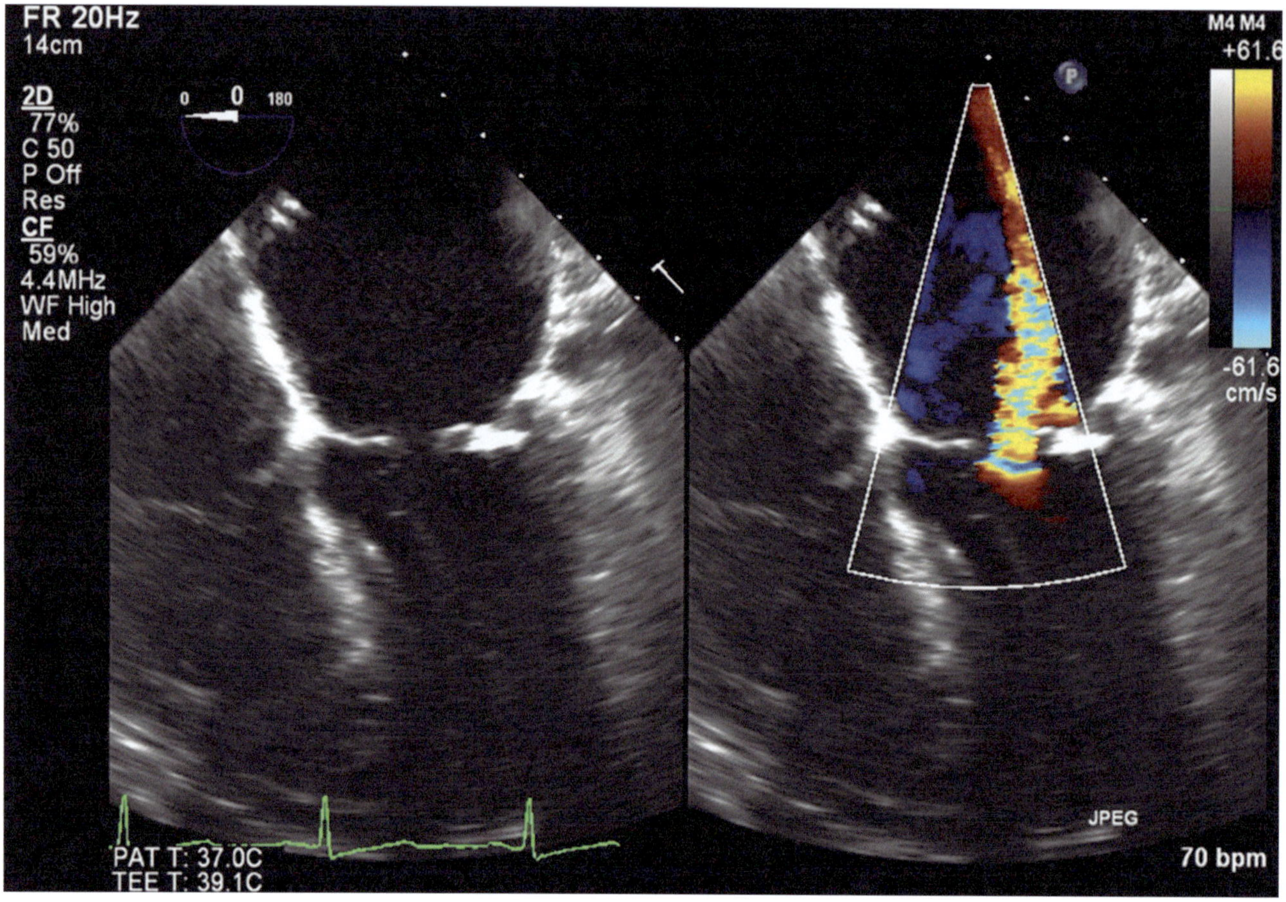

Fig. 19.4 Transesophageal modified four-chamber view showing medial aspect of A2 and P2. The image on the *left* shows a ridge of calcium passing on the ventricular surface of the posterior mitral valve leaflet. The *right* Heart Image is to demonstrate the presence of elevated pulmonary systolic pressure as described in the text. Likely to be secondary to the presence of a degree of mitral stenosis following two clip procedure

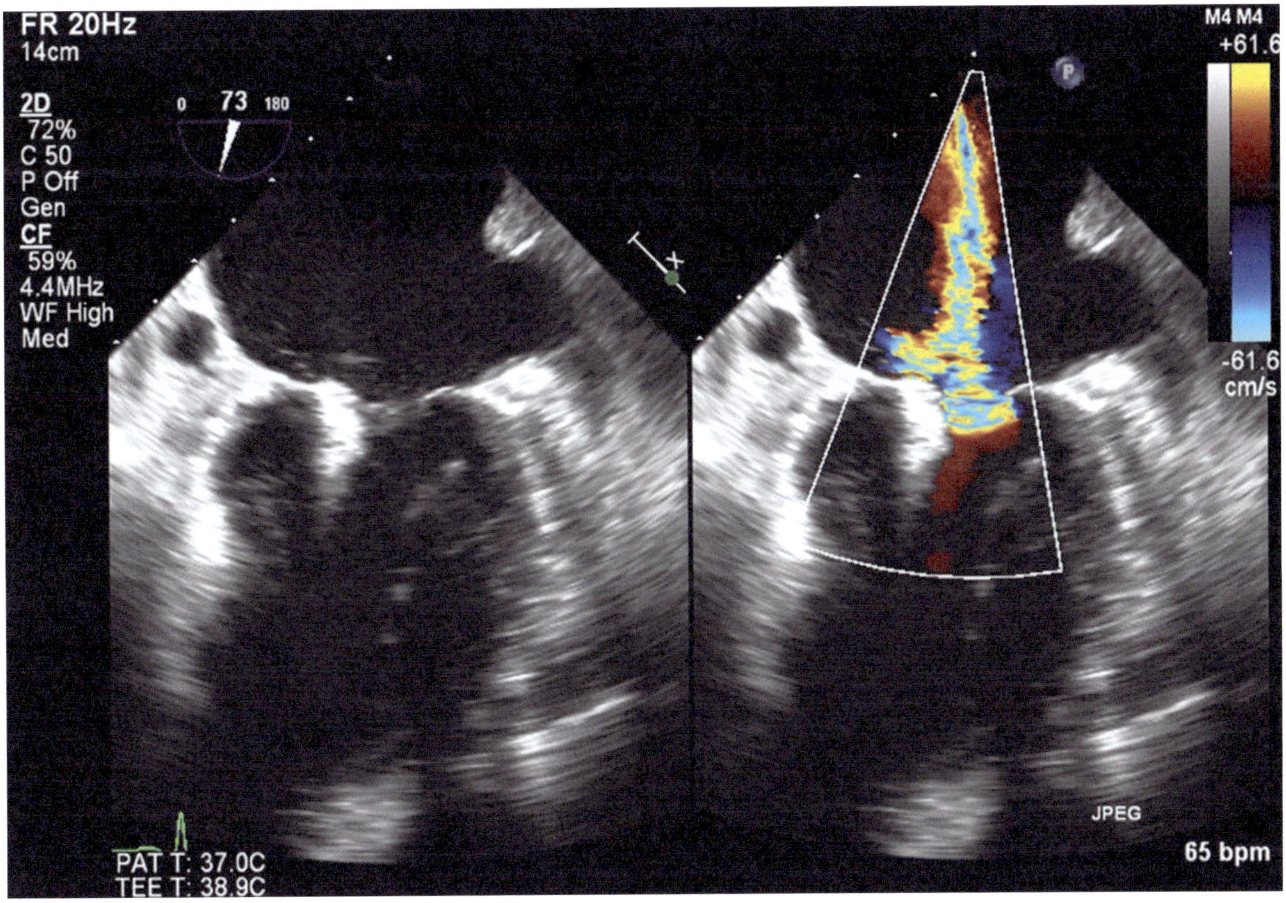

Fig. 19.5 Transesophageal bi-commissural view showing a medially placed first MitraClip resulting in significant reduction in the mitral regurgitation from the medial aspect of the mitral valve (i.e., at lateral aspect of A3/P3). There is a significant jet of mitral regurgitation at the central and lateral aspect of the valve (i.e., A2/P2 and medial aspect of A1/P2)

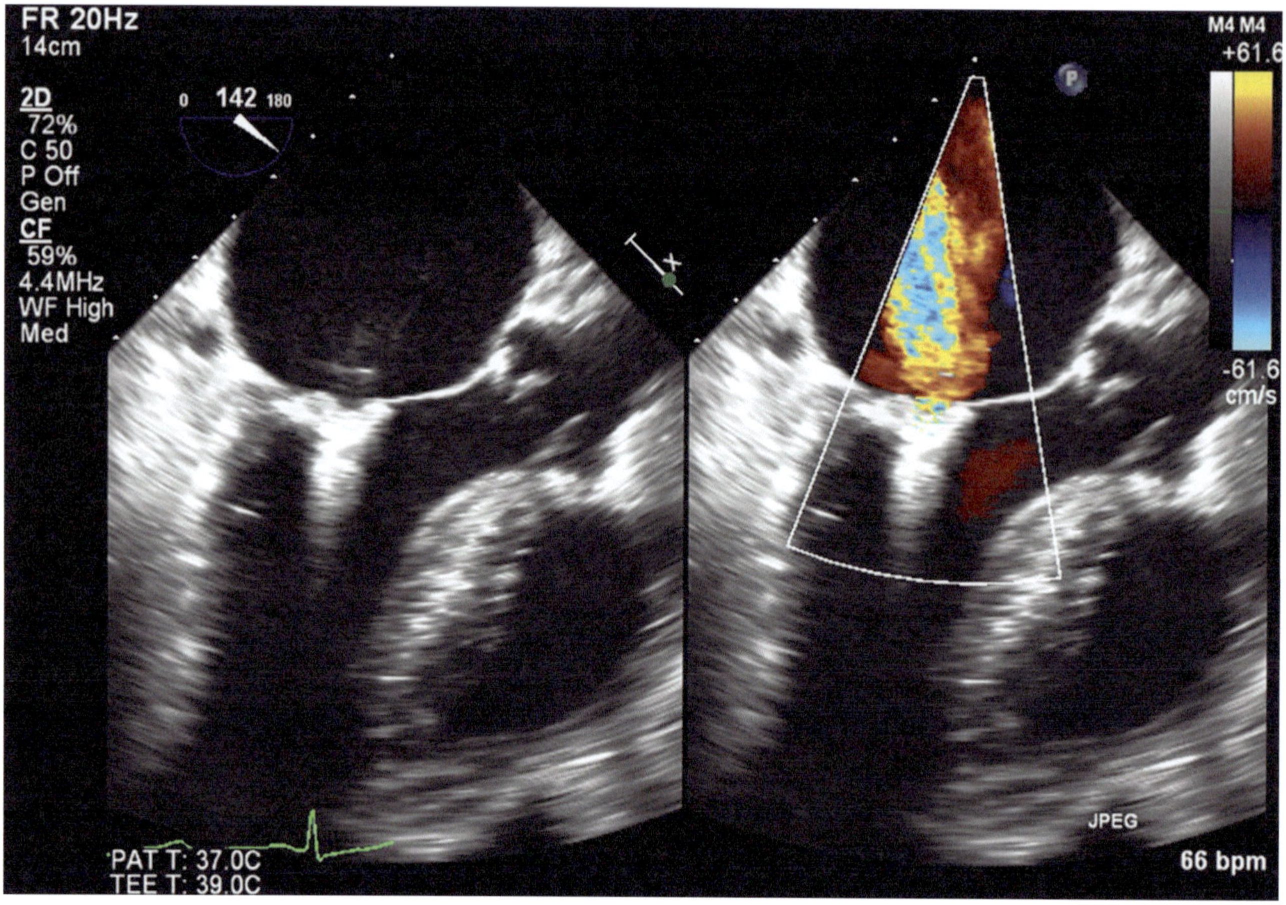

Fig. 19.6 Transesophageal long axis view showing a medially placed first MitraClip resulting in significant reduction in the mitral regurgitation from the medial aspect of the mitral valve (i.e., at lateral aspect of A3/P3). There is a significant jet of mitral regurgitation arising behind the clip from the central aspect of the mitral valve

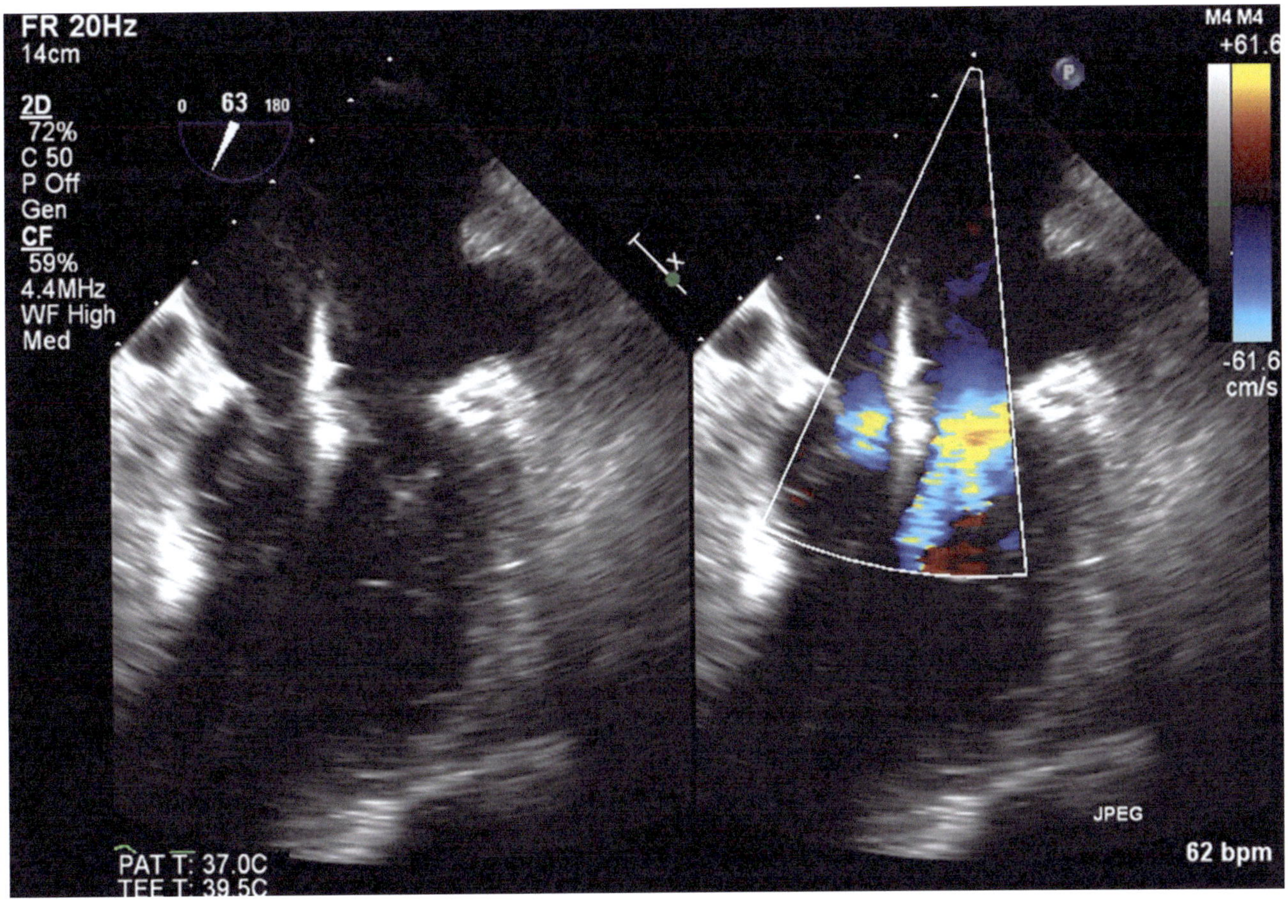

Fig. 19.7 Transesophageal bi-commissural view at 63° in ventricular diastole showing a single MitraClip resulting in a double orifice mitral valve. In this figure, the mitral valve is open with presence of turbulent forward flow across both orifices of the mitral valve

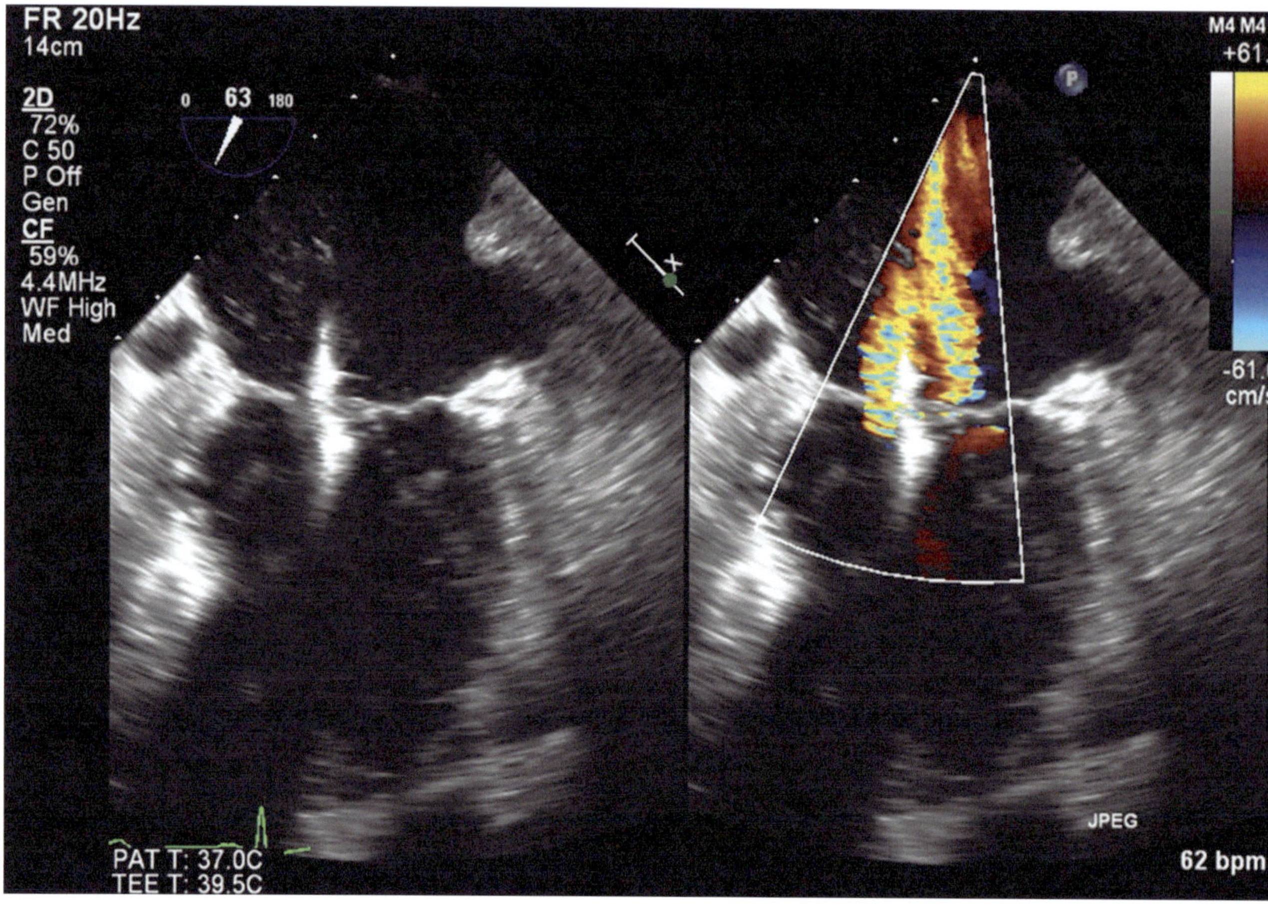

Fig. 19.8 Transesophageal bi-commissural view at 63° in ventricular systole showing a single MitraClip positioned in the lateral aspect of A3/P3 and the medial aspect of A2/P2 resulting reduction of the severity of mitral regurgitation, but there is significant residual mitral regurgitation on the medial aspect of the valve and also requiring a second clip to be placed more laterally

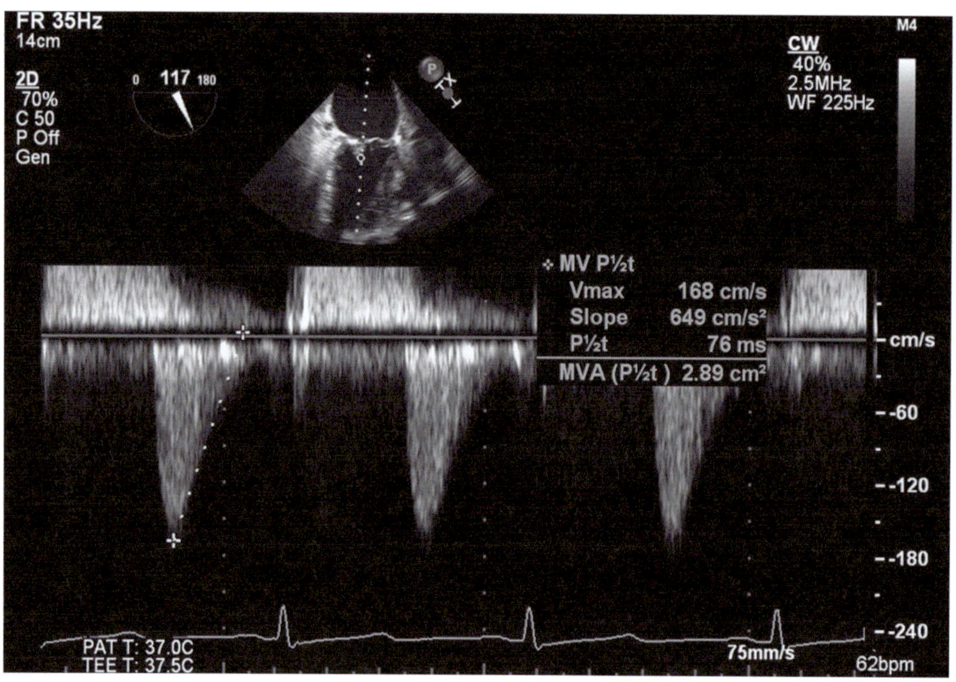

Fig. 19.9 Continuous wave Doppler across one of the orifices of the double lumen mitral valve post single clip placement showing no significant mitral stenosis as suggested by the pressure half time of 76 ms

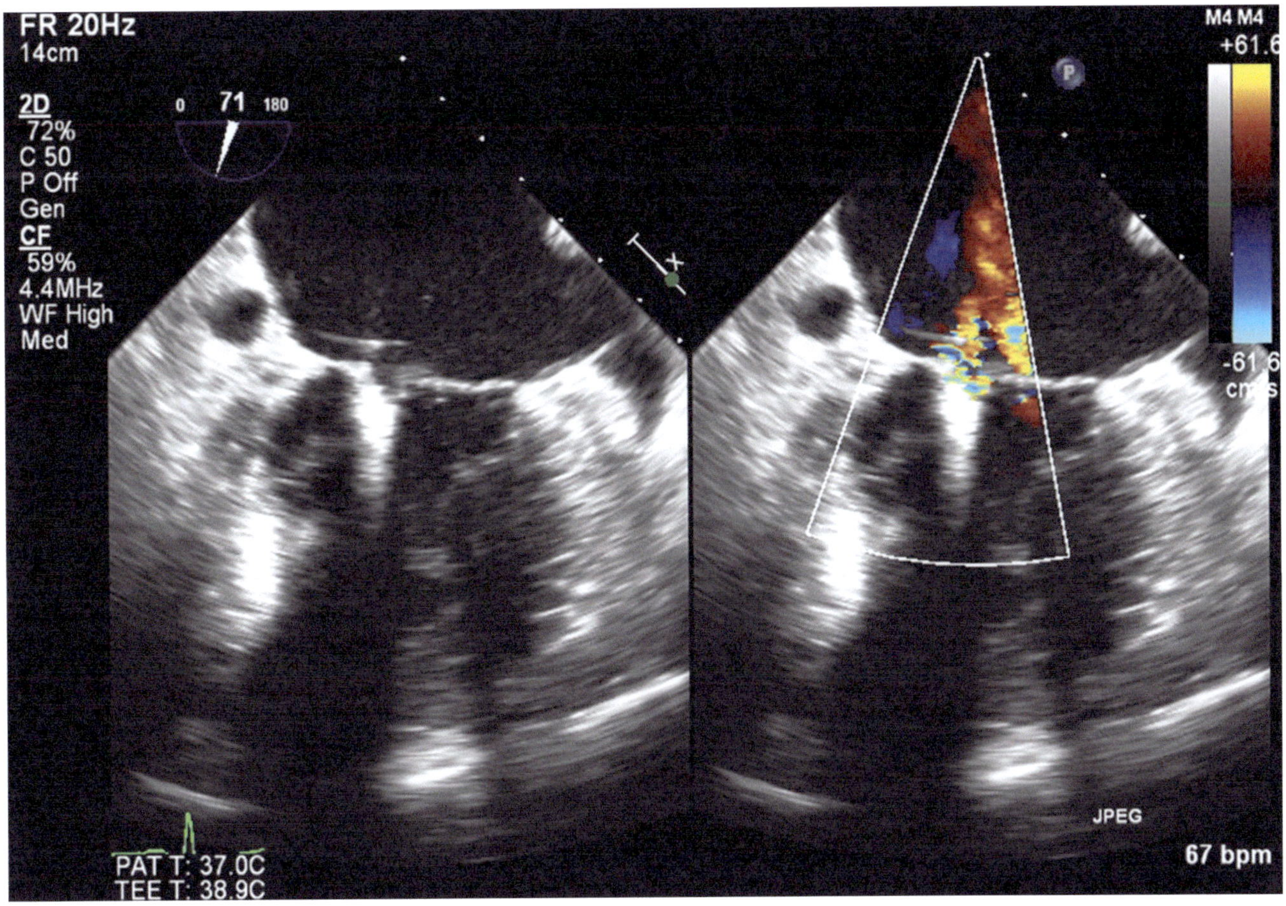

Fig. 19.10 Transesophageal bi-commissural view at 71° showing a single clip in the medial aspect of the mitral valve. In this view, there is good resolution of the mitral regurgitation at the medial aspect of the valve

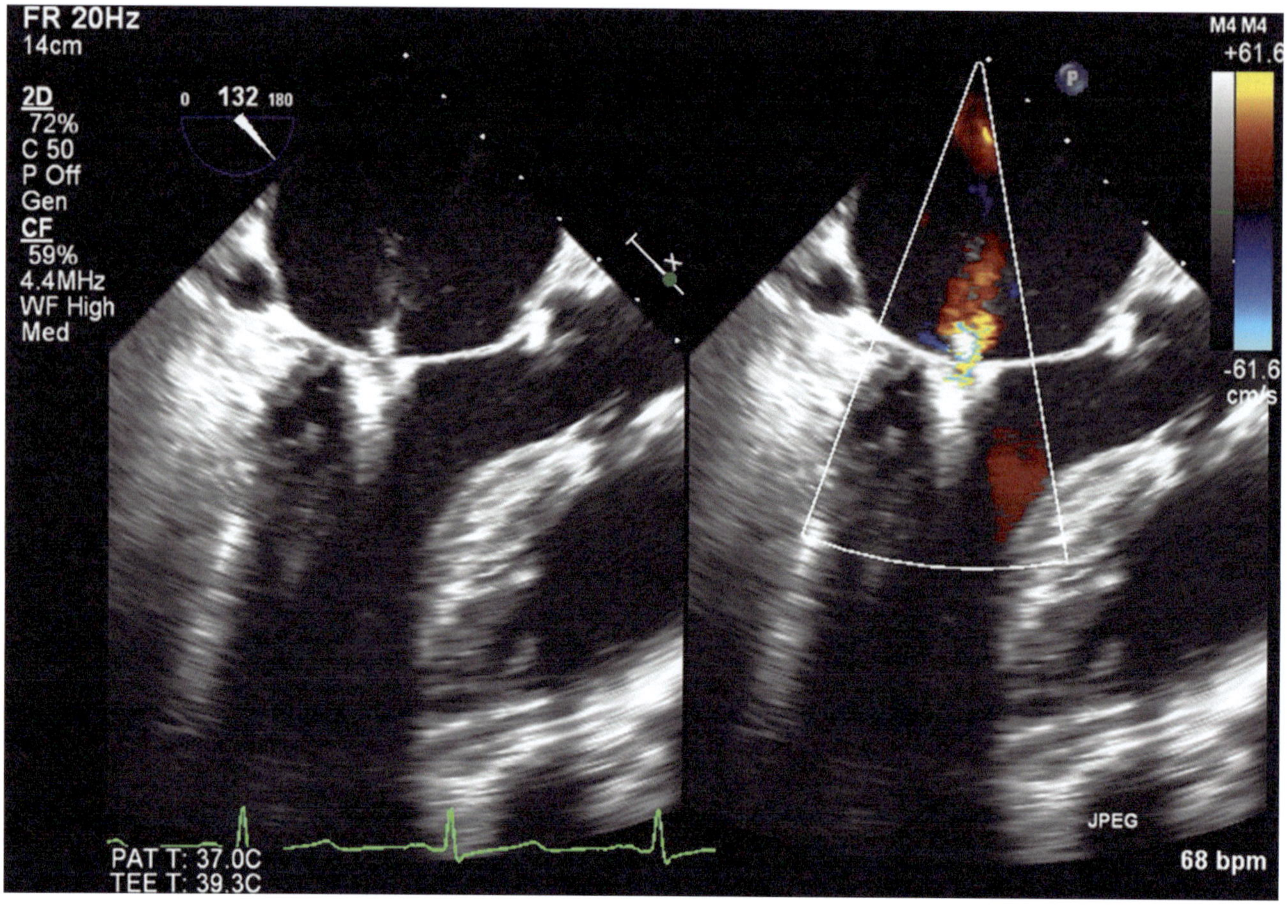

Fig. 19.11 Transesophageal LVOT view showing a single clip with good reduction of the mitral regurgitation

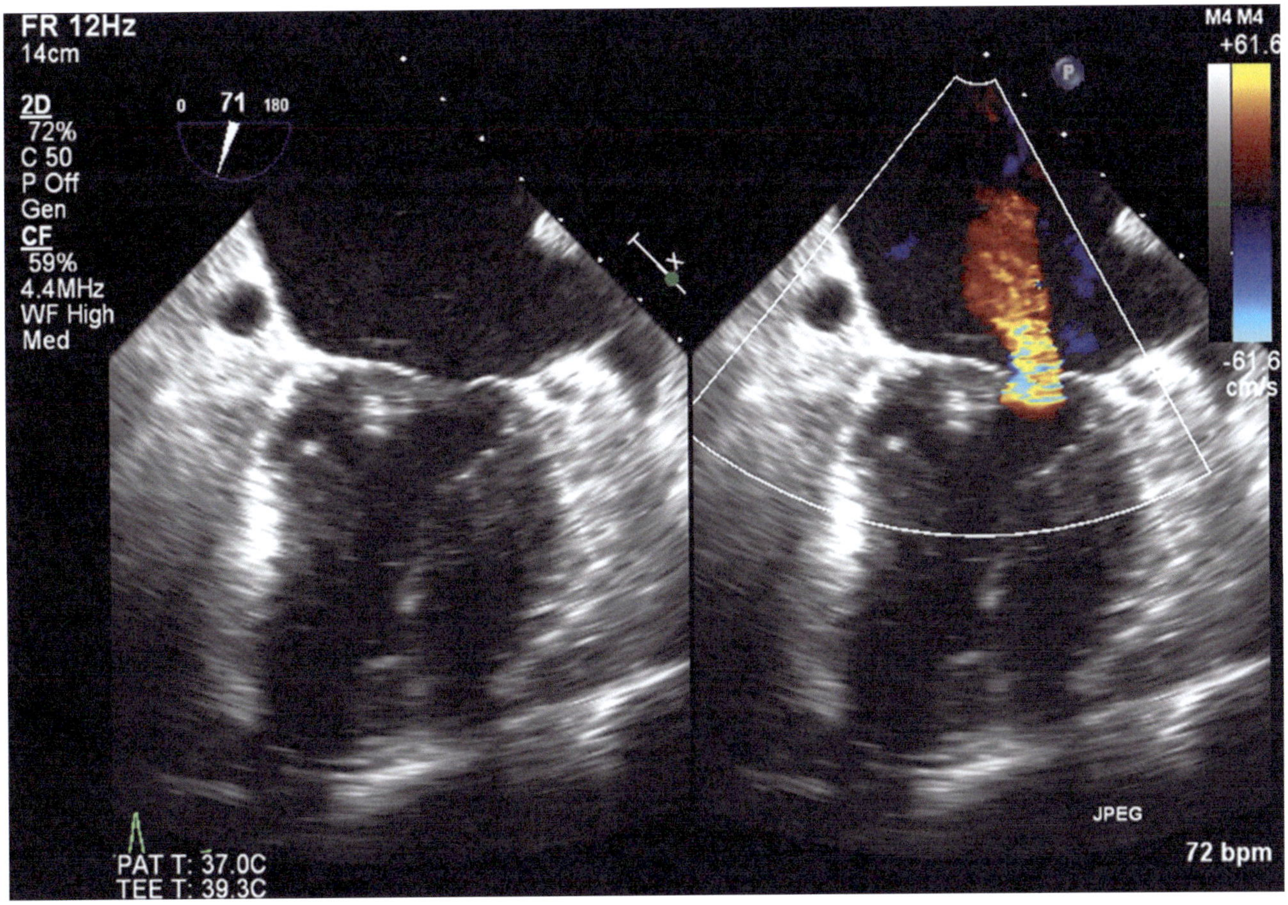

Fig. 19.12 Transesophageal bi-commissural view at 71° showing a single clip in the medial aspect of the mitral valve. In this view, there is good resolution of the mitral regurgitation at the medial aspect of the valve, but significant regurgitation at the central and lateral aspect of the valve

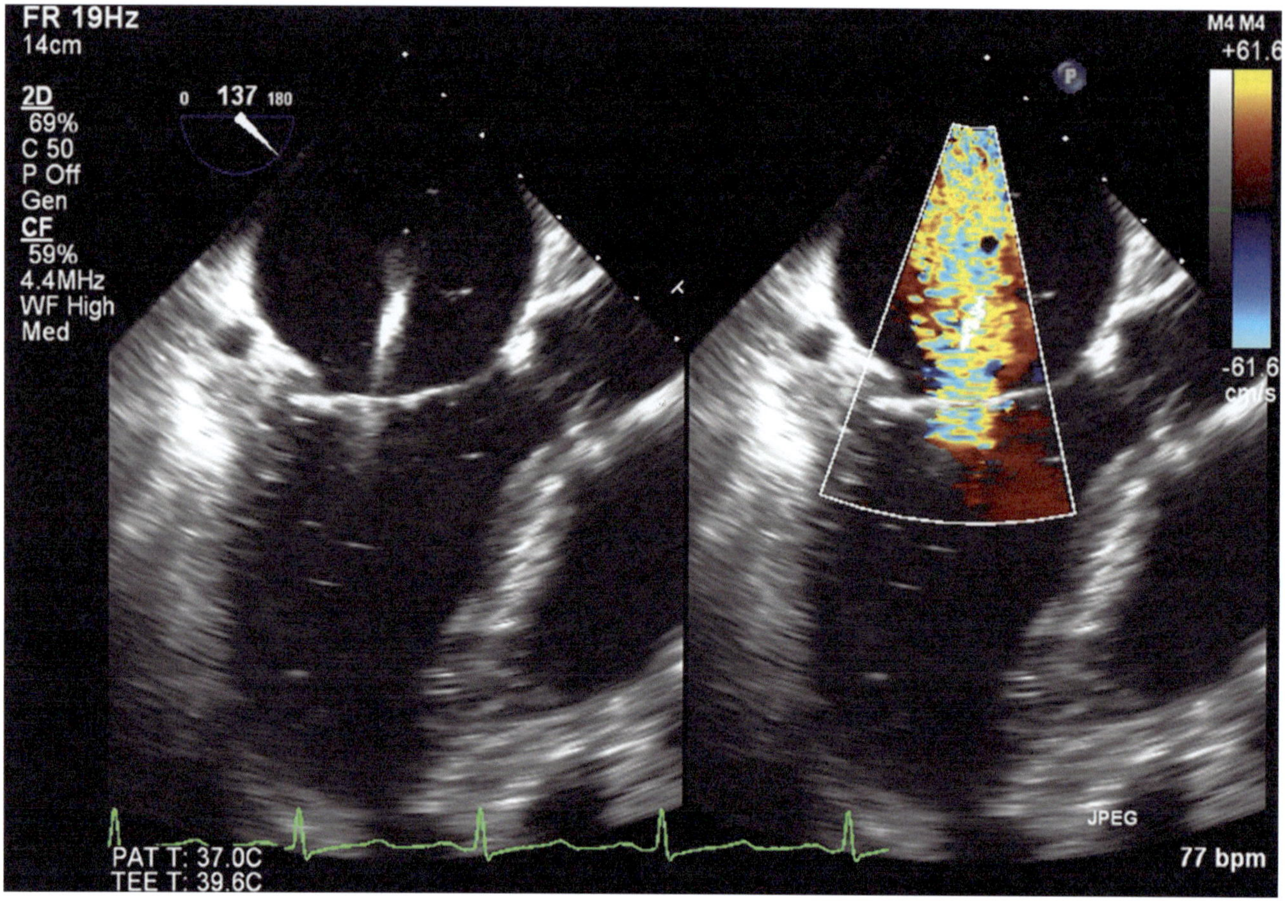

Fig. 19.13 Transesophageal long axis view showing a single clip in the medial aspect of the mitral valve, but there is significant regurgitation at the central and lateral aspect of the valve (i.e., lateral aspect of A2/P2 and medial aspect of A1/P1)

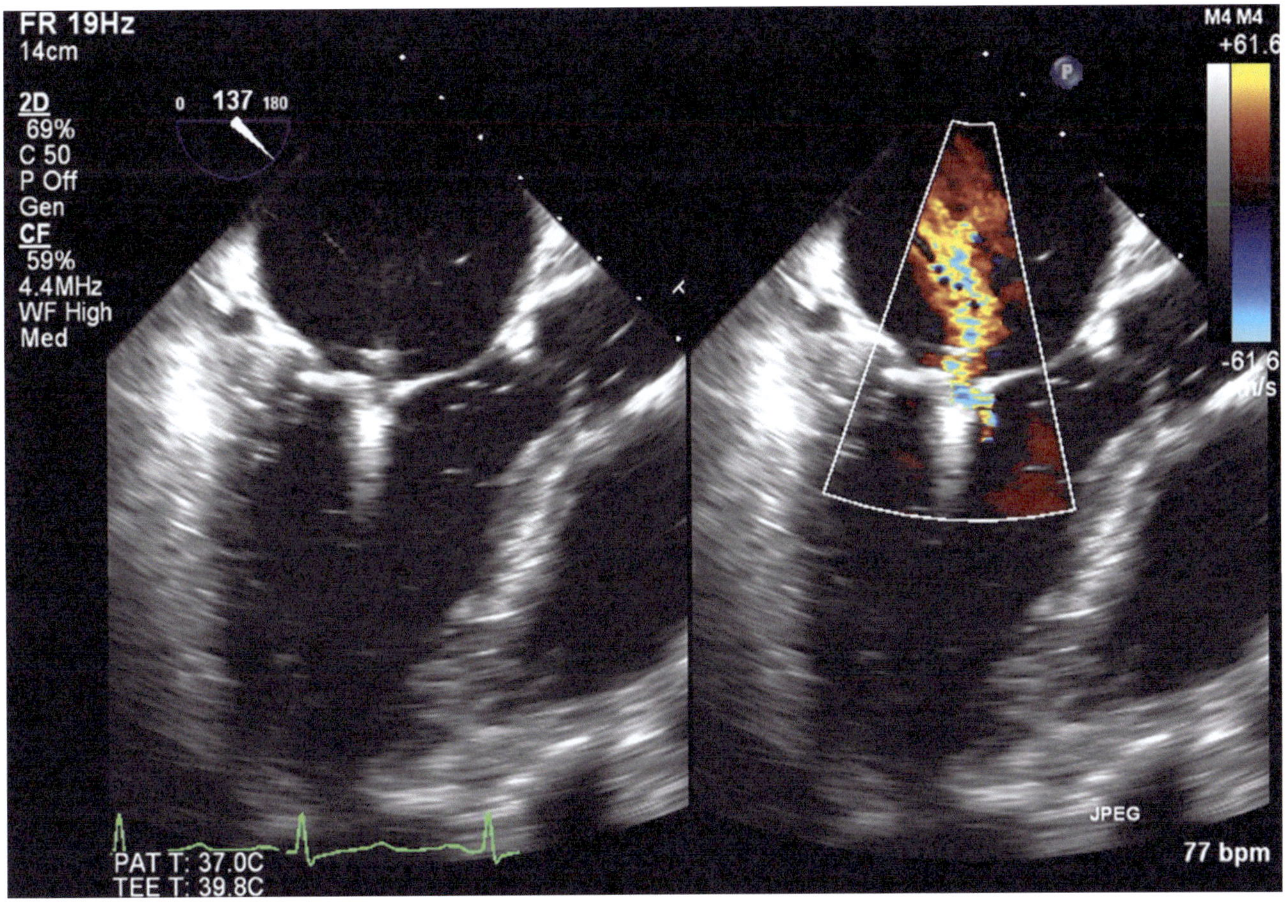

Fig. 19.14 Transesophageal long axis view showing a single clip in the medial aspect of the mitral valve, with significant reduction in mitral regurgitation in the vicinity of the first clip placed in the medial aspect of the mitral valve

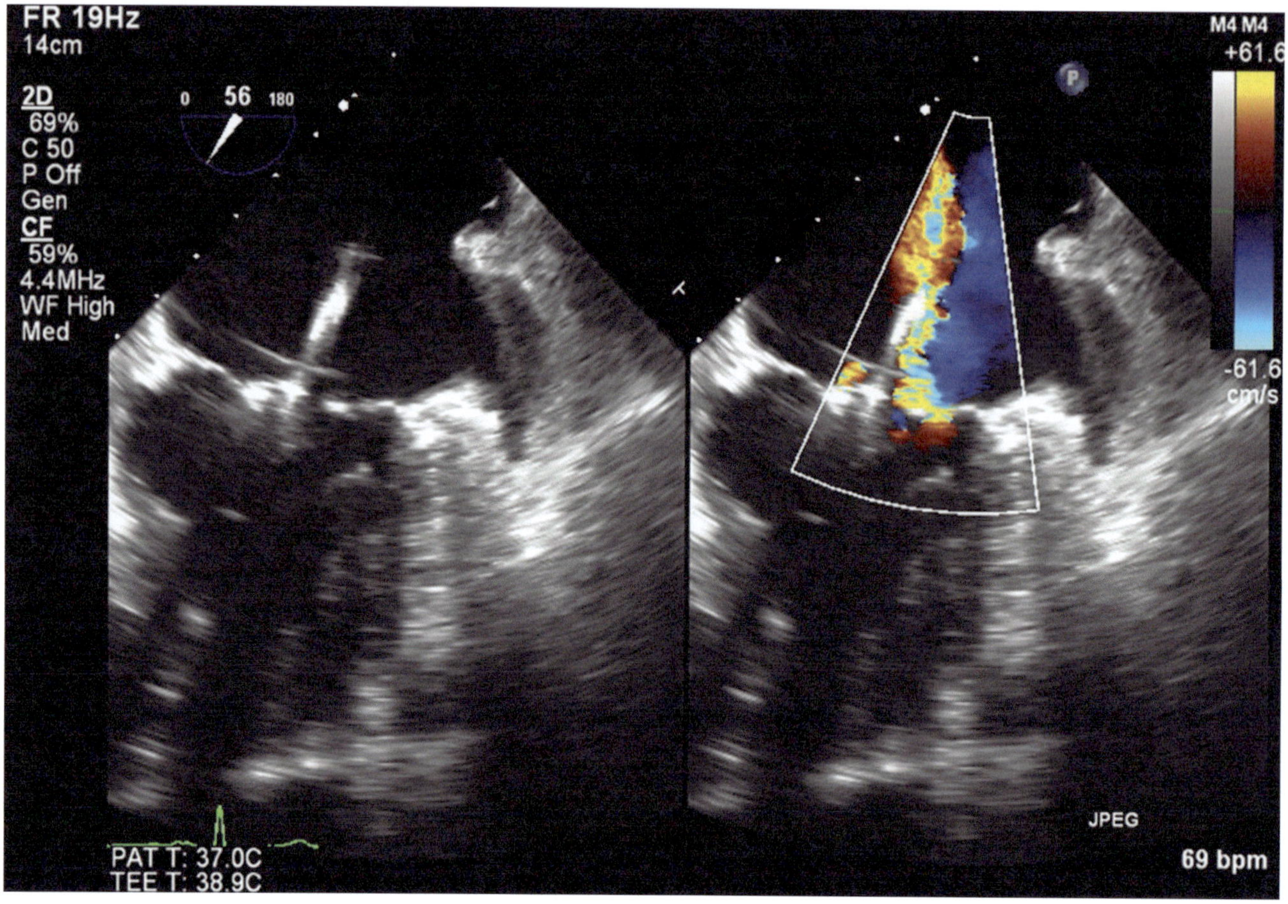

Fig. 19.15 Transesophageal bi-commissural view at 56° showing a second MitraClip position just adjacent to first clip. Lateral to the second clip is a jet of mitral regurgitation arising from the central and lateral aspect of the mitral valve

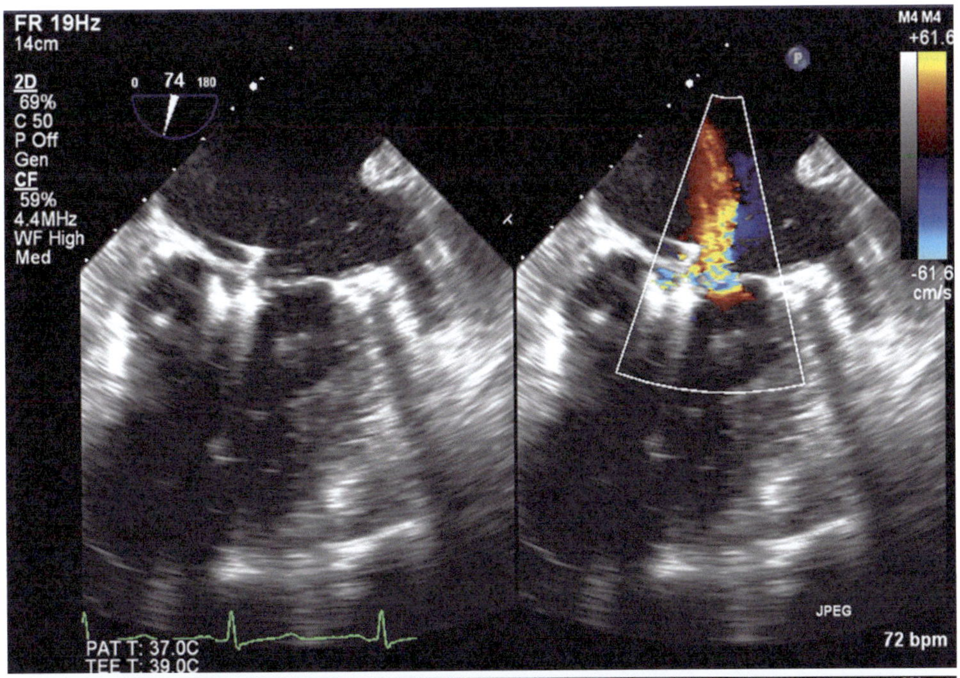

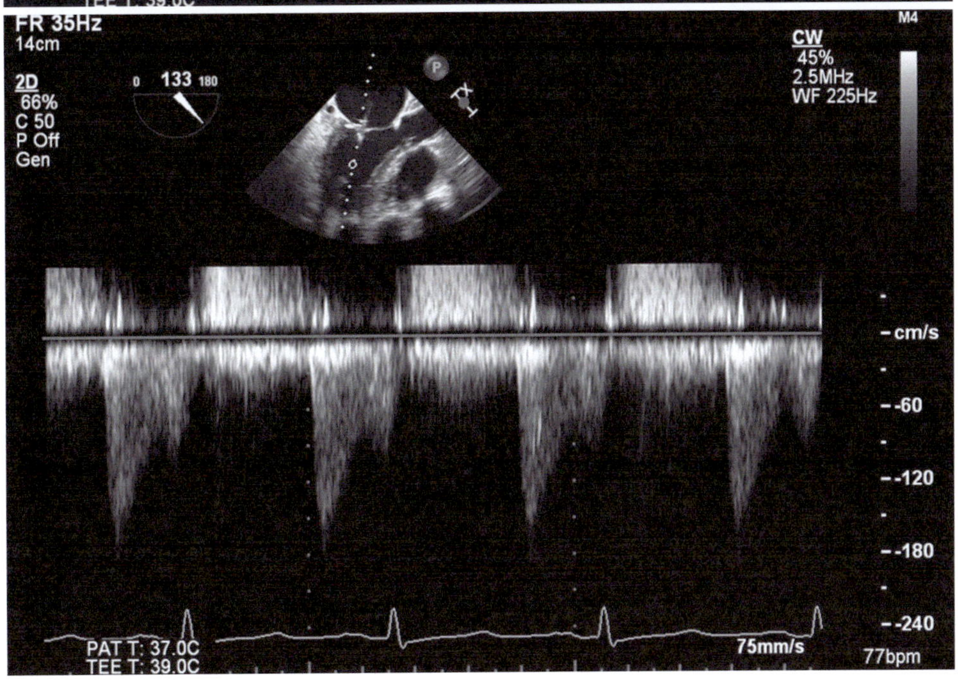

Figs. 19.16 and 19.17 Figure 19.16 shows transesophageal bi-commissural view at 74° showing a second MitraClip positioned just adjacent to first clip. Lateral to the second clip is a significant jet of mitral regurgitation arising from the central and lateral aspect of the mitral valve. If the second clip is positioned here, there will still be a significant degree of residual mitral regurgitation, but no significant mitral stenosis as suggested by the continuous wave Doppler through the mitral valve in Fig. 19.17

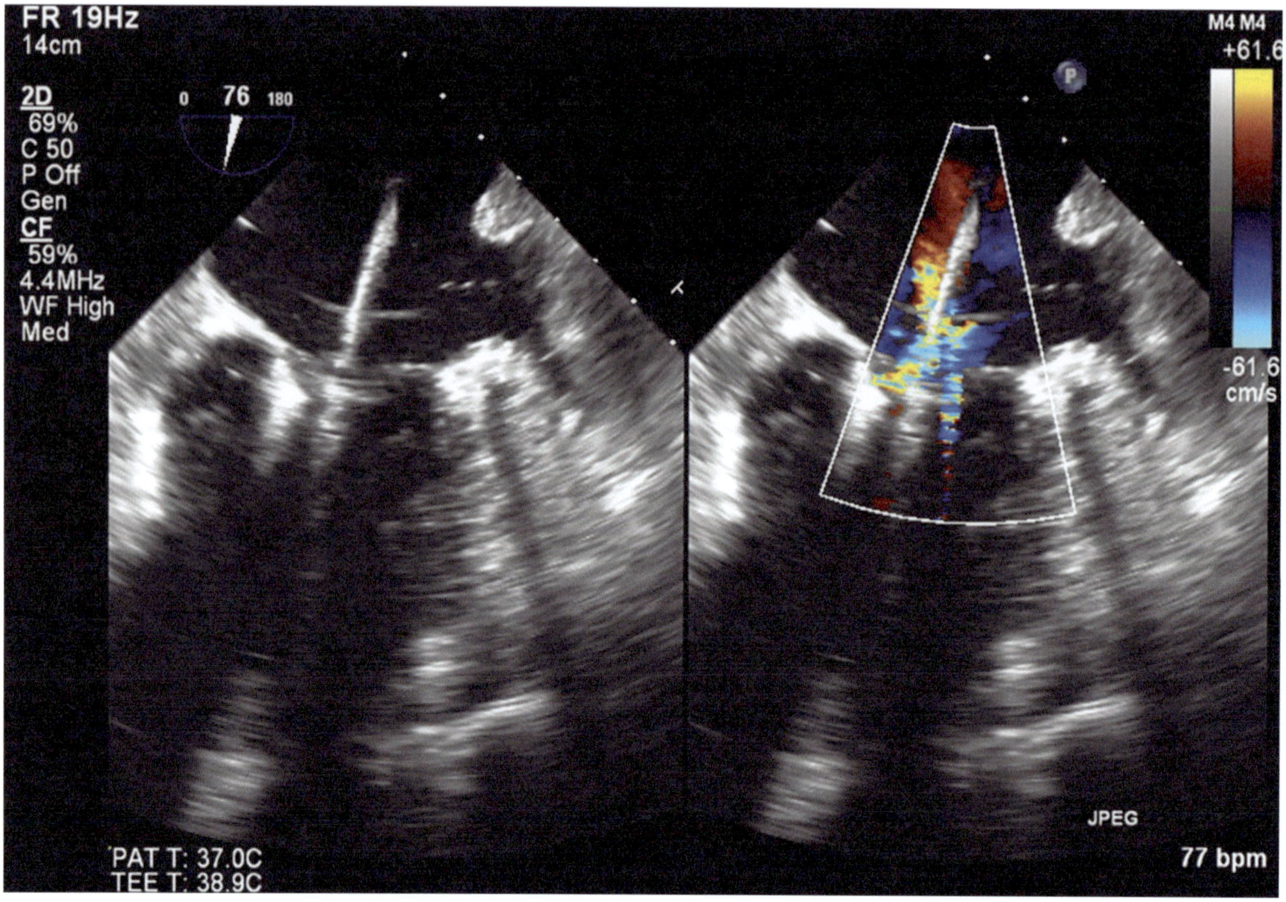

Fig. 19.18 Transesophageal bi-commissural view at 76° showing a second MitraClip positioned just adjacent to first clip, but in a more lateral position as compared to Fig. 19.16. There is more significant reduction in the regurgitation from the central and lateral aspect of the mitral valve

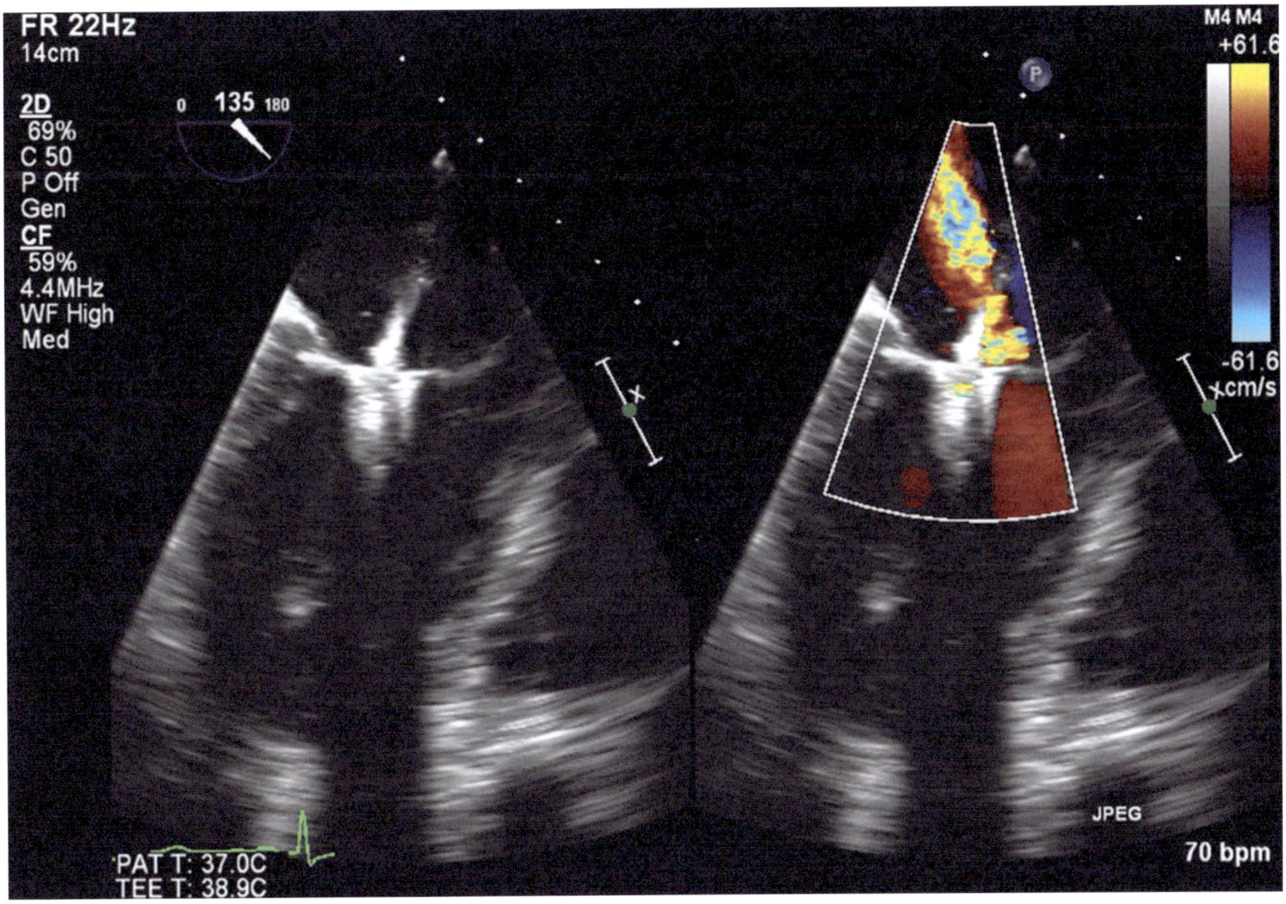

Fig. 19.19 Transesophageal long axis view showing a second MitraClip positioned just adjacent to the first clip, following from Fig. 19.18. There is more significant reduction in the mitral regurgitation

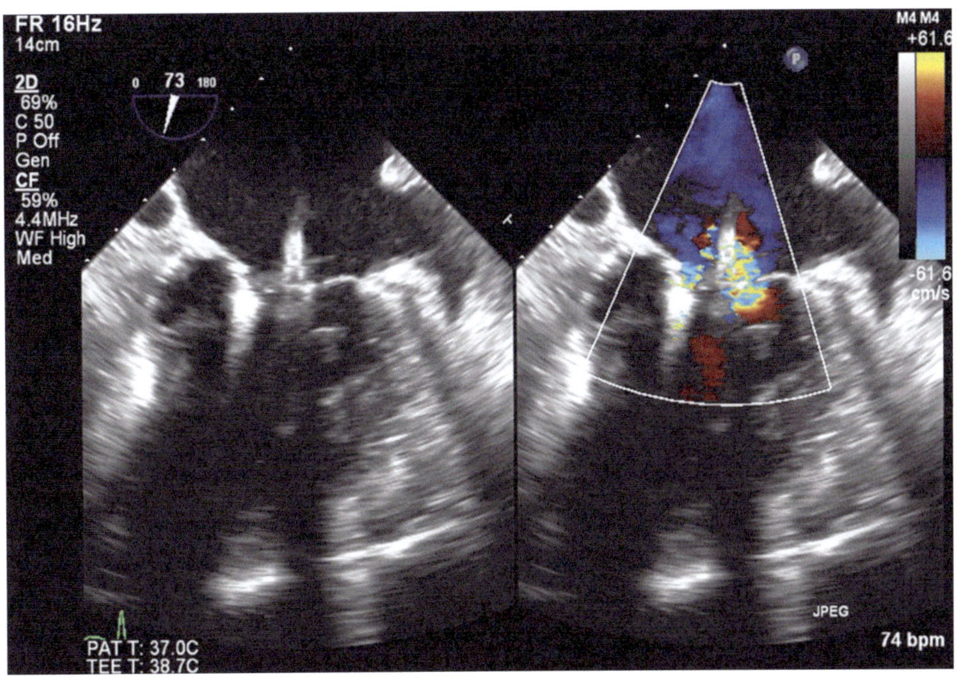

Figs. 19.20, 19.21, and 19.22 Transesophageal bi-commissural view at 73° (Fig. 19.20) and long axis view (Fig. 19.21) showing a second MitraClip position just adjacent to first clip, but the second clip has been repositioned into a more lateral position to have a more effective reduction in the severity of the mitral regurgitation. There is a further reduction in size of the mitral valve orifice as suggested by increase in pressure half time to 96 ms (see Fig. 19.22), as compared to Figs. 19.9 and 19.17

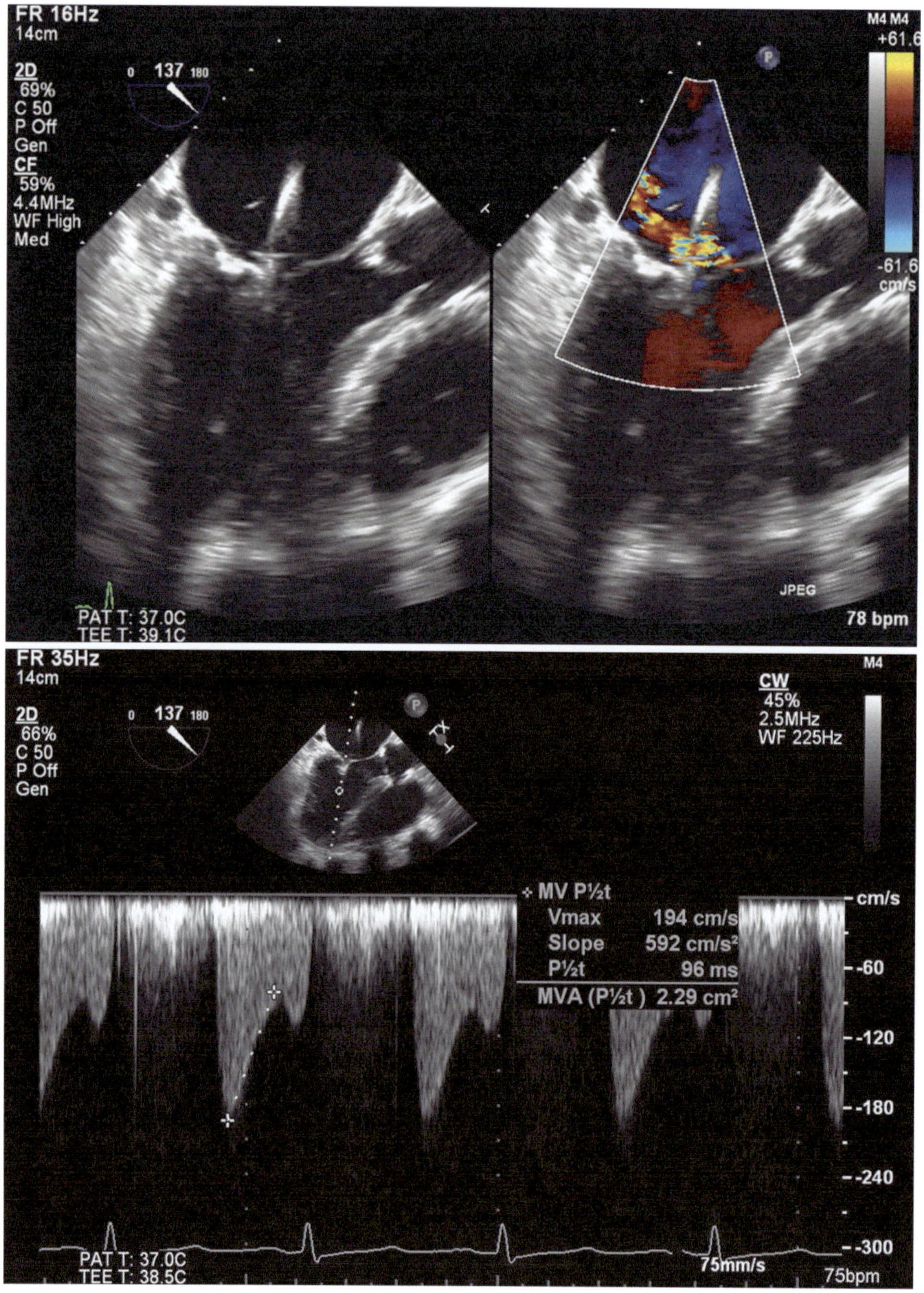

Figs. 19.20, 19.21, and 19.22 (continued)

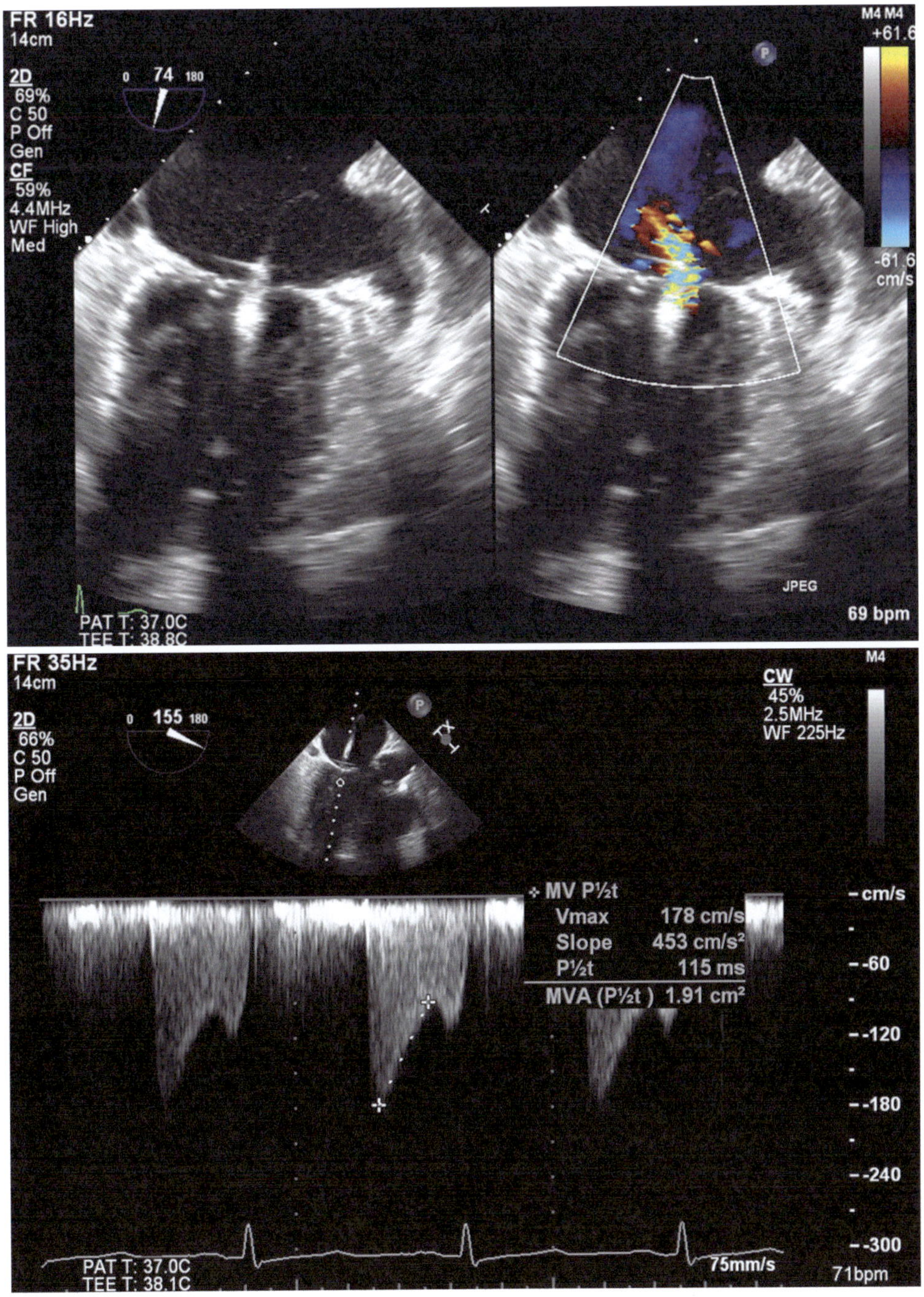

Figs. 19.23, 19.24, 19.25, 19.26, and 19.27 Figure 19.23 Transesophageal bi-commissural view at 74° showing a second MitraClip position just adjacent to first clip, but in a much more lateral position as compared to Figs. 19.20, 19.21, and 19.22, resulting in the most significant reduction in the severity of the mitral regurgitation, but at the cost of further prolonging the mitral valve pressure half time to suggest a degree of mitral stenosis (Figs. 19.24, 19.25, and 19.26). The two clips are at a distance from one another so they appear to have created a triple orifice mitral valve (indicated by *arrows* in Fig. 19.27), with the central orifice located between the two clips seen when the valve is open in ventricular diastole

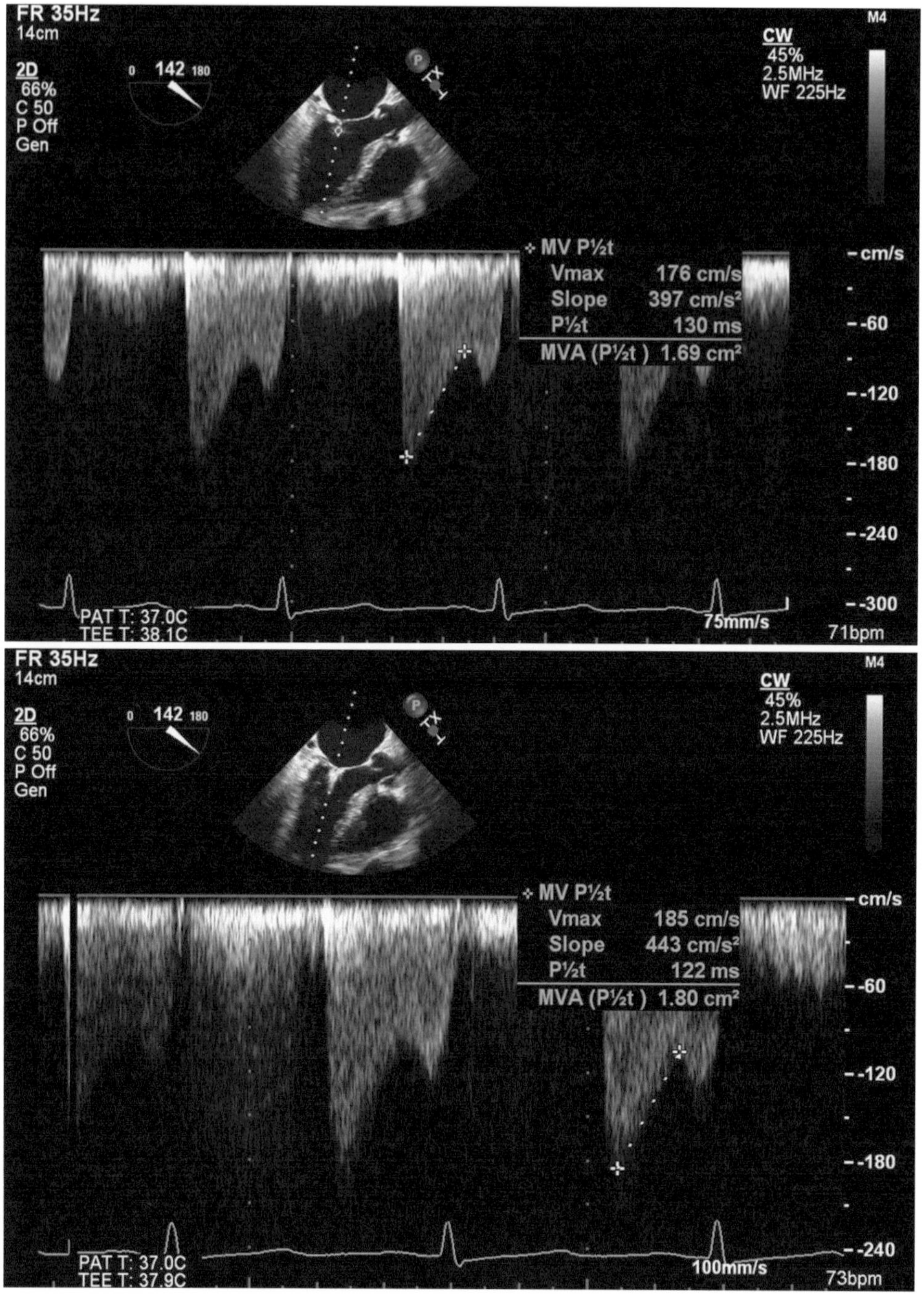

Figs. 19.23, 19.24, 19.25, 19.26, and 19.27 (continued)

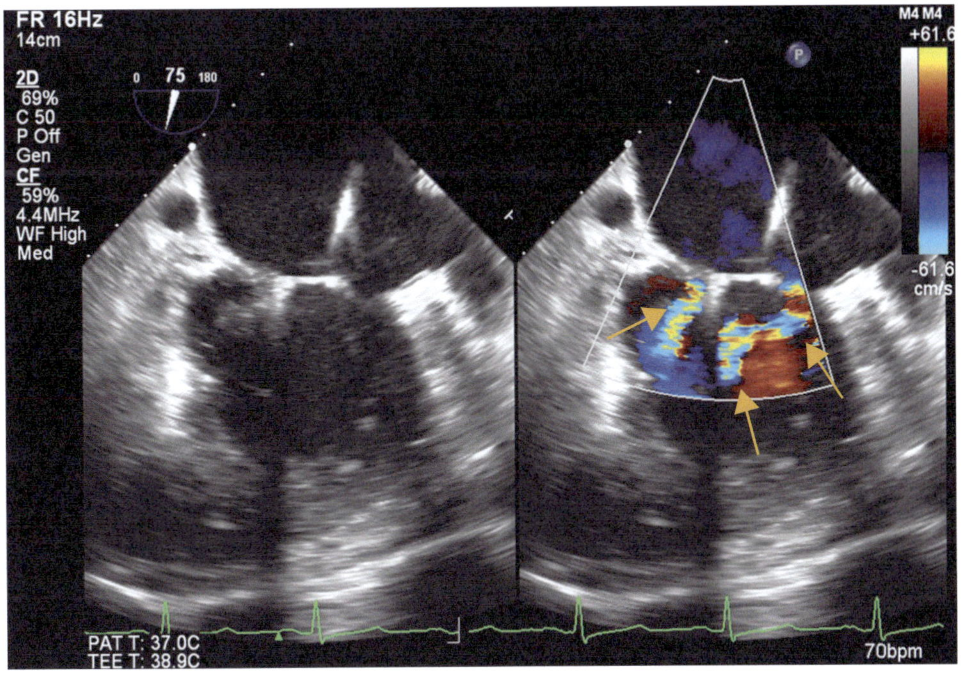

Figs. 19.23, 19.24, 19.25, 19.26, and 19.27 (continued)

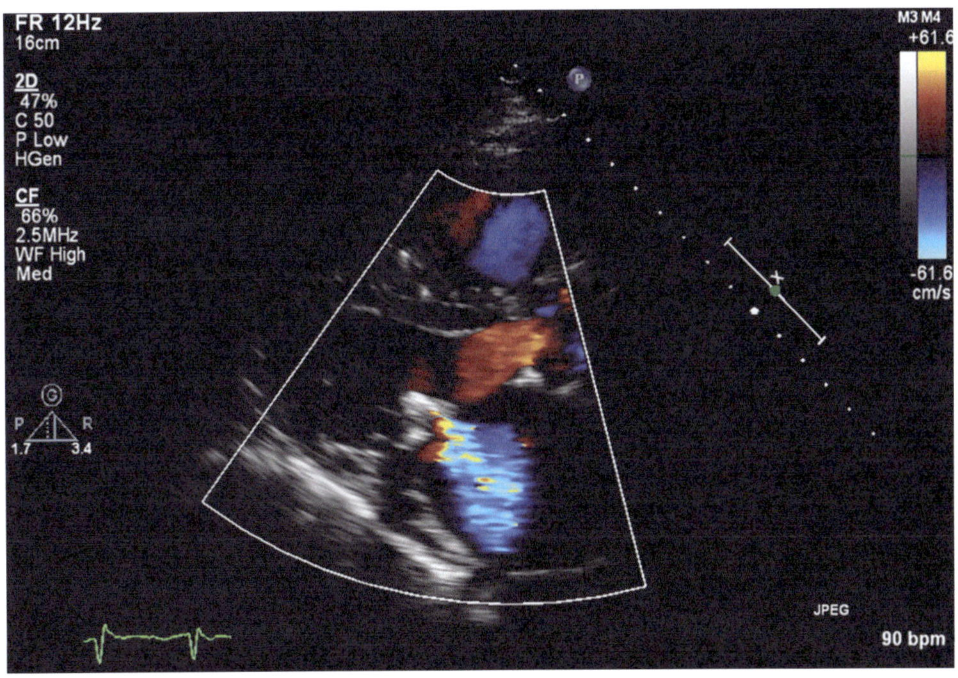

Fig. 19.28 Transthoracic parasternal long axis view showing a MitraClip device in place with at least a moderate degree of mitral regurgitation

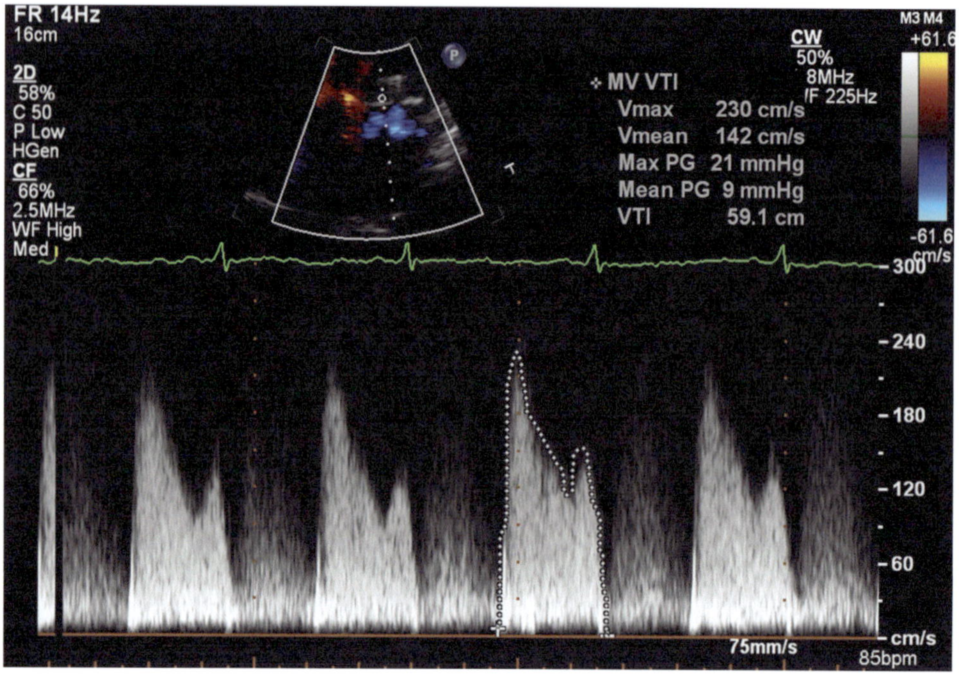

Fig. 19.29 Continuous wave Doppler across the mitral valve in the presence of two MitraClips. It is uncertain which of the three orifices of the mitral valve the Doppler signal is crossing, but there appears to be an increased mean gradient across the valve of 9 mmHg suggestive of at least moderate mitral stenosis

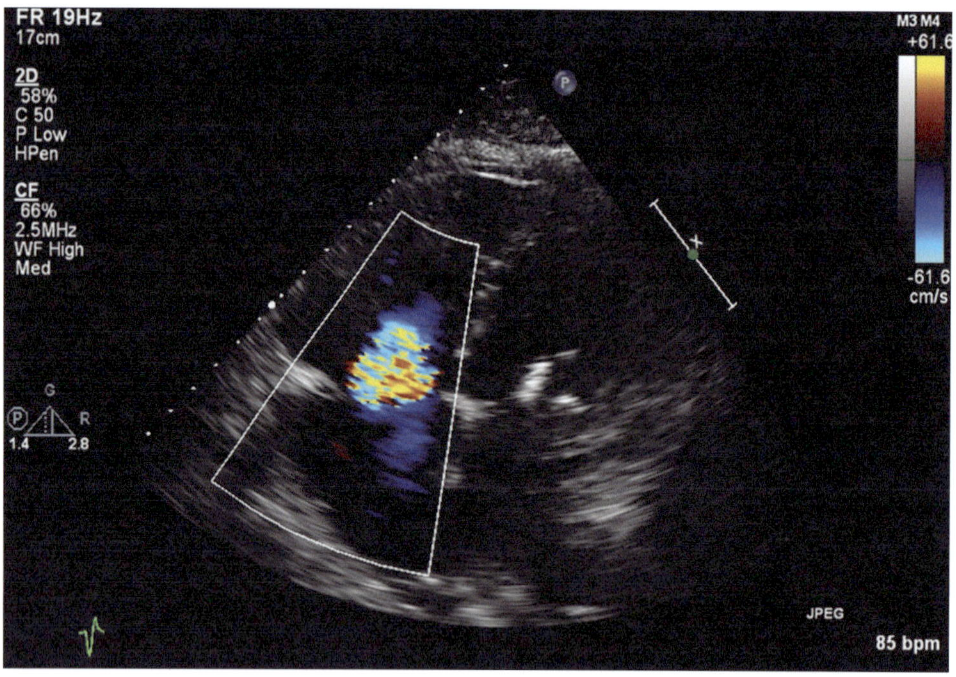

Fig. 19.30 Apical four-chamber view showing severe tricuspid regurgitation on color Doppler across the tricuspid valve

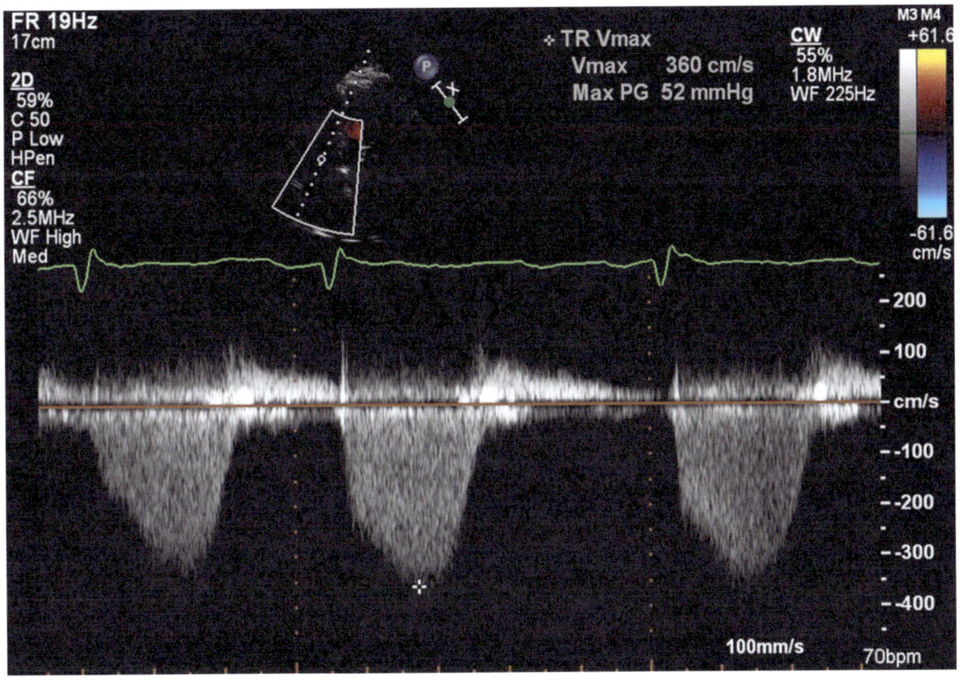

Fig. 19.31 Continuous wave Doppler across the tricuspid valve showing a peak systolic gradient of 52 mmHg suggestive of significant pulmonary arterial hypertension

Infective Endocarditis Associated with the MitraClip

20

Ali Vazir, Olaf Franzen, Neil Eric Moat, and Susanna Price

Abstract

This case describes a patient who had been treated with the MitraClip for severe degenerative mitral regurgitation. He then developed infective endocarditis of the mitral valve associated with the MitraClip more than a year after the index procedure. This was complicated by systemic embolization from the endocarditis

Keywords

Mitral regurgitation • MItraClip • Infective endocarditis

Clinical History

A 67-year-old man with previous bioprosthetic aortic valve replacement for severe aortic regurgitation presented with exertional breathlessness (NYHA III). His echocardiogram confirmed severe mitral regurgitation (4+) secondary to flail A2 segment of the anterior mitral valve leaflet. He underwent coronary angiography as part of his workup. This had shown a significant stenosis in the left circumflex artery, for which he underwent PCI. Despite this, his symptoms persisted. In view of his comorbidities, he was referred for percutaneous edge-to-edge repair with the MitraClip.

Figures 20.1, 20.2, and 20.3 demonstrate the original pathology with severe mitral regurgitation (4+), which was repaired using a single MitraClip placed at A2/P2 (see Fig. 20.4), resulting in significant reduction in the severity of mitral regurgitation (1+) and improvement in symptoms.

Fourteen months later, he developed pain within his left calf pain at rest, and he presented to his local hospital. He was found to have weak left-sided pedal and popliteal pulses, which on CT angiography confirmed blocked left-sided distal popliteal artery. A trans-thoracic echocardiogram was performed at his local hospital that showed a highly mobile mass measuring 1 cm associated with the MitraClip and the mitral valve with worsening of the mitral regurgitation (see Figs. 20.5, 20.6, 20.7, 20.8, 20.9, 20.10, 20.11, 20.12 and Videos 20.1, 20.2, 20.3, 20.4, 20.5, 20.6, 20.7, 20.8). The clip appeared to remain in position.

A. Vazir, MBBS, MRCP, CCDS, Ph.D. (✉)
Department of Cardiology, Royal Brompton Hospital,
Royal Brompton and Harefield NHS Foundation Trust,
Sydney Street, London SW3 6NP, UK

Department of Cardiology, Royal Brompton Hospital, National Heart and Lung Institute, Imperial College, London, UK
e-mail: a.vazir@rbht.nhs.uk, ali.vazir@btinternet.com

O. Franzen, M.D.
Department of Cardiology, The Heart Center, Rigshospitalet,
University of Copenhagen,
Blegdamsvej 9, Copenhagen 2100, Denmark

Royal Brompton Hospital, Royal Brompton and Harefield NHS Foundation Trust, London, UK
e-mail: owfranzen@gmx.de

N.E. Moat, MBBS, MS., FRCS
Department of Cardiac Surgery,
Head of Trans-catheter valve programme, Royal Brompton Hospital,
Sydney Street, London, SW3 6NP, UK
e-mail: n.moat@rbht.nhs.uk

S. Price, MBBS, BSc, MRCP, EDICM, Ph.D., FFICM, FESC
Department of Cardiology, Royal Brompton Hospital,
Sydney Street, London, SW3 6NP, UK
e-mail: s.price@rbht.nhs.uk

Electronic supplementary material The online version of this chapter (doi:10.1007/978-1-4471-4294-2_20) contains supplementary material, which is available to authorized users.

T. Feldman et al. (eds.), *Atlas of Percutaneous Edge-to-Edge Mitral Valve Repair*,
DOI 10.1007/978-1-4471-4294-2_20, © Springer-Verlag London 2013

The patient reported malaise and had a documented temperature with evidence of inflammation (CRP 280, anemia Hb 10 g/dL, white blood cell count 15). Blood cultures revealed alpha-hemolytic streptococcal bacteremia. He was treated with intravenous antibiotics, but despite this, he developed further pains within his buttocks and contralateral calf. Repeat trans-thoracic echocardiography showed that the large mobile mass had disappeared, with a smaller mass associated with the MitraClip (see Figs. 20.13, 20.14, 20.15 and Videos 20.9, 20.10, 20.11), which remained in position. Transesophageal echocardiography demonstrated multiple small masses on the anterior and posterior mitral valve leaflets in the vicinity of the MitraClip (see Figs. 20.16, 20.17, 20.18, 20.19, 20.20, 20.21 and Videos 20.12, 20.13, 20.14, 20.15, 20.16, 20.17), with partial destruction of the anterior mitral valve leaflet, and an increase in the severity of mitral regurgitation.

The case was discussed at the multidisciplinary meeting, regarding high-risk mitral valve replacement surgery for infective endocarditis versus conservative treatment that would involve life-long antibiotics, as the infection would unlikely to be eradicated completely by a 6-week course of intravenous antibiotics alone. The patient remains under review with serial echocardiography.

Learning Points

1. Patients undergoing edge-to-edge repair with the MitraClip device have increased risk of infective endocarditis, similar to those with a valve replacement. They should receive periprocedural antibiotic prophylaxis and should also receive antibiotic prophylaxis prior to dental and other invasive procedures.
2. The risk of endocarditis early post-clip is unknown but is expected to decrease with time as the clip becomes endothelialized.
3. The optimal strategy for management of mitral valve endocarditis in patients who have undergone MitraClip procedure remains unclear but would likely be best approached on a case-by-case basis.

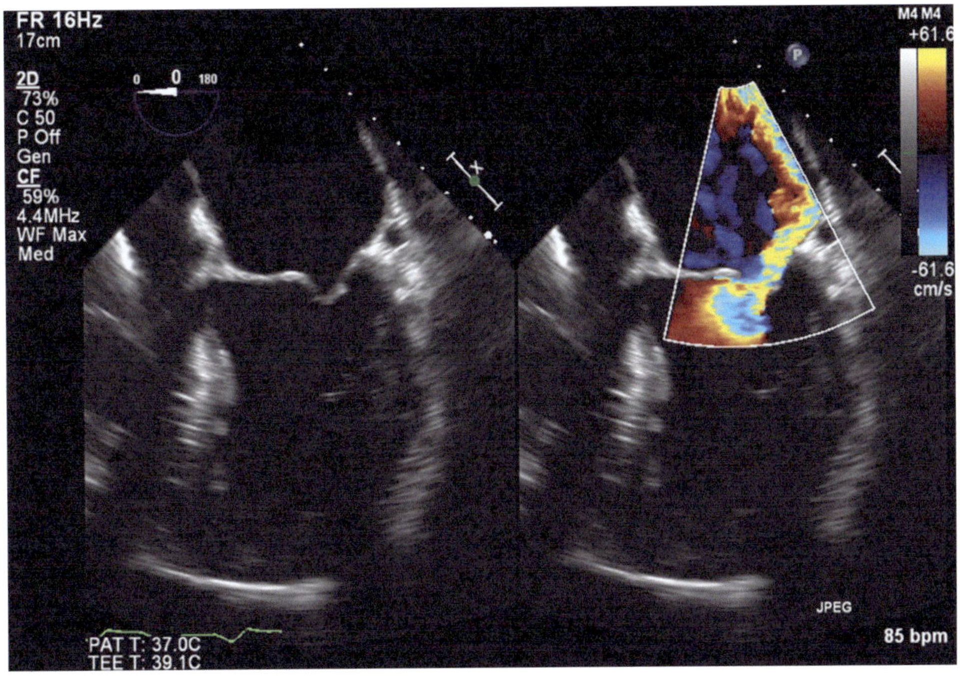

Fig. 20.1 Transesophageal four-chamber view showing prolapsed A2 segment of the anterior mitral valve with severe mitral regurgitation with a posteriorly directed jet

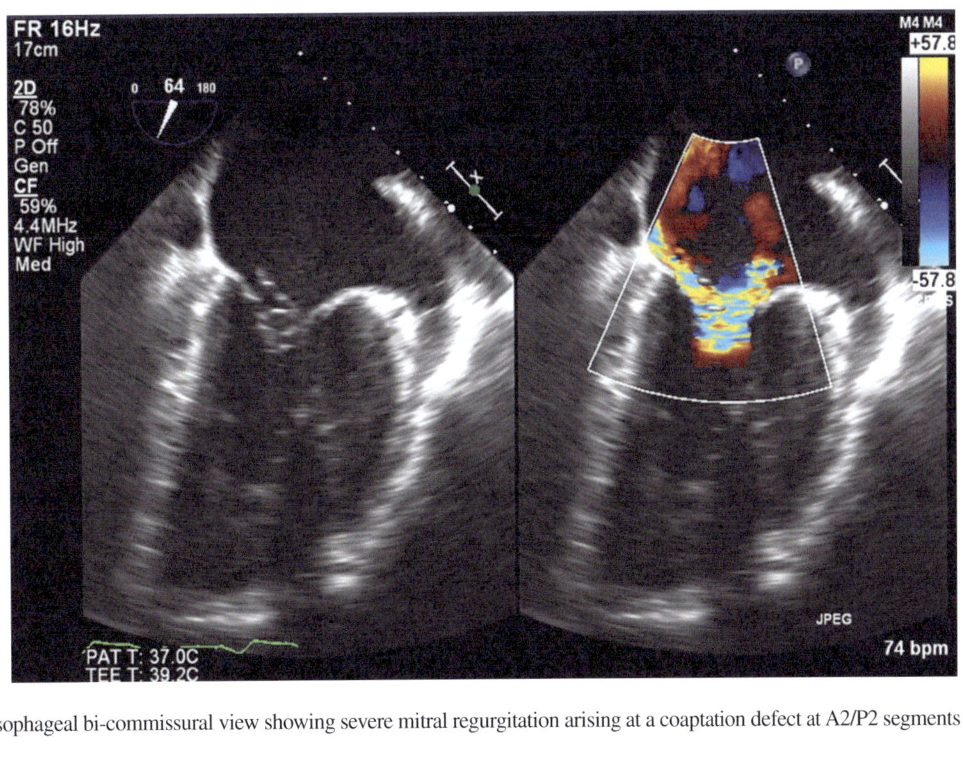

Fig. 20.2 Transesophageal bi-commissural view showing severe mitral regurgitation arising at a coaptation defect at A2/P2 segments of the mitral valve

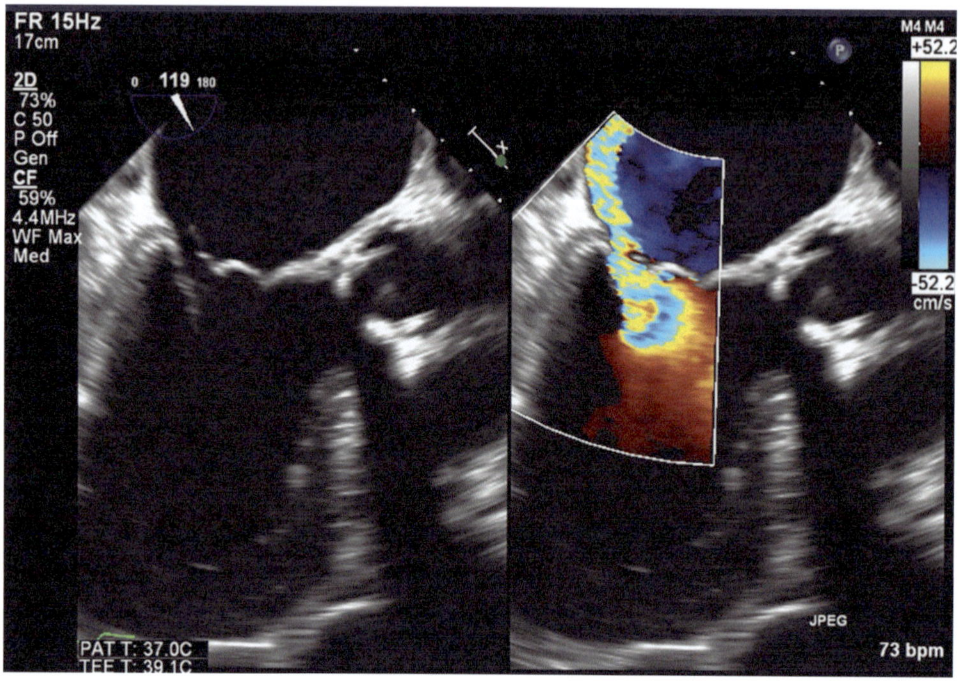

Fig. 20.3 Transesophageal LVOT view showing flail A2 segment of the anterior mitral valve with severe mitral regurgitation with a posteriorly directed jet

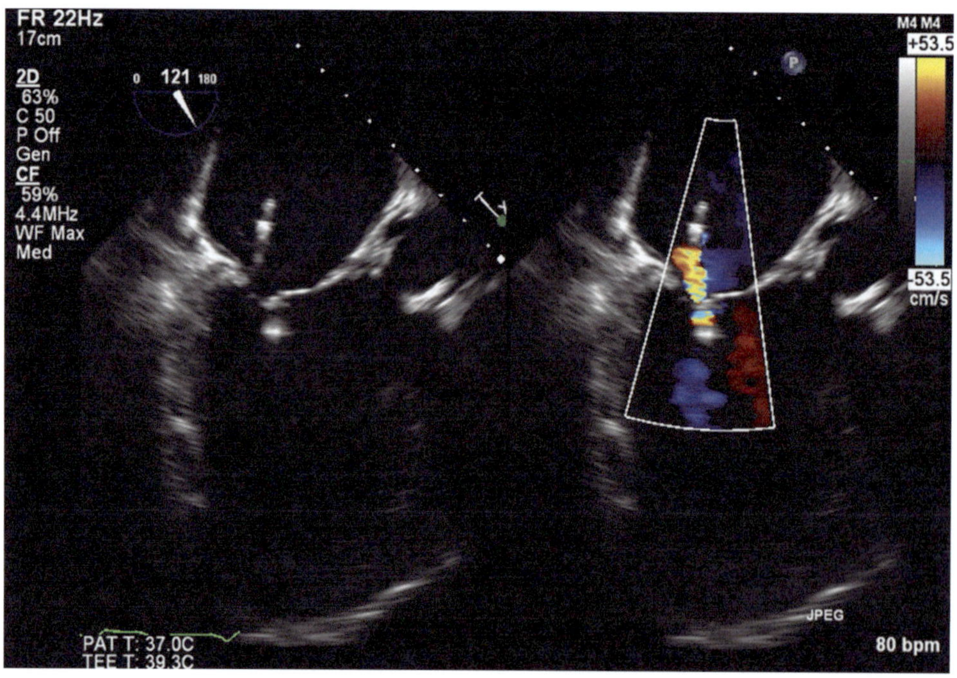

Fig. 20.4 Transesophageal long axis view showing MitraClip positioned at A2/P2 with significant reduction in mitral regurgitation and a mild degree of residual regurgitation

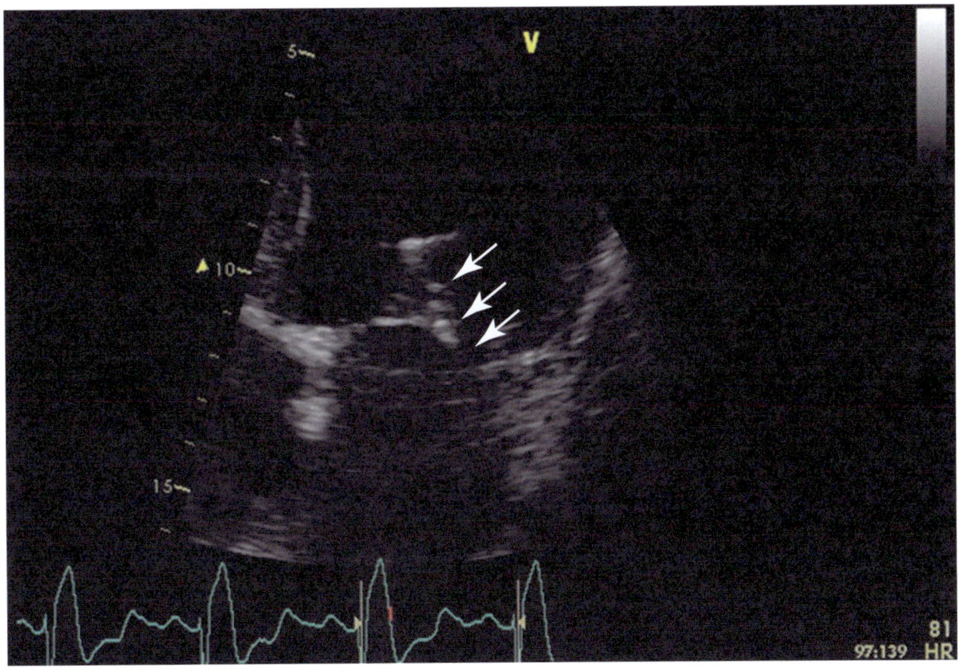

Fig. 20.5 Trans-thoracic apical four-chamber view zoomed on the mitral valve. The clip is seen and is associated with a highly mobile mass suggestive of a vegetation. The mass appears to pass in and out of view in a posterior direction. (*V*) left ventricle

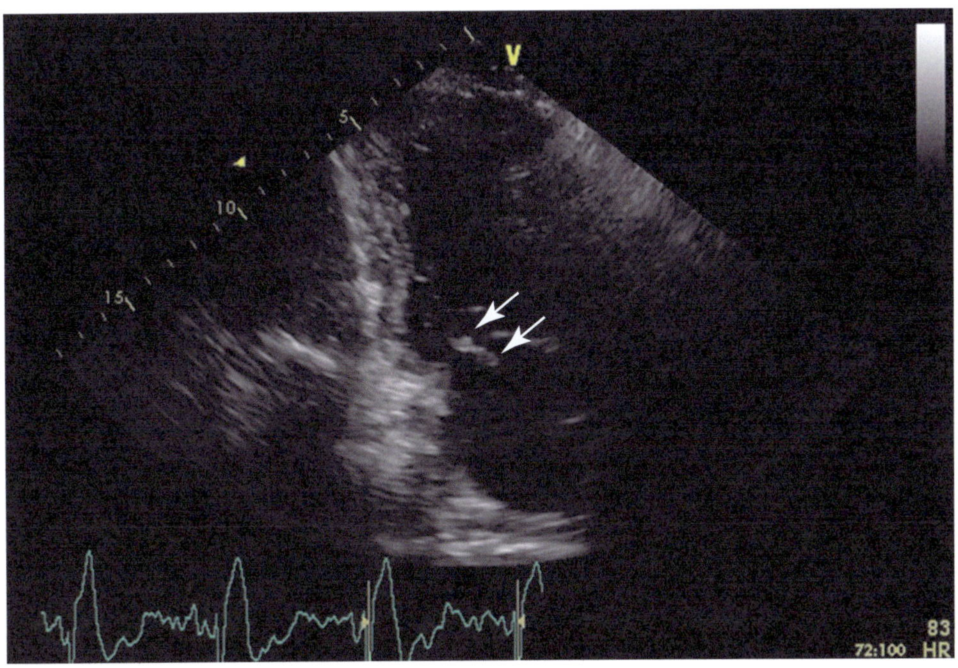

Fig. 20.6 Trans-thoracic apical two-chamber view. The MitraClip is seen and is associated with a highly mobile mass suggestive of a vegetation. The mass appears to pass in and out of view. (*V*) left ventricle

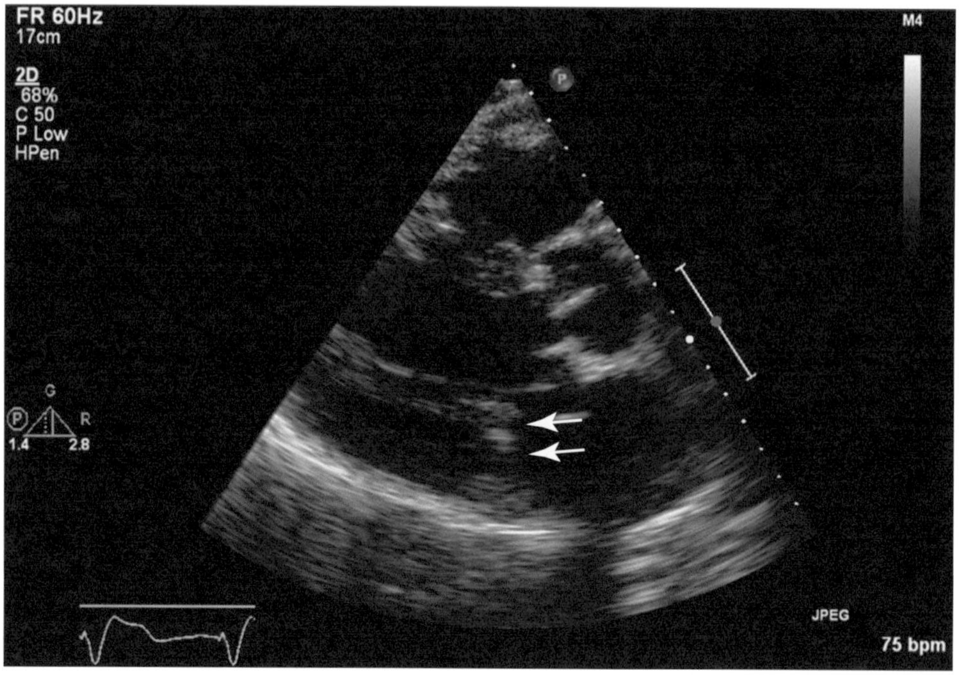

Fig. 20.7 Trans-thoracic parasternal long axis view. The clip is seen and is associated with a highly mobile mass (*arrows*) suggestive of a vegetation. The mass appears to pass in and out of view in a posterior direction

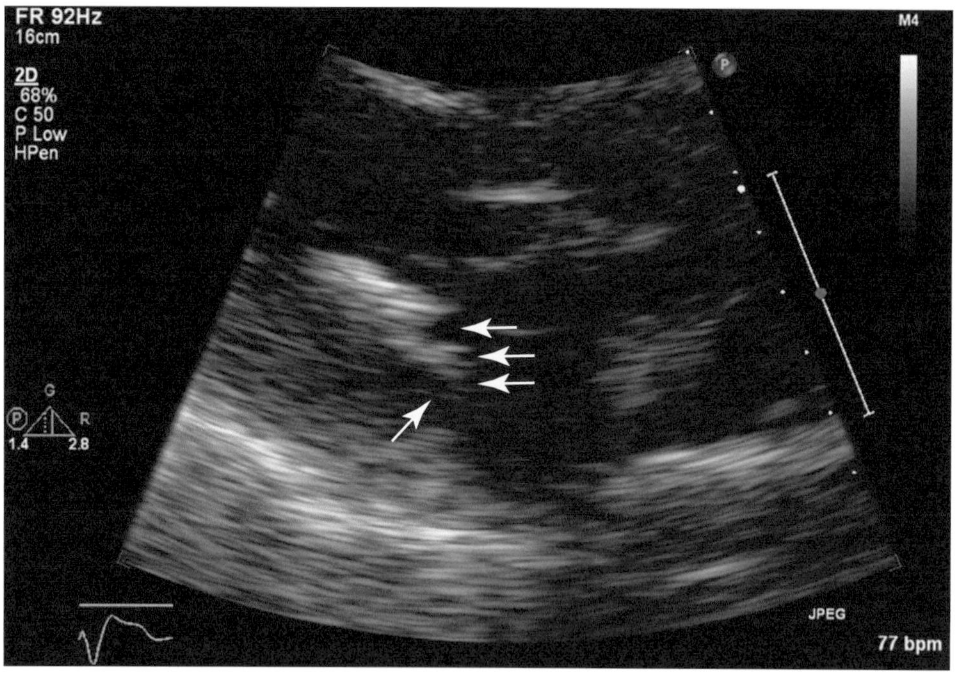

Fig. 20.8 Zooms in on the mitral valve, clip, and the mass seen in Fig. 20.7 (*arrows*)

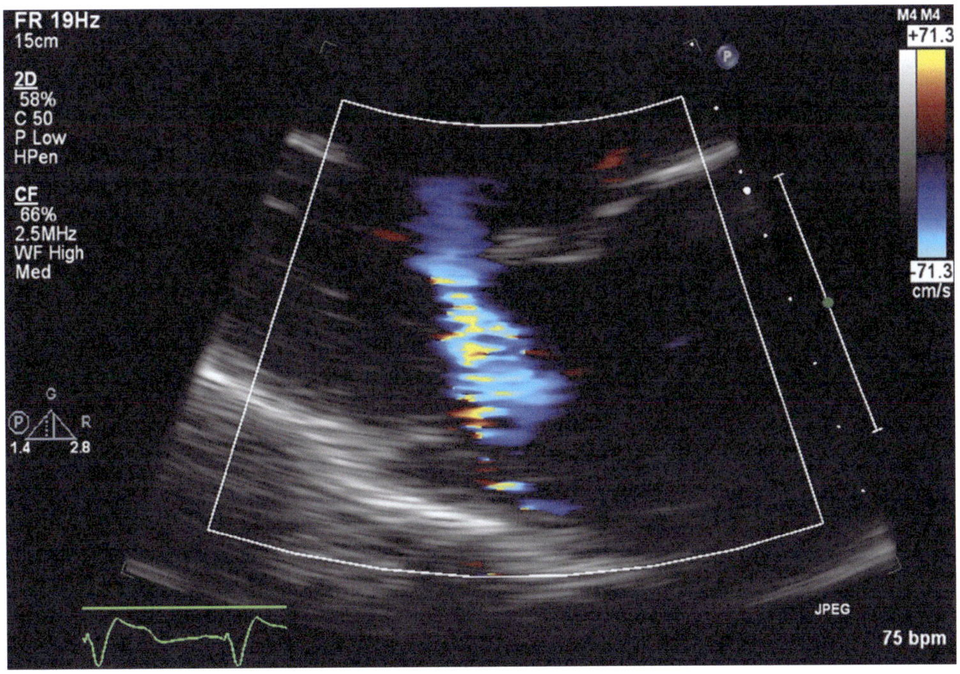

Fig. 20.9 Trans-thoracic parasternal long axis view. The clip is seen and is associated with at least moderate degree of mitral regurgitation with a posteriorly directed jet

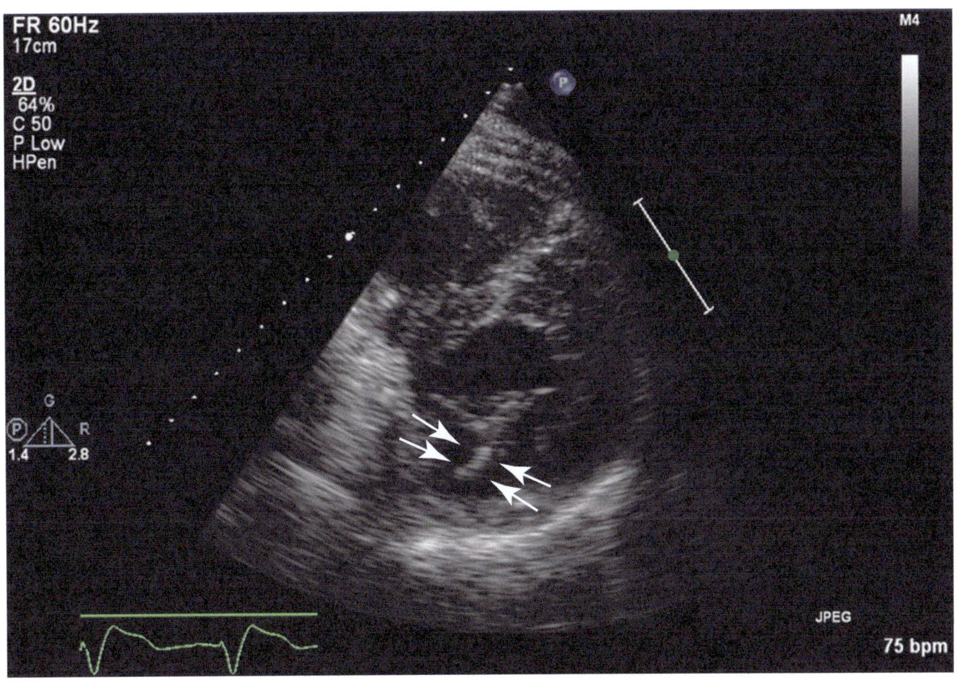

Fig. 20.10 Trans-thoracic parasternal short axis view at the mitral valve level. The clip is seen at central aspect of the mitral valve and is associated with a highly mobile mass suggestive of a vegetation (*arrows*). The mass appears to flick in and out of view in a posterior direction

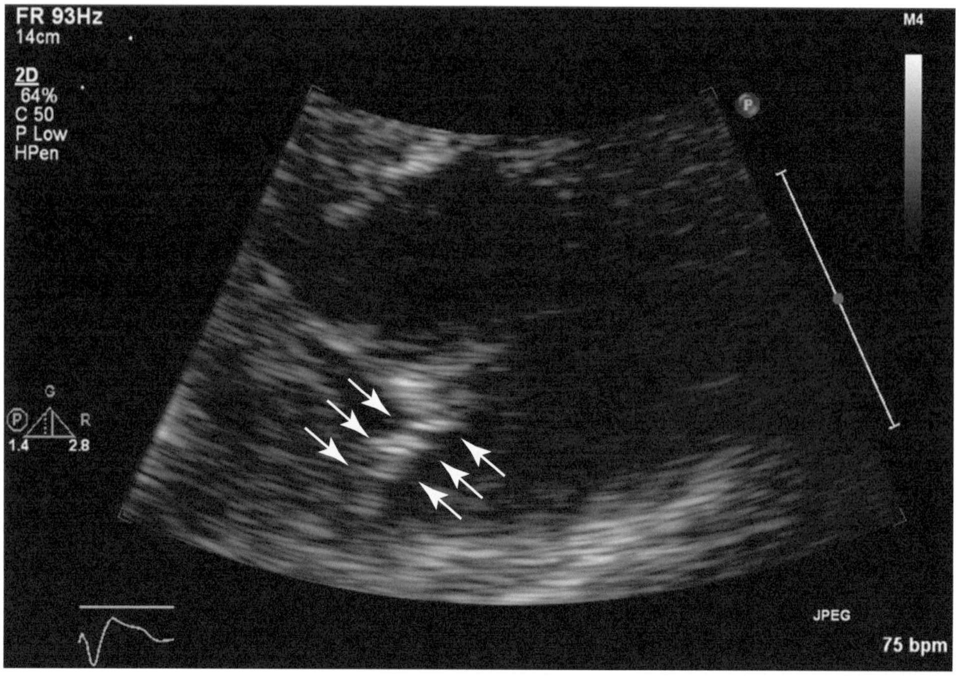

Fig. 20.11 Zooms in on the mitral valve and the mass (*arrows*) seen in Fig. 20.10

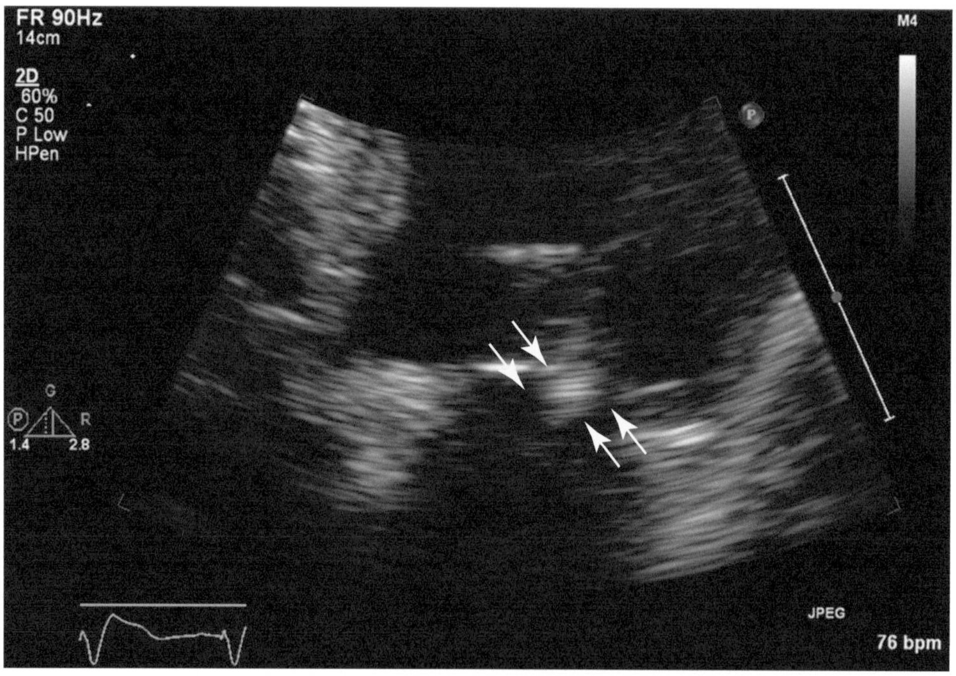

Fig. 20.12 Trans-thoracic apical four-chamber view zoomed on the mitral valve. The clip is seen and is associated with a highly mobile mass suggestive of a vegetation (*arrows*)

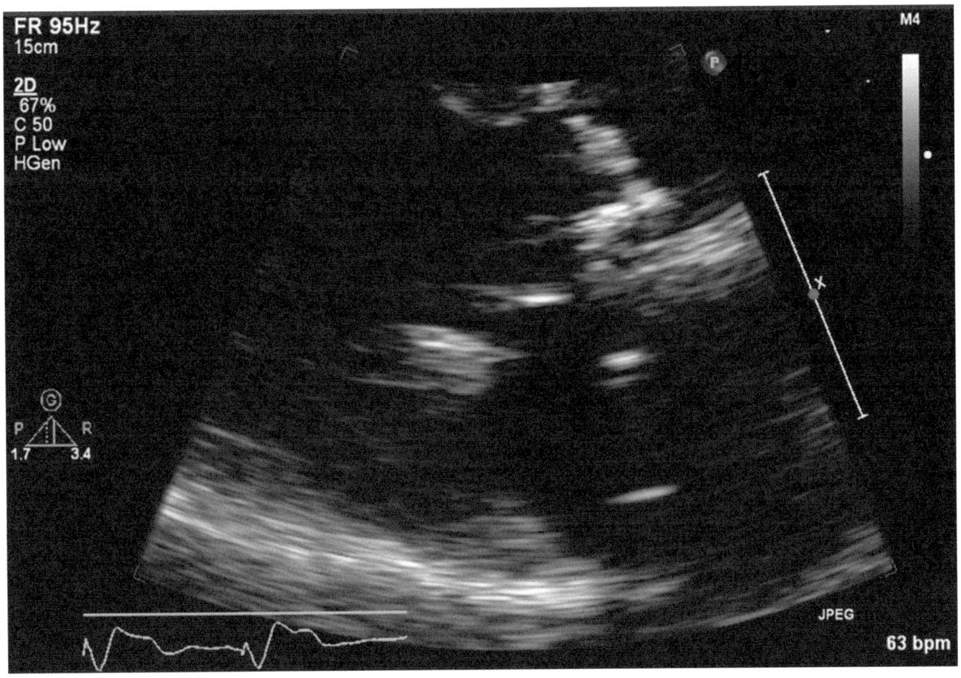

Fig. 20.13 Trans-thoracic parasternal long axis view. The clip is seen, but the large mass is no longer present

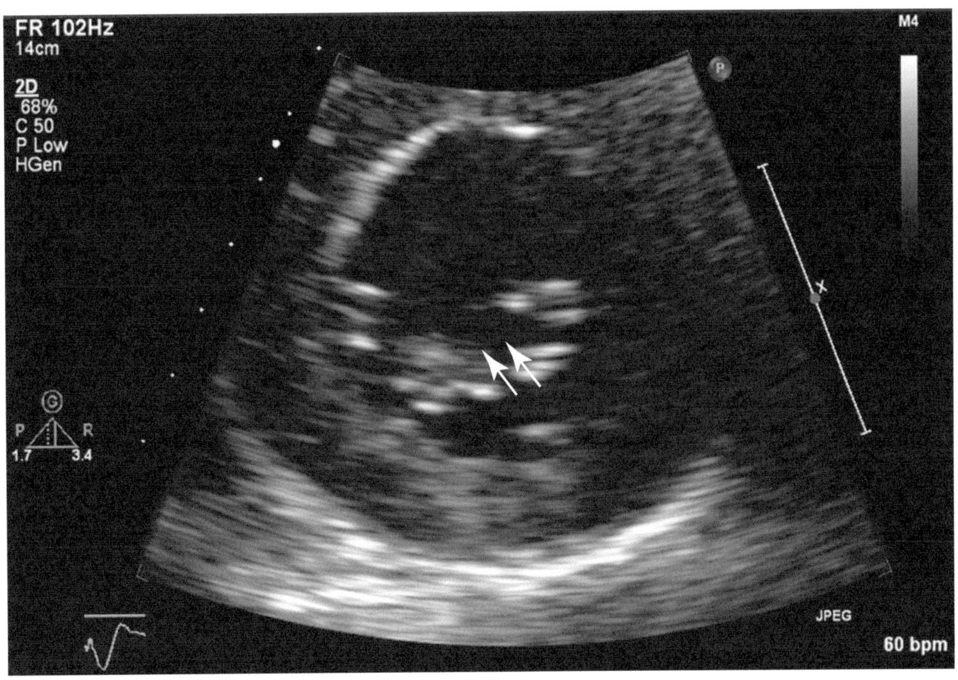

Fig. 20.14 Trans-thoracic parasternal short axis view at the mitral valve level. The clip is seen, but the large mass seen in previous figures is not present, suggesting possible embolization. On close inspection, a small mobile mass is visible in association with the MitraClip on the posterior leaflet of the mitral valve (*arrows*)

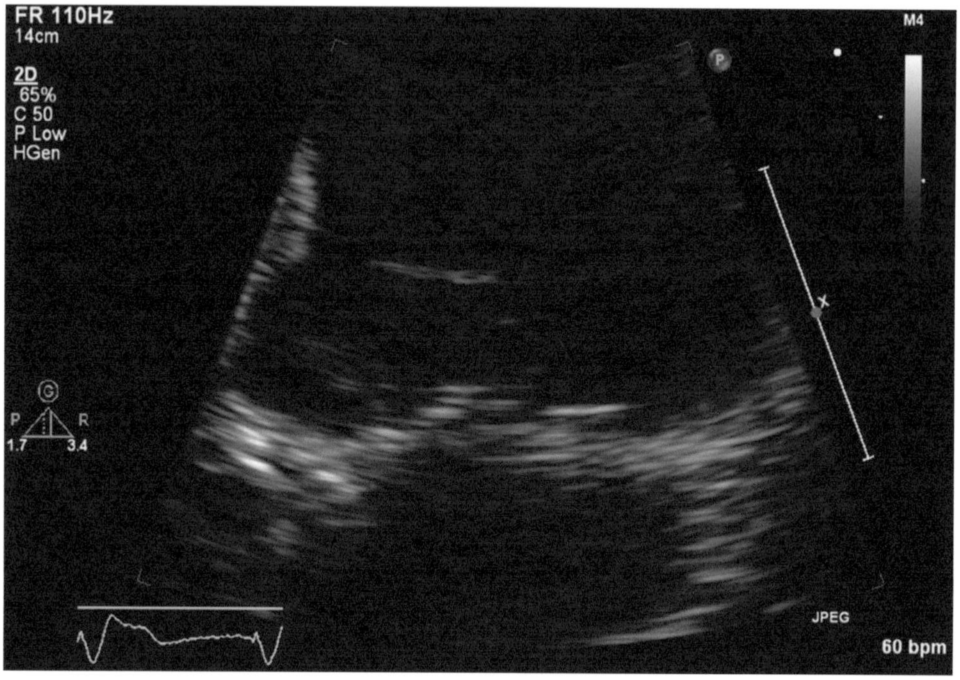

Fig. 20.15 Trans-thoracic apical four-chamber view zoomed on the mitral valve. The clip is seen and is associated with a small mobile mass as oppose to a large mass seen on the previous figures

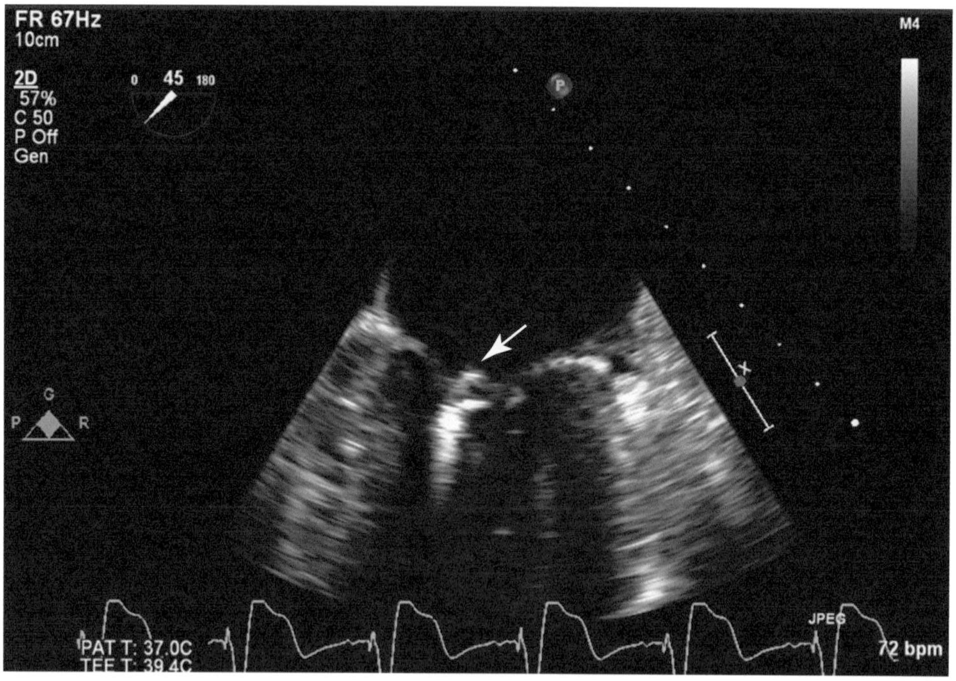

Fig. 20.16 Transesophageal modified bi-commissural view at 45° showing MitraClip at A2/P2 position. There is a small mobile mass (*arrow*) associated with the clip on the atrial surface

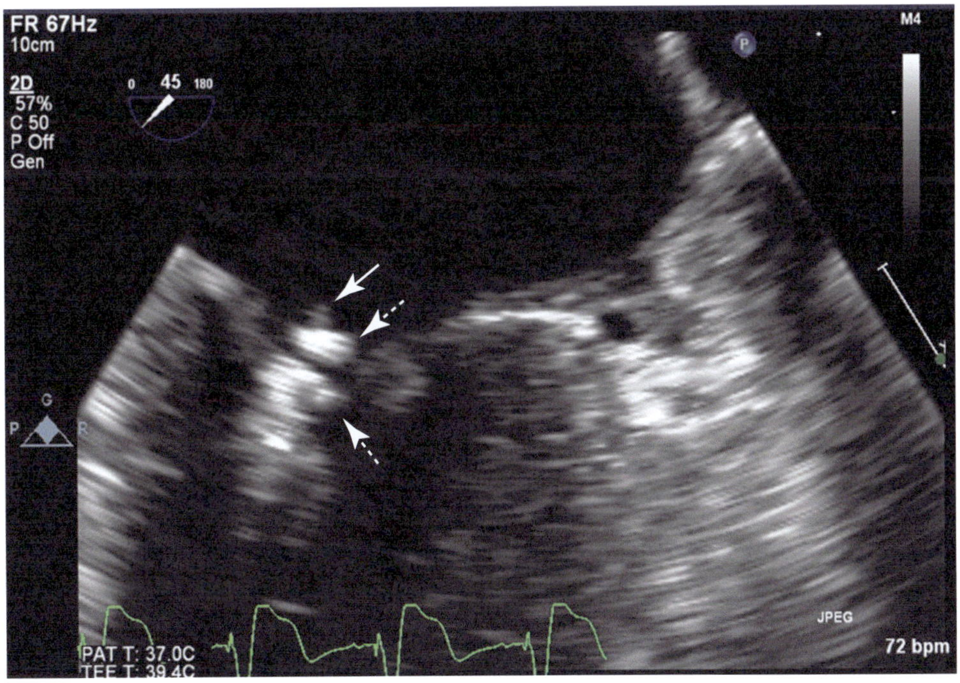

Fig. 20.17 Transesophageal modified bi-commissural view at 45° zoomed in on the mitral valve and showing the MitraClip at A2/P2 position. There is a small mobile mass (*solid arrow*) and two larger calcified mobile masses (*broken arrow*) associated with the clip on the atrial surface of the clip and mitral valve. The presence of *broken arrow* will help differentiate between small mobile mass and the larger calcified masses. This is easier to seen on the video clips of these still images

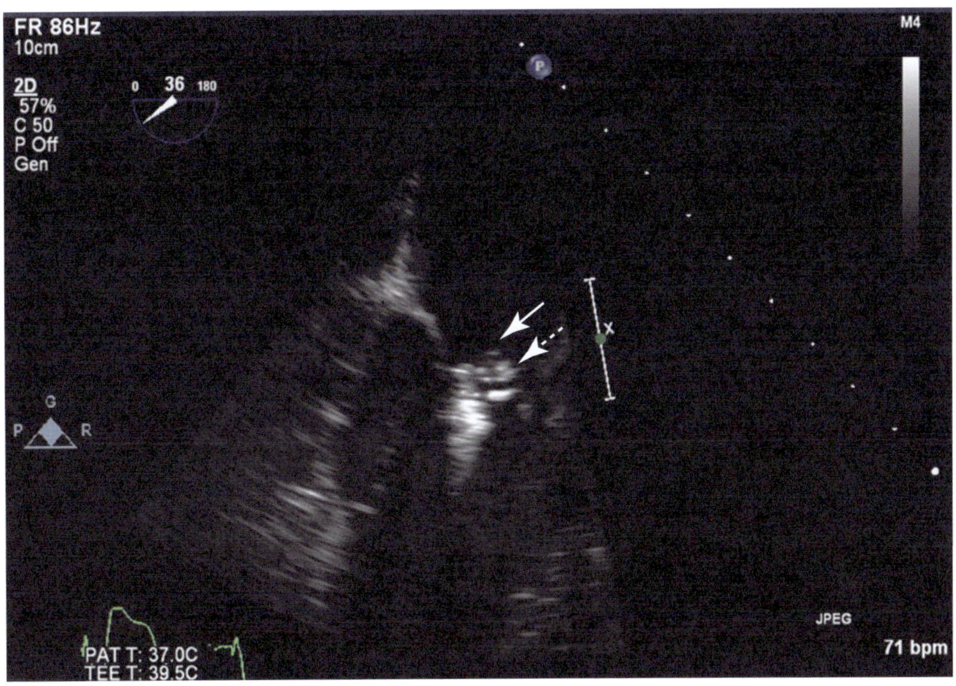

Fig. 20.18 Transesophageal modified bi-commissural view at 36° showing MitraClip at A2/P2 position. There is a small mobile mass (*solid arrow*) and larger calcified mobile mass (*broken arrow*) associated with the clip on the atrial surface of the mitral valve

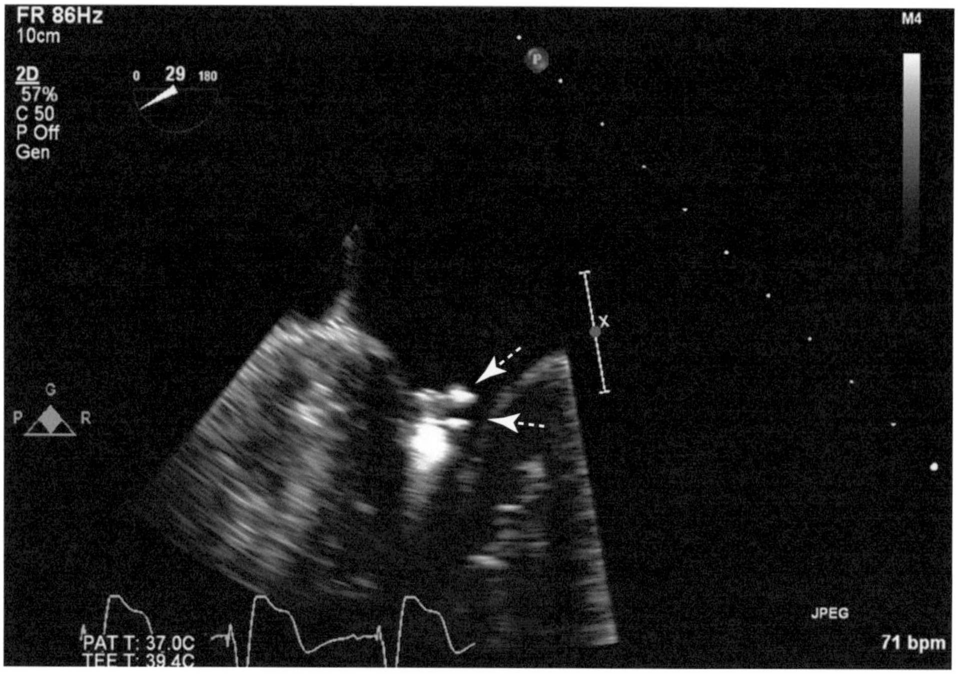

Fig. 20.19 Transesophageal modified bi-commissural view at 29° zoomed in on the mitral valve showing the MitraClip positioned A2/P2 associated with two large (*broken arrows*) mobile calcified masses

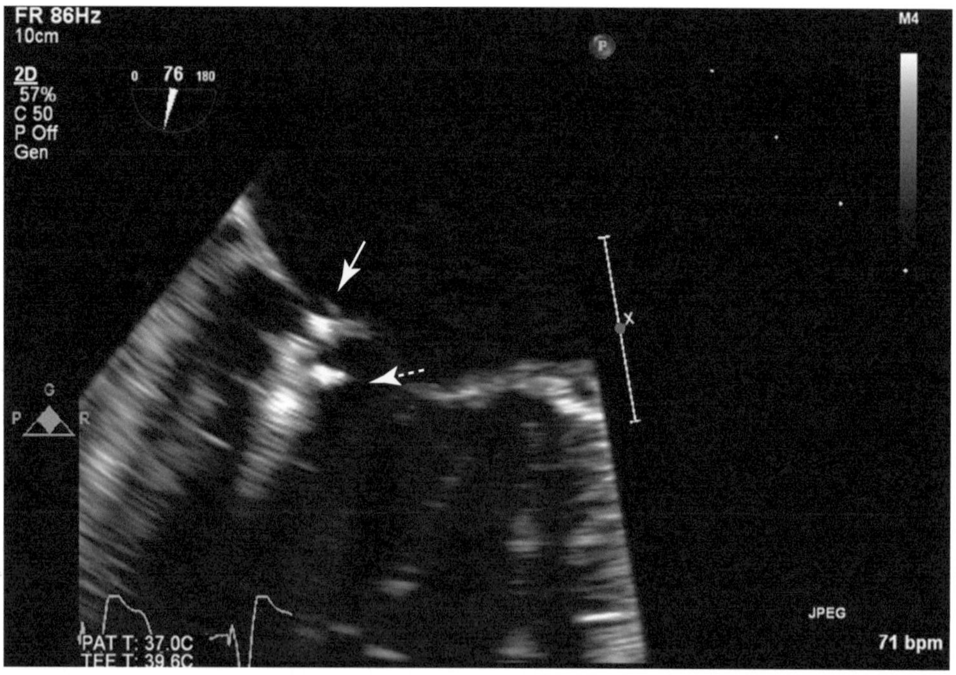

Fig. 20.20 Transesophageal modified bi-commissural view at 76° zoomed in on the mitral valve showing MitraClip at A2/P2 position. There is a small mobile mass (*solid arrow*) and a larger mobile calcified mobile mass (*broken arrow*) associated with the clip on the atrial surface of the clip and the mitral valve

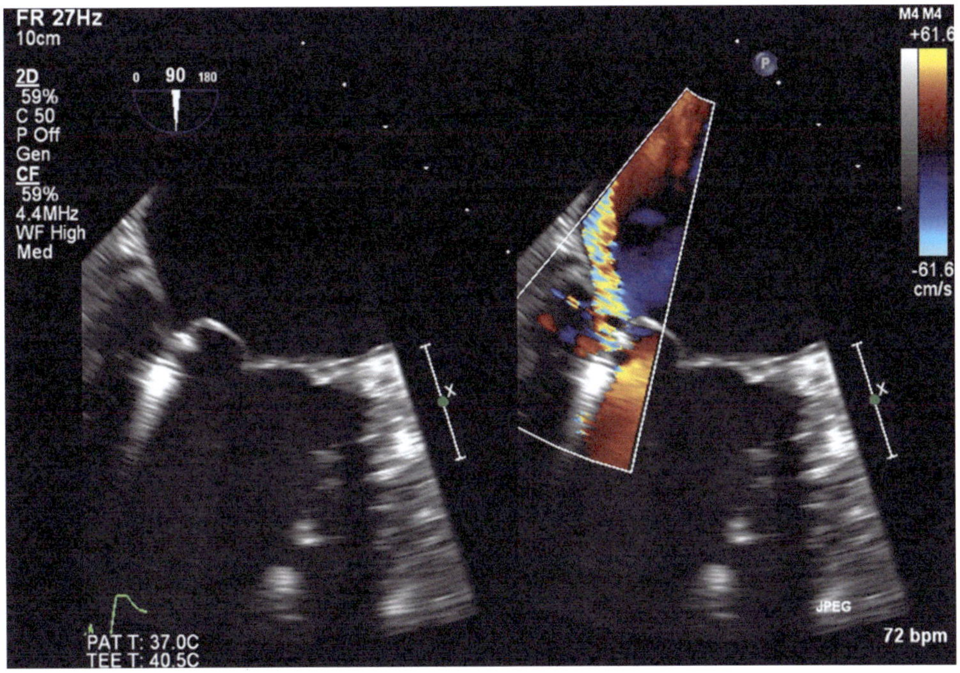

Fig. 20.21 Transesophageal two-chamber view at 90° showing MitraClip at A2/P2 position, with a degree of prolapse of the anterior leaflet resulting in at least moderate regurgitant jet passing posteriorly and hugging the posterior aspect of the atrial wall

EVEREST II MitraClip After Failed Surgical Mitral Valve Repair

21

Scott Lim

Abstract
This case demonstrates the use of the MitraClip to successfully repair severe mitral regurgitation in a patient with prior mitral annuloplasty ring repair. The annuloplasty ring complicated the procedure by causing shadowing artifacts and by limiting movement of the clip. The case also illustrates how transthoracic and intracardiac echocardiography can complement transesophageal echo in the MitraClip procedure.

Keywords
Mitral regurgitation • MitraClip • Annuloplasty ring • Intracardiac echo

Clinical History

A 76-year-old man presented with NYHA Class IV heart failure. He had a history of an ischemic cardiomyopathy with severe functional mitral regurgitation and previously underwent coronary bypass grafting and mitral valve repair with a Medtronic-Duran flexible annuloplasty ring 10 years previously. His course had been complicated by worsening heart failure over the previous 6 months, along with diminishing renal function (estimated glomerular filtration rate of 32 ml/min). His mammary graft and one of his vein grafts remained patent. He also had a history of moderate lung disease with severe pulmonary hypertension and was turned down for repeat cardiac surgery.

S. Lim, M.D.
Department of Cardiology, University of Virginia Medical Center, 1215 Lee Street, Hospital Expansion, Room 4038, Charlottesville, VA 22908, USA
e-mail: sl9pc@virginia.edu

Summary

This case presents several diagnostic and procedural challenges. While the transthoracic echocardiogram demonstrated severe mitral regurgitation from a central jet, the inflow Doppler signal suggested mitral stenosis. Since the mitral orifice area below the ring was planimetered at 5.1 cm^2, it was felt that the inflow gradient was due to the increased flow from severe MR around the mitral ring. This was confirmed by a diagnostic catheterization with transseptal access to the left atrium, in which there was no late diastolic gradient. The procedure was complicated by echocardiographic shadowing from the ring, which limits the ability to visualize leaflet insertion into the MitraClip from the TEE point of view. To assist in imaging in this case, we utilized intraprocedure transthoracic imaging to complement the TEE. In subsequent cases (images shown below), we have utilized left ventricular intracardiac imaging to confirm adequate leaflet insertion. In this particular case, the patient has remained free from significant residual MR at 4 years post procedure.

Electronic supplementary material The online version of this chapter (doi:10.1007/978-1-4471-4294-2_21) contains supplementary material, which is available to authorized users.

T. Feldman et al. (eds.), *Atlas of Percutaneous Edge-to-Edge Mitral Valve Repair*,
DOI 10.1007/978-1-4471-4294-2_21, © Springer-Verlag London 2013

Learning Points

1. Transmitral gradient may overestimate the degree of mitral stenosis if severe mitral regurgitation is present.
2. Transthoracic echocardiography and intracardiac echocardiography may be useful and complement TEE in situations where imaging from TEE is affected by patient or anatomic factors.
3. The MitraClip can be safely performed in patients with a history of mitral annuloplasty ring repair.

Screening Transthoracic Echo

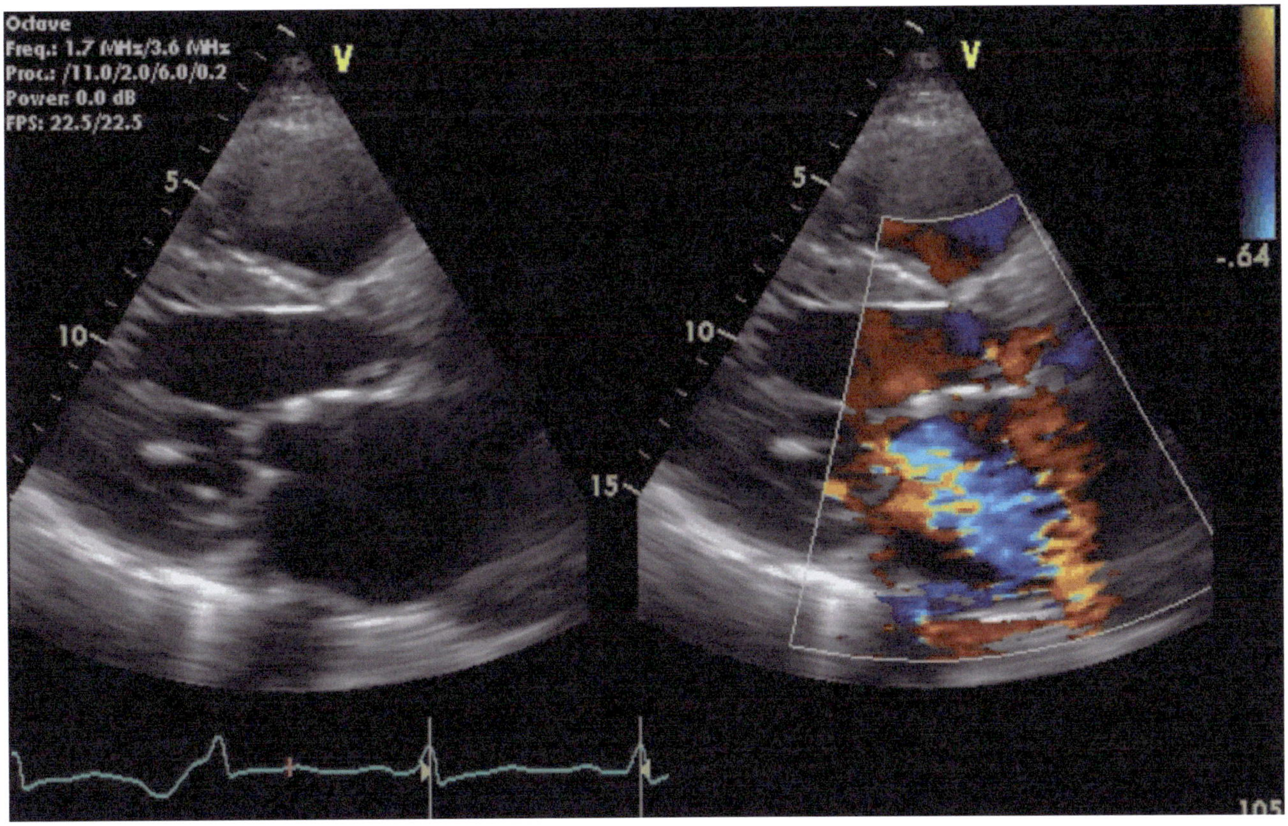

Fig. 21.1 TTE: parasternal LAX w/color. The parasternal long axis demonstrates severe mitral regurgitation with the jet filling the left atrium below the level of the annulus. The annuloplasty ring is visualized restraining the posterior annulus

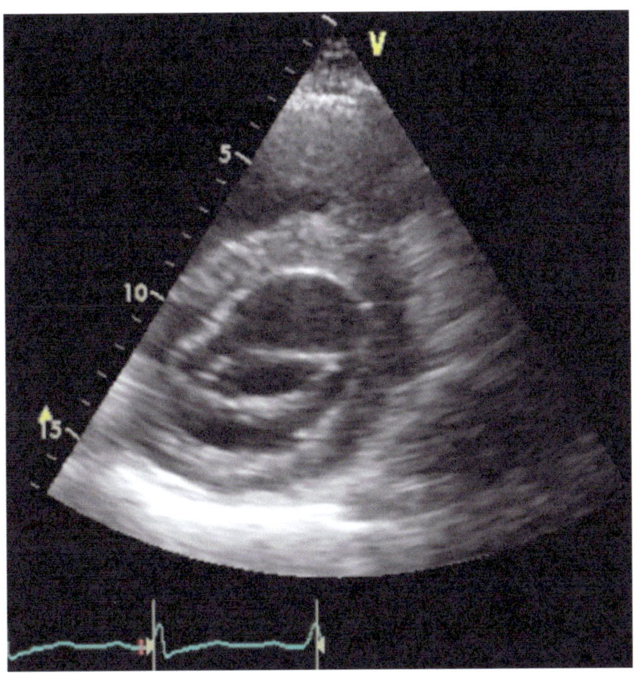

Fig. 21.2 TTE: parasternal SAX. The mitral inflow orifice area is measured by planimetry at 5.1 cm^2

Screening Transthoracic Echo

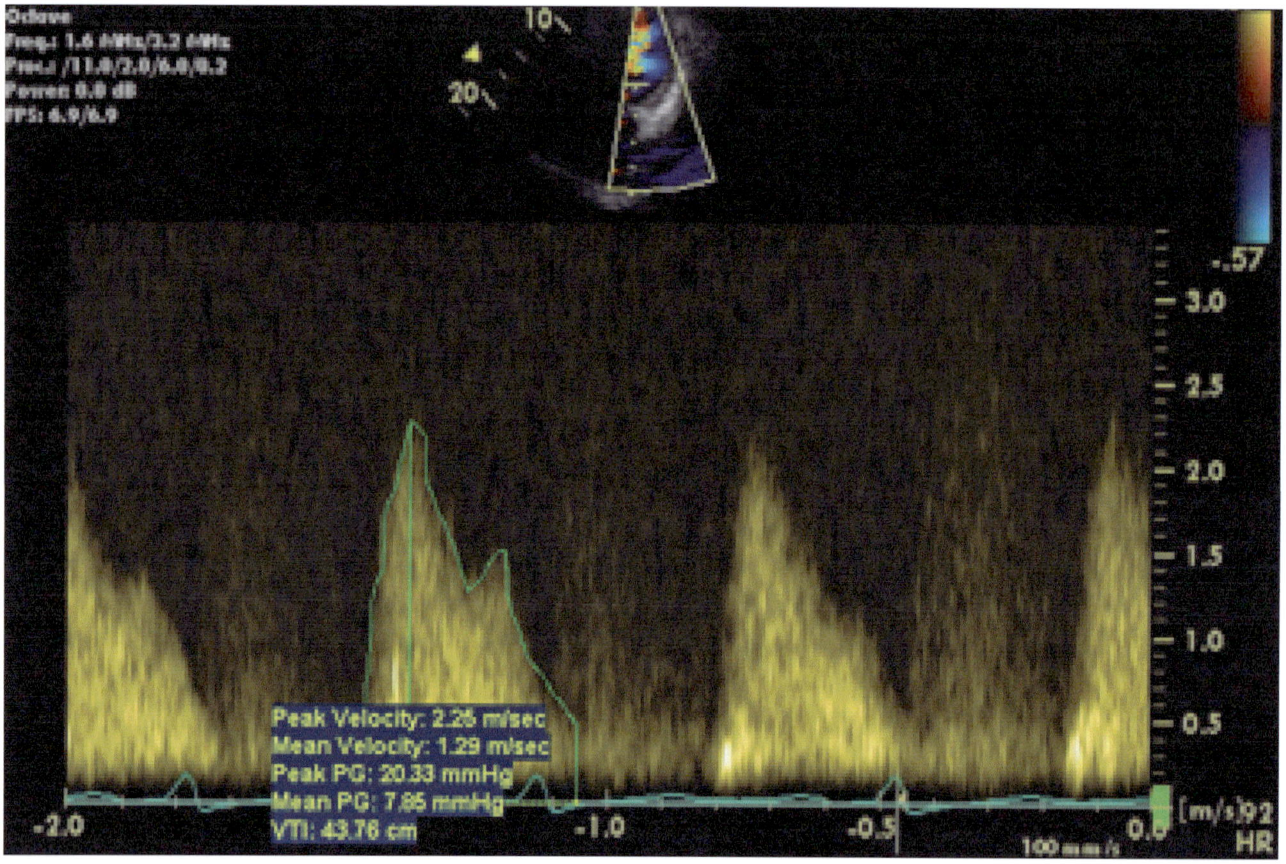

Fig. 21.3 TTE: Doppler mitral inflow. While the Doppler mean gradient across the mitral inflow predicts a mean gradient of 8 mmHg, suggesting mitral stenosis, there is a rapid E wave descent in the presence of severe mitral regurgitation

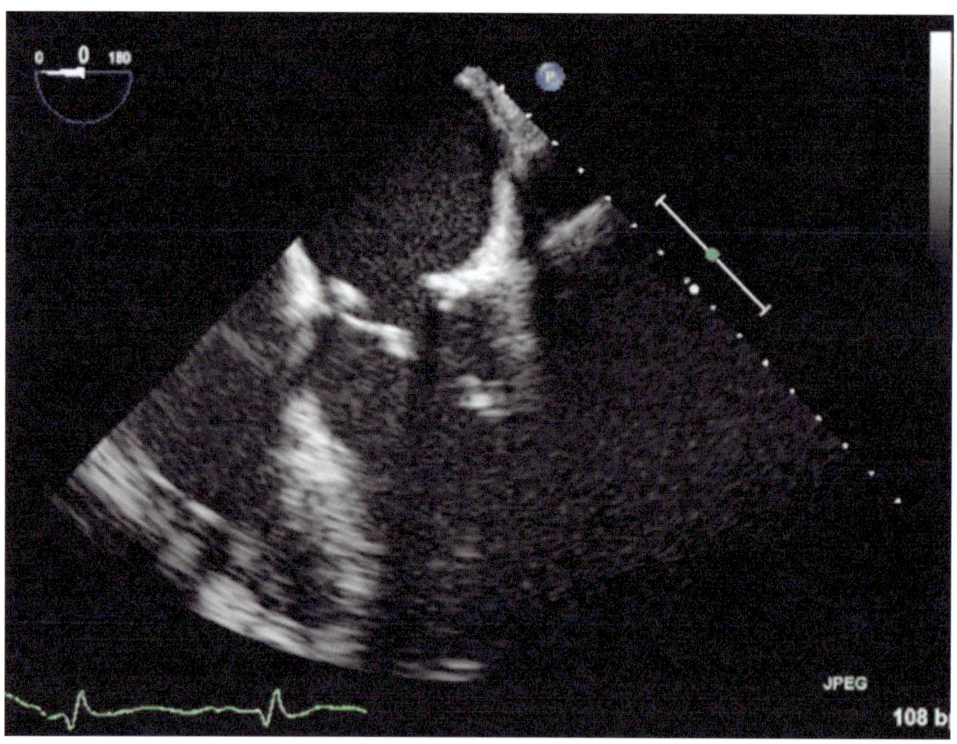

Fig. 21.4 TEE: 4C view. The four-chamber view shows shadowing from the annuloplasty ring obscuring the tips of the anterior and posterior leaflets

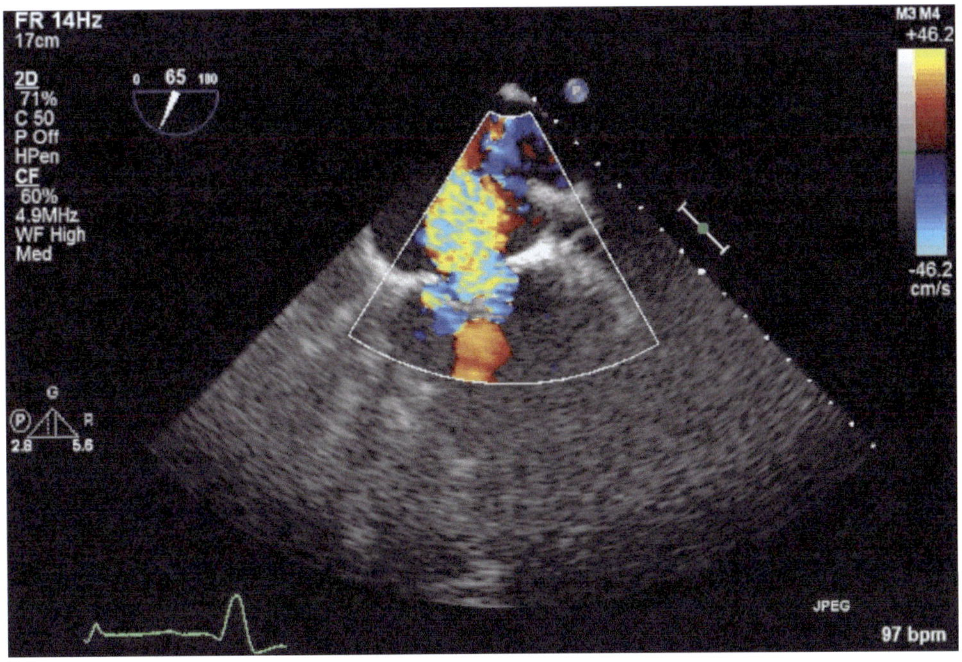

Fig. 21.5 TEE: 2C w/color. In the two-chamber view, the wide PISA is apparent, which is consistent with severe MR

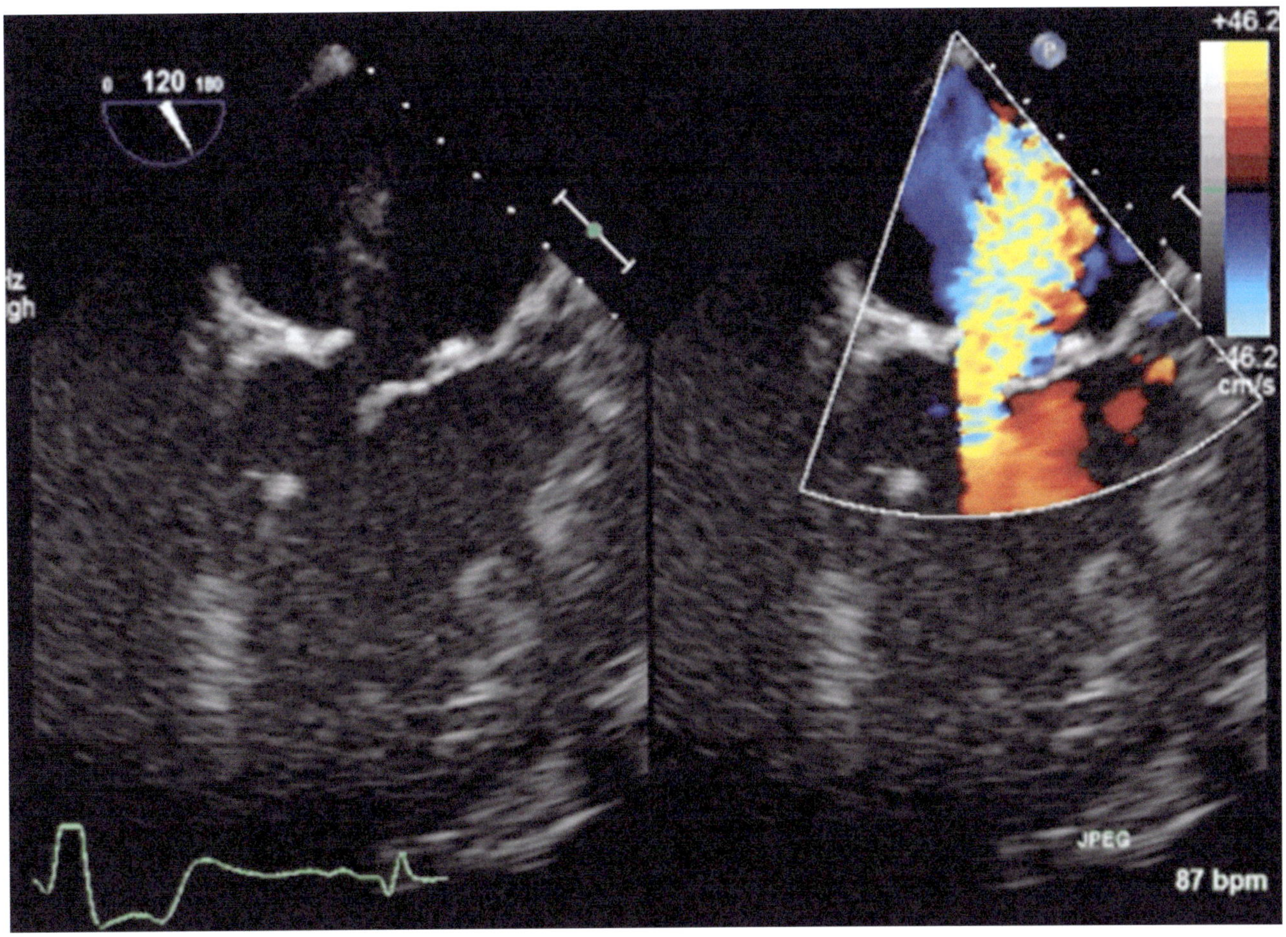

Fig. 21.6 TTE LVOT: w/color. The posterior leaflet is shadowed by the annuloplasty ring, making eventual determination of leaflet insertion into the MitraClip difficult

Intraprocedure TEE and Fluoroscopy

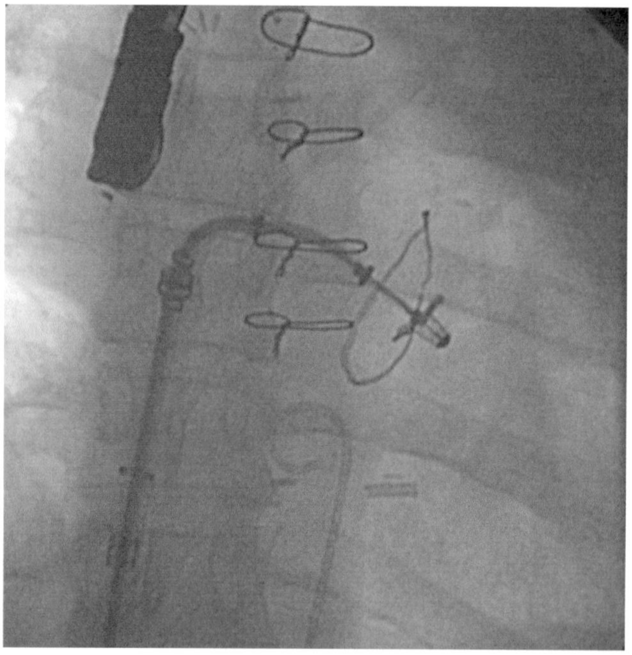

Fig. 21.7 Fluoro. The standard approach of translating the MitraClip into the ventricle with the clip arms open was not possible as the annuloplasty ring obstructed entry of the MitraClip into the LV

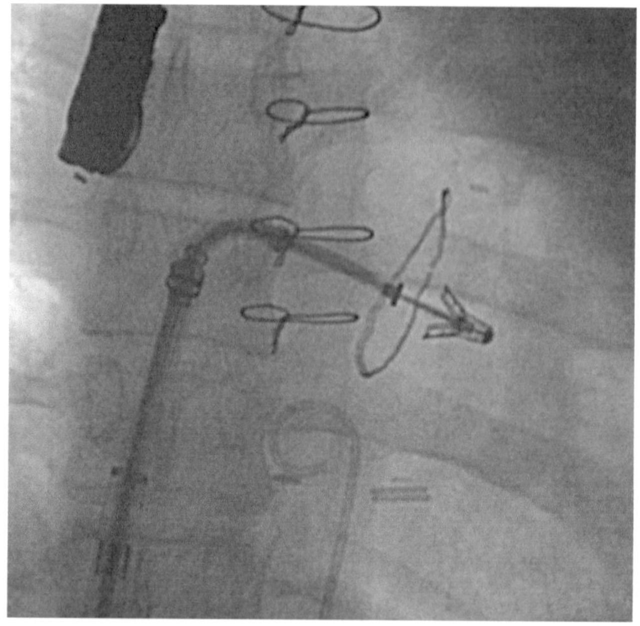

Fig. 21.8 Fluoro. Closing the clip arms to ~60° allowed translation of the clip into the ventricle without getting hung up on the annuloplasty ring

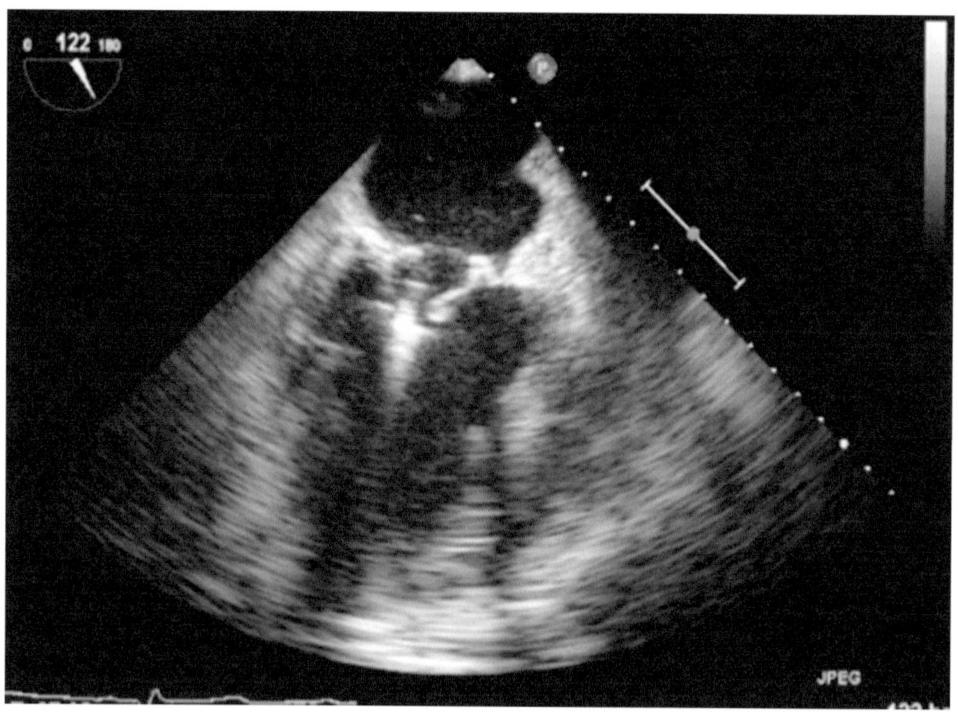

Fig. 21.9 TEE: Intraprocedure. With the MitraClip advanced into the ventricle, shadowing from the annuloplasty ring limits visualization of the clip arms

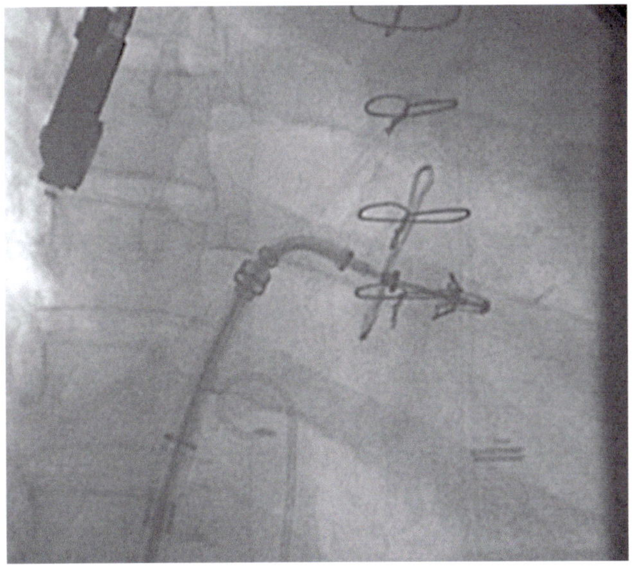

Fig. 21.10 Fluoro. Leaflet grasping with the MitraClip performed

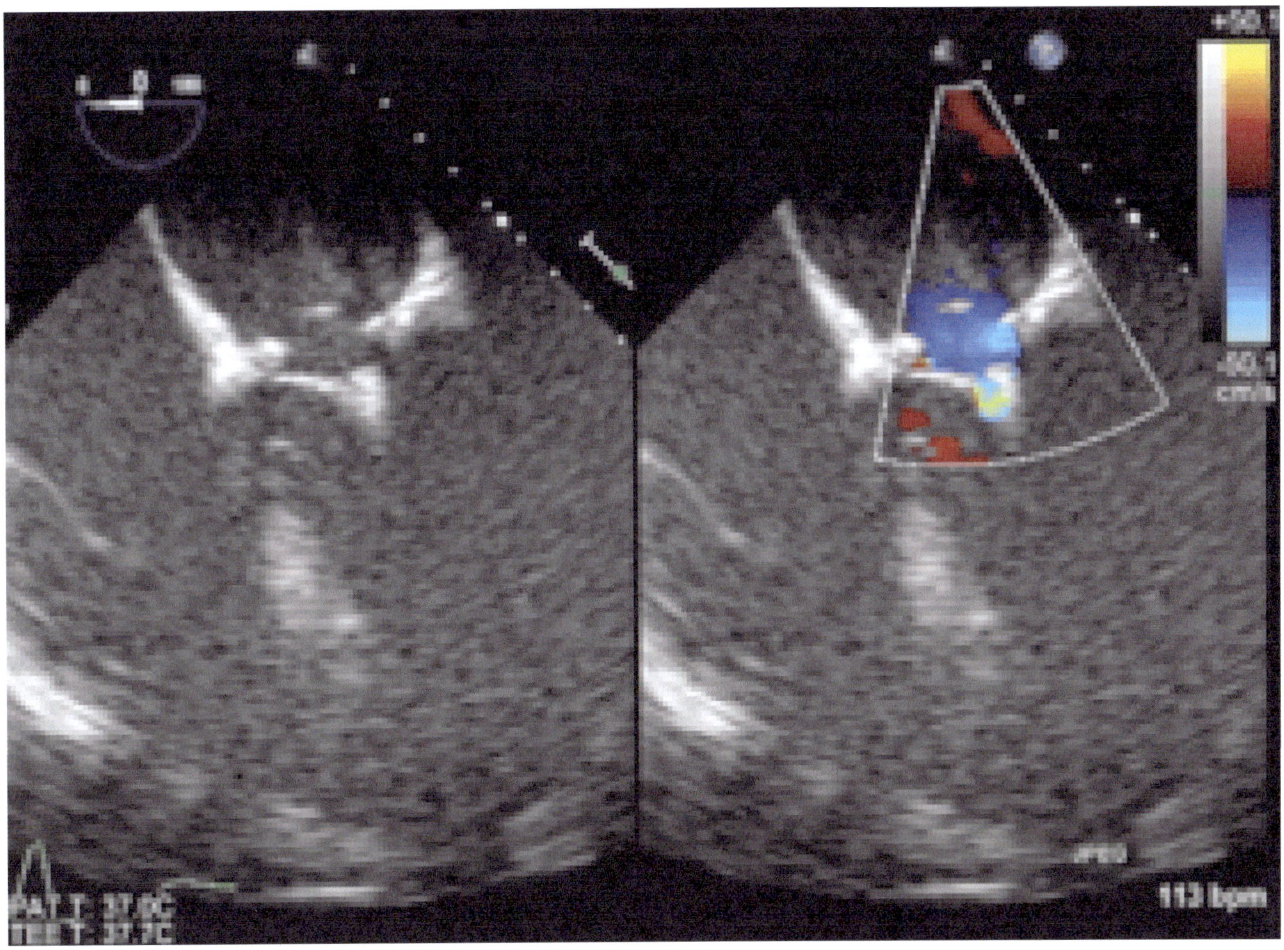

Fig. 21.11 TEE: 4C w/color. The four-chamber view shows significant reduction of the mitral regurgitation after a single clip, but determination of posterior leaflet insertion is difficult

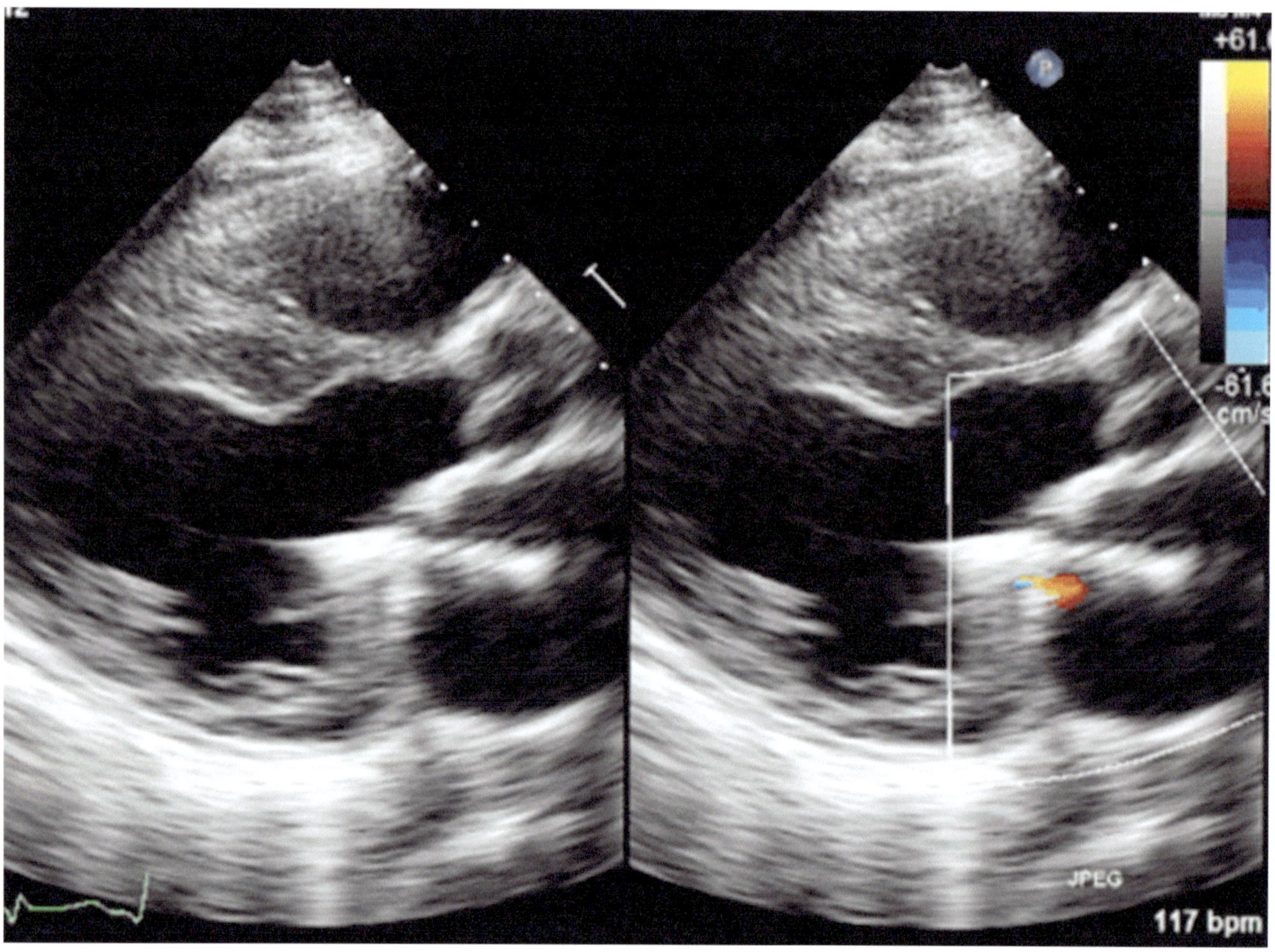

Fig. 21.12 Intraprocedure TTE. The long axis view demonstrates restriction of the anterior leaflet by the clip

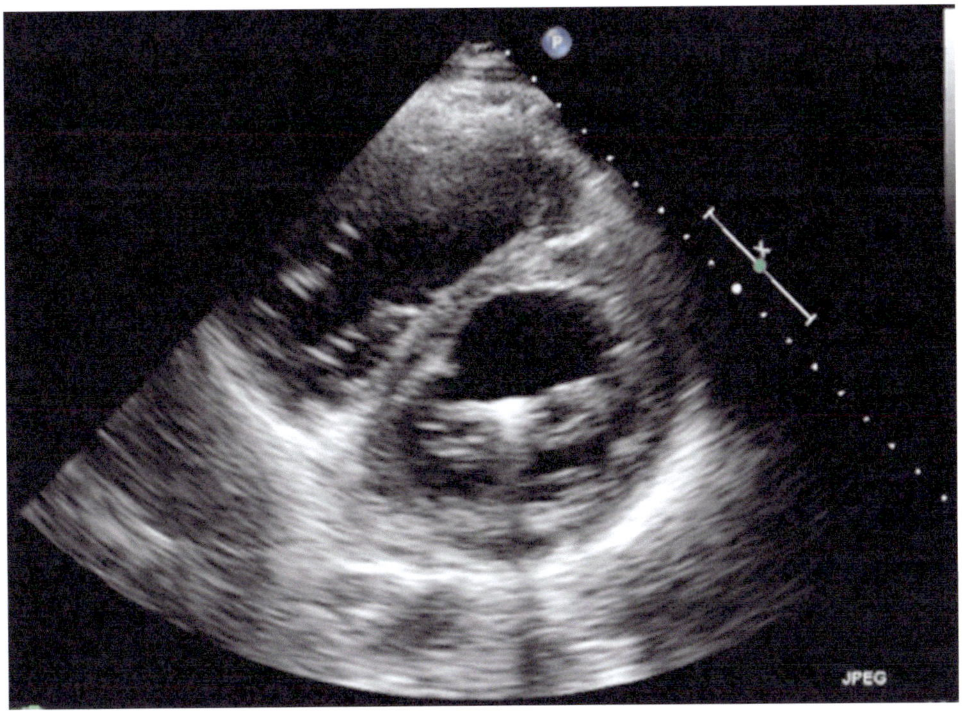

Fig. 21.13 Intraprocedure TTE. The parasternal short axis view demonstrates both anterior and posterior leaflets entering appropriately into the clip arms

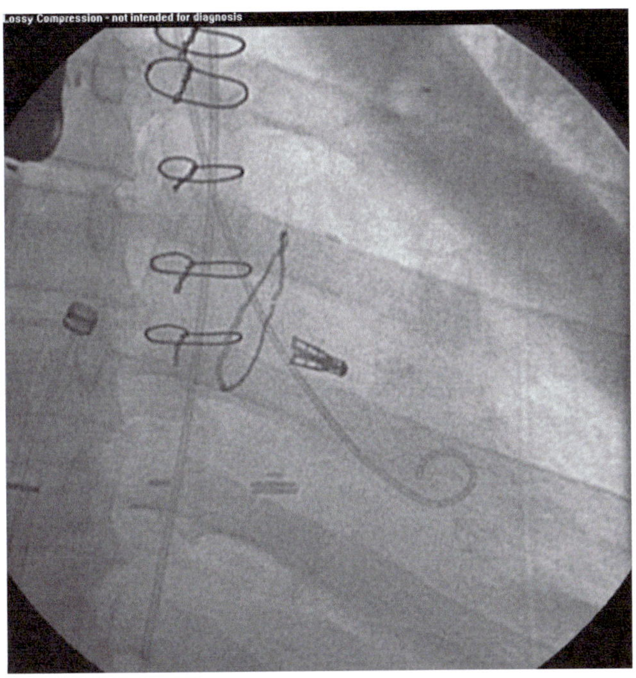

Fig. 21.14 Fluoroscopy. After clip deployment, stable position of the MitraClip relative to the ring is demonstrated

Use of Intracardiac Echo in Left Ventricle

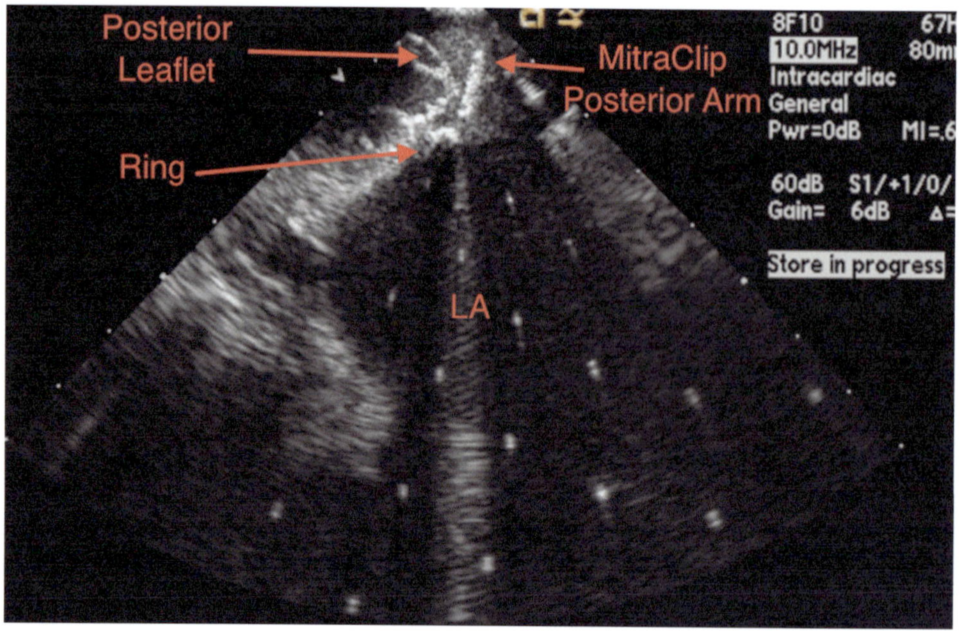

Fig. 21.15 ICE. The intracardiac echo probe has been advanced retrograde to the left ventricle and is positioned in the left ventricular outflow tract. The posterior clip arm is demonstrated below the ring and above the posterior leaflet in this view

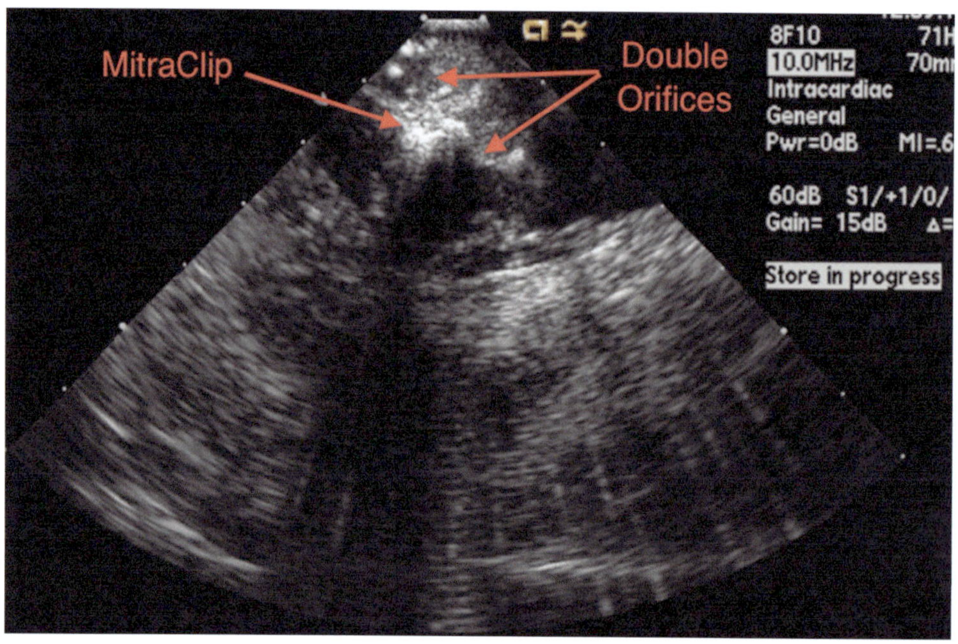

Fig. 21.16 ICE. The ICE probe is angulated 90° while remaining in the LVOT, providing a double orifice view with the MitraClip in the middle. Both anterior and posterior leaflet tissues may be visualized entering the clip appropriately

EVEREST II Functional Mitral Regurgitation

22

Ehrin J. Armstrong, Reginald Low, and Jason Rogers

Abstract

This case example describes in a step-by-step fashion the evaluation and management of severe MR in a patient with functional MR due to an inferior-basal left ventricular aneurysm in the setting of prior inferior myocardial infarction.

Keywords

Mitral regurgitation • MitraClip • Functional mitral regurgitation • Ventricular aneurysm

Clinical History

A 75-year-old man presented with NYHA Class III heart failure. He had a history of inferior ST elevation myocardial infarction treated with primary percutaneous coronary intervention. His postoperative course was complicated by an inferobasal aneurysm and severe mitral regurgitation.

Summary

In this case, the patient developed severe functional mitral regurgitation due to an inferobasal left ventricular aneurysm as a complication of an inferior myocardial infarction (Fig. 22.21 and Video 22.21). The left ventricle tethered the posterior leaflet of the mitral valve, resulting in a restricted posterior leaflet excursion and tenting of the mitral leaflets during systole. The origin of the mitral regurgitation jet was central and located along the P2/A2 interface. Additionally, the moderate coaptation depth and adequate length of leaflet coaptation (>2 mm) made the mitral valve anatomy suitable for MitraClip implantation (Figs. 22.1, 22.2, 22.3, 22.4, 22.5, 22.6, 22.7, 22.8, 22.9, 22.10, 22.11, 22.12, 22.13, 22.14 and Videos 22.1, 22.2, 22.3, 22.4, 22.5, 22.6, 22.7, 22.8, 22.9, 22.10, 22.11, 22.12). After deployment of the first MitraClip, there was a lateral jet of residual mitral regurgitation (Figs. 22.15, 22.16, 22.17, 22.18, 22.19, 22.20, 22.21, 22.22 and Videos 22.13, 22.14, 22.15, 22.16, 22.17). After deployment of the second MitraClip, there was only trace MR (Figs. 22.23, 22.24, 22.25, 22.26, 22.28 and Videos 22.18, 22.19, 22.20, 22.21, 22.22). At follow-up, the patient reported greatly improved exercise tolerance, and follow-up TTE at 6 months showed 1+ MR (Figures 22.23, 22.24, 22.25, 22.26, 22.27, 22.28, 22.29, 22.30, 22.31, 22.32 and Videos 22.23, 22.24, 22.25, 22.26)

Learning Points

This is a step-by-step case example of how a patient with functional MR may be treated with the MitraClip.

E.J. Armstrong, M.D., M.Sc.
Division of Cardiovascular Medicine,
University of California, Davis Medical Center,
4860 Y Street, Suite 2820, Sacramento, CA 95817, USA
e-mail: ehrin.armstrong@ucdmc.ucdavis.edu

R. Low, M.D., FACC • J. Rogers, M.D., FACC, FSCAI (✉)
Department of Cardiovascular Medicine,
University of California, Davis Medical Center,
4860 Y Street, Suite 2820, Sacramento, CA 95817, USA
e-mail: ptcra@aol.com; jason.rogers@ucdmc.ucdavis.edu

Electronic supplementary material The online version of this chapter (doi:10.1007/978-1-4471-4294-2_22) contains supplementary material, which is available to authorized users.

T. Feldman et al. (eds.), *Atlas of Percutaneous Edge-to-Edge Mitral Valve Repair*,
DOI 10.1007/978-1-4471-4294-2_22, © Springer-Verlag London 2013

Screening Transthoracic Echo

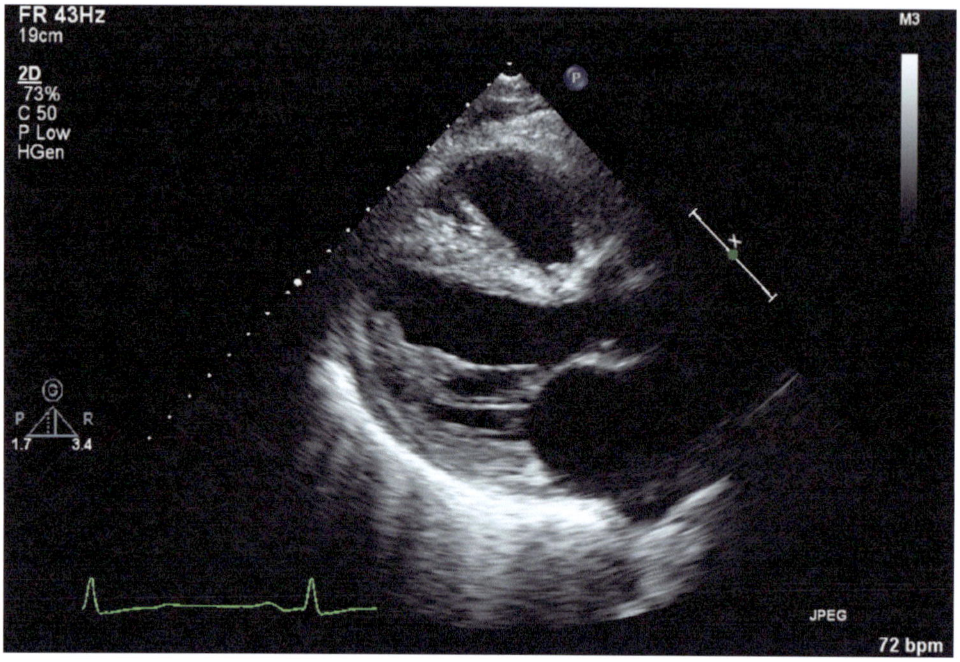

Fig. 22.1 TTE: parasternal LAX w/o color. The parasternal long axis demonstrates significant tenting of the mitral leaflets below the level of the annulus

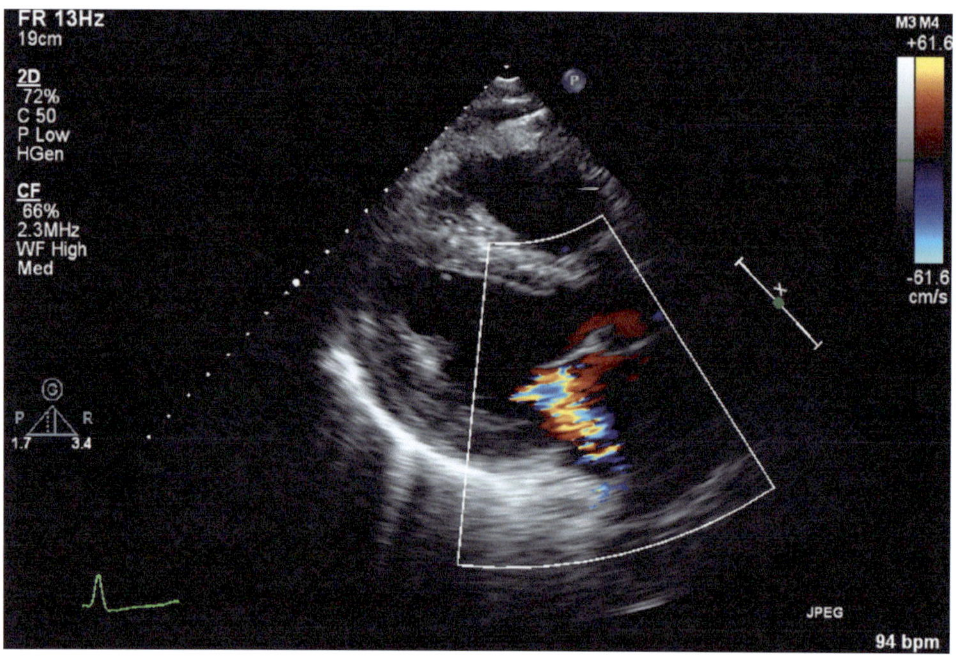

Fig. 22.2 TTE: parasternal LAX w/color. There is a posteriorly directed jet of mitral regurgitation, consistent with functional MR

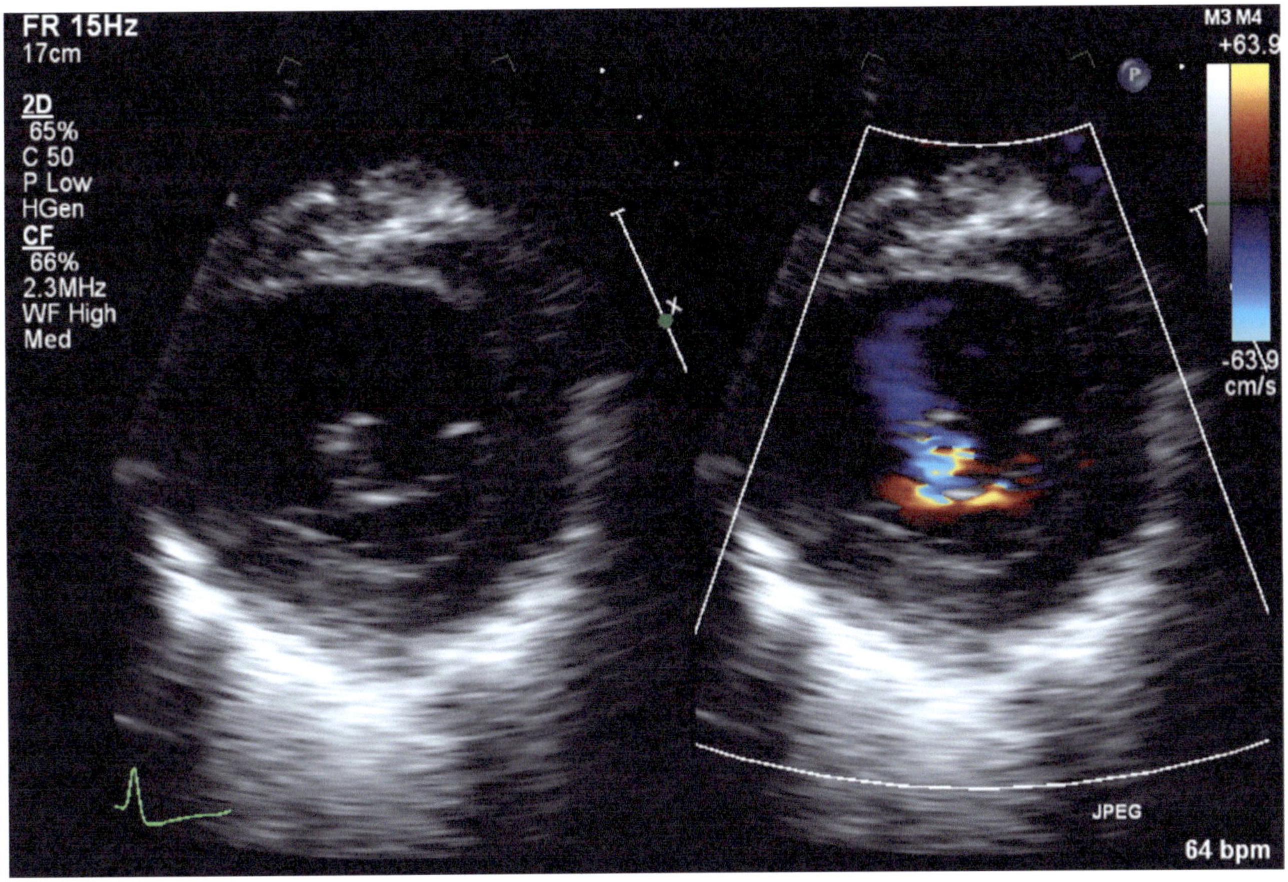

Fig. 22.3 TTE: parasternal SAX. Short axis view shows that the MR has a central origin along the P2/A2 interface

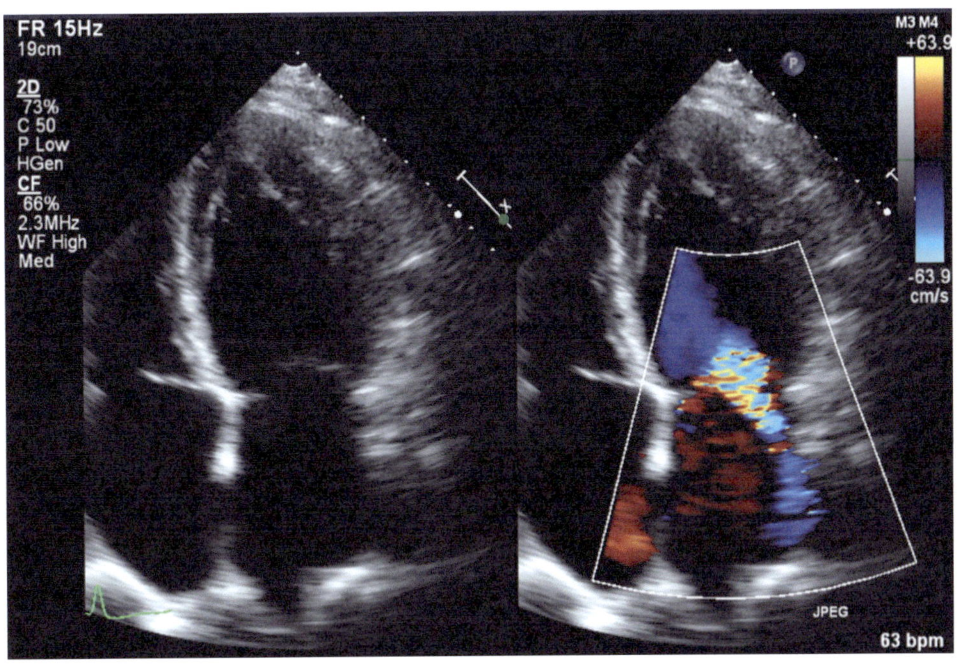

Fig. 22.4 TTE: apical 4C view. The apical four-chamber view shows biatrial enlargement and confirms a posteriorly directed jet of mitral regurgitation resulting from tenting of the posterior leaflet

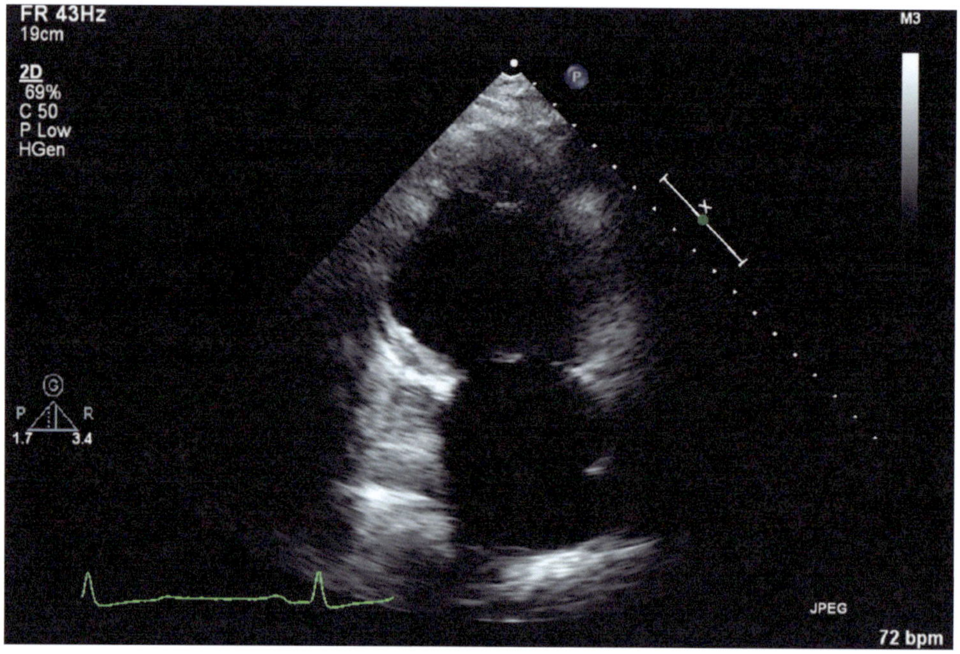

Fig. 22.5 TTE: 2C w/o color. In the apical two-chamber view, the echogenic inferobasal aneurysm is apparent, which is tethering the posterior leaflet

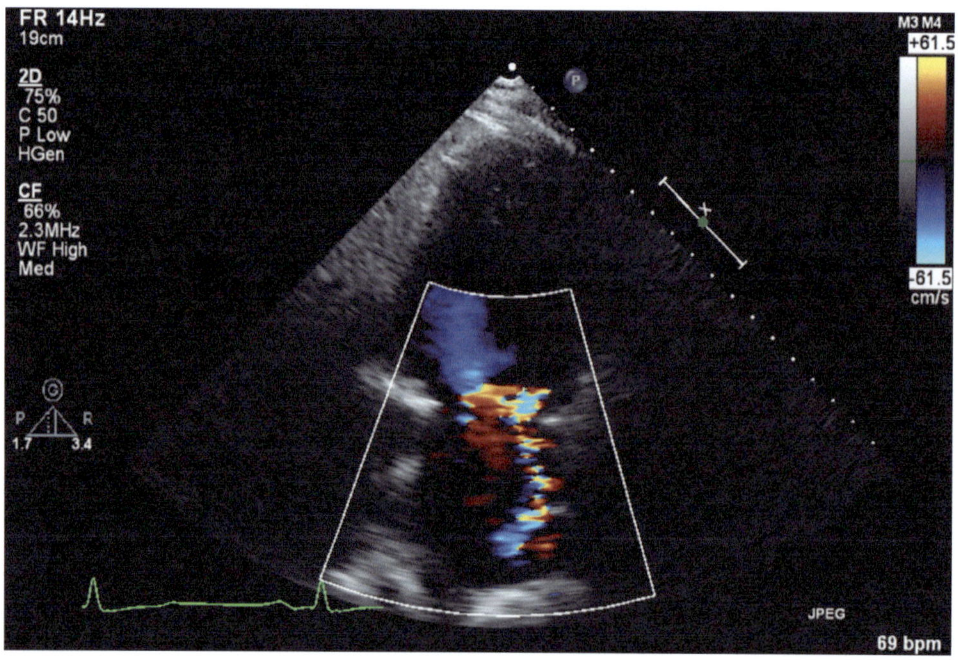

Fig. 22.6 TTE 2C: w/color. The jet of mitral regurgitation is moderate to severe by color Doppler

Screening TEE

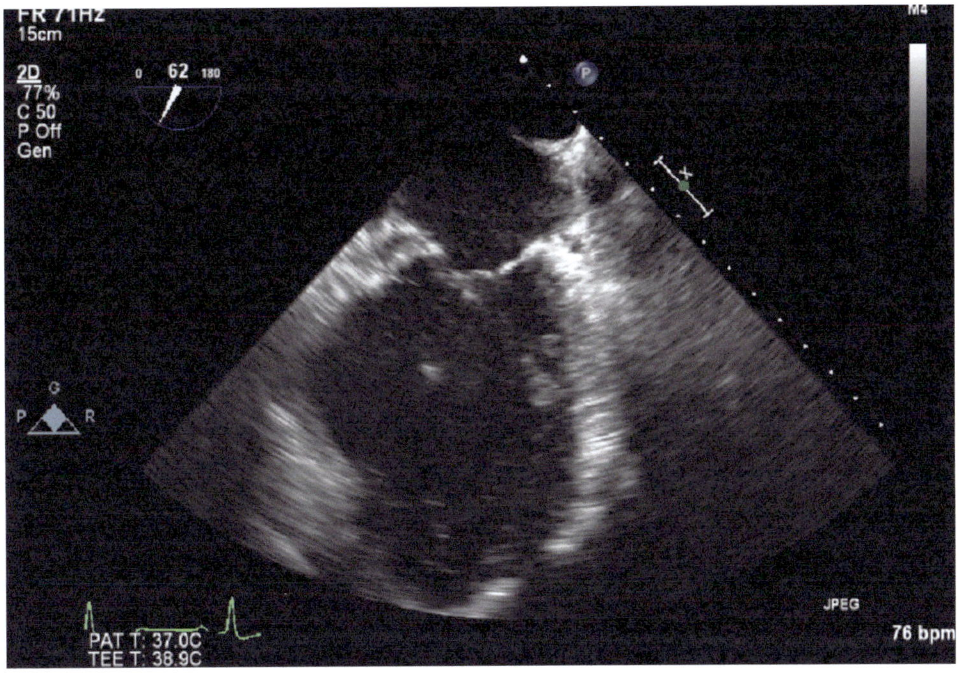

Fig. 22.7 TEE: bicommissural w/o color. The bicommissural view shows the large inferobasal aneurysm

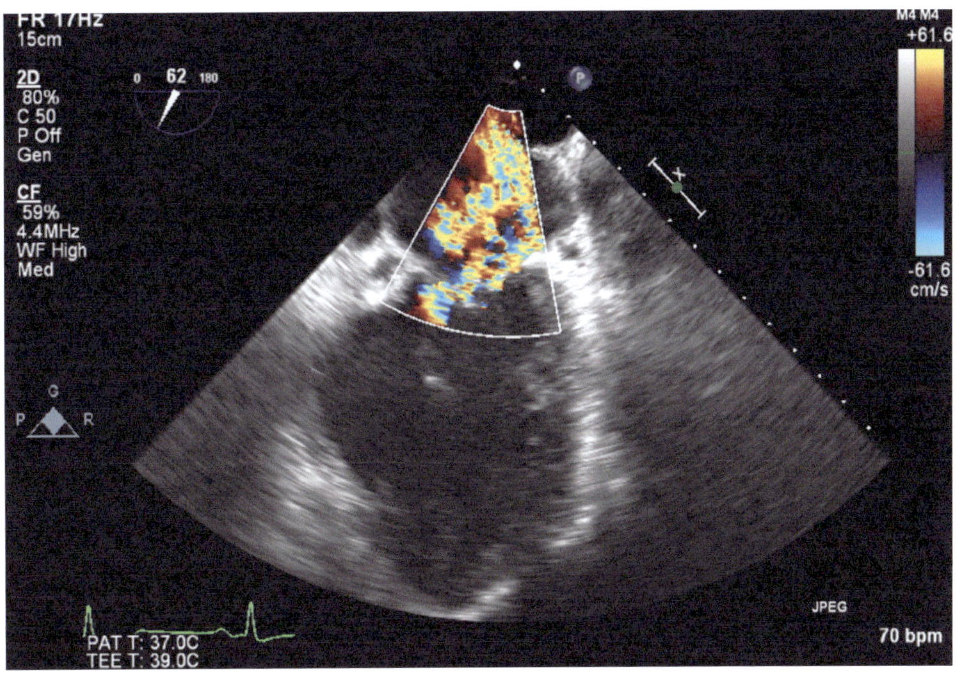

Fig. 22.8 TEE: bicommissural w/color. There is a significant jet of posterior MR resulting from tethering of the leaflets

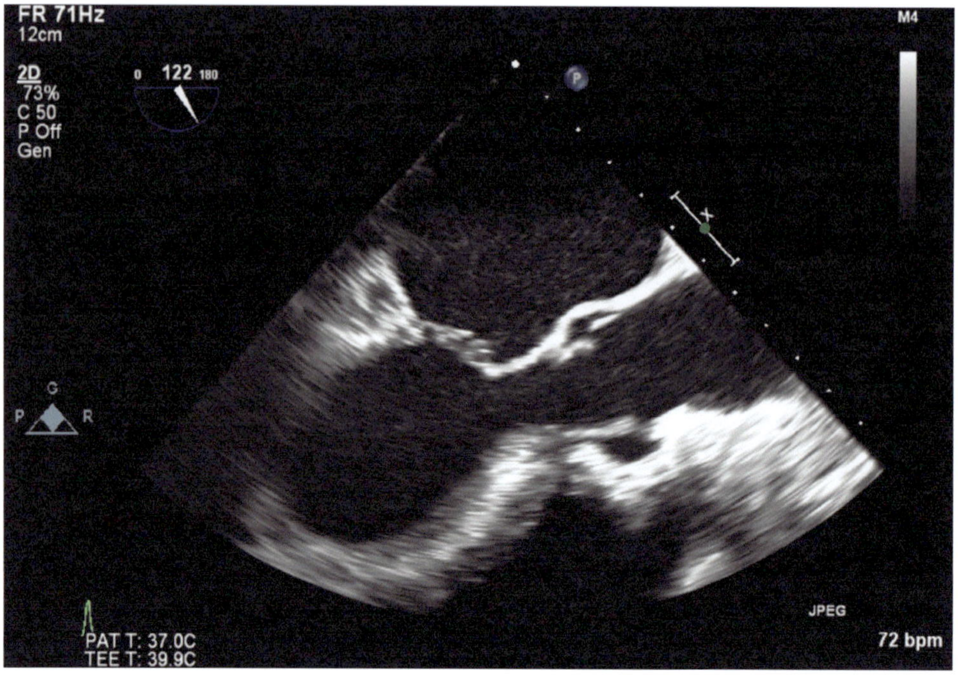

Fig. 22.9 TEE: 3C w/o color. The three-chamber view confirms a posteriorly directed jet originating at the A2/P2 interface

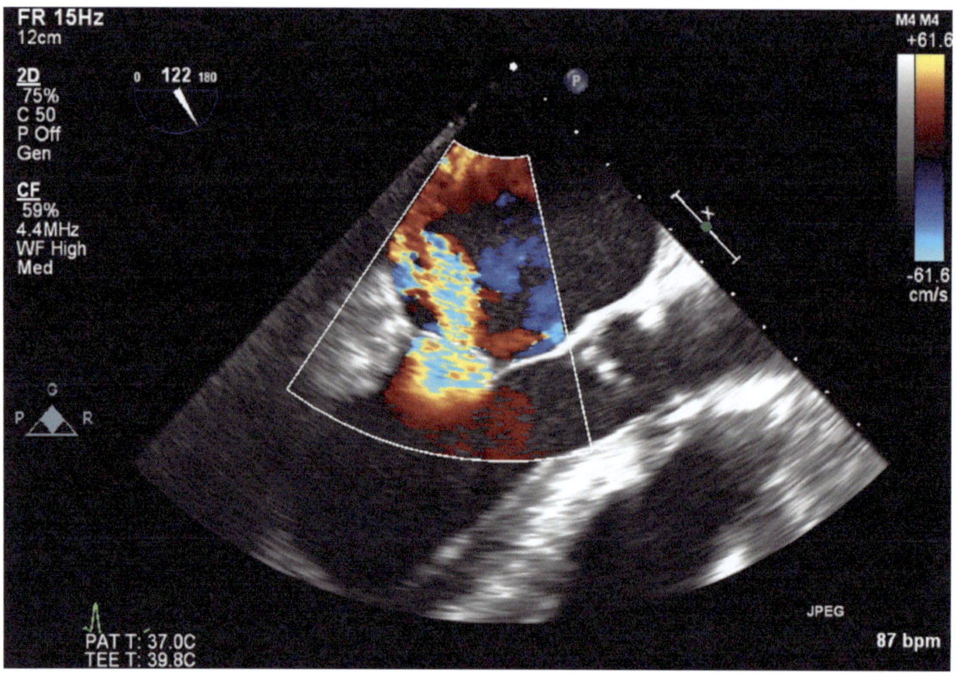

Fig. 22.10 TEE: 3C w/color. There is a large vena contracta and a posteriorly directed jet

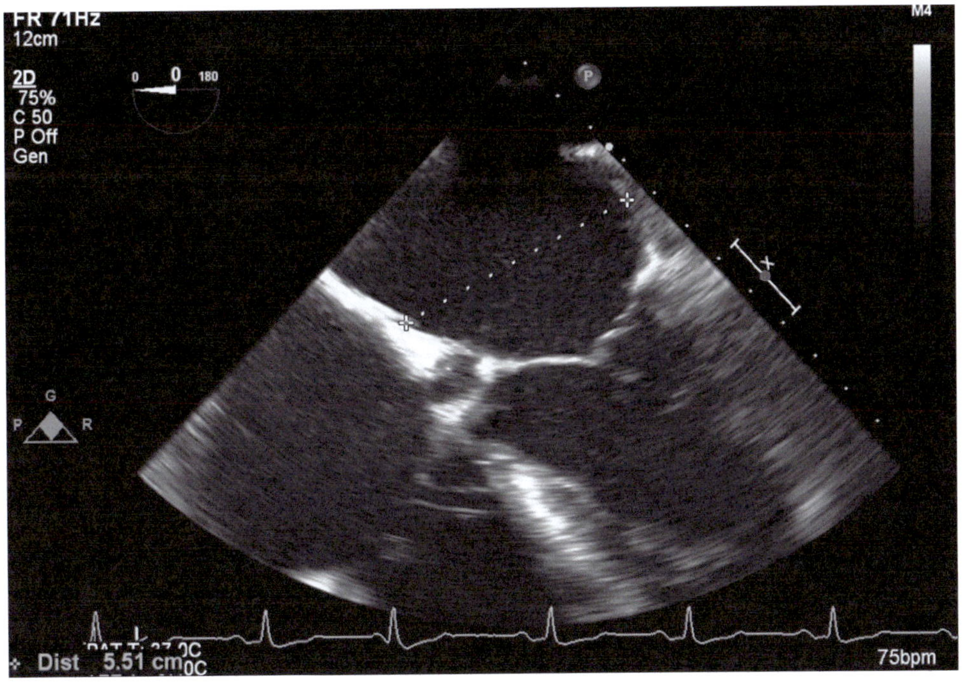

Fig. 22.11 TEE: 4C w/o color. The four-chamber view shows tenting of the mitral valve leaflets. The annulus is also enlarged

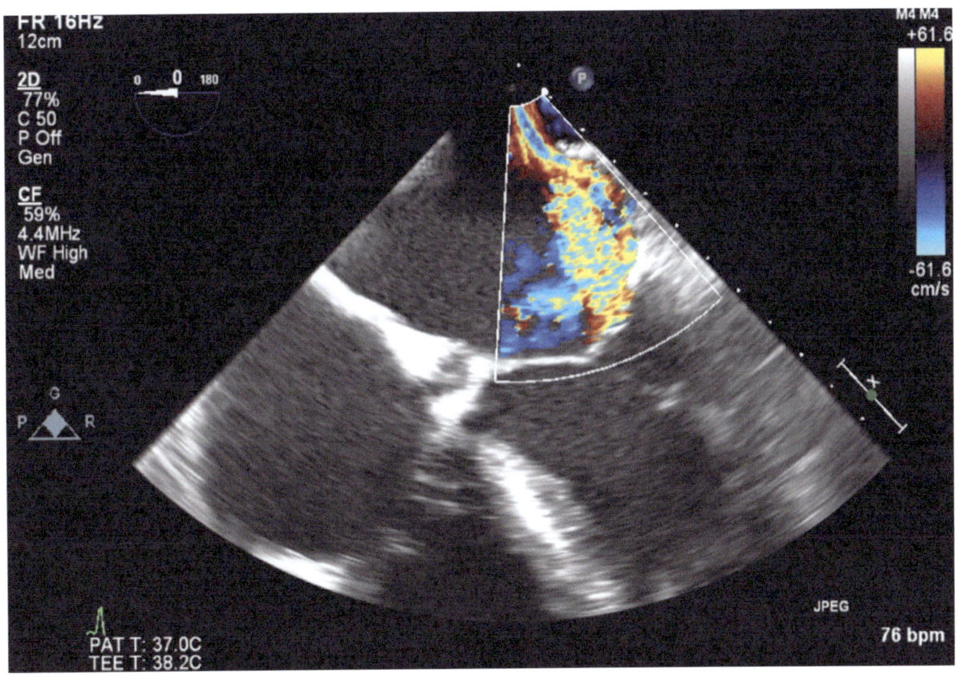

Fig. 22.12 TEE: 4C w/color. The regurgitant jet has a central origin

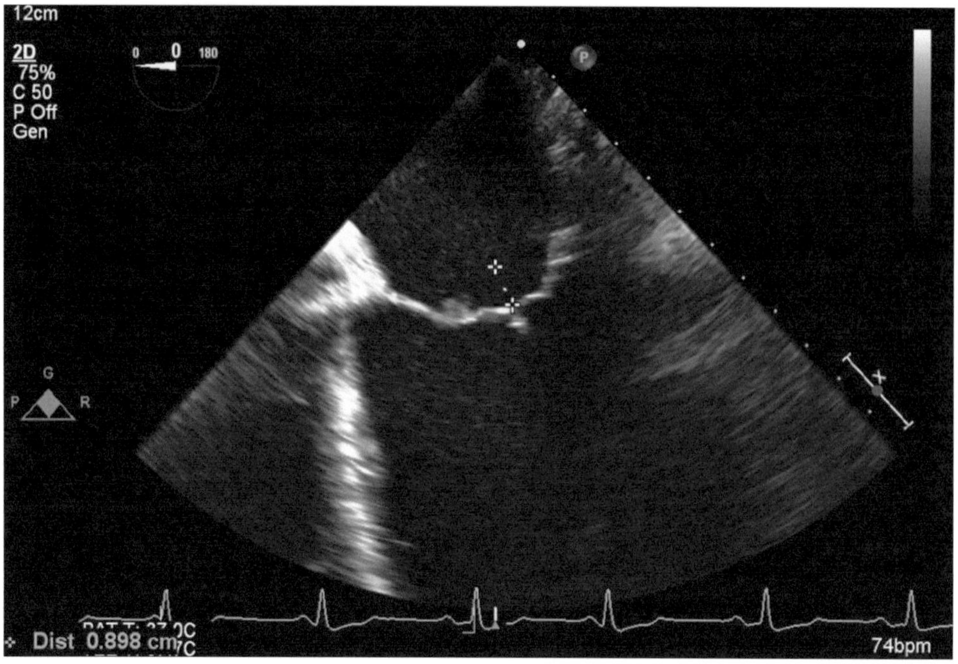

Fig. 22.13 TEE: 4C. The coaptation depth is less than 11 mm

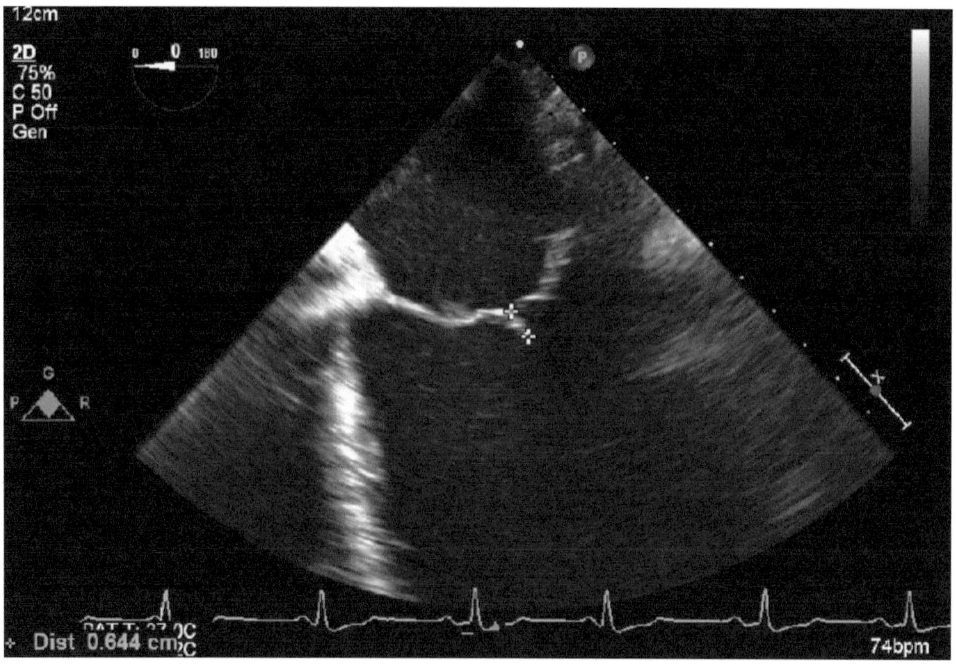

Fig. 22.14 TEE: 4C. The coaptation length is approximately 6 mm, suggesting that the anatomy of the valve apparatus is favorable for MitraClip implantation

Transseptal Puncture

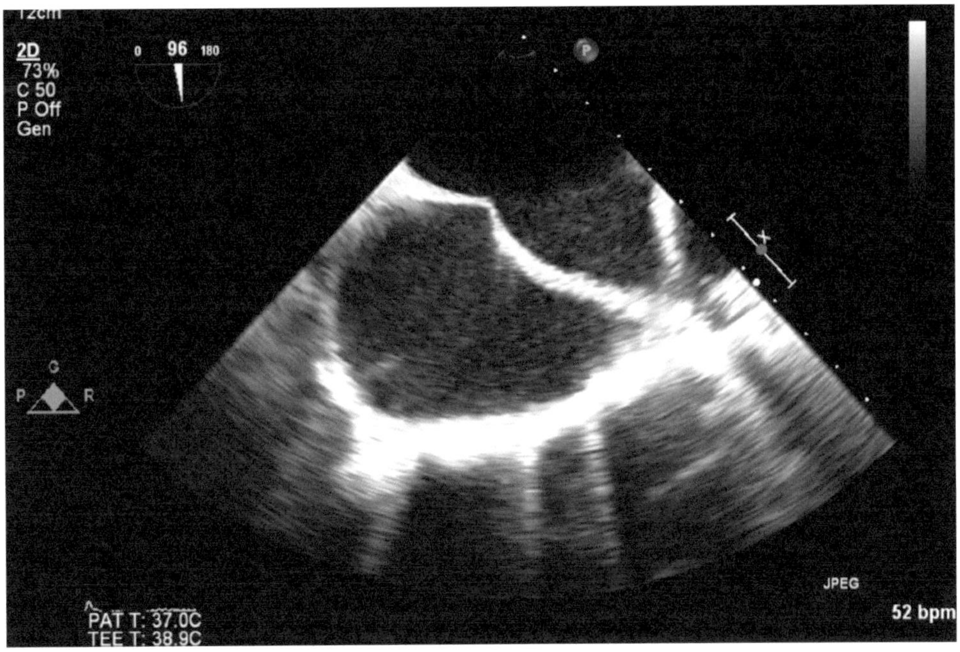

Fig. 22.15 TEE: bicaval view. The transseptal needle is advanced across the interatrial septum in a superior and posterior direction

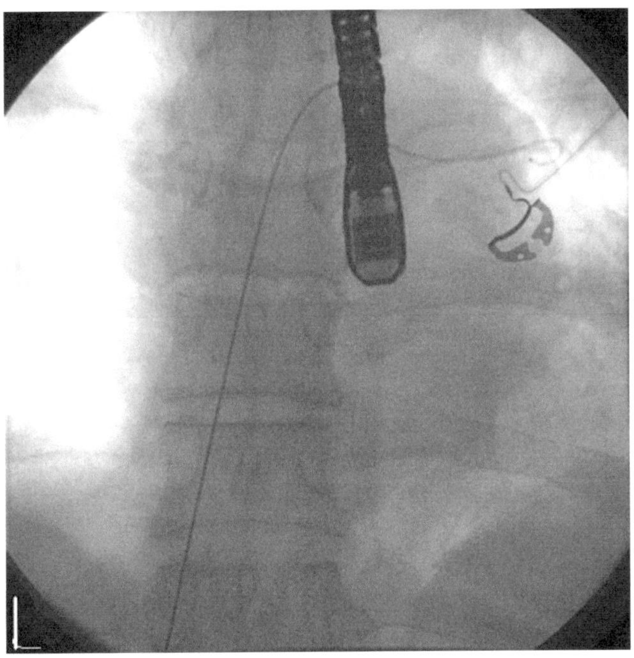

Fig. 22.16 Fluoroscopy. The guidewire is then advanced into the left upper pulmonary vein

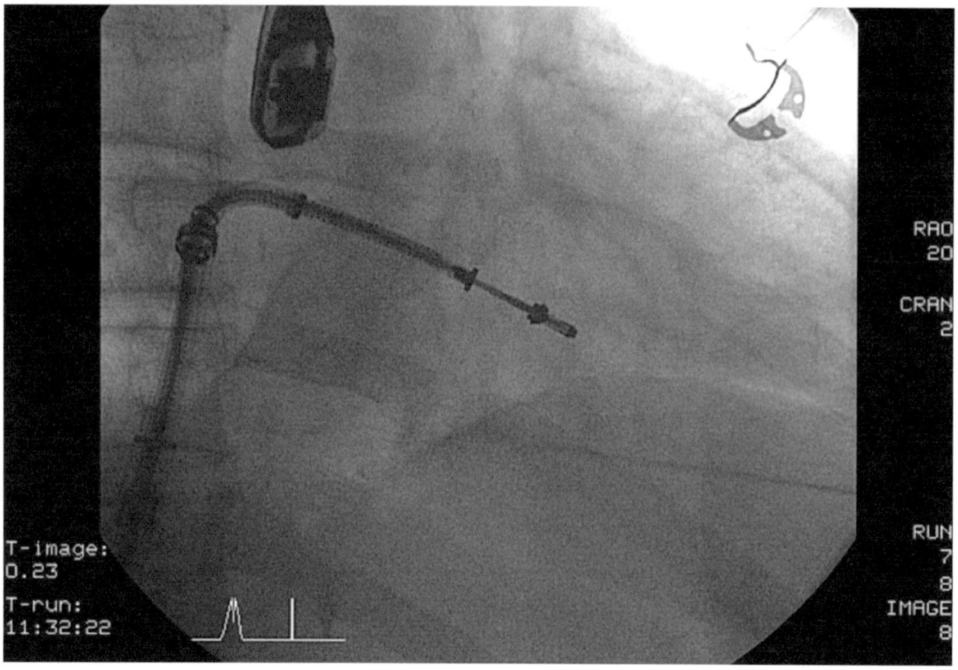

Fig. 22.17 Fluoroscopy. The MitraClip delivery sheath is advanced across the interatrial septum

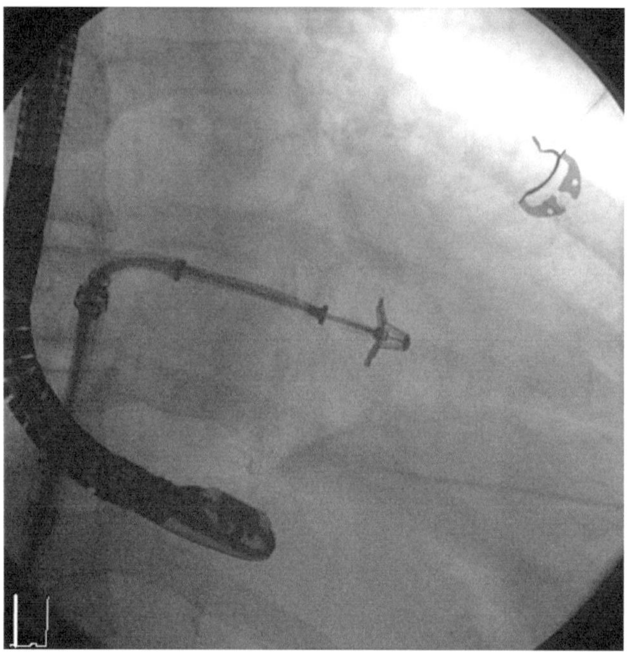

Fig. 22.18 Fluoroscopy. The clip is advanced across the mitral valve, and the clip arms are opened in the left ventricle

Procedural TEE and Fluoro I

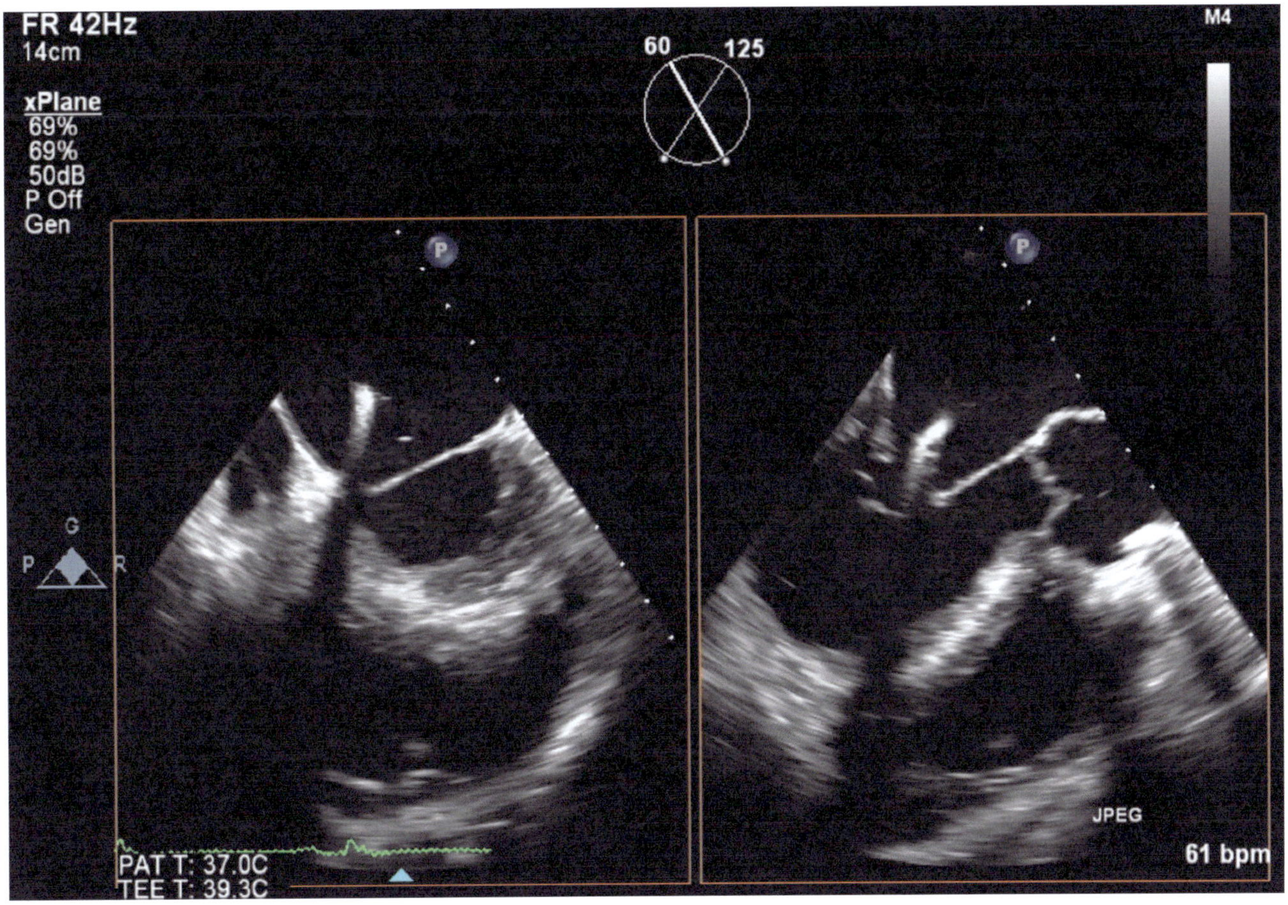

Fig. 22.19 Biplane TEE. The MitraClip is advanced across the mitral valve

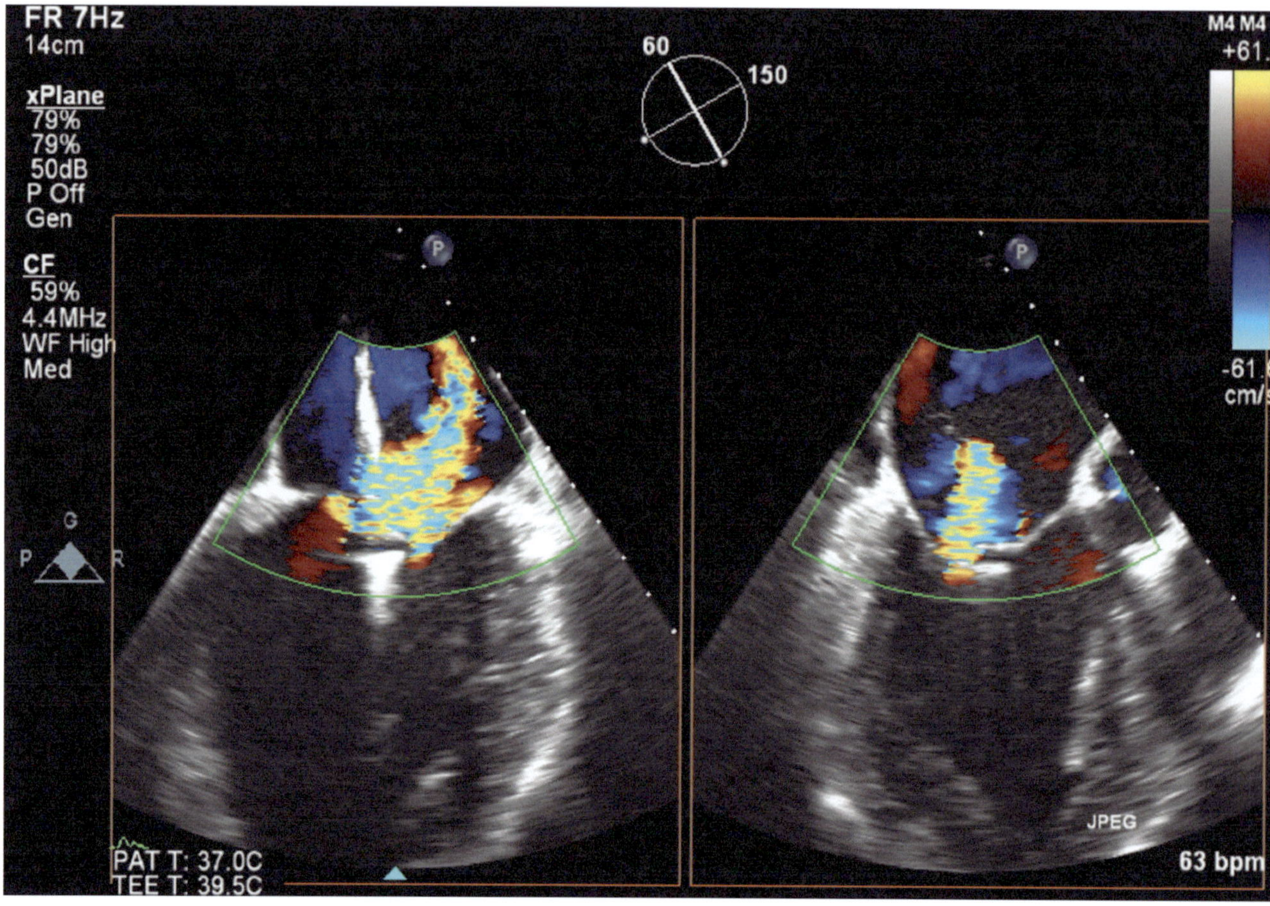

Fig. 22.20 Biplane TEE. Biplane TEE is used to orient the direction of the grasping arms orthogonal to the line of leaflet coaptation

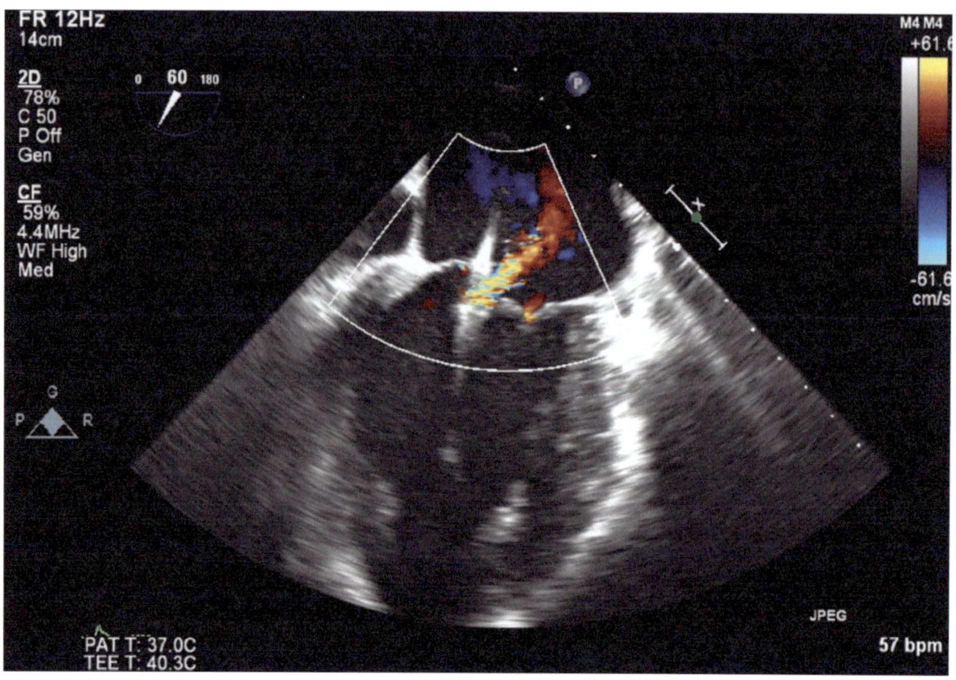

Fig. 22.21 TEE: Bicommissural clip at deployment. Once positioning is confirmed, the device is deployed

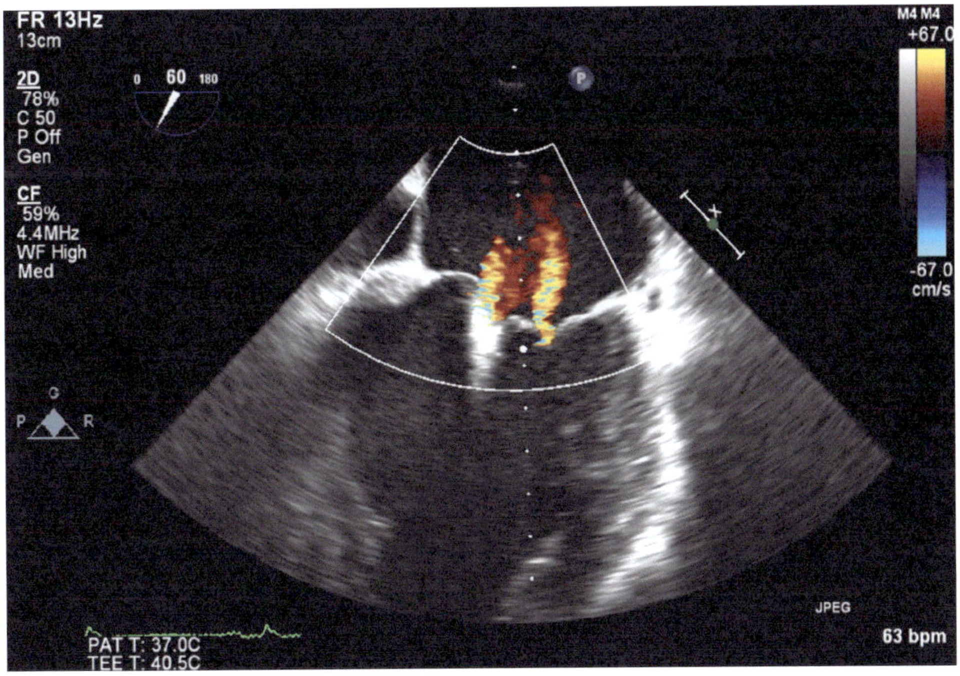

Fig. 22.22 TEE: Bicommissural view after clip deployment. Post-deployment, there is a residual jet of MR lateral to the site of clip attachment

Procedural TEE and Fluoro II

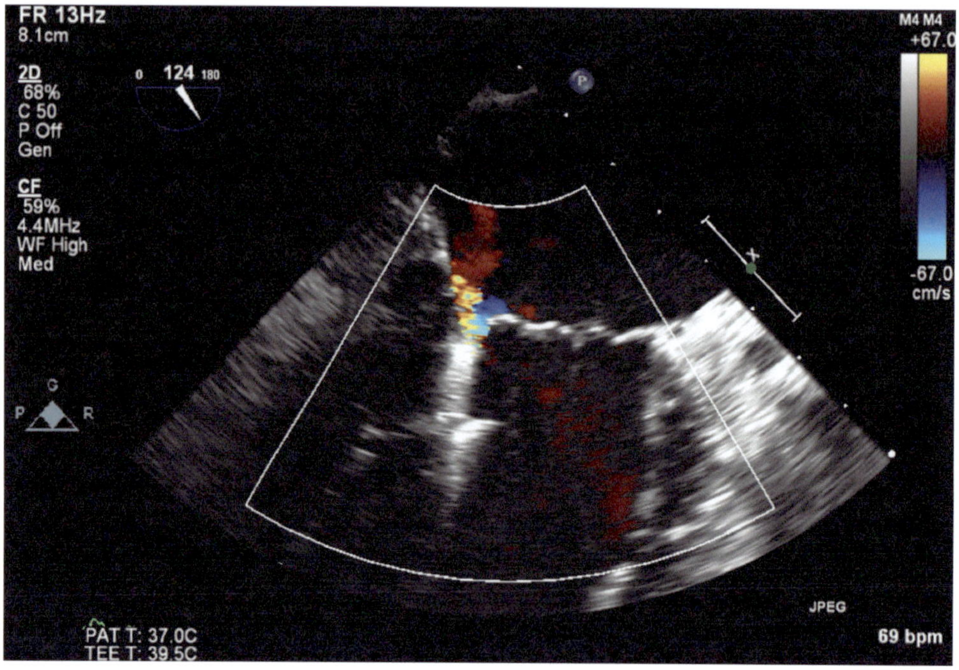

Fig. 22.23 TEE: a second clip is advanced across the mitral valve

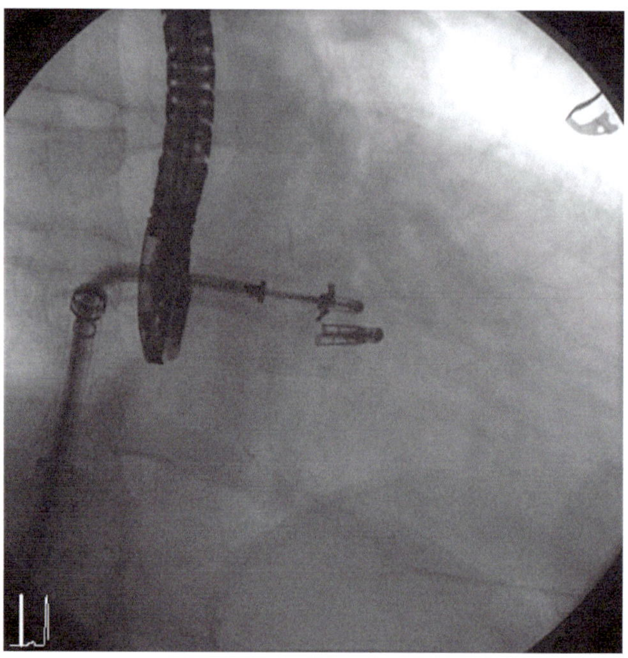

Fig. 22.24 Fluoroscopy. The orientation of the second clip is confirmed with fluoroscopy

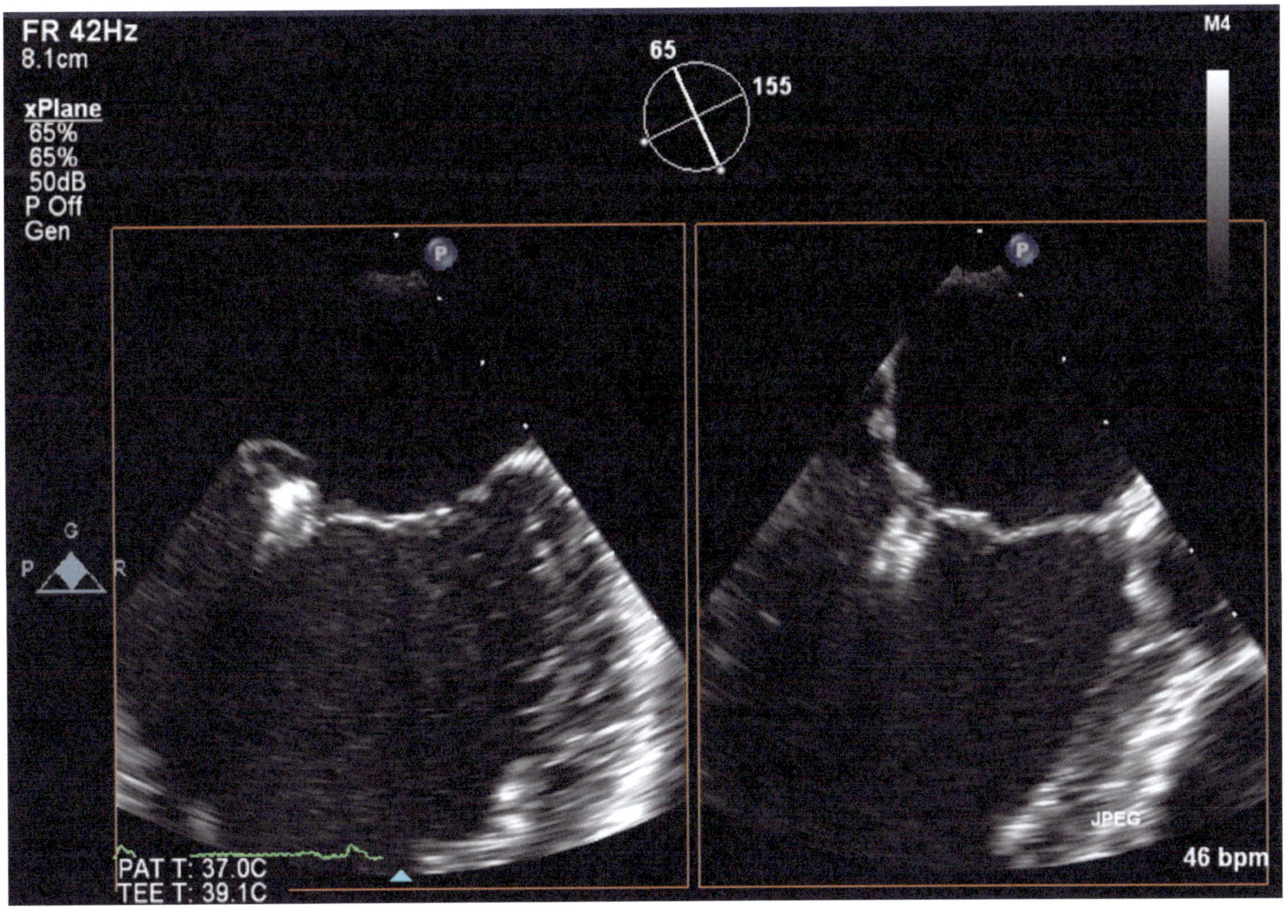

Fig. 22.25 TEE: biplane views. The second clip is deployed slightly lateral to the first clip

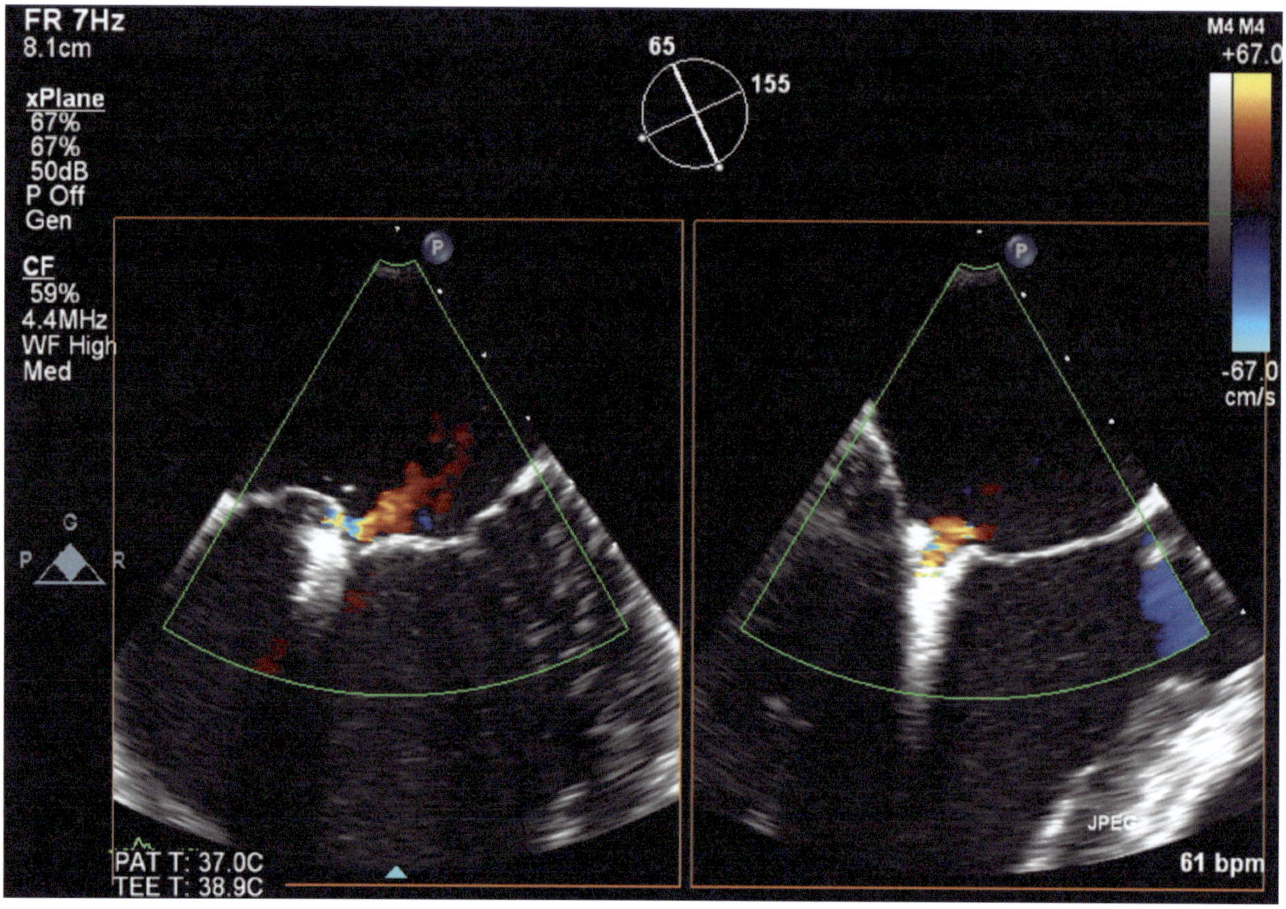

Fig. 22.26 TEE: biplane Doppler views after second clip. Post-deployment, there is trace MR

Procedural TEE and Fluoro III

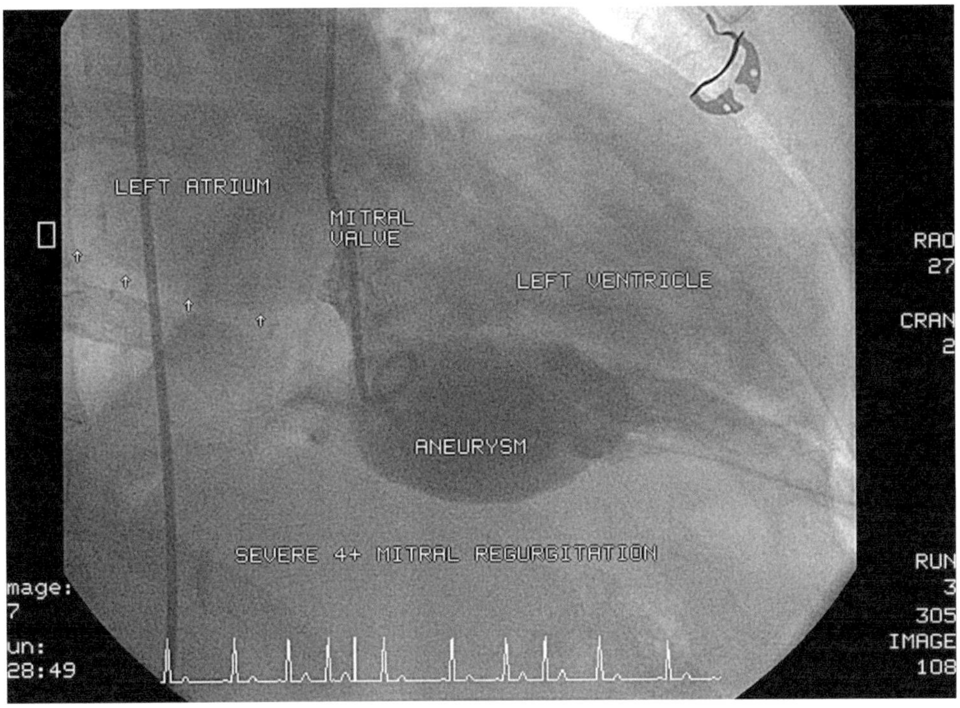

Fig. 22.27 Fluoroscopy. Pre-procedure, there is severe mitral regurgitation with associated severe left atrial enlargement and an inferobasal left ventricular aneurysm

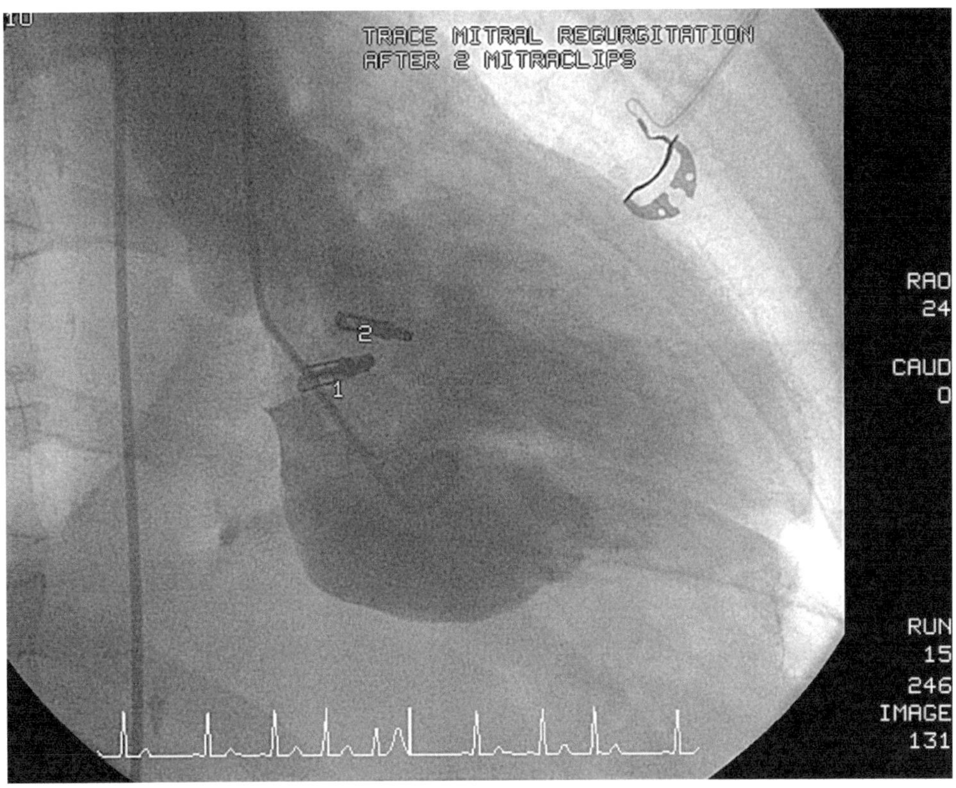

Fig. 22.28 Fluoroscopy. Post-procedure, there is trace MR, and the two MitraClip devices appear well seated on fluoroscopy

Post-procedure TTE

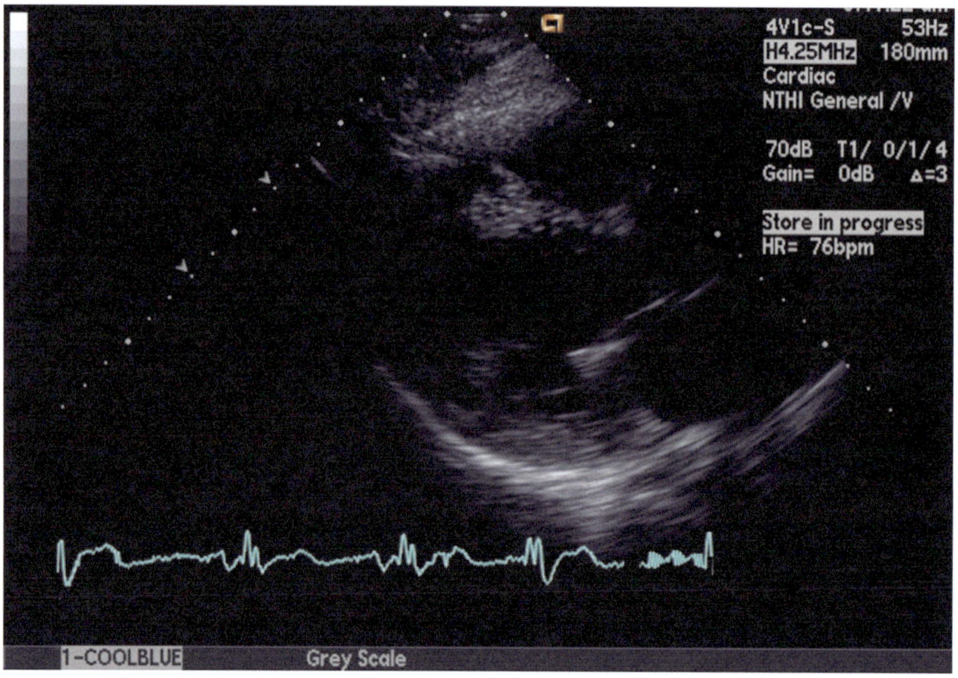

Fig. 22.29 TTE: parasternal LAX. Parasternal long axis view show the MitraClips positioned in the center of the valve

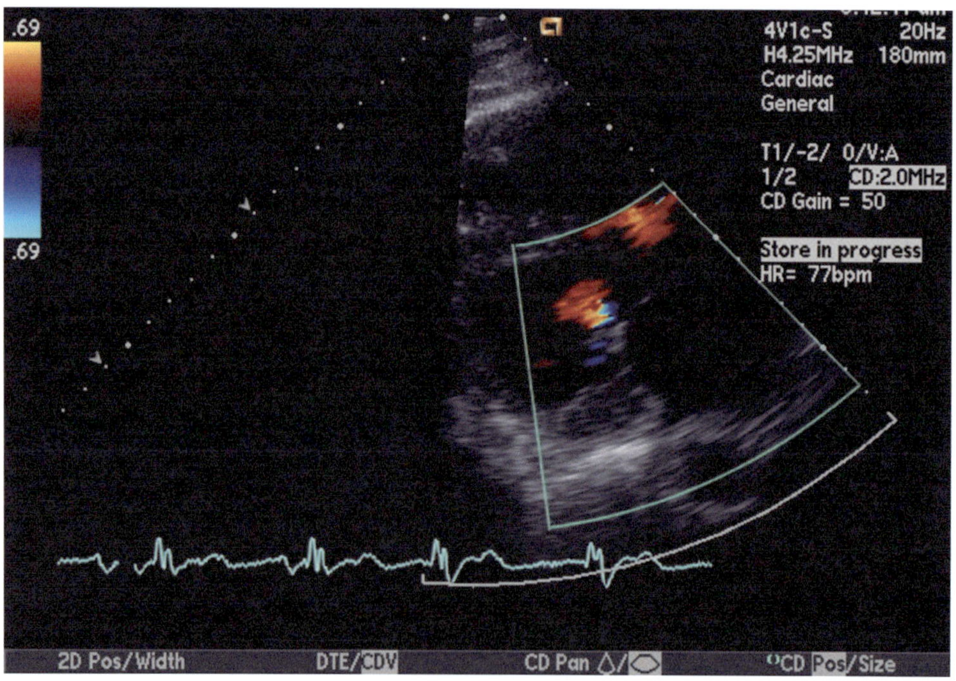

Fig. 22.30 TTE: parasternal LAX w/color. There is trace mitral regurgitation and normal inflow around the MitraClip devices

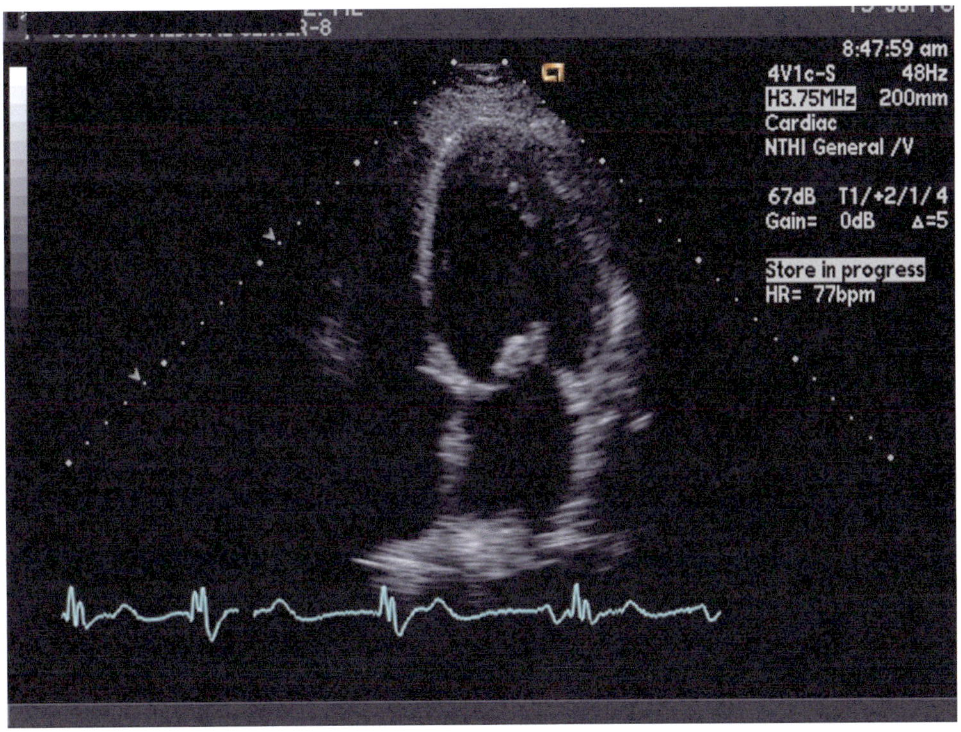

Fig. 22.31 TTE: 4C w/o color. Apical 4C view shows the MitraClips oriented parallel to the mitral inflow

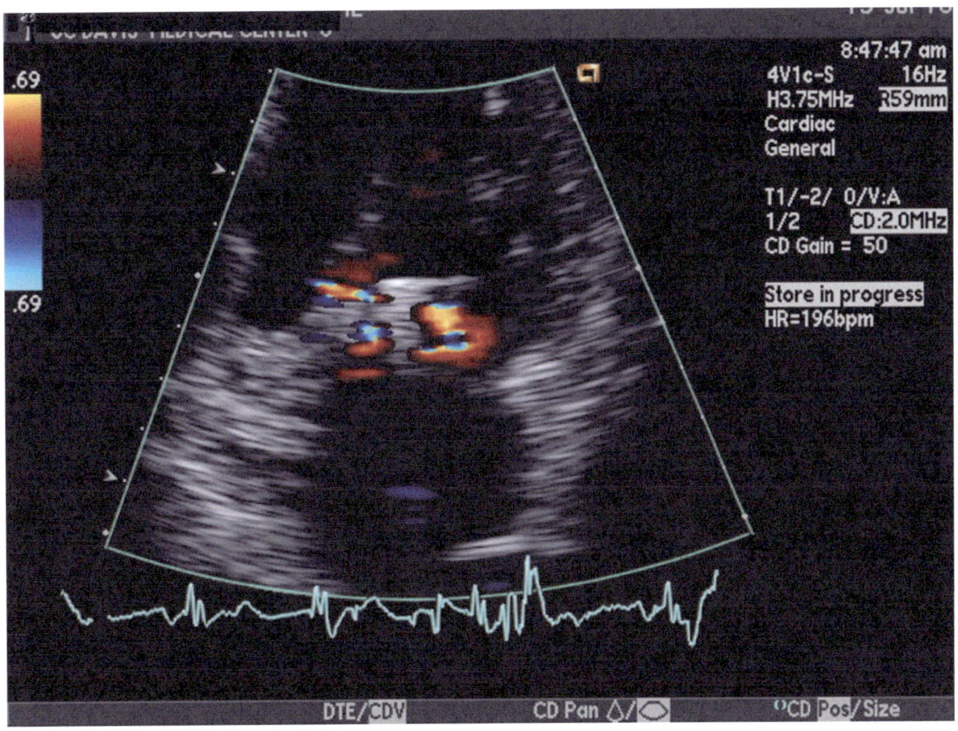

Fig. 22.32 TTE: 4C w color. There is double inlet Doppler flow around the MitraClip devices

23 Chiari Network Complicating a MitraClip Procedure

Khung Keong Yeo, Paul Toon Lim Chiam, Jack Tan, and Zee Pin Ding

Abstract
This case describes an attempted MitraClip procedure that was complicated by a large Chiari network in the right atrium. The Chiari network was trapped by the guide and the stiff wire and dragged into the left atrium where it could not be differentiated from a thrombus. The procedure was aborted, and the guide and Chiari network returned to the right atrium.

Keywords
Mitral regurgitation • MitraClip • Chiari network • Thrombus

Clinical History

A 77-male patient who had severe functional mitral regurgitation (MR) was evaluated for percutaneous MitraClip repair for the MR. He had a history of coronary artery disease and had prior intervention to his right coronary artery. He also had a chronic total occlusion of his circumflex, and a nuclear stress test showed prior infarction in the lateral wall without inducible ischemia. His LVEF was 40 %, and he was NYHA class II. The patient's other comorbidities included hypertension and dyslipidemia.

The patient's baseline transthoracic echocardiography showed a moderately dilated LV cavity with normal LV systolic function the calculated LVEF of 40 % (by modified biplane Simpson's method). There were regional wall motion abnormalities involving the posterior-lateral wall. The LA was severely dilated. The posterior mitral valve leaflet was restricted with tenting. There was severe MR with systolic flow reversal. The estimated pulmonary artery systolic pressure was 35 mmHg. A prominent Chiari network was noted (Fig. 23.1).

The MitraClip procedure was performed according to plan. However, upon removal of the MitraClip guide dilator, it was noted that there was a mobile mass attached to the stiff wire, near the guide tip, which was still parked in the left upper pulmonary vein. It was not possible to differentiate if this mass was a thrombus or a trapped Chiari network (Figs. 23.2, 23.3, and Videos 23.1, 23.2, 23.2). The procedure was aborted, and the guide and wire pulled back into the right atrium. At this time, the Chiari network could be seen flopping back into the right atrium (Figs. 23.4, 23.5, and Video 23.3).

K.K. Yeo, M.B.B.S., FACC, FSCAI (✉)
Department of Cardiology, National Heart Centre Singapore, Mistri Wing, 17 Third Hospital Avenue, Singapore 168752, Singapore

Department of Cardiovascular Medicine, University of California, Davis Medical Center, 4860 Y Street, Suite 2820, Sacramento, CA 95817, USA
e-mail: yeo_kk@yahoo.com, yeo.khung.keong@nhcs.com.sg

P.T. L. Chiam, M.B.B.S. • J. Tan, M.B.B.S. • Z. P. Ding, M.B.B.S.
Department of Cardiology, National Heart Centre Singapore, Mistri Wing, 17 Third Hospital Avenue, Singapore, 168752, Singapore
e-mail: Paul.chiam.t.l@nhcs.com.sg; Jack.tan.w.c@nhcs.com.sg; Ding.zee.pin@nhcs.com.sg

Electronic supplementary material The online version of this chapter (doi:10.1007/978-1-4471-4294-2_23) contains supplementary material, which is available to authorized users.

Learning Points

- In this case of functional MR, the prominent and extensive Chiari network was trapped by the transseptal catheter and wire and dragged into the left atrium. It can be mistaken for thrombus. Even when recognized as a Chiari network in the left atrium, there remains the technical risk of injury and disruption of the Chiari network by the MitraClip during device manipulation. This, in turn, can result in embolization and ischemic end-organ injury, e.g., stroke. Caution should be employed in avoiding the Chiari network during the transseptal puncture and during crossing of the interatrial septum.

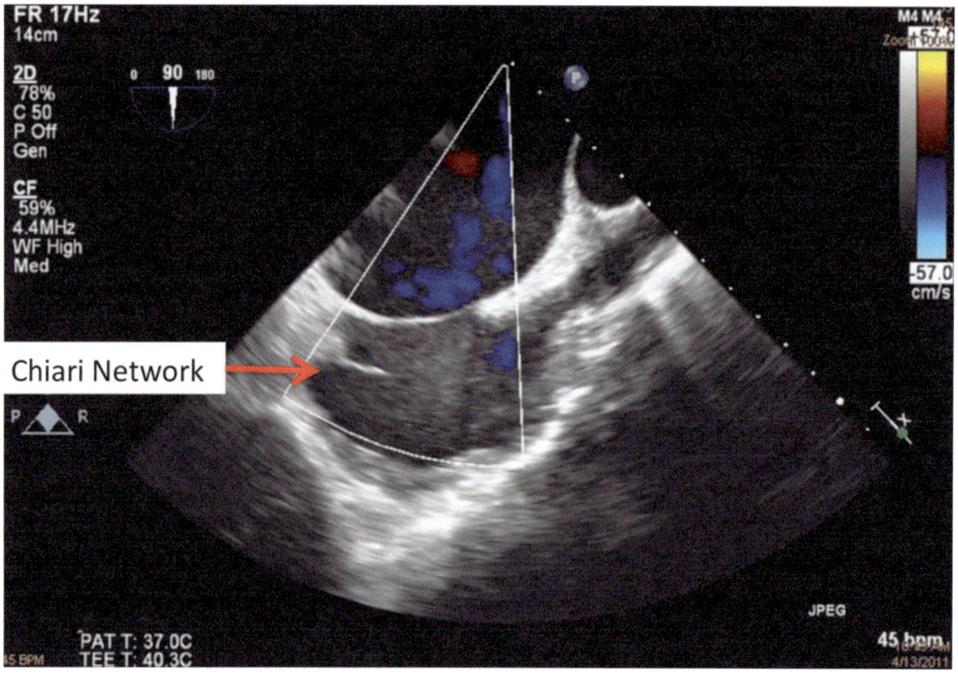

Fig. 23.1 Pre-procedure TEE showing part of the Chiari network

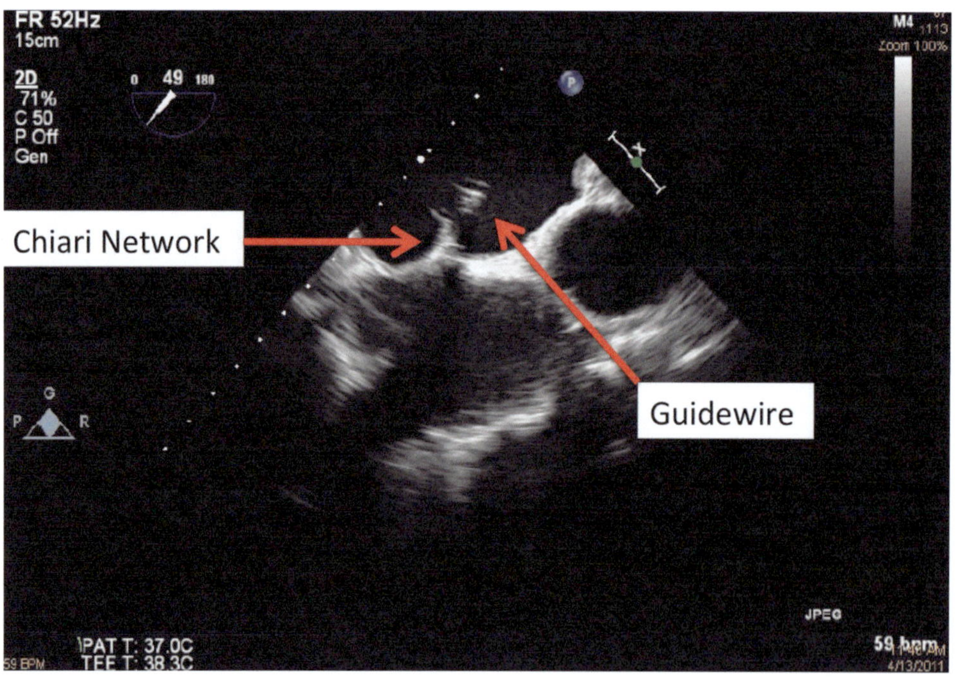

Fig. 23.2 TEE showing the guidewire with the mobile Chiari network attached

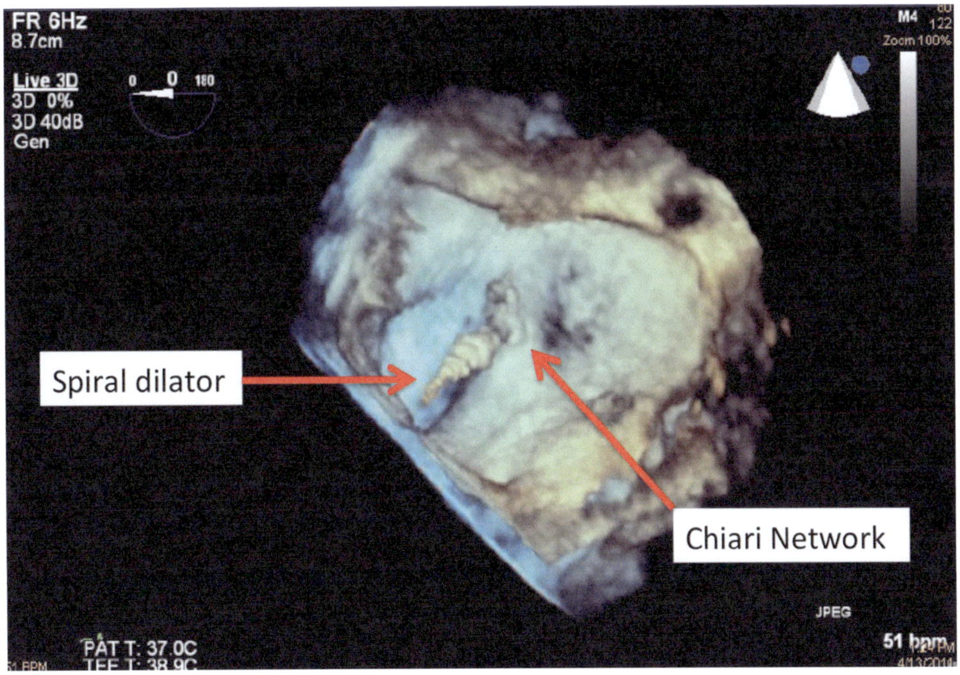

Fig. 23.3 3D TEE view from the left atrium showing the guide with the spiral dilator and the attached Chiari network

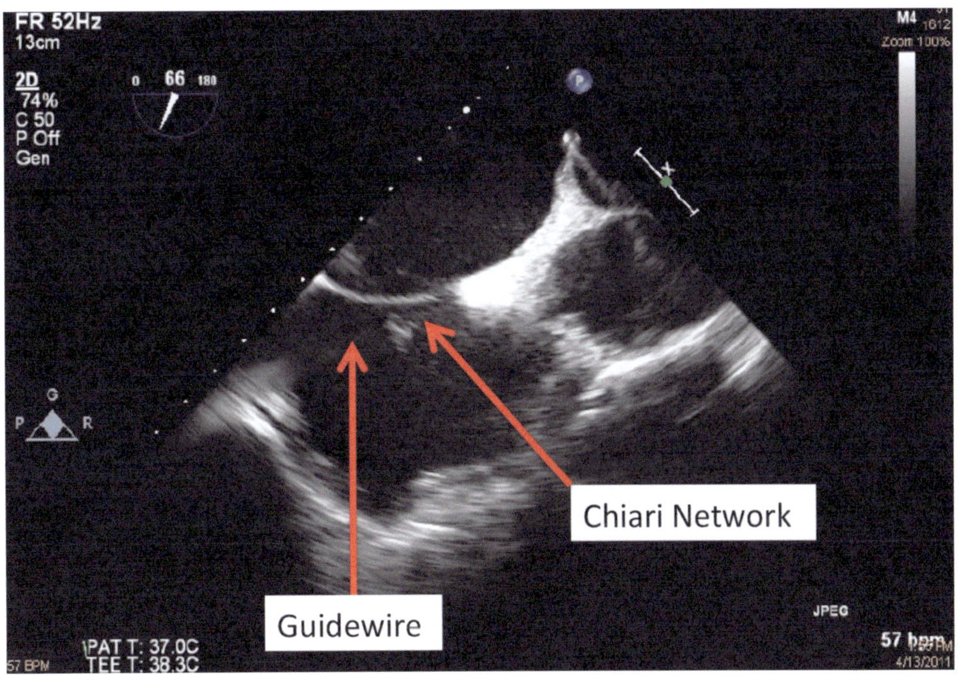

Fig. 23.4 The Chiari network is seen to return to the right atrium as the 0.035 guidewire is withdrawn

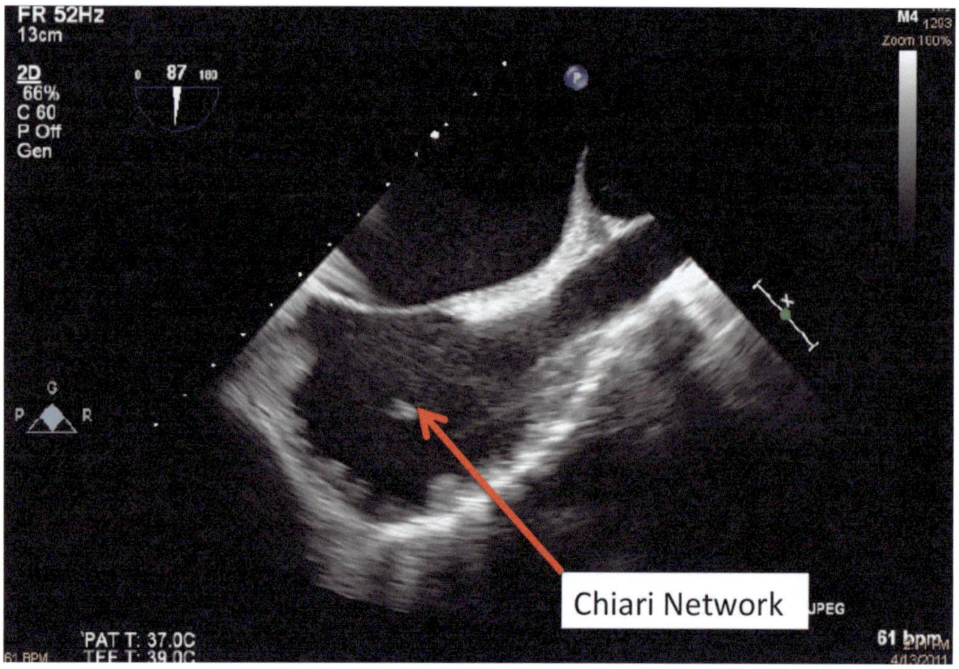

Fig. 23.5 After withdrawal of guide and wire back into the right atrium: Chiari network visualized

24 EVEREST II: Two MitraClip Procedure with Partial Detachment of Second Device

Ehrin J. Armstrong, Khung Keong Yeo, and Jason Rogers

Abstract

An important complication of the MitraClip procedure is single leaflet detachment. This case illustrates such a complication and demonstrates the echocardiographic and fluoroscopic images associated with it.

Keywords

Mitral regurgitation • MitraClip • Single leaflet detachment • Surgery

Clinical History

A 72-year-old woman presented with exertional dyspnea and was found to have severe mitral regurgitation with mild left ventricular enlargement. She qualified for the EVEREST II trial and was randomized to MitraClip therapy.

E.J. Armstrong, M.D., M.Sc.
Division of Cardiovascular Medicine, University of California, Davis Medical Center, 4860 Y Street, Suite 2820, Sacramento, CA 95817, USA
e-mail: ehrin.armstrong@ucdmc.ucdavis.edu

K.K. Yeo, M.B.B.S., FACC, FSCAI
Department of Cardiology, National Heart Centre Singapore, Mistri Wing, 17 Third Hospital Avenue, Singapore, 168752, Singapore

Department of Cardiovascular Medicine, University of California, Davis Medical Center, 4860 Y Street, Suite 2820, Sacramento, CA 95817, USA
e-mail: yeo.khung.keong@nhcs.com.sg

J. Rogers, M.D., FACC, FSCAI (✉)
Department of Cardiovascular Medicine, University of California, Davis Medical Center, 4860 Y Street, Suite 2820, Sacramento, CA 95817, USA
e-mail: jason.rogers@ucdmc.ucdavis.edu

Summary

The patient's pre-procedure echocardiograms demonstrate posterior leaflet prolapse with mild tethering of the anterior leaflet, suggesting a primary degenerative etiology. The origin of the MR was central and met severity and anatomic entry criteria for the randomized EVEREST II trial (Figs. 24.1, 24.2, 24.3, 24.4, 24.5, 24.6, 24.7, 24.8, 24.9, and 24.10). After deployment of the first MitraClip device in a central location, there was a residual jet of MR (Figs. 24.11, 24.12, 24.13, 24.14, and 24.15). Placement of a second device successfully reduced the MR to 1+. Unfortunately, the patient developed minor esophageal trauma from the TEE probe during the procedure, which led to significant post-procedure emesis. The second clip then partially detached, likely due to her periprocedural emesis and inadequate leaflet insertion at the time of initial deployment. Figures 24.11, 24.12, 24.13, 24.14, 24.15, 24.16, 24.17, 24.18, 24.19, 24.20, 24.21, and 24.22 showcase the various steps of the procedure. This case also demonstrates that assessment of leaflet capture by the second

Electronic supplementary material The online version of this chapter (doi:10.1007/978-1-4471-4294-2_24) contains supplementary material, which is available to authorized users.

MitraClip can be difficult given ultrasound shadowing from the adjacent previously deployed device. She subsequently underwent successful surgical explant of the devices and mitral valve repair with only trace residual MR (Figs. 24.23, 24.24, 24.25, 24.26, 24.27, 24.28, 24.29, 24.30, 24.31, and 24.32).

Learning Points

- Inadequate leaflet insertion can lead to single leaflet detachment. Therefore, it is important to do a careful check for adequacy of leaflet insertion after a successful grasping attempt.

Screening Transthoracic Echo

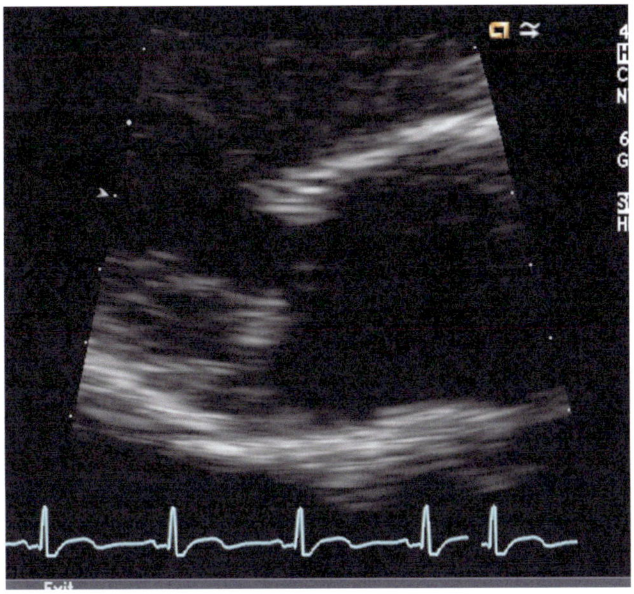

Fig. 24.1 TTE: parasternal LAX w/o color. The parasternal long axis demonstrates mild prolapse of the posterior leaflet with some possible mild restriction of the anterior leaflet during diastole

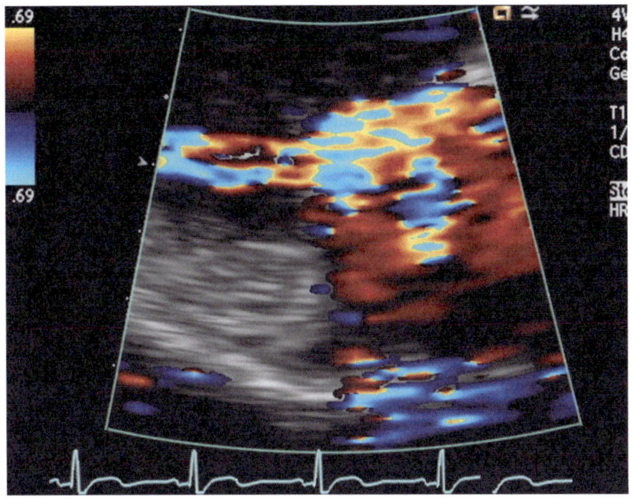

Fig. 24.2 TTE: parasternal LAX w/ color. There is an anteriorly directed jet of mitral regurgitation originating from the site of posterior leaflet prolapse

Screening Transthoracic Echo I

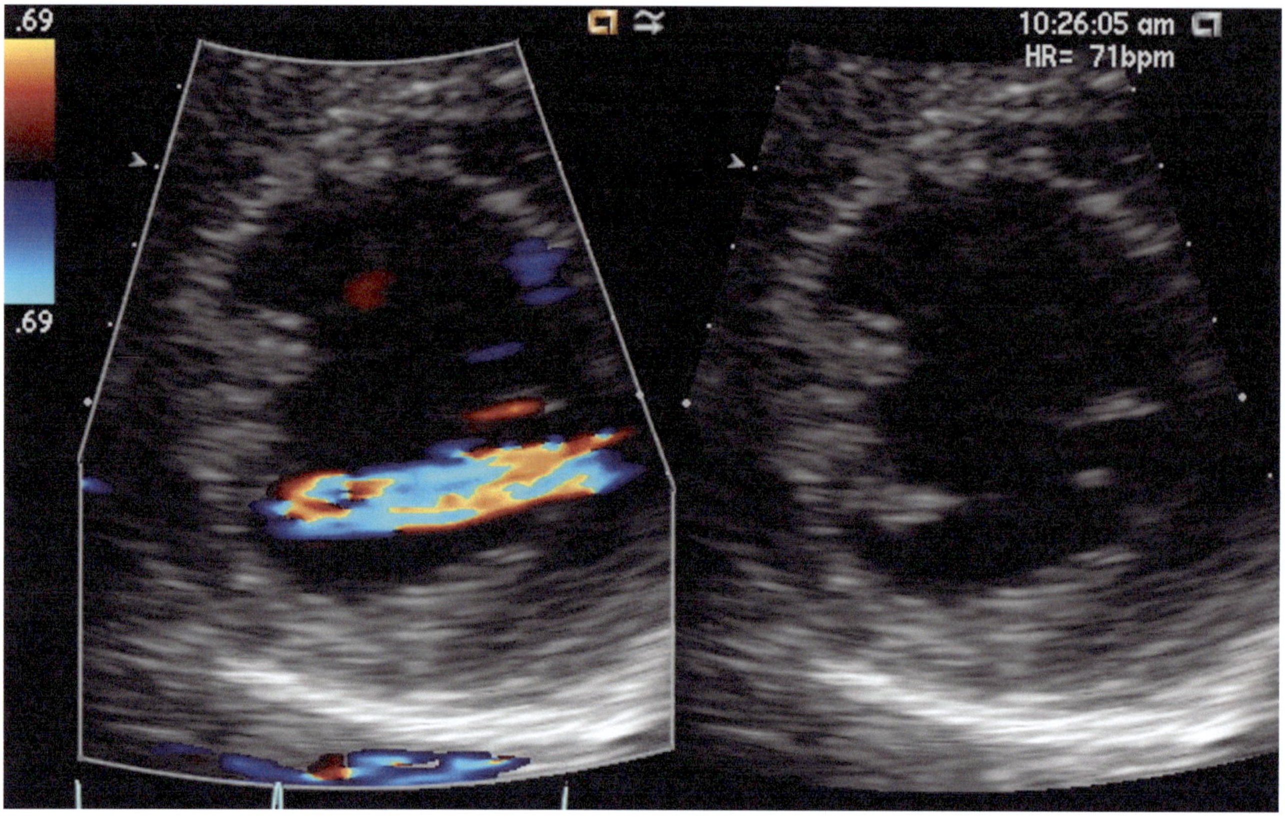

Fig. 24.3 TTE: parasternal SAX. Short axis view shows that the MR has a wide but central jet

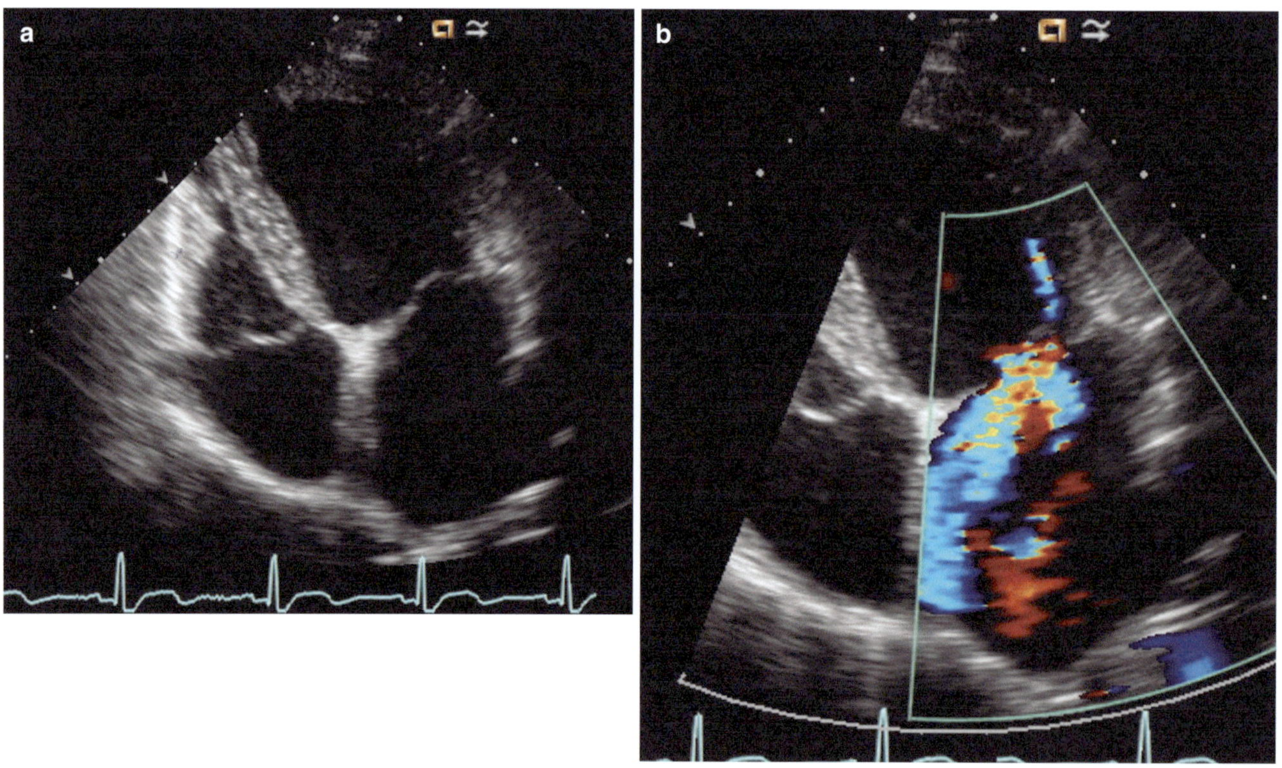

Fig. 24.4 TTE: apical 4C view. The apical four-chamber view shows biatrial enlargement and left ventricular enlargement (**a**). The regurgitant jet originates centrally and is directed anteriorly (**b**)

Screening Transthoracic Echo II

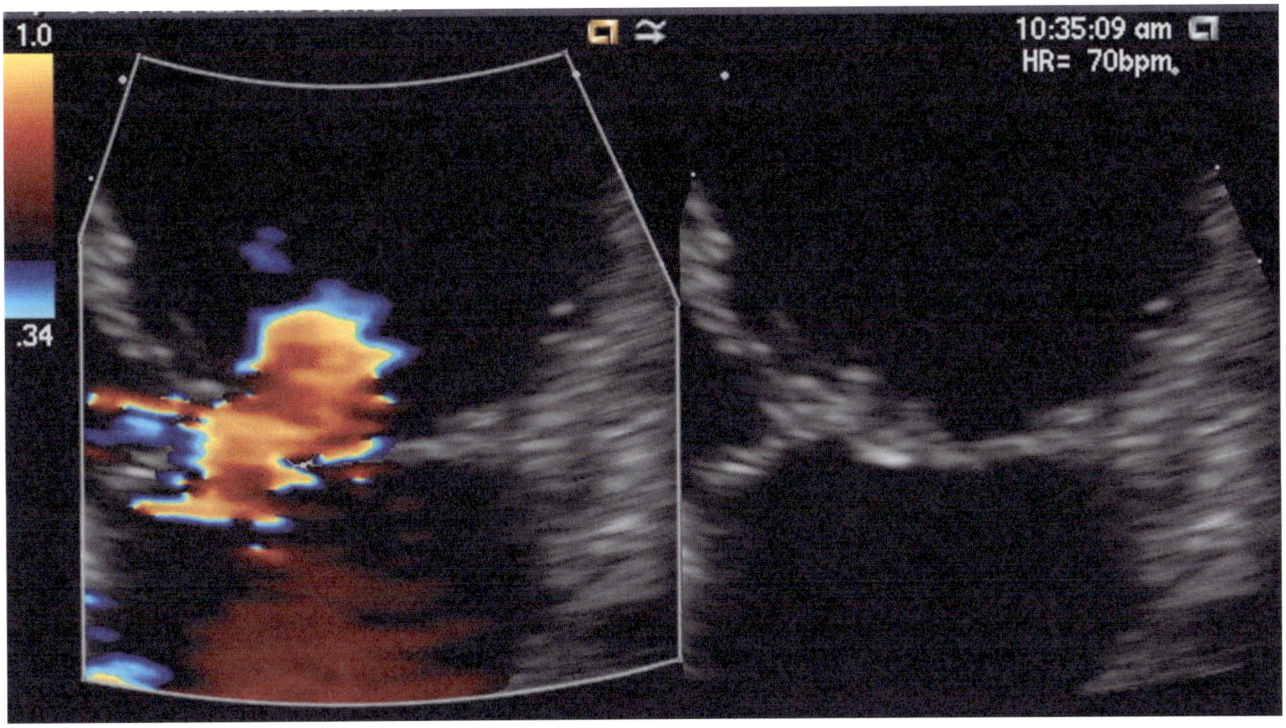

Fig. 24.5 TTE: apical 4C magnified. On magnified apical 4C views with a lower Nyquist limit, the large PISA can be appreciated, as well as the width of the mitral regurgitant jet at the level of the leaflets

Screening TEE

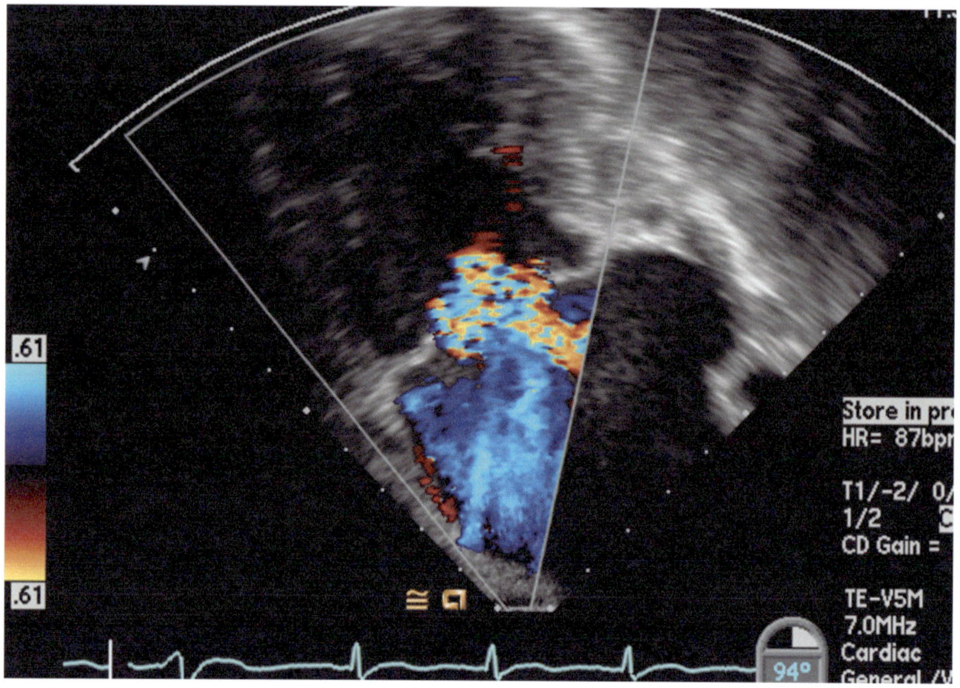

Fig. 24.6 TEE: bicommissural w/ color. The bicommissural view shows a wide central jet

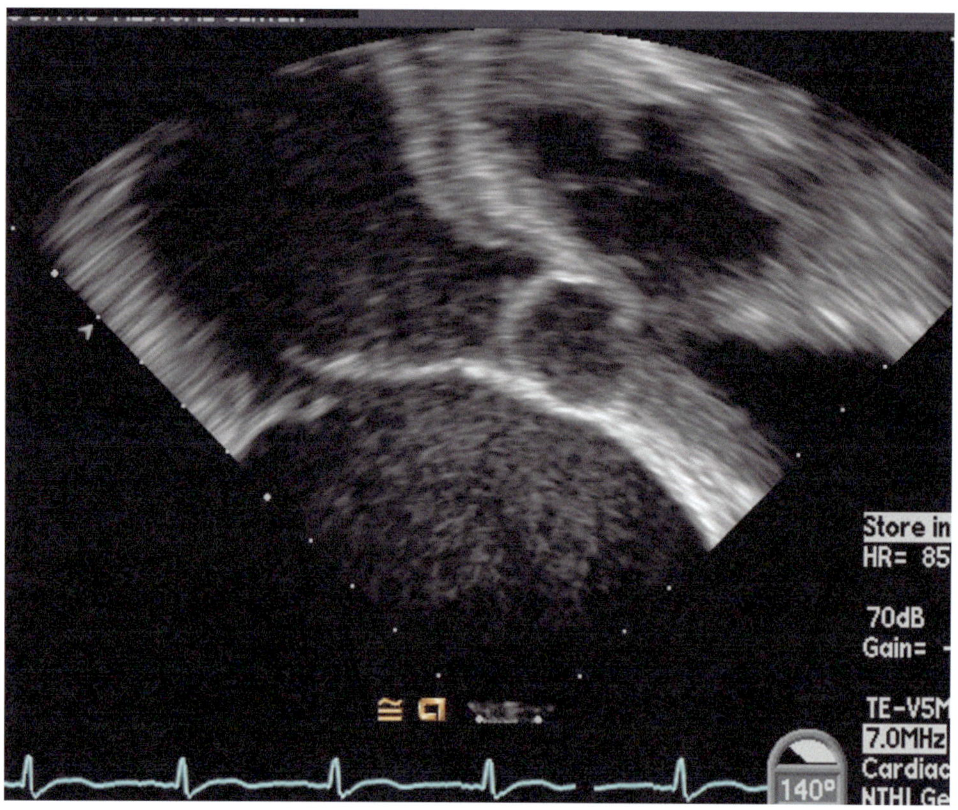

Fig. 24.7 TEE: 3C w/o color. On the three-chamber view, the posterior leaflet prolapse is apparent. There is also mild restriction of the anterior leaflet, suggesting a mixed functional/degenerative etiology

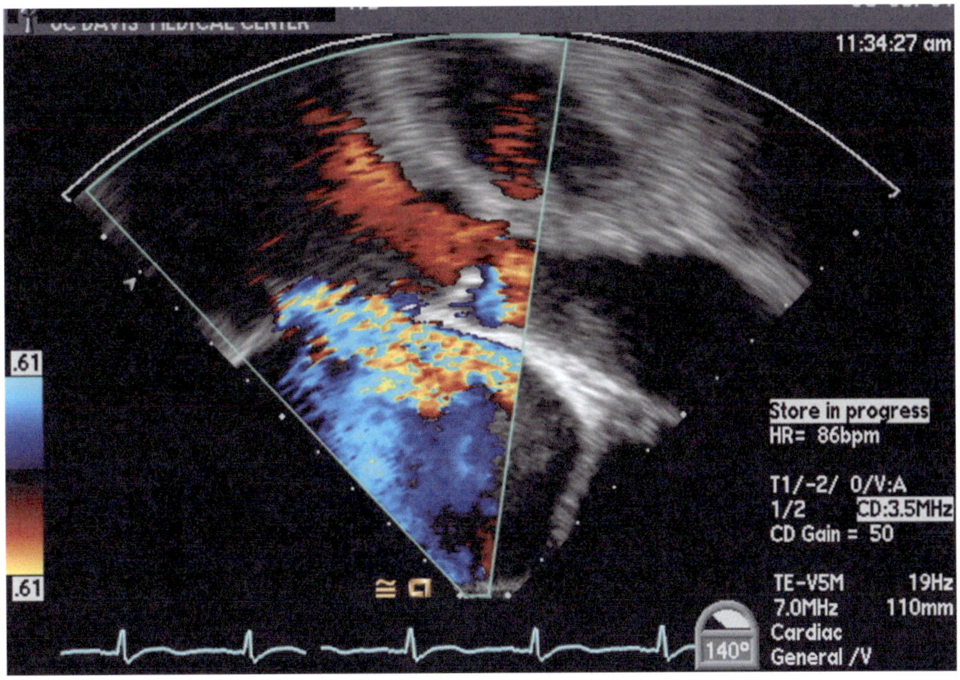

Fig. 24.8 TEE: 3C w/ color. The Doppler imaging shows the origin of the jet at the line of malcoaptation, and that the jet is directed anteriorly

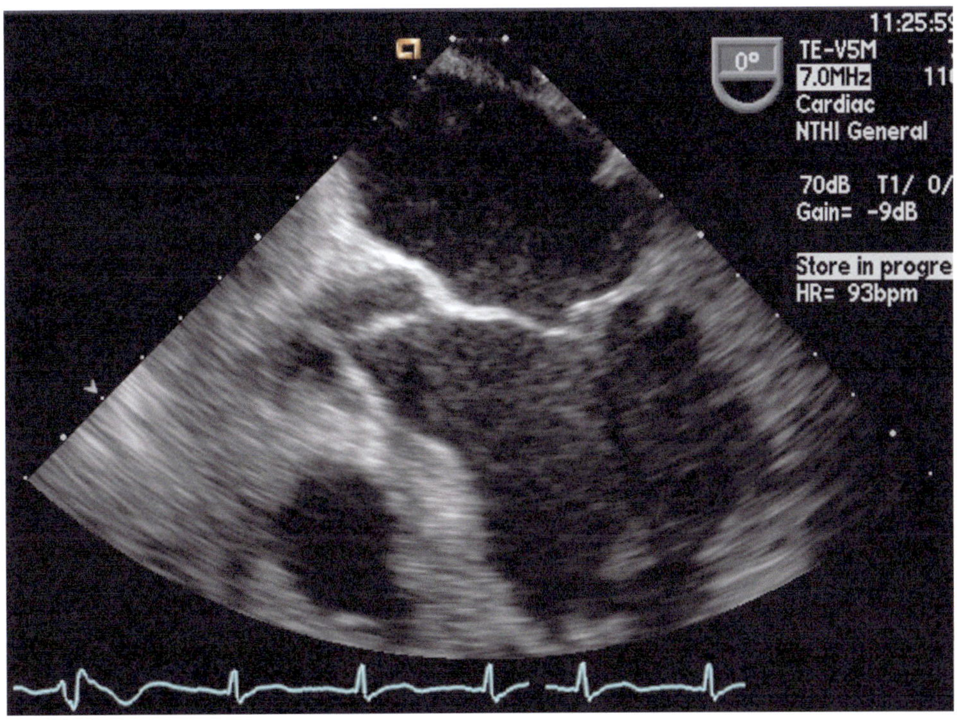

Fig. 24.9 TEE: 4C w/o color. In the four-chamber view, the mild prolapse of P2 is apparent, with concomitant mild tenting of the anterior leaflet

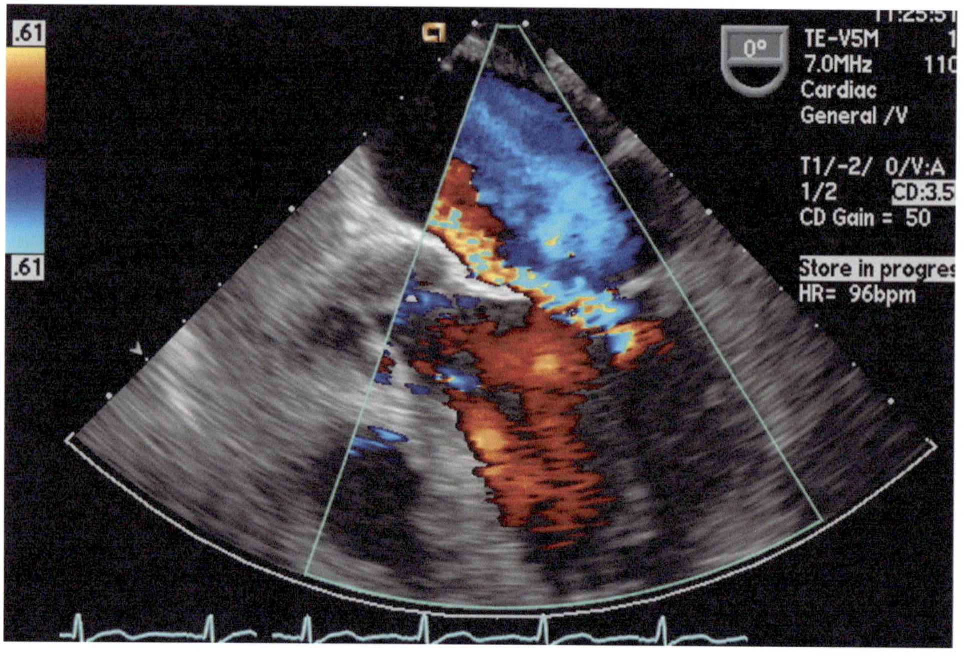

Fig. 24.10 TEE: 4C w/ color. The Doppler regurgitant jet is directed anteriorly

Procedural TEE and Fluoro I

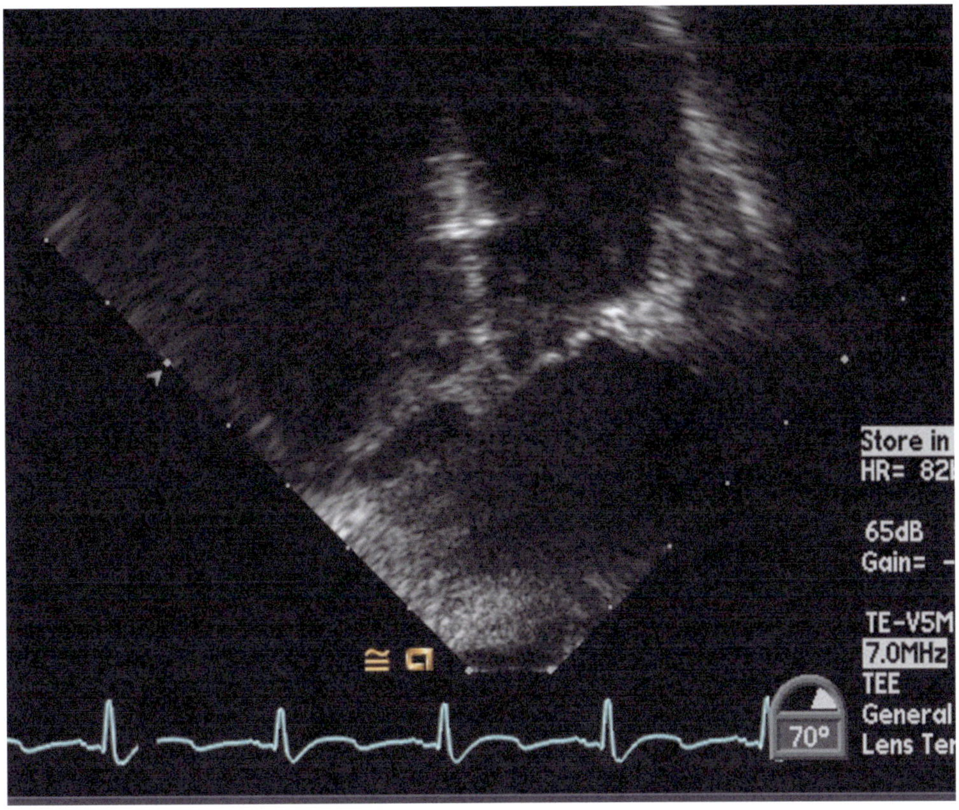

Fig. 24.11 TEE: Bicom view. The first device is advanced across central portion of the valve

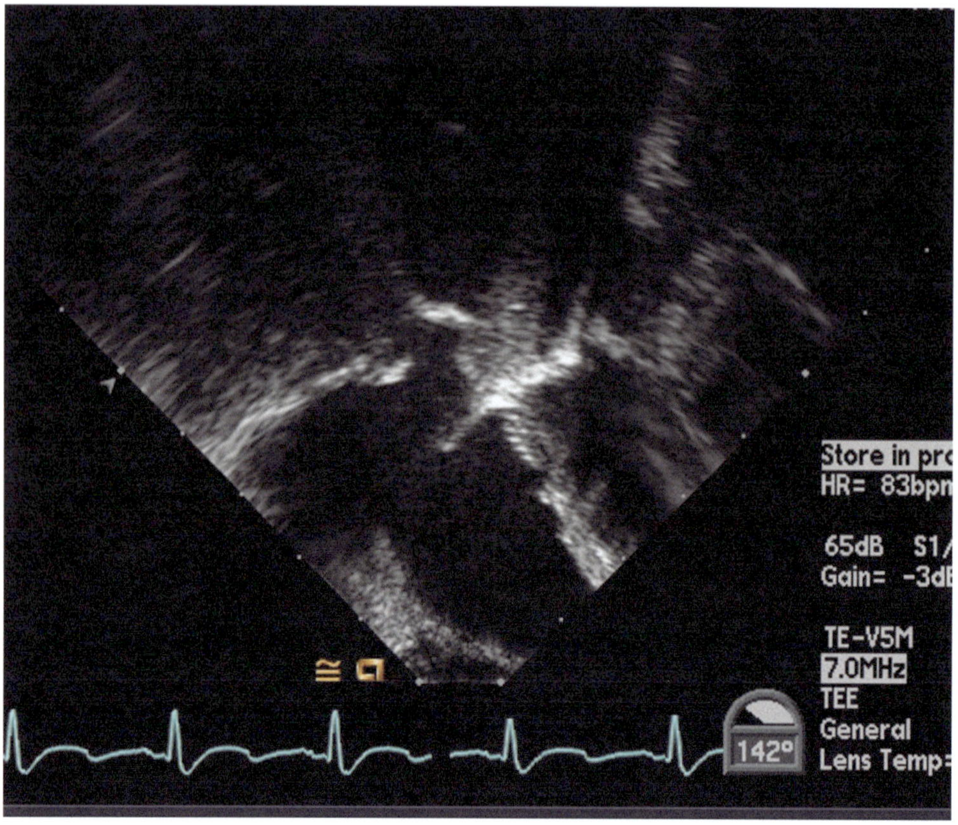

Fig. 24.12 TEE: 3C view. Positioning of the device is confirmed in the 3C view as it is advanced

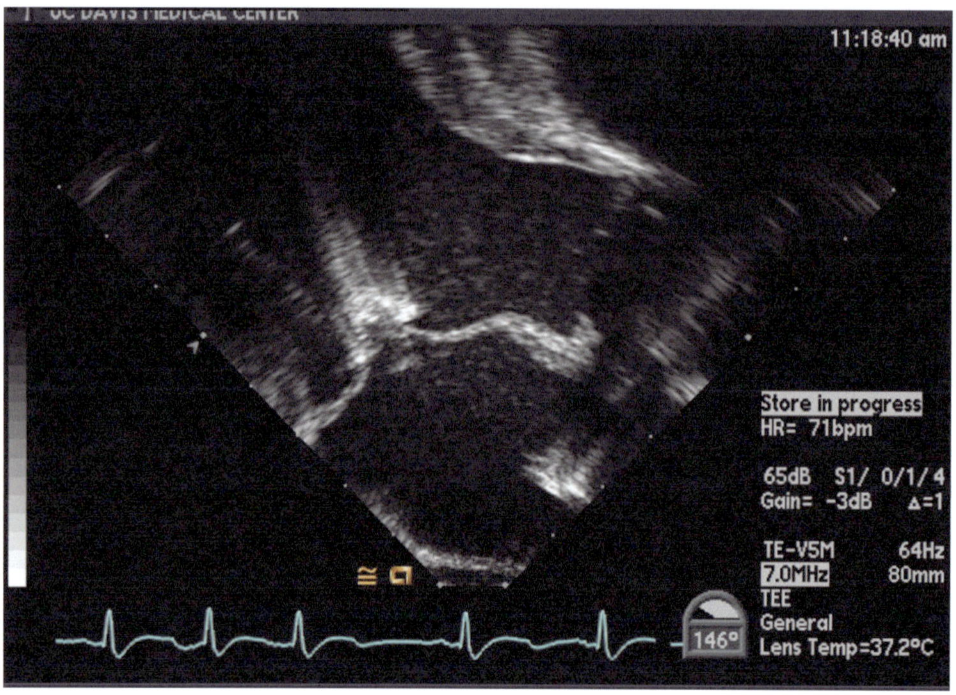

Fig. 24.13 TEE: 3C view. The first device is deployed and grasps the anterior and posterior leaflets in a central location

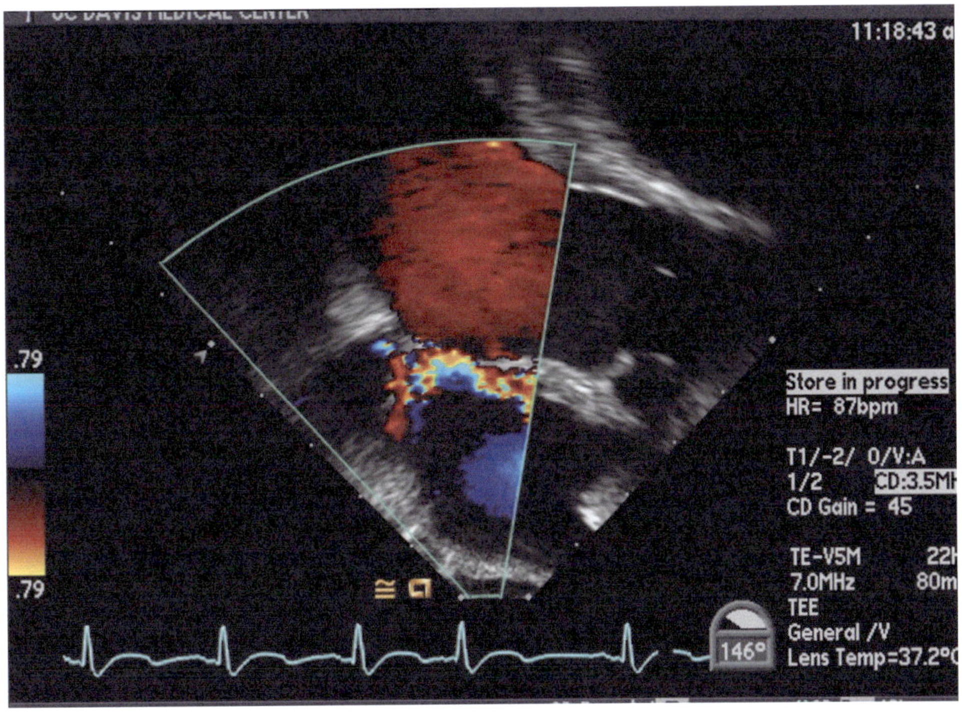

Fig. 24.14 TEE: 3C view with Doppler. There is a persistent anteriorly directed jet of mitral regurgitation after deployment of the first device

Procedural TEE and Fluoro II

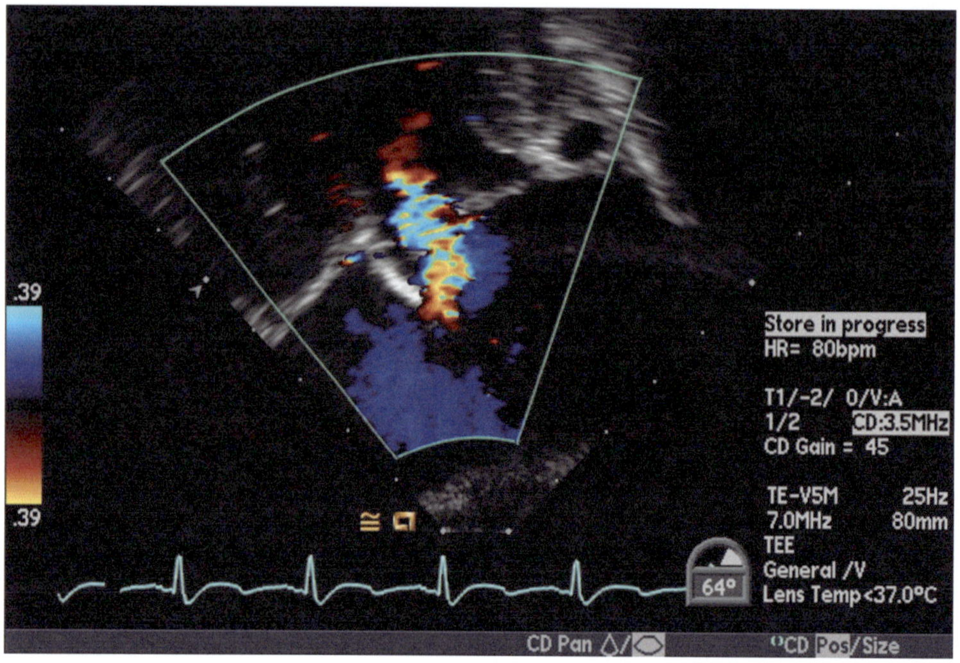

Fig. 24.15 TEE: Bicom view with Doppler. The persistent MR can also be seen in the Bicom view, lateral to the first device

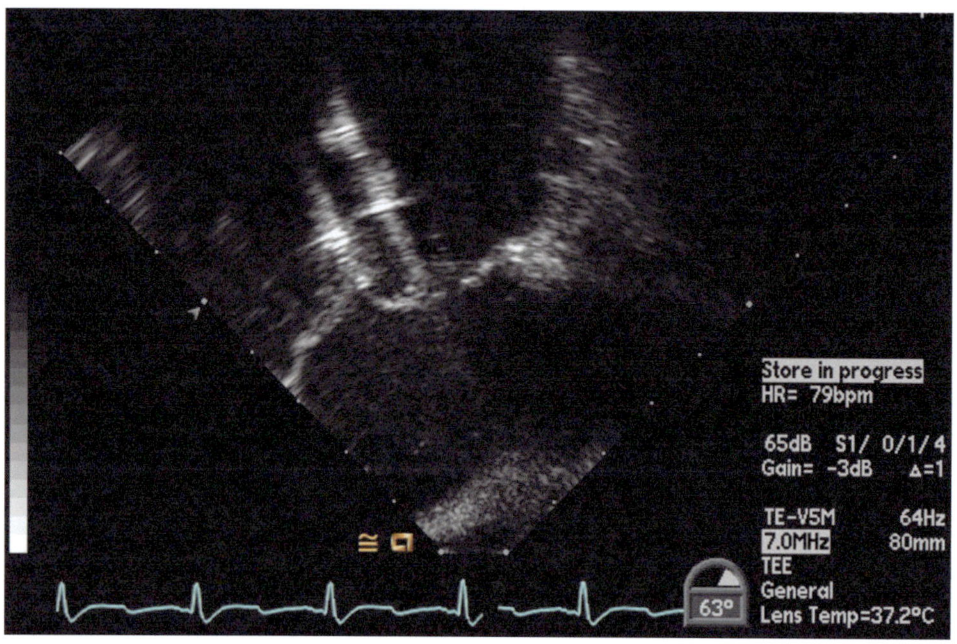

Fig. 24.16 TEE: Bicom view. A second device is advanced across the valve lateral to the first device

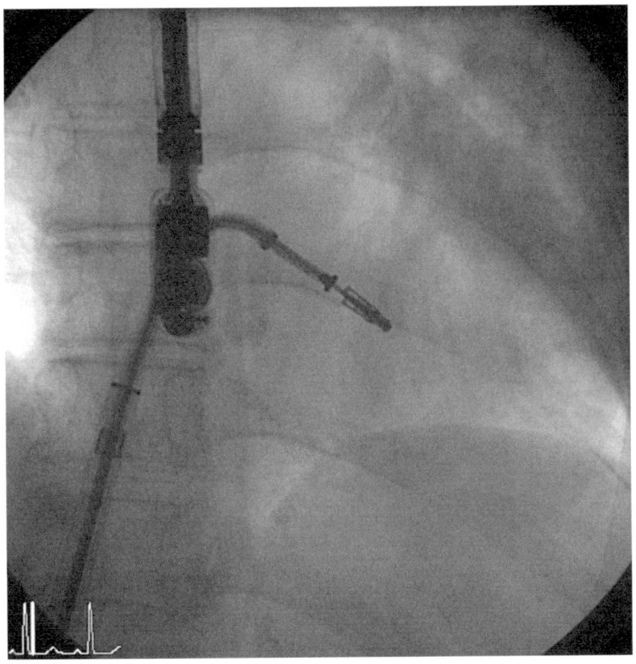

Fig. 24.17 Fluoro: first device alignment. The first device has grasped the mitral leaflets and appears well oriented

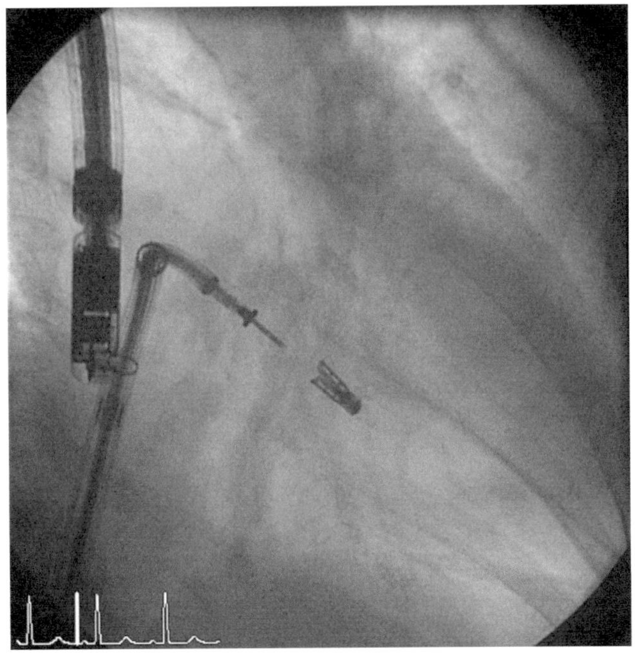

Fig. 24.18 Fluoro: first device deployed. The first device is now detached from the delivery system and has a stable appearance

Procedural TEE and Fluoro III

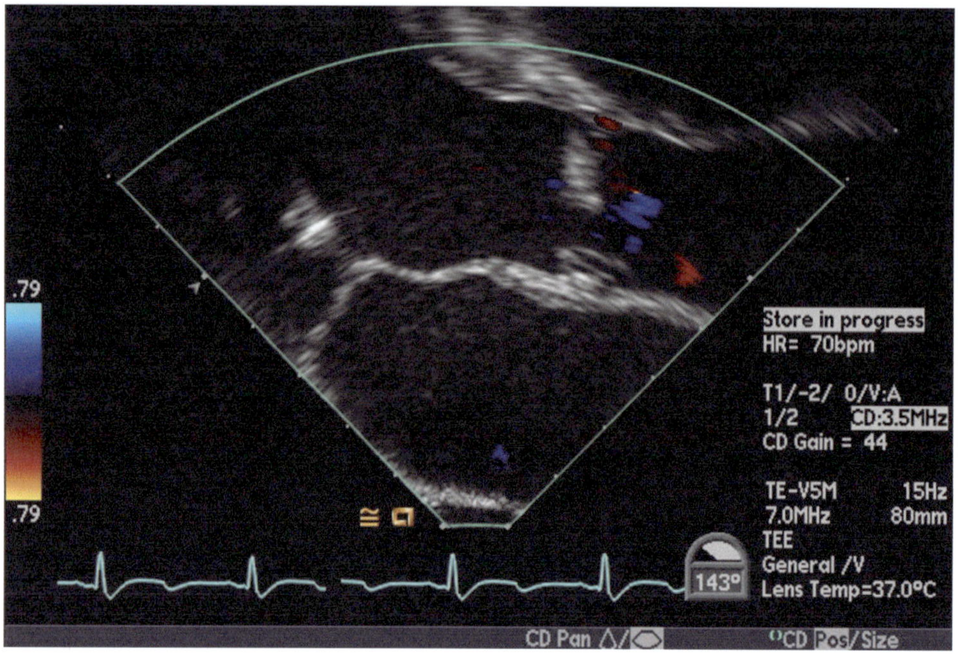

Fig. 24.19 TEE: 3C view with Doppler. Post-deployment of two devices, there is minimal to no MR in the 3C view

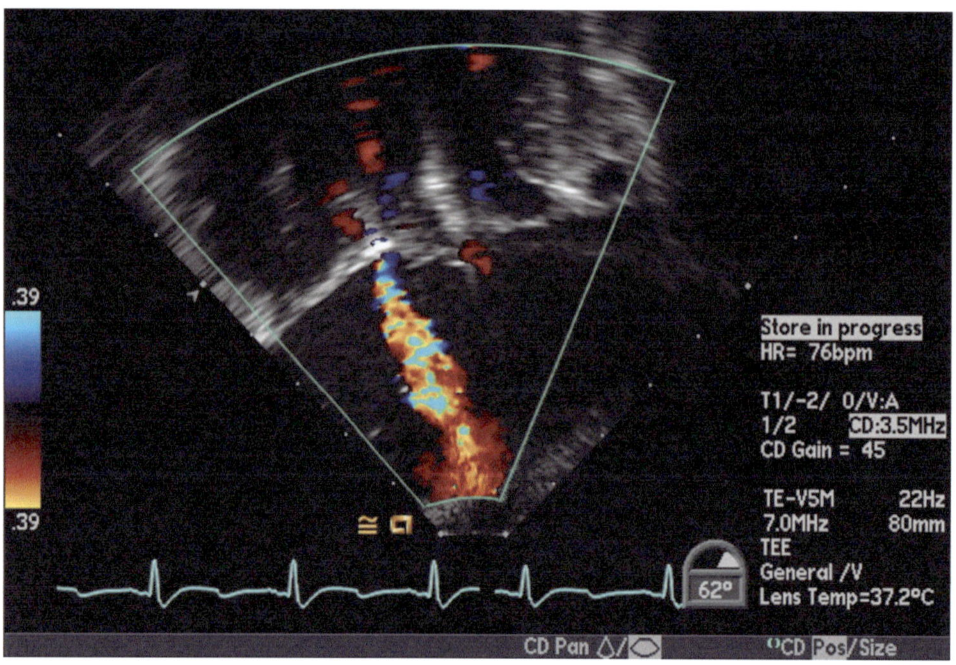

Fig. 24.20 TEE: Bicommissural view after clip deployment. In the bicommissural view, there is a localized jet of persistent MR near the coaptation site of the first device

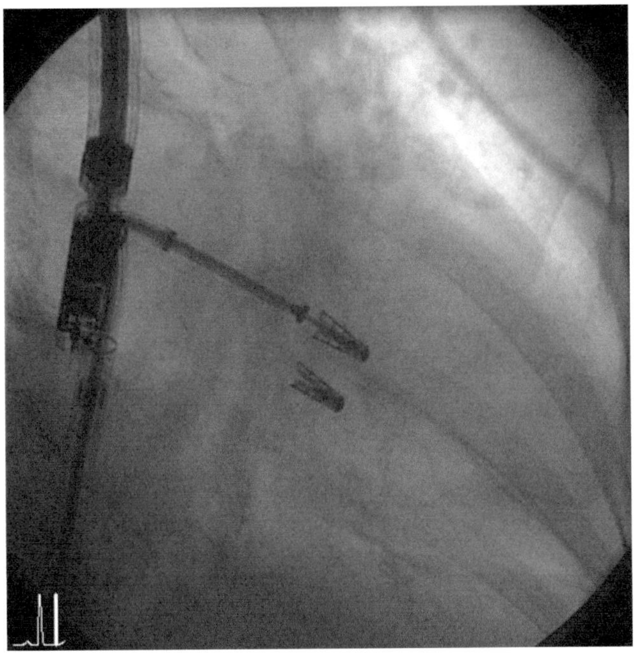

Fig. 24.21 Fluoro: second device deployment. The second device is aligned parallel to the first device

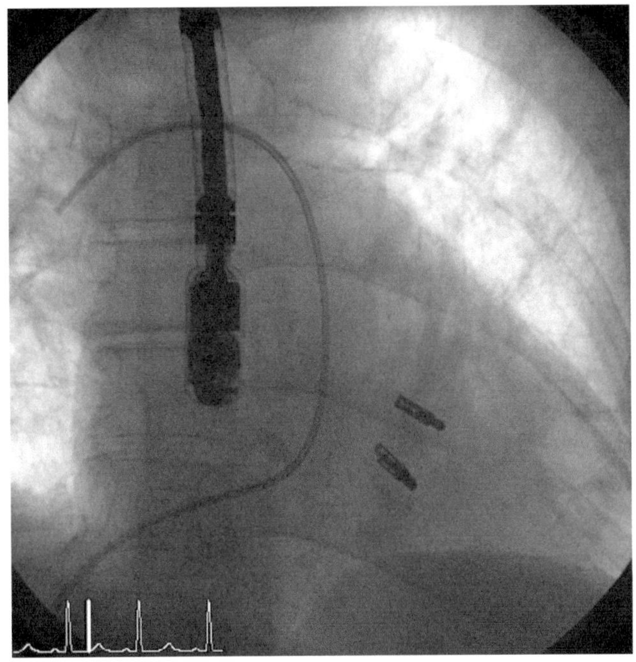

Fig. 24.22 Fluoro: final device position. At the conclusion of the procedure, the device position is stable, and there is 1+ MR

Post-procedure TTE

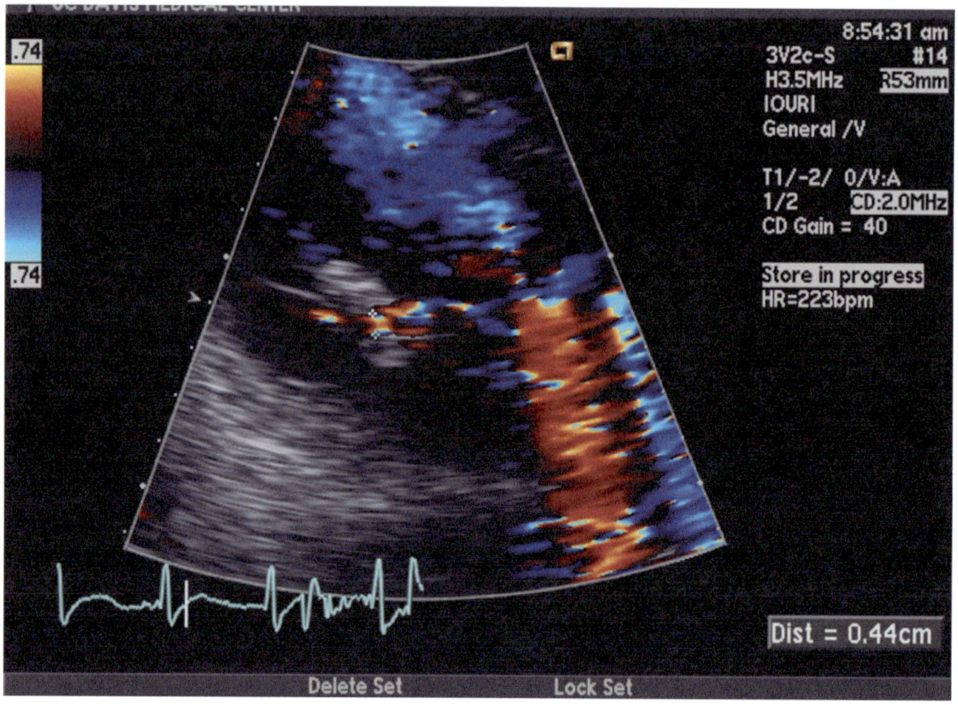

Fig. 24.23 TTE: parasternal LAX w/ color. The parasternal long axis demonstrates recurrent MR with significant aliasing

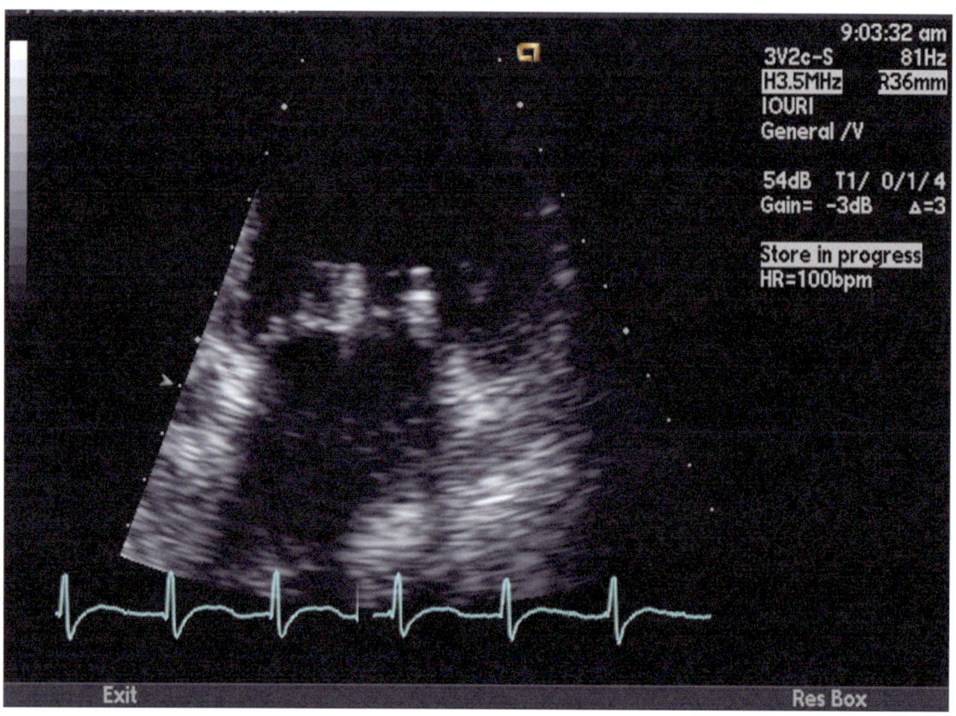

Fig. 24.24 TTE: apical 4C w/o color. In the A4C view during diastole, the devices appear well aligned and parallel

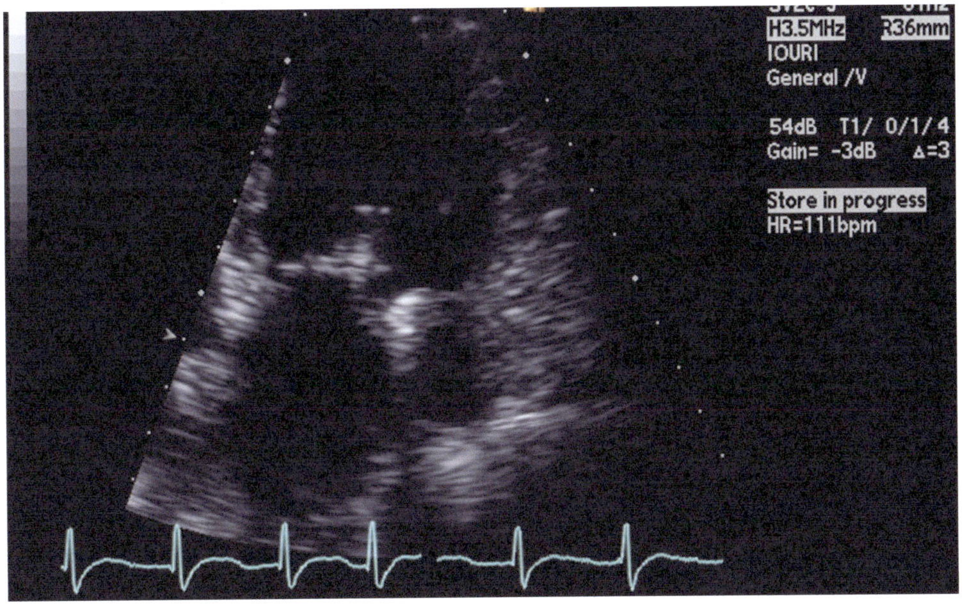

Fig. 24.25 TTE: apical 4C w/o color. In systole, the orientation of the devices has changed, with the more lateral device flipping back into the left atrium. This is consistent with partial clip detachment

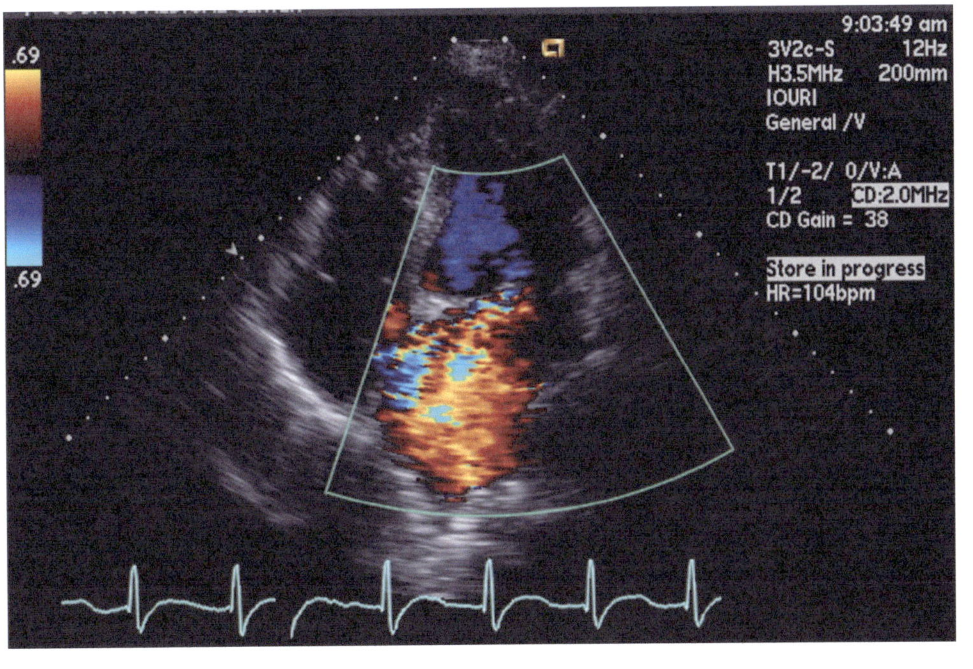

Fig. 24.26 TTE: apical 4-chamber with Doppler. On Doppler imaging, there is a large color jet of recurrent MR

Post-procedure Fluoroscopy

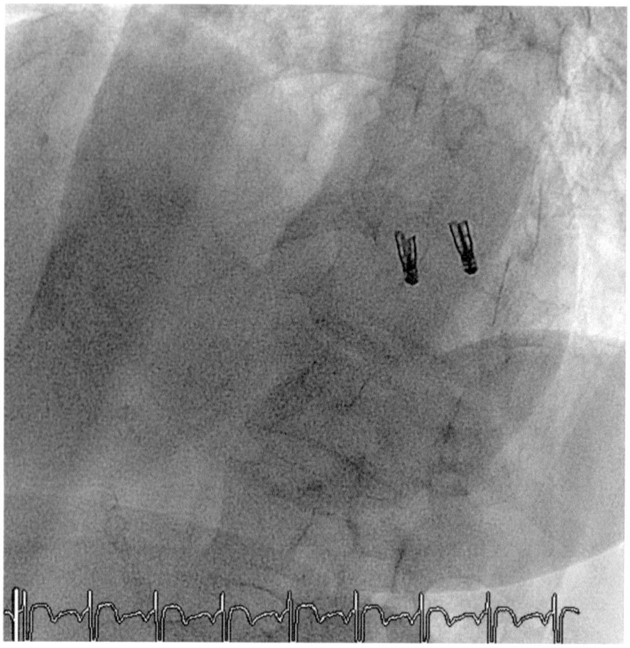

Fig. 24.27 Fluoro: diastole. In LAO cranial view during diastole, the devices appear well oriented in a stable position relative to the mitral valve leaflets

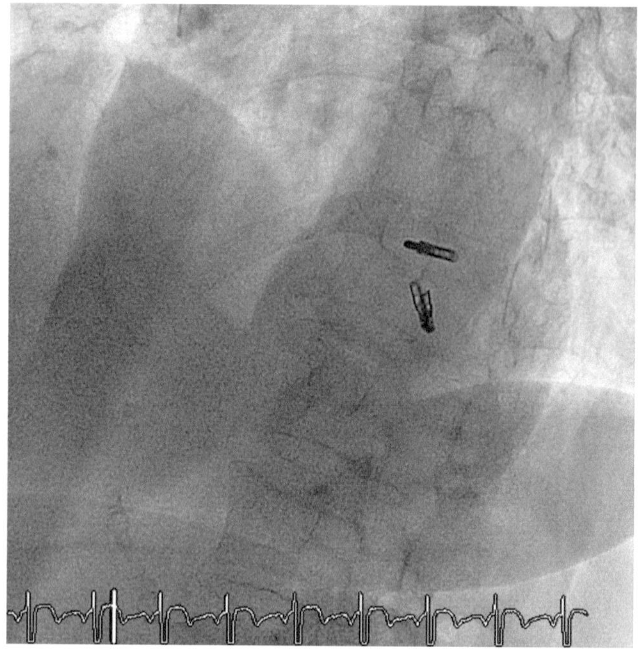

Fig. 24.28 Fluoro: systole. In LAO cranial view during systole, the lateral (second device) changes orientation, consistent with partial clip detachment

Postsurgical Mitral Valve Repair TTE

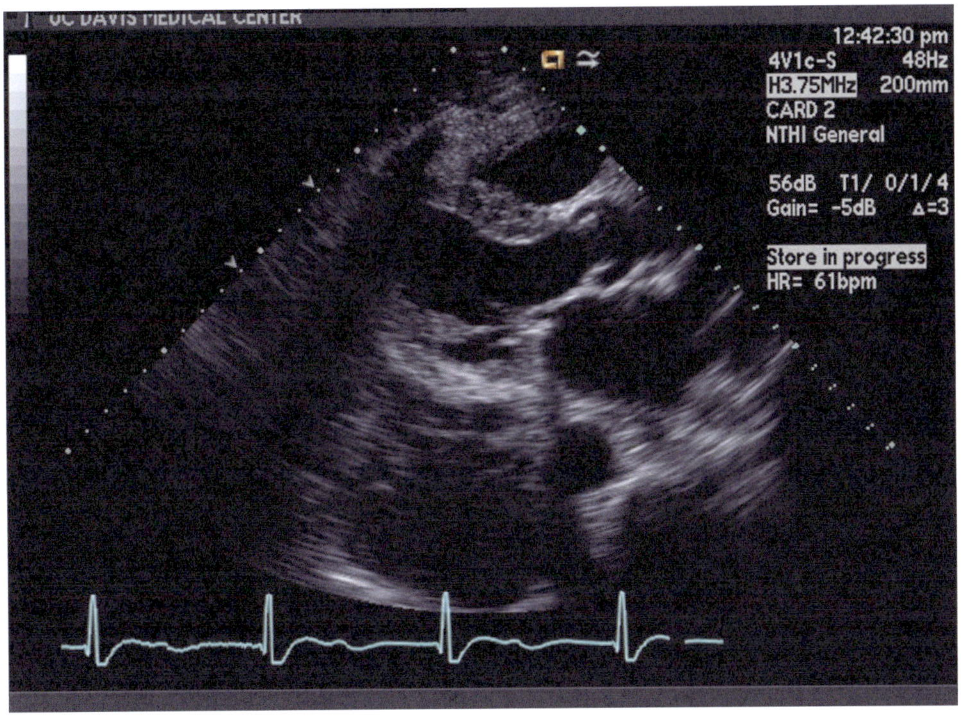

Fig. 24.29 TTE: parasternal LAX w/o color. After device explant and successful surgical mitral valve repair with partial leaflet resection and annular ring placement, there is good coaptation of the anterior and posterior leaflets. There is a postsurgical large pleural effusion

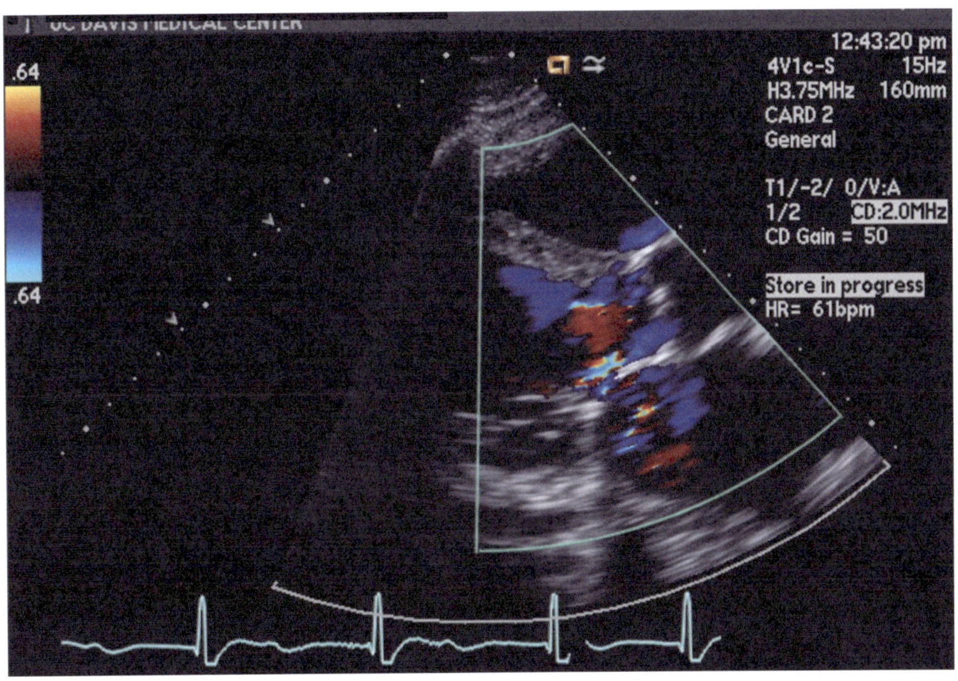

Fig. 24.30 TTE: parasternal LAX w/ color. On Doppler imaging, there is only a trace jet of MR originating near the coaptation of A2 and P2

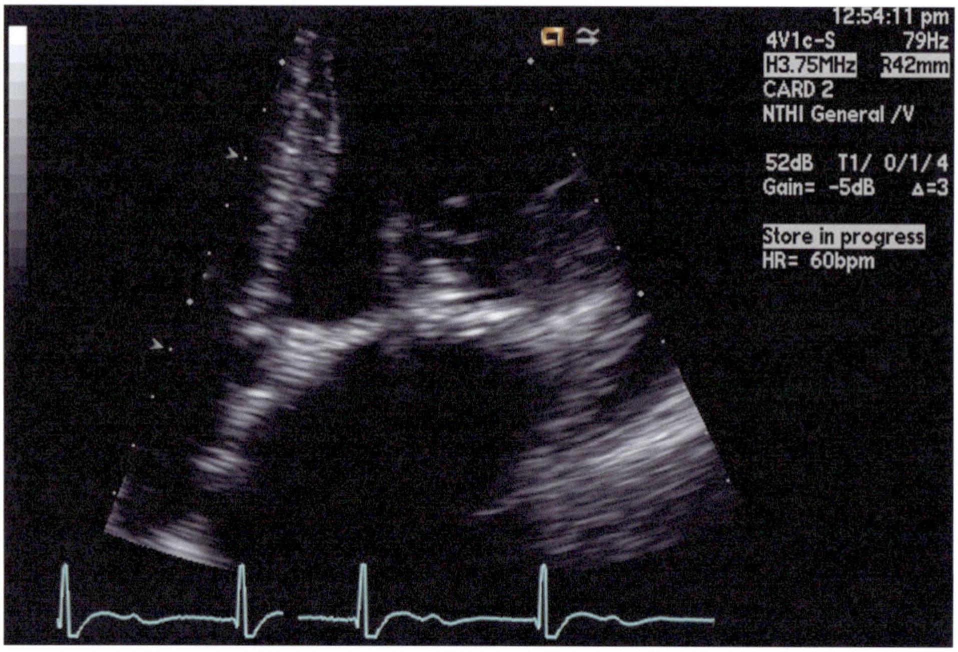

Fig. 24.31 TTE: apical 4C w/o color. A magnified apical 4C view shows the leaflet coaptation after surgical repair

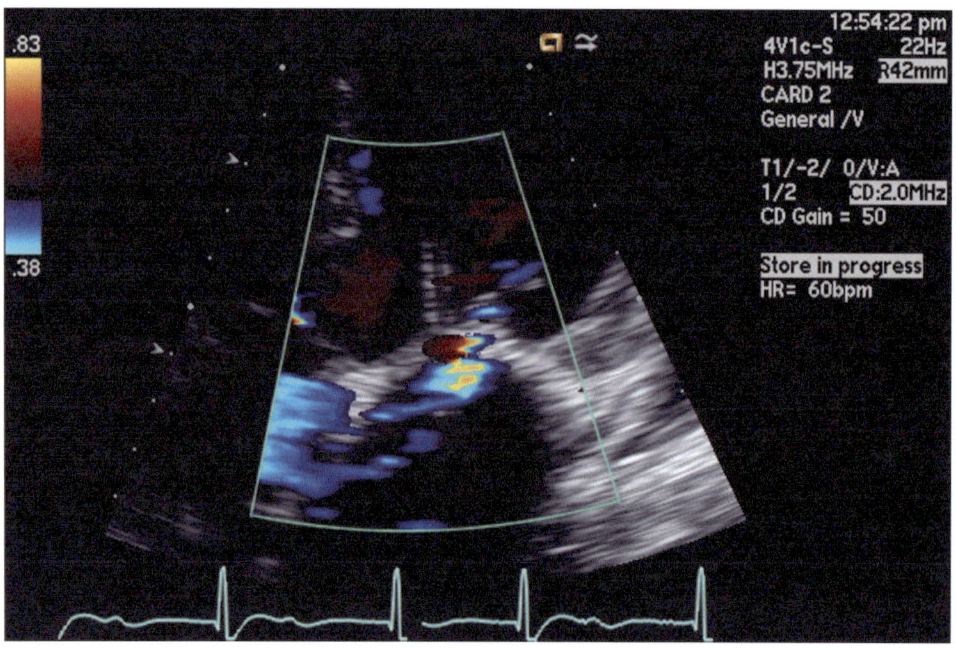

Fig. 24.32 TTE: apical 4C w/ color. There is trace MR by Doppler imaging

MitraClip Procedure in Unusual Heart Position

25

Gian Paolo Ussia, Valeria Cammalleri, Salvatore Scandura, and Corrado Tamburino

Abstract

We describe two cases in which altered thoracic and cardiac anatomy complicated the MitraClip procedure. In the first case, the patient had a prior pneumonectomy which caused rotational displacement of the heart in the mediastinum. The case illustrates the adjustments required for appropriate transseptal puncture. In the second case, transesophageal imaging was adversely affected by a malignancy.

Keywords

Mitral regurgitation • MitraClip • Pneumonectomy • Mesothelioma

The MitraClip procedure is indicated for use in patients at high risk for cardiac surgery. Appropriate patient selection, for clinical indication as well as anatomic eligibility, is of critical importance to ensure a high rate of procedural success. With greater experience and improved skills, patients who are "off label" and not ideal candidates based on anatomical and clinical criteria may be treated with this procedure. The MitraClip device has an important procedural characteristic: It has to be introduced in the left atrium through a transseptal puncture of the interatrial septum and maneuvered in three orthogonal planes into an optimal position perpendicular to the mitral valve plane. The transseptal puncture (TSP) has to be performed at a precise location to allow for adequate manipulation of the catheter delivery system (CDS) for optimal positioning. A TSP site that is too close to the valve plane can increase the complexity of the procedure due to an unfavorable orientation, position, and direction of the delivery CDS in relation to the mitral valve.

Performance of TSP under fluoroscopic guidance alone in cases of abnormal orientation and/or position of the heart, such as scoliosis, is particularly challenging as it is difficult to obtain a safe needle orientation using the standard fluoroscopy landmarks. The use of ancillary imaging modalities like transesophageal echocardiography (TEE) allows the TSP to be performed safely at an appropriate puncture location. The needle tip pressing against the septum creates a tenting artifact that aids in localizing the puncture site and height from the mitral valve (Fig. 25.1). Other chapters in this atlas will further discuss the role of the transseptal puncture. TEE guidance is fundamental to the successful performance of the successive stages of the MitraClip procedure. TSP is performed after identifying a suitable site by TEE that is located posterior and superior to facilitate manipulation and positioning of the CDS above the mitral valve plane. This is followed by navigation of the clip in the left atrium and ventricle, opening the clip and grasping of the mitral valve leaflets. The quality of grasping and degree of reduction in the severity of mitral regurgitation are then evaluated. It is obvious that TEE guidance and monitoring through optimal imaging views is of paramount importance in ensuring a successful procedure and expedient detection of any procedural complications. The following case examples with complex cardiac and thoracic anatomy highlight the importance of the imaging in the MitraClip procedure.

G.P. Ussia, M.D. (✉) • V. Cammalleri • S. Scandura • C. Tamburino
Divisione Clinicizzata di Cardiologia, A.O.U. Policlinico
Vittorio Emanuele, Ospedale Ferrarotto, Universià di Catania,
Via Citelli 1, Catania 95100, Italy
e-mail: gpussia@hotmail.com

T. Feldman et al. (eds.), *Atlas of Percutaneous Edge-to-Edge Mitral Valve Repair*,
DOI 10.1007/978-1-4471-4294-2_25, © Springer-Verlag London 2013

Case 1: Case History

A 74-year-old man with a history of left pneumonectomy for lung cancer and coronary artery disease developed dilated cardiomyopathy and severe functional mitral regurgitation (Fig. 25.2) accompanied with NYHA class III symptoms. The echocardiogram showed a left ventricular ejection fraction of 25 %. The mitral valve anatomy was suitable for MitraClip implantation.

The diagnostic TEE study was technically challenging due to difficulty in obtaining standardized views. A CT scan helped us in understanding the anatomical orientation of the heart, which was rotated clockwise within the thoracic cavity (Fig. 25.3). The procedural steps were planned after integrating imaging data from the TEE and CT images. The technical challenges included: (a) identification of the TSP site; (b) a suitable site for positioning of the stiff wire, the pulmonary veins were inaccessible due to prior ligation in the pneumonectomy; and (c) orientation of the clip above the mitral valve by ensuring a perpendicular alignment of the distal part of the CDS above the mitral valve plane.

The patient was intubated, and a TEE was performed concentrating on the principal views to evaluate mitral valve anatomy and function. The valve was assessed in the long axis (three-chamber view), intercommissural (dual-chamber view), and the trans-gastric short axis view. The TEE probe angulation was adjusted to compensate for cardiac rotation. Hence, the three-chamber view was obtained at 100° angulation, while the normal is 140° (Fig. 25.4a) in order to visualize the mitral valve and enable assessment of mitral regurgitation, and the intercommissural view was obtained at 30°, instead of 60° (Fig. 25.4b).

The transseptal puncture posed some technical challenges. In order to identify correct orientation of the needle in superoinferior and anteroposterior plane as well as height of the puncture above the mitral valve, we obtained a bicaval view, short axis view at the level of the aortic mound (torus aorticus), and a four-chamber view. The TSP was performed in the standard fashion: an 8 F transseptal Mullins sheath was placed over a 0.032 J tip wire in the superior vena cava, the Brockenbrough needle was positioned in the introducer, and the system was rotated in the clockwise direction, while slowly being withdrawn in the right atrium. The height, the posterior orientation of the puncture site, and the tenting of the needle were identified in TEE. The needle required additional clockwise rotation to position it in an adequately posterior orientation. The TEE guidance was critical in ensuring a successful TSP at the required puncture site in the interatrial septum. Once inside the left atrium (LA), an angiogram was performed to ensure the correct position (Fig. 25.5).

The next technical challenge was to position the stiff wire in a suitable location. The standard maneuver consists in advancing a 6-Fr multipurpose catheter (with side holes) over a 0.035 in. wire and placing it in the left upper pulmonary vein (Fig. 25.6). The 0.035 wire is replaced with a superstiff wire, and the catheter is withdrawn. In this particular case, the options were (a) place the wire in the left atrium or (b) in the left ventricle. In general, we prefer not to place any stiff wires in the left atrium unless it is positioned in a pulmonary vein. This is because the atrium is thin and can be damaged, and the length of stiff wire inside the LA may not be enough to provide a safe support for the 24-F guide catheter (GC), especially in a patient who already had a cardiac intervention. In these patients, the atrial septum could be thicker than normal and pose some difficulties in passing through. An Amplatz superstiff wire with 1-cm soft straight tip, shaped into a J tip, was placed in the left ventricle (Fig. 25.7); the TEE in the three-chamber view showed the stiff wire in the LV (Fig. 25.8), the position was stable, and adequate length of the wire was available in the left ventricle, and the 24-Fr GC was safely placed inside the LA (Fig. 25.7b).

The insertion of the CDS has to be strictly monitored with the TEE. The length of GC inside the LA should not exceed 25 mm from the interatrial septum (Fig. 25.9), and the distal tip of the CDS should be advanced under constant visualization to avoid trauma to the atrial wall or the left atrial appendage (Fig. 25.10).

The standard maneuvers utilized in getting optimal orientation of the GC and CDS have to be modified. The operator should be aware of the mitral annular plane and adjust the three knobs: CDS mediolateral, CDS anteroposterior, and GC mediolateral to get the MitraClip as perpendicular to the valve as possible (Fig. 25.11), and the grasp is performed in standard fashion (Fig. 25.12). Small, deliberate movements of the knobs can help in understanding the behavior of the CDS in response to these movements. Each movement needs to be checked in all three spatial axes using multiple 2D imaging planes. The fluoroscopy is used for check the trajectory of the MitraClip and to rule out excessive distortion of the CDS inside the left chambers (Fig. 25.13). These maneuvers are not significantly different from those in a normally oriented heart because the intrinsic relationship of various structures inside the left heart was unaltered after lung surgery. The final result was a mild mitral regurgitation (Fig. 25.14) with the clip placed in the correspondence of A2-P2 scallops (Fig 25.15).

Case 2: Case History

An 82-year-old woman with severe aortic stenosis, severe mitral regurgitation of functional etiology, left ventricular ejection fraction around 30 %, and NYHA class III, considered at high risk for cardiac surgery, was referred for transcatheter valve therapies.

She underwent transcatheter aortic valve implantation with a 26-mm Corevalve Medtronic (Medtronic Inc., USA) and was scheduled for a MitraClip procedure because of persistent severe mitral regurgitation MR despite successful relief of the aortic valve stenosis. Her functional status improved to NYHA class I–II, but the mitral insufficiency remained grade III–IV necessitating high-dose diuretics. The pre-procedural chest X-ray showed mild widening of the mediastinum; after intubation, the TEE probe was placed in the esophagus, but the echocardiographic window was worse in comparison with the initial TEE study performed 3 months earlier. At fluoroscopy (Fig 25.16), the TEE probe was completely deviated from its standard position. The procedure was discontinued, and the patient underwent a CT scan of the thorax with evidence of new mesothelioma (Fig. 25.17).

Learning Points

1. In patients with unusual rotation or position of the heart secondary to a thoracic abnormality (Fig. 25.18), i.e., scoliosis or prior surgery, the TSP is a challenge that is easily surmounted with the appropriate use of TEE. The first case had a clear clockwise rotation of the heart within the thorax (Fig. 25.18a), more evident when compared to a normal patient (Fig. 25.18b). For this reason, the transseptal needle had to be extrarotated in clockwise direction, while the height was similar; in fact, both the inferior and superior vena cava positions were unaltered as noted in the sagittal view of patient CT scan (Fig. 25.19a) compared to the normal (Fig. 25.19b).
2. Despite the altered cardiac orientation, the procedural steps of the MitraClip procedure remain essentially similar to a standard implant procedure. The only difference is the angulation of the TEE probe for visualizing the principal views, with some adjustment to account for the underlying cardiac rotation.
3. It is essential to have an anatomical proximity between the esophagus and the heart to enable adequate visualization of the mitral valve and left ventricle under TEE. Worsening of imaging windows should alert the operator to the possibility of an interceding mass between the esophagus and the heart. In Case 2, the procedure is not safe because of inadequate visualization of the interatrial septum and of the left heart structures.

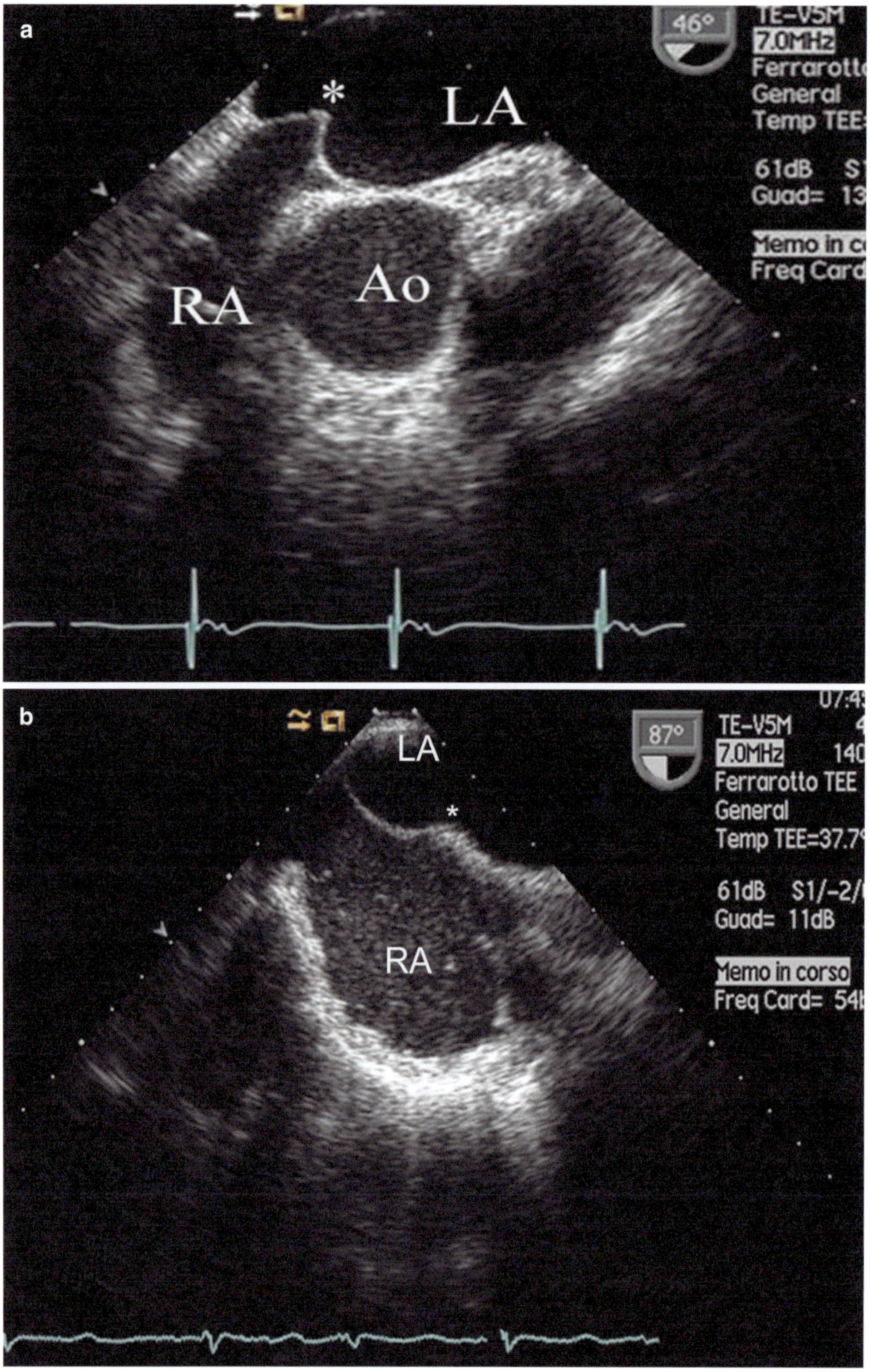

Fig. 25.1 Transesophageal echocardiographic guidance during the transseptal puncture. The tenting created by the needle tip pressing on the septum is evident (*asterisk*), both in mid-esophageal short axis (**a**) and bicaval (**b**) view. The short axis view is useful to guide the puncture localization in an anteroposterior axis, whereas the bicaval window is used to guide the superoinferior orientation of the needle. *LA* left atrium, *RA* right atrium, *Ao* aorta

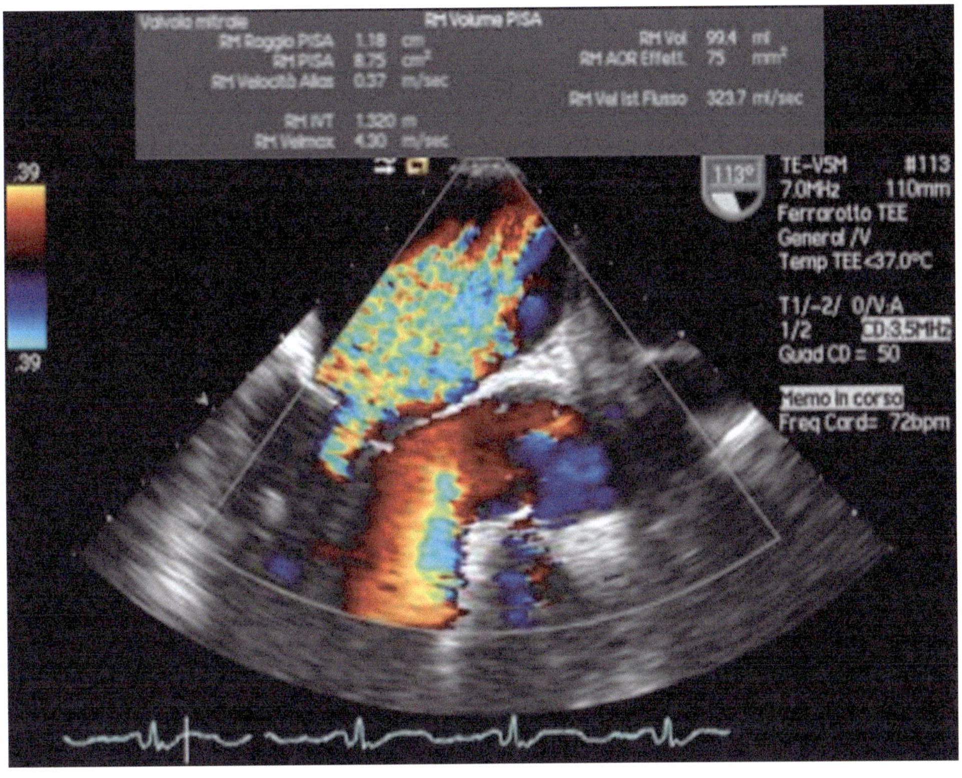

Fig. 25.2 Diagnostic transesophageal echocardiogram. Severe functional mitral regurgitation due to a bi-leaflet tethering in a dilated cardiomyopathy. The effective orifice area and the regurgitant volume, using the proximal isovelocity surface area (*PISA*) method, were calculated

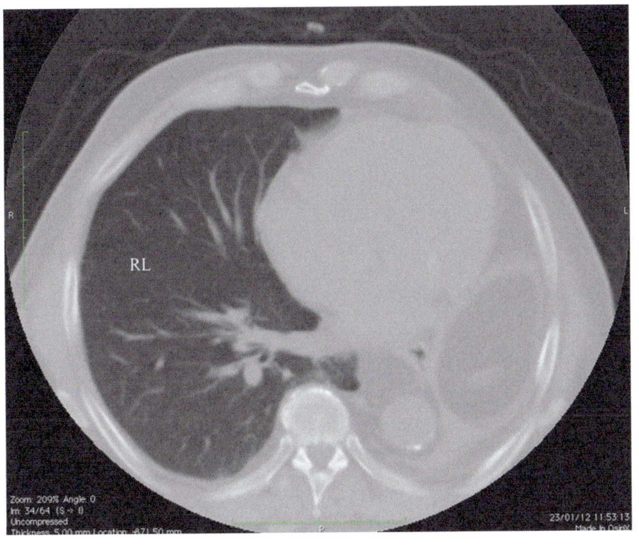

Fig. 25.3 (**a**)Thoracic CT scan without contrast. We note the absence of the left lung, the cardiac silhouette is rotated in clockwise direction, and the right lung (*RL*) is overexpanded.

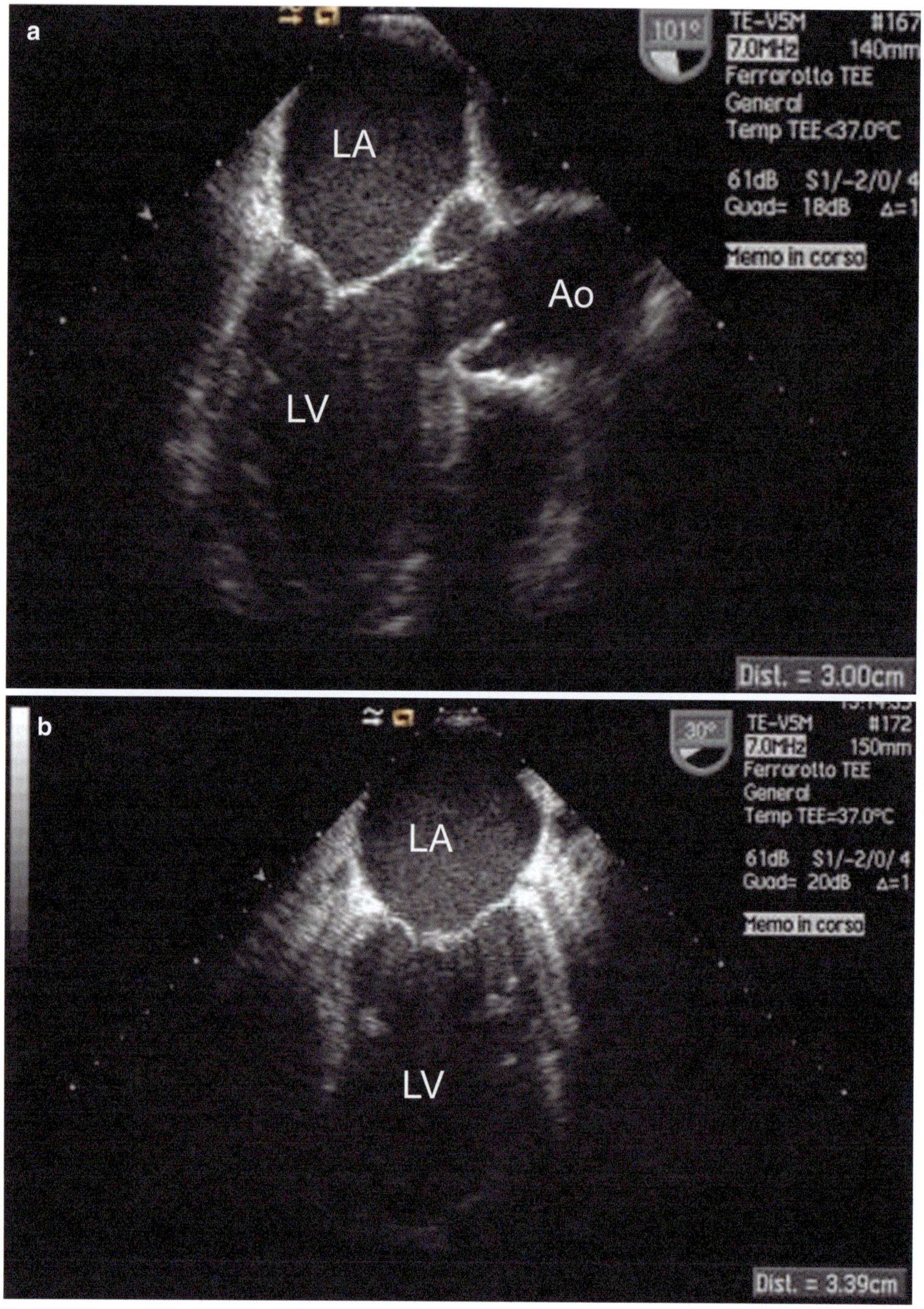

Fig. 25.4 Diagnostic transesophageal echocardiogram. (**a**) The three-chamber view (left ventricular outflow tract (*LVOT*)) is best visualized at a plane angulation of 101°. This view is used for the MitraClip orientation and trajectory testing, for anteroposterior orientation of the MitraClip and the actual leaflet grasping maneuver. (**b**) The intercommissural view is obtained at an angulation of 30°, instead of the normal 60°. This view is used for checking the position on the mediolateral axis. *LA* left atrium, *LV* left ventricle, *Ao* aorta

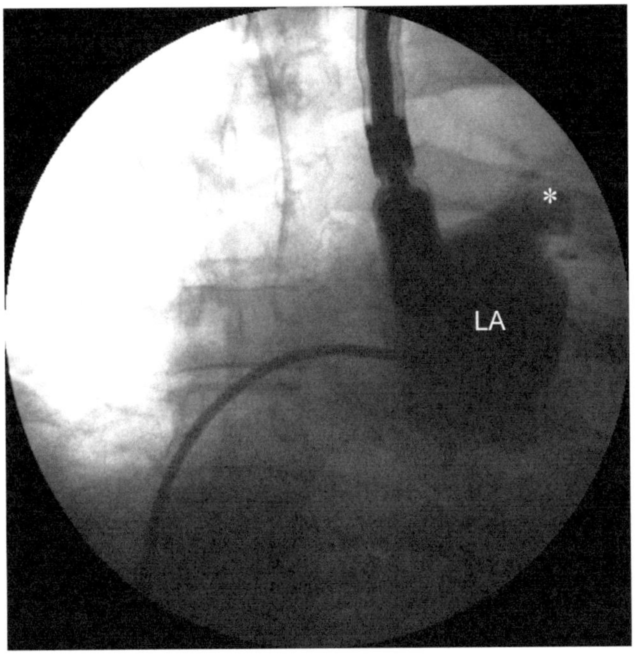

Fig. 25.5 Anteroposterior projection. After the transseptal puncture, an angiography with small amount of contrast medium is performed for checking the correct position of the 8 F introducer in the left atrium (*LA*); the left atrial appendage is also visualized (*). We can use this angiogram for the navigation of the delivery clip system in the *LA*

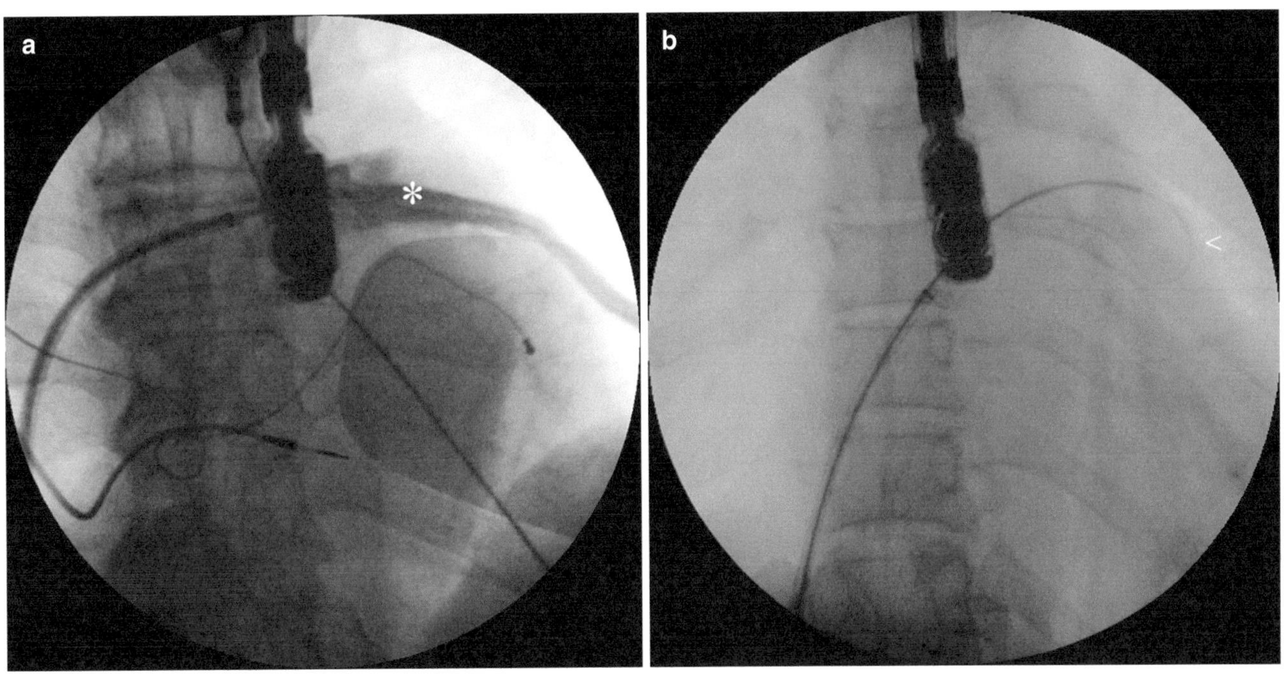

Fig. 25.6 In the standard patient (not this patient) with normal pulmonary venous return, the left upper pulmonary vein (*) is engaged with a 6 F multipurpose catheter with side holes and visualized with angiography (**a**). Then, an exchange superstiff wire is positioned in the pulmonary vein (*the white arrow*), obtaining a good stability for the 24 F guiding catheter insertion (**b**)

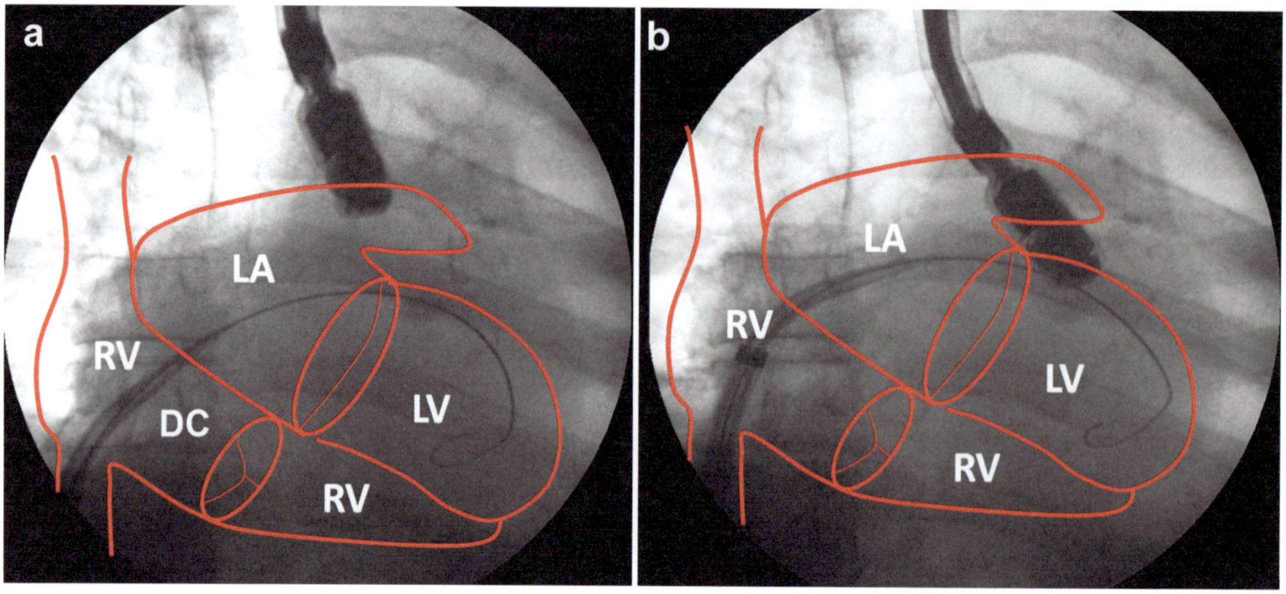

Fig. 25.7 Right anterior oblique projection. The cardiac silhouette is represented in *red*. It is possible to appreciate the superstiff wire placed in the left ventricle (**a**). The tip is J shaped for reducing the trauma on the left ventricular wall and reducing ectopic ventricular beats. The 24-F guiding catheter is passing through the interatrial septum without any trauma on the thin left atrial wall (**b**). *DC* delivery catheter *RA* right atrium, *RV* right ventricle, *LA* left atrium, *LV* left ventricle

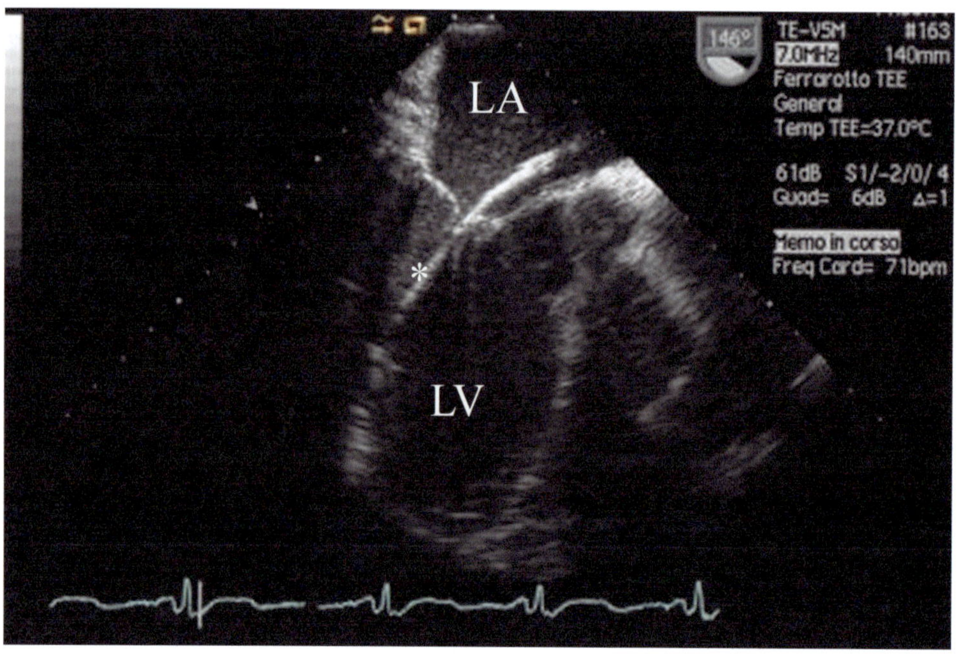

Fig. 25.8 Three-chamber transesophageal echocardiographic view. Note the stiff wire (*) which from the left atrium (*LA*) goes to the left ventricle (*LV*)

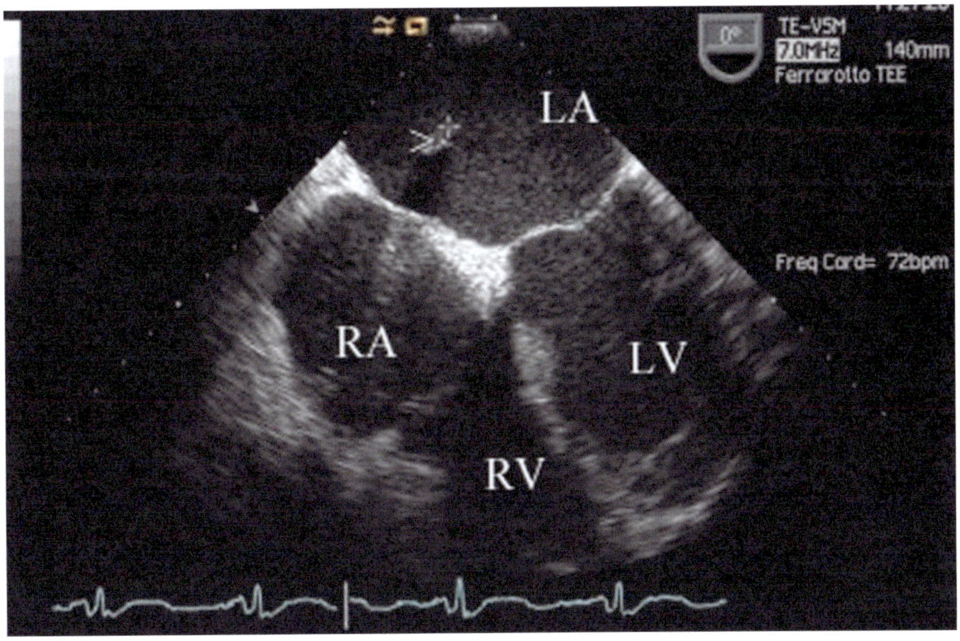

Fig. 25.9 Four-chamber transesophageal echocardiographic view. The distance between the interatrial septum and the tip of the 24-F guiding catheter (*white arrow*) should not be more than 25 mm

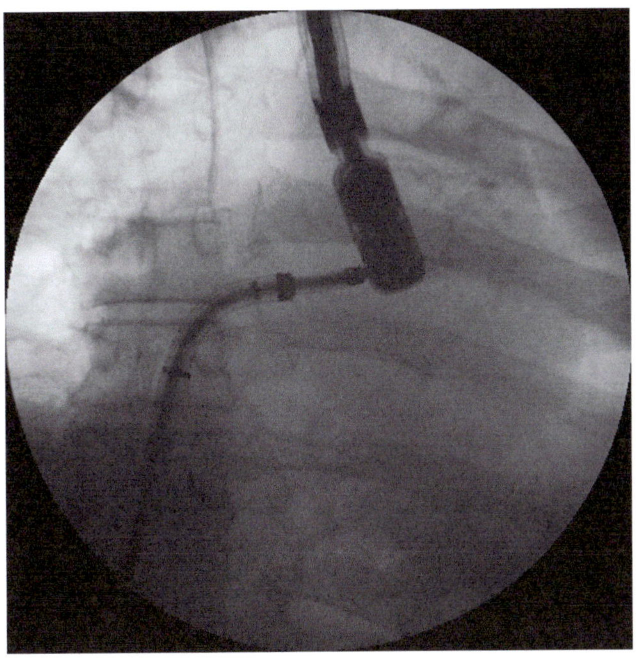

Fig. 25.10 Right anterior oblique projection. The delivery catheter system (*DCS*) is entered inside the left atrium, and the tip is noted to be too close to the left atrial appendage. This undesired position can be appreciated by the abnormal upward direction of the distal part of the DCS

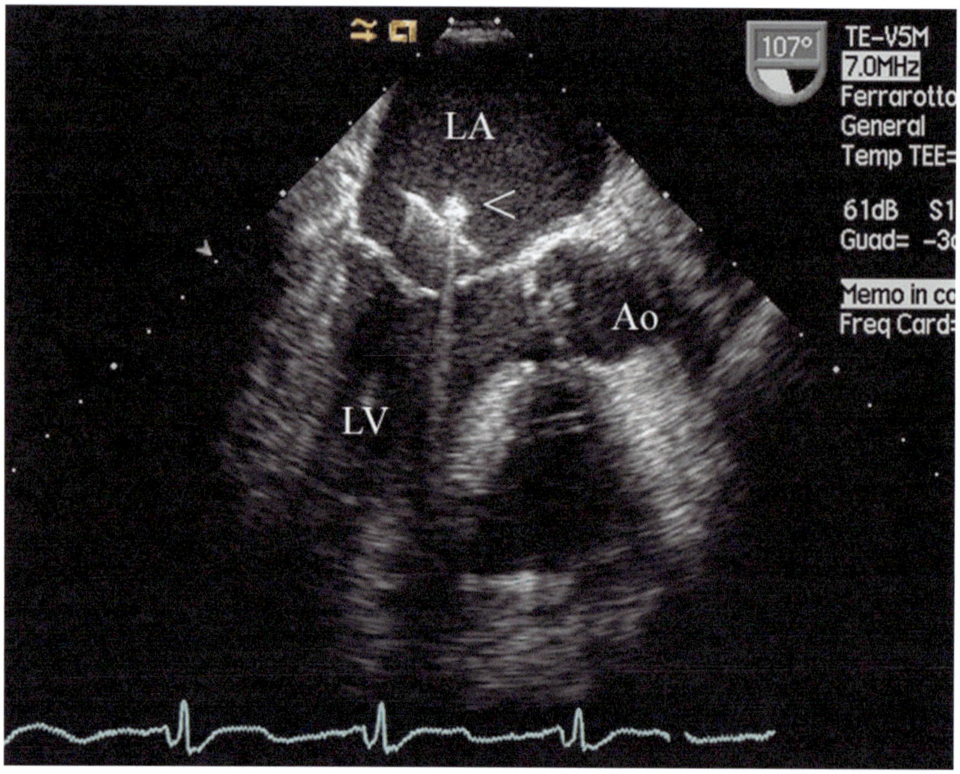

Fig. 25.11 LVOT echocardiographic view. The maneuver of correct orientation of the clip (with *arrow*) with respect to the mitral valve is performed under TEE monitoring without any particular problem. *LA* left atrium, *LV* left ventricle, *Ao* aorta

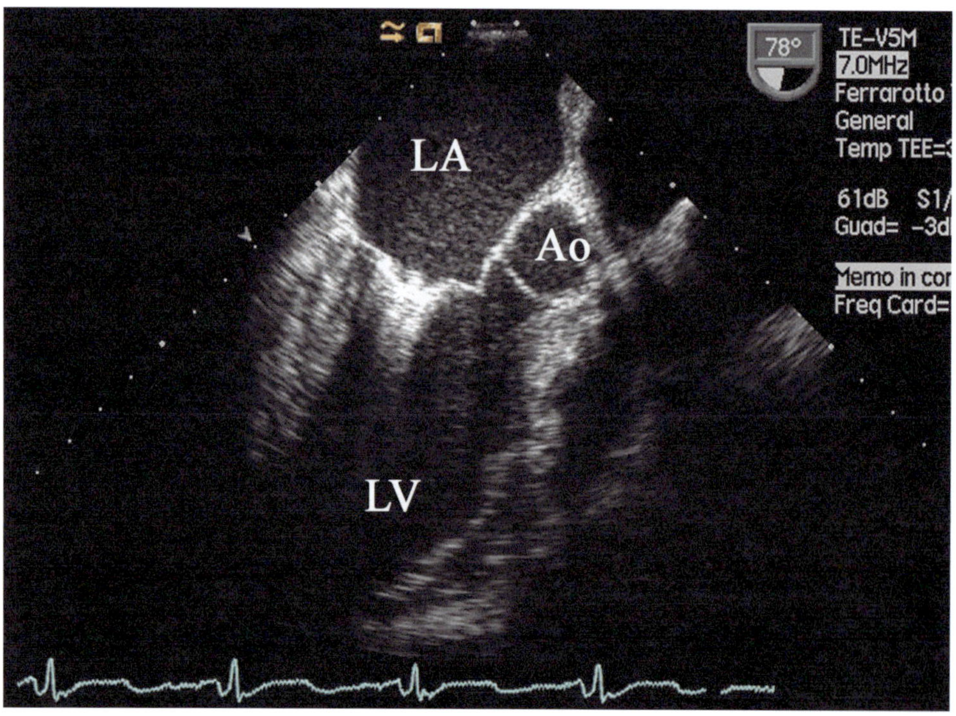

Fig. 25.12 LVOT echocardiographic view. The first grasp is attempted with success. *LA* left atrium, *LV* left ventricle, *Ao* aorta

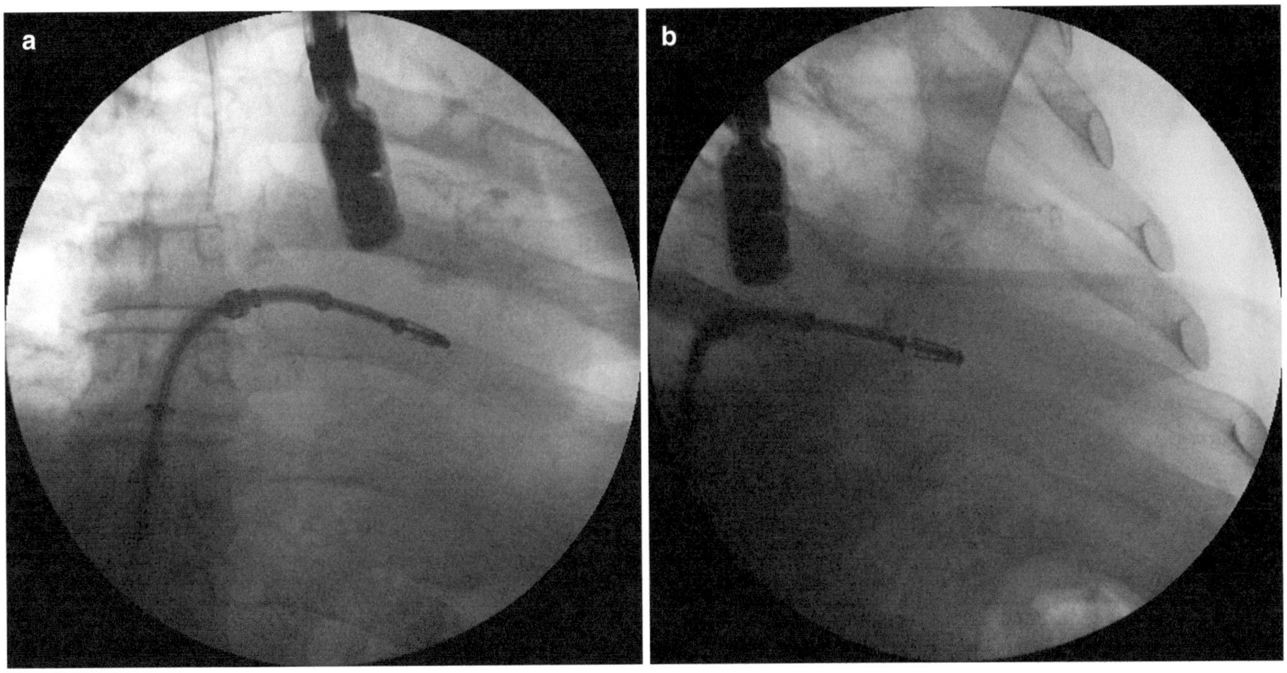

Fig. 25.13 (**a**) Right anterior oblique projection. The MitraClip is closed after the grasp; the direction seems to point more posteriorly than usual. (**b**) In the left anterior oblique projection, the MitraClip is better displayed, and we can check the arms during the release phases

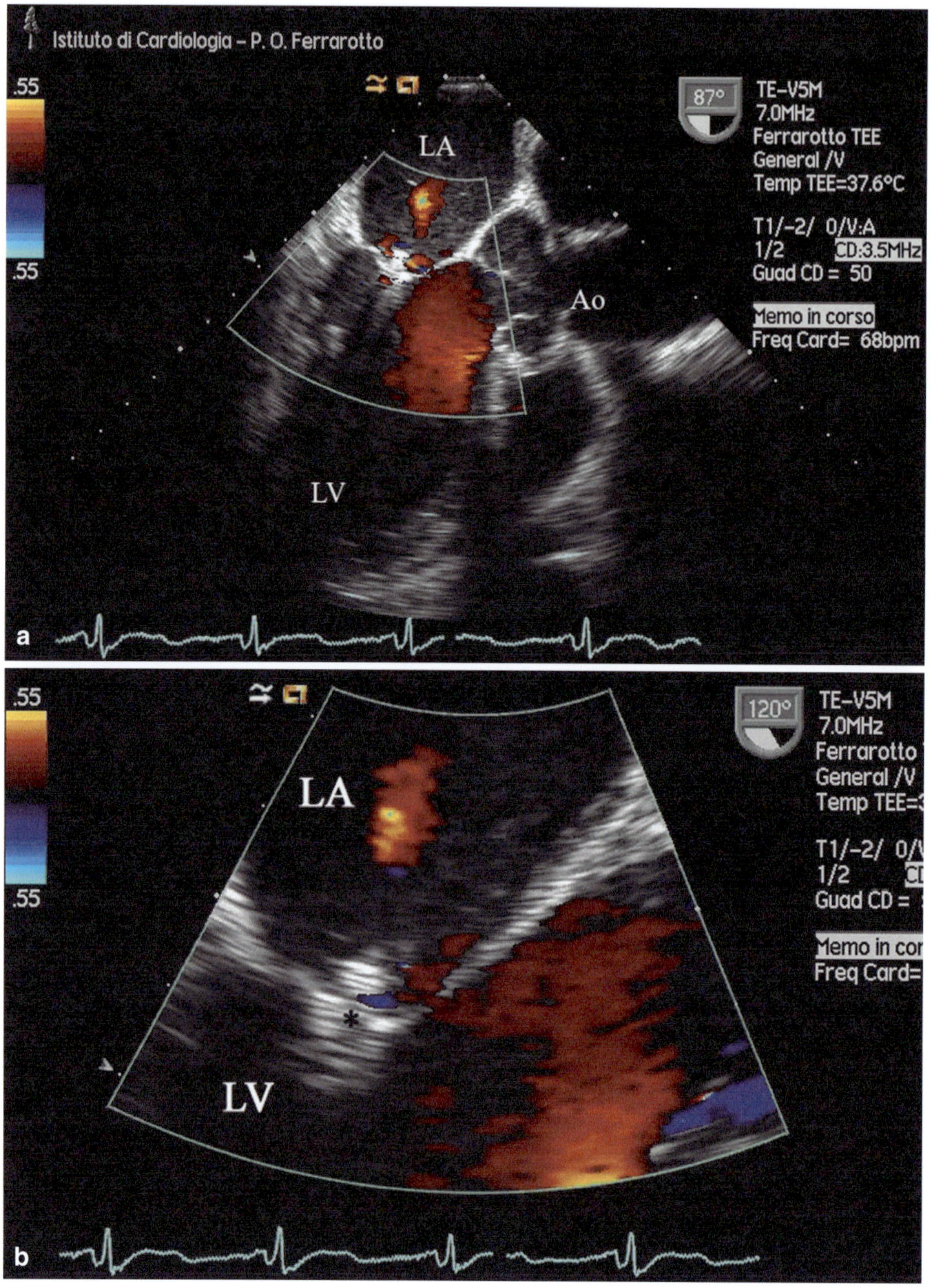

Fig. 25.14 LVOT echocardiographic view. (**a**) After clip release, the residual mitral regurgitation is mild. (**b**) The MitraClip (*) is in good position; it seems that enough tissue, of both leaflets, has been grasped. *Ao* aorta *LA* left atrium, *LV* left ventricle

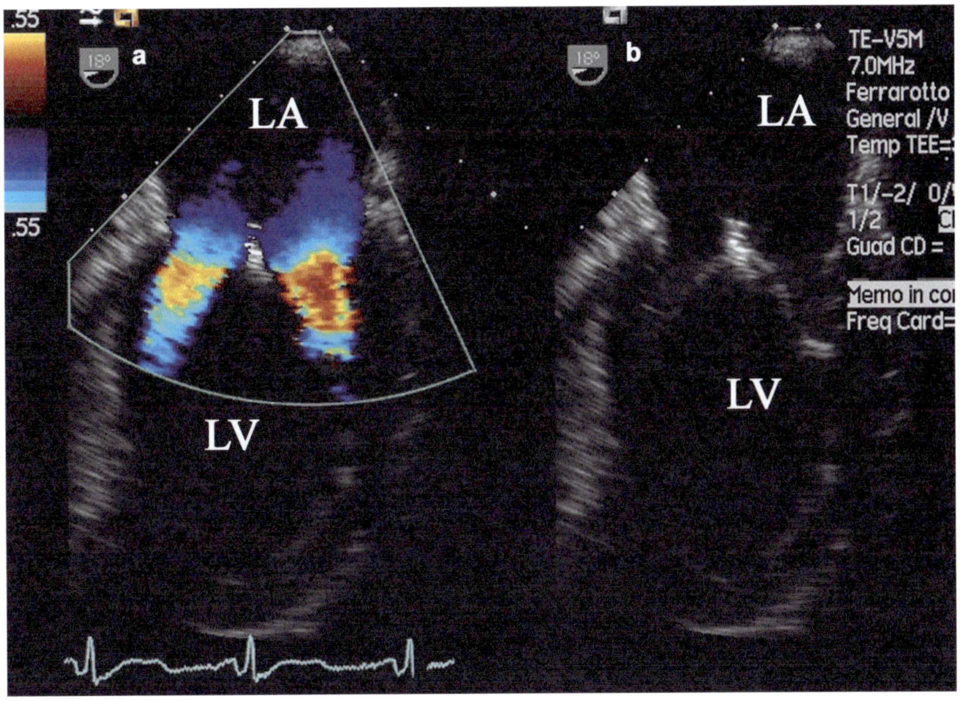

Fig. 25.15 Intercommissural view after MitraClip release. The device has been positioned in the center of the valve, obtaining a double orifice mitral valve. *LA* left atrium, *LV* left ventricle

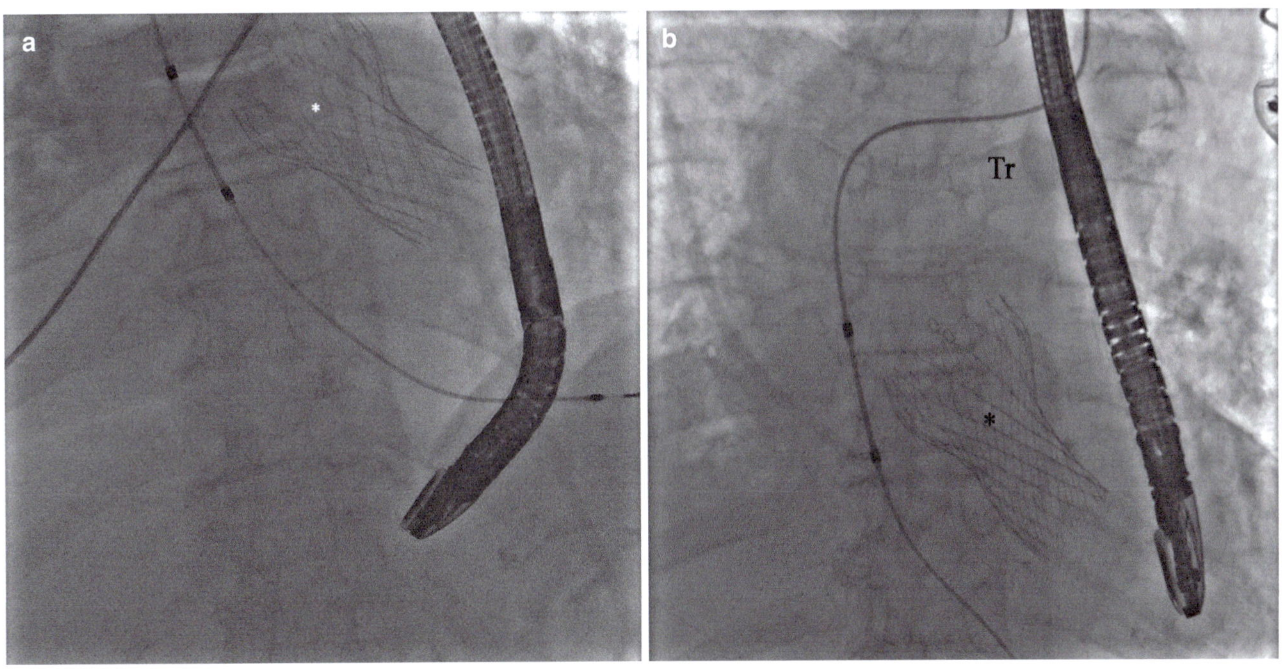

Fig. 25.16 After Corevalve (*) implantation for severe aortic stenosis, a mitral regurgitation reduction with MitraClip is attempted. The transesophageal echocardiographic (*TEE*) window is very poor; at fluoroscopy, the TEE probe has an unusual position with respect to the heart silhouette (**a**, **b**) displaced to the left hemithorax. *Tr* trachea

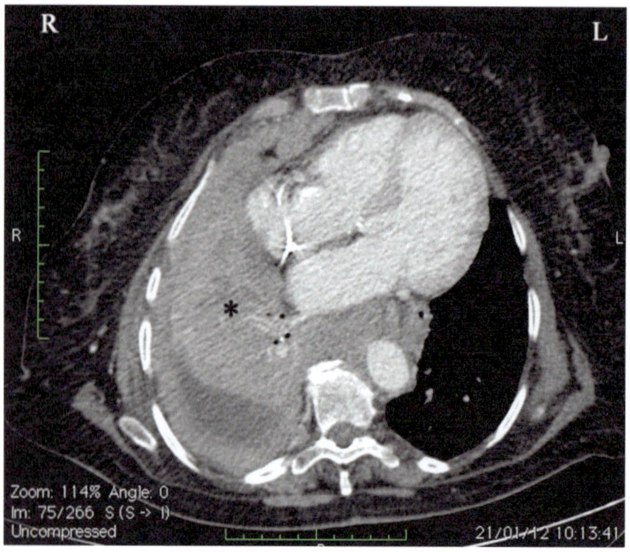

Fig. 25.17 Thoracic CT scan with contrast medium shows that there is a mass (*) which displaces the heart anterior to the left. The esophagus is compressed and deviated

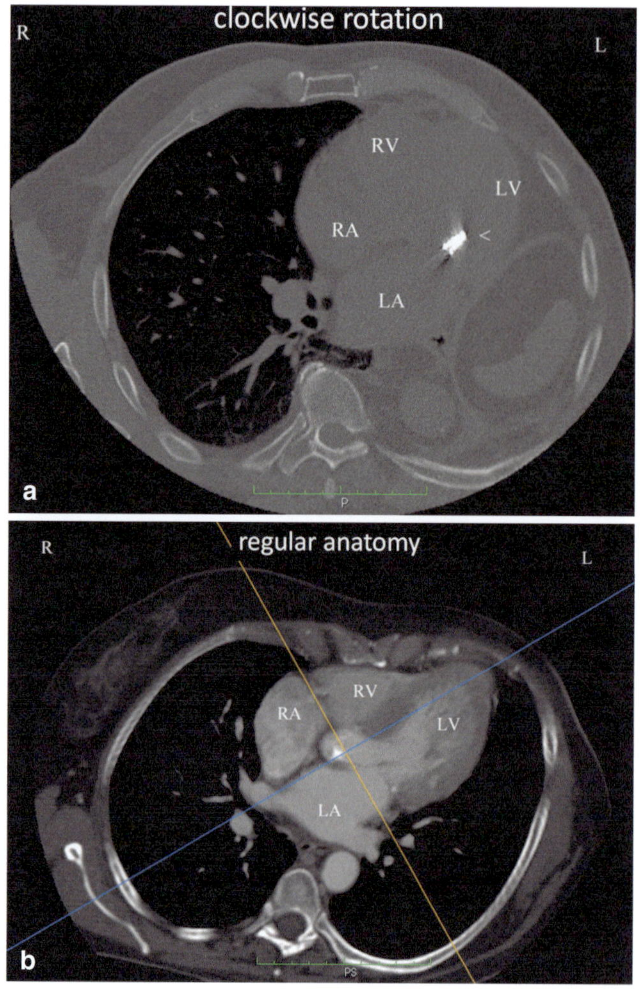

Fig. 25.18 (**a**) Thoracic CT scan of the patient with left lung resection after MitraClip implantation (with *arrow*). The heart appears rotated clockwise direction. The cardiac chambers displacement is better appreciated when compared with CT scan of a subject with normal anatomic relationships (**b**). *LA* left atrium, *LV* left ventricle, *RA* right atrium, *RV* right ventricle

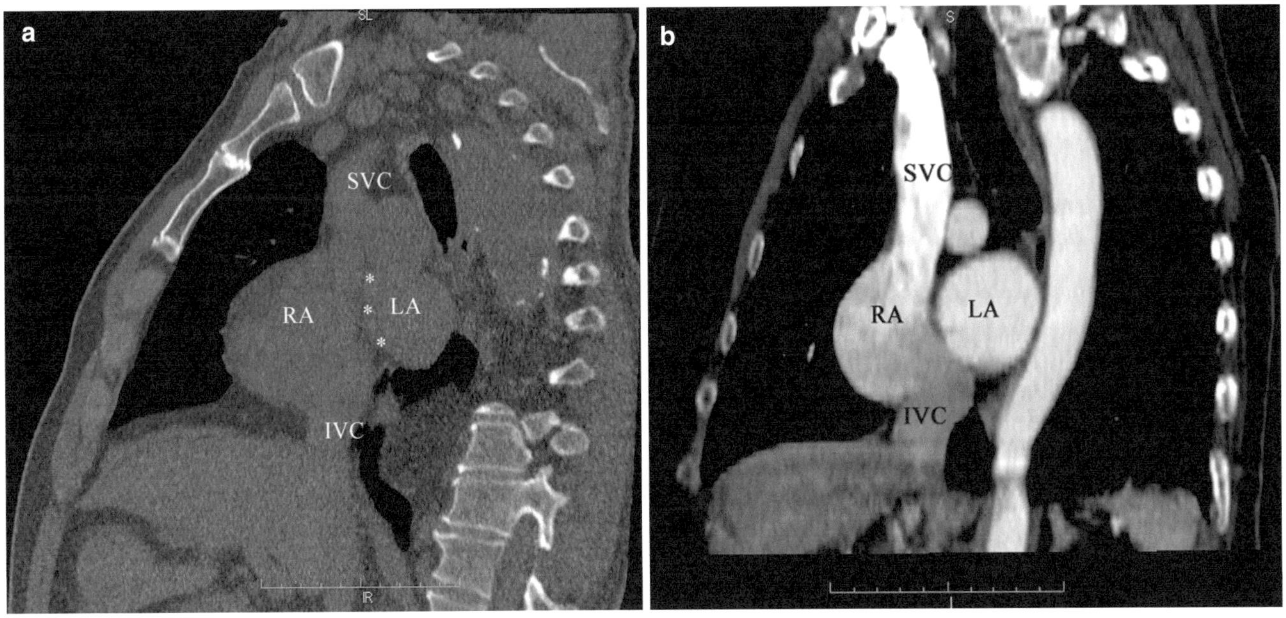

Fig. 25.19 Sagittal view of thoracic CT Scan of the patient with left pneumonectomy (**a**). The anatomic relationship between the venae cavae, interatrial septum (*) and left atrium are not modified respect to the normal (**b**). *LA* left atrium, *RA* right atrium, *SVC* superior vena cava, *IVC* inferior vena cava

Interatrial Septal Tear: A Rare Complication During MitraClip Procedure and Successful Transcatheter Closure

26

Takashi Matsumoto, Wen-Loong Yeow, and Saibal Kar

Abstract

Patients with severe mitral regurgitation and are at high risk for surgery may benefit from a percutaneous leaflet repair with the MitraClip device (Abbott Vascular, Santa Clara, California). Interatrial tear during device manipulation is a rare complication and can be closed percutaneously with an Amplatzer septal occluder (AGA Medical, Plymouth, MN) at the conclusion for the procedure.

Keywords

Percutaneous closure • MitraClip • Amplatzer septal occluder • Interatrial septal tear

Introduction

Surgical repair or replacement remains the treatment of choice for patients with severe mitral regurgitation (MR). Percutaneous repair with the MitraClip device (Abbott Vascular, Santa Clara, California) may be offered if the patient is considered high surgical risk and eligible for study inclusion [1–4]. In this entry, we describe one such patient but developed an interatrial tear, manifested by hypoxia and sudden clip delivery system malposition. As the patient was hemodynamically compromised, the MitraClip was deployed quickly. The tear was then closed with an Amplatzer septal occluder (AGA Medical, Plymouth, MN), and the patient's hemodynamic parameters rapidly stabilized.

Although interatrial tears are not uncommon (e.g., they can happen with balloon sizing during percutaneous atrial septal defect closure), this is the first such case in the current literature associated with the MitraClip device.

T. Matsumoto, M.D. • W. Yeow, M.D., M.B.B.S., FRACP
S. Kar, M.B.B.S., M.D. (✉)
Heart Institute, Cedars-Sinai Medical Center,
8631 W. Third Street, Suite 415E, Los Angeles, CA 90048, USA
e-mail: takashi.matsumoto@cshs.org; wenloong.yeow@cshs.org; saibal.kar2@cshs.org, karsk@cshs.org

Clinical History

An 85-year-old man presented with shortness of breath on mild exertion, with New York Heart Association (NYHA) class III symptoms. He had percutaneous coronary intervention in 1998 for unstable angina, permanent pacemaker implantation in 2008 for complete heart block, and an infrarenal abdominal aortic aneurysm. On transthoracic (TTE) and transesophageal (TEE) echocardiography, there was severe functional mitral regurgitation and severe tricuspid regurgitation. Of note, there was bulging of the interatrial septum toward the left atrium. In consultation with the attending cardiothoracic surgical team, the consensus was to perform percutaneous mitral valve repair using MitraClip system due to his high surgical risk.

The procedure was performed under general anesthesia with TEE guidance. The right femoral vein (RFV) access was pre-closed using two Perclose Proglide devices (Abbott Vascular Devices, CA, USA). The right heart catheterization (RHC) was performed from the right jugular vein; the mean right atrium (RA) pressure was 15 mmHg, the mean pulmonary artery (PA) pressure was 31 mmHg, and the mean pulmonary capillary wedge pressure (PCWP) was 20 mmHg. A transseptal puncture was performed in the standard manner, and the 24-F MitraClip delivery catheter was advanced across the atrial septum into the left atrium (LA) without

T. Feldman et al. (eds.), *Atlas of Percutaneous Edge-to-Edge Mitral Valve Repair*,
DOI 10.1007/978-1-4471-4294-2_26, © Springer-Verlag London 2013

incident (Fig. 26.1a, b). As the MitraClip was orientated in the LA, the height above mitral valve was lost, and the patient became hypoxic with arterial saturations dropping gradually from 98 to 86 %. TEE revealed a tear in the interatrial septum, extending from superior to inferior with significant bidirectional shunt (Fig. 26.2a). The position of a guide catheter and a clip delivery system was reestablished, and the MitraClip was repositioned and deployed without further incidents. The MR grade improved to 2+. Although placement of a second clip would be ideal, the patient remained hemodynamically compromised with an arterial saturation of 85 %. The consensus decision was to remove the delivery system and proceed to close the interatrial septal tear. The tear was slit-like, measuring up to 24 mm in length (Fig. 26.2b). As the tear did not involve surrounding structures and there was a sufficient rim, a 24-mm Amplatzer septal occluder (AGA Medical, Plymouth, MN) was chosen to close the tear. Once the device was deployed, the arterial saturation improved from 86 to 98 %. There was no residual shunt across the tear (Fig. 26.2c). On the final RHC, the mean RA pressure was 16 mmHg, the mean PA pressure was 28 mmHg, and the mean PCWP was 17 mmHg.

The patient was discharged 3 days after procedure without further incidents. At 1-month follow-up, his symptoms had improved (NYHA class II). The MR remained grade 2+, and there was no shunt across the interatrial septum.

Discussion

A residual atrial septal defect (ASD) is usually of no consequence after a MitraClip procedure. On rare occasions, a tear in the septum or in the setting of raised right atrial pressure, there may be significant right to left interatrial shunting. In this case, hemodynamic compromise was secondary to elevated right atrial pressure.

The likely mechanism of interatrial tear relates to both patient and device factors. If the interatrial septum is particularly thin or aneurysmal, then tearing following transseptal puncture and dilatation can occur. Excessive leverage forces on the delivery system could put direct pressure on the ASD edge and cause a tear.

Depending on the type of procedure, most residual ASDs are small in size and are hemodynamically insignificant [5–7]. On the other hand, interatrial tears are usually large in size, complex in shape, and hemodynamically significant [8, 9]. Surgical repair had been required in most of these cases. Also, transcatheter closure can be utilized. The key issue of this technique is to correctly detect a rim and to recognize the shape of interatrial tear and to deploy appropriate-sized septal occluder device. Hence, it should be examined from multiple angles using 2D echocardiogram, and the use of real-time 3D echocardiogram should be considered. In addition, careful tug test and TEE before device release is essential to avoid both device dislodgement and residual shunt.

In this case report, we have presented an interatrial tear occurring during the MitraClip procedure. In this case, the interatrial tear was repaired safely and successfully using transcatheter techniques.

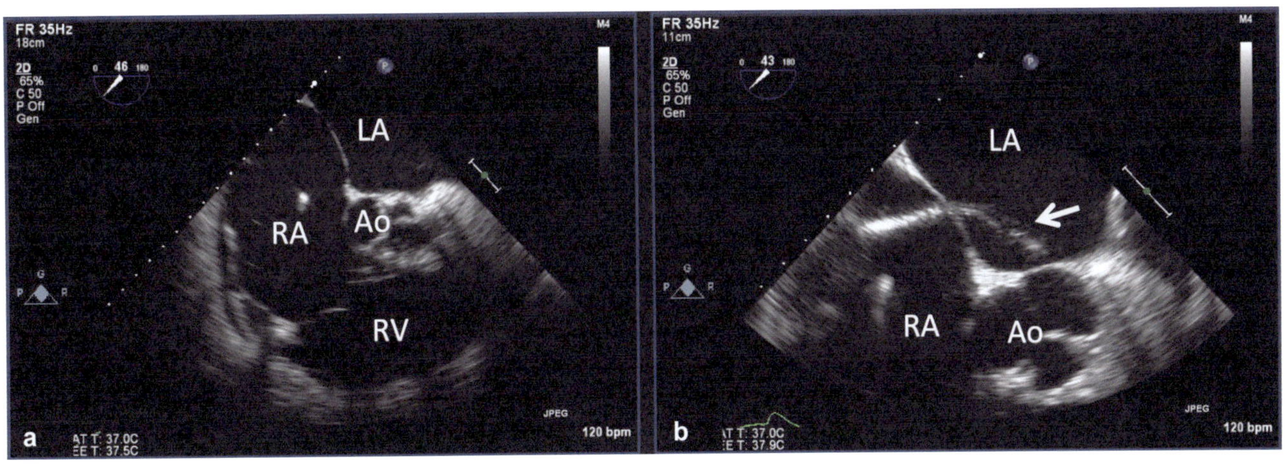

Fig. 26.1 (**a**) TEE image before transseptal puncture showing atrial septum bowing toward the LA. (**b**) TEE image after transseptal puncture showing a 24-F guide catheter (*white arrow*) across the atrium septum. *RA* right atrium, *RV* right ventricle, *LA* light atrium, *Ao* aorta

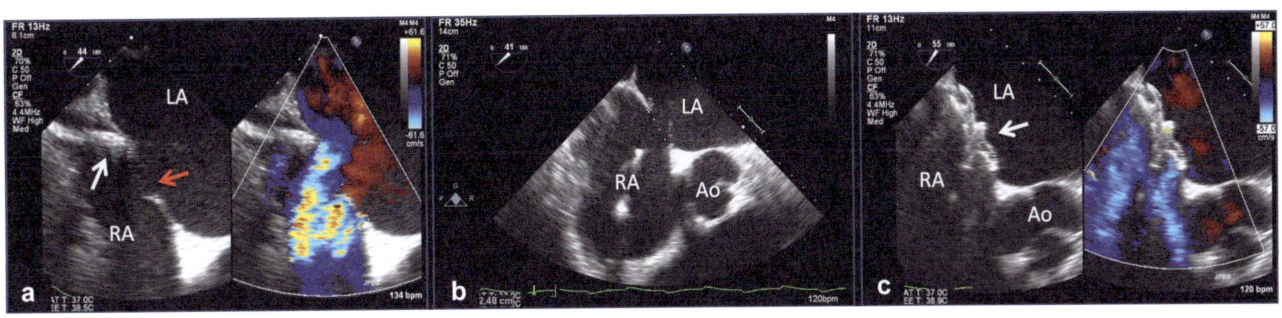

Fig. 26.2 (**a**) TEE image with color Doppler showing interatrial tear (*red arrow*) and a 24-F guide catheter (*white arrow*). (**b**) TEE measurement of the tear showing approximately 24-mm length. (**c**) TEE image with color Doppler showing no significant residual shunt across a 24-mm Amplatzer septal occluder (*white arrow*). *RA* right atrium, *LA* light atrium, *Ao* aorta

References

1. Feldman T, Wasserman HS, Herrmann HC, et al. Percutaneous mitral valve repair using the edge-to-edge technique: six-month results of the EVEREST Phase I Clinical Trial. J Am Coll Cardiol. 2005;46:2134–40.
2. Feldman T, Kar S, Rinaldi M, et al. Percutaneous mitral repair with the MitraClip system: safety and midterm durability in the initial EVEREST (Endovascular Valve Edge-to-Edge REpair Study) cohort. J Am Coll Cardiol. 2009;54:686–94.
3. Feldman T, Foster E, Glower DG, Kar S, et al. Percutaneous repair or surgery for mitral regurgitation. N Engl J Med. 2011;364: 1395–406.
4. Whitlow PL, Feldman T, Pedersen WR, Lim DS, Kipperman R, Smalling R, Bajwa T, Herrmann HC, Lasala J, Maddux JT, Tuzcu M, Kapadia S, Trento A, Siegel RJ, Foster E, Glower D, Mauri L, Kar S, EVEREST II Investigators. Acute and 12-month results with catheter-based mitral valve leaflet repair: the EVEREST II (Endovascular Valve Edge-to-Edge Repair) High Risk Study. J Am Coll Cardiol. 2012;59(2):130–9.
5. Yoshida K, Yoshikawa J, Akasaka T, Yamaura Y, et al. Assessment of left-to-right atrial shunting after percutaneous mitral valvuloplasty by transesophageal color Doppler flow-mapping. Circulation. 1989;80:1521–6.
6. Cequier A, Bonan R, Serra A, Dyrda I, et al. Left-to-right atrial shunting after percutaneous mitral valvuloplasty. Incidence and long-term hemodynamic follow-up. Circulation. 1990;81:1190–7.
7. Rillig A, Meyerfeldt U, Birkemeyer R, Treusch F, et al. Persistent iatrogenic atrial septal defect after pulmonary vein isolation: incidence and clinical implications. J Interv Card Electrophysiol. 2008;22:177–81.
8. Harikrishnan S, Narayanan NK, Sivasubramonian S. Sizing balloon-induced tear of the atrial septum. J Invasive Cardiol. 2005;17(10):546–7.
9. Alsaileek AA, Omran A, Godman M, Najm HK. Echocardiographic visualization of laceration of atrial septum during balloon sizing of atrial septal defect. Eur J Echocardiogr. 2007;8(2):155–7.

Percutaneous Double-Valve Treatment in a Patient with Degenerative Aortic Stenosis and Functional Mitral Regurgitation

27

Volker Rudolph and Stephan Baldus

Abstract

We describe a case in which an 82-year-old patient had severe symptomatic aortic stenosis and severe functional mitral regurgitation. He had very high surgical risk and underwent successful transcatheter aortic valve replacement with a CoreValve and, in the same setting, underwent a successful MitraClip procedure. This case example illustrates the technical feasibility of performing two procedures together.

Keywords

Mitral regurgitation • MitraClip • Aortic stenosis • Transcatheter aortic valve replacement • CoreValve

Clinical History

An 82-year-old male patient presented with NYHA Class III heart failure. He had a history of severe three-vessel coronary heart disease (prior PCI), stroke without residual neurological deficits, and permanent atrial fibrillation. Cardiac risk factors were hypertension, hyperlipidemia, and insulin-dependent diabetes mellitus type II.

At admission, echocardiography revealed severely impaired left ventricular function with an ejection fraction of 29 %, severe degenerative aortic stenosis with a planimetered aortic valve area of 1.0 cm^2, and functional moderate-to-severe mitral regurgitation grade III+ (ERO: 0.30 cm^2) due to severe left ventricular dilation with mild sclerotic posterior leaflet restriction (Fig. 27.1). On coronary angiography, no significant coronary stenosis was detected.

The heart team opted against surgery because of the high perioperative risk (logistic EuroScore 28.5) for combined mitral and aortic surgery, and a decision was made for combined transcatheter aortic valve implantation and percutaneous mitral valve repair using the MitraClip during one procedure.

An 18-F sheath was inserted into the right femoral artery, a temporary pacer was placed into the right ventricle via the left femoral vein, and a 6-F sheath was placed in the left femoral artery. Uncomplicated aortic valve balloon dilatation was performed during adenosine-induced third degree AV block. Thereafter, a 29-mm CoreValve™ prosthesis was deployed with a residual grade I paravalvular aortic regurgitation. However, MR remained grade III despite the reduction in afterload (Fig. 27.2). Accordingly, the arterial 18-F sheath was removed, the arteriotomy closed using a ProStar closure device and an 18-F sheath was inserted into the right femoral vein. Following transesophageal (TEE)-guided transseptal puncture, a MitraClip was positioned in the A2/P2 segment of the mitral valve, where the maximal vena contracta was observed. Given significant residual mitral regurgitation after deployment of the first clip, a second clip was implanted laterally of the first clip yielding reduction of MR to grade II (Figs. 27.3 and 27.4). The patient had a stable postprocedural course.

V. Rudolph, M.D. (✉)
Department of General and Interventional Cardiology, University Heart Center, Hamburg, Germany

Department of Cardiology, Heart Center, University Hospital Cologne, Kerpener Str. 62, Cologne, 50937, Germany
e-mail: volker.rudolph@uk-koeln.de

S. Baldus, M.D.
Department of General and Interventional Cardiology, University Heart Center, Hamburg, Germany
e-mail: baldus@uke.de

T. Feldman et al. (eds.), *Atlas of Percutaneous Edge-to-Edge Mitral Valve Repair*,
DOI 10.1007/978-1-4471-4294-2_27, © Springer-Verlag London 2013

Summary

Bivalvular transcatheter treatment is a promising new treatment strategy for patients with aortic stenosis, in whom concomitant mitral regurgitation remains severe even after transcatheter aortic valve implantation. The fact that MitraClip therapy usually does not provoke any hemodynamic instability allows for treatment of both valves within the same procedure. Additional studies are required to address who may derive the most long-term benefit from these complex and costly procedures.

Learning Points

The MitraClip procedure is a safe procedure that can be performed together in the same setting with transcatheter aortic valve replacement if clinically indicated.

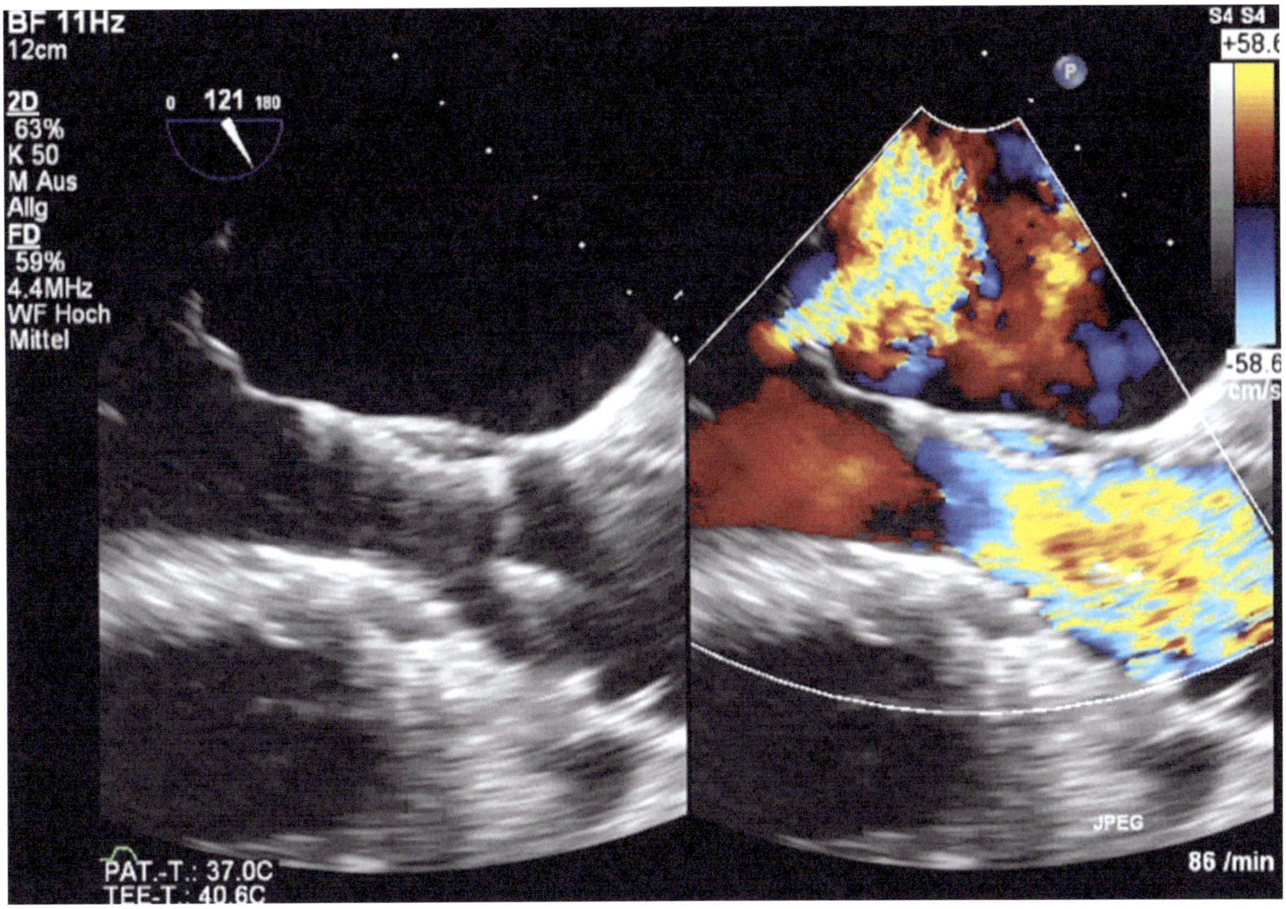

Fig. 27.1 TEE three-chamber color Doppler view showing the mitral regurgitation following deployment of the transcatheter aortic valve

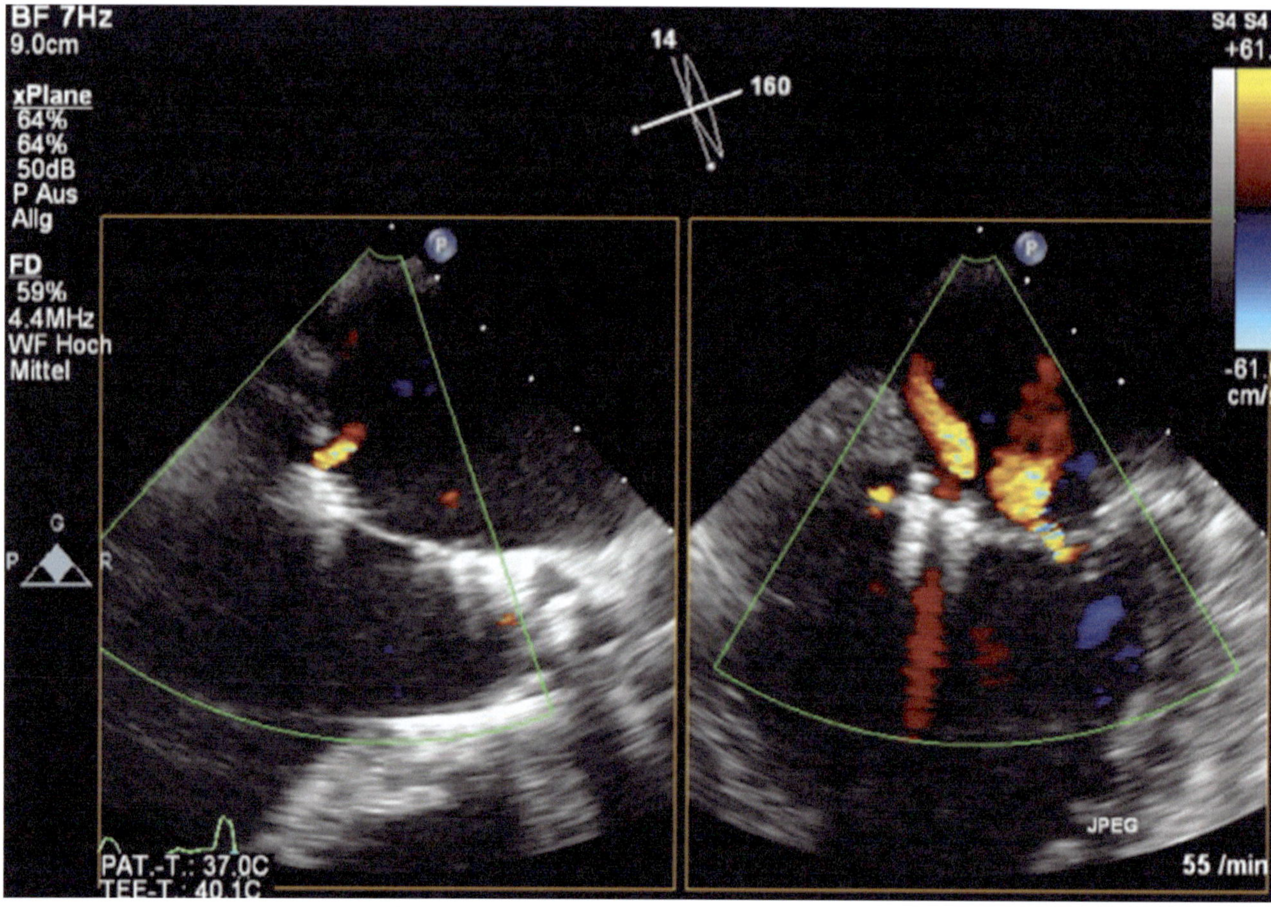

Fig. 27.2 X-plane view™ showing simultaneous LVOT- and intercommissural color Doppler views after implantation of two clips in the same patient

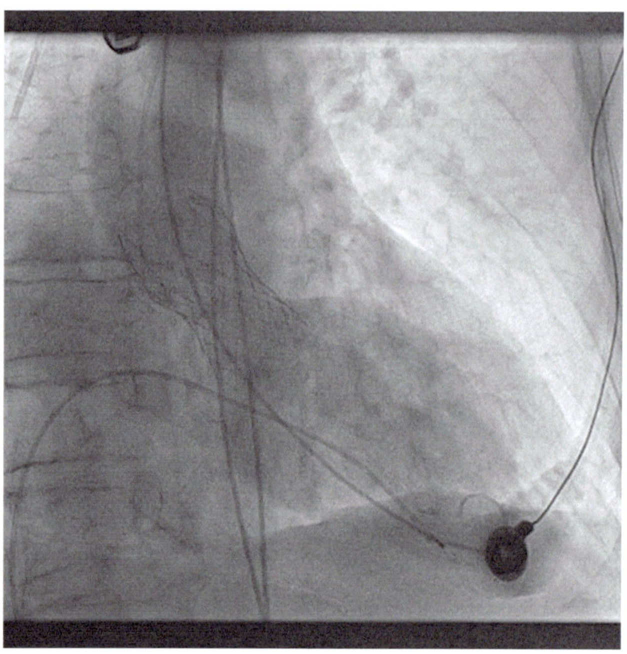

Fig. 27.3 Ventriculography showing severe mitral regurgitation following CoreValve™ implantation

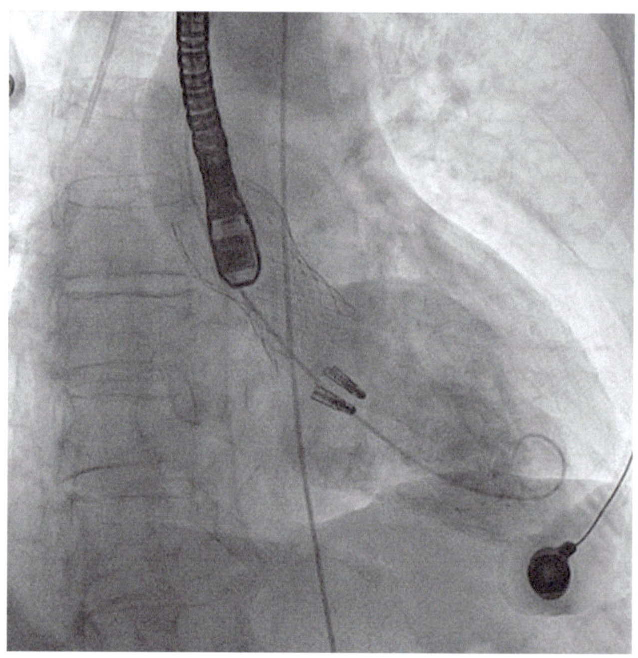

Fig. 27.4 Ventriculography following simultaneous transcatheter aortic valve replacement and percutaneous mitral valve repair

Percutaneous Mitral Valve Repair After Previous Mitral Valve Reconstruction

28

Volker Rudolph and Stephan Baldus

Abstract

This case describes the MitraClip procedure for recurrent mitral regurgitation in a patient with a history of Libman-Sacks endocarditis and prior mitral annuloplasty. The mechanism of the recurrent mitral regurgitation was ring dehiscence. Surgery was felt to be very high risk due to multiple comorbidities.

Keywords

Mitral regurgitation • MitraClip • Libman-Sacks endocarditis • Mitral annuloplasty • Ring dehiscence

A 71-year-old female patient with previous mitral valve reconstruction (30-mm physio ring) and tricuspid valve reconstruction (36-mm Edwards ring) due to residual severe mitral regurgitation following Libman-Sacks endocarditis presented with recurrent heart failure symptoms despite optimal heart failure medication 1 year after mitral valve surgery.

Besides her diagnosis for systemic lupus erythematosus, the patient had chronic obstructive lung disease (FEV1 35 %), paroxysmal atrial fibrillation, and history of stroke. A dual chamber pacemaker was implanted in 2010 for symptomatic sick sinus syndrome. Significant coronary artery disease was excluded.

Echocardiography revealed moderately impaired left ventricular systolic function and moderate-to-severe mitral regurgitation grade III+ (ERO: 0.41 cm^2) due to leaflet malcoaptation caused by ring dehiscence (Fig. 28.1 and Videos 28.1, 28.2).

Because of the high perioperative risk, the decision was made for percutaneous mitral valve repair. Mitral clip implantation was performed by carefully navigating the clip through the reconstructed annulus. 3D echocardiography proved helpful in steering the clip into the central part of the line of coaptation (Fig. 28.2). After successful implantation of a single clip, mitral regurgitation was reduced to grade I (Figs. 28.3 and 28.4).

V. Rudolph, M.D. (✉)
Department of General and Interventional Cardiology, University Heart Center, Hamburg, Germany

Department of Cardiology, Heart Center, University Hospital Cologne, Kerpener Str. 62, Cologne, 50937, Germany
e-mail: volker.rudolph@uk-koeln.de

S. Baldus, M.D.
Department of General and Interventional Cardiology, University Heart Center, Hamburg, Germany
e-mail:baldus@uke.de

Electronic supplementary material The online version of this chapter (doi:10.1007/978-1-4471-4294-2_28) contains supplementary material, which is available to authorized users.

T. Feldman et al. (eds.), *Atlas of Percutaneous Edge-to-Edge Mitral Valve Repair*, DOI 10.1007/978-1-4471-4294-2_28, © Springer-Verlag London 2013

Summary

MitraClip therapy in patients who have previously undergone mitral annuloplasty is a novel and potentially important adjunct treatment strategy for patients, in whom conventional reoperation carries a high perioperative risk. However, the mechanism of recurrent mitral regurgitation must be carefully evaluated on TEE. In addition, the quality of the leaflet must be assessed prior to the procedure.

Learning Points

Recurrent mitral regurgitation after mitral annuloplasty may be treated successfully with the MitraClip depending on the mechanism of the recurrent mitral regurgitation

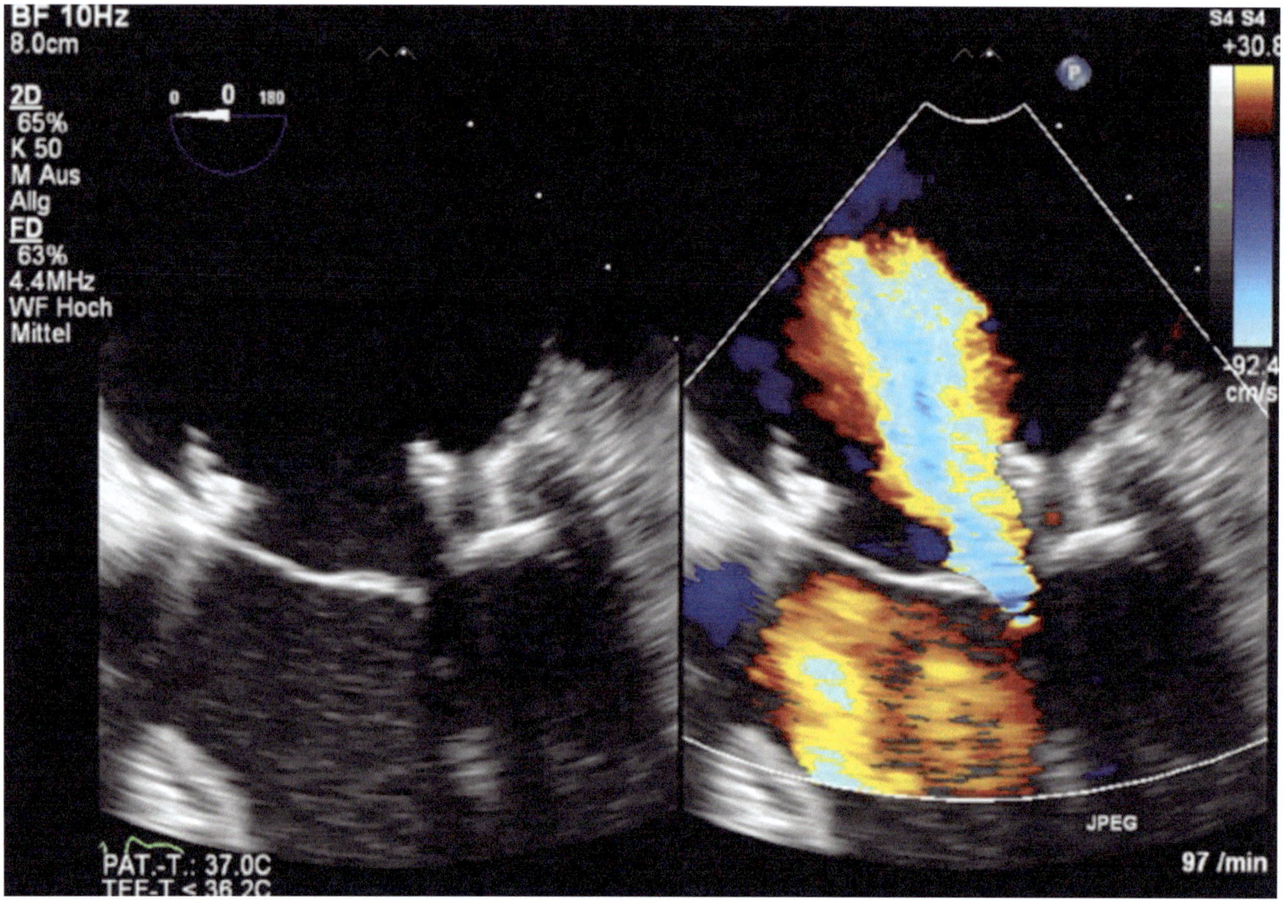

Fig. 28.1 Intraprocedural transesophageal four-chamber color Doppler view of the mitral regurgitation prior to percutaneous valve repair

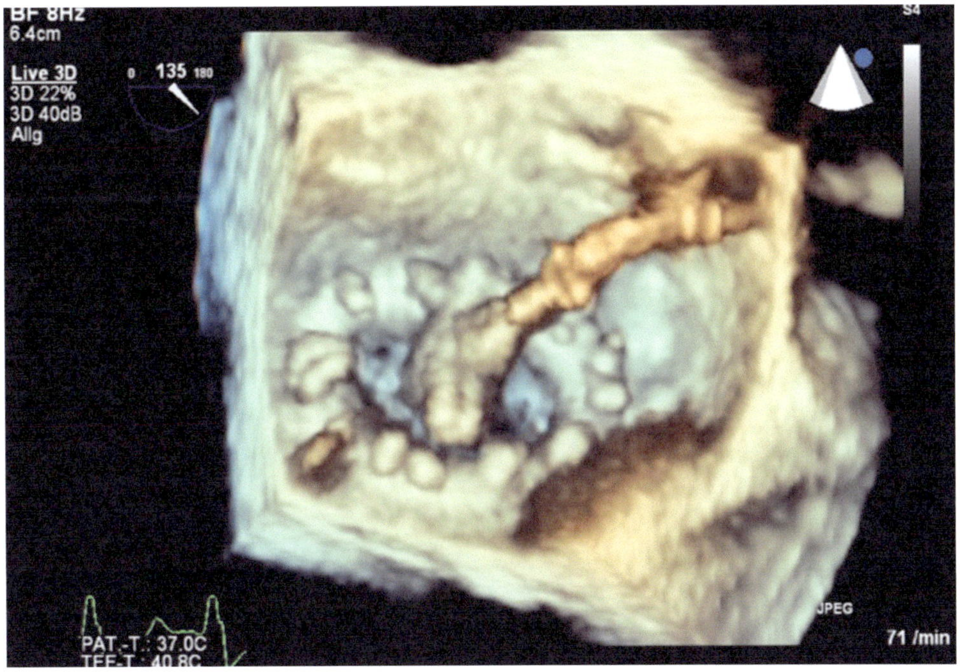

Fig. 28.2 3D view showing perpendicular alignment of the MitraClip prior to passing through the valve

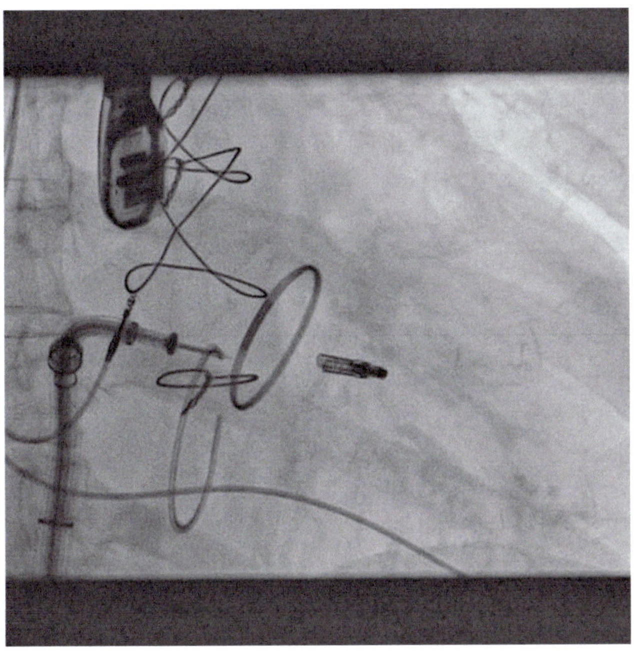

Fig. 28.3 Fluoroscopic image after deployment of the clip

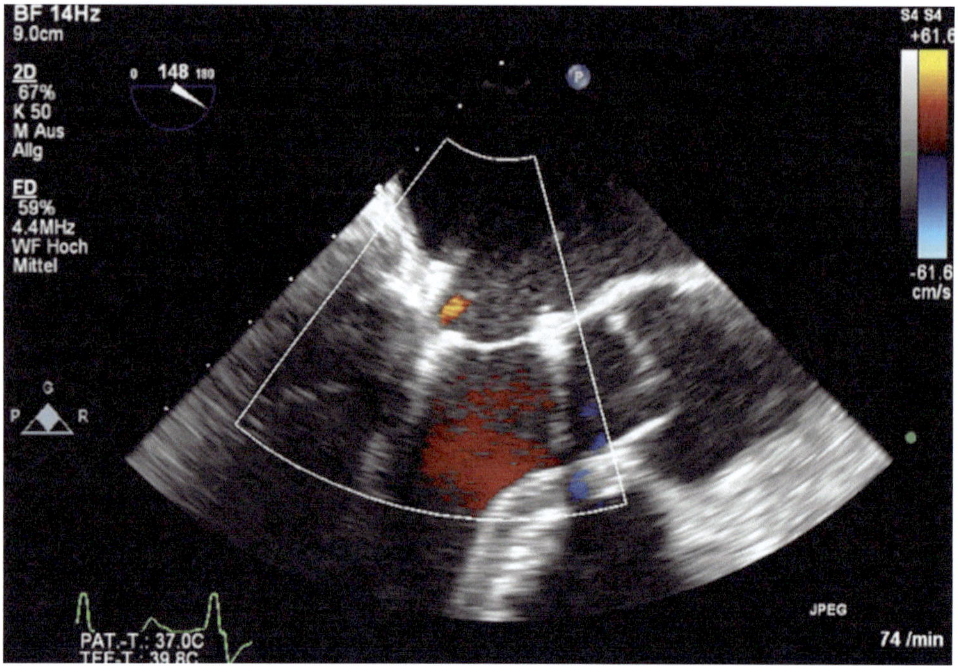

Fig. 28.4 Transesophageal three-chamber view showing the minimal residual mitral regurgitation following implantation of one clip

Case Examples: (1) Delayed Functional Mitral Regurgitation in a High Risk Patient, and (2) Complex Degenerative Mitral Regurgitation (Anterior Leaflet Prolapse) with Commissural Impingement

29

Francesco Maisano, Maurizio Taramasso, Iryna Arendar, and Giovanni La Canna

Case 1: Delayed Functional Mitral Regurgitation in a High Risk Patient

Abstract

In this case, a patient underwent MitraClip repair of severe functional MR. He subsequently developed recurrent severe MR. A successful repeat MitraClip procedure was performed with the second clip placed lateral to the first clip.

Keywords

Mitral regurgitation • MitraClip • Recurrence

Background

Functional mitral regurgitation (FMR) is frequently observed in heart failure patients with postischemic or idiopathic dilated cardiomyopathy due to left ventricular (LV) dysfunction and remodeling [1]. Perioperative mortality after mitral surgery for FMR is not negligible, and a large number of patients with FMR are rejected for open heart surgery because of predicted high surgical risk or comorbidities [2]. Percutaneous edge-to-edge technique with MitraClip implantation has been used to treat FMR in high risk end-stage patients with favorable safety and efficacy results [3–5].

MitraClip implantation can be repeated in case of delayed recurrent MR. We report the case of a patient with end-stage heart failure who had delayed recurrent FMR 10 months after the first MitraClip procedure who underwent successful repeat MitraClip implantation.

F. Maisano, M.D., FESC (✉) • M. Taramasso, M.D.
I. Arendar, M.D. • G. La Canna, M.D.
Cardiothoracic Department, San Raffaele University Hospital, Via Olgettina 58, Milan 20132, Italy
e-mail: maisano.francesco@hsr.it; taramasso.maurizio@hsr.it; arendar.iryna@hsr.it; lacanna.giovanni@hsr.it

Clinical History

A 67-year-old man with a previous history of percutaneous coronary revascularization underwent MitraClip implantation to treat severe ischemic FMR. Comorbidities included chronic renal failure (preoperative serum creatinine was 2.0 mg/dl). The patient was in NYHA functional class II heart failure. Biventricular ICD-CRT was previously implanted. Early outcome of MitraClip implantation was considered acceptable with a discharge echocardiography showing residual moderate MR (2+). Ten months after the procedure, recurrent severe MR was diagnosed. The main regurgitant jet was located in the lateral orifice. After multidisciplinary discussion, a second MitraClip implantation was planned.

Preoperative transesophageal echocardiography showed severe FMR due to residual tethering in correspondence of the lateral orifice, with severe systolic dysfunction (LVEF 20 %); LVEDV and LVESV were 150 and 100 ml, respectively. Severe pulmonary hypertension was documented (PASP 75 mmHg). Total mitral valve area was 3.2 cm^2.

Although several echo views are performed, the three key views are: the intercommissural two-chamber view (See Fig. 29.1a), the LVOT view (Fig. 29.1b), and the transgastric short axis view (Fig. 29.1c, d). Color compare visualization is the key to properly identify the target. Transgastric view (Fig. 29.1d) demonstrates that the main regurgitant jet is located in the lateral orifice.

Two asymmetric orifices were evident at 3D preoperative echocardiography (Fig. 29.2a), and 3D color Doppler documented a double regurgitant jet with main component from the lateral orifice (Fig. 29.2b).

Proper location of the transseptal puncture is critical to ensure a smooth procedure. The transseptal puncture may be particularly challenging in case of thick septum (as in case of postcardiotomy patients), large left or right atrium, in presence of bulging septum and in presence of intracardiac pacing leads. Possible complications due to suboptimal puncture are "aorta hugging" (too anterior puncture), inability to cross

T. Feldman et al. (eds.), *Atlas of Percutaneous Edge-to-Edge Mitral Valve Repair*, DOI 10.1007/978-1-4471-4294-2_29, © Springer-Verlag London 2013

the mitral valve (too high puncture), inability to pull back the clip and tether the leaflets (too low puncture), and perforation (too posterior puncture).

Initially, the bicaval view is used to determine the superior-inferior level of the puncture. As tenting is evident on the bicaval view (Fig. 29.3a), the echo probe is moved to obtain a short axis at the base view (Fig. 29.3b). The aim of this view is to provide information on the position of the needle tip on the anteroposterior axis. The ideal location of the tenting in this view is posterior, along the projected coaptation line. Before the puncture, final check by a four-chamber view incorporating the septum and the free edge of the mitral valve at the site of regurgitation is performed. Ideally, the distance between the tenting and the mitral valve should be between 3.5 and 4.5 cm in the four-chamber view, in correspondence of the superior side of the fossa ovalis. In the present case, transseptal puncture was performed in the optimal position, 3.9 cm above the mitral annulus in the four-chamber view (Fig. 29.3c). Interestingly, at 10 months after the previous procedure, no residual shunt was visible. The correct position allowed us to move the delivery system above the mitral valve leaflets in a perpendicular fashion during the procedure. Radiofrequency puncture helped us to improve the safety and the precision of the puncture (Fig. 29.3d shows the appearance of microbubbles in the left side of the atrium subsequent to septal crossing).

The delivery system was then advanced in the left atrium and steered toward the mitral valve (Fig. 29.4a). The clip was oriented perpendicular to the coaptation line, laterally to the first clip, in correspondence of the lateral orifice and close to the previously implanted clip (Fig. 29.4b, c). Therefore, it was advanced in the LV (Fig. 29.4d).

The clip was then pulled back, and the leaflets fell spontaneously into the clip; tethering was observed, and the grippers were dropped (Fig. 29.5a). The clip was closed to 60° to secure the leaflets between grippers and clip arms. This step is important to determine leaflets insertion. Proper assessment is performed using x-plane technique to adequately image the second clip (Fig. 29.5b). The clip was then fully closed, and acute reduction of MR jet was observed (Fig. 29.5c). The clip was released. Final judgment about the procedural result has to be done only after the final release because the tension of the delivery system can distort the final result. Final result after clip release showed mild residual MR (Fig. 29.5d).

Figure 29.6a, b show the comparison between 3D echocardiography before (Fig. 29.6a) and after the second (Fig. 29.6b) clip implantation. No significant mitral stenosis was present at the end of the procedure (Fig. 29.6c). Total valve area was 2.1 cm^2. Mean gradient was 3 mmHg. No complications occurred. Total duration of the procedure was 75 min, and the patient was discharged to home 3 days after the procedure.

Three-dimensional reconstruction of the mild residual regurgitant jet (Fig. 29.7a); double diastolic flow during diastolic phase showing minimal acceleration of flow, and no significant stenosis(Fig. 29.7b).

At 6 months follow-up, the patient was asymptomatic (NYHA I) and in good clinical conditions, with optimal quality of life. No re-hospitalization occurred. Transthoracic echocardiography showed the absence of MR (Fig. 29.8a, b); LVEF improved to 35 % and PASP dropped to 50 mmHg.

Learning Points

1. The ongoing LV remodeling process may lead to recurrent FMR after MitraClip.
2. In cases of delayed recurrent MR, if the residual mitral valve area is adequate, a second MitraClip procedure can be performed.

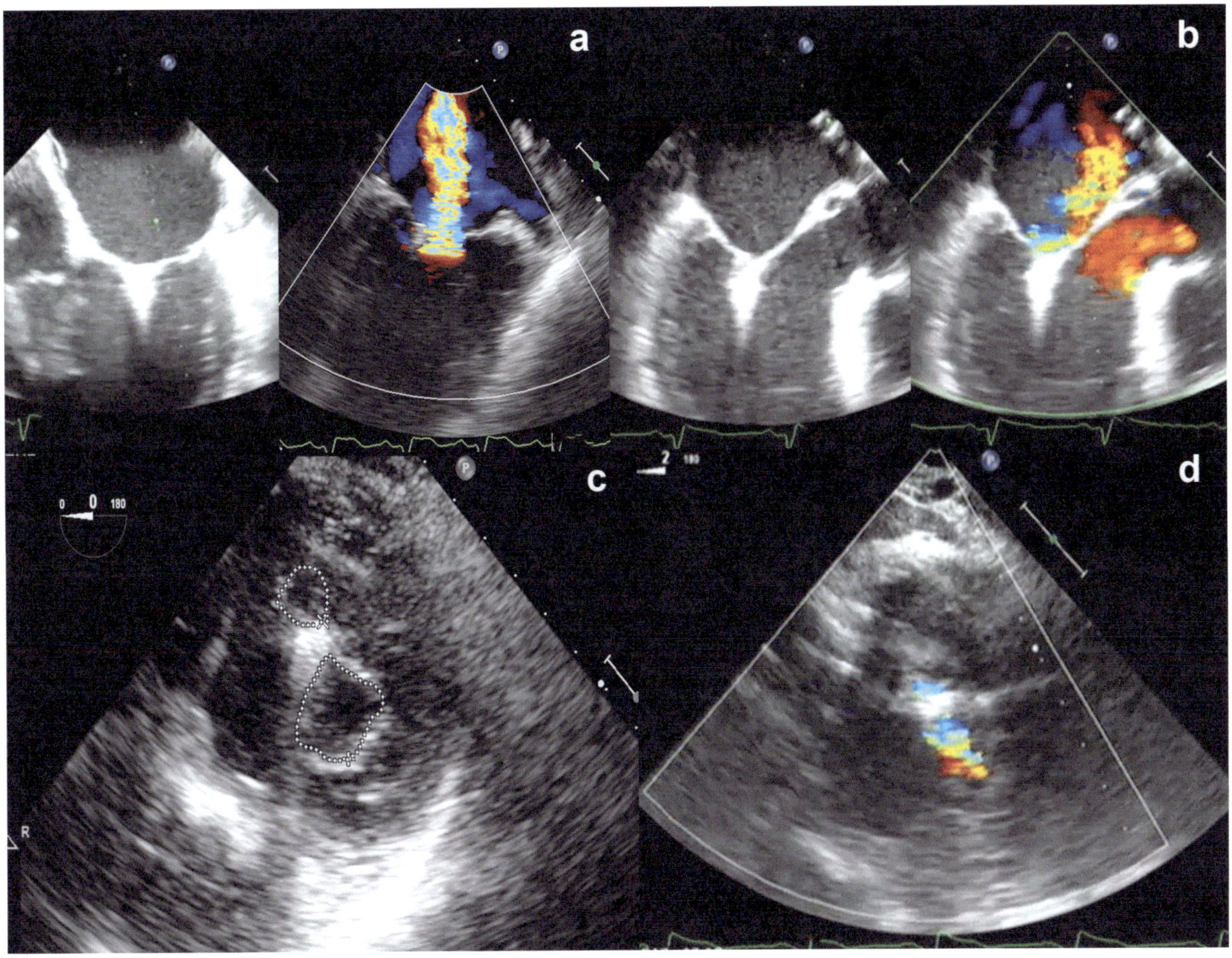

Fig. 29.1 Color compare visualization of intercommissural two-chamber view (**a**), LVOT view (**b**), and the transgastric short axis view (**c**, **d**)

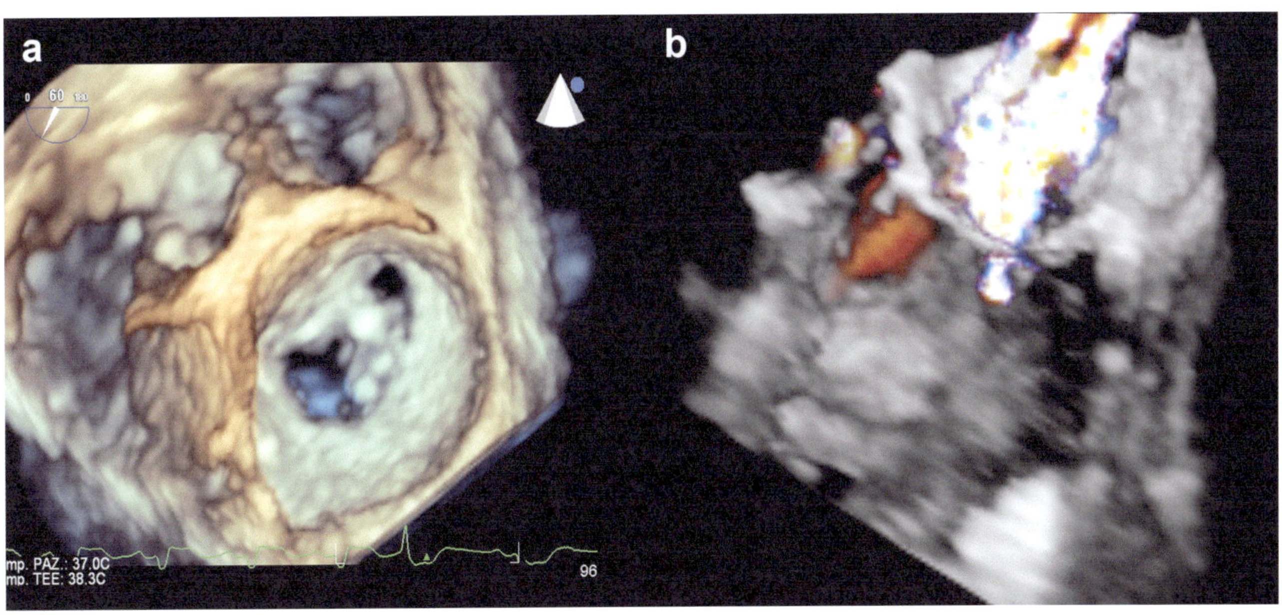

Fig. 29.2 3D preoperative echocardiography (**a**) and 3D color Doppler (**b**)

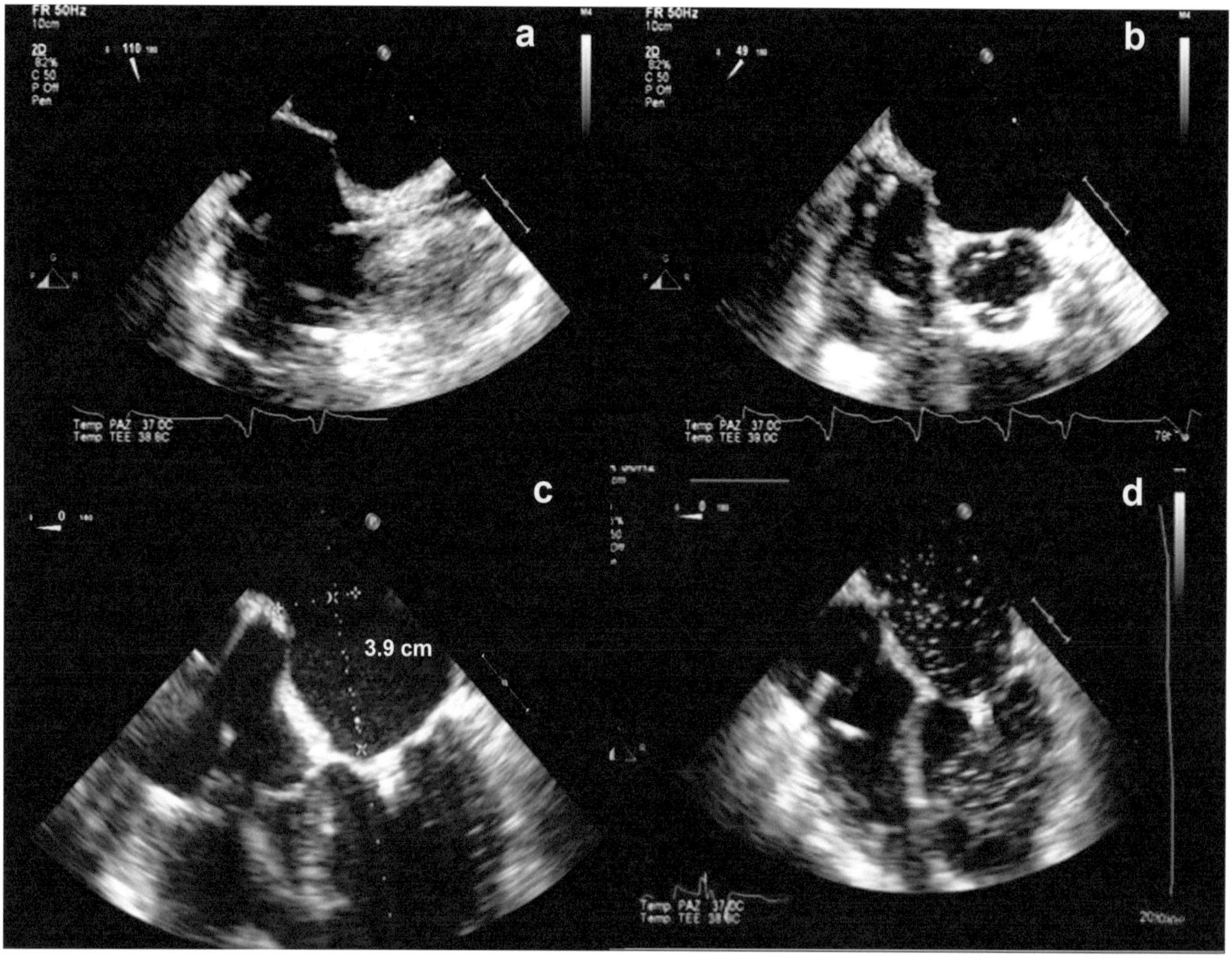

Fig. 29.3 Transseptal puncture: evidence of tenting on the bicaval view (**a**) and short axis at the base view (**b**). Check by a 4-chamber view: in this case transseptal puncture was performed 3.9 cm above the mitral annulus (**c**); appearance of microbubbles in the left side of the atrium subsequent to septal radiofrequency crossing (**d**)

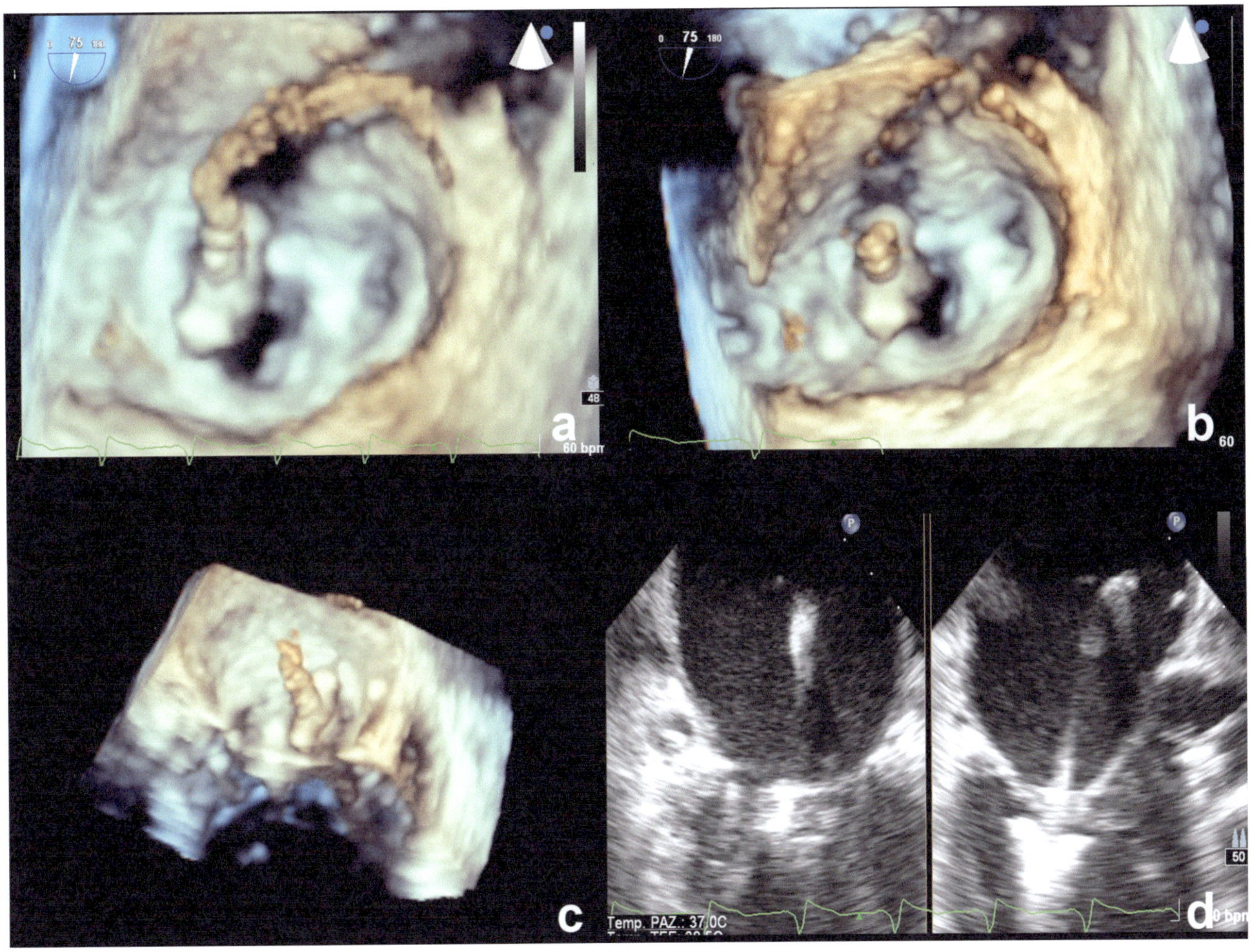

Fig. 29.4 Advance of the delivery system in the left atrium (**a**); orientation of the clip, in correspondence of the anterolateral orifice, close to the previously implanted clip (**b**, **c**); advancement of the clip in the LV (**d**)

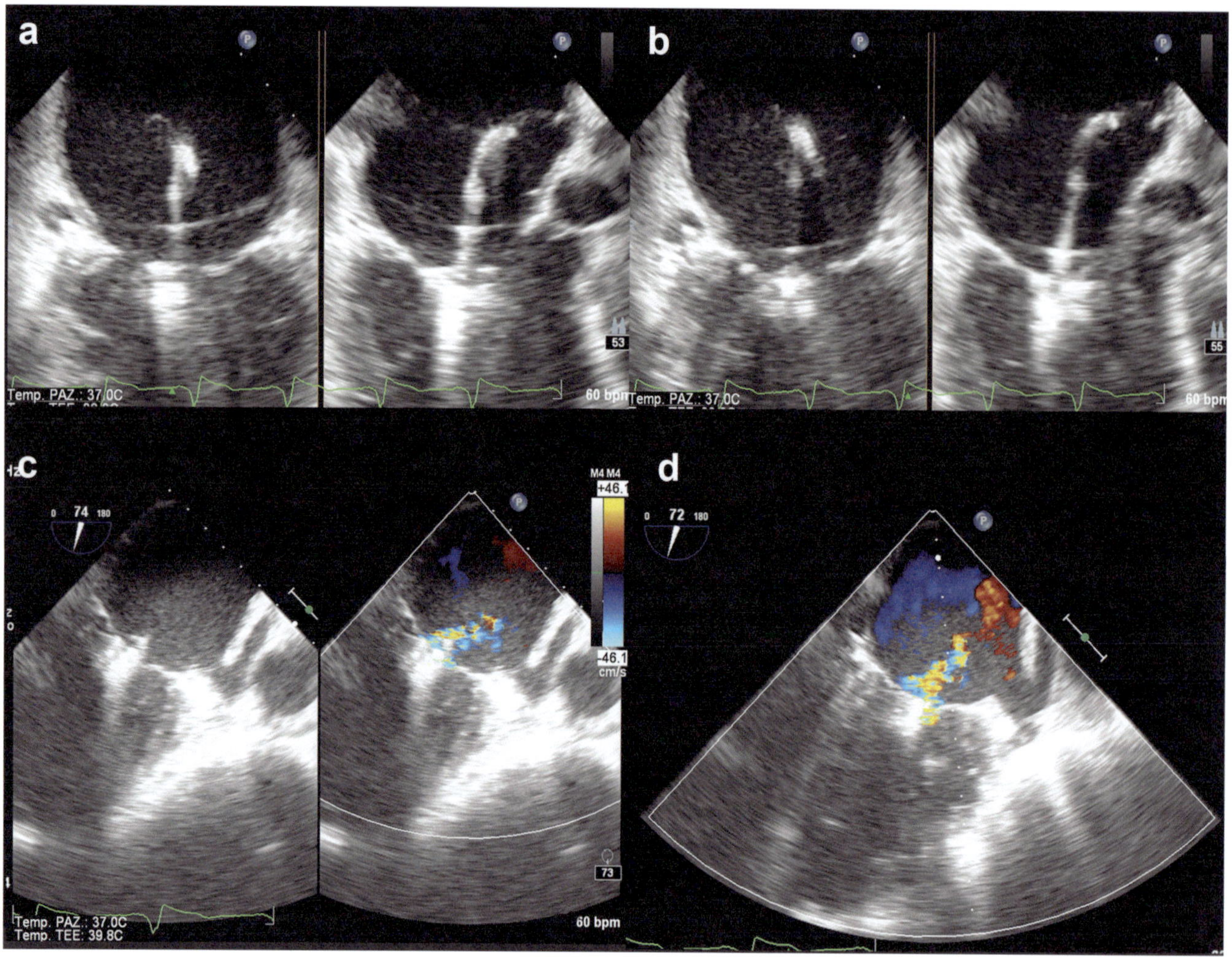

Fig. 29.5 Leaflet grasping: the clip is pulled back; the grippers are dropped (**a**); closure of the clip to 60° to secure the leaflets between grippers and clip arms (**b**); full closure with acute reduction of MR (**c**); final result after clip release (**d**)

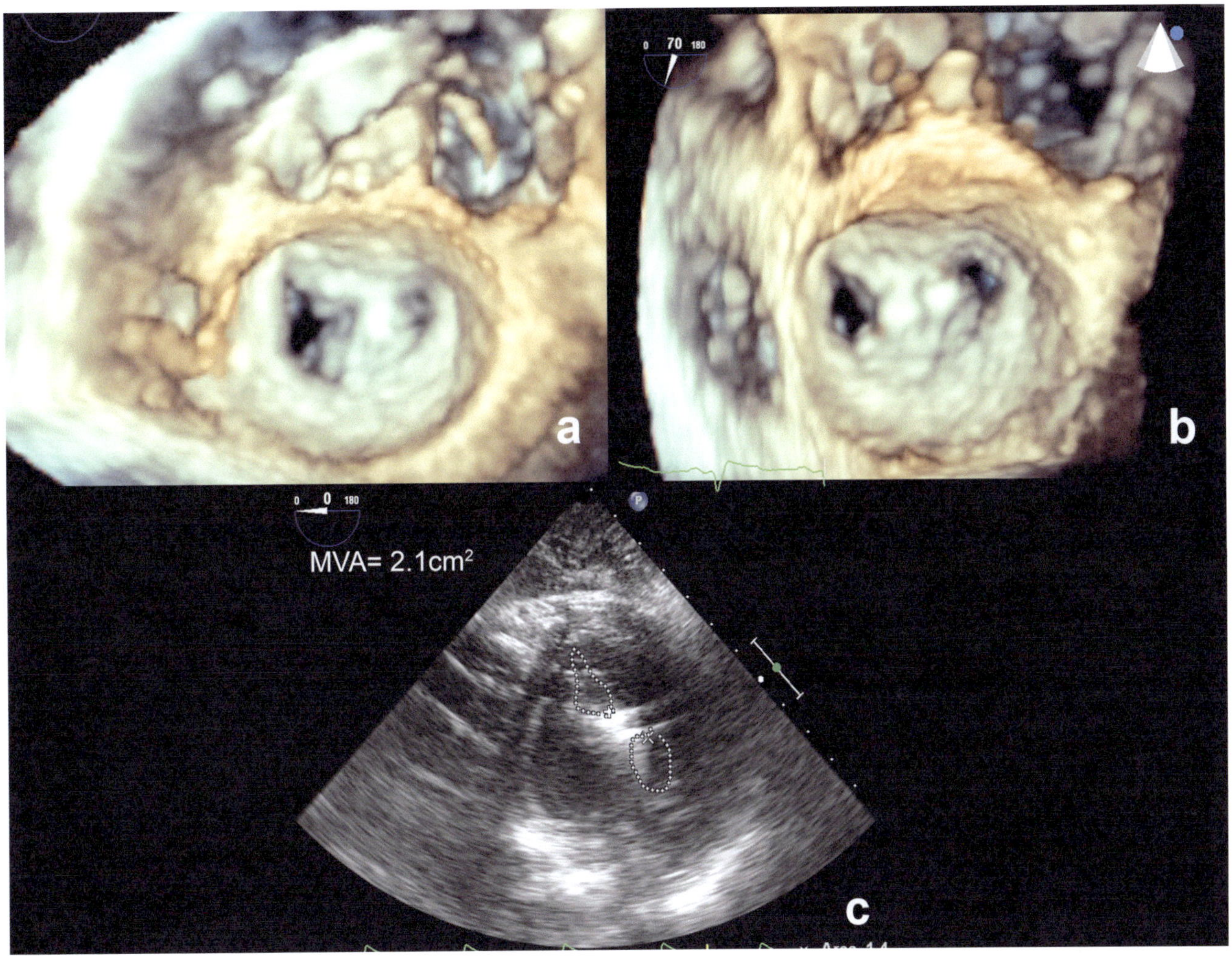

Fig. 29.6 Comparison between 3D echocardiography before (**a**) and after the second (**b**) clip; no mitral stenosis is present (**c**)

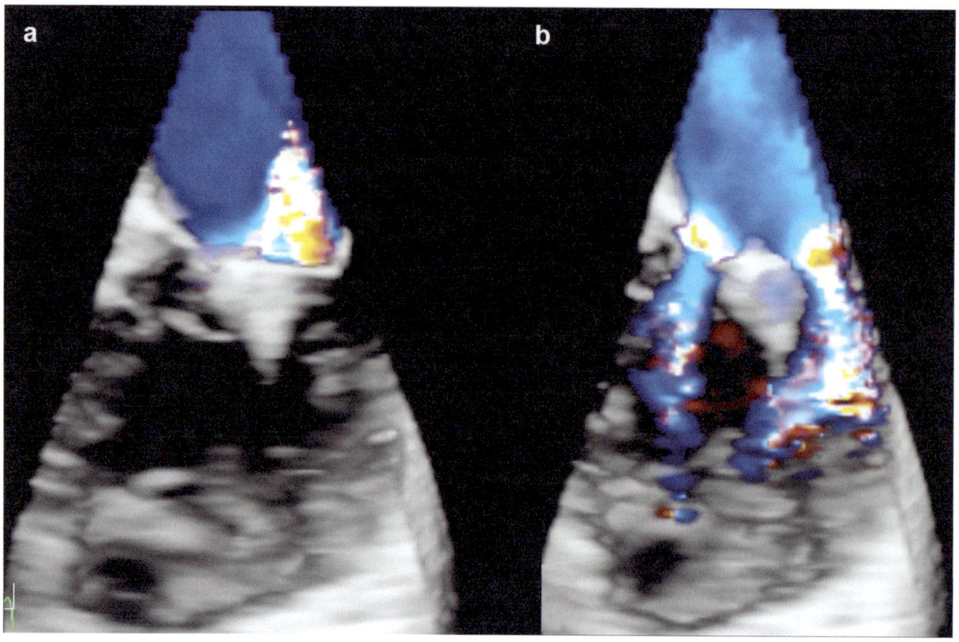

Fig. 29.7 3D reconstruction of the mild residual regurgitant jet (**a**); minimal acceleration of flow during diastolic phase without significant stenosis (**b**)

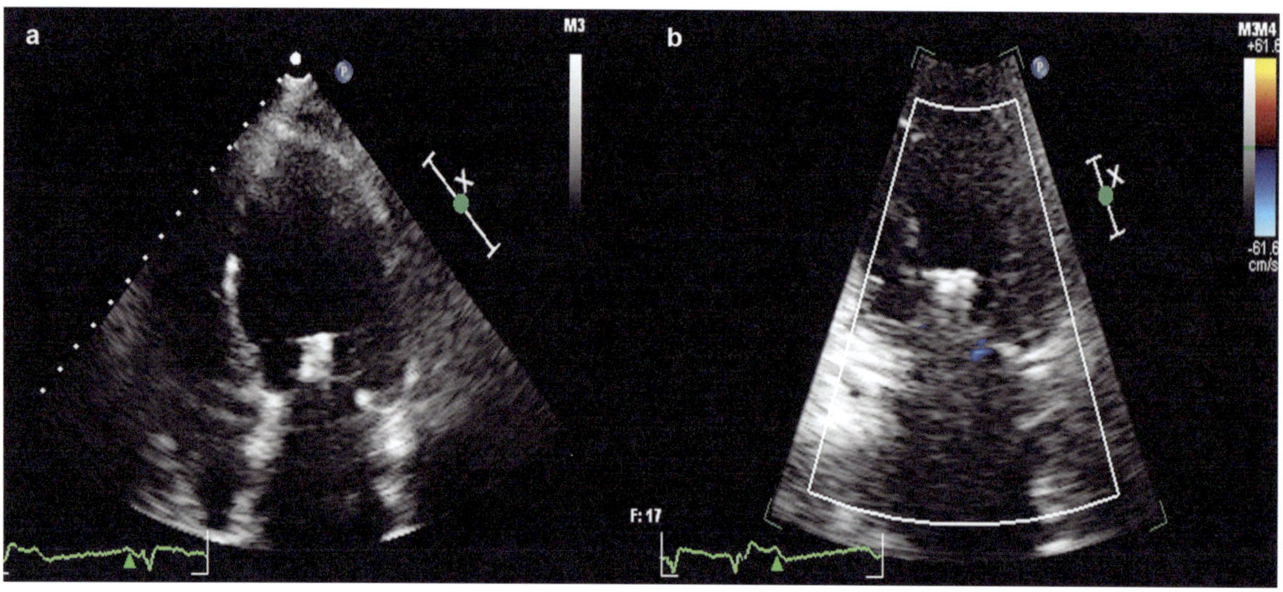

Fig. 29.8 Absence of MR 6-month follow-up transthoracic echocardiography (**a**, **b**)

Case 2: Complex Degenerative Mitral Regurgitation (Anterior Leaflet Prolapse) with Commissural Impingement

Abstract

This case illustrates the successful use of the MitraClip in a patient with degenerative mitral regurgitation that exceeds the constraints of the EVEREST II trial criteria. It also highlights the common procedural pitfall of entanglement in the chordae tendineae and the steps taken to extricate from that situation.

Keywords

Mitral regurgitation • Degenerative mitral valve • MitraClip • Chordae tendineae

Background

Surgical edge-to-edge procedure has been used with excellent result for the treatment of complex degenerative mitral regurgitation (DMR), such as anterior or bileaflet prolapse [6, 7]. Similarly, MitraClip system has been applied to a wide spectrum of degenerative mitral regurgitation (DMR), with good results even in patients with suboptimal anatomy, extending beyond the EVEREST II trial criteria [8].

We here report the case of a patient with a complex DMR who underwent successful MitraClip implantation in our institution.

Clinical History

An 81-year-old man with a past medical history of surgical myocardial revascularization was admitted to our institution because of heart failure (NYHA functional class III) secondary to degenerative mitral regurgitation. Logistic EuroScore was 35.4 %, so a MitraClip procedure was planned because of the prohibitive surgical risk.

Preoperative transesophageal echocardiography showed severe mitral regurgitation due to anterior leaflet flail (A2 segment); flail gap was 3 mm, and flail width was 15 mm. LV function was moderately depressed (LVEF is 40 %). LVEDD and LVESD were 65 and 40 mm, respectively; PASP was 55 mmHg. Figure 29.9a, b show intercommissural views with and without color demonstrating that the MR jet is central. Figure 29.9c, d show LVOT views with and without color demonstrating the characteristics of the lesion (A2 flail with short flail gap). Figure 29.10 shows the 3D surgical view of the valve.

Transseptal puncture was challenging because of the presence of a convex floppy septum, with thick muscular portion (Fig. 29.11a); it was performed 4.0 cm above the mitral plane (Fig. 29.11b).

A possible complication of the MitraClip procedure is the impingement of the clip in the subvalvular mitral apparatus. This complication is particularly frequent when the clip is advanced inadvertently into the commissural area. This occurs when the operators focus on the clip rather than on the target during echo guidance (Fig. 29.12a, b). In most cases, the clip can be retracted without complications after the complete opening of the clip arms. However, proper management of clip delivery system is necessary to avoid this complication. Key elements are the following: (1) stable echo image focusing on the target, (2) avoid rotations of the clip in the commissural area, (3) always check the trajectory during the advancement into LV, and (4) stop ventilation during the maneuver.

In the present case, the clip remained entangled within the chordae tendineae in the commissural area (Fig. 29.12c). After clip eversion (Fig. 29.12d), the clip was released and retracted in the left atrium, without structural damages to the mitral valve.

Subsequently, the clip was properly aligned to the regurgitant jet and advanced into the LV. The clip was pulled back, and the leaflets spontaneously fell into the clip (Fig. 29.13a). The clip was closed to 60° to secure the leaflets between grippers and clip arms and to check for leaflet insertion (Fig. 29.13b). After the complete closure, reduction of MR jet is observed (Fig. 29.13c), and the clip is released with mild residual jets on both sides of the clip (Fig. 29.13d). The patient had uneventful postoperative course and was discharged to home 4 days after the intervention. Predischarge echocardiography showed residual mild to moderate MR (1–2+). At 30 days follow-up, the patient was in excellent clinical conditions (NYHA class I).

Learning Points

1. Procedural success can be achieved in patients with complex degenerative mitral disease, such as anterior leaflet prolapse.
2. Although the incidence of intraprocedural complications is low, such complications may be catastrophic, and a prompt diagnosis with appropriate management is important.
3. It is important to have procedural discipline and follow the key steps of the MitraClip procedure so as to avoid complications such as entanglement in the chordae tendineae.
4. Early recognition of entanglement of the MitraClip in the chordae tendineae is important and can be treated by eversion of the clip and withdrawal back into the left atrium.

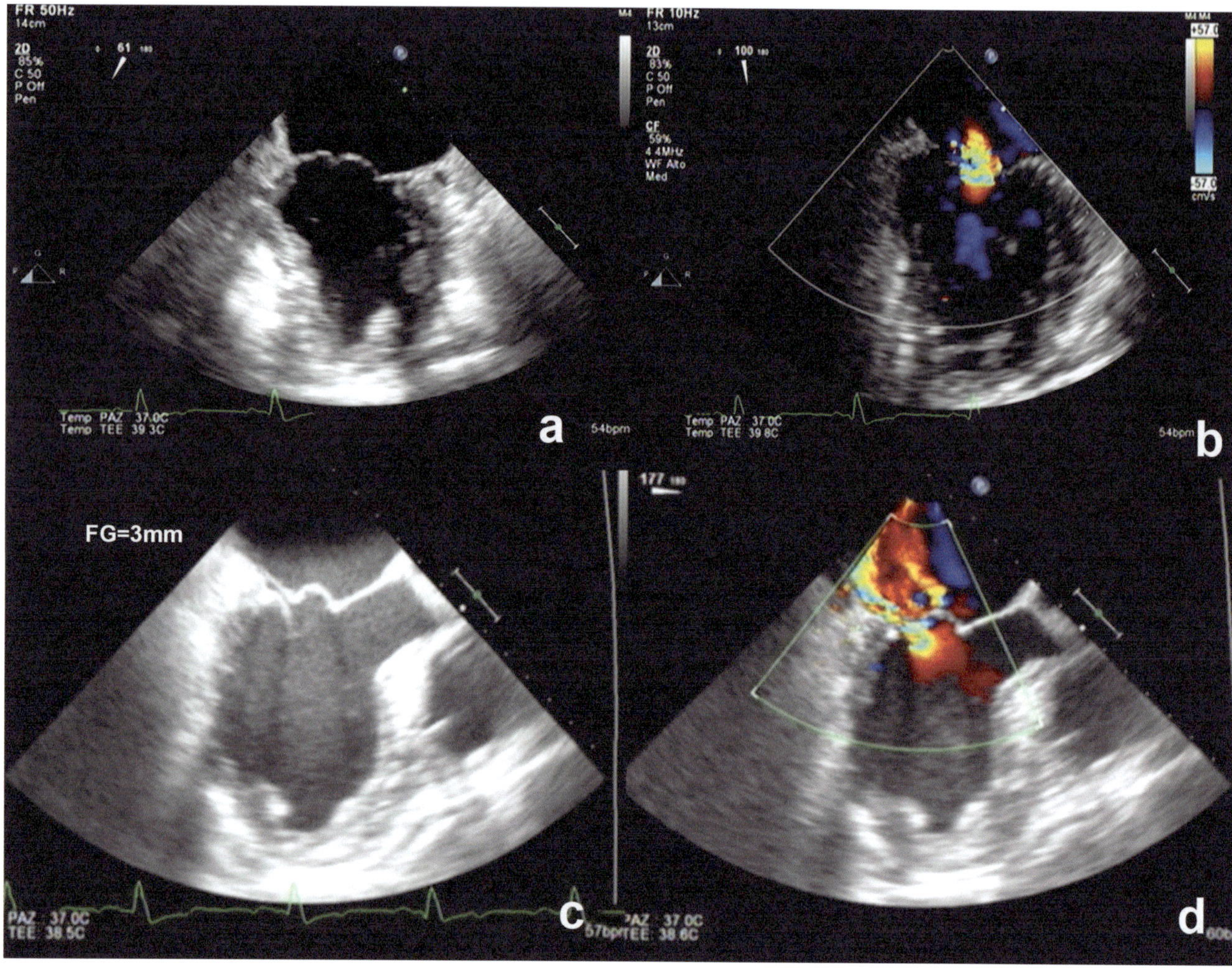

Fig. 29.9 Color compare intercommissural images showing central jet (**a**, **b**); color compare images of the LVOT view demonstrating the characteristics of the lesion (**c**, **d**)

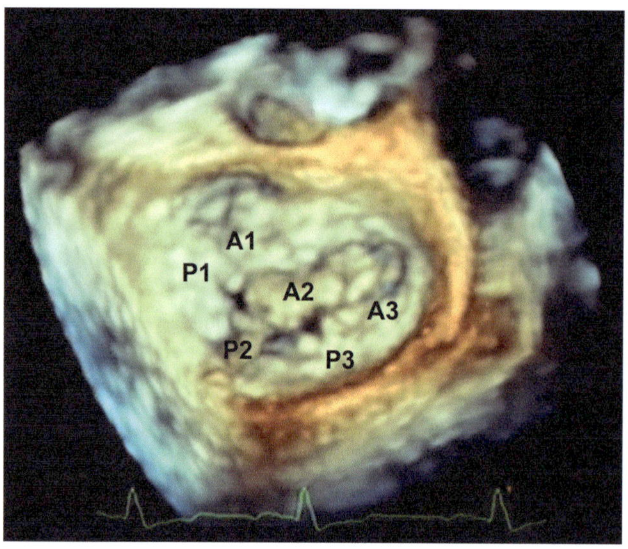

Fig. 29.10 3D surgical view of the valve

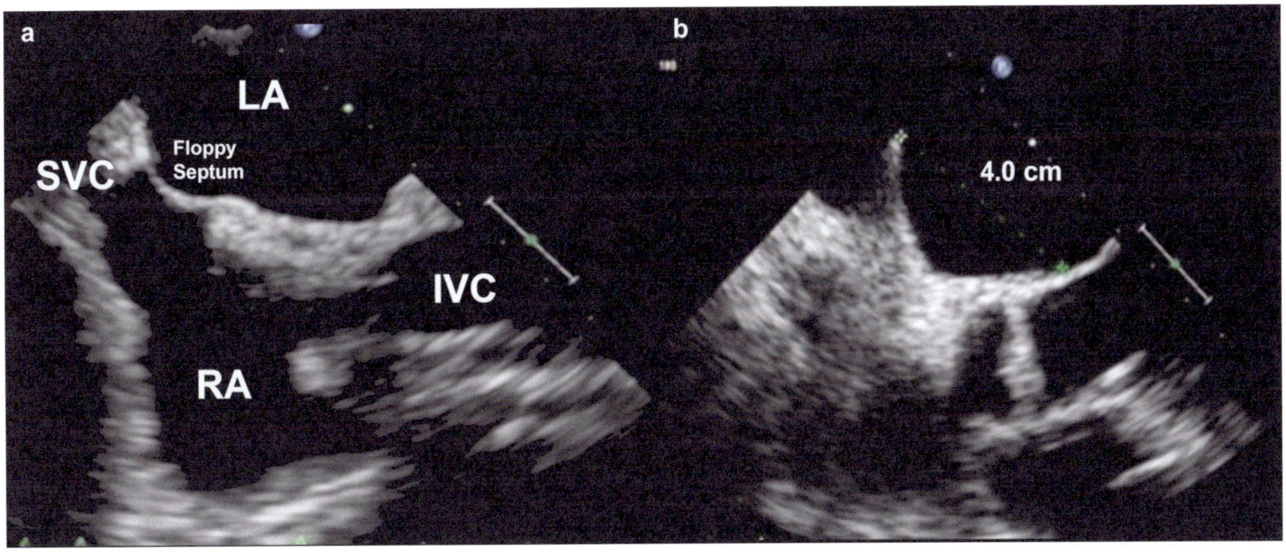

Fig. 29.11 Presence of a convex floppy septum, with thick muscular portion (**a**); puncture is performed 4.0 cm above the mitral plane (**b**). *LA* left atrium, *RA* right atrium, *SVC* superior vena cava, *IVC* inferior vena cava

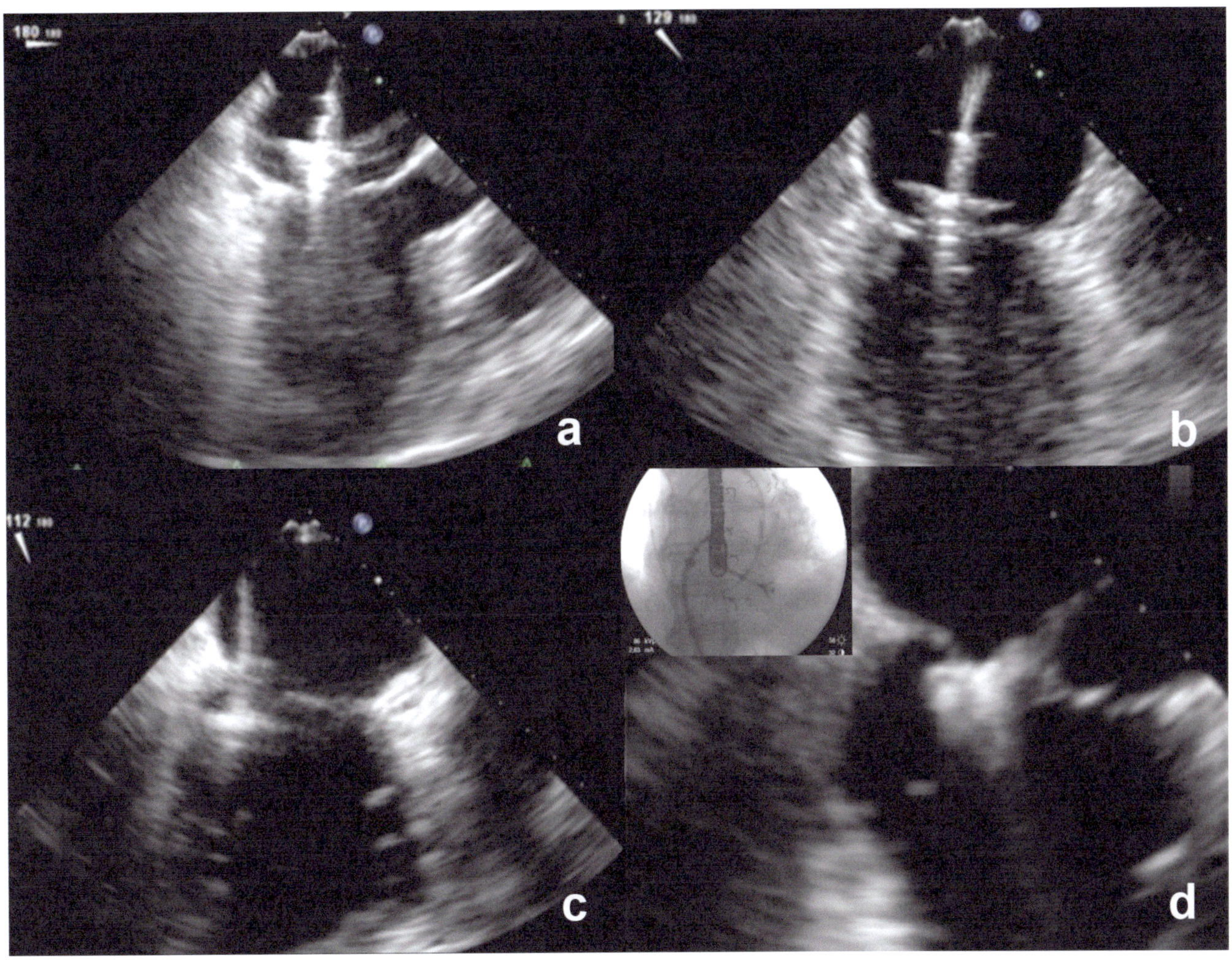

Fig. 29.12 Focus on the clip rather than on the target during echo guidance (**a**, **b**) with subsequent impingement of the clip in the subvalvular mitral apparatus in the commissural area (**c**); release of the clip after complete clip reversal (**d**)

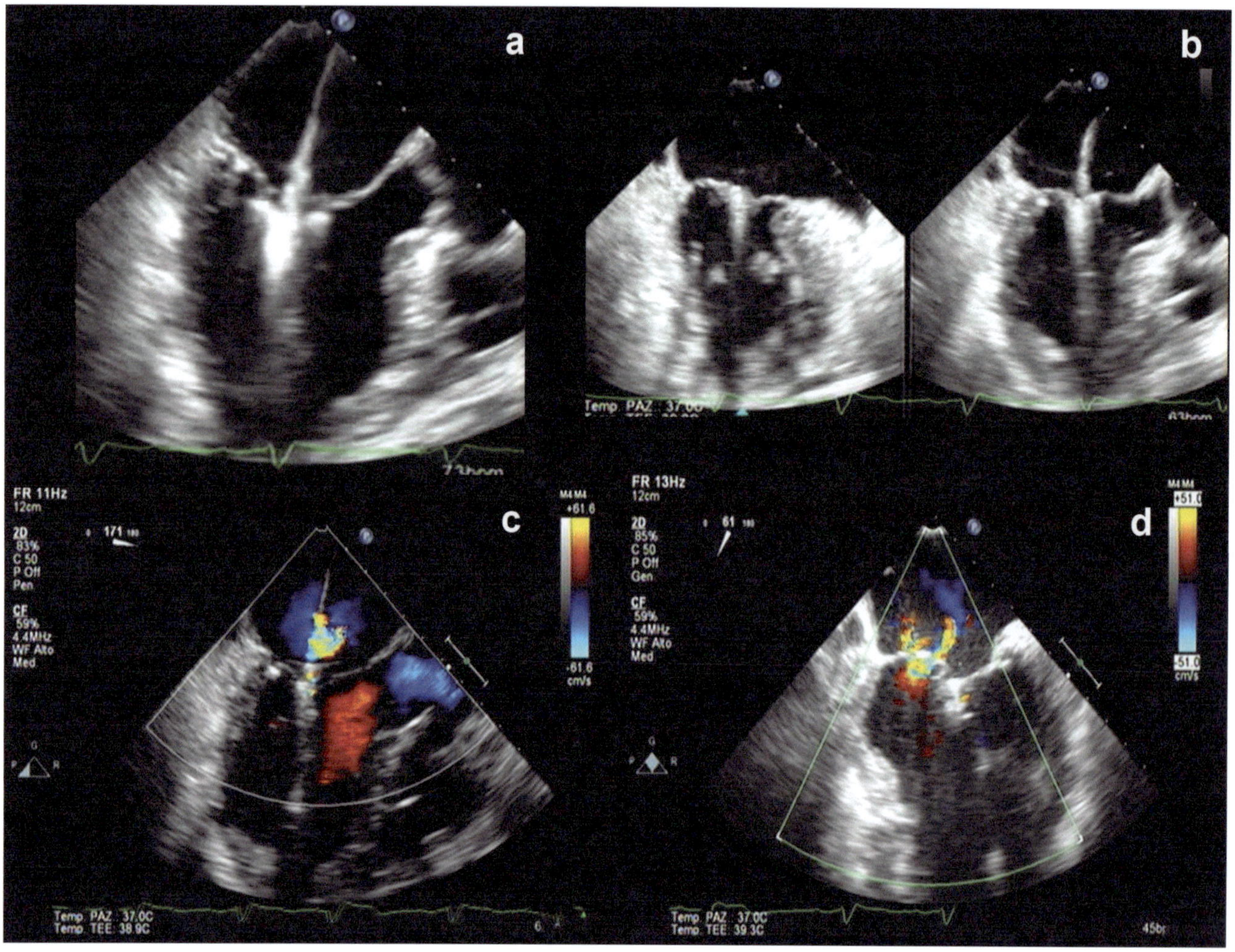

Fig. 29.13 A new clip is advanced in the LV, pulled back, and the leaflets spontaneously fell into the clip (**a**); closure to 60 to check for leaflet insertion (**b**); reduction of MR jet after complete clip closure (**c**); complete clip release with mild residual jets (**d**)

References

1. Yiu SF, Enriquez-Sarano M, Tribouilloy C, Seward JB, Tajik AJ. Determinants of the degree of functional mitral regurgitation in patients with systolic left ventricular dysfunction: a quantitative clinical study. Circulation. 2000;102:1400–6.
2. Mirabel M, Iung B, Baron G, Messika-Zeitoun D, Détaint D, Vanoverschelde JL, Butchart EG, Ravaud P, Vahanian A. What are the characteristics of patients with severe, symptomatic, mitral regurgitation who are denied surgery? Eur Heart J. 2007;28:1358–65.
3. Tamburino C, Ussia GP, Maisano F, Capodanno D, La Canna G, Scandura S, Colombo A, Giacomini A, Michev I, Mangiafico S, Cammalleri V, Barbanti M, Alfieri O. Percutaneous mitral valve repair with the MitraClip system: acute results from a real world setting. Eur Heart J. 2010;31:1382–9.
4. Franzen O, van der Heyden J, Baldus S, Schlüter M, Schillinger W, Butter C, Hoffmann R, Corti R, Pedrazzini G, Swaans MJ, Neuss M, Rudolph V, Sürder D, Grünenfelder J, Eulenburg C, Reichenspurner H, Meinertz T, Auricchio A. MitraClip® therapy in patients with end-stage systolic heart failure. Eur J Heart Fail. 2011;13:569–76.
5. Franzen O, Baldus S, Rudolph V, Meyer S, Knap M, Koschyk D, Treede H, Barmeyer A, Schofer J, Costard-Jäckle A, Schlüter M, Reichenspurner H, Meinertz T. Acute outcomes of MitraClip therapy for mitral regurgitation in high-surgical-risk patients: emphasis on adverse valve morphology and severe left ventricular dysfunction. Eur Heart J. 2010;31:1373–81.
6. Maisano F, Schreuder JJ, Oppizzi M, Fiorani B, Fino C, Alfieri O. The double-orifice technique as a standardized approach to treat mitral regurgitation due to severe myxomatous disease: surgical technique. Eur J Cardiothorac Surg. 2000;17:201–5.
7. De Bonis M, Lorusso R, Lapenna E, Kassem S, De Cicco G, Torracca L, Maisano F, La Canna G, Alfieri O. Similar long-term results of mitral valve repair for anterior compared with posterior leaflet prolapse. J Thorac Cardiovasc Surg. 2006;131:364–70.
8. Franzen O, Baldus S, Rudolph V, Meyer S, Knap M, Koschyk D, Treede H, Barmeyer A, Schofer J, Costard-Jackle A, Schluter M, Reichenspurner H, Meinertz T. Acute outcomes of MitraClip therapy for mitral regurgitation in high-surgical-risk patients: emphasis on adverse valve morphology and severe left ventricular dysfunction. Eur Heart J. 2010;31:1373–81.

Severe Functional Mitral Regurgitation with Missing Leaflet Coaptation

30

Antti Saraste, Juha Lund, Markku Saraste, Matti Luotolahti, Juhani Airaksinen, and Olaf Franzen

Abstract

This case illustrates the use of the MitraClip in a patient with severe functional mitral regurgitation. The mitral valve anatomy was unfavorable, but the procedure was successfully performed using a stepwise approach using two clips to improve coaptation of the leaflets.

Keywords

Mitral regurgitation • MitraClip • Functional

Clinical History

The patient is 71-year-old male who used to exercise regularly until he had an acute ST elevation myocardial infarction of the inferior wall. Urgent coronary artery bypass graft surgery for total occlusion in the middle right coronary artery and ostial stenosis in the left circumflex artery was performed. Postoperative echocardiography showed myocardial infarct scar in the basal inferior wall, mildly reduced left ventricular systolic function, and moderate-to-severe mitral valve regurgitation. The patient responded well to intensive therapy for heart failure, and reoperation for the mitral regurgitation was not considered necessary. Six years later, the patient was referred for reevaluation due to worsening of heart failure symptoms to NYHA class 3–4 despite optimal medical therapy. Coronary angiography showed no significant stenosis, and the patient was referred for evaluation of the mitral regurgitation.

Transthoracic echocardiography (TTE, Fig. 30.1) shows aneurysmal infarct scar in the basal inferior wall and moderately reduced left ventricular systolic function (ejection fraction of 35–40 %). Central mitral valve regurgitation jet directed toward posterior wall was present. Consistent with severe regurgitation, effective regurgitant orifice area (EROA) was 0.5 cm^2 based on the PISA method. Transesophageal echocardiography (TEE, Fig. 30.2) of the mitral valve revealed wide regurgitation jet and a 4-mm gap between the leaflets due to annular dilatation (up to 50 mm) and restricted motion of the posterior leaflet. The patient was considered high risk for surgery due to previous cardiac surgery, poor

A. Saraste, M.D., Ph.D. • J. Lund, M.D.
J. Airaksinen, M.D., Ph.D. (✉)
Department of Medicine, Turku University Hospital, Kiinamyllynkatu 4-8, Turku, 20520, Finland
e-mail: antti.saraste@utu.fi; juha.lund@tyks.fi; juhani.airaksinen@tyks.fi

M. Saraste, M.D.
Department of Medicine, Turku University Hospital, Turku, Finland

Department of Clinical Physiology, Nuclear Medicine and PET, Turku University Hospital, Kiinamyllynkatu 4-8, Turku, 20520, Finland
e-mail: markku.saraste@tyks.fi

M. Luotolahti, M.D., Ph.D.
Department of Clinical Physiology, Nuclear Medicine and PET, Turku University Hospital, Kiinamyllynkatu 4-8, Turku, 20520, Finland

Heart Centre, Rigshospitalet, University of Copenhagen, Copenhagen, Denmark
matti.luotolahti@tyks.fi

O. Franzen, M.D.
Department of Cardiology, The Heart Center, Rigshospitalet, University of Copenhagen, Blegdamsvej 9, Copenhagen, 2100, Denmark

Royal Brompton Hospital, Royal Brompton and Harefield NHS Foundation Trust, London, UK
e-mail: owfranzen@gmx.de

T. Feldman et al. (eds.), *Atlas of Percutaneous Edge-to-Edge Mitral Valve Repair*,
DOI 10.1007/978-1-4471-4294-2_30, © Springer-Verlag London 2013

left ventricular systolic function, reduced lung capacity, and advanced heart failure. Therefore, the patient was referred for MitraClip therapy to correct the functional mitral regurgitation despite unfavorable valve anatomy.

Because of the challenging anatomy, our plan was to correct the regurgitation "gradually" with two clips. The procedure started with implantation of the first clip oriented at the site of maximal regurgitation jet slightly laterally (Fig. 30.3). Successful leaflet capture and grasp was possible after some attempts (Fig. 30.3). Perpendicularity of the clip was confirmed in transgastric view. Implantation of the first clip resulted in a considerable reduction of the coaptation gap and regurgitant jet, but as expected, a significant residual jet was present medial to the first clip, and a second clip was implanted at this site (Fig. 30.3). Implantation of the second clip resulted in marked reduction of the regurgitant jet with mild residual jet (Fig. 30.4). On the next day, two MitraClips and only a minor regurgitant jet were seen by TTE (Fig. 30.4). Symptoms of heart failure were immediately relieved, and the patient was discharged on the second postoperative day. Anticoagulation therapy with warfarin was continued due to atrial fibrillation.

Learning Points

This case illustrates that it may be possible to correct large functional mitral regurgitation with a stepwise technique of two adjacent MitraClips even in the presence of missing coaptation between the leaflets in a severely symptomatic patient.

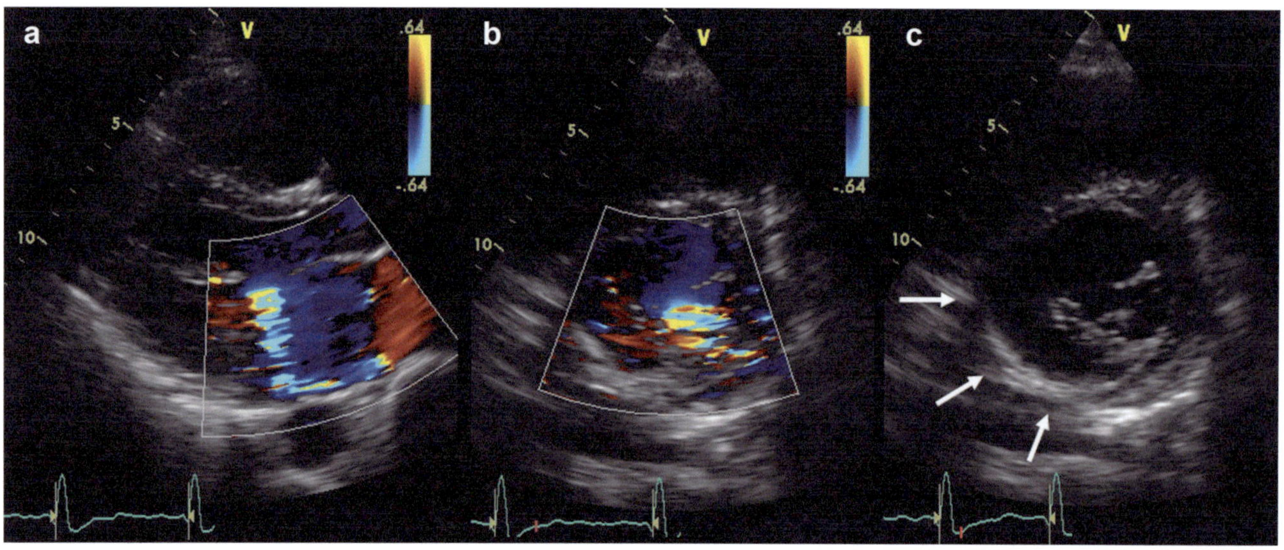

Fig. 30.1 Transthoracic echocardiography (*TTE*) images with color Doppler showed central and posteriorly directed mitral valve regurgitation jet in parasternal long axis view (**a**) and short axis view (**b**). Note the presence of aneurysmatic infarct scar (*arrows*) in the basal inferior wall in the short axis view (**c**)

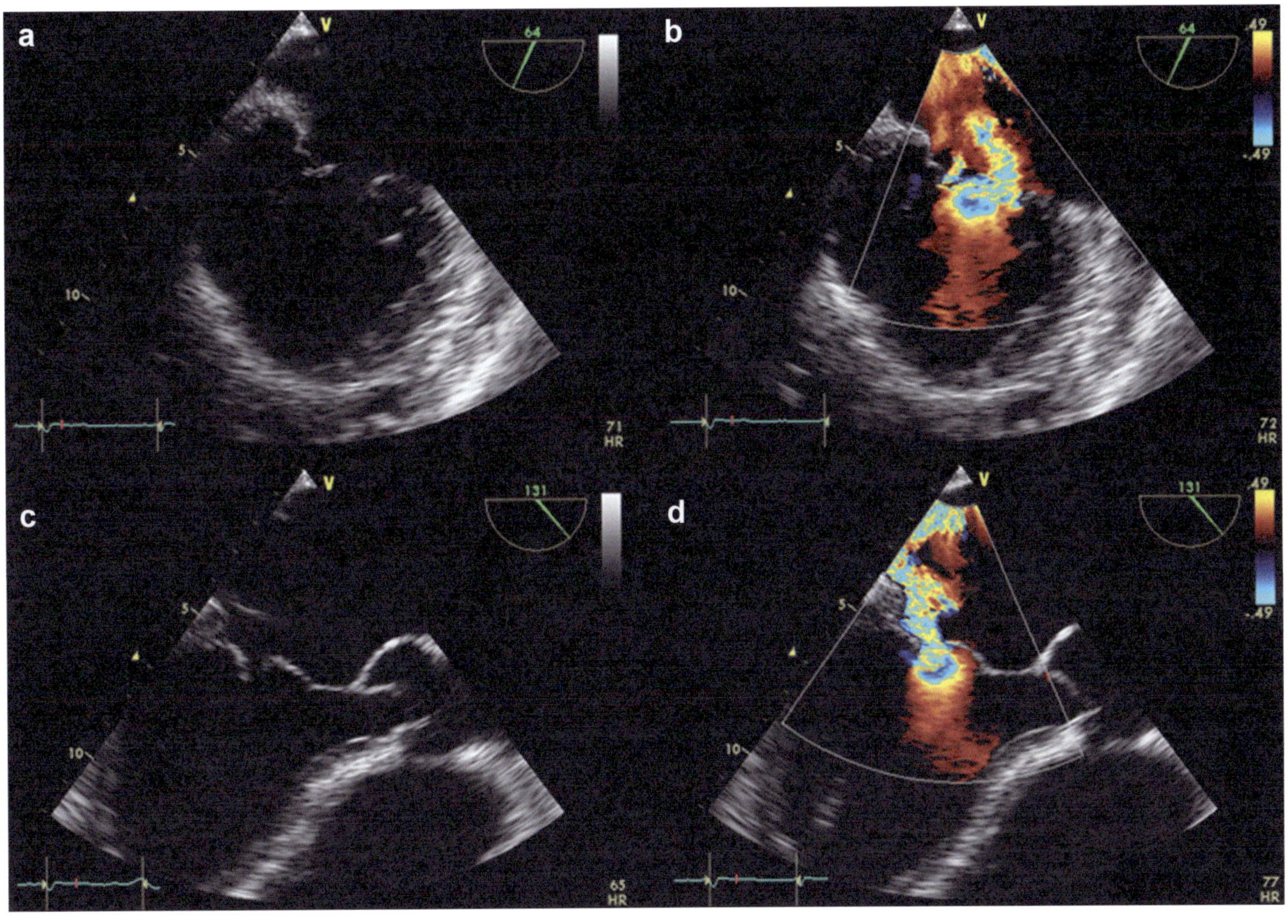

Fig. 30.2 Transesophageal echocardiography (*TEE*) images of the mitral valve with (**b**, **d**) and without (**a**, **c**) color Doppler showing wide regurgitation jet and a gap of 4 mm between the leaflets due to dilated annulus and restricted motion of the posterior leaflet in intercommissural (**a**, **b**) and long axis (**c**, **d**) views

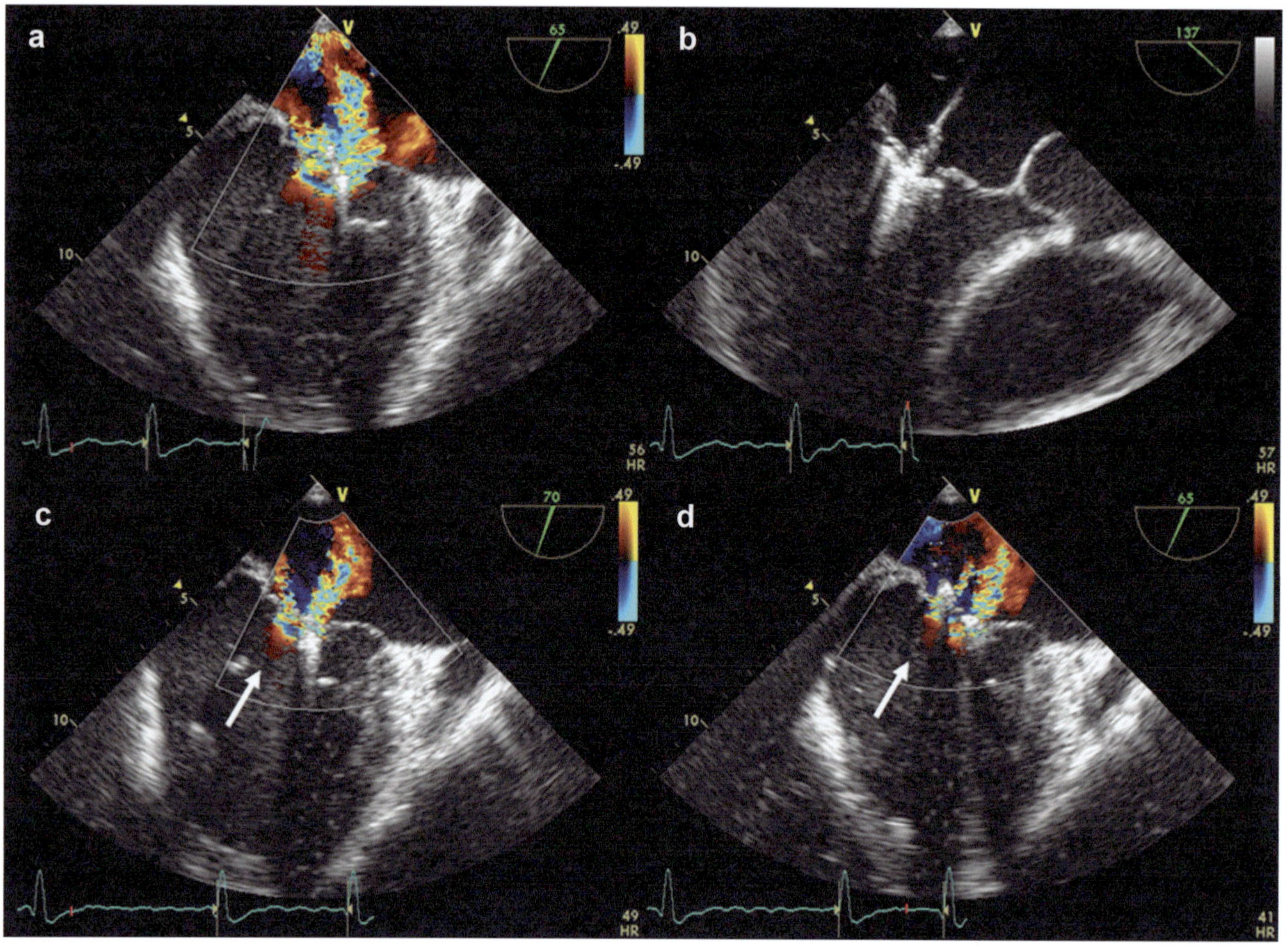

Fig. 30.3 TEE images showing positioning of the first MitraClip at the site of the largest regurgitant jet (**a**), successful leaflet grasp (**b**), and reduction in the coaptation gap and regurgitant jet after closure of the clip arms (**c**) enabling the positioning of the second clip at the site of residual jet (*arrows*) medial to the first clip (**c**, **d**)

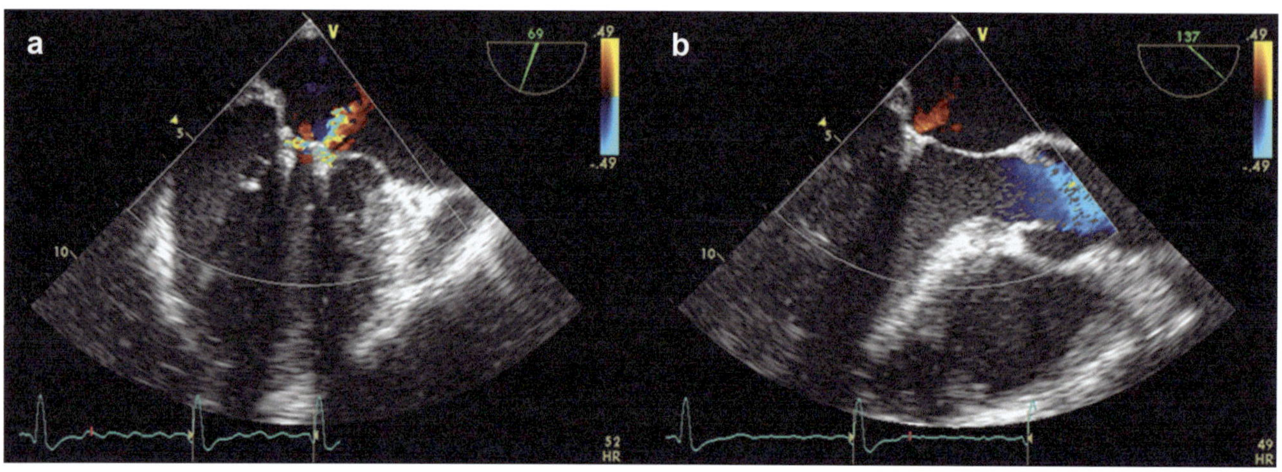

Fig. 30.4 TEE images with color Doppler showing only a small residual jet after implantation of two MitraClips in intercommissural (**a**) and long axis (**b**) views

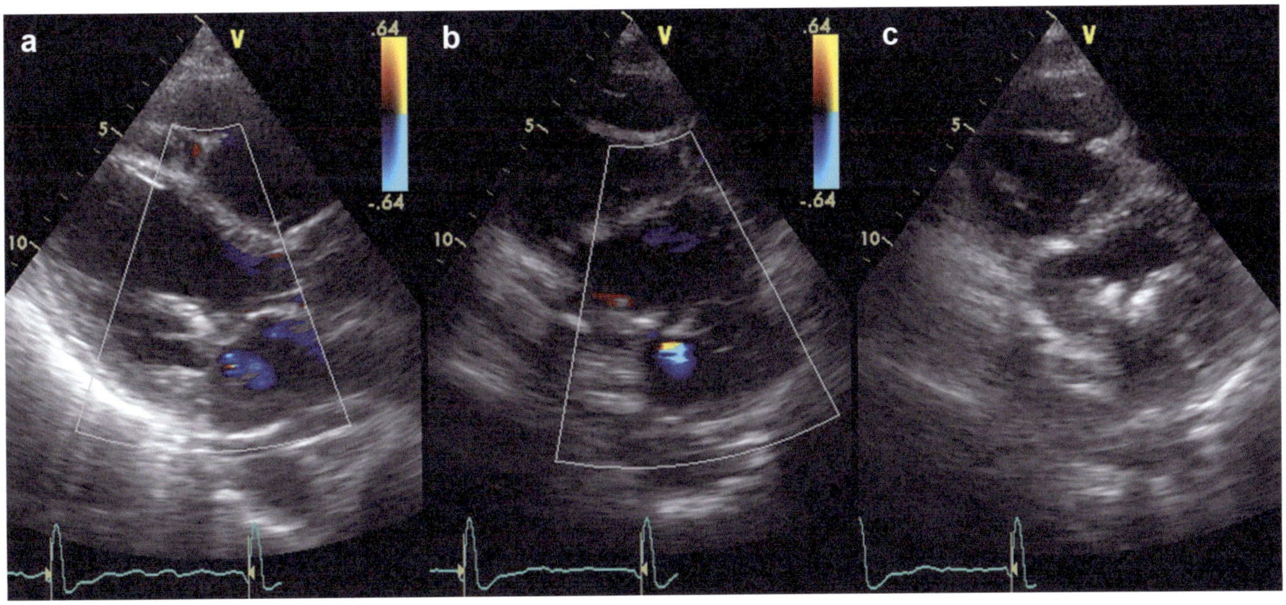

Fig. 30.5 TTE images showed two clips in position and only minor residual mitral valve regurgitant jets on the postoperative day in parasternal long axis view with color (**a**) and short axis views with (**b**) and without color Doppler (**c**)

Severe Ischemic Heart Failure with Functional Improvement After MitraClip Therapy

31

Janne M. Rapola

Abstract
In this case, an intra-aortic balloon pump was required to stabilize a patient with severe left ventricular dysfunction and severe functional mitral regurgitation during a MitraClip procedure. Despite residual moderate mitral regurgitation, the patient had significant functional improvement from NYHA class III to class I.

Keywords
Mitral regurgitation • MitraClip • Intra-aortic balloon pump

Clinical History

A previously healthy 61-year-old man was referred because of tiredness and shortness of breath. One month earlier, he had experienced chest pain and a feeling of general illness but had not seen a doctor then. Since his condition did not improve, he visited a general practitioner, who observed signs and symptoms of heart failure, with significant Q-waves on the ECG, and referred him to a university hospital.

On initial examination, he was hemodynamically stable, but with clear symptoms (dyspnea, orthopnea) and signs (rales, edema in lower extremities, tachycardia) and findings (chest X-ray, Fig. 31.1, proBNP 5,429 ng/l) of heart failure. On initial echocardiogram, large posterolateral hypokinesis was observed along with moderate ischemic-type mitral regurgitation (MR).

The patient underwent coronary angiography, which revealed a total occlusion of the circumflex artery (Fig. 31.2). Revascularization was planned, but scintigraphy revealed a large scar with very little residual ischemia (Fig. 31.3). Thus, no revascularization was performed.

The patient was discharged after medical treatment for heart failure. During follow-up, despite optimal medical therapy, the patient remained symptomatic NYHA III with persistent orthopnea. Echocardiography showed severe (grade 3+) functional mitral regurgitation. His 6-min walk distance was 457 m and proBNP level 3,756 ng/l. Right heart catheterization revealed high filling pressures with a marked v-wave (mean PCW 30 mmHg, v-wave 44 mmHg). Significant tricuspid regurgitation and elevated right-sided pressures were also observed (mean pulmonary artery pressure was 45 mmHg). Global ejection fraction on echo was estimated at 25–30 %. Surgery was considered, but with a poor EF and no evidence of ischemia, the patient was referred for the MitraClip procedure. Preoperative TTE in Fig. 31.4 demonstrates severe MR. This was confirmed on perioperative transesophageal echocardiography, where a wide coaptation gap was seen (Figs. 31.5, 31.6, and 31.7)

MitraClip implantation itself was uneventful. The first clip reduced the regurgitation only slightly, so a second clip was placed. Despite satisfactory clip placement, there was still grade 2 MR after the procedure (Figs. 31.8, 31.9, 31.10, and 31.11). At the end of the procedure, the patient was hypotensive with reduced cardiac output, and an intra-aortic balloon pump (IABP) was placed. Due to low output, the patient was 4 days in intensive care. He was gradually weaned from IABP and made a rapid recovery. He was discharged from the hospital on the tenth postoperative day.

In follow-up, his functional class was NYHA I; he had restarted his work and reported taking long walks with no symptoms. At 6 months, his 6-min walking distance had

J.M. Rapola, M.D., Ph.D.
Department of Cardiology, Helsinki University Hospital,
340, Helsinki, 00029, HUS, Finland
e-mail: janne.rapola@hus.fi

T. Feldman et al. (eds.), *Atlas of Percutaneous Edge-to-Edge Mitral Valve Repair*,
DOI 10.1007/978-1-4471-4294-2_31, © Springer-Verlag London 2013

increased to 575 m, and his pro BNP had decreased to 1,895 ng/l. On echo, the MR was still grade II and the EF around 30–40 % (Fig. 31.12).

Discussion

This is a typical patient with ischemic MR and poor LV function. Since he had no need for revascularization, he was referred for the MitraClip procedure. Though the echocardiographic result regarding decrease of MR was modest and he had an extended postoperative convalescence, his functional class returned to near-normal. Walking distance increased and pro BNP halved from the immediate preoperative value. In patients who are treated with the MitraClip, there may be significant clinical benefit despite moderate residual regurgitation.

Learning Points

1. In patients with severe left ventricular dysfunction, temporary hemodynamic support with an intra-aortic balloon pump may be required for the MitraClip procedure.
2. There may be significant medium to long-term clinical benefits even if MR remains moderate after the MitraClip.

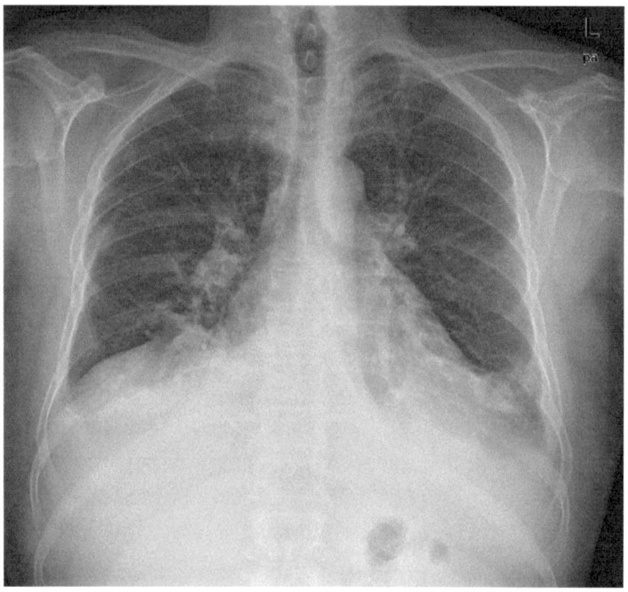

Fig. 31.1 Chest X-ray at admission shows decompensation and pleural effusion

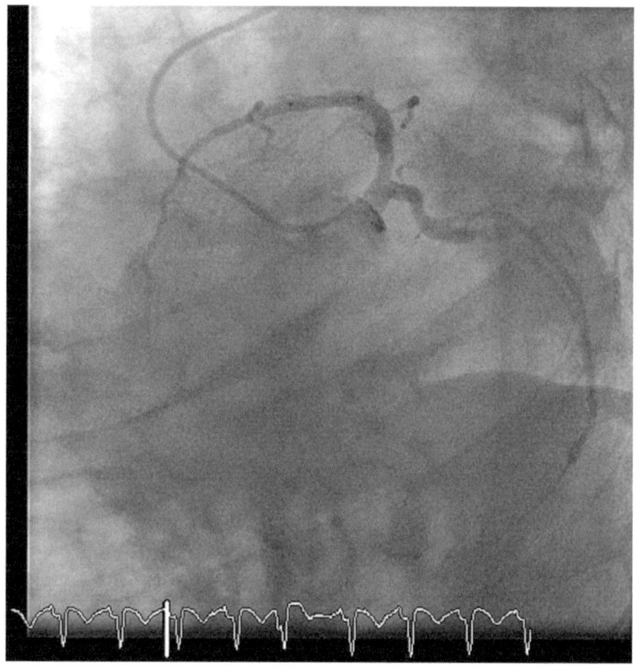

Fig. 31.2 Coronary angiogram with total occlusion of the circumflex artery

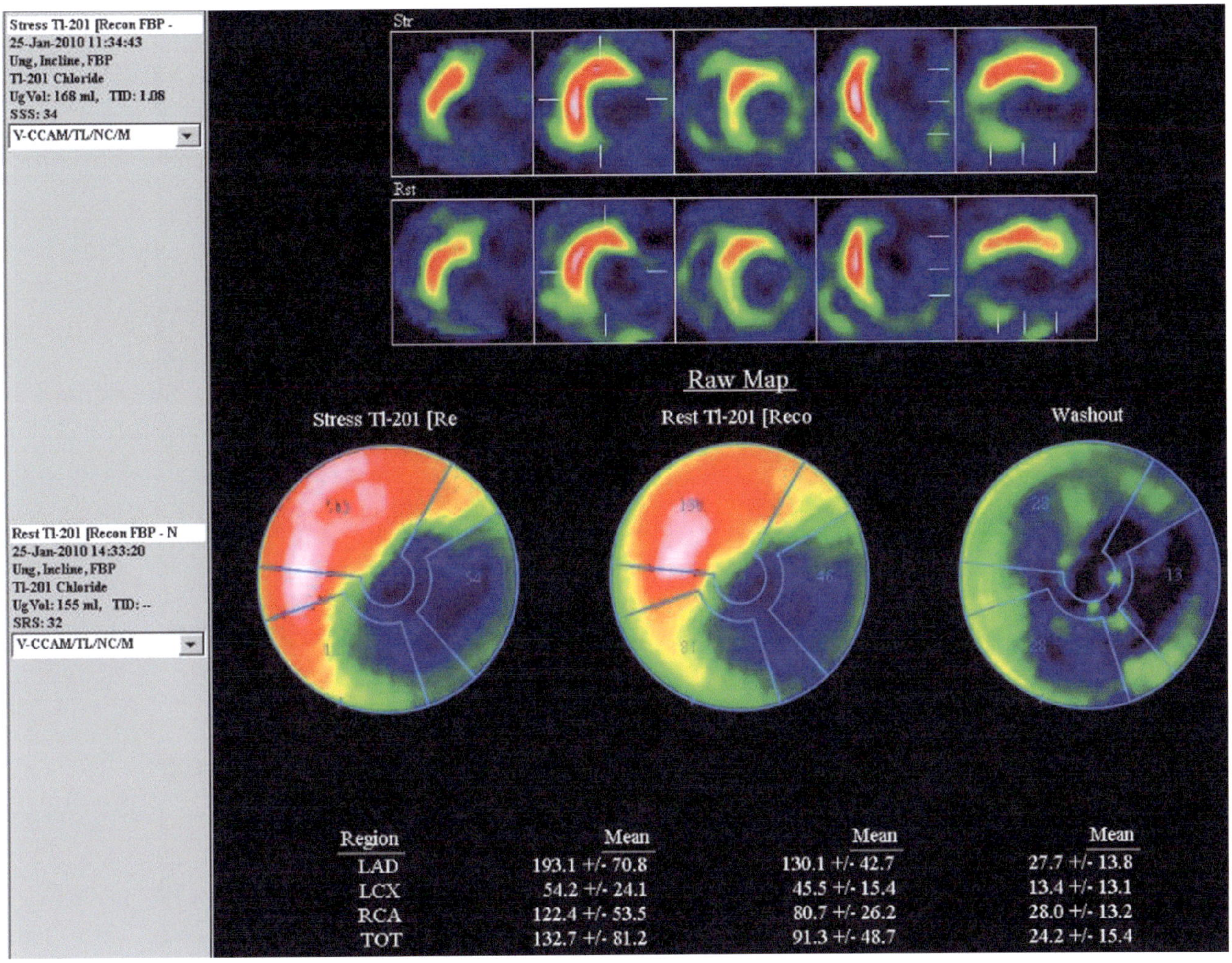

Fig. 31.3 Large fixed perfusion defect on scintigraphy

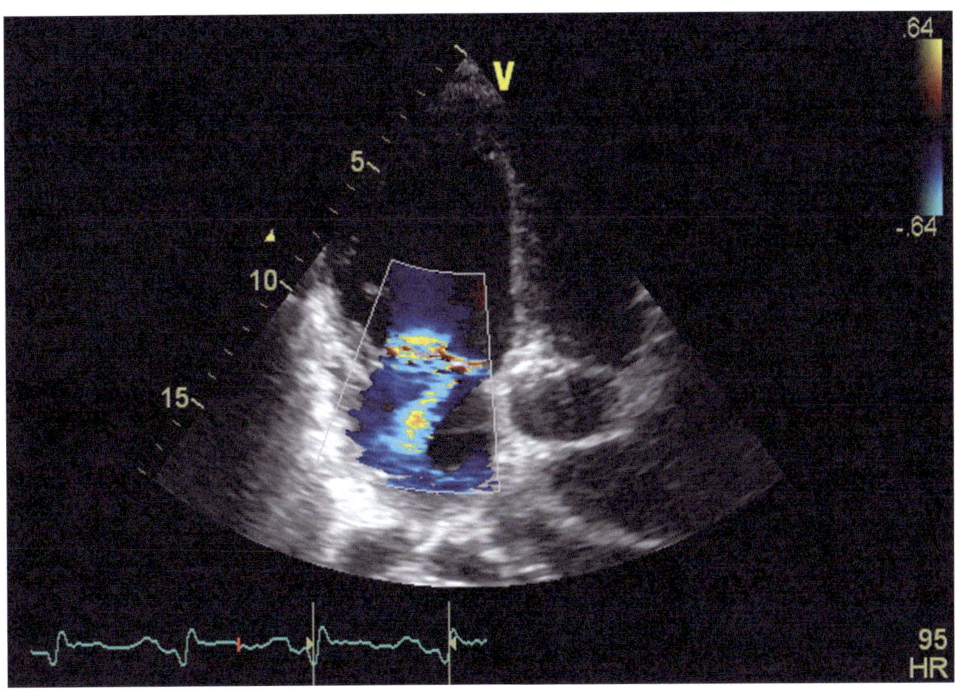

Fig. 31.4 Apical view demonstrating severe MR

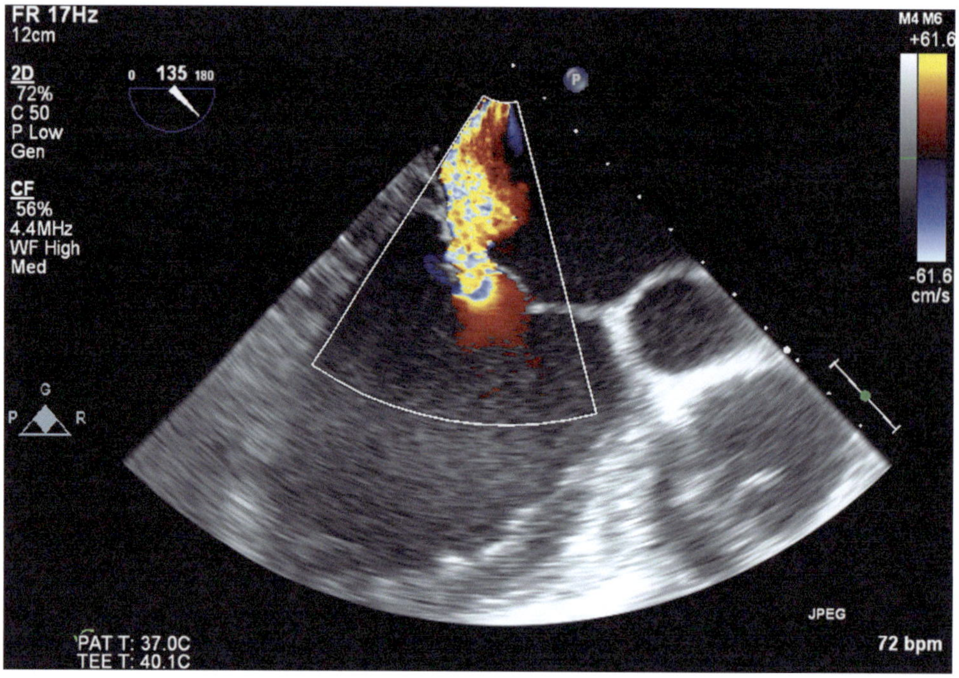

Fig. 31.5 TEE image shows severe MR at the A2-P2 area in an LVOT view

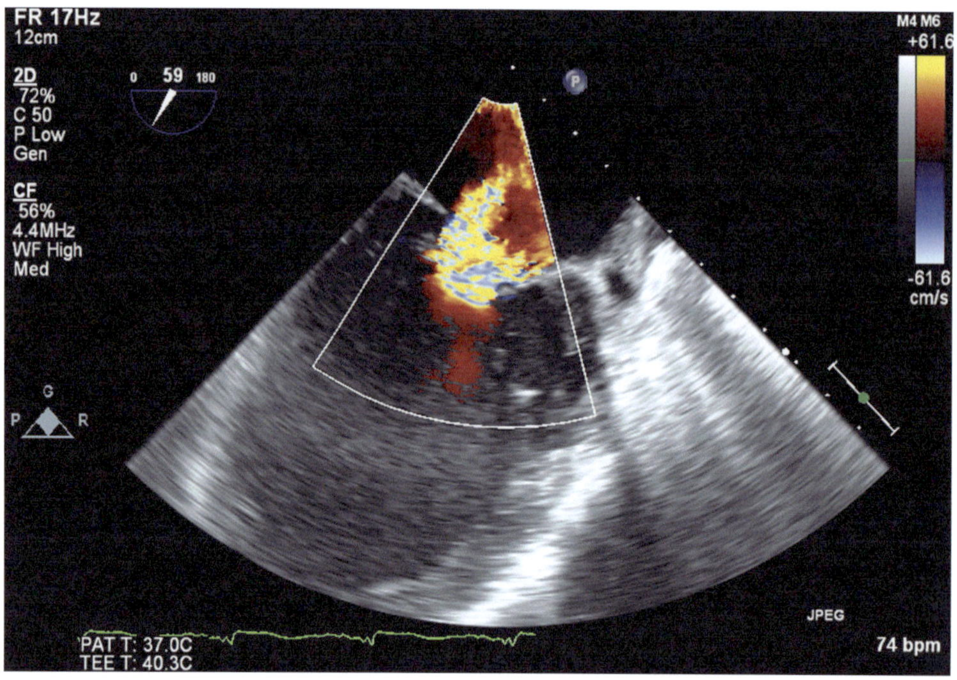

Fig. 31.6 The intercommissural view confirms severe central MR

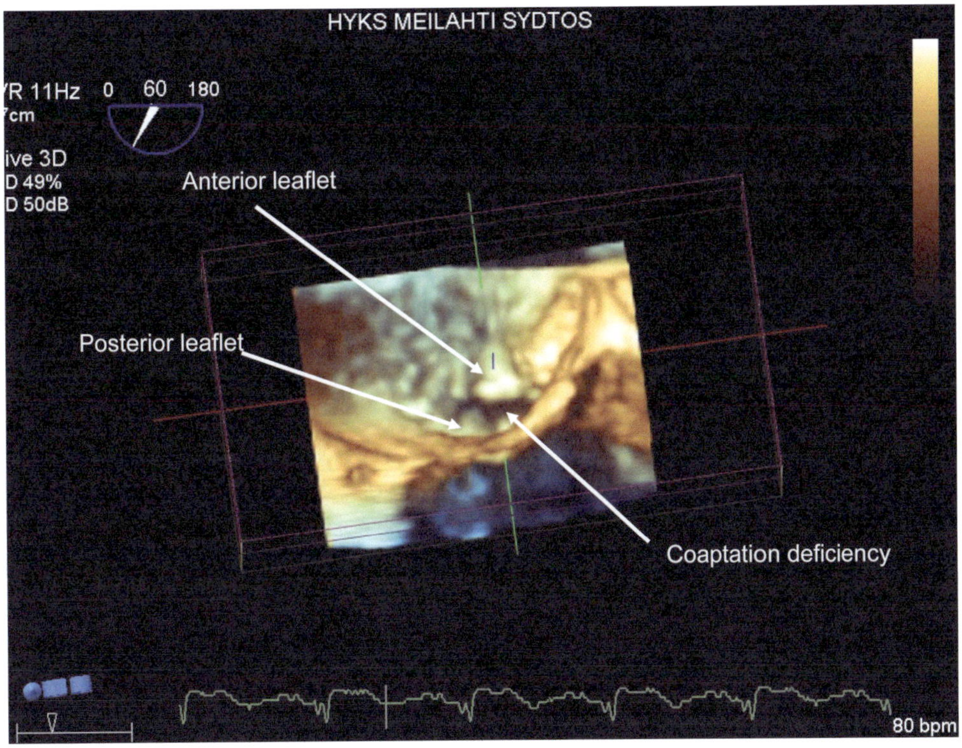

Fig. 31.7 3D echo view toward the mitral orifice from the left atrium shows a marked coaptation deficiency in systole

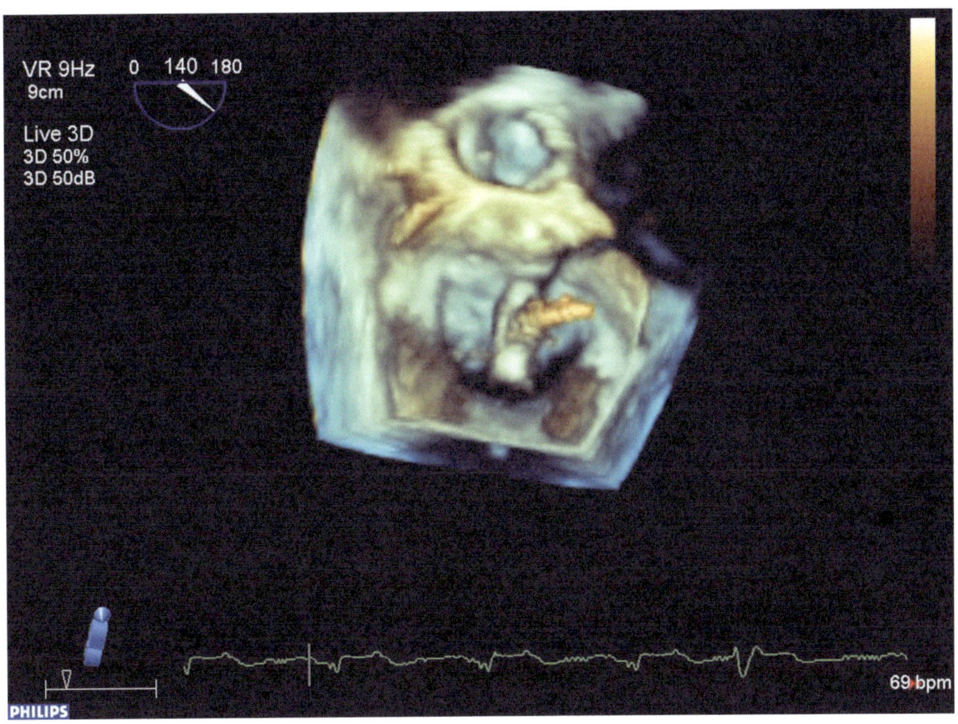

Fig. 31.8 First clip heading toward the mitral valve. All 3D images are from the left atrium

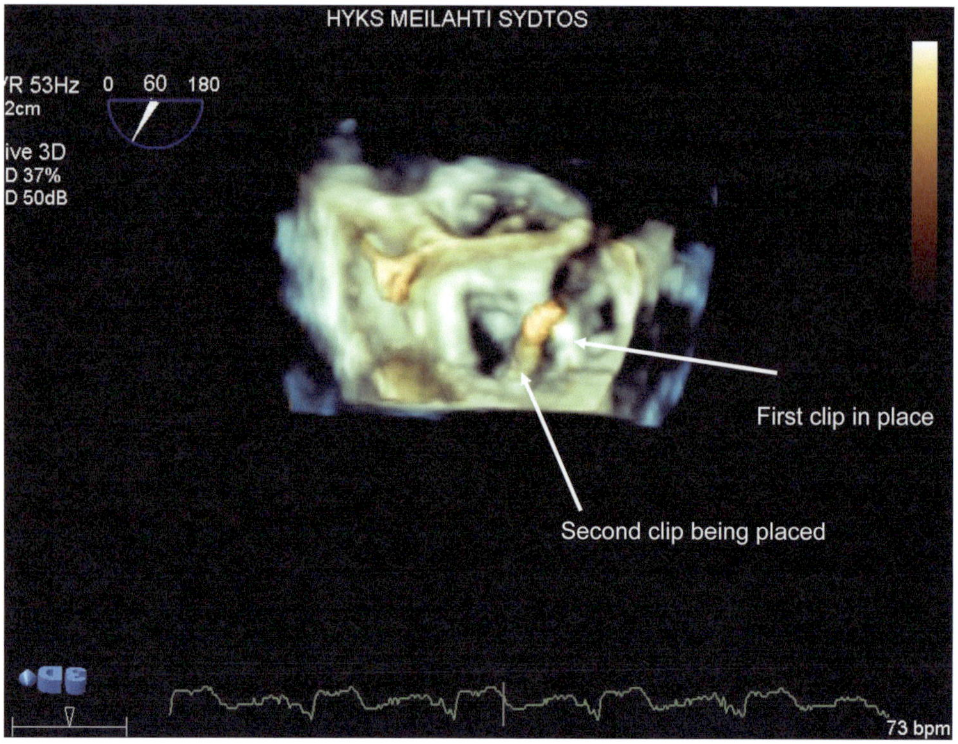

Fig. 31.9 Second clip being placed laterally (to the *left side* on the image) to the first clip

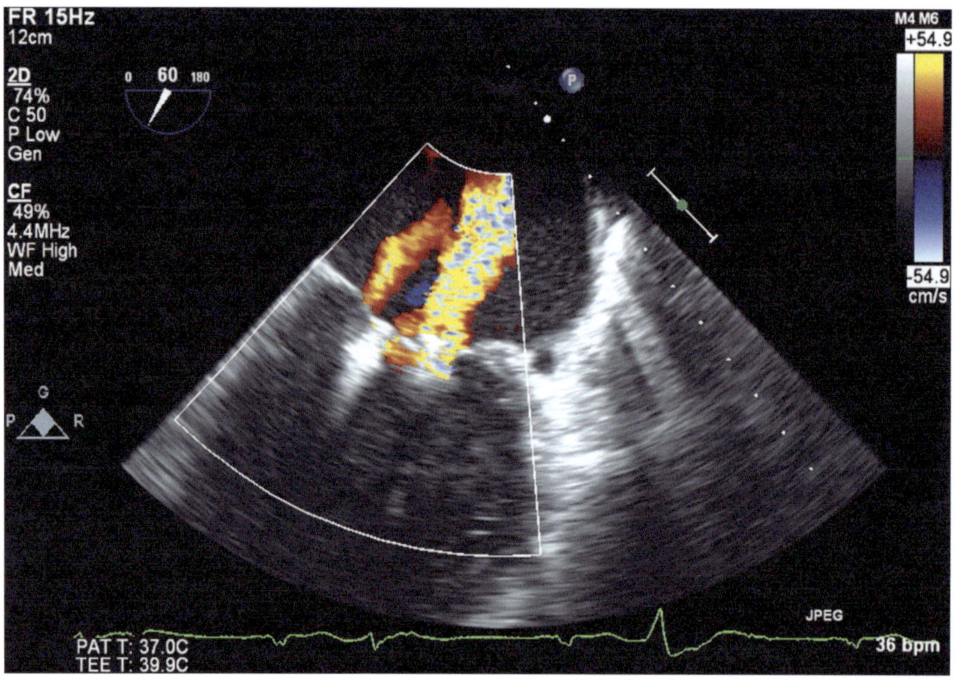

Fig. 31.10 After two clips, there is still moderate (grade 2) MR left

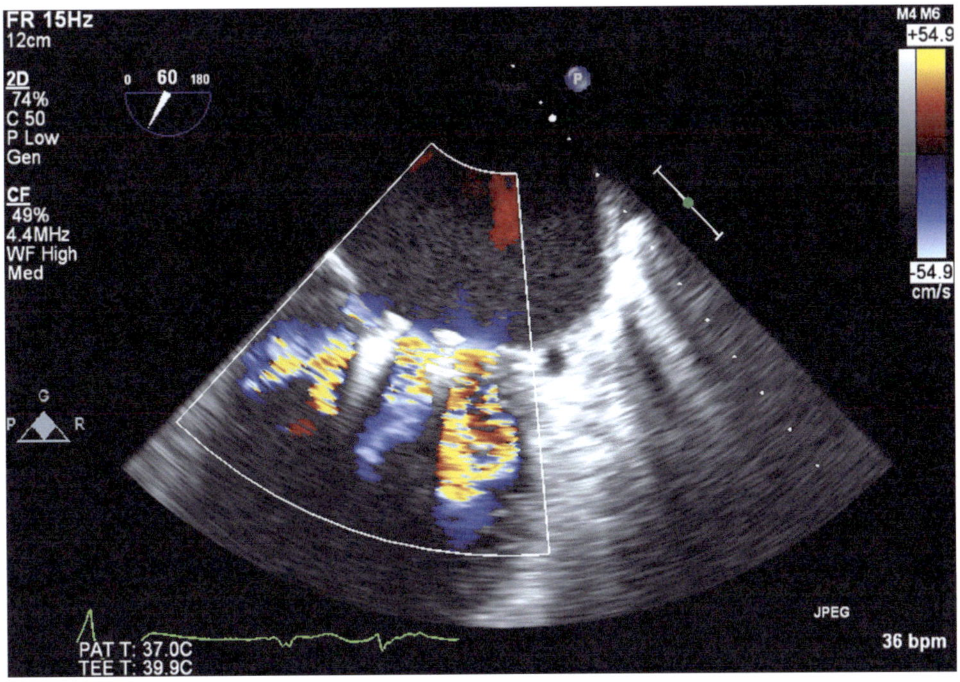

Fig. 31.11 Mitral inflow in the double orifice. There is slight inflow between the clips, almost like a triple orifice

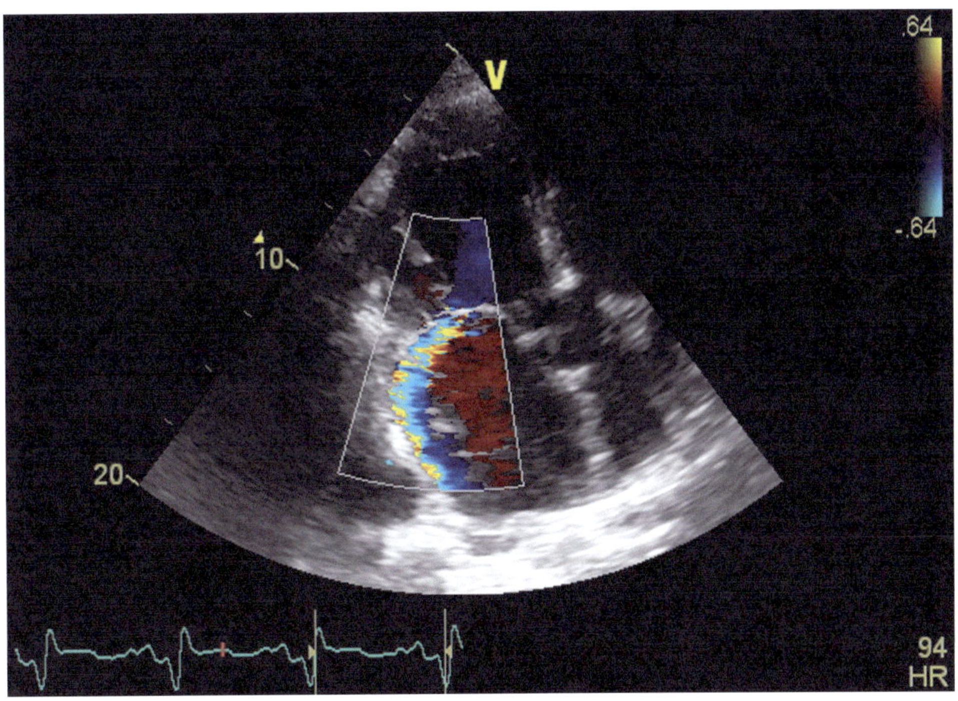

Fig. 31.12 At 6-month follow-up, there is still moderate eccentric MR present

Severe Left-to-Right Shunting from Iatrogenic Atrial Septal Defect

32

Mark Hünlich, Miriam Puls, and Wolfgang Schillinger

Abstract

Pulmonary hypertension may persist after MitraClip repair of mitral regurgitation. The iatrogenic atrial septal defect (ASD) created by the MitraClip guide may result in significant left-to-right shunting and aggravate the pulmonary hypertension. In this case example, a patient with persistent pulmonary hypertension and severe left-to-right shunting from the iatrogenic ASD was treated with an atrial septal occluder at the end of the MitraClip procedure.

Keywords

Mitral regurgitation • MitraClip • Atrial septal defect • Atrial septal occluder • Pulmonary hypertension

Background

Right heart failure and pulmonary hypertension are common sequelae of chronic severe mitral valve insufficiency. Unfortunately, the regression of pulmonary hypertension after mitral valve surgery or repair, respectively, is often delayed and incomplete. In addition, the transseptal access for the MitraClip system may result in a persistent atrial septal defect (ASD) which may lead to additional volume overload of the right heart. We report a case of an atrial septal defect closure after MitraClip implantation with a significant regression of pulmonary hypertension.

M. Hünlich, M.D. (✉) • M. Puls, M.D.
Abteilung für Kardiologie und Pneumologie,
Herzzentrum, Universitätsmedzin, Georg-August-Universität
Göttingen, Robert-Koch-Straβe 40, Göttingen 37099, Germany
e-mail: huenlich@med.uni-goettingen.de;
dr.m.puls@med.uni-goettingen.de

W. Schillinger, M.D.
Abteilung für Kardiologie und Pneumologie, Herzzentrum,
Universitätsmedzin, Georg-August-Universität Göttingen,
Robert-Koch-Straβe 40, Göttingen 37099, Germany

Department of Cardiology and Pneumology,
University Medical Center Göttingen, Heart Center Göttingen,
Robert-Koch-Strasse 40, Göttingen 37075, Germany
e-mail: schiwolf@med.uni-goettingen.de

Clinical History

An 84-year-old Caucasian man underwent MitraClip mitral valve repair because of severe functional mitral regurgitation with left heart failure, New York Heart Association (NYHA) class III. Pre-intervention transthoracic echocardiography showed a moderate depressed LV function, severe left atrium and ventricle dilatation, and severe pulmonary hypertension (systolic pulmonary pressure 55 mmHg, diastolic 39 mmHg, mean 45 mmHg) in addition to severe tricuspid valve insufficiency.

Pulmonary pressures were monitored continuously during the procedure by a Swan-Ganz catheter. MitraClip implantation was performed, and mitral insufficiency was reduced from severe to trace. Simultaneously, mean pulmonary pressure decreased by 4 mmHg. A severe left-to-right shunt was seen beside the guide by transesophageal echocardiogram (Fig. 32.1). Therefore, the iatrogenic atrial septal defect was closed with an Amplatzer 14-mm septal occluder. An Amplatz extra-stiff guide wire was advanced in the upper left pulmonary vein, and the

T. Feldman et al. (eds.), *Atlas of Percutaneous Edge-to-Edge Mitral Valve Repair*,
DOI 10.1007/978-1-4471-4294-2_32, © Springer-Verlag London 2013

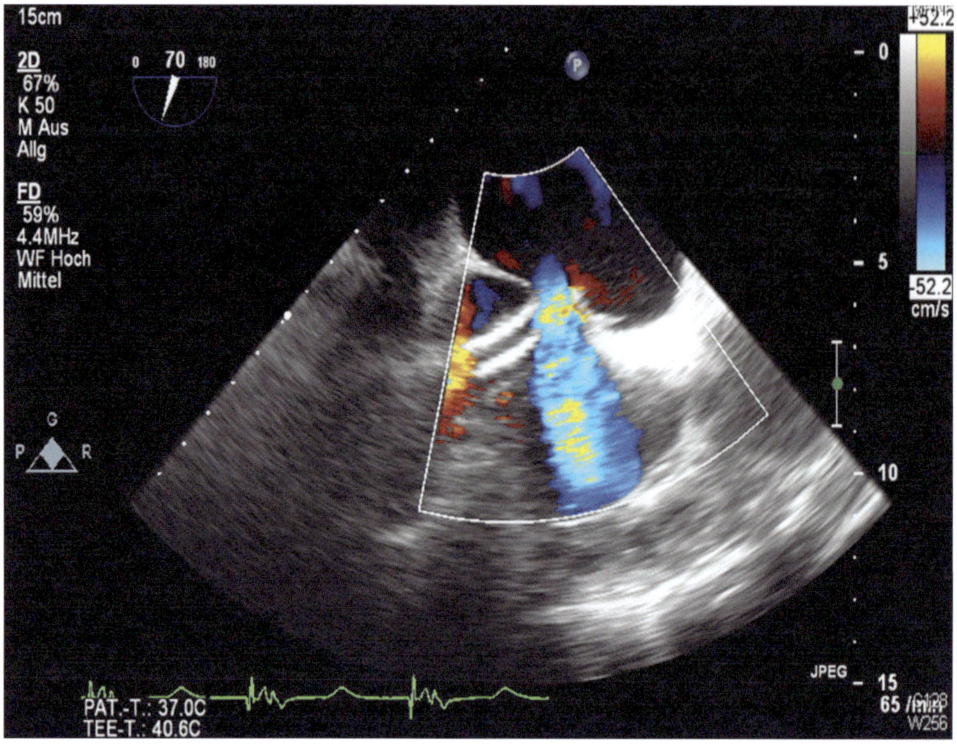

Fig. 32.1 Severe left-to-right shunt beside the guide

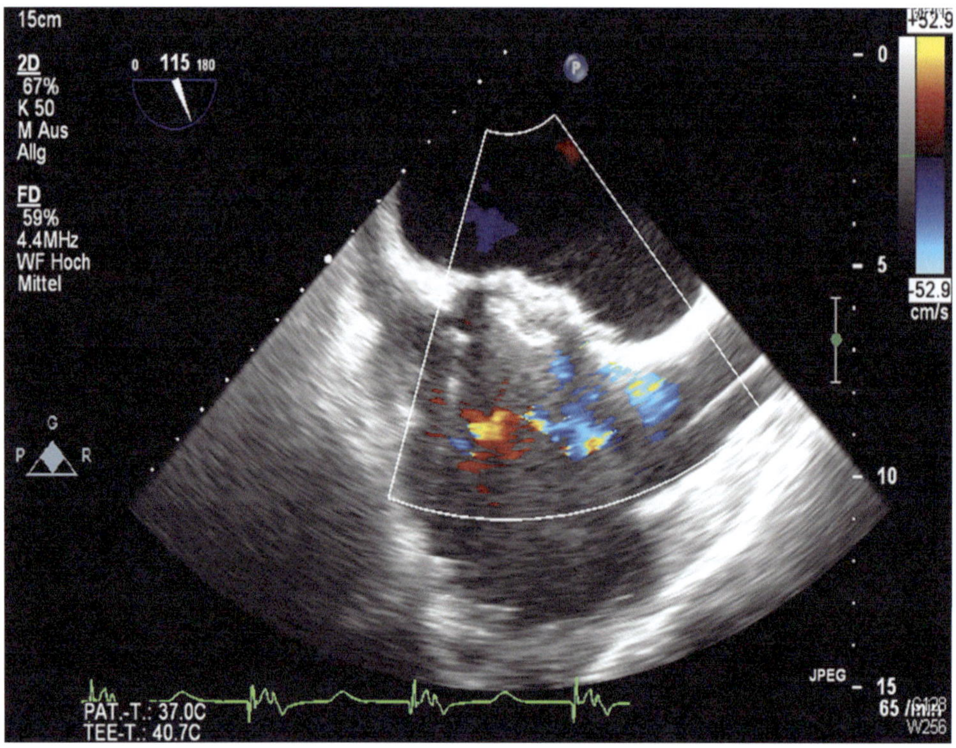

Fig. 32.2 Amplatzer ASD occluder in place with no residual shunt

MitraClip guide was switched to the 9-F TorqVue 45° delivery sheath. Then the Amplatzer septal occluder was placed with no residual shunt (Fig. 32.2). An immediate additional decline of the mean pulmonary pressure by 3 mmHg was noted. The patient improved clinically and was discharged in NYHA class I–II 2 days later. Echo-measured mean pulmonary pressure was approximately 35 mmHg predischarge.

Discussion

Transcatheter mitral valve repair and transcatheter closure of ASD can be successfully performed in selected patients. In a recent publication from the EVEREST investigators, pulmonary artery pressure and pulmonary capillary wedge pressure were unchanged after successful mitral valve repair with MitraClip [1]. The same was found in more than 50 % of the patients after surgical valve repair. In two surgical cohorts, patients had persistent pulmonary hypertension 1–2 years after surgery associated with a poor prognosis [2, 3]. Gaemperli et al. [4] documented the most significant changes in pulmonary pressure immediately after mitral repair with MitraClip. In parallel with these results, we observed a relevant reduction in mean pulmonary pressure but still persistent pulmonary hypertension after MitraClip.

Right ventricular overload is decreased after ASD closure with improvements of right heart cavity dimensions and reduced pulmonary pressure as seen in patients with moderate to severe pulmonary hypertension [5]. But many patients do not have complete normalization of pulmonary pressure and right heart dimensions similar to subjects with mitral valve repair. These findings might be caused by myocardial and pulmonary remodeling due to long-term volume overload [6].

Thus, the severe left-to-right shunt due to transseptal puncture observed in our patient was closed by Amplatzer 14-mm ASD occluder in an attempt to reduce right ventricular volume overload.

In conclusion, patients with symptomatic congestive heart failure and persistent pulmonary hypertension may persist despite MitraClip repair of severe mitral regurgitation. Although most patients have only a small residual iatrogenic ASD after the MitraClip procedure that closes over time, there may be selected patients that benefit from closure of a larger iatrogenic atrial septal defect. It is important to note that closure of the ASD with a septal occluder may preclude additional treatment with another MitraClip procedure. However, the timing and effects of concurrent closure of the iatrogenic ASD after MitraClip implantation as a therapeutic strategy require further study.

References

1. Siegel RJ, Biner S, Rafique AM, Rinaldi M, Lim S, Fail P, Hermiller J, Smalling R, Whitlow PL, Herrmann HC, Foster E, Feldman T, Glower D, Kar S, EVEREST Investigators. The acute hemodynamic effects of MitraClip therapy. J Am Coll Cardiol. 2011;57(16):1658–65.
2. Goldstone AB, Chikwe J, Pinney SP, Anyanwu AC, Funt SA, Polanco A, Adams DH. Incidence, epidemiology, and prognosis of residual pulmonary hypertension after mitral valve repair for degenerative mitral regurgitation. Am J Cardiol. 2011;107(5): 755–60.
3. Walls MC, Cimino N, Bolling SF, Bach DS. Persistent pulmonary hypertension after mitral valve surgery: does surgical procedure affect outcome? J Heart Valve Dis. 2008;17:1–9.
4. Gaemperli O, Moccetti M, Surder D, Biaggi P, Hurlimann D, Kretschmar O, Buehler I, Bettex D, Felix C, Luscher TF, Falk V, Grunenfelder J, Corti R. Acute haemodynamic changes after percutaneous mitral valve repair: relation to mid-term outcomes. Heart. 2012;98(2):126–32.
5. Balint OH, Samman A, Haberer K, Tobe L, McLaughlin P, Siu SC, Horlick E, Granton J, Silversides CK. Outcomes in patients with pulmonary hypertension undergoing percutaneous atrial septal defect closure. Heart. 2008;94(9):1189–93.
6. Patel A, Lopez K, Banerjee A, Joseph A, Cao QL, Hijazi ZM. Transcatheter closure of atrial septal defects in adults > or =40 years of age: immediate and follow-up results. J Interv Cardiol. 2007; 20(1):82–8.

33

MitraClip Implantation in Chronic Degenerative Mitral Regurgitation with Extensive Calcification

Miriam Puls, Mark Hünlich, and Wolfgang Schillinger

Abstract

Calcification of the mitral valve and the mitral subvalvular apparatus can potentially complicate the MitraClip procedure by affecting leaflet grasp and increasing the risk of chordal or papillary muscle rupture. This case example shows a successful MitraClip procedure in a patient with extensive calcification of the mitral apparatus.

Keywords

Mitral regurgitation • MitraClip • Papillary muscle • Chordae tendineae • Calcification

Clinical History

We report on an 86-year-old man who was repeatedly admitted to a local hospital because of congestive heart failure, stage NYHA IV, due to severe mitral regurgitation (MR). In 2006, he underwent coronary artery bypass grafting. Furthermore, he suffered from pulmonary hypertension, chronic renal failure, and peripheral vascular disease (EuroSCORE II: 12.72 %; log. EuroSCORE I: 35.17 %). Conventional surgery was denied because of very advanced age, previous bypass surgery with patent grafts, and comorbidities. Finally, the patient was referred to our center for evaluating the suitability for percutaneous mitral valve repair with MitraClip.

Pre-procedural transesophageal echocardiography revealed extensive calcification of the posterior mitral annulus, the posterior leaflet, and the chordae tendineae (possibly with chordal fusions) (Fig. 33.1a, b). The calcification of the chordae led to an asymmetric restriction of the leaflet motion (Fig. 33.2a, b) in both systole and diastole. In addition, there was a small P2 prolapse in this patient resulting in severe eccentric mitral regurgitation along the anteroseptal wall of the left atrium (Carpentier II and IIIa [1]) (Fig. 33.3a–d). The heavy calcifications of the leaflets and the subvalvular apparatus were felt to make MitraClip implantation more risky, including the possibility of chordal or papillary rupture. However, the patient was accepted for the procedure due to severe symptoms with recurrent cardiac decompensation and the lack of other treatment options.

Figures 33.4, 33.5, and 33.6 demonstrate the MitraClip implantation procedure. A first clip was placed directly into the PISA zone of the MR jet (Fig. 33.4a, b) creating a double orifice (Fig. 33.4c) with significant reduction of regurgitation grade (Fig. 33.4d). However, because of significant residual MR, a second clip was placed lateral to the first one

M. Puls, M.D. (✉) • M. Hünlich, M.D.
Abteilung für Kardiologie und Pneumologie, Herzzentrum, Universitätsmedzin, Georg-August-Universität Göttingen, Robert-Koch-Straβe 40, Göttingen 37099, Germany
e-mail: dr.m.puls@med.uni-goettingen.de; huenlich@med.uni-goettingen.de

W. Schillinger, M.D.
Abteilung für Kardiologie und Pneumologie, Herzzentrum, Universitätsmedzin, Georg-August-Universität Göttingen, Robert-Koch-Straβe 40, Göttingen 37099, Germany

Department of Cardiology and Pneumology, University Medical Center Göttingen, Heart Center Göttingen, Robert-Koch-Strasse 40, Göttingen 37075, Germany
e-mail: schiwolf@med.uni-goettingen.de

T. Feldman et al. (eds.), *Atlas of Percutaneous Edge-to-Edge Mitral Valve Repair*,
DOI 10.1007/978-1-4471-4294-2_33, © Springer-Verlag London 2013

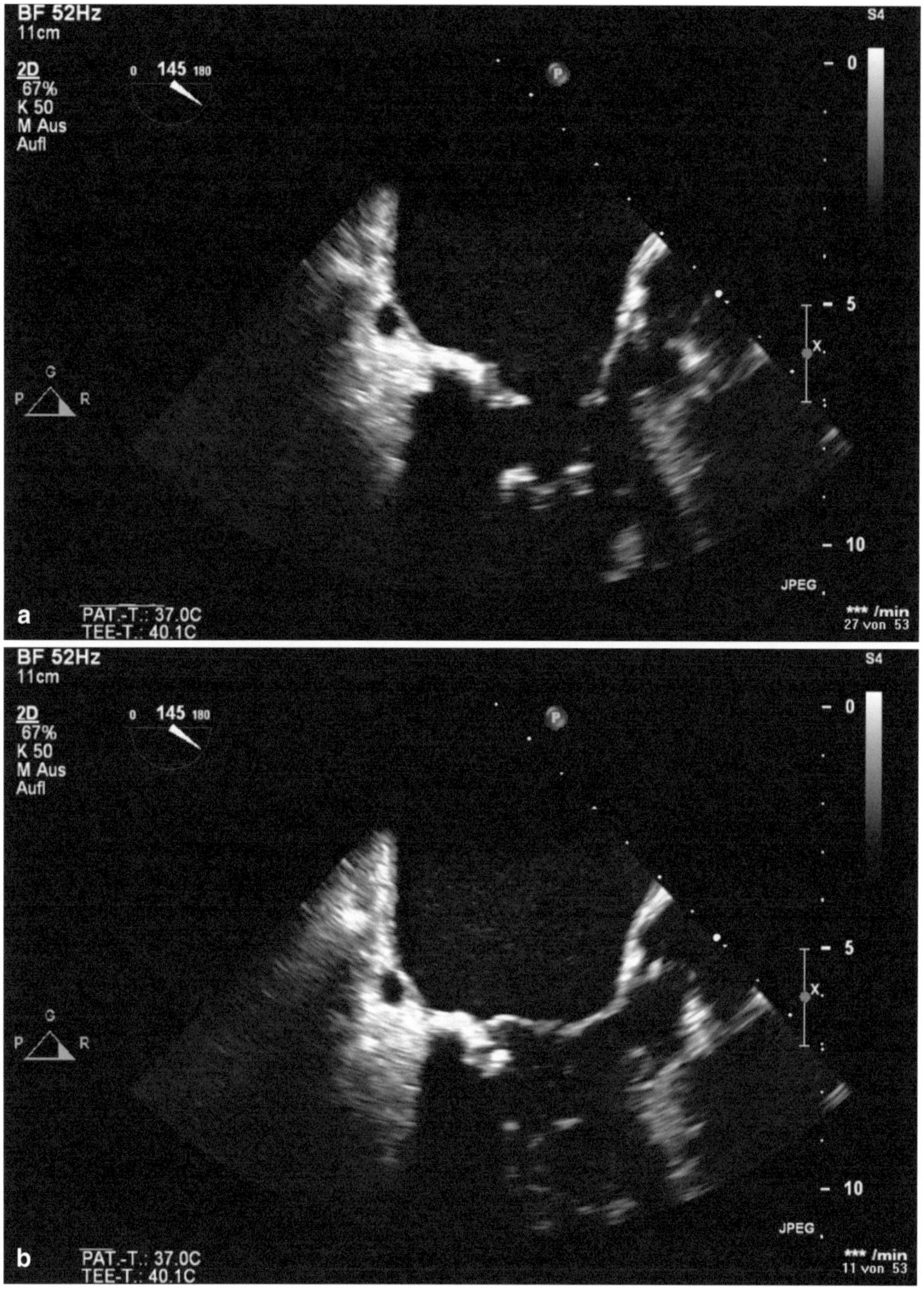

Fig. 33.1 Transesophageal three-chamber views in diastole (**a**) and systole (**b**) demonstrating extensive calcification of the posterior mitral annulus, the posterior leaflet, the chordae tendineae (possibly with chordal fusions), and the heads of the papillary muscles

(Fig. 33.5a). The mean gradient after implantation of the second clip was acceptable (5 mmHg), with reduction of regurgitation grade to mild MR (Fig. 33.6a, b). The patient was discharged 4 days after the procedure, with no periprocedural complications.

At 1-year follow-up, the patient reported a good quality of life and denied any symptoms of congestive heart failure. The 6-min walk test had increased from 240 m pre-procedural to 300 m at follow-up. TTE demonstrated only mild mitral regurgitation (Fig. 33.7).

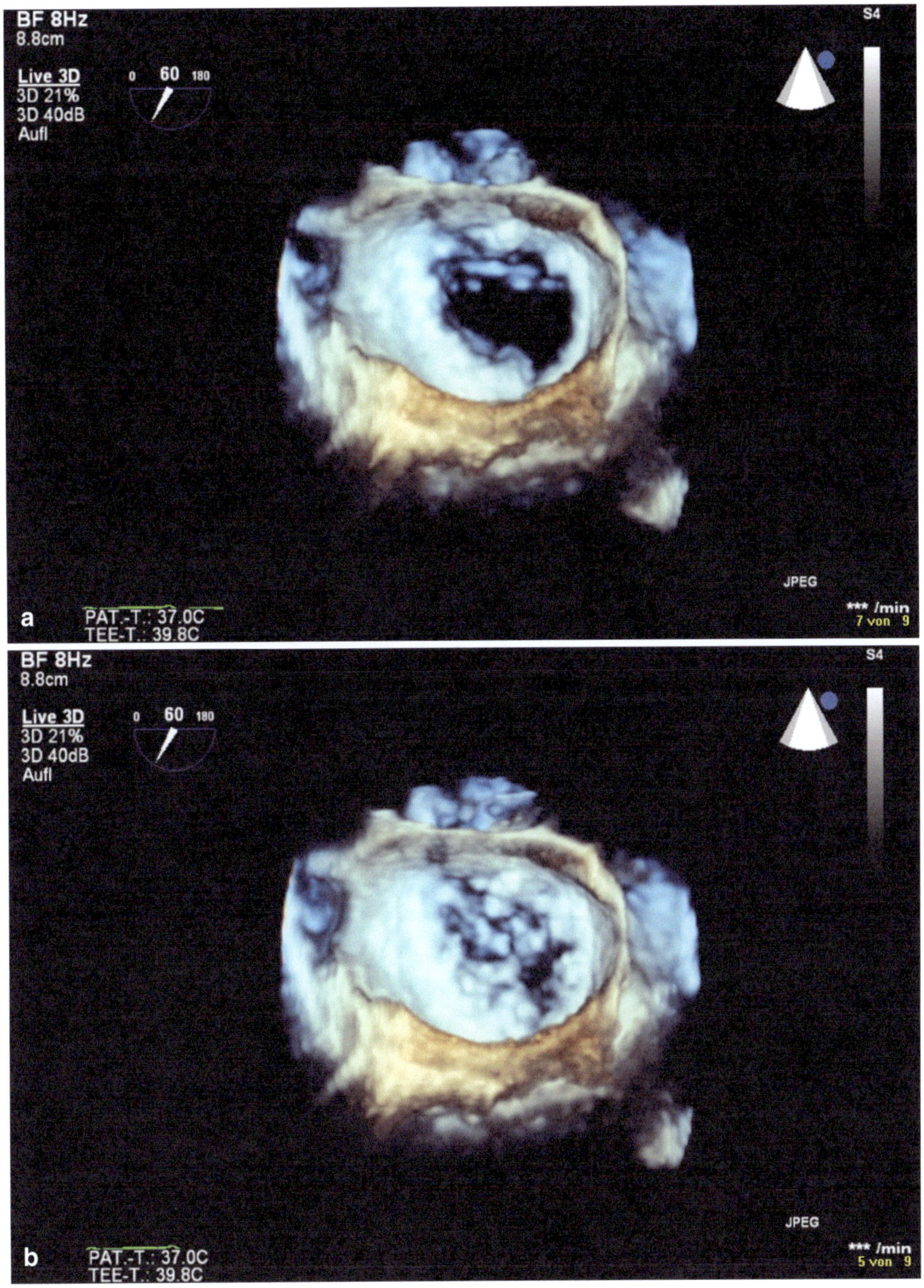

Fig. 33.2 3D images of the mitral valve in diastole (**a**) and systole (**b**). Focal leaflet calcification is visible. The chordal calcifications provoke an asymmetric restriction of leaflet motion leading to poor leaflet coaptation in systole and a small P2 prolapse (**b**)

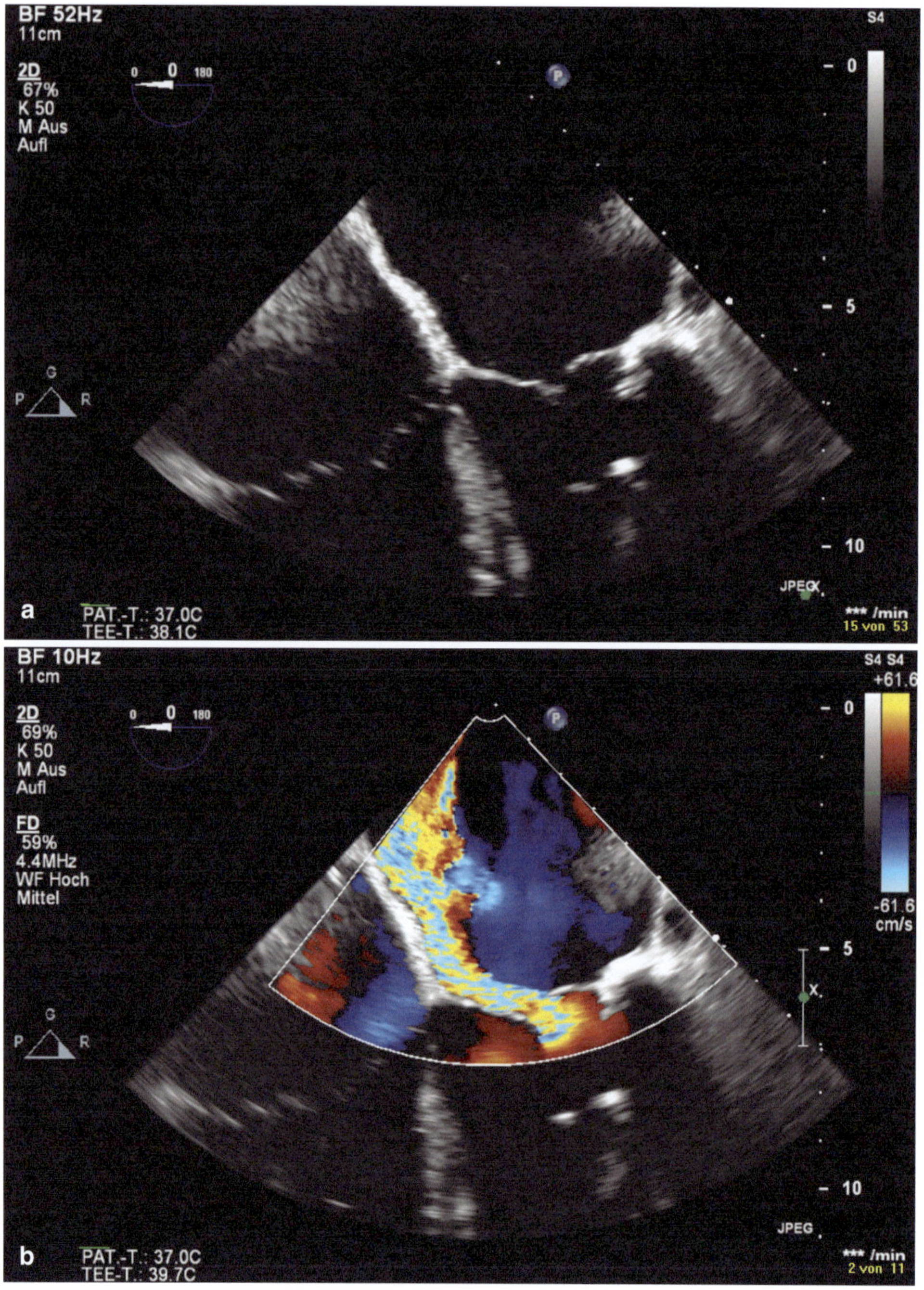

Fig. 33.3 Transesophageal four-chamber views (**a**, **b**) and three-chamber views (**c**, **d**) with (**b**, **d**) and without (**a**, **c**) color Doppler show severe eccentric mitral regurgitation along the anteroseptal wall of the left atrium

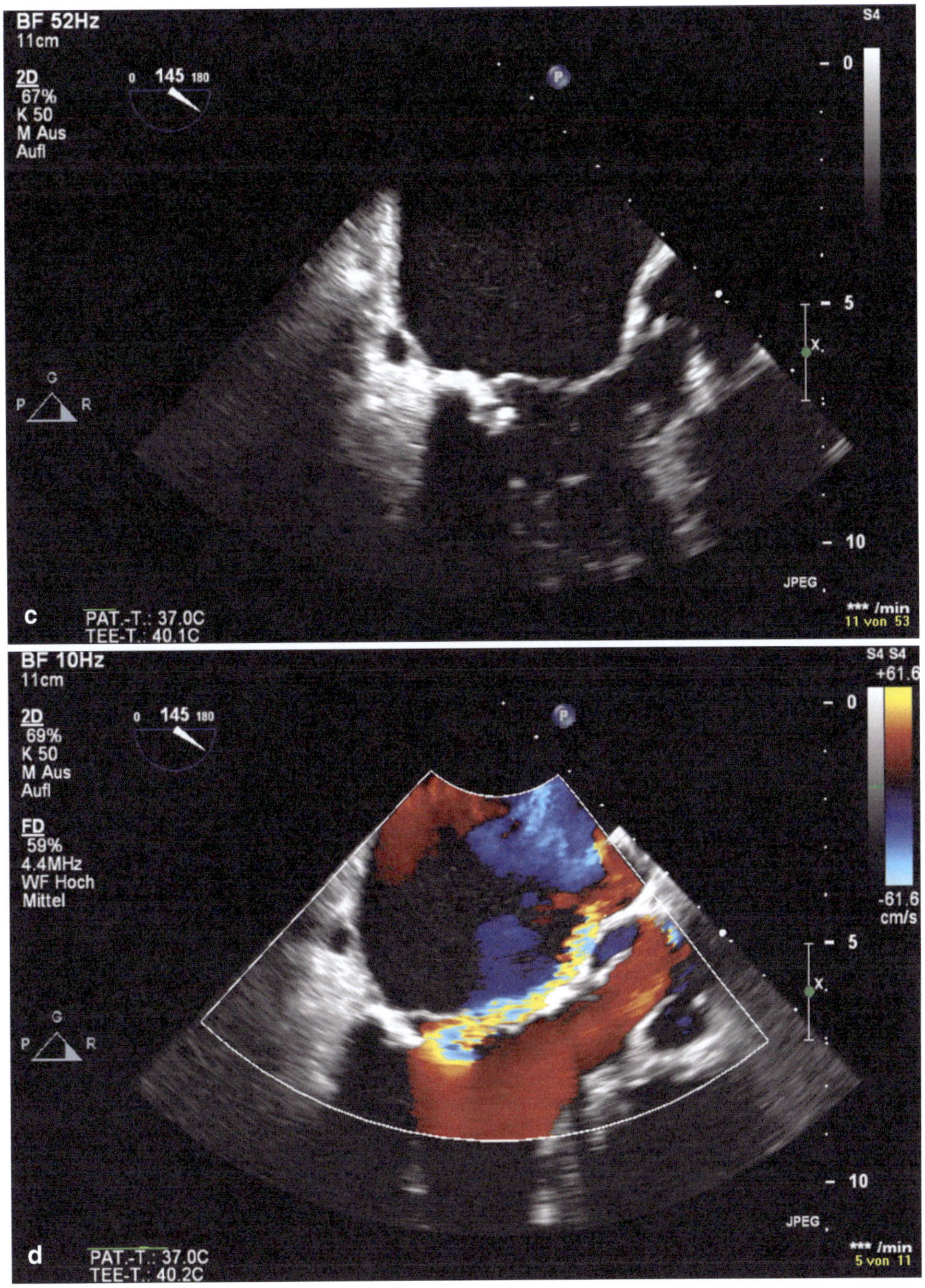

Fig. 33.3 (continued)

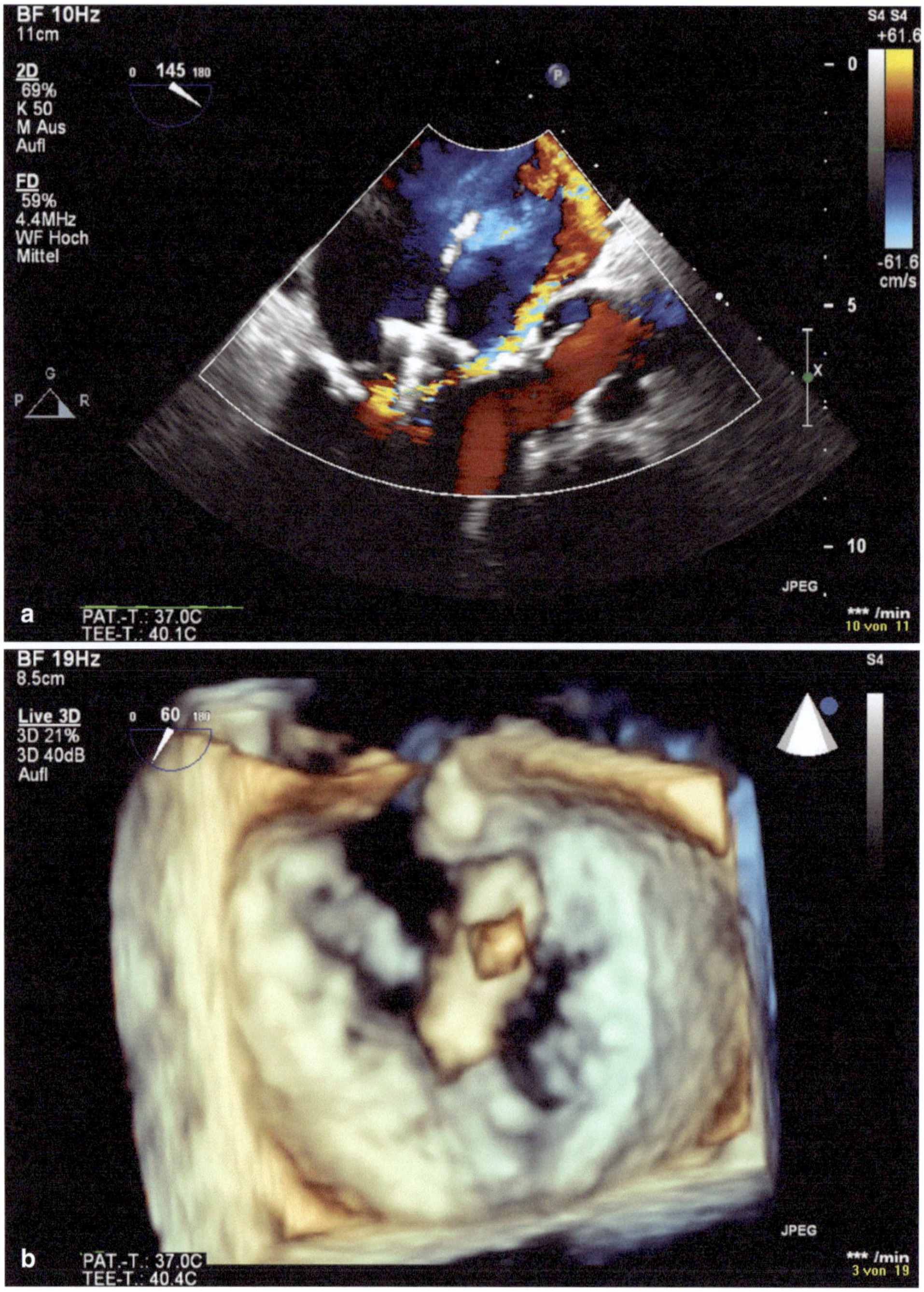

Fig. 33.4 Placement of a first MitraClip directly into the PISA zone of the MR jet (**a**, **b**) creating a double orifice (**c**) with visible MR reduction (**d**)

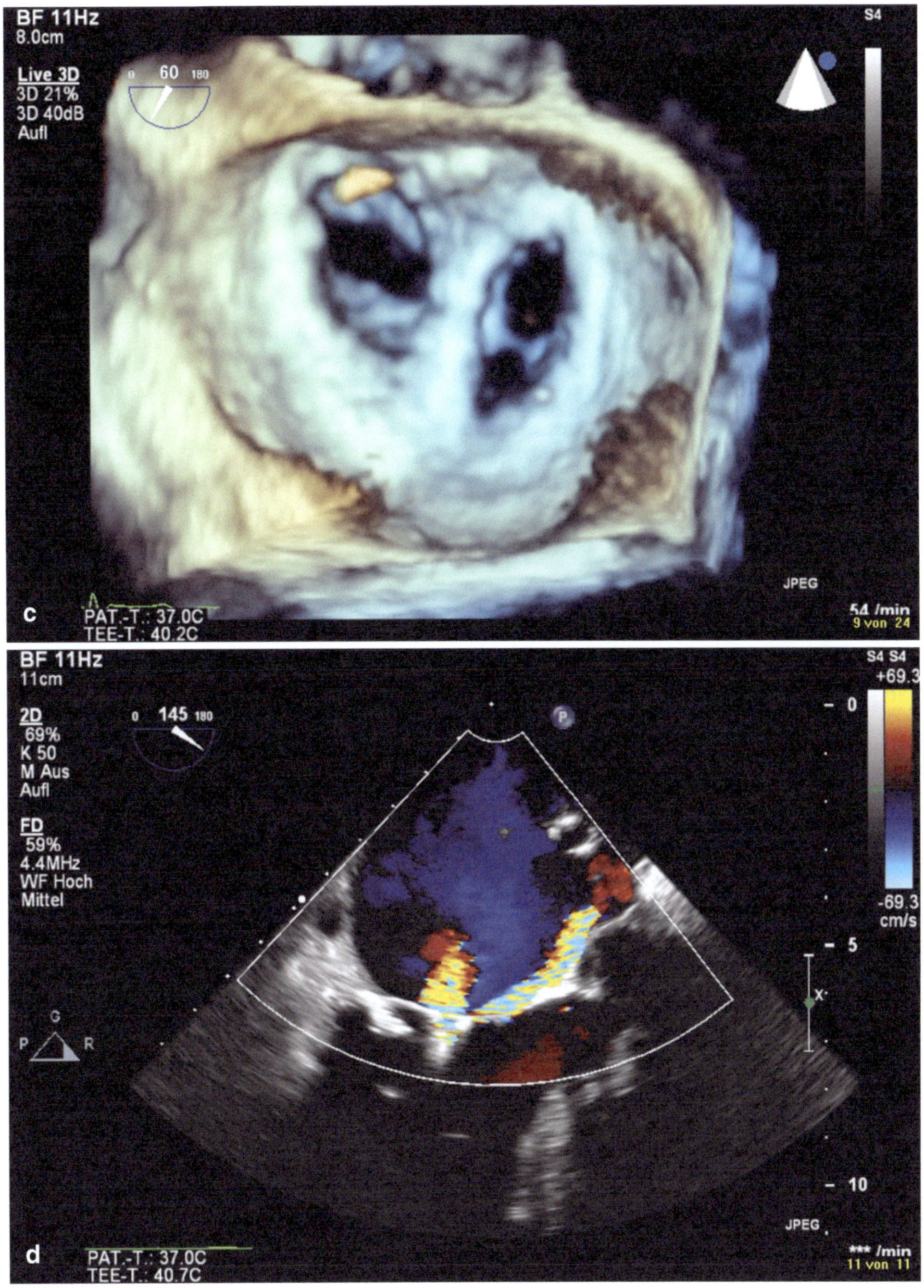

Fig. 33.4 (continued)

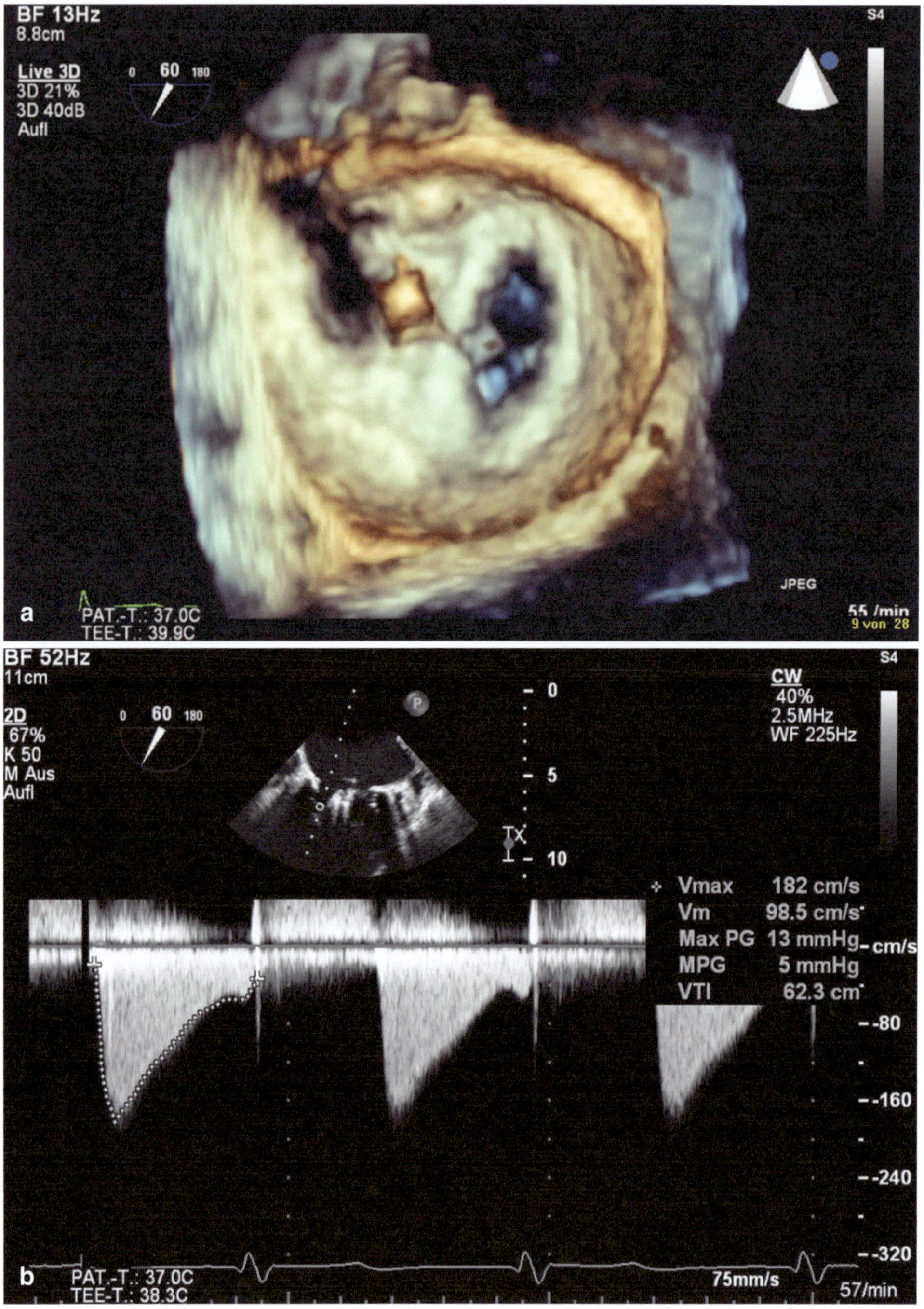

Fig. 33.5 Placement of a second clip lateral from the first one (**a**) with a post-procedural mean gradient of 5 mmHg (**b**)

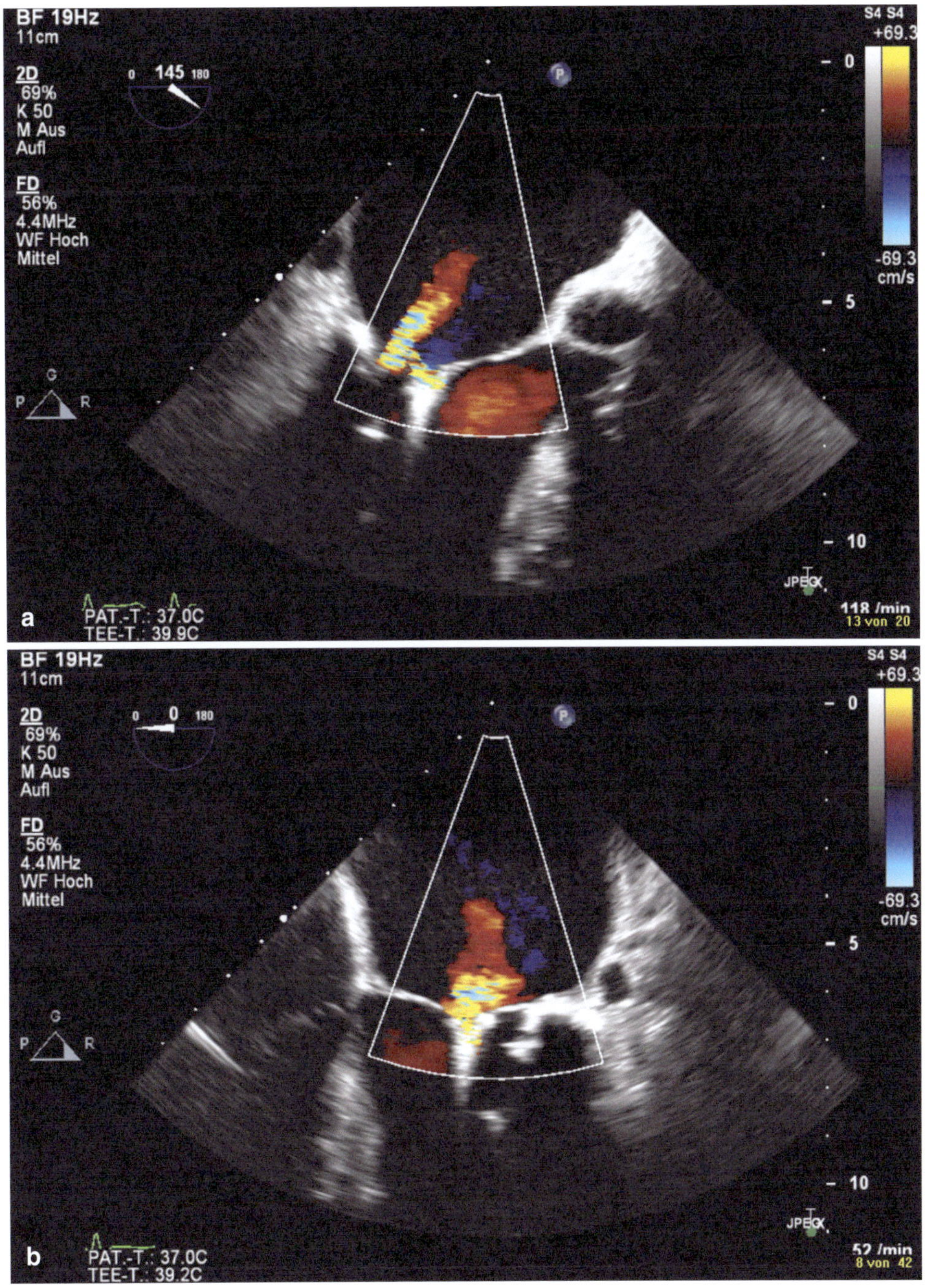

Fig. 33.6 Color Doppler images demonstrate only mild residual MR (**a**: three-chamber view; **b**: four-chamber view)

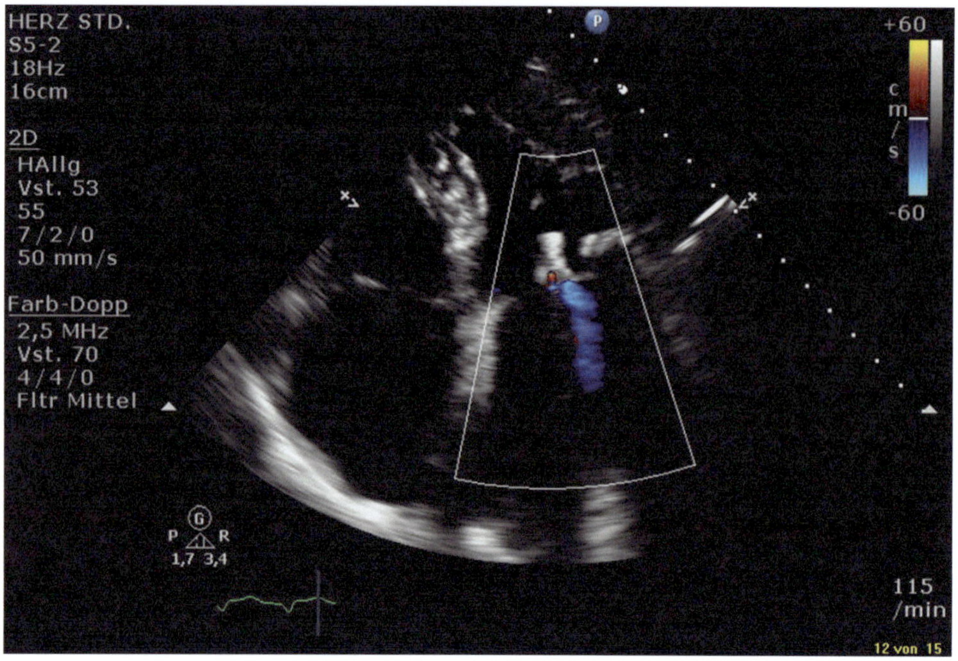

Fig. 33.7 TTE (four-chamber view) at 12-months follow-up confirms the presence of only mild MR

34 3D Transesophageal Echo-Guided MitraClip Treatment of P3 Mitral Valve Prolapse

Martin J. Swaans and Jan A.S. Van der Heyden

Abstract

This case highlights the use of 3D transesophageal echo imaging to guide the placement of a MitraClip for treatment of P3 prolapse. In such cases, the usual 2D views may not adequately allow for assessment of clip perpendicularity. Real-time 3D imaging allows for assessment of perpendicularity and should be used in cases with either very medial (A3/P3) or lateral (A1/P1) prolapse.

Keywords

Mitral regurgitation • MitraClip • Three-dimensional • Mitral valve prolapse

Clinical History

A 70-year-old male with asymptomatic severe mitral valve regurgitation (MR) was referred to discuss his therapeutic options. The patient had severe MR due to mitral valve prolapse involving the P3 scallop (Fig. 34.1). In this particular case, the patient himself was a thoracic surgeon, who was well aware of the different techniques available, both surgical and percutaneous. In our institution, only patients who are refused for surgery are referred for percutaneous mitral valve repair. Although surgery would be the first choice for this patient since he had no significant comorbidities and a normal left ventricular ejection fraction, we deviated from our institutional protocol. First, the patient himself did not want to undergo any procedure requiring extracorporeal circulation, arguing that he was in a position to assess the periprocedural risks. Second, we believed that a percutaneous approach could be successful if we would be able to acquire the proper 3D transesophageal echo views (TEE) of the prolapse in the P3 segment [1]. The latter is crucial when deciding to treat a prolapse in the P3 area using the MitraClip. This is because assessing perpendicularity of the clip in the P3 area (or P1 area) is often difficult to assess with 2D TEE alone. In cases where the clip should be placed in a lateral (A1–P1) or medial (A3–P3) position, 3D TEE can be extremely helpful. In these cases, the clip is not visible in the left ventricular outflow tract (LVOT) or intercommissural view (the clip is not in these planes) in which normally perpendicularity is assessed [2]. As can be appreciated in the figures (Figs. 34.1, 34.2, 34.3, and 34.4), the acquired images were very useful and allowed for procedural guidance of the clip (Fig. 34.3). We achieved a complete reduction of the MR using one MitraClip, which was sustained at the 1-year follow-up (Fig. 34.4).

Learning Points

In cases of very medial (A3/P3) or lateral (A1/P1) mitral valve prolapse, 3D TEE imaging is a very helpful tool, especially in evaluating for perpendicularity.

M.J. Swaans, M.D. (✉) • J.A.S. Van der Heyden, M.D.
Department of Cardiology, St. Antonius Hospital,
Koekoekslaan 1, Nieuwegein 3434CM, The Netherlands
e-mail: m.swaans@antoniusziekenhuis.nl;
jvdheijden@antoniusziekenhuis.nl

T. Feldman et al. (eds.), *Atlas of Percutaneous Edge-to-Edge Mitral Valve Repair*,
DOI 10.1007/978-1-4471-4294-2_34,

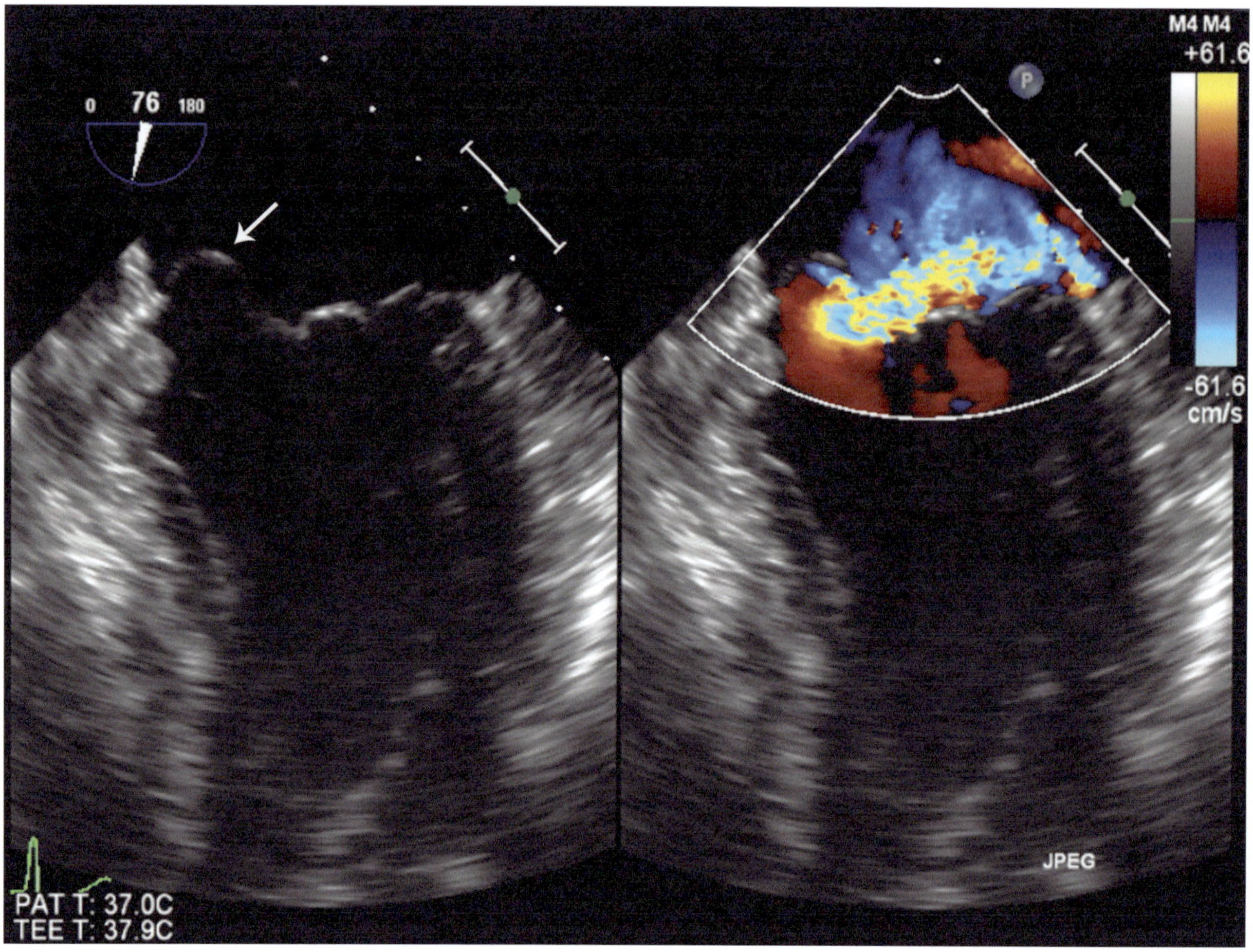

Fig. 34.1 Two-dimensional transesophageal echocardiography intercommissural view with and without color showing prolapse of the P3 segment (*arrow*) with a severe eccentric (toward the lateral wall) mitral valve regurgitation

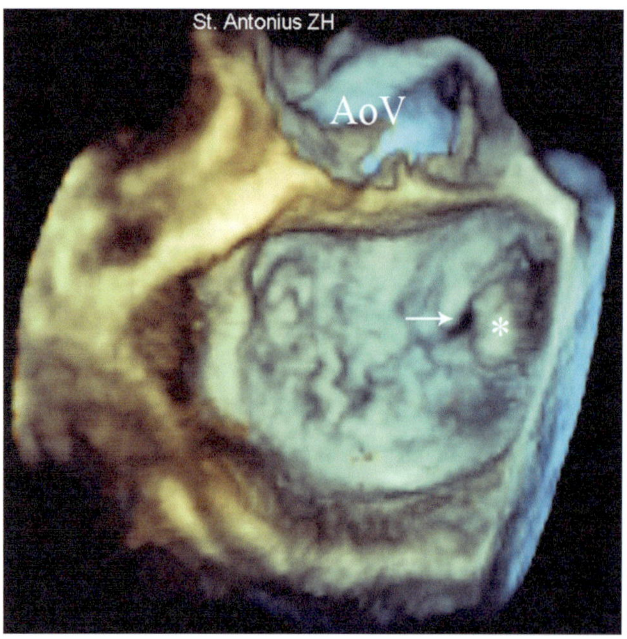

Fig. 34.2 Three-dimensional transesophageal echocardiography, left atrial view, showing prolapse of the P3 segment (*asterisk*) and the regurgitant orifice (*arrow*) of the mitral valve; *AoV* aortic valve

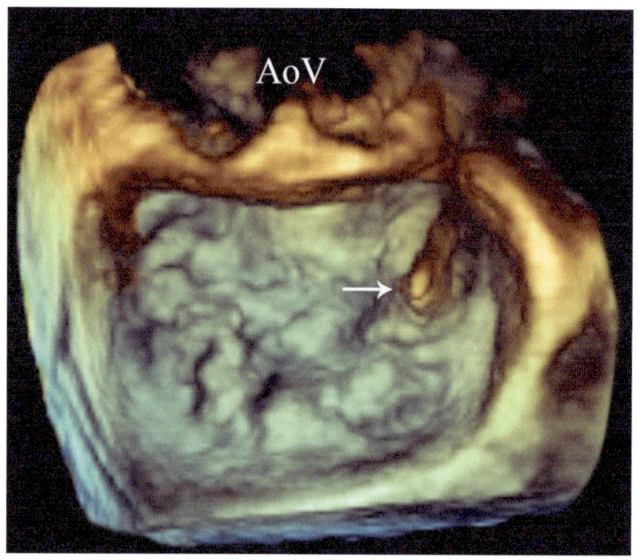

Fig. 34.3 Three-dimensional transesophageal echocardiography, left atrial view, during the procedure with the clip (*arrow*) still attached to the clip delivery system after grasping the P3-segment prolapse; *AoV* aortic valve

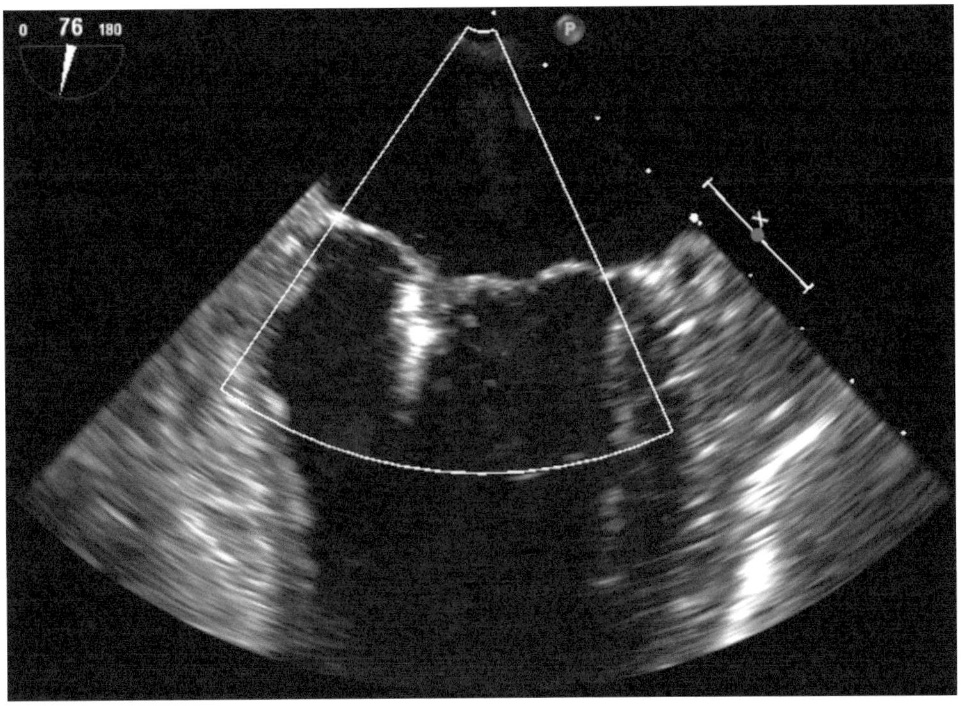

Fig. 34.4 Two-dimensional transesophageal echocardiography intercommissural view with color after the procedure. The prolapsing P3 segment is grasped with complete disappearance of the mitral regurgitation

References

1. Swaans MJ, Van den Branden BJ, Van der Heyden JA, et al. Three-dimensional transoesophageal echocardiography in a patient undergoing percutaneous mitral valve repair using the edge-to-edge clip technique. Eur J Echocardiogr. 2009;10(8):982–3.
2. Swaans MJ, Van den Branden BJ, Post MC, Van der Heyden JA. The percutaneous mitral valve repair procedure – the role of echocardiographic guidance. Eur Cardiol. 2011;7(3):175–8.

35 Failure and Complications of MitraClip® Implantation for Severe Functional Mitral Regurgitation: A Combination of Unexpected Findings and Early Experience

Nicolas Dumonteil, Mathieu Gautier, Nicolas Boudou, Bertrand Marcheix, and Didier Carrié

Abstract

This case illustrates the importance of a well-placed transseptal puncture and appreciation of the mitral subvalvular apparatus. In this case, the procedure was complicated by rupture of a chord resulting in worsened mitral regurgitation. This may have been prevented by an appreciation of the unusual chordal and papillary structures seen on the initial transthoracic echocardiogram.

Keywords

Mitral regurgitation • MitraClip • Functional mitral regurgitation • Cardiomyopathy • Complication • Chordae tendineae • Papillary muscle

Clinical History

A 67-year-old man with a history of ischemic dilated cardiomyopathy was referred to our institution because of end-stage systolic heart failure with refractory symptoms (NYHA class IV) despite optimal medical treatment and cardiac resynchronization therapy. Transthoracic echocardiography (TTE) revealed severe left ventricular (LV) dilatation (LV end-diastolic diameter 88 mm, LV end-diastolic volume 350 ml), severely impaired LV ejection fraction (LVEF 20 %), and severe functional mitral regurgitation (FMR) (ERO 40 mm^2, RVol 45 ml/b) (Fig. 35.1). Due to age the patient was considered to be a non-optimal candidate for heart transplantation, and he rejected the proposal of LV assist device implantation. The risk of surgical mitral valve (MV) annuloplasty was considered prohibitive, and the patient was suggested for MitraClip therapy. The mitral valve was deemed to be suitable for MitraClip therapy.

The procedure was performed under general anesthesia, in the catheterization laboratory, under fluoroscopic and transesophageal echocardiography (TEE) guidance with real-time three-dimensional capability. We were at the beginning of our learning curve with MitraClip® procedures, and this patient was the second in our experience.

Steering was difficult due to an anterior transseptal puncture (Fig. 35.2). Nevertheless, coaxiality to the cardiac long axis and perpendicularity of the clip arms in relation to the line of mitral leaflet coaptation was finally achieved with the usage of the + knob of the steerable guide, and a first grasp was attempted. The grasp was in the medial part of P2 and

N. Dumonteil, M.D. (✉) • N. Boudou, M.D. • D. Carrié, M.D., Ph.D. • M. Gautier, M.D.
Pôle CardioVasculaire et Métabolique, Rangueil University Hospital, Toulouse, France
e-mail: dumonteil.n@chu-toulouse.fr; boudou.n@chu-toulouse.fr; carrie.didier@chu-toulouse.fr; e-mail: gautier.m@chu-toulouse.fr

B. Marcheix, M.D., Ph.D.
Pôle CardioVasculaire et Métabolique, Rangueil University Hospital, Toulouse France

Department of Cardiovascular Surgery, CHU Rangueil, 1 avenue du Pr Jean Poulhès, Toulouse 31059, France
e-mail: marcheix.b@chu-toulouse.fr

Electronic supplementary material The online version of this chapter (doi:10.1007/978-1-4471-4294-2_35) contains supplementary material, which is available to authorized users.

resulted in insufficient MR reduction after complete closure of the clip (Fig. 35.3). Multiple unsuccessful grasps in this region were performed. Finally we tried to capture the mitral leaflets in a more central A2/P2 position. After almost 6 h, no simultaneous grasp of anterior and posterior mitral leaflets in the central area of P2 could be achieved. In TEE, an oval, echolucent structure (3 × 1.5 cm) was found in the left atrium, visible in different echocardiographical views. The structure was judged to be a thrombus rather than an artifact (Fig. 35.4 and Video 35.3). Even though the peri-procedural ACT had been monitored every 30 min and was kept above 250 s, the length of the procedure made a thrombus formation plausible. Additionally TEE also demonstrated a torn mitral chord at the origin of the first grasp accompanied by an increase of MR severity (Fig. 35.5).

Considering this possible thrombus in the left atrium and the risk of its embolization, and the increase of mitral regurgitation due to the chordal rupture and the inability to implant the clip in a correct position, we decided to convert the procedure to open-heart surgery. It was planned to remove the MitraClip® system from the left atrium under direct vision.

No thrombus was found in the left atrium during surgery. The MitraClip was cut and removed (Fig. 35.6a). The surgeon noticed an abrasion on the atrial side of the posterior mitral leaflet and a rupture of a medial P2 chord (Fig. 35.6b, c). The valve was successfully repaired and a surgical ring implanted. Weaning of cardiopulmonary bypass was difficult and required inotropic and vasopressor support. The patient was extubated a few hours after cardiac surgery. However, he developed a refractory cardiogenic shock with multiple organ failure and died after 6 days.

Discussion

A careful review of the case was done. Some critical points could be identified. The anterior puncture made the steering difficult. Retrospectively the transgastric short axis view of the TEE revealed an echogenic structure close to the posterior wall and an echogenic structure attached to opposing AML. This finding was judged to be sclerosed heads of a high posteromedial papillary muscle group giving rise to one head just close to the indentation between segment P2 and P3 and one head to the opposing AML (Fig. 35.7 and Video 35.1). Alternatively, the finding could be sclerosed and fused chords possibly in combination with an accessory posterior papillary muscle. The short chords arising from this posterior structure were supporting the leaflet adjacent to the indentation between P2 und P3. In this area the first grasp was attempted (Video 35.2). This unfavorable anatomic finding in combination with the very large left ventricle might have induced extreme tension on the mitral chords during the several grasps, finally leading to a chordal rupture. Additionally it is obvious that in some occasions, the differentiation between an intracardiac mass and an artifact from the MitraClip device can be very difficult. An unfortunate combination of adverse findings and difficult echocardiographic interpretation can make the MitraClip procedure unexpectedly difficult.

Learning Points

- Careful localization of the transseptal puncture is crucial for a smooth and successful MitraClip procedure.
- The subvalvular apparatus of the mitral valve needs to be carefully evaluated for the MitraClip procedure.
- Chordal structures and papillary muscle may be damaged during the MitraClip procedure.

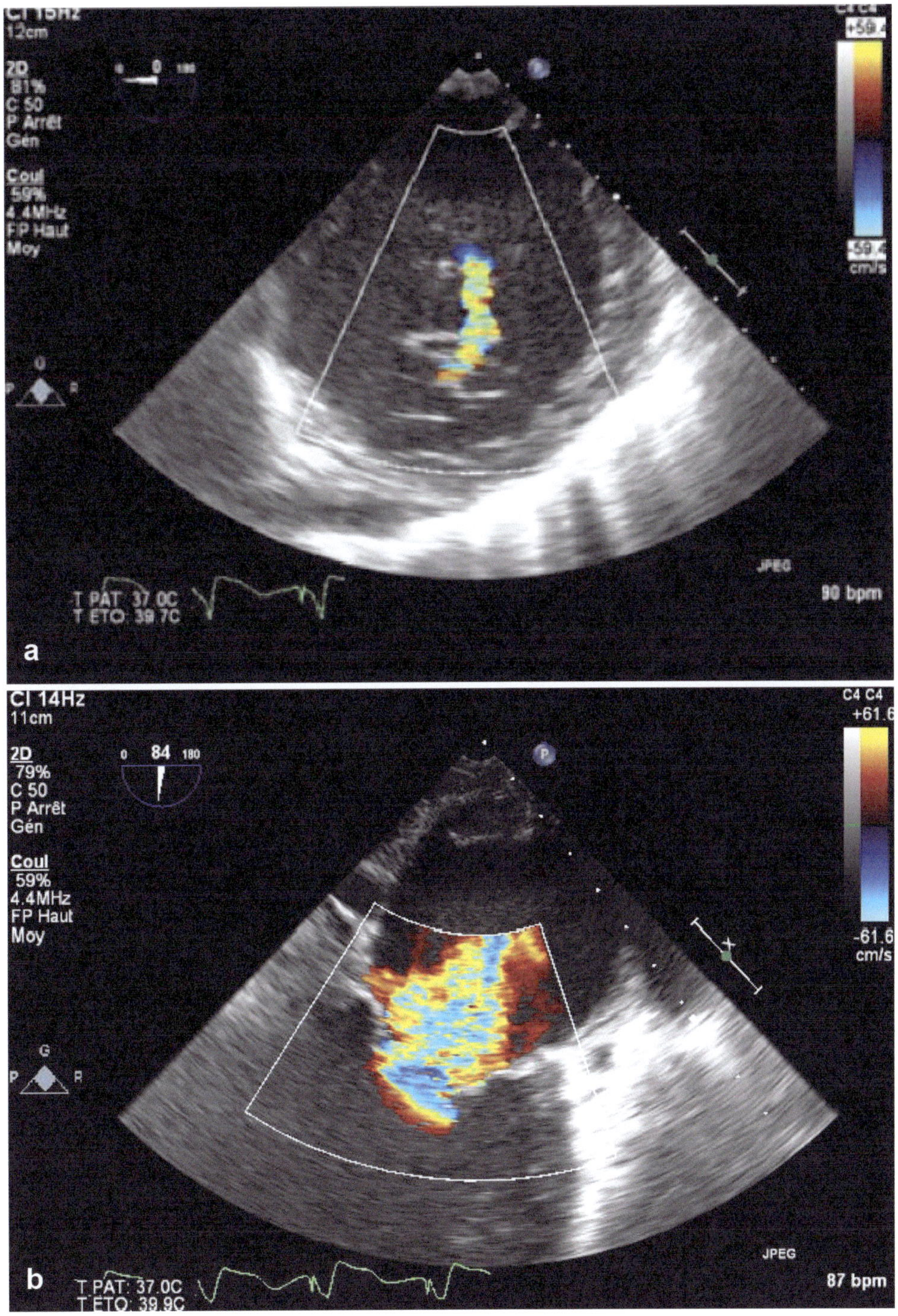

Fig. 35.1 Preoperative TEE showing severe FMR with color-Doppler imaging. (**a**) Transgastric view. (**b**) Bi-commissural view

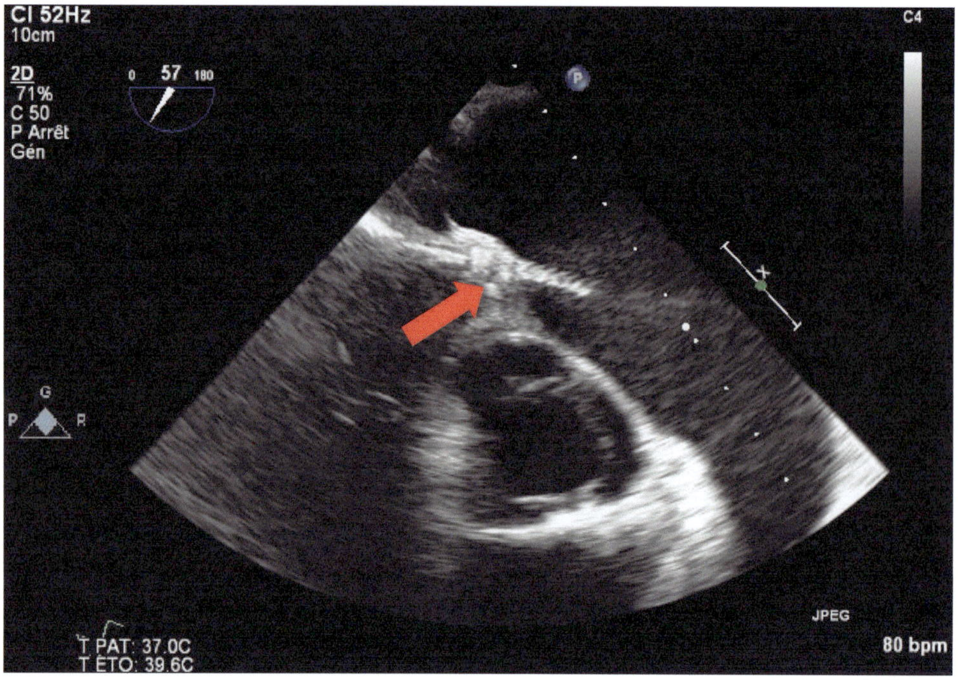

Fig. 35.2 Intraoperative TEE. Short-axis view showing an anterior transseptal puncture and insertion of the guide (*arrow*)

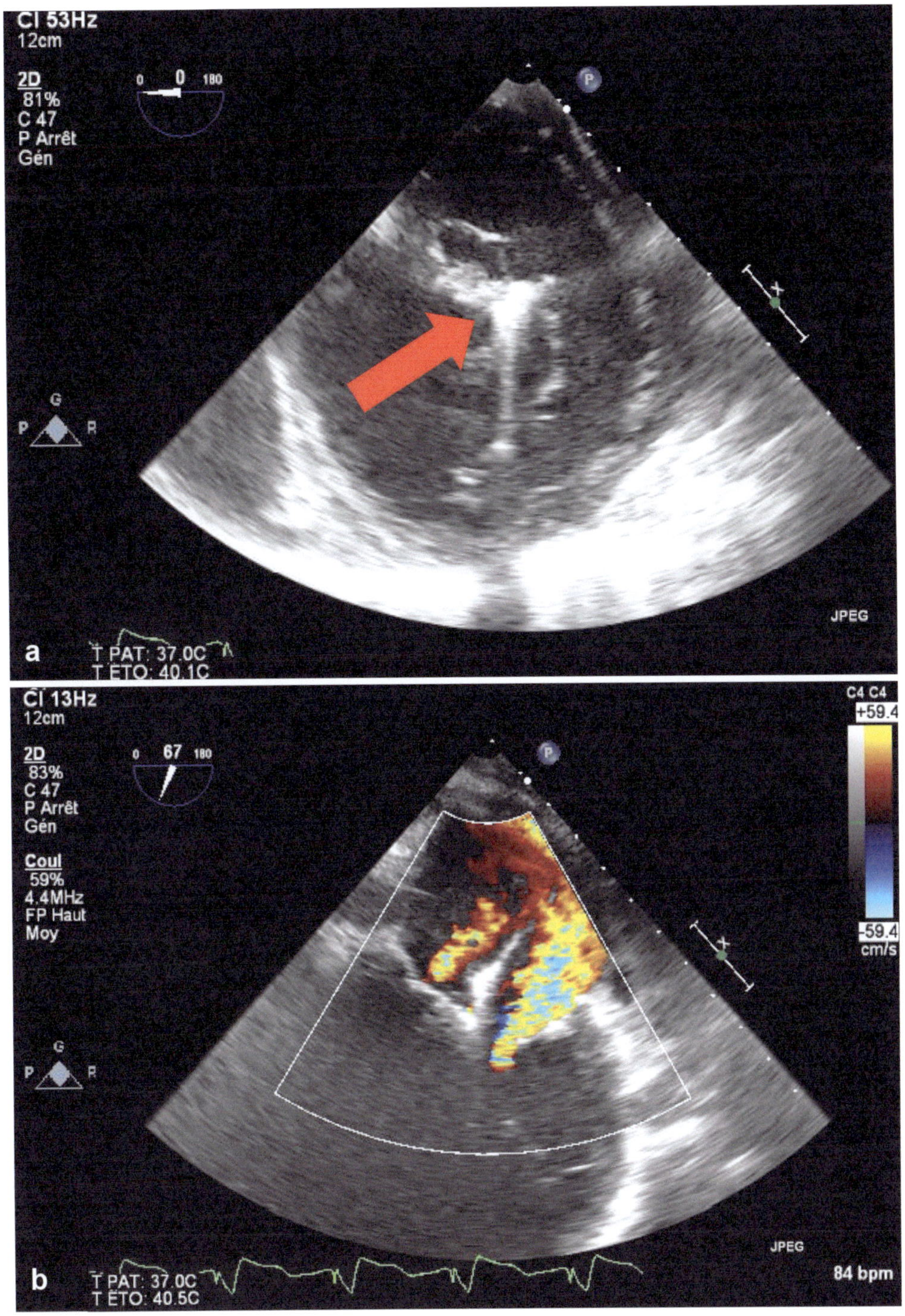

Fig. 35.3 Intraoperative TEE. (**a**) Transgastric view showing too medial MitraClip® (*red arrow*) implantation. (**b**) Bi-commissural view with color-Doppler imaging showing severe residual MR despite leaflet grasping

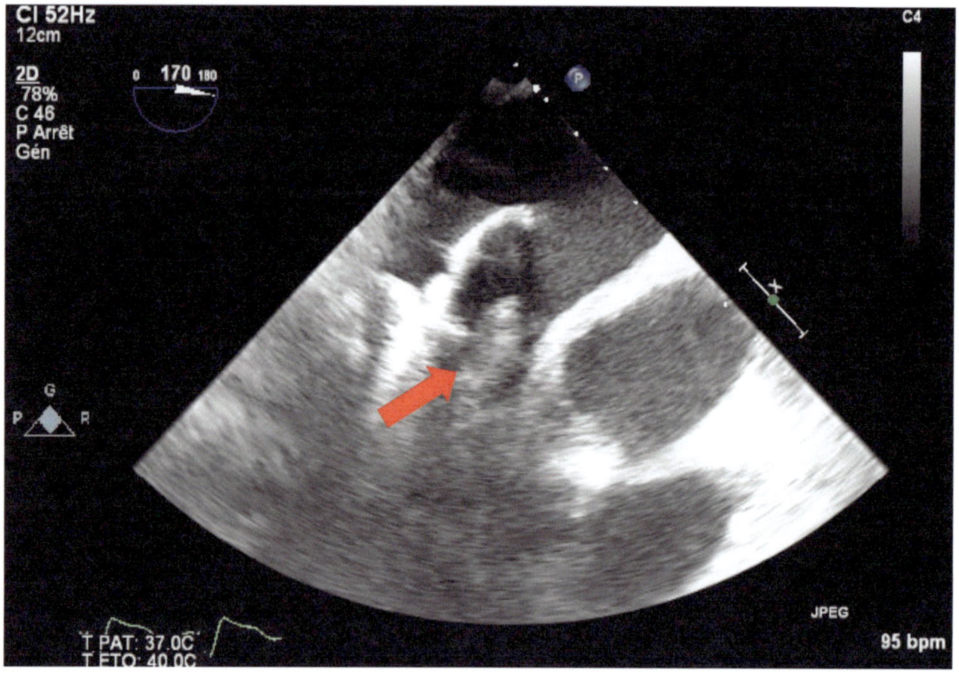

Fig. 35.4 Intraoperative TEE showing oval, echolucent image (3 × 1.5 cm) appearing in the left atrium, visible in all incidences, assumed to be a thrombus (*red arrow*) rather than an artifact

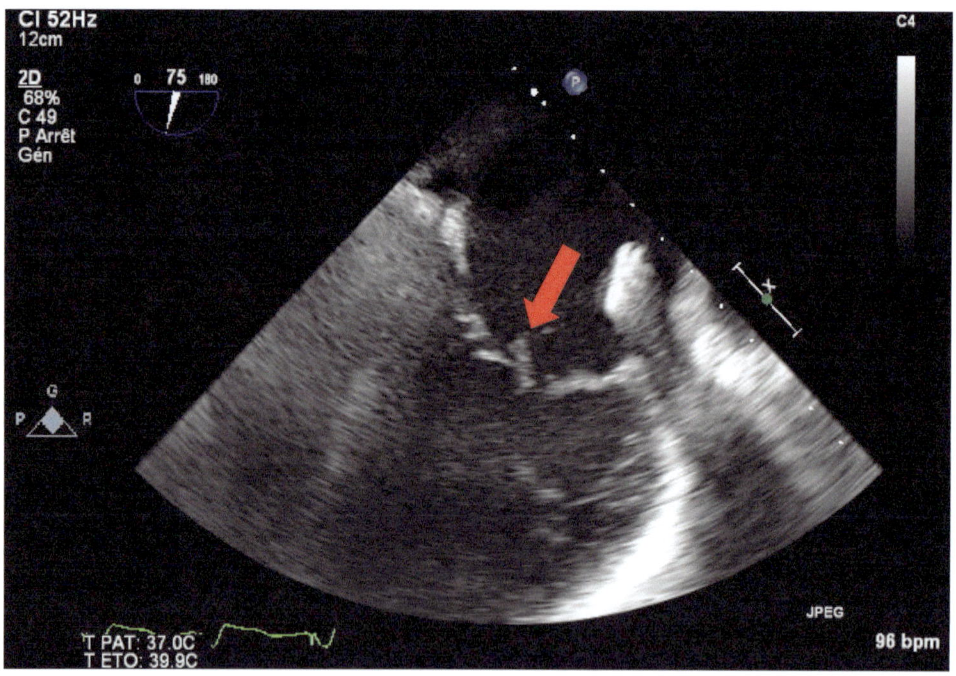

Fig. 35.5 Intraoperative TEE showing in bi-commissural view a torn P2 mitral chord (*red arrow*)

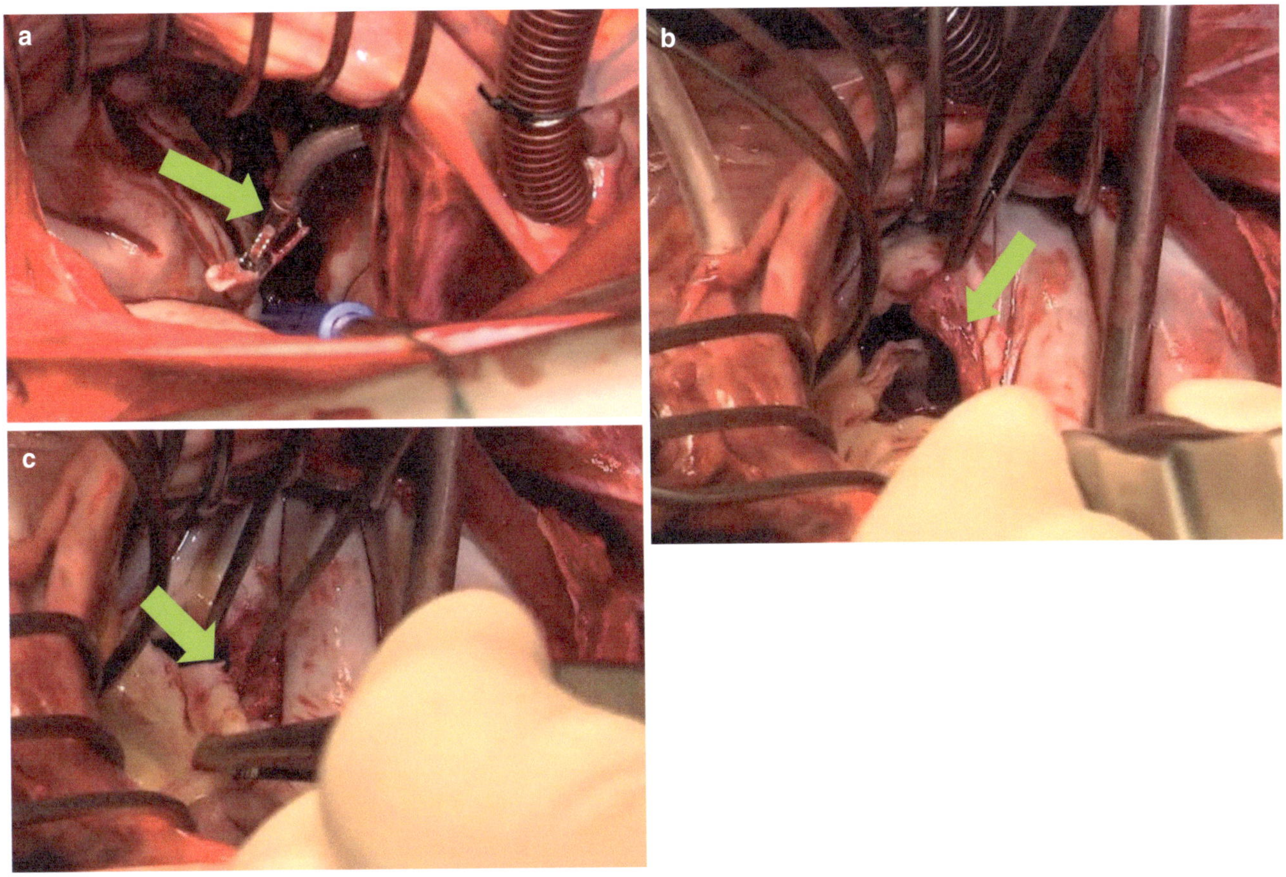

Fig. 35.6 Surgical view of mitral valve. (**a**) MitraClip® in place in left atrium (*arrow*). (**b**) Atrial side abrasion of PML (*arrow*), and below to the left, thickened chord. (**c**) P2 chord rupture (*arrow*)

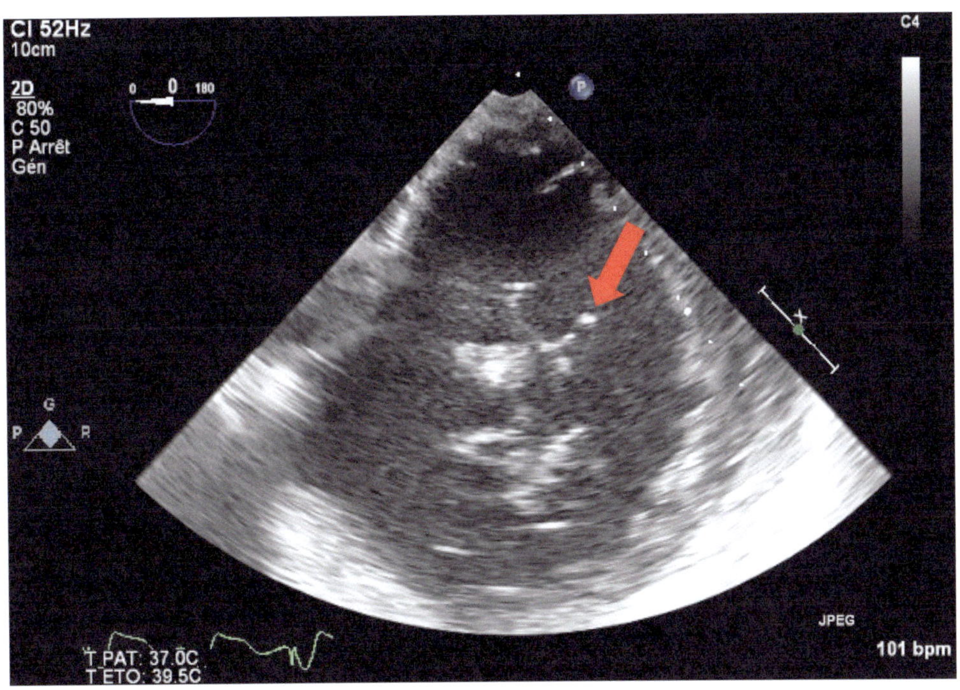

Fig. 35.7 Intraoperative TEE showing in transgastric view, a short chord arising from an accessory papillary muscle or the head of a high papillary muscle close to the indentation between segment P2 and P3 (*red arrow*)

Mitral Valve Repair Using the MitraClip System in a Patient with Severe Mitral Regurgitation in the A3/P3 Region due to Chordae Rupture During Transapical TAVI

36

Magnus Settergren, Per-Herman Jacobsen, Magnus Bäck, and Reidar Winter

Abstract

This case describes the use of the MitraClip in a patient with a ruptured chord which had occurred during a transapical transcatheter aortic valve replacement procedure. The ruptured chord resulted in anterior mitral valve prolapse in the A3 segment. This was successfully repaired using the MitraClip. This case highlights the importance of transesophageal echo, especially 3D imaging in localizing the regurgitant jet and in guiding the procedure.

Keywords

Mitral regurgitation • MitraClip • Ruptured chord

Clinical History

A 76-year-old male with hypertension, atrial fibrillation, congestive heart failure, previous coronary bypass surgery, aortic valve replacement, and percutaneous coronary interventions underwent transapical TAVI due to degeneration of the biological aortic valve prosthesis. A rupture of a chorda tendinea to the anterior mitral valve leaflet complicated the procedure. Postoperative transesophageal echocardiogram (TEE) could confirm the ruptured chorda to the anterior mitral valve leaflet causing a severe mitral regurgitation (MR) originating in the A3/P3 region (Fig. 36.1a–d).

The patient's symptoms rapidly deteriorated, and after a few months, he had progressed to New York Heart Association (NYHA) functional class IV and was accepted for a MitraClip intervention as compassionate use.

In the EVEREST I and II trials, the MR had to be central, i.e., in the A2/P2 region, and accordingly intervention in pathologies outside of this region is generally not recommended. However, there is growing experience in experienced centers of procedures outside of the A2/P2 region.

When performing the MitraClip intervention in pathologies that originates from the AI/P1 or A3/P3 region, certain changes to how that procedure is performed compared to when the pathology lies within the A2/P2 region has to be made.

Firstly, it is even more important to use color Doppler when steering the clip down toward the valve, since the origin of the MR is noncentral (Fig. 36.2).

Secondly, the 3D TEE "en face" view is especially useful when adjusting the clip perpendicular to the line of coaptation since the angle of the clip will be completely different when it is perpendicular in the A3/P3 region compared to a clip that is perpendicular in the A2/P2 region (Fig. 36.3).

Thirdly, the 3D en face view is very helpful in choosing/determining the correct view for grasping, which due to the curvature of the line of coaptation is different from the LVOT view used for grasping in the A2/P2 pathology cases.

Finally, it is more likely to get caught in chordae when grasping outside of the A2/P2 region, and one should

M. Settergren, M.D., Ph.D. (✉)
Department of Cardiology, Unit for PCI/GUCH, Karolinska University Hospital, Stockholm 17176, Sweden
e-mail: magnus.settergren@karolinska.se

P. Jacobsen, M.D.
Department of Cardiology, Unit of GUCH, Karolinska University Hospital, Stockholm 17176, Sweden
e-mail: per-herman.jacobsen@karolinska.se

M. Bäck, M.D. Ph.D. • R. Winter, M.D., Ph.D.
Department of Cardiology, Karolinska University Hospital, Huddinge, Stockholm 17176, Sweden
e-mail: magnus.back@ki.se; reidar.winter@karolinska.se

T. Feldman et al. (eds.), *Atlas of Percutaneous Edge-to-Edge Mitral Valve Repair*,
DOI 10.1007/978-1-4471-4294-2_36, © Springer-Verlag London 2013

therefore always be prepared to invert the clip and retract back to the left atrium.

In the current case, we were able to grasp the leaflets in the A3/P3 region (Fig. 36.4), and when closing the clip under continuous color Doppler, we could appreciate the MR reduction from grade 3+ to trace (Fig. 36.5a–d).

The patient was discharged after 3 days in the hospital, and at 1-month follow-up, he is now in NYHA class 1–2, having an active lifestyle.

Learning Points

- The MitraClip procedure can be performed when the pathology is outside of the A2/P2 region. This intervention should be performed in experienced centers.
- The guidance of live 3D TEE is strongly recommended.
- The operator should be aware of the greater risk of getting caught in the chordae.

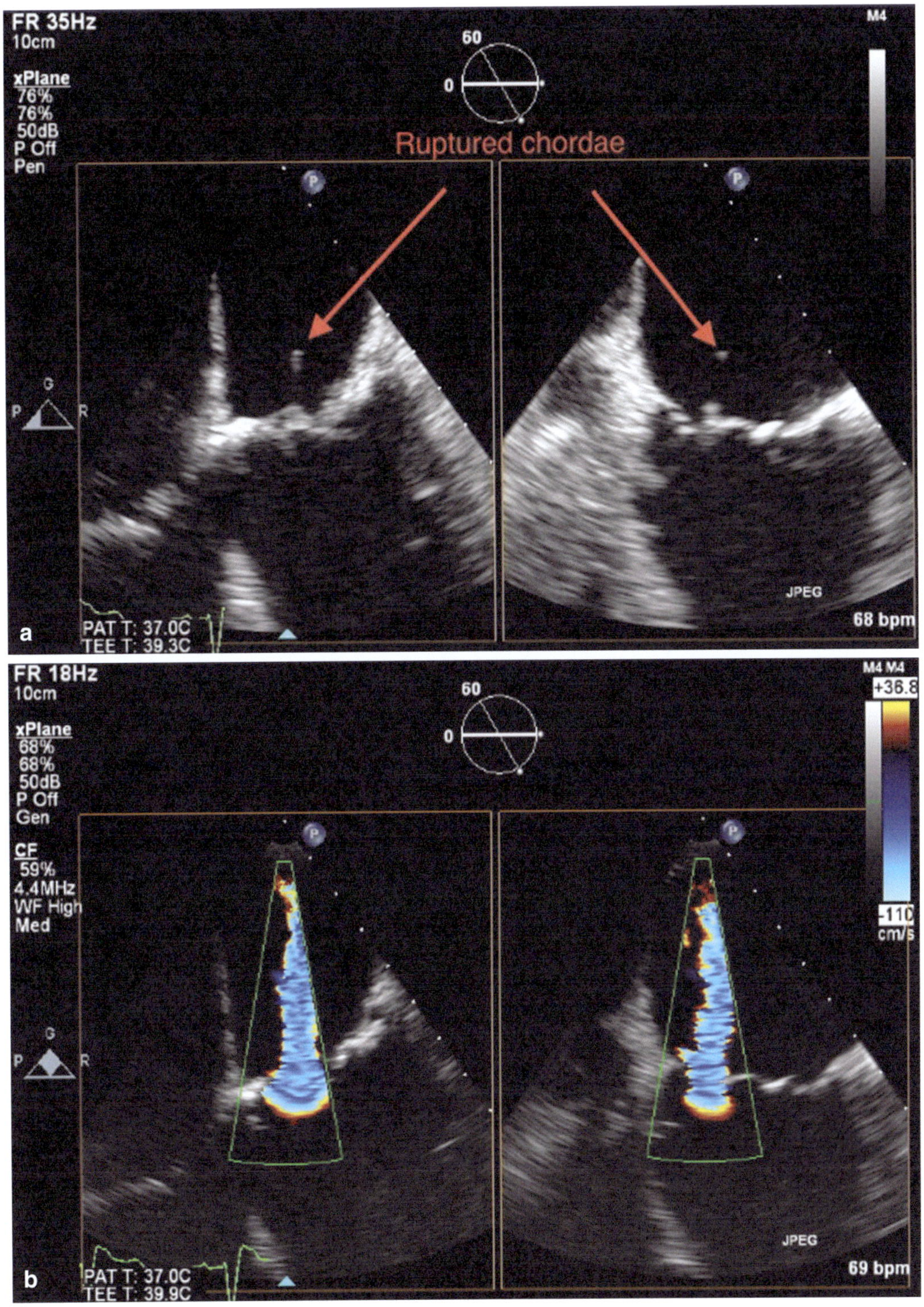

Fig. 36.1 (**a**–**d**) X-plane TEE reveals the ruptured chordae from the anterior leaflet (**a**) causing a severe medial mitral regurgitation (**b**). The exact location of the defect is best visualized using 3D TEE (**c**–**d**)

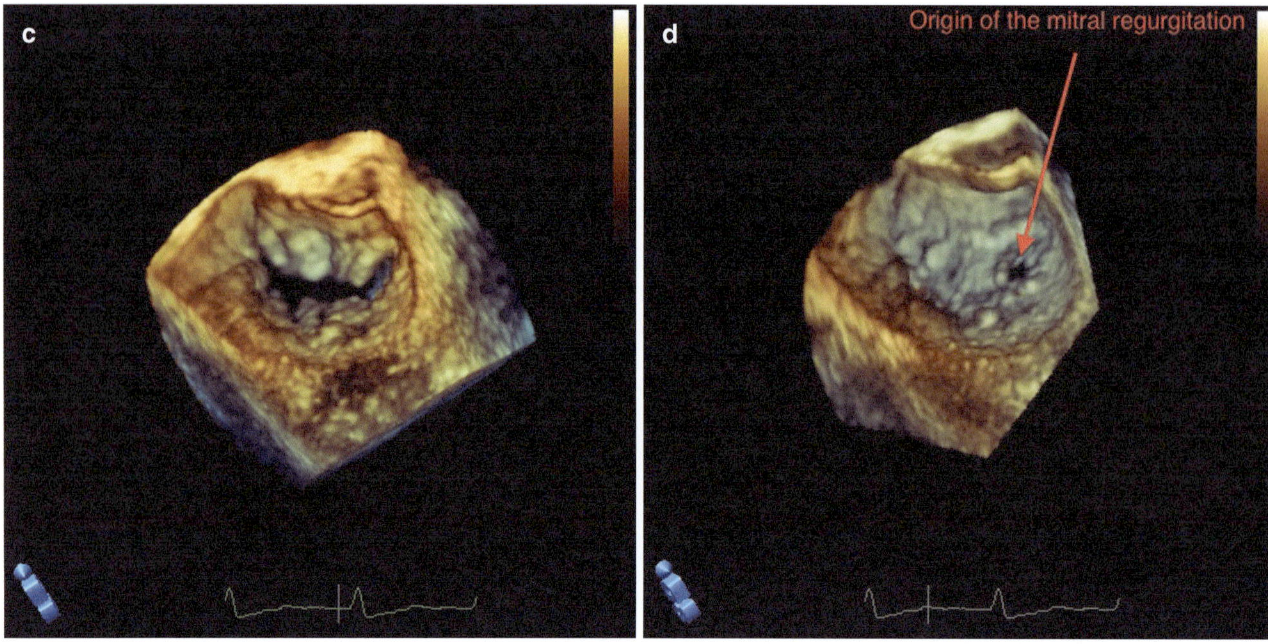

Fig. 36.1 (continued)

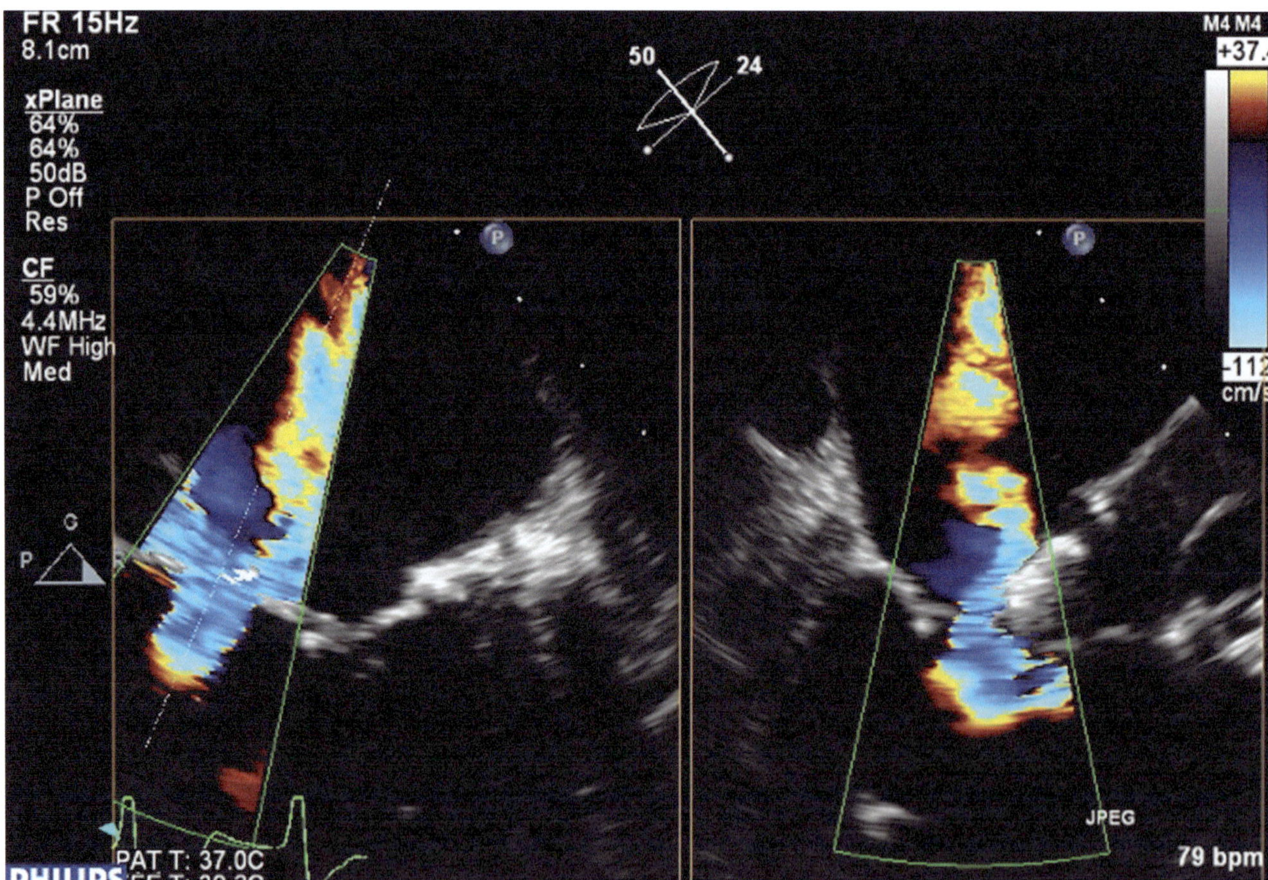

Fig. 36.2 X-plane TEE with color Doppler. The clip is positioned directly above the MR that is located in the A3/P3 region

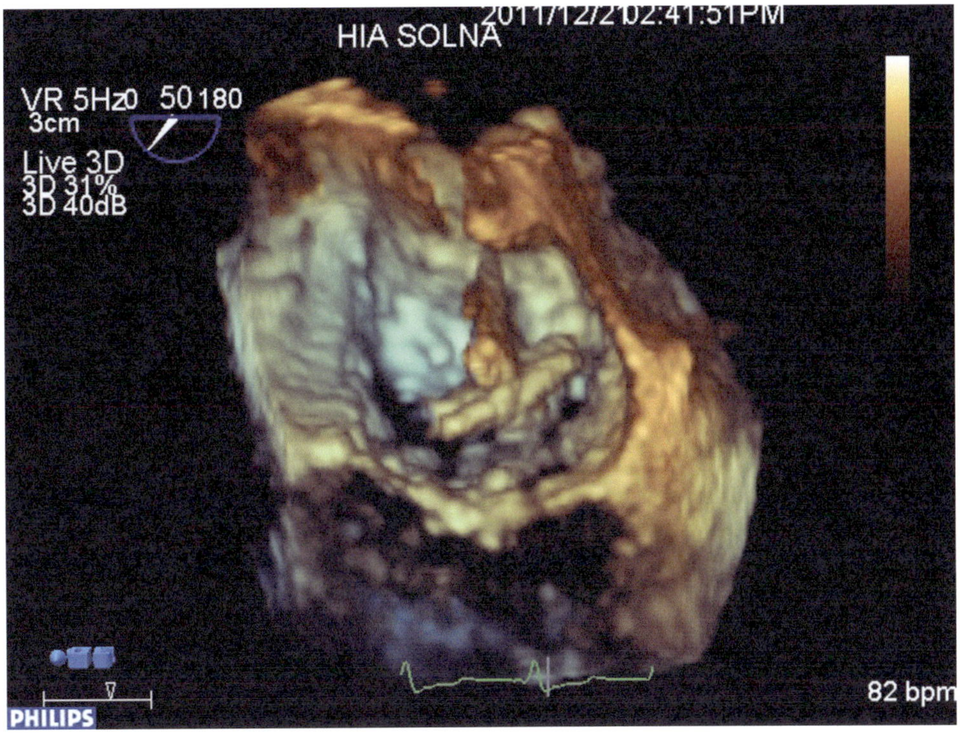

Fig. 36.3 Live 3D TEE. Demonstrating an incorrect angle of the clip to line of coaptation

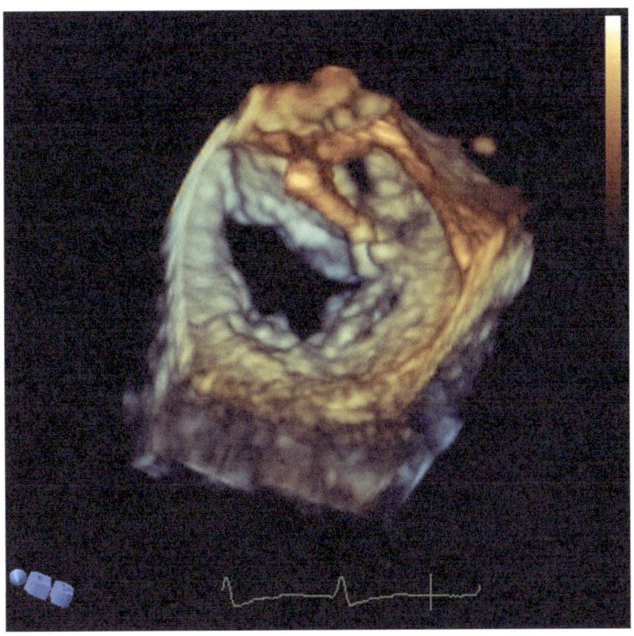

Fig. 36.4 Live 3D TEE. The clip has grasped the leaflets in the A3/P3 region and is still attached to the clip delivery system

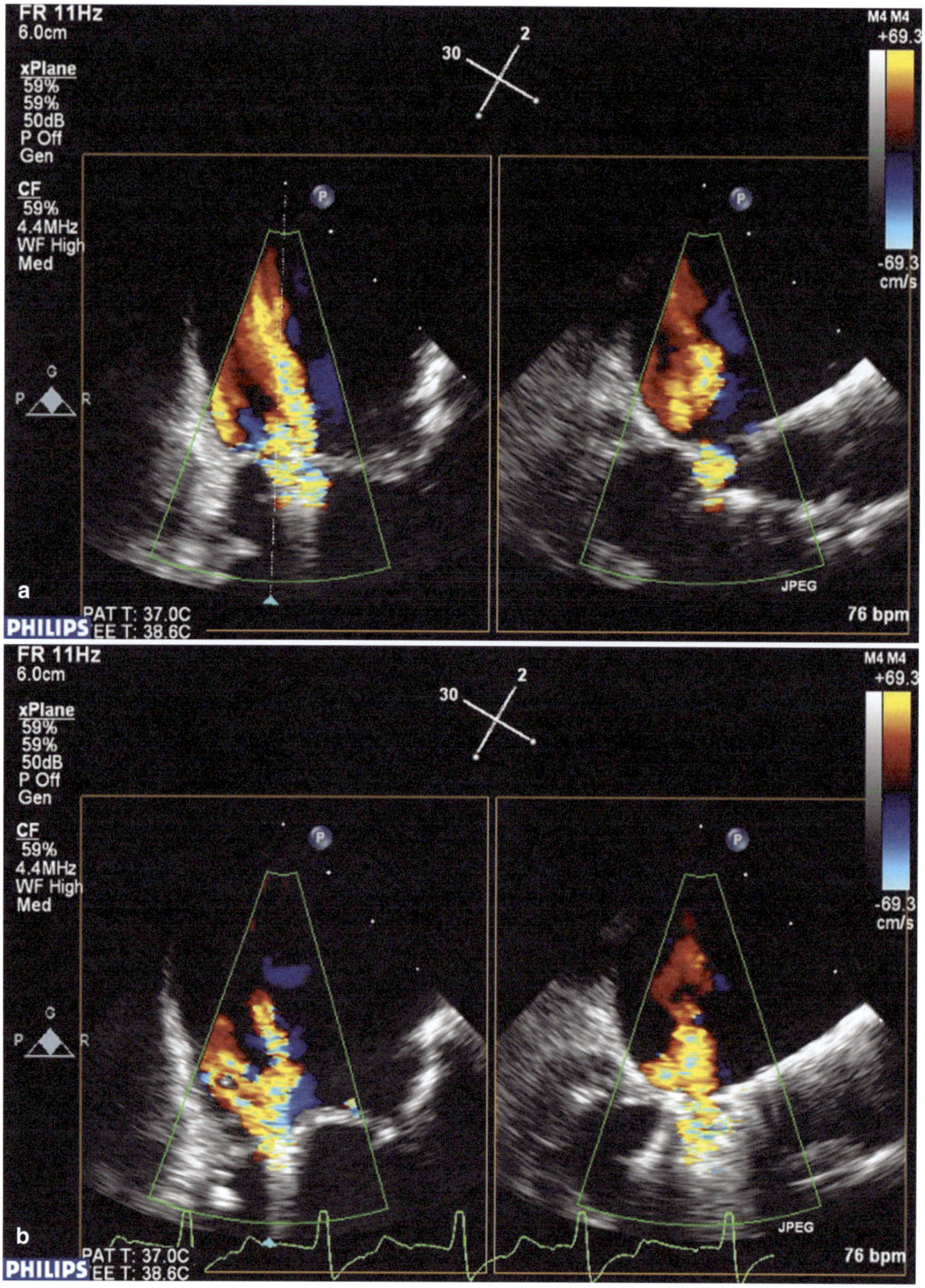

Fig. 36.5 (**a**–**d**) X-plane TEE. Closing of the clip with continuous color Doppler showing the reduction in MR from grade 3+ to trace

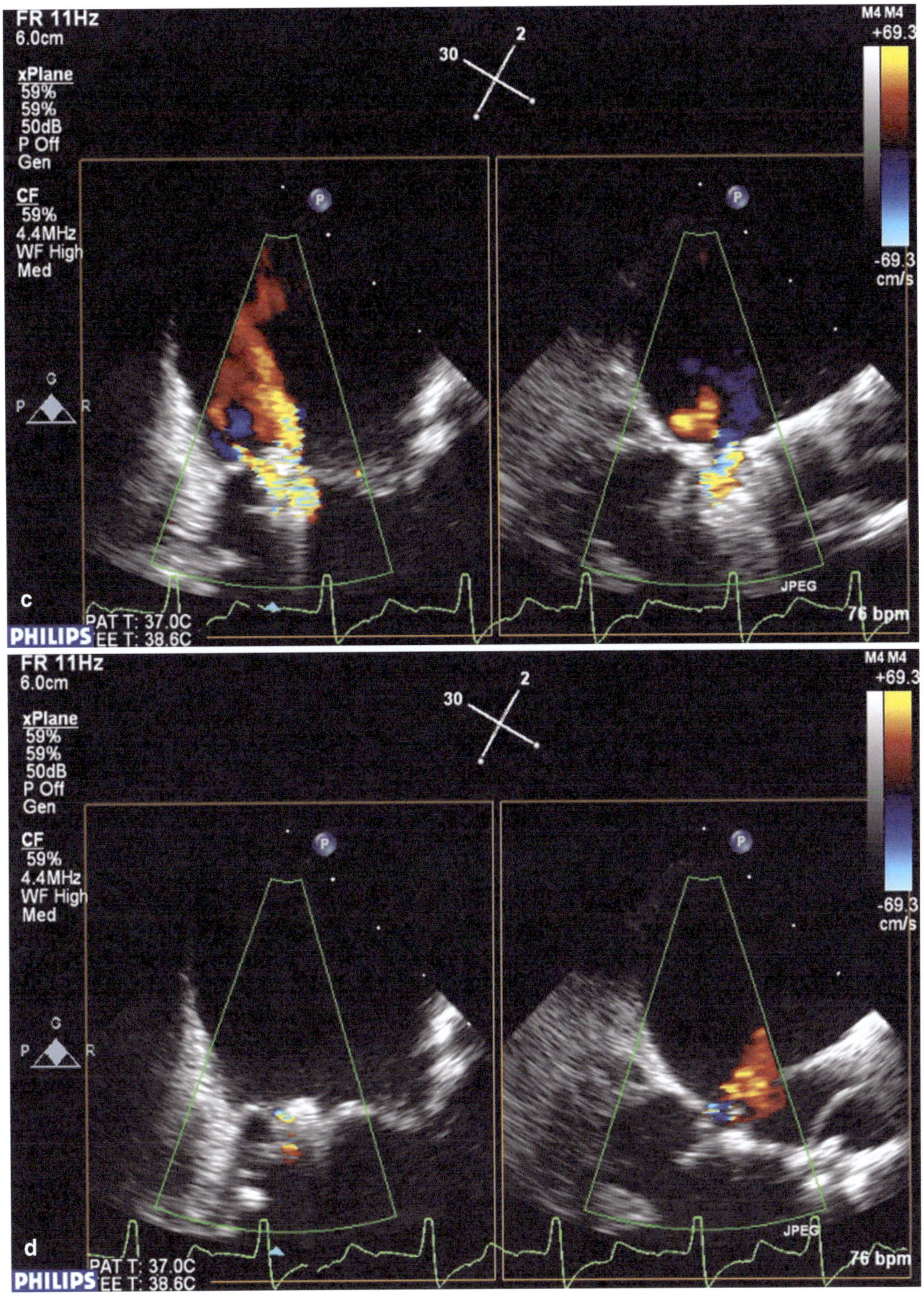

Fig. 36.5 (continued)

MitraClip Implantation in a Patient with Severe Mitral Annular Calcification and a Small Orifice Area

37

Philipp C. Lurz, Norman Mangner, Stephan Blazek, Gerhard Schuler, and Holger Thiele

Abstract

The MitraClip may be performed safely even in high-surgical-risk patients. This case describes the treatment of a high-surgical-risk patient who has a borderline mitral valve area and heavy annular and leaflet calcification. With a single clip, the mitral regurgitation was reduced from 4+ to 1+. The mitral valve area decreased from 3.6 to 2.4 cm^2. The patient had clinical improvement in NHYA functional class from III to I–II. Although there was no clinical evidence of stroke, the patient's MRI scan showed microembolic events.

Keywords

Mitral regurgitation • MitraClip • Mitral stenosis • Calcification • Microemboli

Clinical History

An 80-year-old woman with two previous episodes of acute cardiac decompensation and hospitalization was referred to our hospital for further noninvasive and invasive diagnostics. At the age of 75, this woman underwent triple vessel coronary artery bypass grafting combined with aortic valve replacement (biological prosthesis) for severe aortic stenosis. The patient has also a history of arterial hypertension, type II diabetes mellitus, severe chronic renal failure, and restrictive lung disease.

At the time of hospital admission, she reported shortness of breath on minimal exertion (New York Heart Association (NYHA) class III), loss of 15 kg of body weight within 6 months suggesting cardiac cachexia, and dramatic reduction in subjective cardiopulmonary capacity.

She underwent coronary angiography, which revealed a good result after coronary artery bypass grafting with patency of all grafts. Transthoracic and transesophageal echocardiography demonstrated a left ventricular ejection fraction of 60 % and severe central mitral regurgitation due to tethering of the anterior leaflet and prolapsing of the posterior leaflet. The mitral valve annulus appeared to be heavily calcified with some degree of leaflet calcifications (Figs. 37.1 and 37.2).

Importantly, the effective mitral valve area (MVA), as determined by planimetry, was measured as 3.6 cm^2 (pressure half-time calculation 3.7 cm^2). A dilated left atrium (50 × 55 mm), severe mitral regurgitation with systolic flow reversal in all pulmonary veins, and moderate to severe tricuspid regurgitation with a right ventricular systolic pressure of 75 mmHg was also noted in this study. The aortic prosthetic valve was found to be functioning well.

Due to the MVA of <4.0 cm^2 and the heavy annular calcifications, the anatomy was initially deemed to be unfavorable for the MitraClip® procedure. However, after interdisciplinary discussion of this patient's case within the "Heart Team," open-heart surgery was considered to be at too high risk (EuroScore = 40.9 %; Society of Thoracic Surgeons (STS) score = 16.1 %). Thus, a MitraClip® procedure was planned in this lady with borderline anatomy.

With the patient under general anesthesia and using fluoroscopic and transesophageal echocardiographic guidance, the MitraClip® device was advanced via the transseptal

P.C. Lurz, M.D., Ph.D. (✉) • N. Mangner, M.D.
S. Blazek, M.D. • G. Schuler, M.D. • H. Thiele, M.D.
Department of Internal Medicine/Cardiology,
Heart Centre, University of Leipzig,
Strümpellstraße 39, 04289 Leipzig, Germany
e-mail: philipp.lurz@gmx.de; norman.mangner@med.uni-leipzig.de; stephan.blazek@med.uni-leipzig.de; gerhard.schuler@med.uni-leipzig.de; thielh@medizin.uni-leipzig.de

T. Feldman et al. (eds.), *Atlas of Percutaneous Edge-to-Edge Mitral Valve Repair*,
DOI 10.1007/978-1-4471-4294-2_37,

route across the mitral annulus into the left ventricle. Without any specific technical issues, a clip could be implanted, grasping the anterior and posterior leaflet at the A2/P2 segments. Transesophageal echocardiography demonstrated a significant reduction of mitral regurgitation grade from III+ to I. Furthermore, analysis of transmitral flow patterns just before releasing the clip revealed a mean gradient across the mitral valve of 5 mmHg, excluding relevant left ventricular inflow obstruction in this patient with an MVA of <4.0 cm^2 prior to the procedure (Fig. 37.3).

Echocardiography performed 4 days after the intervention confirmed marked reduction in mitral regurgitation (to grade I+) with loss of pulmonary vein flow reversal and decrease of pulmonary artery pressure from 75 to 47 mmHg. MVA was reduced from 3.7 to 2.4 cm^2, with a corresponding mean transmitral pressure gradient of 7.3 mmHg. During the post-interventional course, NYHA functional class improved from III to I–II (Fig. 37.4).

Due to the annular and leaflet calcifications, there were some concerns regarding the risk of stroke secondary to cerebral emboli. Clinically, there was no evidence for neurological impairment after the procedure. This is supported by similar scores of the Montreal Cognitive Assessment (MOCA) before and after the procedure (score 18 vs. 17 out of 30). Cerebral magnetic resonance imaging, however, revealed some diffuse new microemboli (Fig. 37.5).

Discussion

Here we present a case of MitraClip® implantation in a patient with borderline anatomy for this intervention: firstly, MVA before implantation was found to be <4.0 cm^2; secondly, heavy annular calcifications in addition to some degree of leaflet calcifications were present.

In general, percutaneous edge-to-edge mitral valve repair is recommended in patients with an MVA of >4.0 cm^2 only to minimize the risk of mitral stenosis post procedure. Although certainly not advised in all patients, this case suggests that this procedure can be considered in selected patients with a smaller MVA on a case-by-case basis.

A calcified annulus or leaflet of the mitral valve can cause problems during clip application. Apart from technical issues during the procedure, there is a risk of cerebral emboli. Although clinically silent, magnetic resonance imaging demonstrated some cerebral microemboli, which may be attributable to the procedure. Wider application of magnetic resonance for assessment of the incidence of procedure-related cerebral emboli should help to improve our understanding of the clinical relevance of these findings and might refine patient selection.

Learning Points

- The MitraClip is a relatively safe procedure that can be performed even in high-surgical-risk patients.
- In patients with mitral valve areas <4.0 cm^2, the MitraClip may still be considered as a therapeutic procedure if the clinical benefits outweigh the risk of mitral stenosis.
- Extensive annular and leaflet calcification may predispose to cerebral microemboli. However, the clinical significance of this remains unclear.

Transthoracic Echocardiographic Assessment Prior to the Intervention

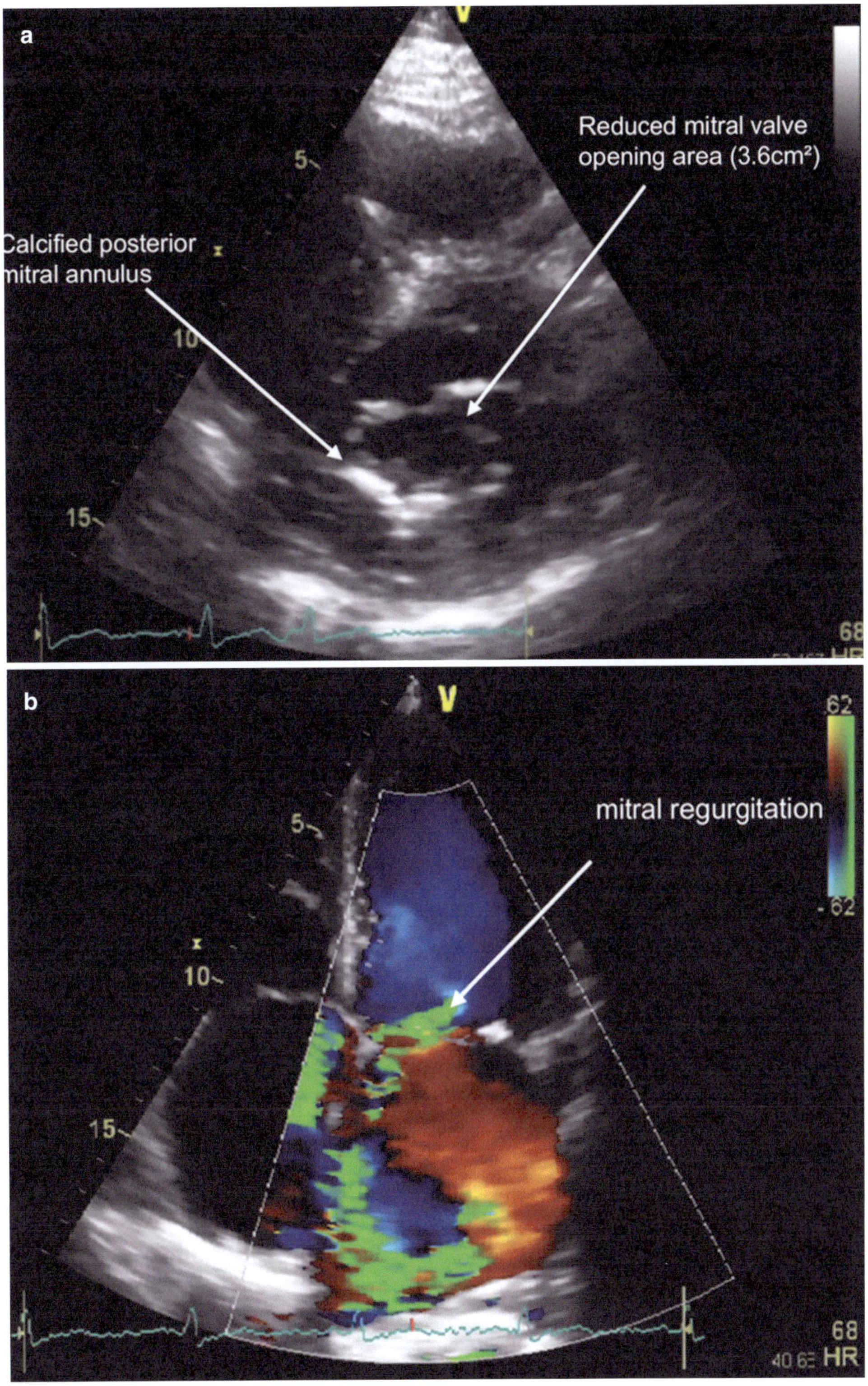

Fig. 37.1 Transthoracic echocardiography before MitraClip® Implantation showed heavy calcifications of the posterior mitral annulus as well as some degree of leaflet calcifications (**a**). Importantly, planimetric assessment of the effective mitral valve orifice area revealed an opening area of <4.0 cm² (3.6 cm²). Color flow Doppler imaging indicated severe mitral regurgitation with an eccentric regurgitant jet toward the septum (**b**)

Transesophageal Echocardiographic Assessment Prior to the Intervention

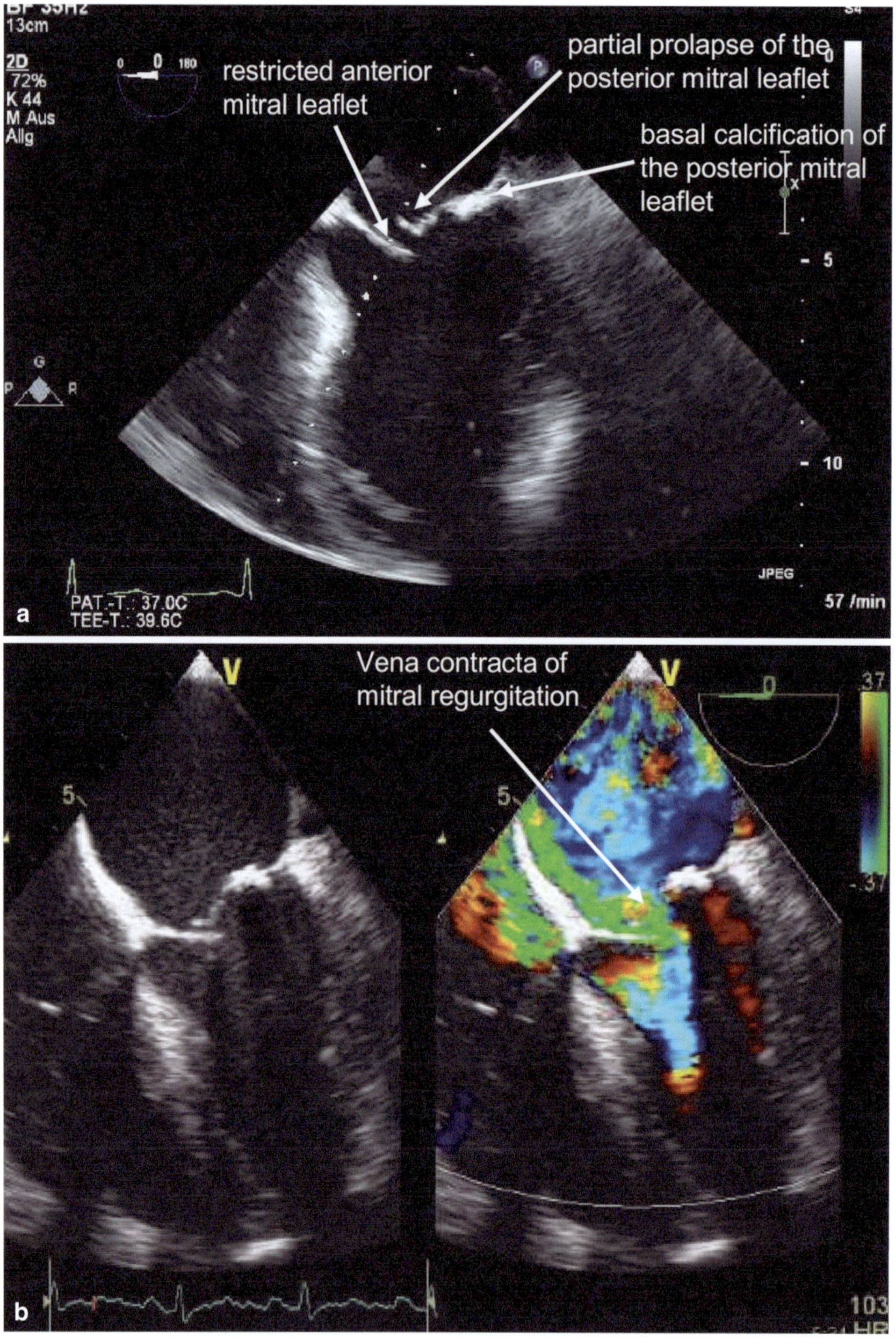

Fig. 37.2 Transesophageal echocardiographic long axis view demonstrates the mechanism of severe mitral regurgitation: a restrictive anterior mitral leaflet due to tethering and prolapsing of the posterior leaflet with heavy annular calcifications, resulting in an apparent coaptation gap (**a**). Color flow Doppler imaging shows severe mitral regurgitation (**b**) and systolic flow reversal in all pulmonary veins

Periprocedural Transesophageal Echocardiographic Assessment

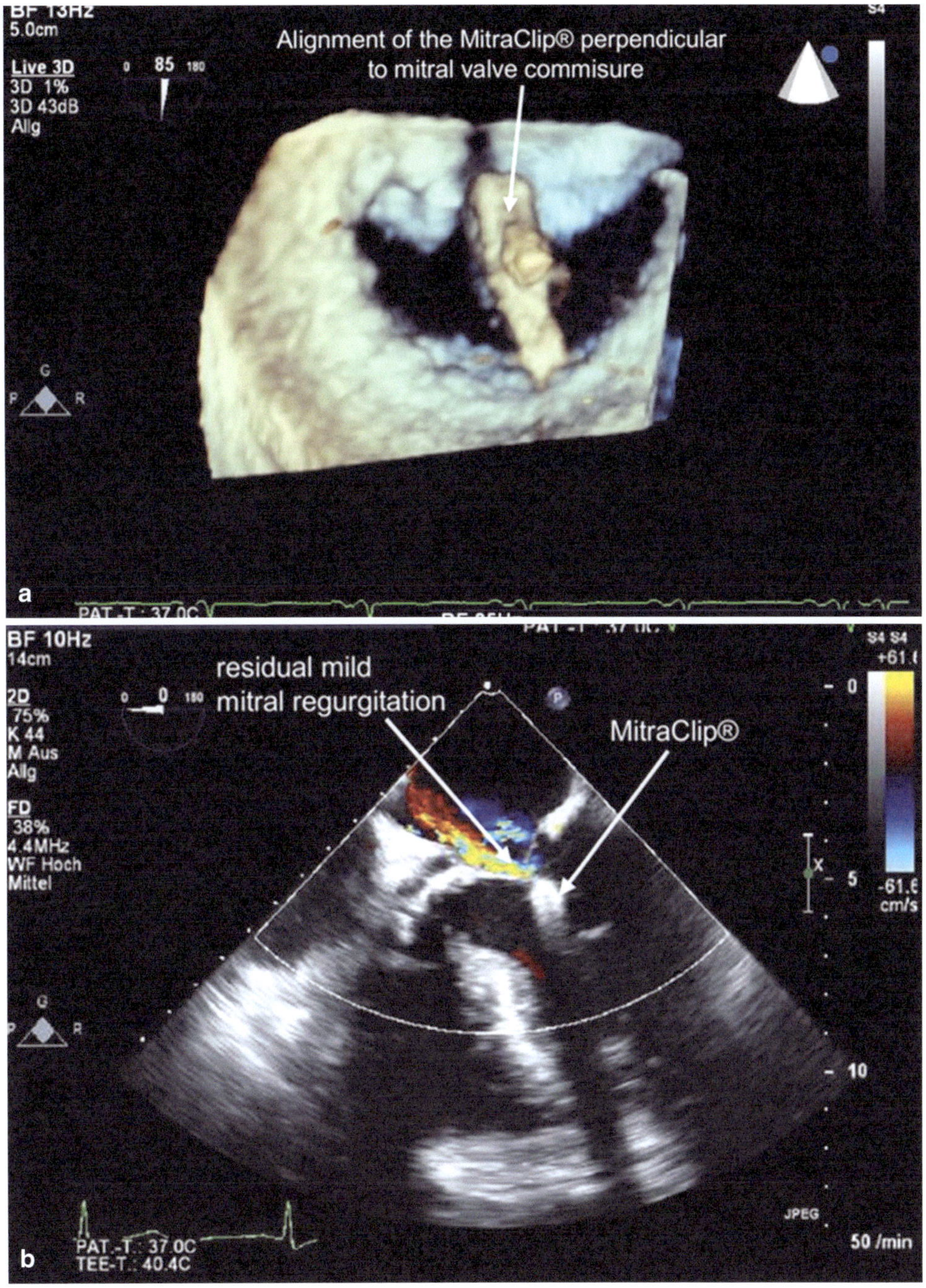

Fig. 37.3 (**a**) Periprocedural transesophageal echocardiography using three-dimensional imaging provides good visualization of the MitraClip® perpendicularly aligned to the mitral commissures in an "en face" view. (**b**) Color Doppler flow imaging shows reduction in mitral regurgitation down to grade I after positioning of the clip. (**c**) Analysis of transmitral flow patterns on continuous pulsed wave Doppler imaging reveals no increase in mean gradient across the mitral valve 5 mmHg just before releasing the clip

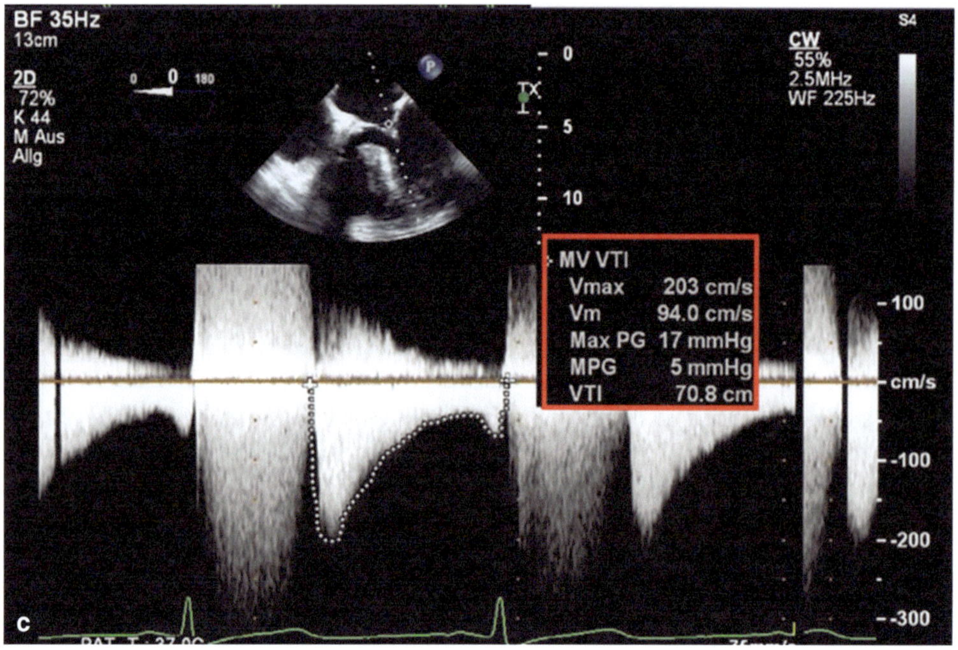

Fig. 37.3 (continued)

Post-procedural Transthoracic Echocardiographic Evaluation

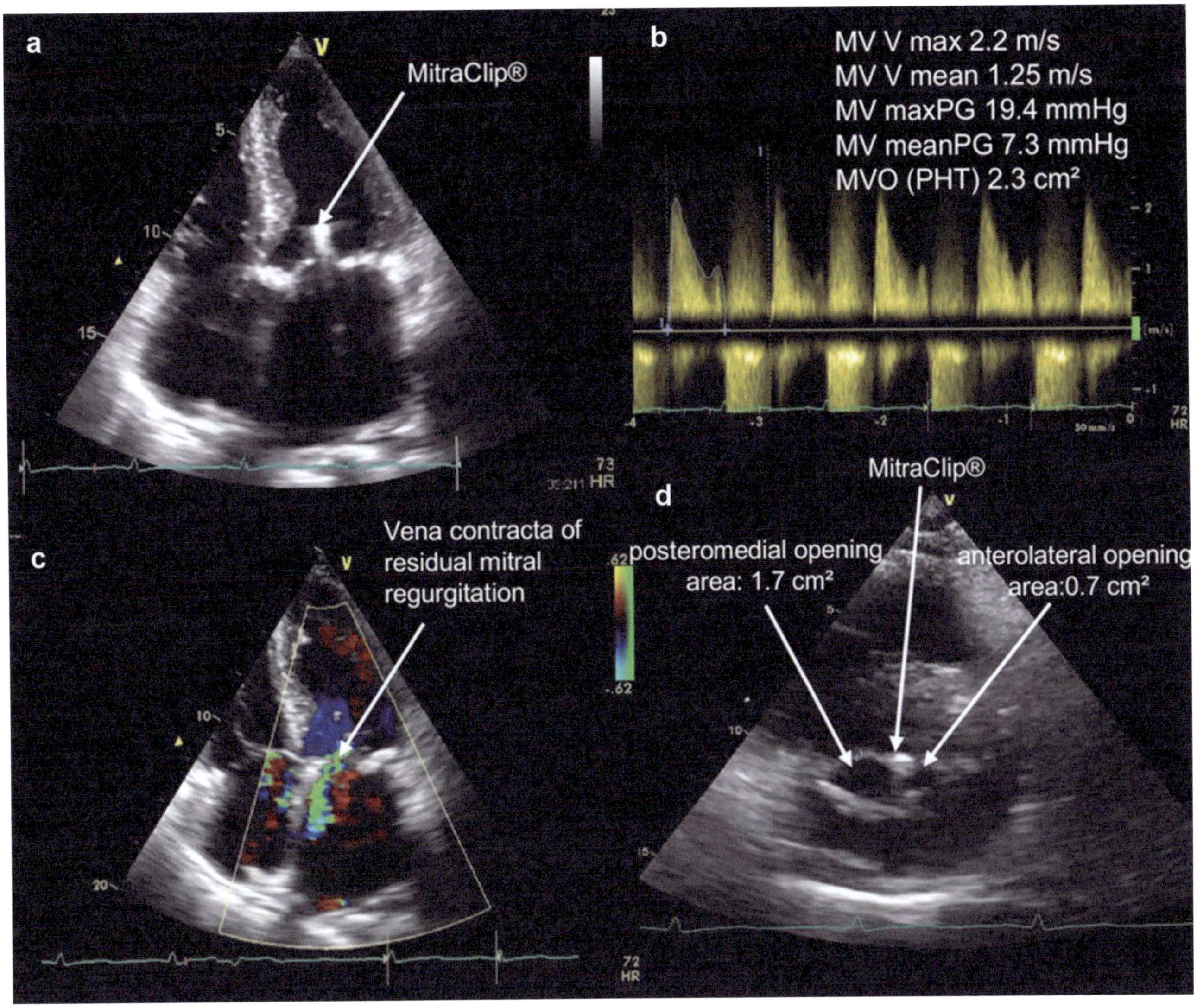

Fig. 37.4 (**a**) Four-chamber view depicting the MitraClip® in correct position. (**b**) Pulsed wave Doppler imaging demonstrates no relevant left ventricular inflow tract obstruction with a mean transmitral pressure gradient of 7.3 mmHg in this lady with an effective mitral orifice area of only 3.6 cm^2 before intervention. (**c**) Color flow imaging showing mild residual mitral regurgitation. (**d**) This short-axis "en face" view of the mitral valve illustrates the recreated double orifice mitral valve with an opening area of 2.4 cm^2

Diffusion-Weighted Magnetic Resonance Imaging of the Brain

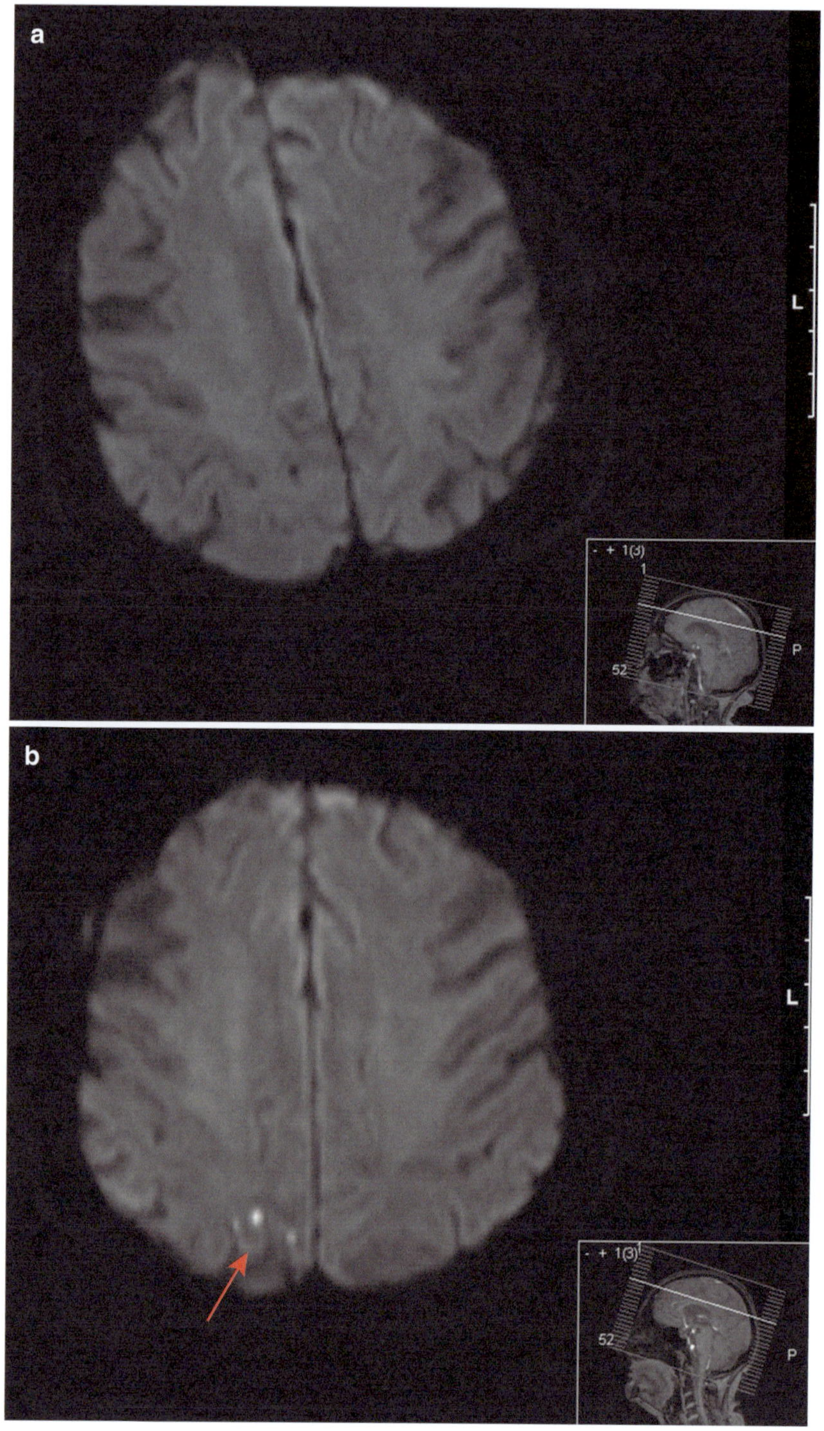

Fig. 37.5 Diffusion-weighted magnetic resonance imaging of the brain before (*panel a*) and after MitraClip® Implantation *panel b*. Note the presence of microemboli in the right occipital lobe (*red arrow*) detected on the post-procedural scan

Conflicts of Interest None

Functional Mitral Regurgitation Treatment with MitraClip: Difficult Transseptal Puncture with Anterior Approach Complicated by Right Atrial Thrombus

38

Genco Yucel and Alpay Sezer

Abstract

This case describes a challenging MitraClip case in which there were technical difficulties with the transseptal puncture. This was further complicated by the presence of a right atrial thrombus, which was successfully aspirated and removed. The difficult transseptal puncture led to an "aorta-hugger" scenario which was successfully managed by advanced steering techniques.

Keywords

Mitral regurgitation • MitraClip • Thrombus • Advanced steering

Clinical History

A 68-year-old man with a history of coronary bypass surgery, chronic obstructive pulmonary disease, diabetes mellitus, and atrial fibrillation was admitted multiple times with congestive heart failure over a few months. He was in NYHA Class III–IV heart failure despite optimal medical therapy, including high dose of diuretics. Echocardiography showed dilated left ventricle with EF of 38 % and severe 4+ functional mitral regurgitation (Figs. 38.1 and 38.2). There was a large central jet, which was measured to have PISA of 11 mm, vena contracta of 7 mm, and ERO of 0.59 cm^2, and regurgitant volume was measured to be 96 ml. There was tethering of both leaflets. Coaptation length was 3.6 mm, and the depth was 8 mm. Mitral valve area was measured to be 5.1 cm^2.

The patient was referred for the MitraClip procedure, and this was performed in the cardiac cath laboratory under general anesthesia. There was significant difficulty in creating good contact with transseptal needle at the posterior part of the fossa. Despite multiple attempts for more than 1 h with differently bent and angulated transseptal needles, the only reliable contact with fossa was obtained at the anterior portion where a PFO would have been, with adequate height from mitral annulus (Figs. 38.3, 38.4, 38.5, and 38.6)

Following a successful puncture and exchanging for an extra stiff wire, a mobile mass was noted on the wire on the right side of the septum (Figs. 38.7 and 38.8). A decision was made to aspirate the presumed thrombus. The deflectable MitraClip guide was advanced over the wire very close to the septum, and suction was applied with a 50 cc syringe. This successfully removed the thrombus (Fig. 38.9).

The guide was then placed in the left atrium (LA), and the clip delivery system (CDS) was advanced close to the tip of the catheter. Because of the anterior location of the transseptal puncture, it was difficult to advance the clip into the LA without touching the aorta (Figs. 38.10 and 38.11).

Deflecting the guide with the (+) knob without straddling and rotating the guide clockwise (posteriorly) to move away from aorta was done (Figs. 38.12, 38.13, and 38.14). The clip was then advanced outside the sheath (which was deflected (+) at maximum), and by rotating the guide back counter-clockwise (anteriorly) and by using small movements of M/L and A/P knob, the clip was successfully steered toward the valve and aligned (Figs. 38.15 and 38.16). Grasping with standard techniques was successfully performed (Fig. 38.17). However, before grasping

G. Yucel, M.D. (✉) • A. Sezer, M.D.
Department of Cardiology, American Hospital Istanbul, Guzelbahce str. No 20s, Nisantasi, Istanbul 34365, Turkey
e-mail: gencoy@amerikanhastanesi.org; alpays@amerikanhastanesi.org

T. Feldman et al. (eds.), *Atlas of Percutaneous Edge-to-Edge Mitral Valve Repair*,
DOI 10.1007/978-1-4471-4294-2_38, © Springer-Verlag London 2013

it was noted that the clip lock mechanism was tensioned, and the clip could not be opened more than 180°. As locking of the clip could not be confirmed, the clip was unlocked and pulled out. The second clip was advanced using the same maneuvers, and mitral leaflets were grasped again successfully (Figs. 38.18 and 38.19). This time, the locking mechanism remained intact, and the clip was released successfully. The MR severity improved by two grades (Fig. 38.20), and the procedure successfully concluded (Fig. 38.21). The patient was discharged on second postoperative day. On the third month follow-up post procedure, the patient is in NYHA Class II–III. His echocardiography shows 3+ MR with significant but half of the original regurgitant volume of 50 ml, with same medications as pre-procedure.

Learning Points

- A prolonged transseptal puncture attempt may result in thrombus formation. Operators and echocardiologists have to be mindful of thrombus developing. Regular aspiration and flushing of the transseptal system should be performed. Low-dose heparin may be considered on a case-by-case basis if the transseptal puncture takes a long time, but this has to be balanced against the risk of uncontrolled bleeding if perforation occurs.
- An anteriorly biased transseptal puncture will make the rest of the MitraClip procedure difficult but not impossible. Stress placed on the system because manipulation of the guide before the CDS straddles the guide markers may damage the clip system.

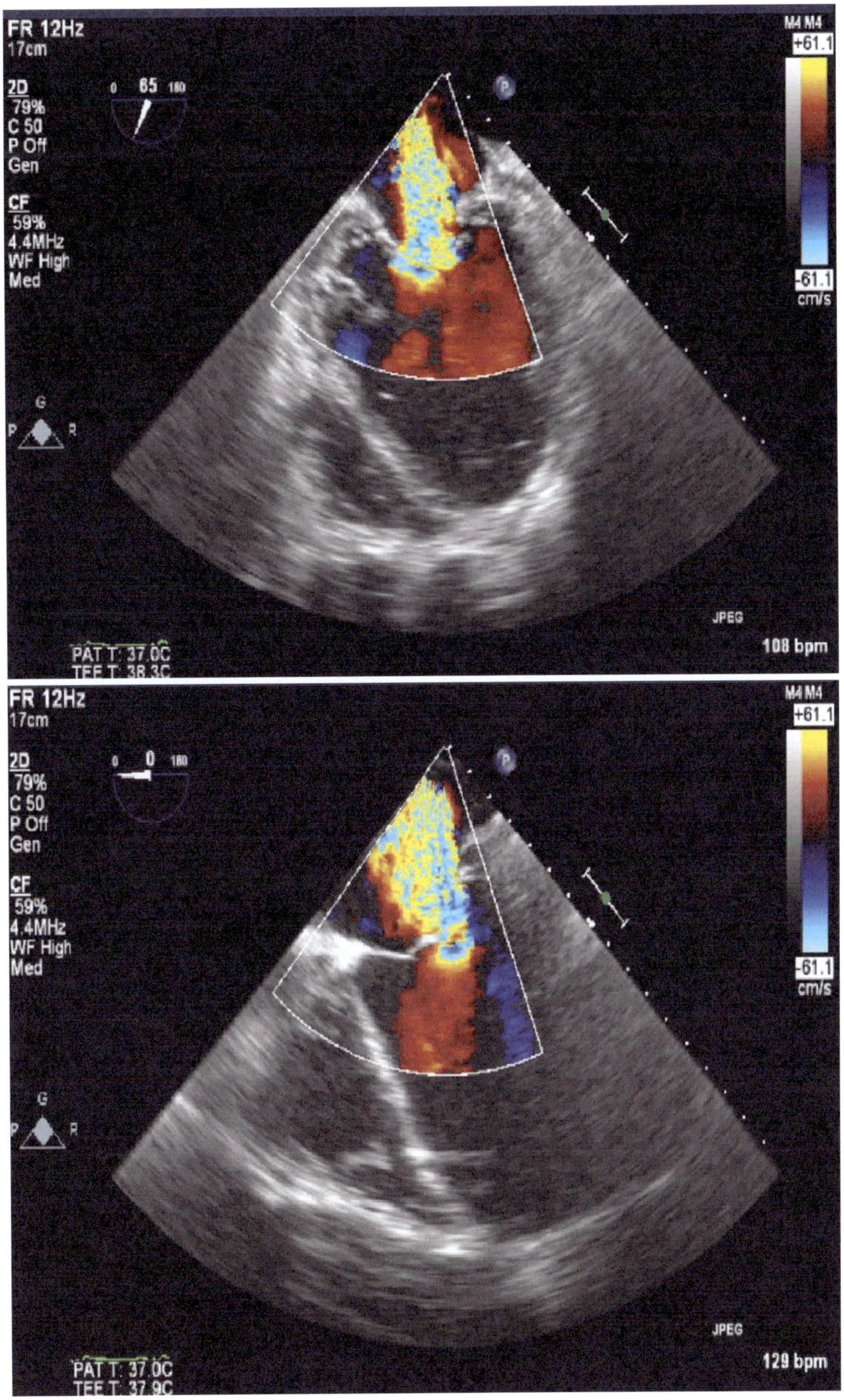

Figs. 38.1 and 38.2 Large wide central MR jet

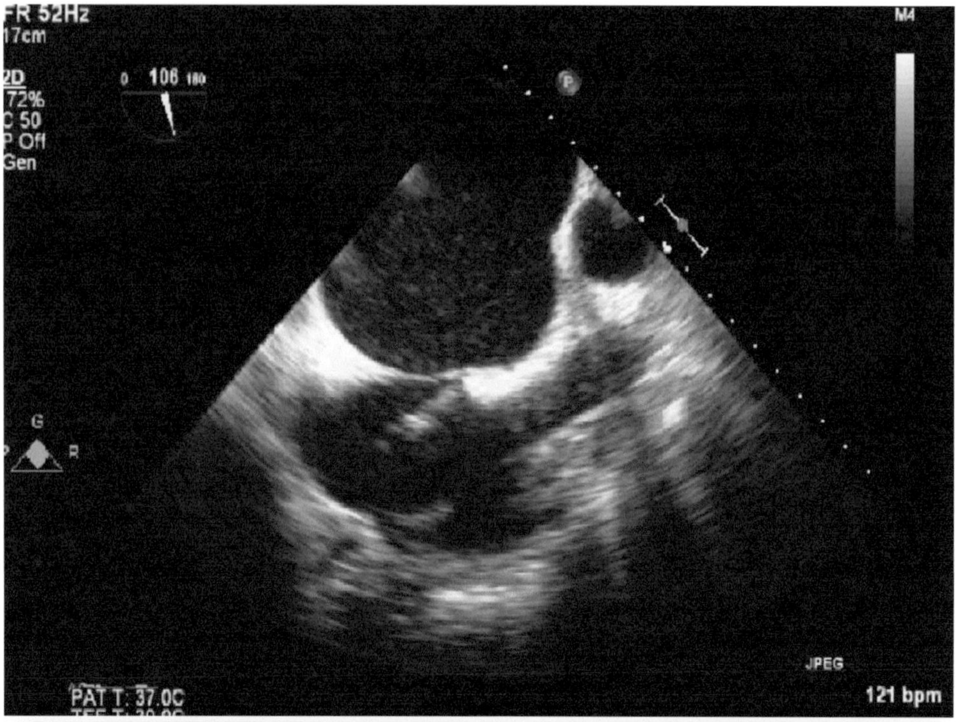

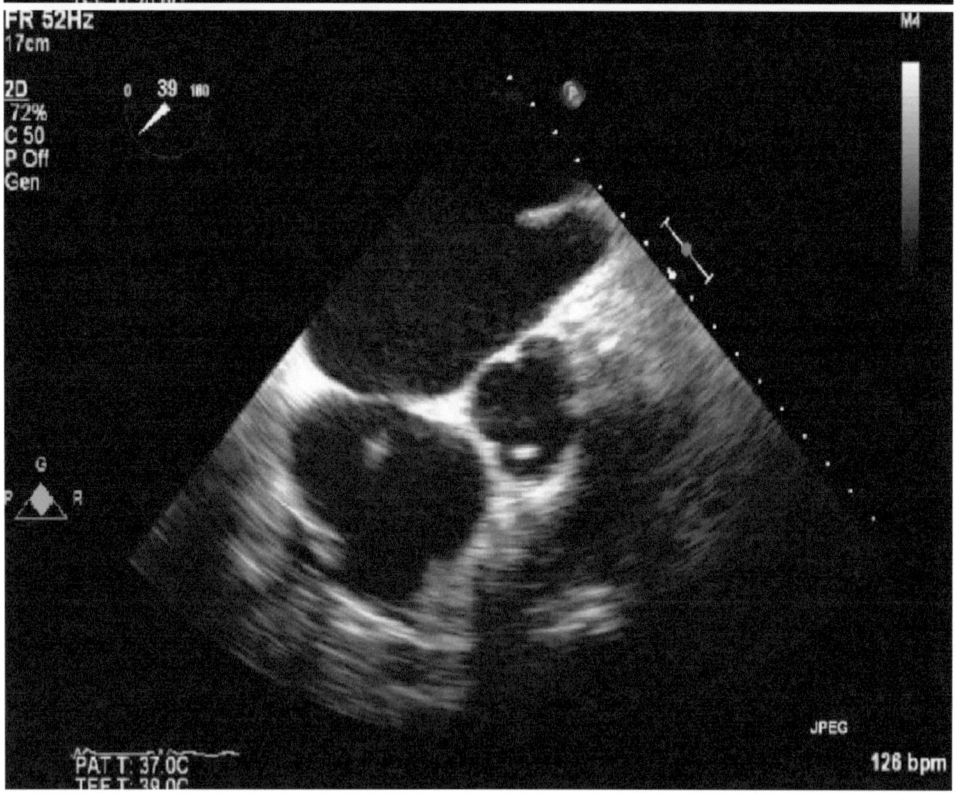

Figs. 38.3 and 38.4 Only position within fossa with good contact during transseptal approach, needle pointing anterior

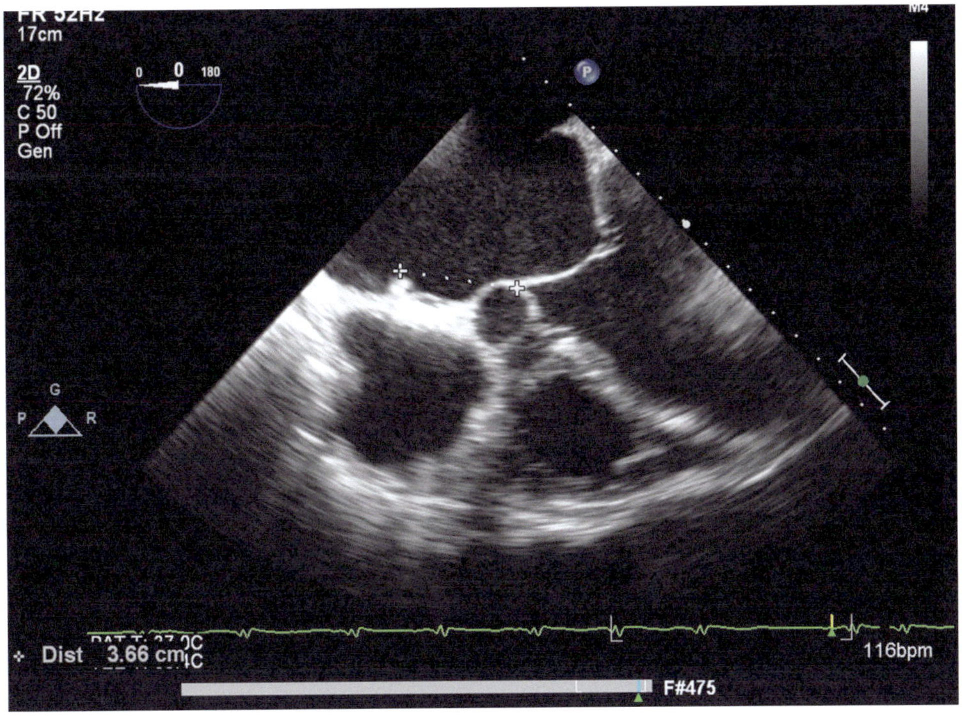

Fig. 38.5 Sufficient height from mitral annulus at the transseptal puncture site

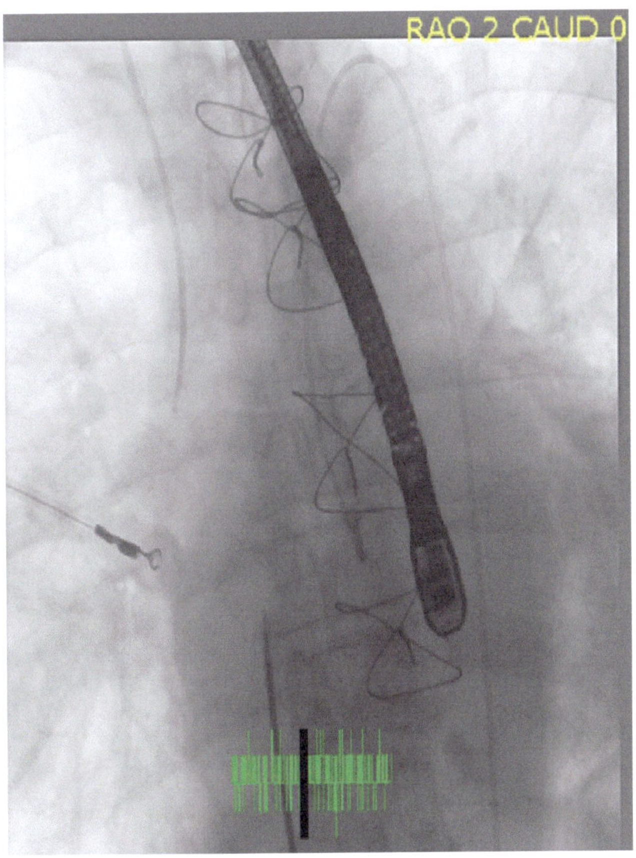

Fig. 38.6 Site of transseptal puncture fluoroscopically

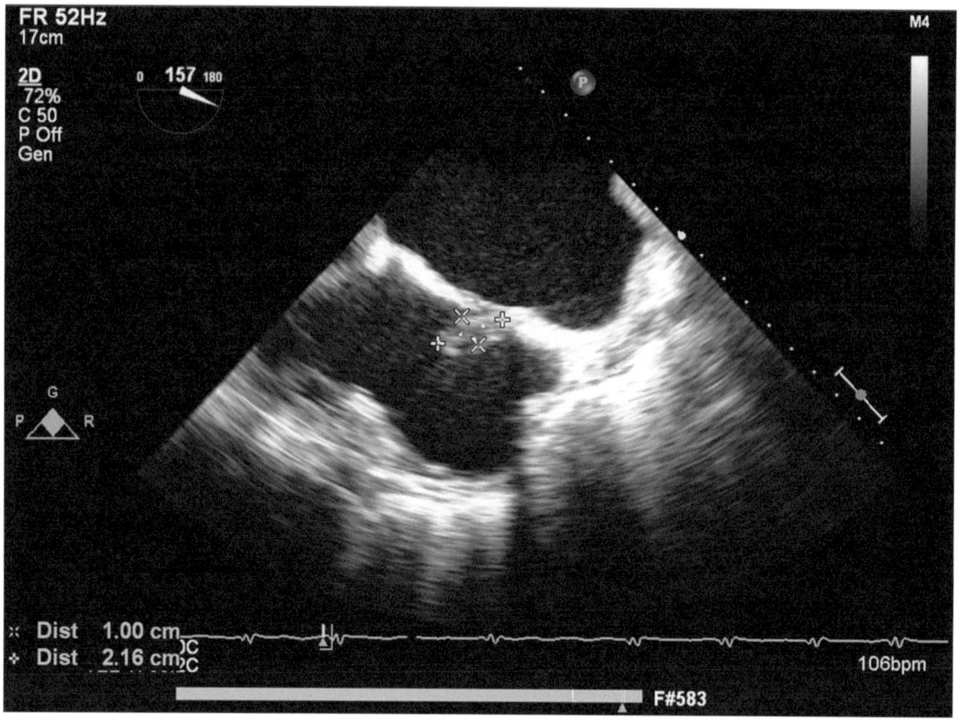

Fig. 38.7 Mobile mass consistent with fresh thrombus on the right side of the atrial septum, on the wire crossing into the left atrium

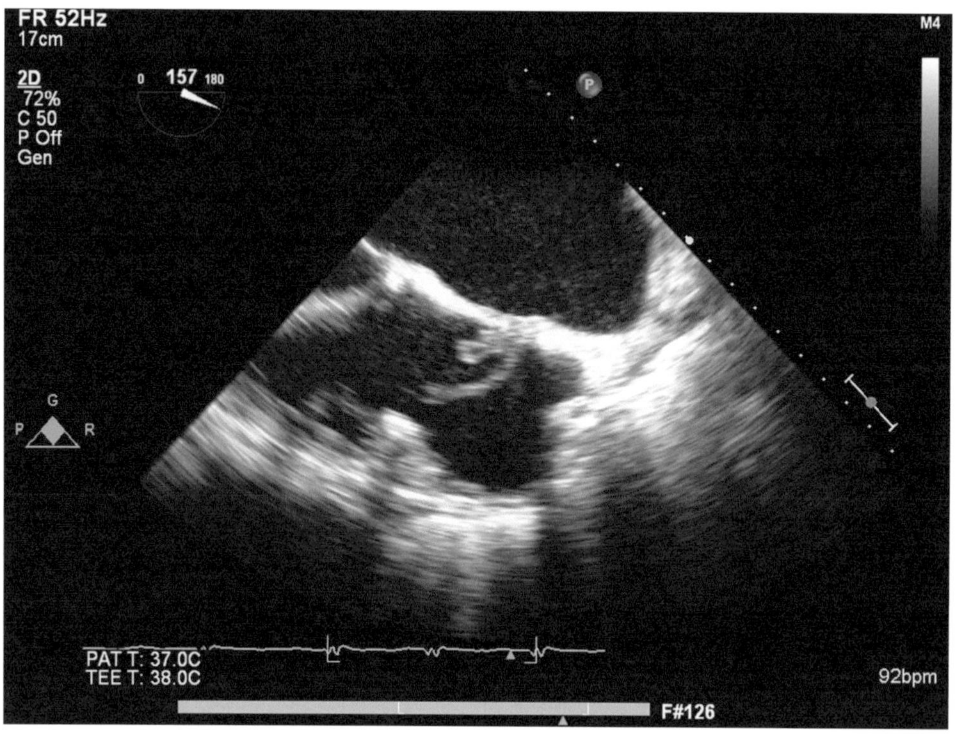

Fig. 38.8 Mobile mass consistent with fresh thrombus on the right side of the atrial septum

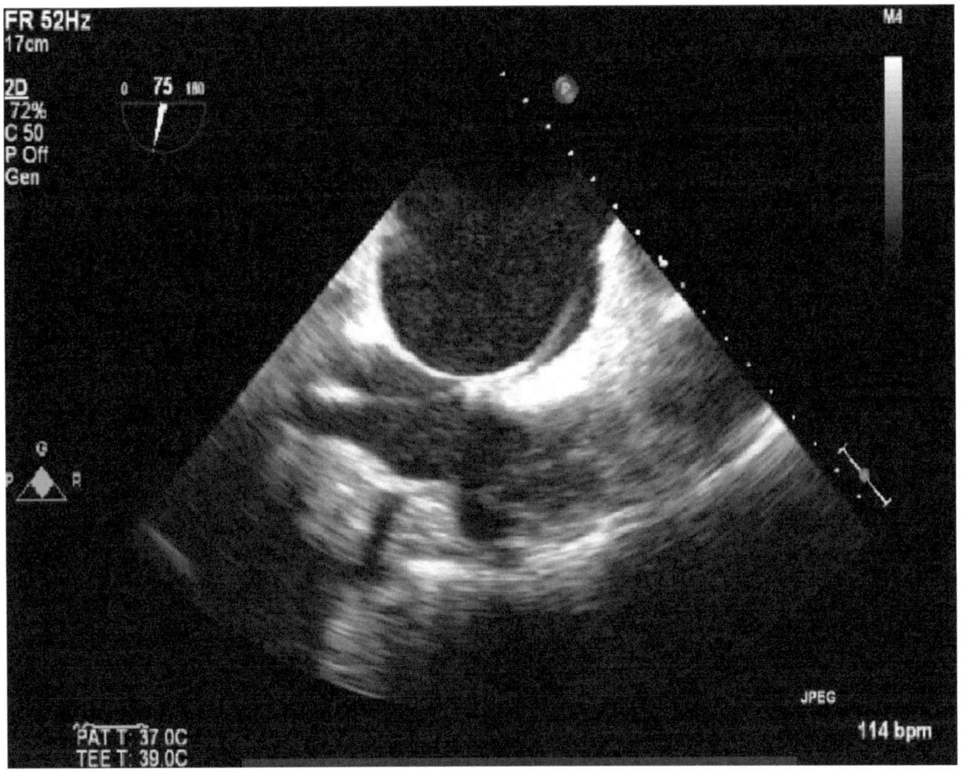

Fig. 38.9 Deflectable sheath tip close to septum to suck the thrombus

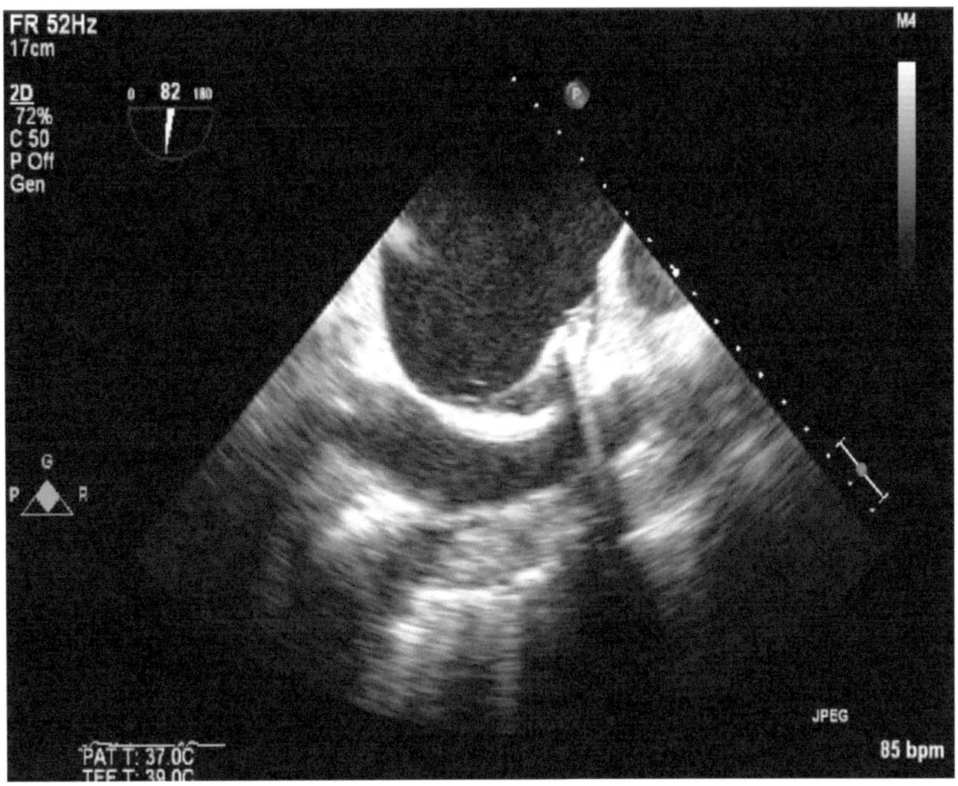

Fig. 38.10 Sheath and clip almost touching the aorta

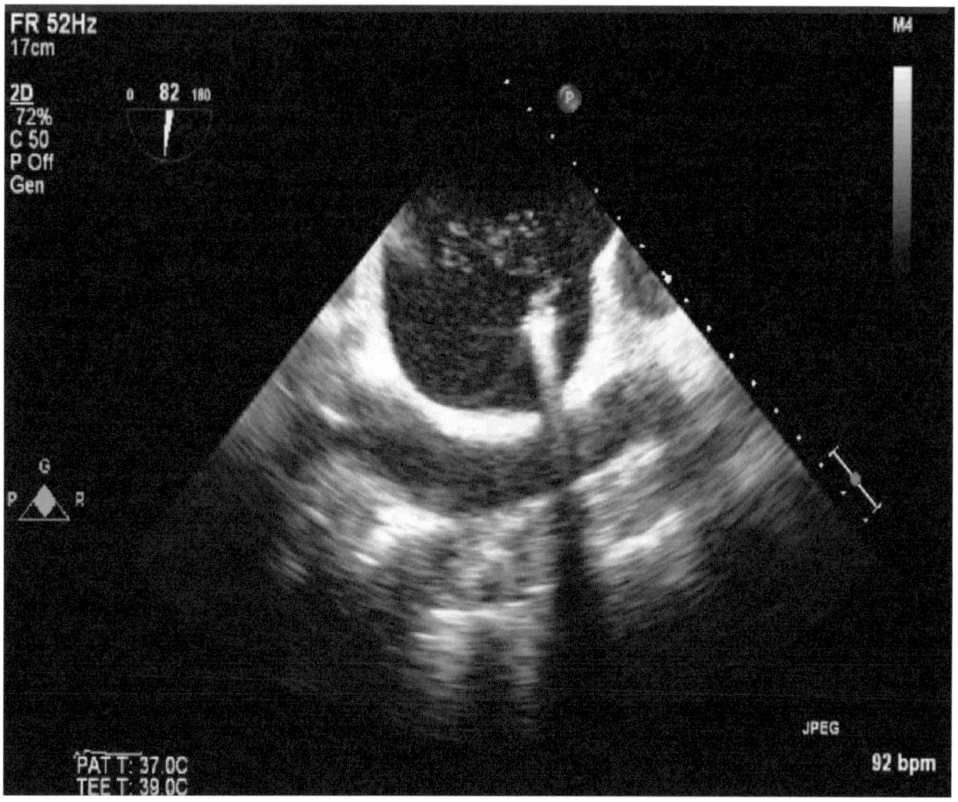

Fig. 38.11 Sheath and clip moving away from the aorta with posterior rotation and some (+) deflection. Clip is being advanced out of the sheath

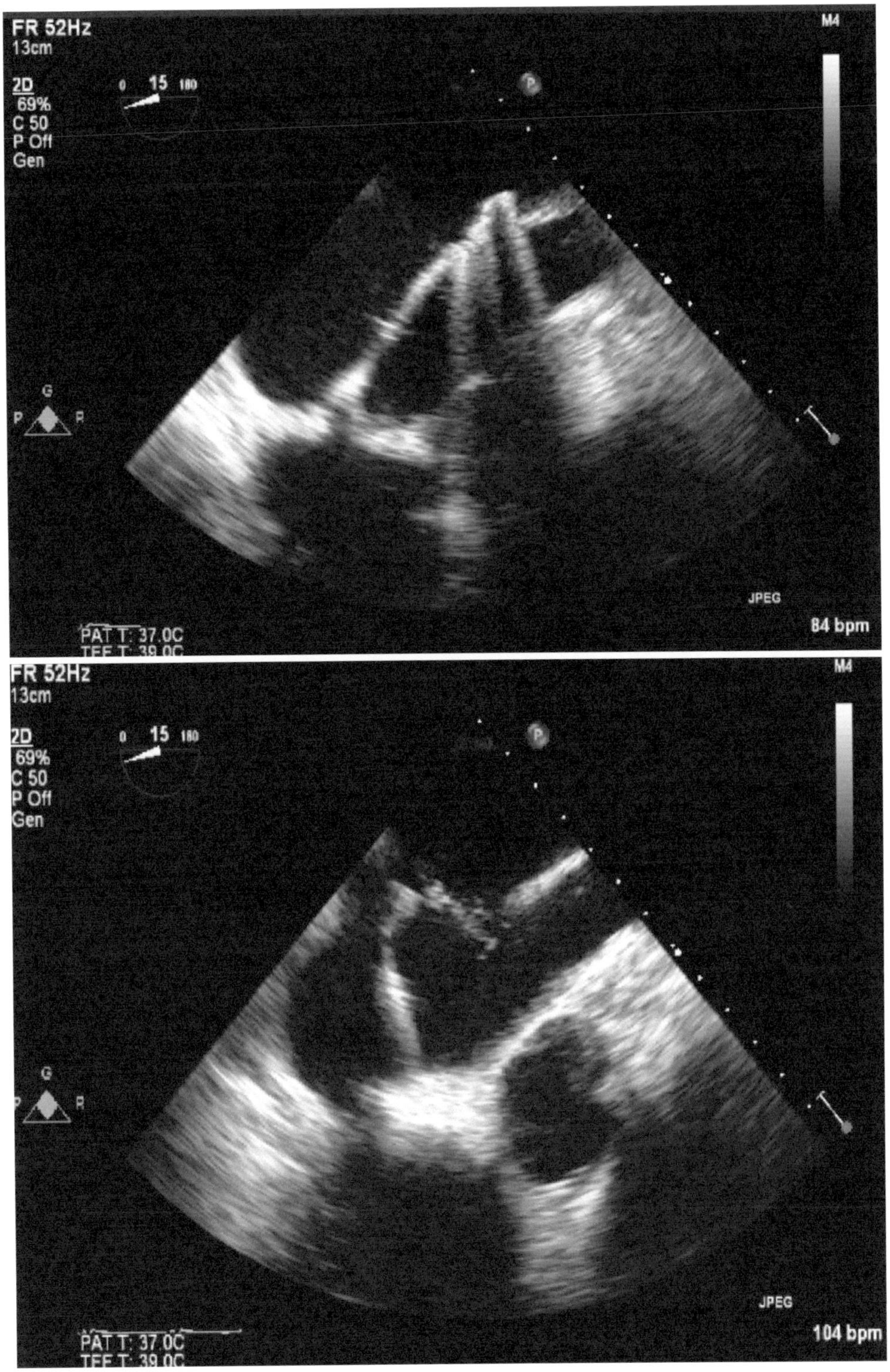

Figs. 38.12, 38.13, and 38.14 Clip advanced out of sheath, posterior rotation and (+) deflection to get away from the left atrial appendage ridge

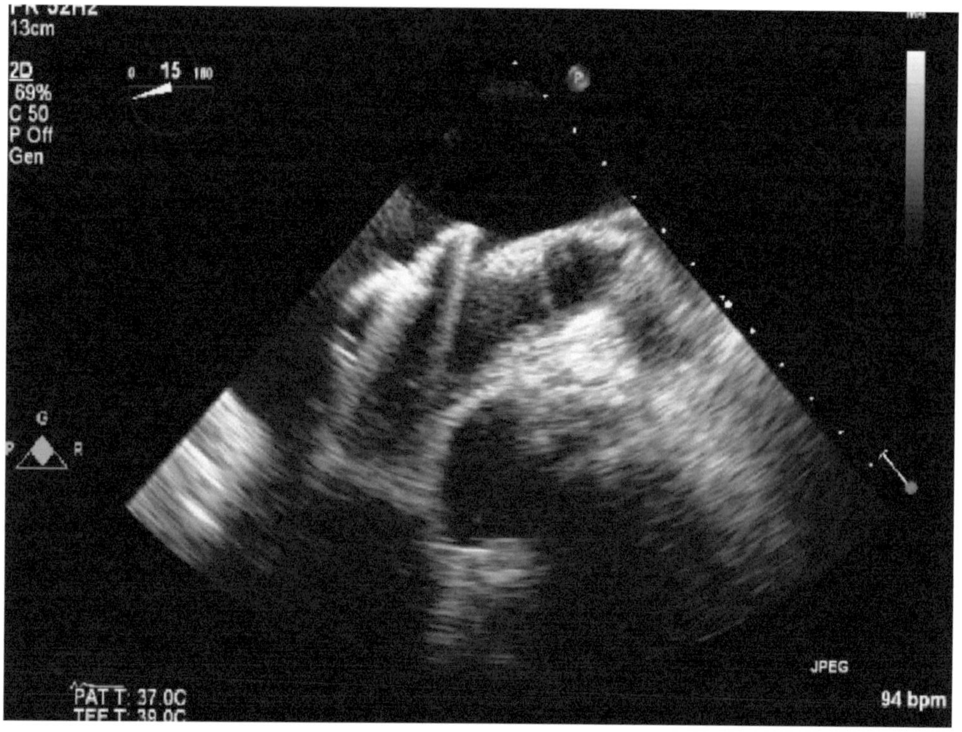

Figs. 38.12, 38.13, and 38.14 (continued)

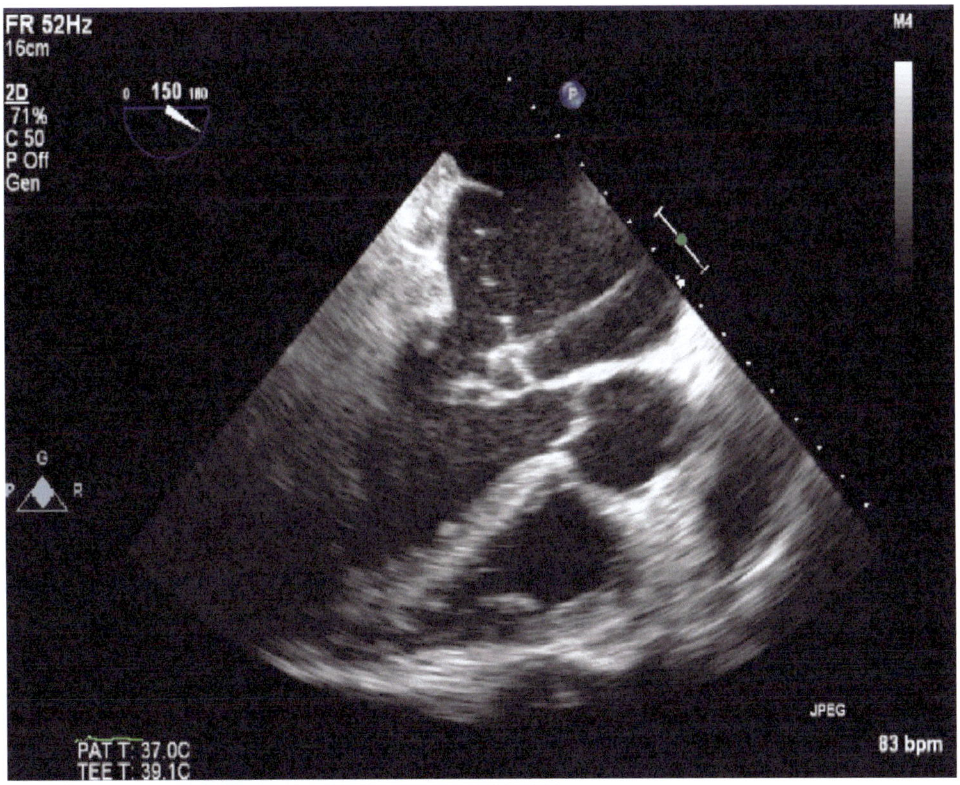

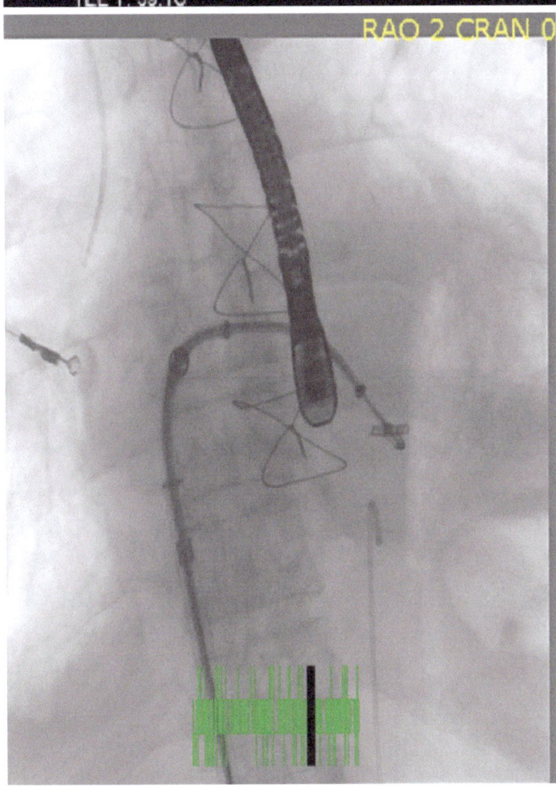

Figs. 38.15 and 38.16 Clip arms are open above the mitral leaflets

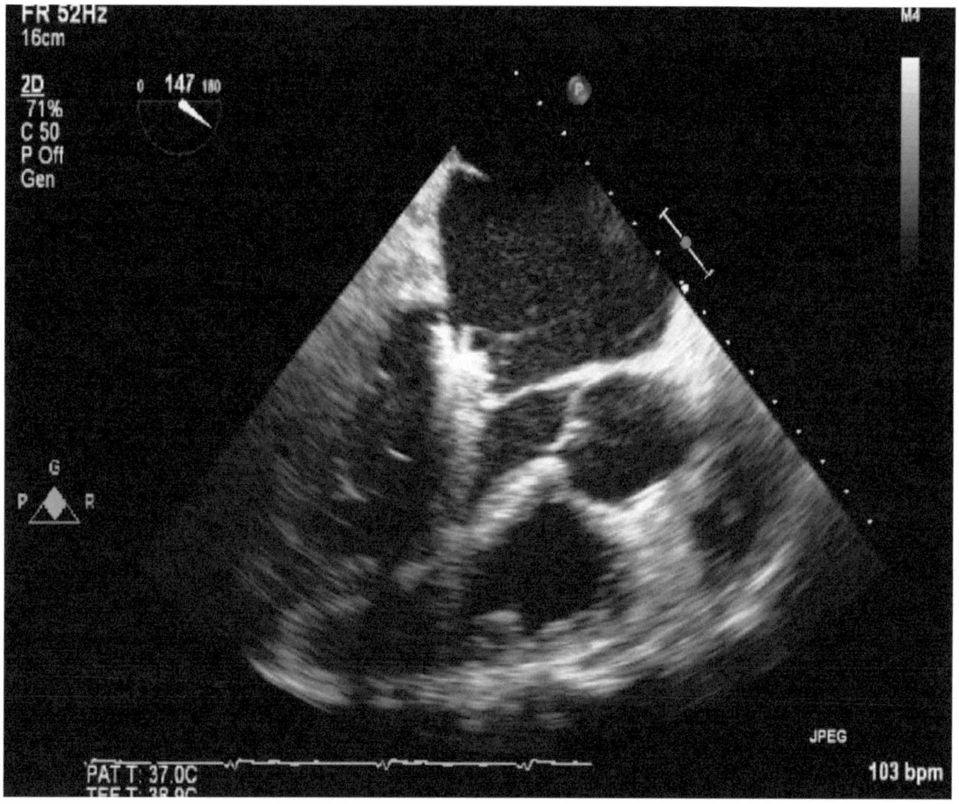

Fig. 38.17 Mitral leaflets are being grasped

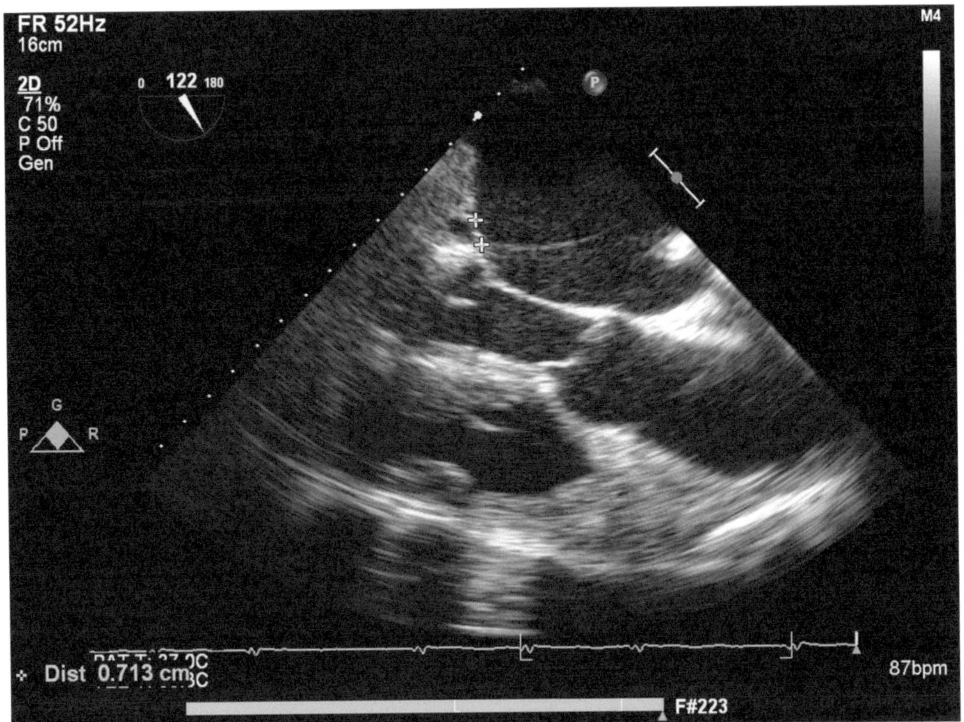

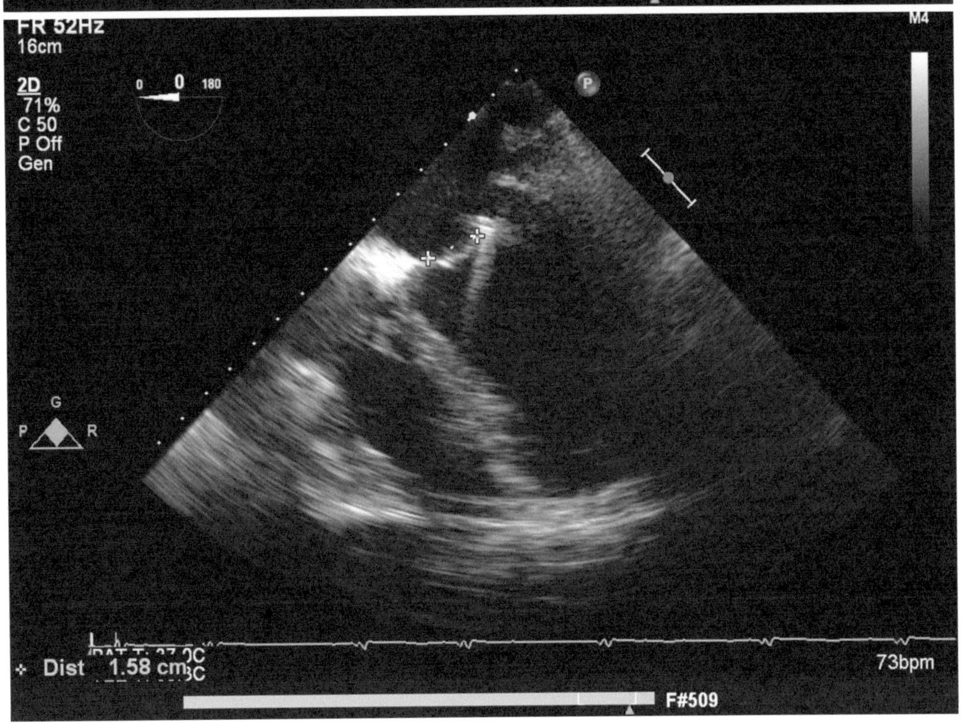

Figs. 38.18 and 38.19 Sufficient mitral leaflet tissue grasped

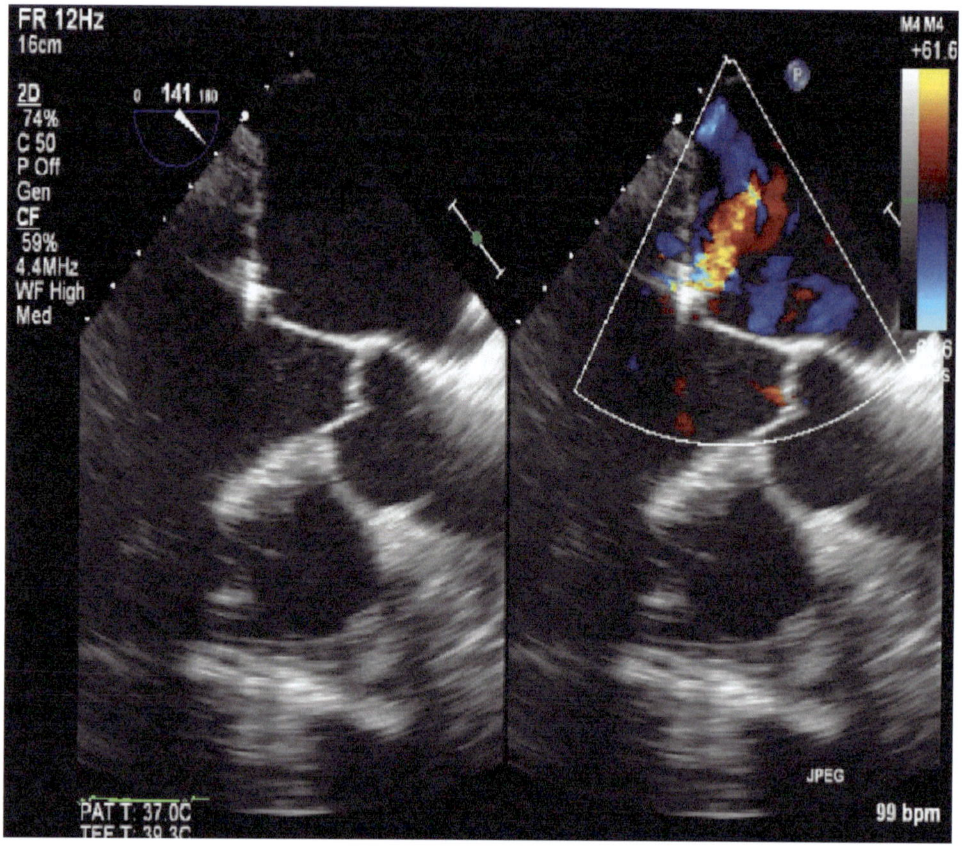

Fig. 38.20 Clip released with decreased mitral regurgitation

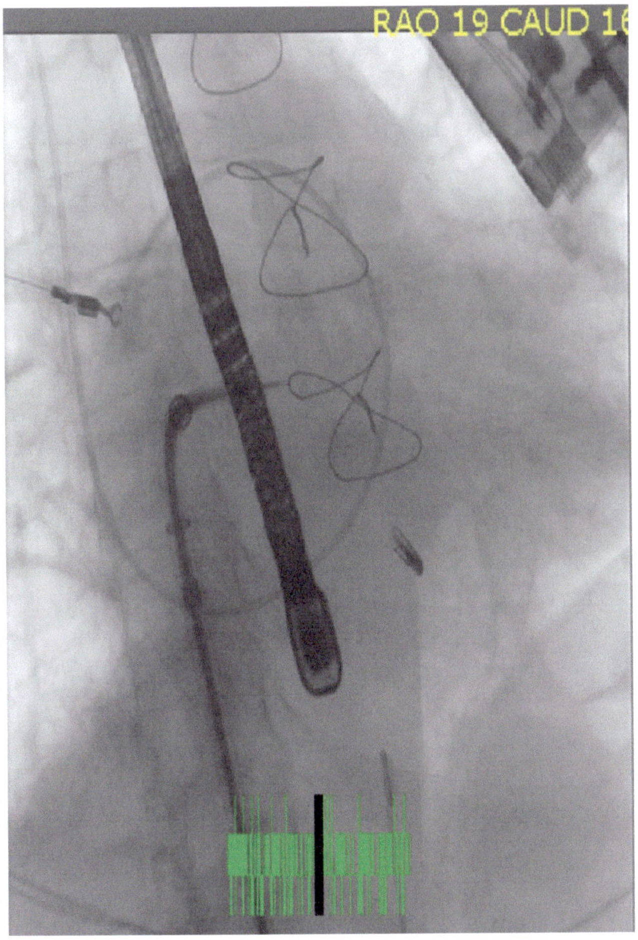

Fig. 38.21 Clip released successfully

MitraClip in a Patient with Dextrocardia and Scoliosis Complicated by Delayed Clip Detachment

39

Niels Erik Nielsen, Jacek Baranowski, Gabriella Boano, Eva Nylander, and Lars Wallby

Abstract

A patient with dextrocardia, scoliosis, restrictive lung disease, severe degenerative mitral regurgitation (MR), and with NYHA Class III heart failure was referred for the MitraClip after unsuccessful surgery. The procedure was complicated by difficult visualization of cardiac anatomy requiring adjunctive imaging with intracardiac echo. Although there was successful leaflet grasp with reduction of MR, the patient deteriorated a few days later with complete clip detachment and return of severe MR.

Keywords

Mitral regurgitation • MitraClip • Scoliosis • Dextrocardia • Intracardiac echo • Clip detachment • Clip embolization

Clinical History

A 68-year-old man was referred for percutaneous mitral valve repair with the MitraClip. He had a history of dextrocardia, previous rickets, scoliosis (Fig. 39.1) with significant lung function impairment since childhood, hypertension, and paroxysmal atrial fibrillation. In 2007, he underwent unsuccessful surgery for severe mitral regurgitation secondary to prolapse of the anterior mitral leaflet (AML). During surgery with median sternotomy, it was impossible to get anatomic access to the atria because of the anatomy, and the patient became hemodynamically unstable during the efforts to do so, and the operation was terminated. A right-sided thoracotomy was discussed, but a decision was made for percutaneous mitral valve repair in the future.

When referred for the MitraClip procedure, he was in NYHA class III. During the procedure it was difficult to visualize the entire atrial septum by transesophageal echo (TEE), and intracardiac echo (ICE) was used for adjunctive imaging (Videos 39.1 and 39.2). Transseptal puncture was done in the superior-posterior rim of the fossa ovalis. The

N.E. Nielsen, M.D., Ph.D. (✉) • L. Wallby, M.D., Ph.D.
Seldinger Unit, Heart Centre, University Hospital, Linköping, Sweden

Department of Cardiology, Heart Centre, University Hospital, Linköping 58185, Sweden
e-mail: niels-erik.nielsen@lio.se; lars.wallby@lio.se

J. Baranowski, M.D., Ph.D.
Seldinger Unit, Heart Centre, University Hospital, Linköping, Sweden

Department of Clinical Physiology, Heart Centre, University Hospital, Linköping 58185, Sweden
e-mail: jacek.baranowski@lio.se

G. Boano, M.D.
Seldinger Unit, Heart Centre, University Hospital, Linköping, Sweden

Department of Thoracic Surgery, Heart Centre, University Hospital, Linköping S-58185, Sweden
e-mail: gabriella.Boano@lio.se

E. Nylander, M.D., Ph.D.
Seldinger Unit, Heart Centre, University Hospital, Linköping, Sweden

Department of Clinical Physiology, Faculty of Health Sciences, Heart Centre, University Hospital, Linköping 58185, Sweden
e-mail: eva.nylander@lio.se

Electronic supplementary material The online version of this chapter (doi:10.1007/978-1-4471-4294-2_39) contains supplementary material, which is available to authorized users.

T. Feldman et al. (eds.), *Atlas of Percutaneous Edge-to-Edge Mitral Valve Repair*, DOI 10.1007/978-1-4471-4294-2_39, © Springer-Verlag London 2013

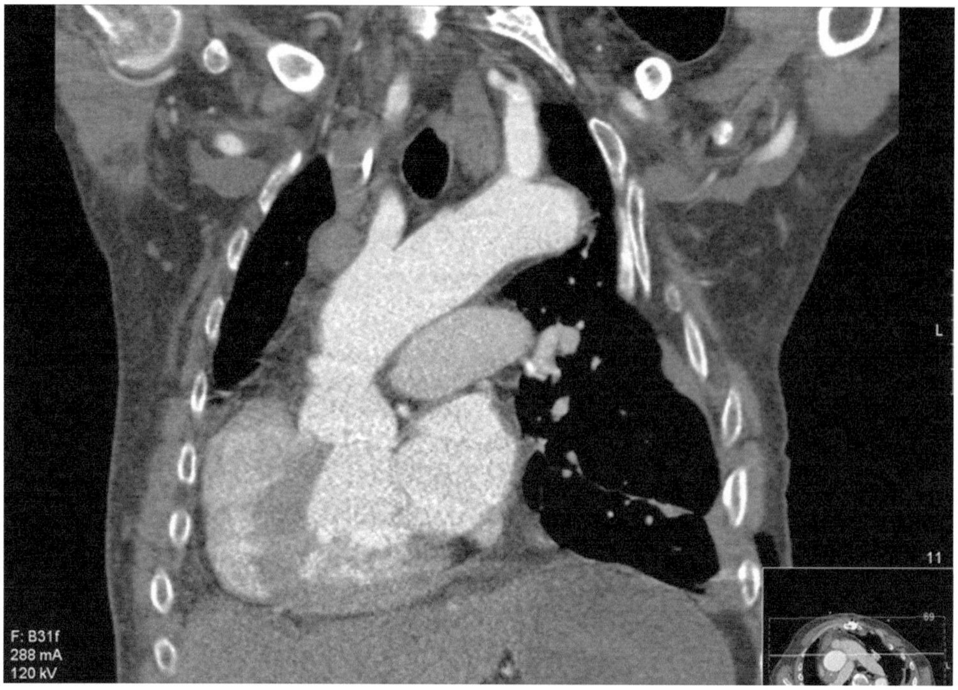

Fig. 39.1 Dextrocardia and scoliosos

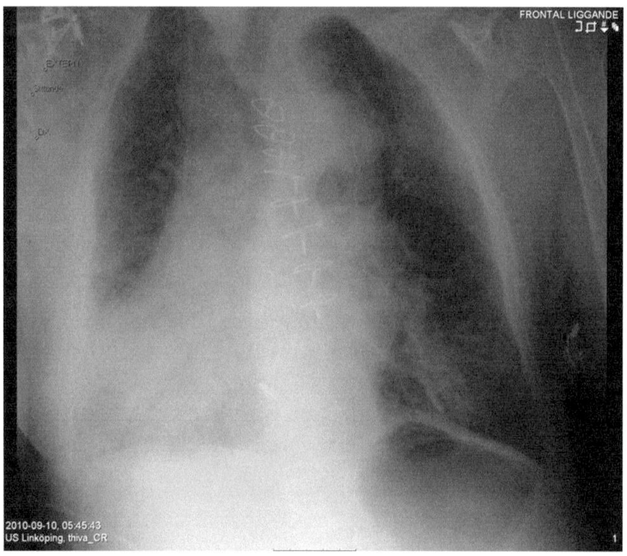

Fig. 39.2 MitraClip in expected position in patient with dextrocardia day 1 post-implant

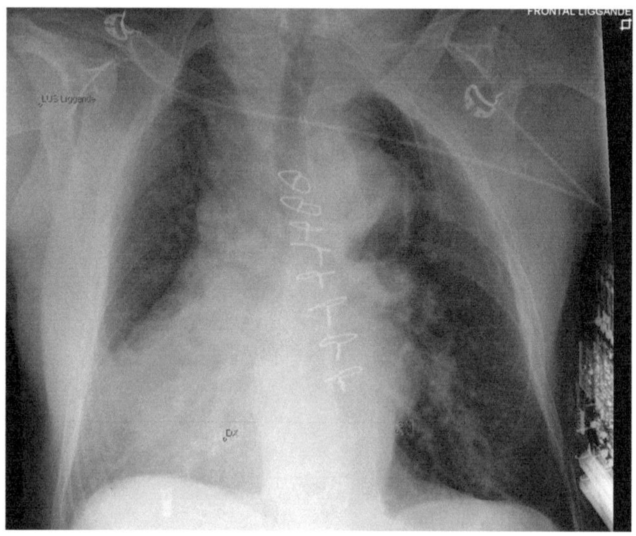

Fig. 39.3 The detached MitraClip is seen at the apex of the heart

MitraClip system was introduced in the usual way, but all through the procedure, the steering of the system was difficult because of the anatomy, and the visualization on echo and fluoro was markedly different from usual. Because of this we had great difficulty in grasping both leaflets. Finally we succeeded with only a small regurgitant jet left. After clip release there was some bulging of the AML, but no prolapse and no clip detachment (Videos 39.3 and 39.4). The result was judged as good, and no further clip was introduced.

Echocardiography the following day showed a somewhat greater mitral regurgitation than immediately after the procedure, and the clip was more mobile (Video 39.5). X-ray showed the clip to be in the expected position with regard to the patient's anatomy (Fig. 39.2). However, the patient was better with less dyspnea. Two days later the patient started to deteriorate with dyspnea. Echocardiography showed severe mitral regurgitation and no clip visible in the valve (Videos 39.6 and 39.7), and chest X-ray revealed the clip lying in the apex of the left ventricle (Fig. 39.3).

The patient rapidly deteriorated with hemodynamic instability and was put on ventilator. A decision was taken to try to retrieve the clip with a snare and place a new MitraClip. The patient was taken to the cath lab. Fluoro showed that the

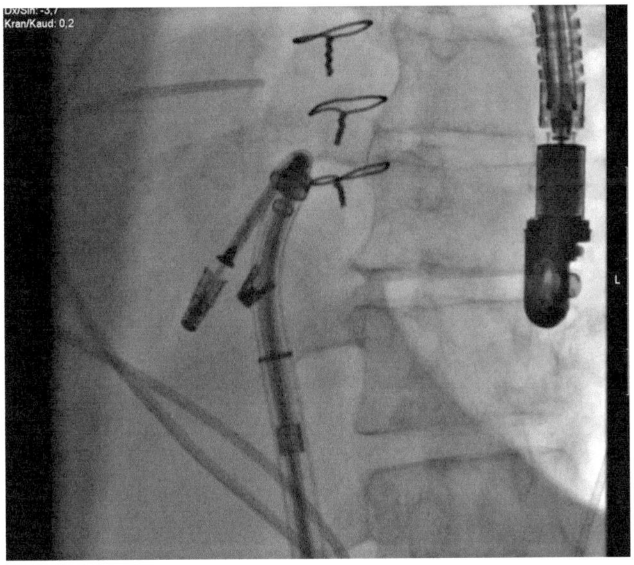

Fig. 39.4 Note the unusual CDS position in the patient with dextrocardia

detached clip was now in the left atrial appendage. We decided to leave it there and instead place a new clip. This was placed laterally in the valve, with some reduction but still significant mitral regurgitation was seen (Video 39.8). We decided to leave this clip and put in another MitraClip for further reduction of the MR and for stabilization of the first clip. The second clip was placed more medially, and a significant reduction of the MR was seen, and TEE showed grasping of both AML and PML, and the clip was released (Video 39.9 and Fig. 39.4). However, few minutes later TEE showed return of significant MR, and the reason being that the second clip had detached from the AML (Videos 39.10 and 39.11).

All through the procedure the patient was hemodynamically very unstable and several times external heart compression was performed to keep up a reasonable circulation. Even after the placement of the second clip the patient had very low cardiac output, and after the second clip detached the patient deteriorated rapidly with biventricular failure in spite of aggressive pharmacological treatment and died in cath lab.

Discussion

This was a very difficult case with a very challenging anatomy. This made the MitraClip procedure and TEE visualization very difficult technically. This, in combination with poor leaflet quality, which can be a problem in some patients with degenerative MR, may be the explanation for the tragic outcome in this patient. As leaflet quality is difficult to judge by any imaging method, the threshold for applying two clips for security should probably be rather low. In retrospect, placing a second clip after the first clip may help stabilize the first clip but this is speculative.

Learning Points

- Unusual anatomy can complicate a MitraClip procedure. This is because the MitraClip procedure is dependent on imaging, predicate standard views, and restricted control of the device once in the body.
- Mitral valve leaflet quality can affect stability of the clip grasp and should be evaluated carefully.
- In patients with poor leaflet quality, a two-clip strategy should be considered.

Massive Air Embolism During MitraClip Insertion

40

Niels Erik Nielsen, Jacek Baranowski, Gabriella Boano, Eva Nylander, and Lars Wallby

Abstract

This case describes massive air embolism occurring a MitraClip procedure. This most likely occurred when the guide catheter was against the left atrial wall, resulting in external air entrainment. There was air embolism to the right coronary artery causing acute myocardial ischemia and ventricular fibrillation. The patient was successfully rescued and recovered. She underwent a successful MitraClip procedure subsequently.

Keywords

Mitral regurgitation • MitraClip • Air embolism

N.E. Nielsen, M.D., Ph.D. (✉) • L. Wallby, M.D., Ph.D.
Seldinger Unit, Heart Centre, University Hospital, Linköping, Sweden

Department of Cardiology, Heart Centre, University Hospital, Linköping, 58185, Sweden
e-mail: niels-erik.nielsen@lio.se, lars.wallby@lio.se

J. Baranowski, M.D., Ph.D.
Seldinger Unit, Heart Centre, University Hospital, Linköping, Sweden

Department of Clinical Physiology, Heart Centre, University Hospital, Linköping, 58185, Sweden
e-mail: jacek.baranowski@lio.se

G. Boano, M.D.
Seldinger Unit, Heart Centre, University Hospital, Linköping, Sweden

Department of Thoracic Surgery, Heart Centre, University Hospital, Linköping, S-58185, Sweden
e-mail: gabriella.boano@lio.se

E. Nylander, M.D., Ph.D.
Seldinger Unit, Heart Centre, University Hospital, Linköping, Sweden

Department of Clinical Physiology, Faculty of Health Sciences, Heart Centre, University Hospital, Linköping, 58185, Sweden
e-mail: eva.nylander@lio.se

Clinical History

A 75-year-old woman with myelodysplastic syndrome and chronic atrial fibrillation was referred for progressive dyspnea on exertion. She was NYHA III heart failure and could only walk slowly for 100 m before stopping. Echocardiography showed significant mitral regurgitation (MR) secondary to left ventricular dilatation and dysfunction, restricted posterior mitral leaflet (PML) motion, and a dilated mitral annulus with consequent leaflet malcoaptation. The surgeons felt she was a poor surgical candidate given her myelodysplasia, and she was referred for the MitraClip.

An uncomplicated septal puncture was performed with insertion of the steerable guide catheter (SGC) to the left atrium (LA). The dilator and extra stiff guidewire were extracted during continuous aspiration as usual. The clip system was introduced into the SGC to the tip of the SGC during continuous infusion of saline. At that time, air was seen in the ascending aorta (AA) on transesophageal echo (TEE), and air was sucked into the right coronary artery (RCA) (Video 40.1). ST elevation was seen on ECG, and the patient's systolic BP dropped to 50 mmHg. The right ventricle became

Electronic supplementary material The online version of this chapter (doi:10.1007/978-1-4471-4294-2_40) contains supplementary material, which is available to authorized users.

T. Feldman et al. (eds.), *Atlas of Percutaneous Edge-to-Edge Mitral Valve Repair*,
DOI 10.1007/978-1-4471-4294-2_40, © Springer-Verlag London 2013

dilated with marked reduced systolic function. A pigtail catheter was introduced through the left femoral artery to the AA, and through the pigtail catheter, large amount of air was aspirated from the AA. The pigtail catheter was switched to a right Judkins catheter, and contrast injection showed that RCA was filled with air (Fig. 40.1 and Video 40.2). Large quantities of air were then sucked out from RCA. Contrast injection now showed filling of RCA, but the patient went into ventricular fibrillation, and she needed defibrillation and external heart compressions. Left-sided coronary angiography showed no air embolism. Because of continuous low BP in spite of good blood flow in RCA, an intra-aortic balloon pump (IABP) was inserted. The procedure was discontinued, and the patient was taken to ICU.

In the following days, the patient initially had signs of multiorgan failure but then improved clinically as well as on echocardiography. The IABP was removed after 3 days, and she was extubated after 5 days. She had no signs of cerebral damage. After 2½ weeks in the hospital, she was discharged.

Six weeks later the patient came for an outpatient visit. She was feeling quite well although still in NYHA III. On echocardiography the RV had recovered. The patient was very persistent to give it another try with MitraClip, "It cannot happen twice," she said. Two months later, the patient underwent another MitraClip procedure without any complications, and at 6 weeks follow-up, she reported a significant physical improvement.

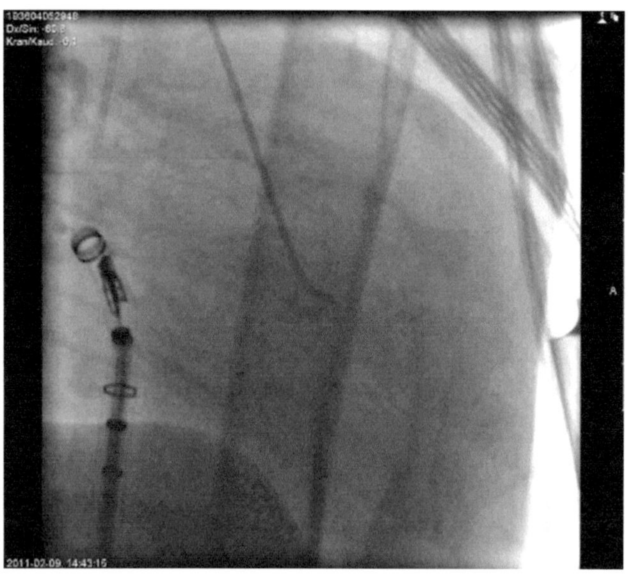

Fig. 40.1 RCA was filled with air

Discussion

After the procedure the entire MitraClip system was thoroughly investigated without any positive findings of leakage. However, when occluding the tip of the SGC and at the same time aspirating through the system, we were able to suck in air through the valve in the SGC. We think that the most probable cause of the air embolism was that the tip of the SGC was too far into the LA, and when we started to retract the guide dilator during aspiration, the tip of the SGC was sucked to the wall of the LA (Video 40.3). This created a negative pressure in the system. We were able to aspirate blood from the distal part of the system, but at the same time, air was sucked in through the valve. When we introduced the MitraClip, we pushed air in front of the MitraClip into the LA.

The MitraClip system is a large caliber, which infers a potential risk for air trapping in the system. The system has limited possibilities for simultaneous pressure recording from the LA, which would be very helpful for judging the effect of the treatment and for discovering if occlusion occurs somewhere in the system. This case highlights the fact that it is crucial throughout the entire procedure to have a very close overview of the system in the LA. It is very easy to "want to be secure" and advance the system too far into the LA, but at the cost of increased risk of serious complications, in this case, air embolism. Another risk may be perforation of the atrial wall.

Learning Points

- Air embolism is a potential serious complication.
- Air embolism can occur if the SGC is against the wall of the LA and air is entrained when blood is aspirated.
- The operator and echocardiologist must be watchful for the SGC being advanced too far into the LA and impinging against the LA wall.
- The echocardiologist has a very crucial role in observing for any unexpected anomalies occurring during the procedure (in this case, air in the ascending aorta).
- Immediate actions to aspirate air from the aorta and coronary arteries, and an intra-aortic balloon pump may be lifesaving.

41 The Degree and Type of Mitral Regurgitation Present at the Baseline Is Not Always a Good Predictor of the Procedural Technical Needs or of the Final Result

Antonio Colombo, Cosmo Godino, and Eustachio Agricola

Abstract
This case describes a case of severe functional mitral regurgitation in which there appeared to be two jets, one central and one at the posteromedial commissure. However, with one central clip, the overall MR was markedly reduced with 1+. This case highlights the strategy of using a central clip first in patients with functional MR and reassessing residual MR after that.

Keywords
Mitral regurgitation • Functional mitral regurgitation • MitraClip

Clinical History

The patient is a 70-year-old male with a history of hypertension, dyslipidemia, chronic renal failure, and prior coronary artery disease. He had a prior inferior MI and had undergone coronary artery bypass surgery, multiple percutaneous coronary interventions, and al so has a defibrillator. He presented with recurrent hospitalizations for NYHA Class III heart failure. His echo showed a depressed LVEF of 35 % with severe mitral regurgitation. His logistic EuroSCORE was 21 % and his STS risk of mortality 6 %.

His echo showed severe functional mitral regurgitation (vena contracta 0.67 cm) with asymmetrical tethering involving the posterior leaflet (Figs. 41.1 and 41.2). The MR was a double jet: an eccentric paracommissural (jet with posteromedial direction, Fig. 41.1, red-dashed border) and a second jet central location (Fig. 41.1, green-dashed border). The leaflet coaptation depth was 1.1 cm; coaptation length was 0.47 cm; and left posterior mitral leaflet residual tissue motion was 1 cm. The left ventricular diastolic diameter was 62 mm with an akinetic inferior and posterior wall. The estimated PA systolic pressure was 40 mmHg.

The patient was referred for the MitraClip procedure in view of the symptomatic severe functional MR. Considering the characteristics of the baseline mitral regurgitation with two jets, one central and one located posteromedially, the need for two clips in a relatively complex procedure was foreseen. To our surprise, the placement of a central clip, inducing a double orifice (Fig. 41.3), reduced both the central jet and the paracommissural jet as well (Videos 41.1 and 41.2) to an MR grade of 1+. This finding highlights a certain degree of unpredictability in which way the final result will be reached. The possibility to add a second or a third clip, in case of persistent mitral

A. Colombo, M.D. (✉)
Cardio-Thoracic-Vascular Department, San Raffaele Institute (IRCCS), Via Olgettina 60, Milan 20132, Italy

Cardiac Catheterisation Laboratory, EMO-GVM Centro Cuore Columbus, Via Michelangelo Buonarroti 48, Milan 20145, Italy
e-mail: info@emocolumbus.it

C. Godino, M.D. • E. Agricola, M.D.
Cardio-Thoracic-Vascular Department, San Raffaele Institute (IRCCS), Via Olgettina 60, Milan 20132, Italy
e-mail: cosmogodino@gmail.com; agricola.eustachio@hsr.it

Electronic supplementary material The online version of this chapter (doi:10.1007/978-1-4471-4294-2_41) contains supplementary material, which is available to authorized users.

regurgitation, gives the MitraClip procedure further options if the initial clip did not have a good result. In other words, what appears complex can became simple, and what appears simple can became complex. A careful and thoughtful conduct of the procedure will lead to a desirable outcome.

Learning Points

- In patients with functional MR, although it can appear that there are multiple jets potentially requiring multiple clips, one central clip may result in reduction of all areas of MR.

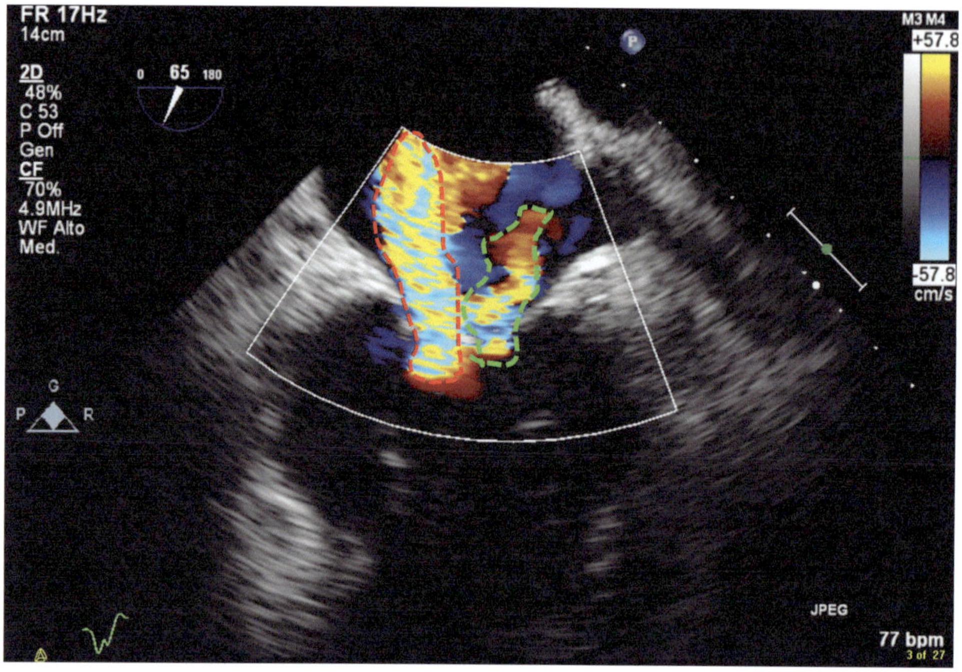

Fig. 41.1 Transesophageal echocardiography (*TEE*) two-chamber view. The picture shows severe mitral regurgitation consists of two jets, one posteromedial (*red-dashed border*) and one central (*green-dashed border*)

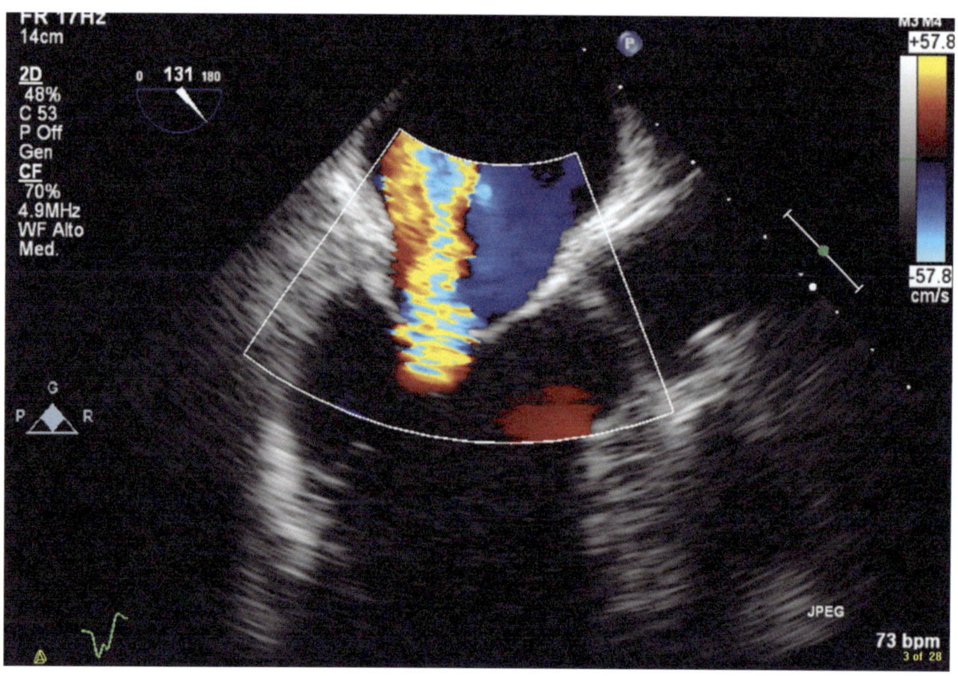

Fig. 41.2 Transesophageal echocardiography (*TEE*) long-axis view. The picture shows severe ischemic mitral regurgitation (vena contracta 0.67 cm)

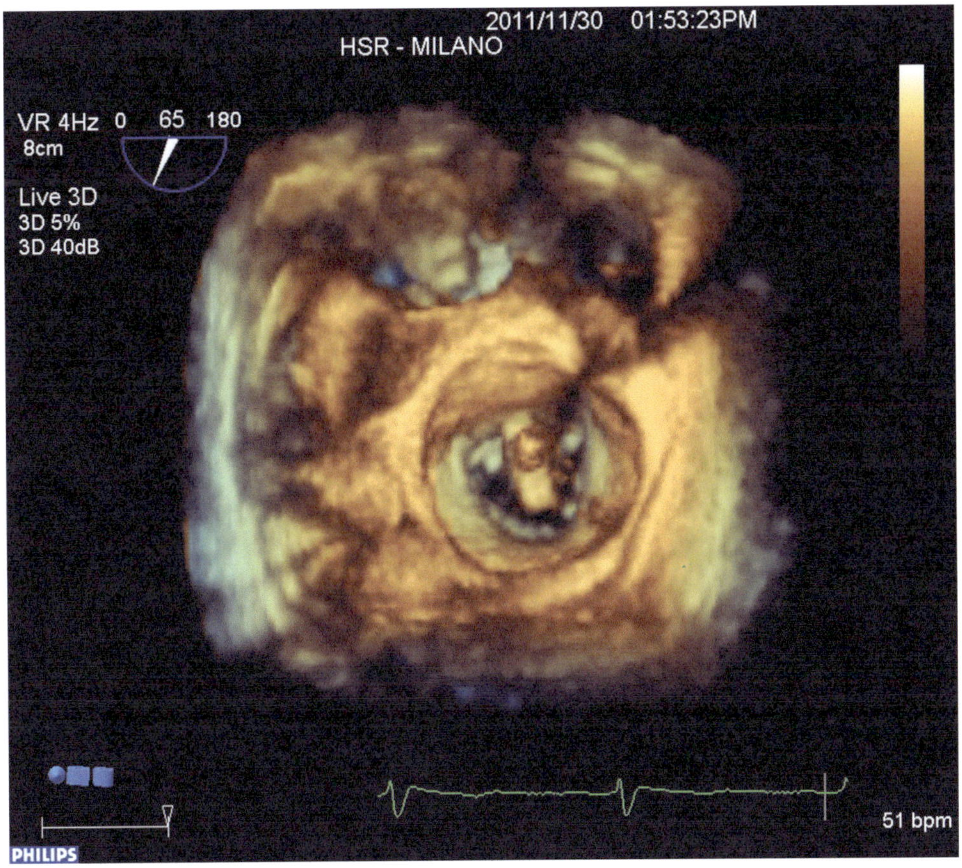

Fig. 41.3 3D TEE with the "surgeon's" view. The picture shows the precise orientation and positioning of the MitraClip in the central part of the mitral annulus

42 Functional Mitral Regurgitation with a Wide Extension of the Central Regurgitant Jet

Gry Dahle, Kai A. Andersen, Magne Brekke, and Kjell Arne Rein

Abstract
In this case, a patient with severe and extensive functional MR was treated with two MitraClips® with dramatic improvement in the MR severity and functional status. The two MitraClips® were placed some distance from each other because of the wide and extensive nature of the regurgitation, creating a three-orifice mitral valve.

Keywords
Mitral regurgitation • MitraClip® • Functional mitral regurgitation • Triple orifice

Introduction

The surgical edge-to-edge technique making a double orifice [1] is a versatile procedure for mitral valve repair and at present is also emulated percutaneously with the MitraClip® system [2, 3]. A triple-orifice technique has also been reported for surgical repair of the scarred, retracted mitral leaflets, creating three instead of two openings through the valve. This might give improved hemodynamics [4]. In some small series, this triple-orifice technique for treating mitral regurgitation (MR) has been used with good outcomes [5–7]. We demonstrate a patient with a wide extension of a central, functional mitral regurgitation with residual leakage following the first clip application. This regurgitation was considerably reduced upon placement of a second MitraClip® at some distance from the first, creating a triple orifice appearance of the mitral valve.

G. Dahle, M.D. (✉) • K.A. Andersen, M.D., Ph.D.
• K. A. Rein, M.D., Ph.D.
Department of Cardiothoracic Surgery,
Rikshospitalet, Oslo University Hospital,
Sognsvannsvein 20, Oslo 0855, Norway
e-mail: gdahle@ous-hf.no, g_dahle@hotmail.com;
kanderse@ous-hf.no; kjrein@ous-hf.no

M. Brekke, M.D.
Department of Radiology, Ullevål, Oslo University Hospital,
Kirkevn 166, Oslo 0450, Norway
e-mail: magbre@ous-hf.no

Clinical History

A 55-year-old man with a severe ischemic MR was admitted to the local hospital for severe congestive heart failure in July 2011. He had undergone several PCI treatments during the last 10 years as well as CRTD implantation in 2007. He had a dilated left ventricle with an EF of 20 %, MR grade IV, and was in NYHA functional class IV. Angiography showed no new stenoses, and his stents were patent. Heart transplantation was not an option due to social issues, and he was considered a high surgical risk for conventional mitral valve repair surgery. Following careful echo evaluation he was accepted for MitraClip® implantation.

The patient underwent successful MitraClip® repair with two clips as shown in the following Figs. 42.1, 42.2, 42.3, 42.4, and 42.5. At follow-up, he is in good clinical condition, going from NYHA class IV to NYHA class II. The quality of life has ameliorated, and he performs the daily work without any hesitation.

T. Feldman et al. (eds.), *Atlas of Percutaneous Edge-to-Edge Mitral Valve Repair*,
DOI 10.1007/978-1-4471-4294-2_42, © Springer-Verlag London 2013

Learning Points

- Two or more MitraClips® are often used to eliminate mitral regurgitation. Most often these are placed parallel to each other and close together. In some cases of central regurgitation with great extension, the use of two Mitraclips® separated by some distance may be useful to create a triple orifice mitral valve. This can be done with good hemodynamics and low gradient as long as the opening area of the valve is big enough (>4 cm^2).

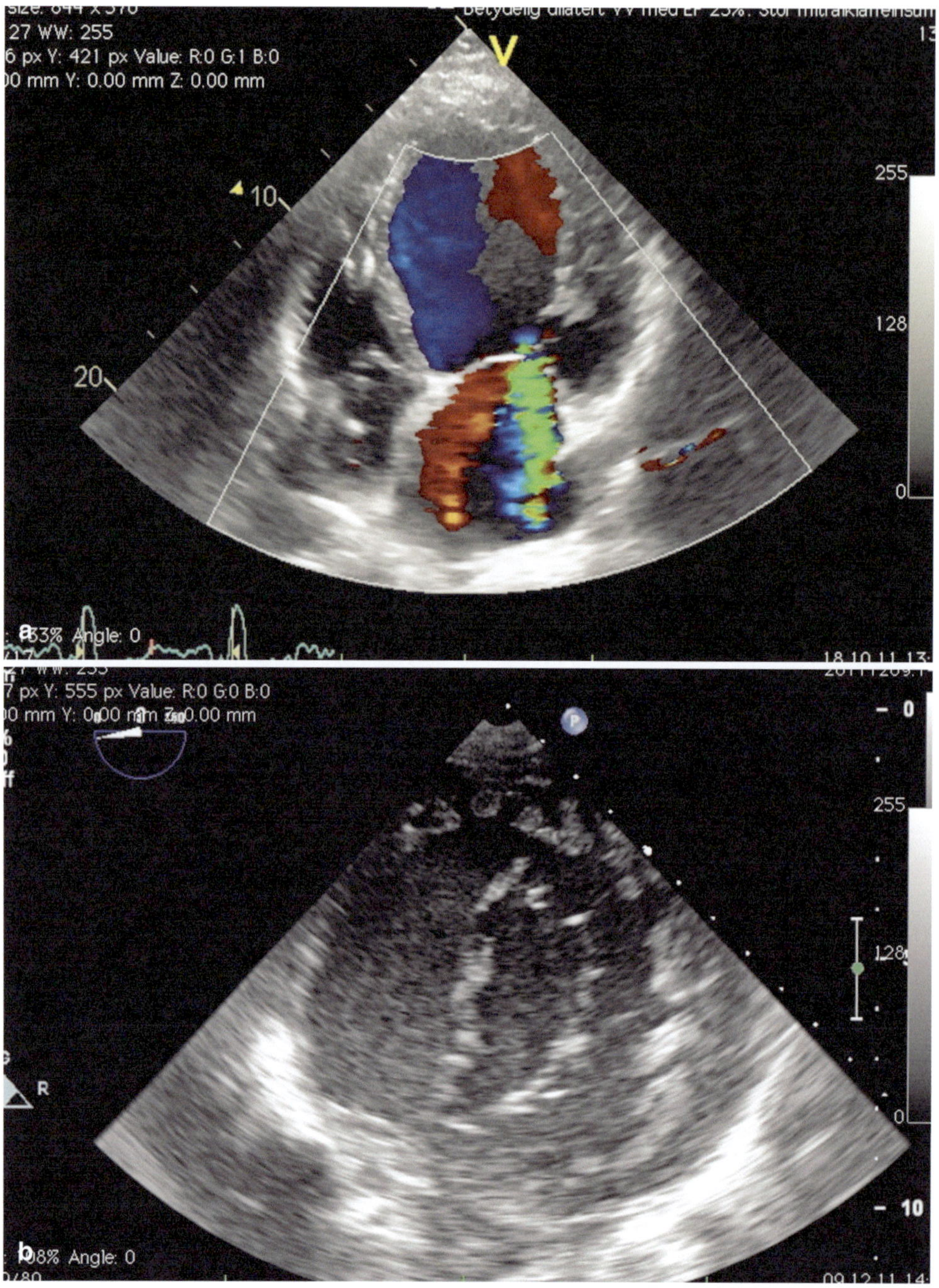

Fig. 42.1 Transesophageal echo demonstrated very extensive mitral regurgitation located centrally between A2 and P2, dilated mitral annulus (4.4 × 4.8 cm) with mal-coaptation of leaflets due to tenting of the leaflets. Coaptation depth 13 mm, coaptation length 2 mm. Four-chamber view (**a**) showing a very large, central mitral regurgitation reaching the roof of the left atrium. In the transgastric, short axis view (**b**) we measured the opening area of the mitral orifice to be more than 4 cm^2. In the intercommissural two-chamber view with color (**c**) and without color (**d**), we perceived two separate jets. This was mainly due to the wide extension of the regurgitation and the angulation of the echo probe, making an overly anterior transection across the anterior mitral leaflet

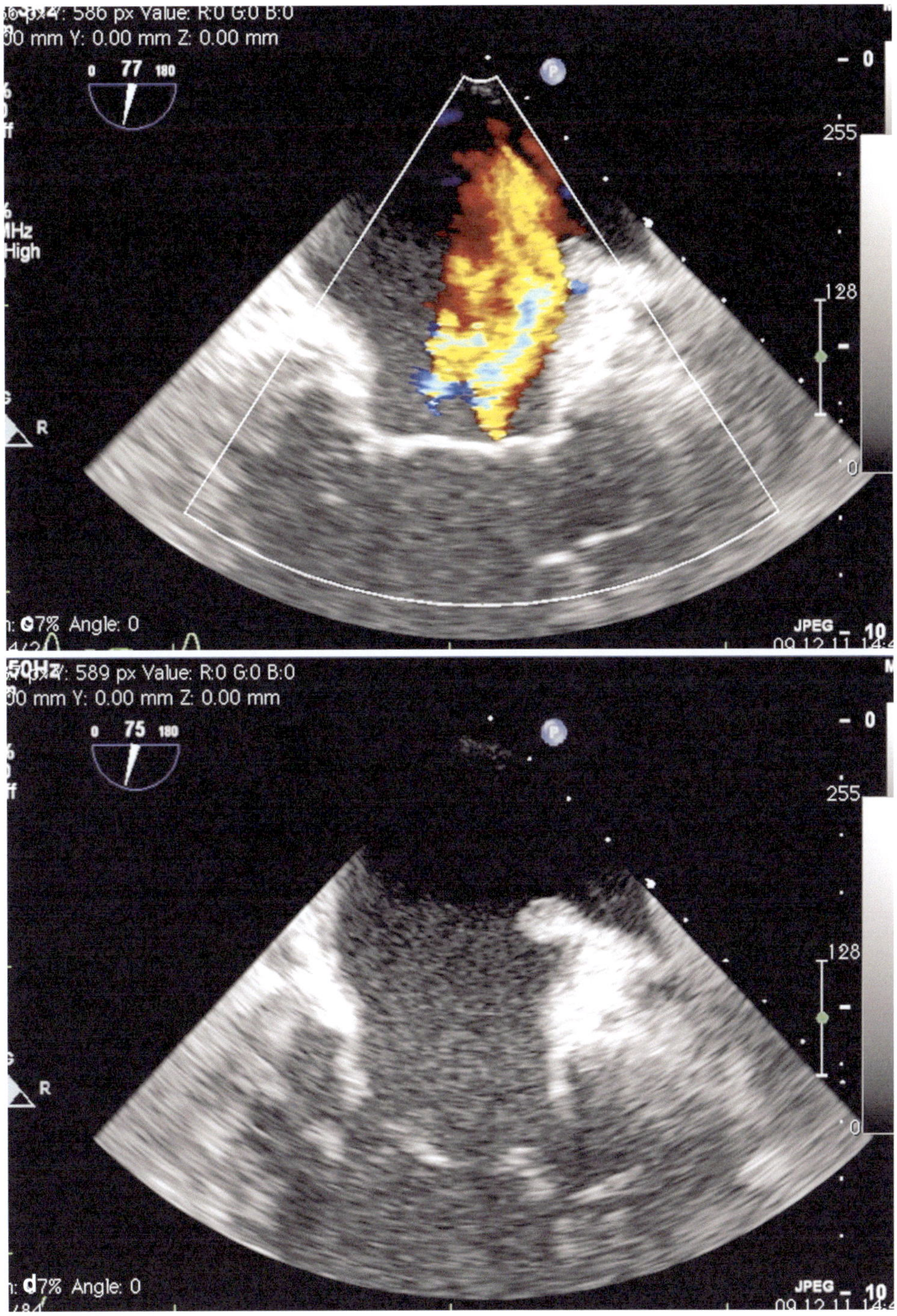

Fig. 42.1 (continued)

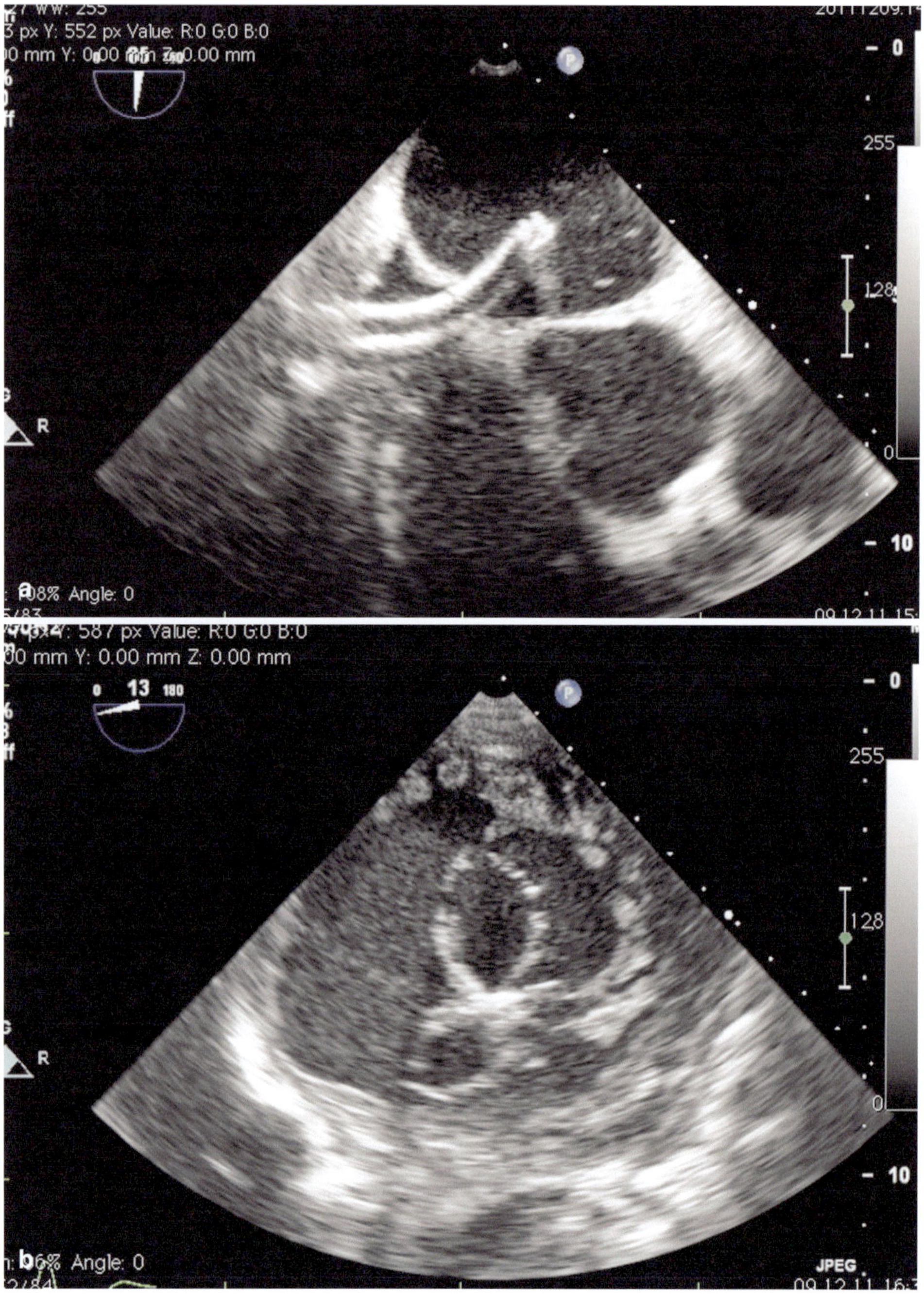

Fig. 42.2 The first clip was placed centrally creating the usual double orifice configuration of the valve. Due to the extensive regurgitation, one clip was not sufficient. (**a**) The Steerable Guide Catheter (*SG*) containing the Clip Delivery System (*CDS*) punctured through the septum some few millimeters into the left atrium. (**b**) A transgastric, short axis view with the double orifice appearance after implantation of one single clip. (**c**) The intercommissural, two-chamber view showing still significant regurgitation in the lateral part of the A2/P2 segments

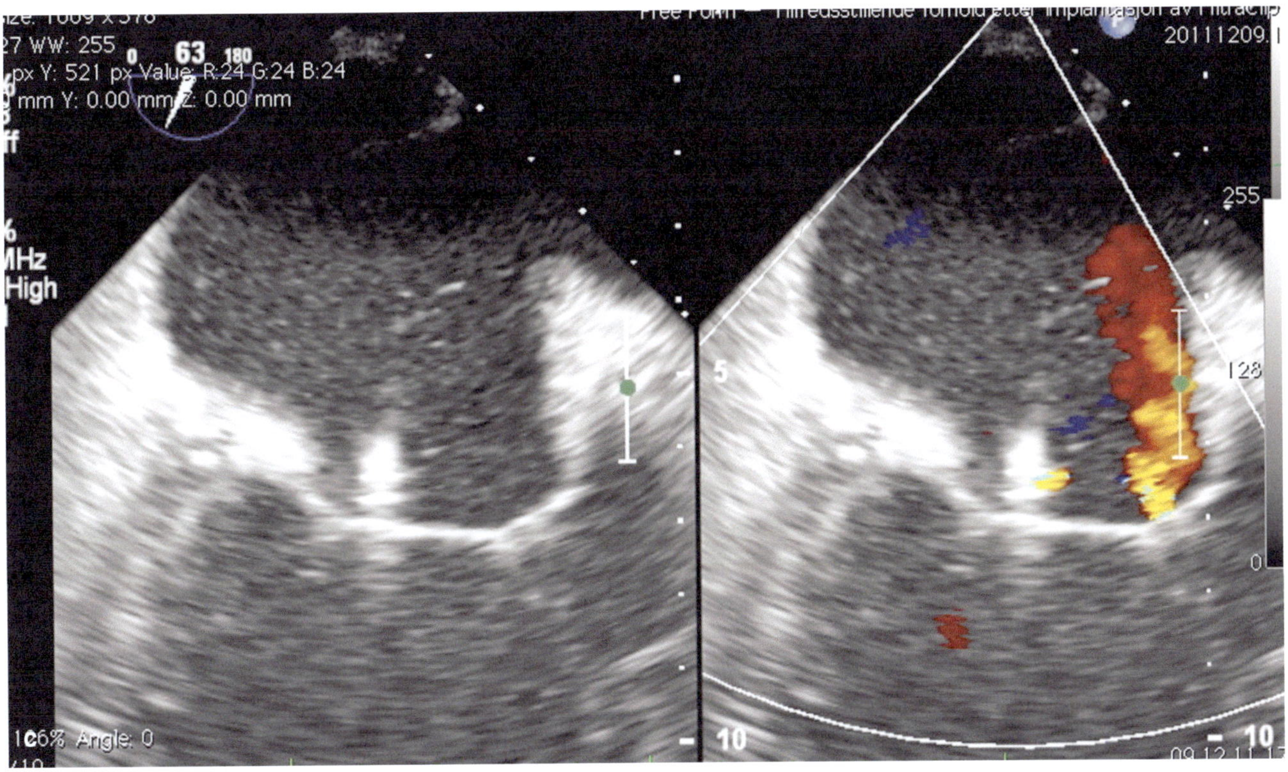

Fig. 42.2 (continued)

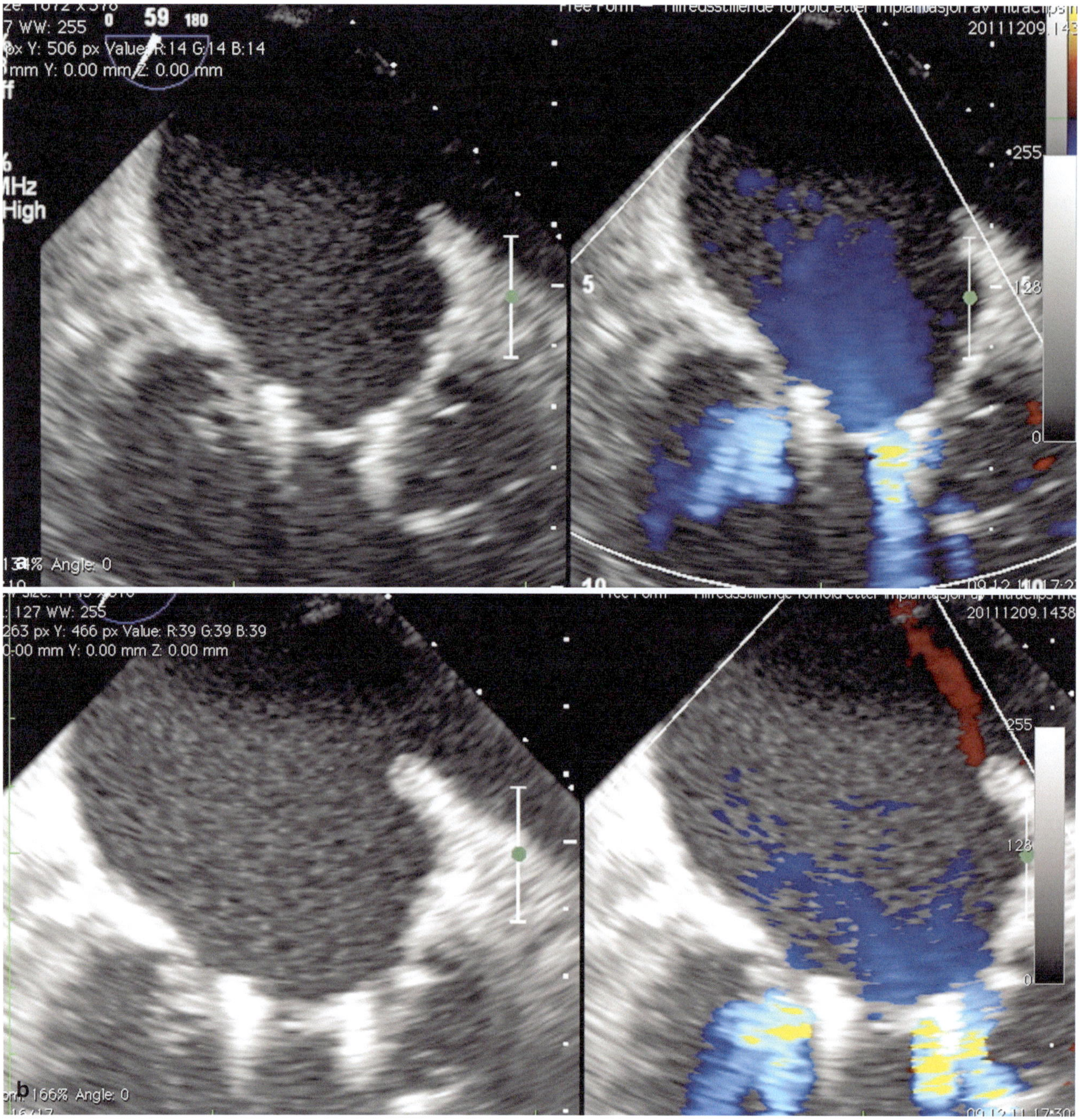

Fig. 42.3 A second clip was placed more laterally at some distance from the first one, where the residual regurgitant jet was most pronounced (**a**). The regurgitation was thereby reduced from grade 4 to only trace. The overall mitral gradient was less than 3 mmHg. Importantly, one could observe antegrade flow in all the three orifices (**a**, **b**) demonstrating the triple orifice opening of the mitral valve

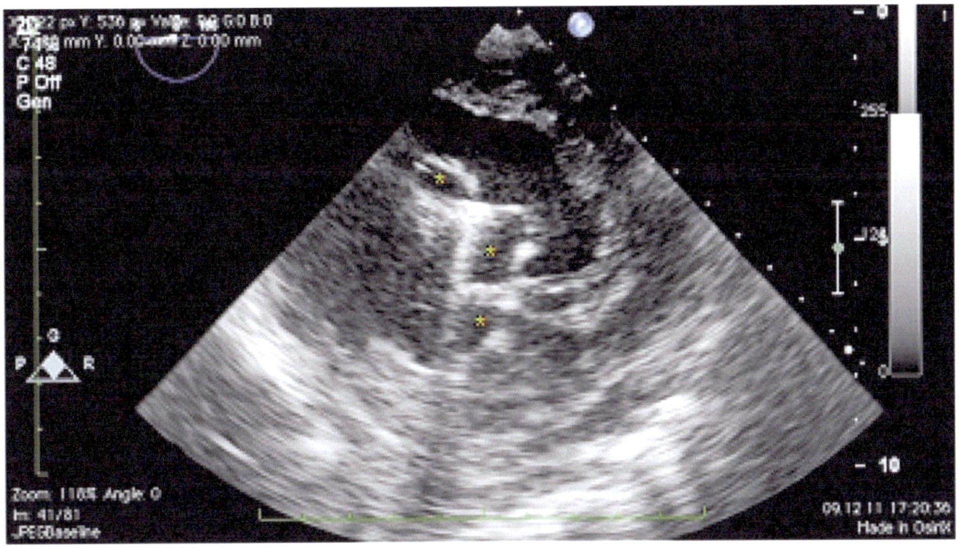

Fig. 42.4 This triple orifice appearance of the mitral valve like a clover was also demonstrated in the transgastric, short axis view. The asterisk depicts the three orifices

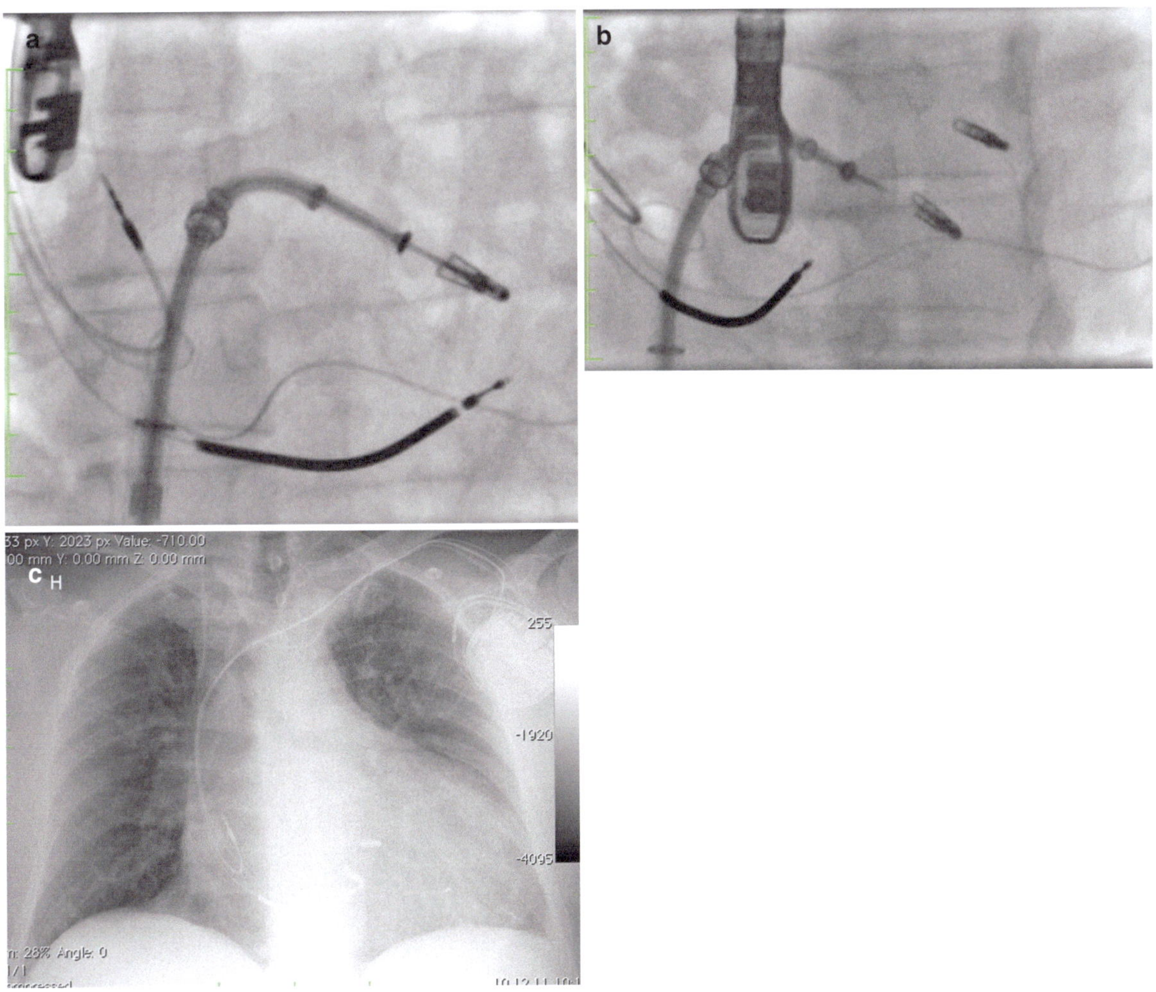

Fig. 42.5 Following the first clip deployment (**a**) shown on fluoroscopy, the second clip was implanted at quite a distance from the first one (**b**), where on echocardiography, the maximal residual regurgitant jet was observed. The distance between the two MitraClips® was also recorded on a chest X-ray the following day (**c**)

References

1. Maisano F, Schreuder JJ, Oppizzi N, Fiorani B, Fino C, Alfieri O. The double-orifice technique as a standardized approach to treat mitral regurgitation due to severe myxomatous disease: surgical technique. Eur J Cardiothorac Surg. 2000;17(3):201–5.
2. Tamburino C, Ussia GP, Maisano F, Capodanno D, La Canna G, Scandura S, Colombo A, Giacomini A, Michev I, Mangiafico S, Cammalleri V, Barbanti M, Alfieri O. Percutaneous mitral valve repair with the MitraClip system: acute results from a real world setting. Eur Heart J. 2010;31(11):1382–9.
3. Maisano F, La Canna G, Colombo A, Alfieri O. The evolution from surgery to percutaneous mitral valve interventions. J Am Coll Cardiol. 2011;58(21):2174–82.
4. Aaron BL, Lower RR. Advantages of open mitral commissurotomy using a triple-orifice technique. Ann Thorac Surg. 1975;19(6):654–8.
5. Fucci C, Faggiano P, Nardi M, D'Aloia A, Coletti G, De Cicco G, Latini L, Vizzardi E, Lorusso R. Triple-orifice valve repair in severe Barlow disease with multiple-jet mitral regurgitation: Report of mid-term experience. Int J Cardiol. (2012) (In Press).
6. Cianciulli TF, Lax JA, Saccheri MC, Morita LA, Picone VP, Prezioso HA. Echocardiographic evaluation of mitral valve repair by modified "edge to edge" technique. Echocardiography. 2006;23(9):771–3.
7. Faletra F, Grimaldi A, Pasotti E, Klimusina J, Evangelista A, Alfieri O, Moccetti T, Pedrazzini G. Real-time 3-dimensional transesophageal echocardiography during double percutaneous mitral edge-to-edge procedure. JACC Cardiovasc Imaging. 2009;2:1031–3.

Percutaneous Edge-to-Edge Mitral Valve Repair for Functional Mitral Regurgitation in a High-Surgical-Risk Patient

43

Dominique Himbert, Eric Brochet, David Messika-Zeitoun, Gregory Ducrocq, Jean Michel Juliard, Bernard Iung, and Alec Vahanian

Abstract

This case describes the use of the MitraClip to treat severe functional MR in an acutely decompensated high-surgical-risk patient.

Keywords

Mitral regurgitation • MitraClip • Functional mitral regurgitation • High surgical risk

Clinical History

An 87-year-old woman was admitted due to recurrent episodes of acute pulmonary edema. In January 2011, she suffered an anterior acute myocardial infarction, which was treated by late revascularization of the left anterior descending artery. Myocardial infarction was complicated by congestive heart failure and atrioventricular block, which required a permanent pacemaker. During the next few months, several episodes of congestive heart failure occurred in conjunction with left ventricular dysfunction and dilatation and severe functional mitral regurgitation (MR). Ventricular resynchronization was then performed. However, despite resynchronization and optimal medical therapy, heart failure worsened. At admission, her hemodynamic condition was unstable, with daily pulmonary edema requiring noninvasive ventilation. Physical examination showed signs of severe mitral regurgitation with clear congestive heart failure. Chest X-ray showed cardiac enlargement and pulmonary edema. Transthoracic (TTE) and transesophageal echocardiography (TEE) (Fig. 43.1a) showed severe functional MR with left ventricular dysfunction (ejection fraction 30 %) (Fig. 43.1b) and pulmonary hypertension (systolic pulmonary artery pressure 80 mmHg) (Fig. 43.1c). Due to the prohibitive surgical risk (EuroSCORE 80 %), an edge-to-edge percutaneous mitral repair was considered by consensus of a medical-surgical team. TEE showed anatomical mitral characteristics compatible with the technique (Fig. 43.2 and Videos 43.1, 43.2).

The procedure was performed on January 10, 2012. It was technically simple and clinically uneventful. It succeeded in achieving a dramatic reduction of MR volume after implantation of one MitraClip (Figs. 43.3, 43.4, 43.5, 43.6 and Videos 43.3, 43.4). The postoperative period was not complicated; there was an immediate improvement in the hemodynamic condition, and no recurrent pulmonary edema occurred. Predischarge TTE showed the MitraClip in good position with mild residual MR (Fig. 43.6), stable left ventricular ejection fraction, and normalization of pulmonary pressures (Figs. 43.7 and 43.8). The patient was discharged at day 7 post procedure. At 1-month follow-up, there was no clinical event, and the patient remained asymptomatic.

D. Himbert, M.D. (✉) • E. Brochet, M.D. • D. Messika-Zeitoun, M.D.
G. Ducrocq, M.D. • J.M. Juliard, M.D. • B. Iung, M.D., Ph.D.
A. Vahanian, M.D., Ph.D.
Department of Cardiology, AP-HP, Bichat Hospital,
46 Rue Henri Huchard, Paris 75018, France
e-mail: dominique.himbert@bch.aphp.fr; eric.brochet@bch.aphp.fr; david.messika-zeitoun@bch.aphp.fr; gregory.ducrocq@bch.aphp.fr; jean-michel.juliard@bch.aphp.fr; bernard.iung@bch.aphp.fr; alec.vahanian@bch.aphp.fr

Electronic supplementary material The online version of this chapter (doi:10.1007/978-1-4471-4294-2_43) contains supplementary material, which is available to authorized users.

T. Feldman et al. (eds.), *Atlas of Percutaneous Edge-to-Edge Mitral Valve Repair*,
DOI 10.1007/978-1-4471-4294-2_43, © Springer-Verlag London 2013

Summary

This case illustrates the safety and the effectiveness of the edge-to-edge mitral repair, using the MitraClip device, in selected high-risk patients who are not candidates for surgery, with severe functional MR, responsible for unstable hemodynamic condition and requiring urgent intervention.

Learning Points

- The MitraClip can be safely performed at relatively low risk even in high-surgical-risk patients with severe functional MR.

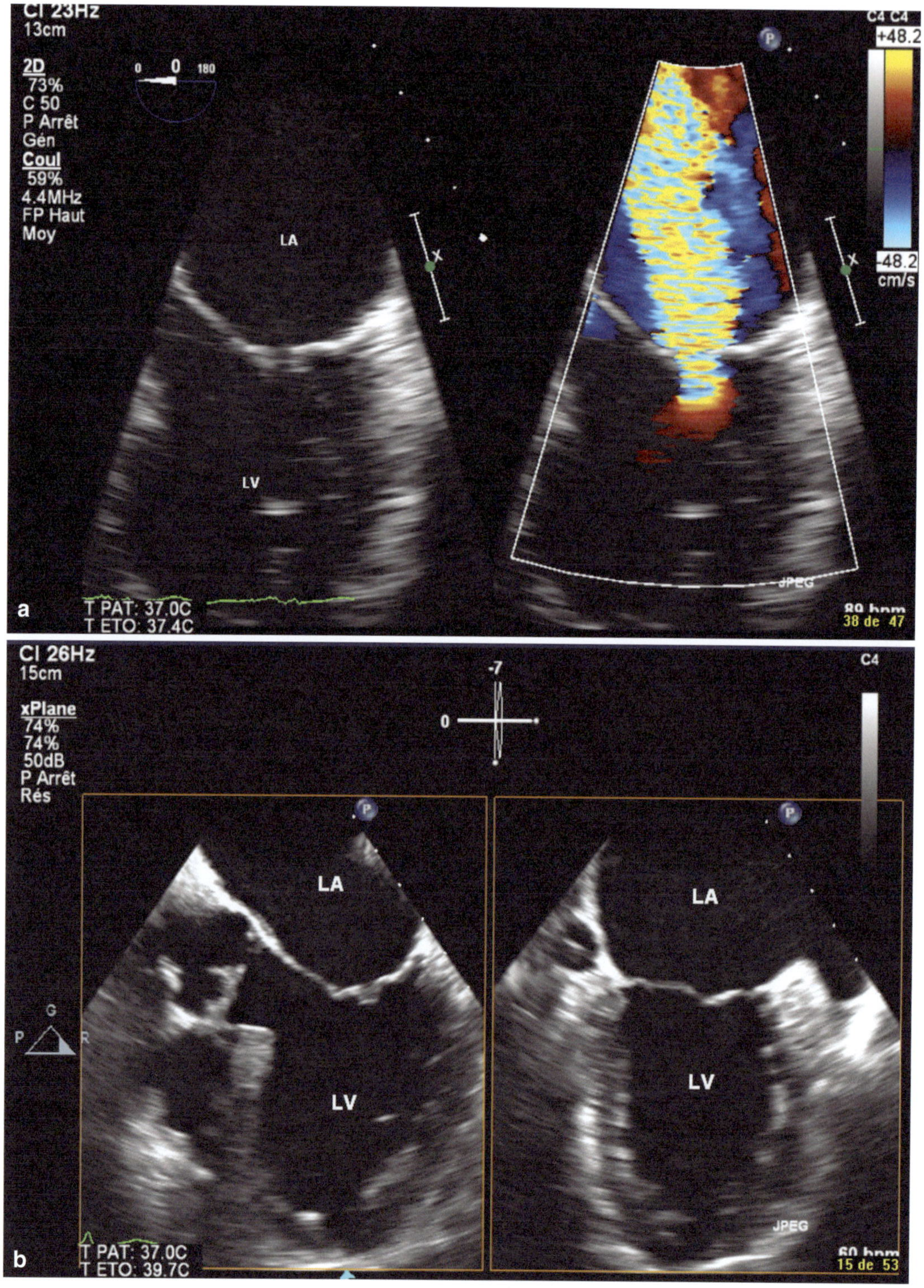

Fig. 43.1 (**a**) 2-D TEE. Severe functional mitral regurgitation . Tenting of both mitral leaflets and large central MR jet. (**b**) Biplane 2-D TEE. LV enlargement and LV dysfunction. (**c**) Tricuspid regurgitation. Severe pulmonary hypertension

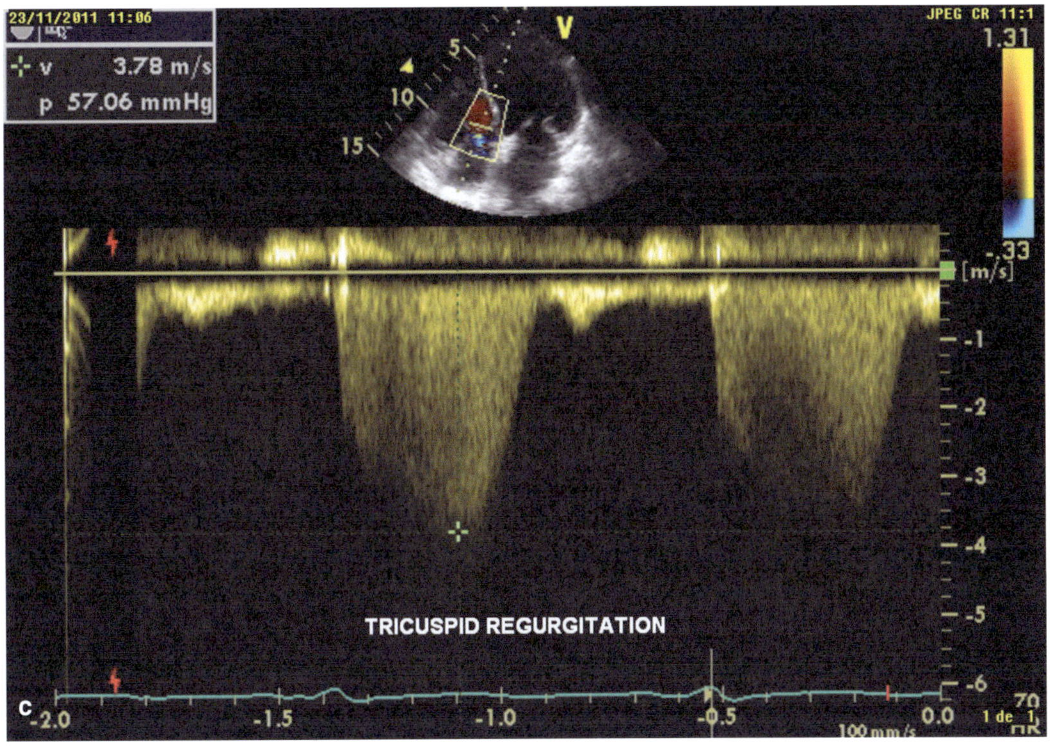

Fig. 43.1 (continued)

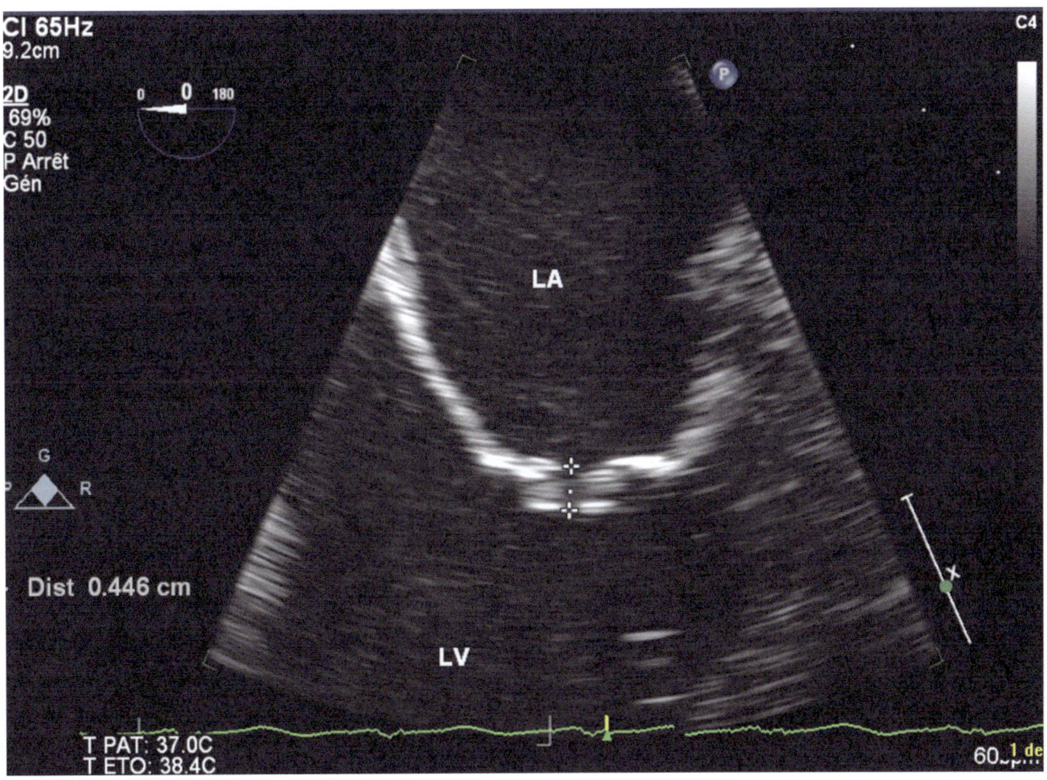

Fig. 43.2 2-D TEE. Tenting height 10 mm. Coaptation length 4 mm

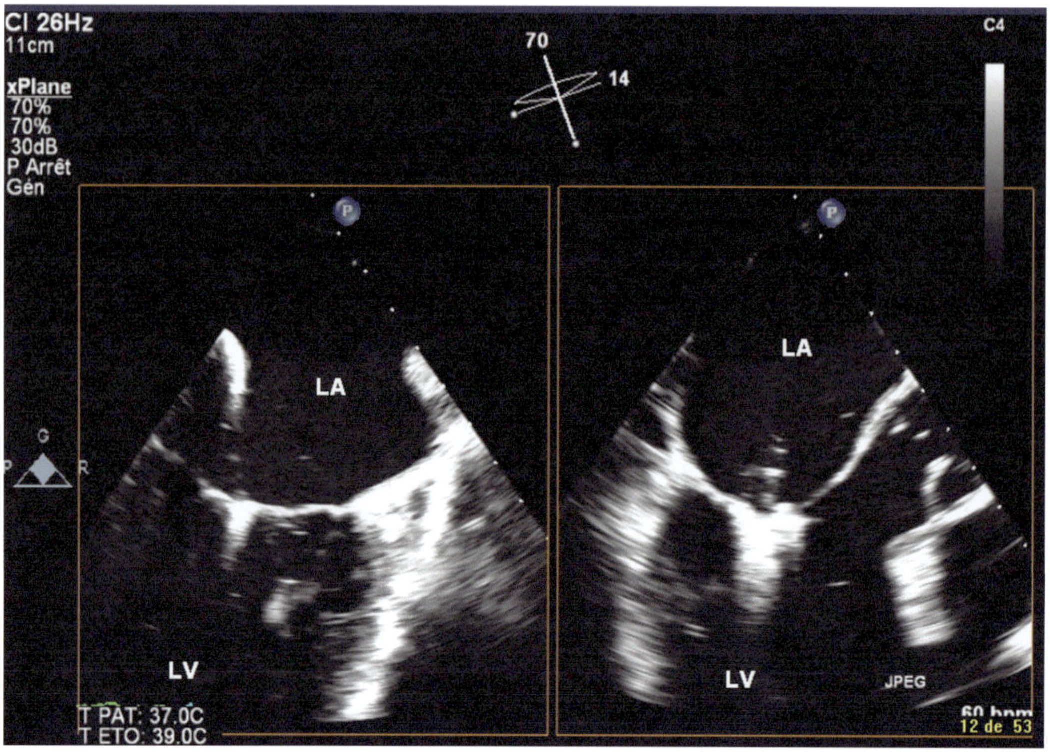

Fig. 43.3 2-D TEE guidance during the procedure. MitraClip opened below the mitral valve

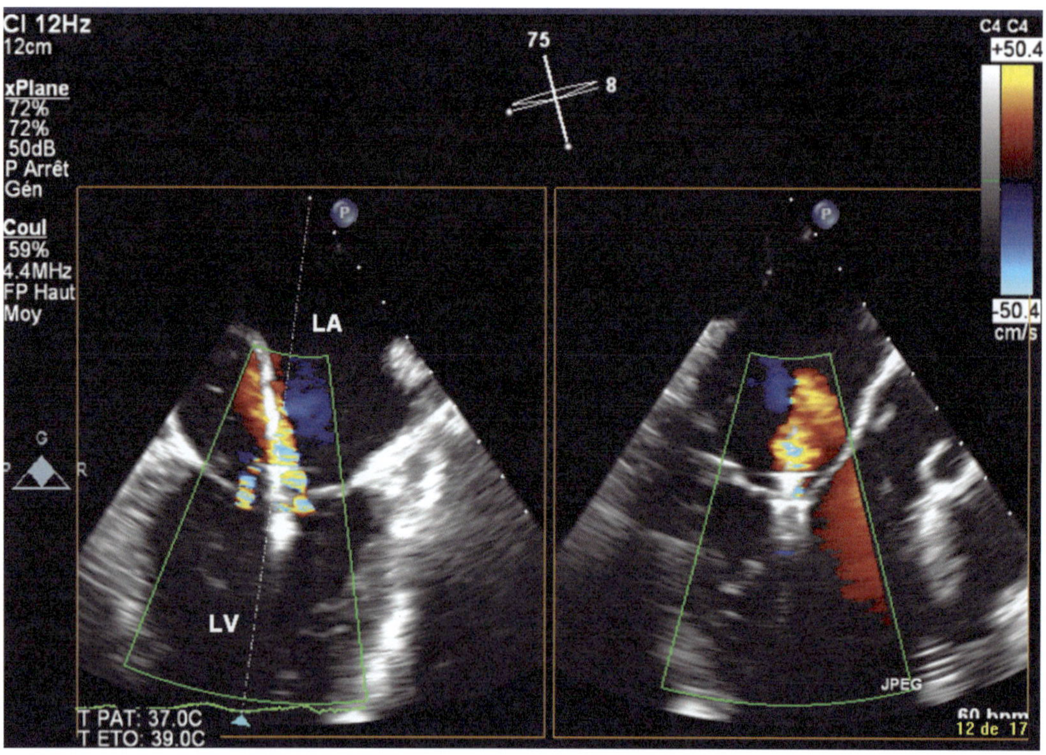

Fig. 43.4 Biplane 2-D TEE guidance during the procedure. Reduction of MR with color Doppler before and after closure of the clip

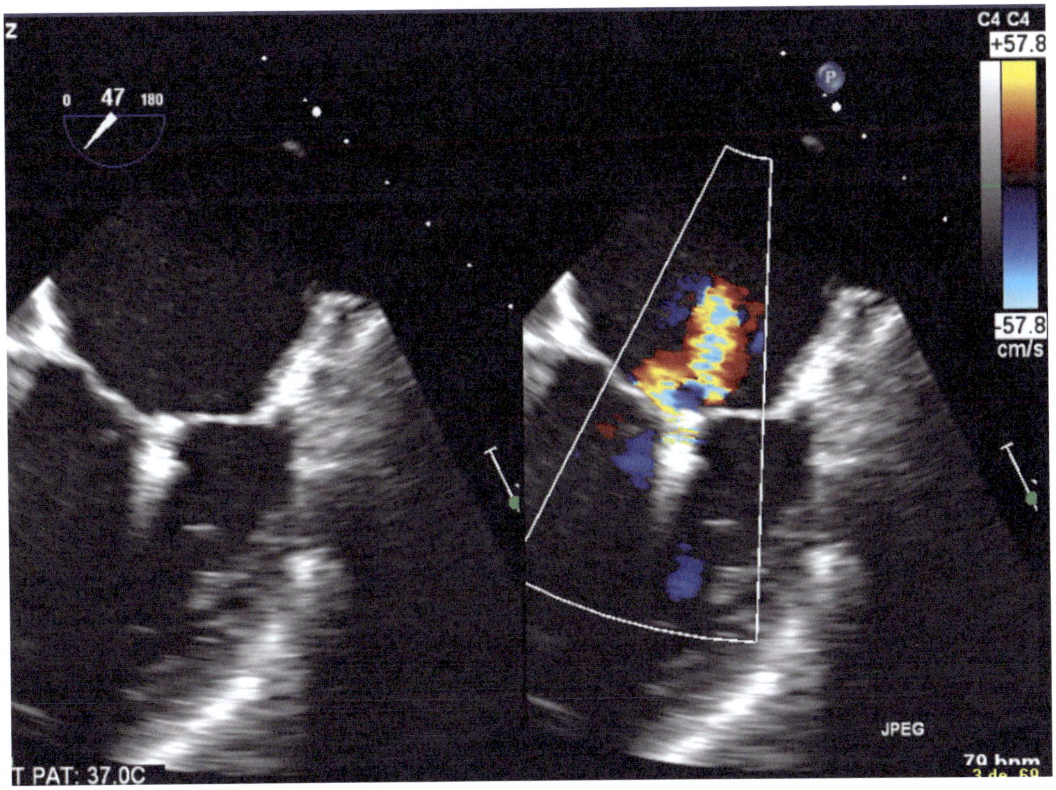

Fig. 43.5 2-D TEE guidance during the procedure. Residual MR assessment after clip release

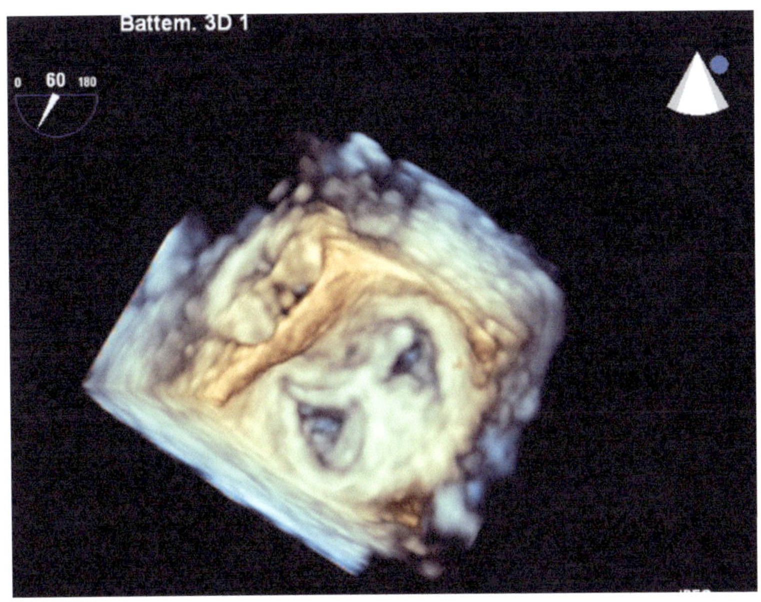

Fig. 43.6 Real-time 3-D TEE en face view of the double mitral orifice after clip release

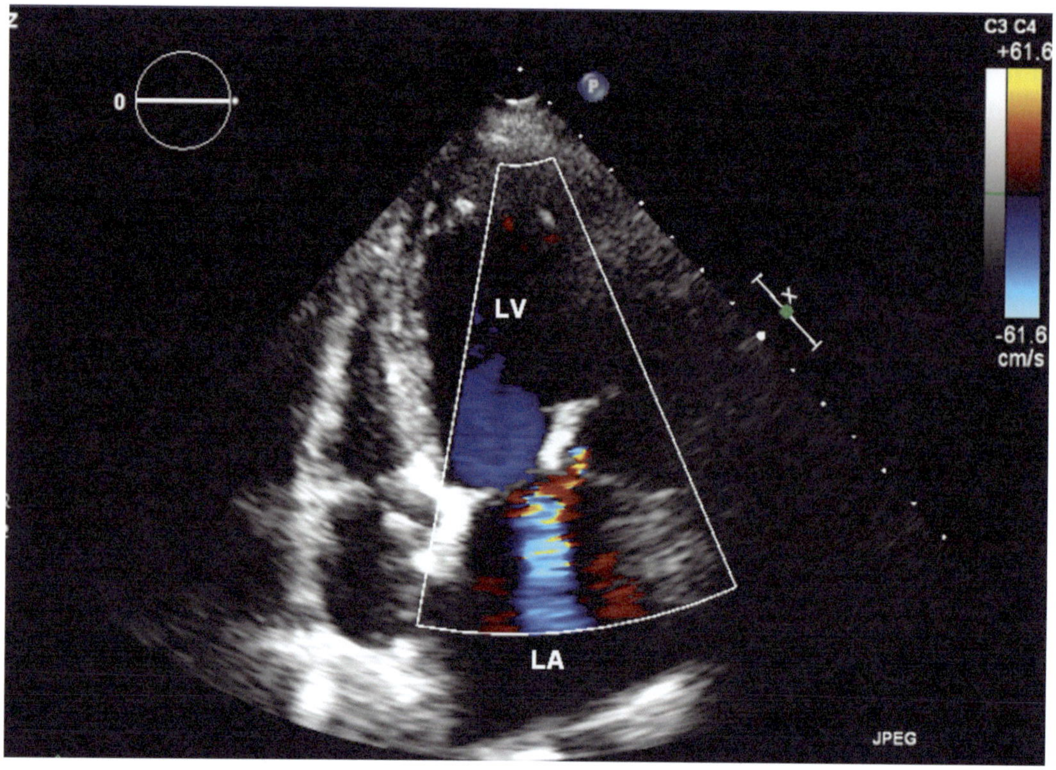

Fig. 43.7 TTE before discharge. Mild residual MR with color Doppler

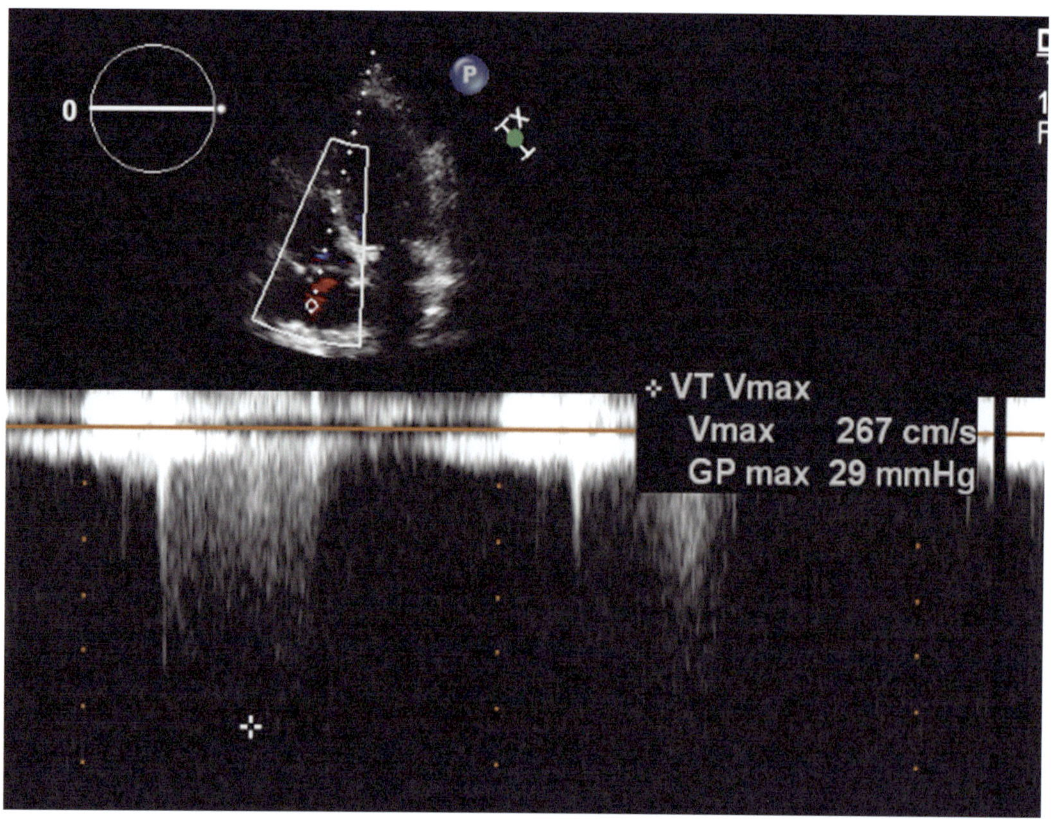

Fig. 43.8 TTE before discharge. Tricuspid regurgitation. Normalization of pulmonary pressures

Mitral Stenosis After MitraClip Therapy and a Partial Solution for Treatment

44

Ulrich Schäfer, Christian Frerker, Felix Kreidel, and Kuck Karl-Heinz

Abstract

This case showcases the use of the MitraClip in a patient with degenerative mitral regurgitation due to a prolapsed A2 segment. Although technically successful, the procedure was complicated by the development of mitral stenosis which worsened with time after the procedure. The operators proceeded to perform careful balloon valvuloplasty of each orifice of the dual-orifice mitral valve with some improvement in gradient.

Keywords

Mitral regurgitation • MitraClip • Mitral valve prolapse • Mitral stenosis • Mitral valvuloplasty

Introduction

Mitral valve regurgitation due to different etiologies is the leading cause of structural valvular heart disease. Currently, transcatheter mitral valve repair using the MitraClip (Abbott Laboratories, Abbott Park, IL, USA) device is the most commonly used percutaneous procedure to treat mitral valve regurgitation (MR). The procedure can be performed to treat MR due to degenerative disease or to functional MR. In the past, morphological criteria with suitable or non-suitable anatomies have been established according to the EVEREST trials. In general, pathoanatomical understanding in catheter-based heart valve therapies is of fundamental importance for treatment success. Usually, it is advisable to exclude patients with small anatomical mitral surface areas and severe mitral valve tethering and/or very little coaptation. In addition, avoidance of suboptimal clip placement (partial leaflet grasping with resultant risk of acute or late clip embolization/detachment) is especially important in patients with prolapsing or flail leaflets. Ideally, the gap between the free edges of the leaflets (flail gap) should be small to achieve capture of both leaflets and adequate tissue grasping.

U. Schäfer, M.D. (✉) • C. Frerker, M.D. • F. Kreidel, M.D.
K. Karl-Heinz, M.D.
Department of Cardiology, Asklepios Clinics St. Georg, Lohmühlenstrasse 9, Hamburg 20099, Germany
e-mail: ul.schaefers@klepios.com; c.frerker@asklepios.com; f.kreidel@asklepios.com; k.kuck@asklepios.com

Clinical History

We report a 76-year-old patient with moderate to severe mitral valve regurgitation (NYHA functional class 3), with increased risk for conventional open-heart surgery (logistic EuroScore 28.2 %: previous aortic valve replacement, chronic atrial fibrillation, pulmonary hypertension with restrictive pulmonary disease, calcific pleuritis (Figs. 44.21, 44.22, 44.23, and 44.24), and impaired renal function). Pre-procedural echocardiographic evaluation demonstrated prolapse of the A2 segment (Figs. 44.1, 44.2, and 44.3), in a suitable but overall small valve (mitral valve orifice area 4.1 cm2, anterior–posterior diameter 2.6 cm, see Figs. 44.4, 44.5, and 44.6). In addition, transseptal puncture was deemed feasible.

The MitraClip procedure was performed in a stepwise manner with TEE guidance, including transseptal puncture, steering of the guide catheter and the clip within the mitral valve (Fig. 44.7), and closing of the clip (Fig. 44.8). Functional assessment of the reduction of mitral regurgitation (Figs. 44.8 and 44.9) revealed a good result, and most importantly, assessment of leaflet insertion showed very

T. Feldman et al. (eds.), *Atlas of Percutaneous Edge-to-Edge Mitral Valve Repair*,
DOI 10.1007/978-1-4471-4294-2_44, © Springer-Verlag London 2013

tensioned mitral leaflets (Fig. 44.8). In fact, there was significant shortening of the anterior–posterior diameter, explained by the fact that the clip was too large for this particular small anatomy (Fig. 44.7). Accordingly, a significant gradient was immediately observed (Fig. 44.10). Thus, the clip was reopened and tentatively placed deeper inside the left ventricle to reduce the amount of leaflet tissue inside the clip arms (Fig. 44.11). With this approach, reduction of mitral regurgitation was similar effective (Figs. 44.12 and 44.13), and the gradient was significant less (Fig. 44.14). Invasive recordings after clip deployment revealed a similar but borderline high transmitral gradient (Fig. 44.15).

Unfortunately, subsequent TTE and TEE examinations at 1 week after implantation demonstrated the development of a severe transmitral gradient (Fig. 44.16) due to mitral stenosis (Fig. 44.17 and 44.18), and the patient started to cough blood while he developed pneumonia. After 10 days of antibiotic treatment, the patients' condition improved, but the gradient remained high at 2 and 4 weeks (not shown). Three months later, the patient was referred again to our hospital because of further aggravation of his dyspnea, and subsequent TEE examinations demonstrated an even worse gradient, with more severe mitral stenosis (Figs. 44.19 and 44.20). The patients' condition was judged again to be too poor for open-heart surgery, and the patient was taken to the hybrid OR for sequential valvuloplasty of both mitral orifices. Left ventricular angiography (Fig. 44.21) and TEE examinations revealed only mild mitral regurgitation before the procedure. After establishment of a long wire loop (arterial-venous circuit) across the lateral orifice of the mitral valve, sequential opening with a PTA balloon (6×40 mm) followed by a larger balloon (12×40 mm, Fig. 44.22) was performed under rapid right ventricular pacing (140 bpm). Subsequently, the same was done inside the medial orifice (Fig. 44.23). The reason for using the wire loop in conjunction to a steerable sheath (Agilis NxT, SJM) was to start with the opening of the balloon at each commissural site within the mitral valve. In general, the PTA balloon was gently inflated to 6–8 atm to obtain a final surface area of 1.1 cm^2 at each individual orifice. Left ventricular angiography after valvuloplasty did not reveal a significant increase in mitral regurgitation (Fig. 44.24), which was confirmed by TEE color Doppler studies (Figs. 44.25 and 44.26). In addition, a modest decrease of the transmitral gradient was found (Fig. 44.27), and the procedure was terminated. Invasive hemodynamic recordings before and after valvuloplasty using a stimulation protocol (intrinsic HR around 45–60 bpm and RV-pacing 120 bpm) revealed a modest decrease of the invasively measured transmitral gradient (Figs. 44.28, 44.29, 44.30, and 44.31), with a lower increase in pulmonary arterial pressures during pacing with 120 bpm (PAP before at 120 bpm: 56/31/41 mmHg and PAP after at 120 bpm: 46/26/34 mmHg). Despite this slightly reduced mitral stenosis, the patients' condition improved slightly, and on retrospect, it was questionable if his underlying pulmonary disease was underestimated before he underwent the mitral clipping procedure.

Summary

Despite the fact that a borderline acceptable gradient was found initially after mitral clip deployment, we found an early and significant increase in the transmitral gradient after 1 week. In retrospect, the patient was not an ideal candidate for mitral clipping, and caution in these small anatomies cannot be emphasized enough. The role of careful valvuloplasty of each mitral orifice after the MitraClip remains unclear but may provide at least palliation in nonsurgical candidates in whom there is significant mitral stenosis.

Learning Points

- Assessment of the mitral valve anatomy is critical prior to the procedure. Patients with a small valve area are at risk of developing mitral stenosis.
- Balloon valvuloplasty of each orifice of the mitral valve after the MitraClip is technically possible, but its utility, safety, timing, and benefits remain unclear.

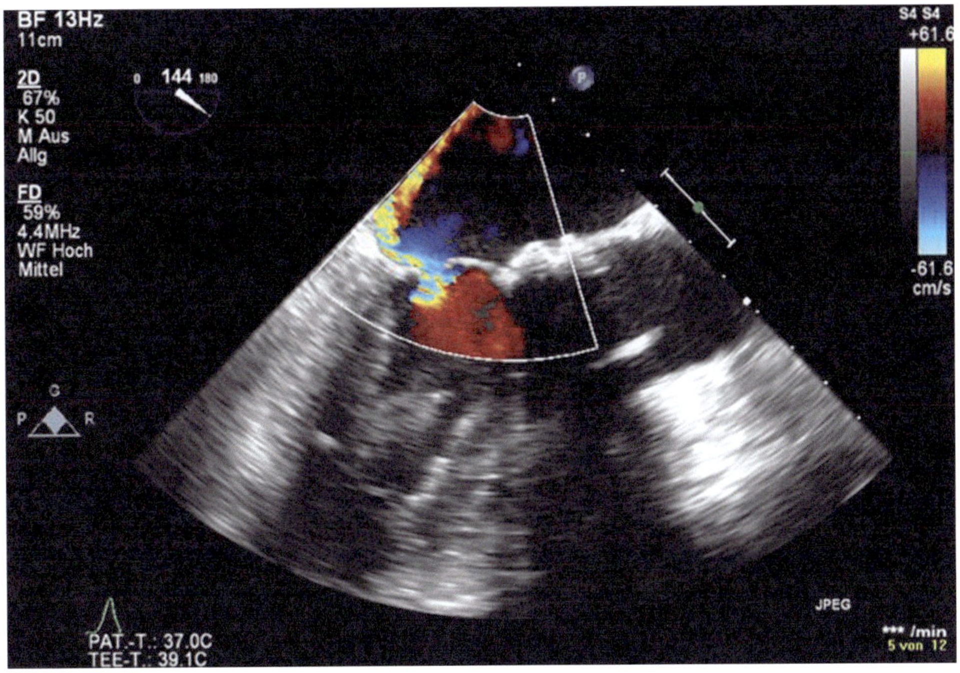

Fig. 44.1 TEE color Doppler with LVOT view

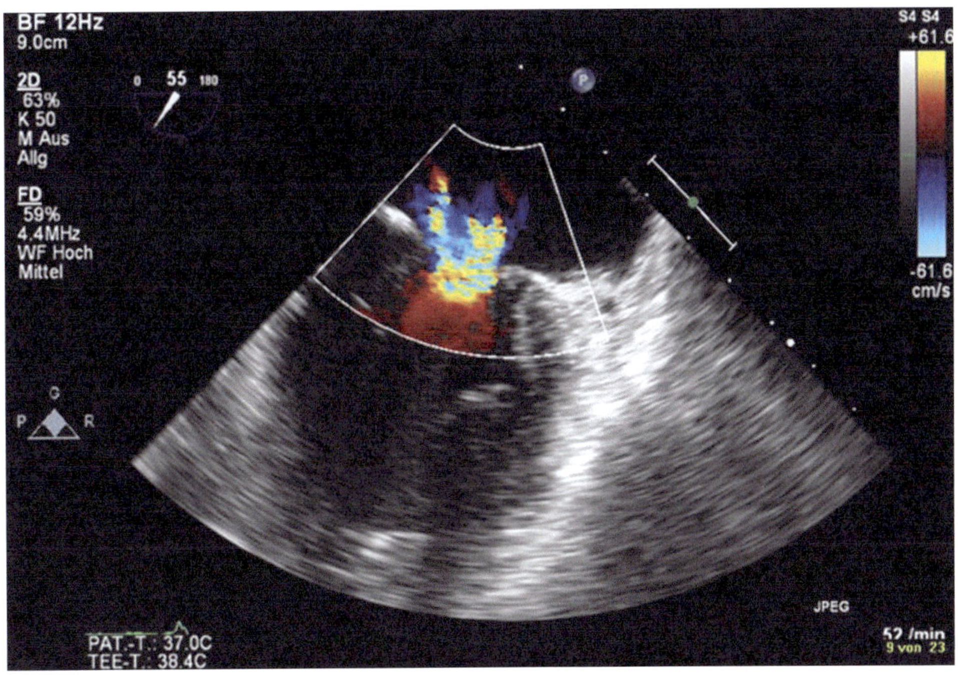

Fig. 44.2 TEE color Doppler with intercommissural view

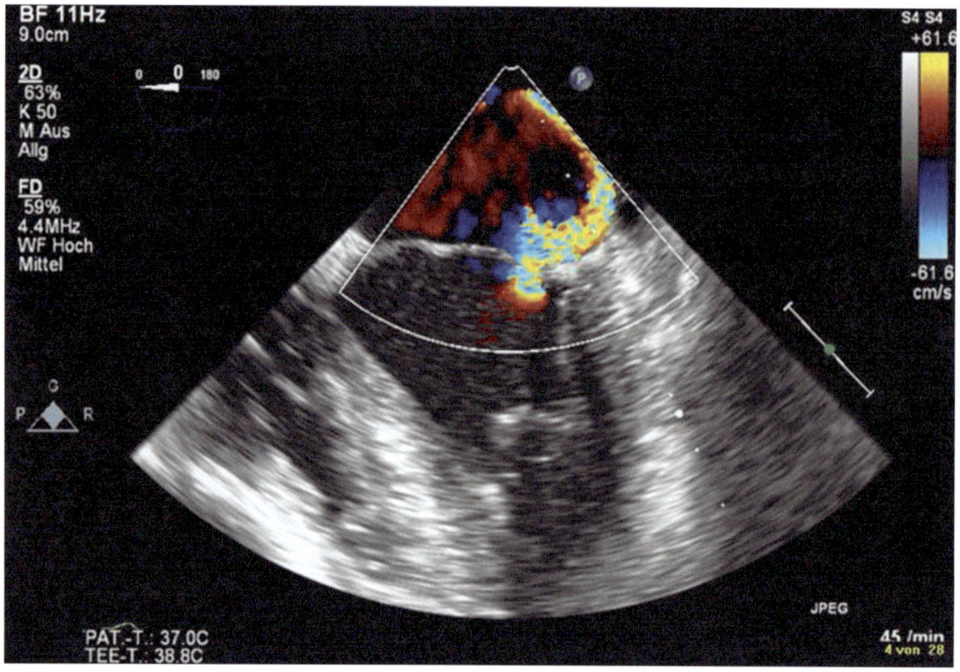

Fig. 44.3 TEE color Doppler with four-chamber view

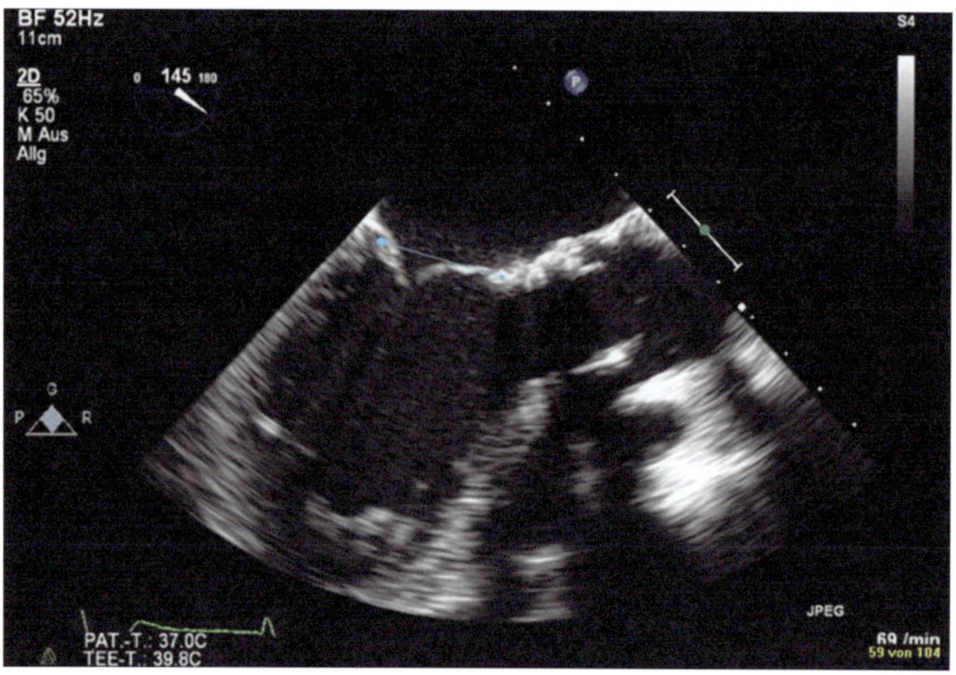

Fig. 44.4 TEE anterior-posterior diameter with LVOT view demonstrating a small orifice (anterior – posterior diameter 2.6 cm)

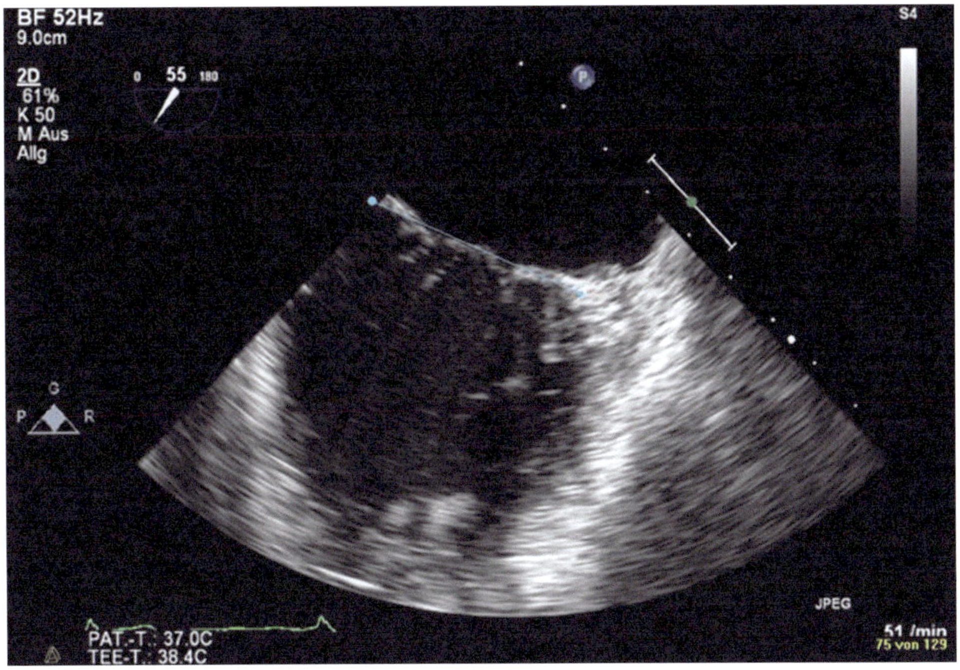

Fig. 44.5 TEE lateral-medial diameter with intercommissural view demonstrating a small orifice anatomy (medial-lateral diameter 3.8 cm)

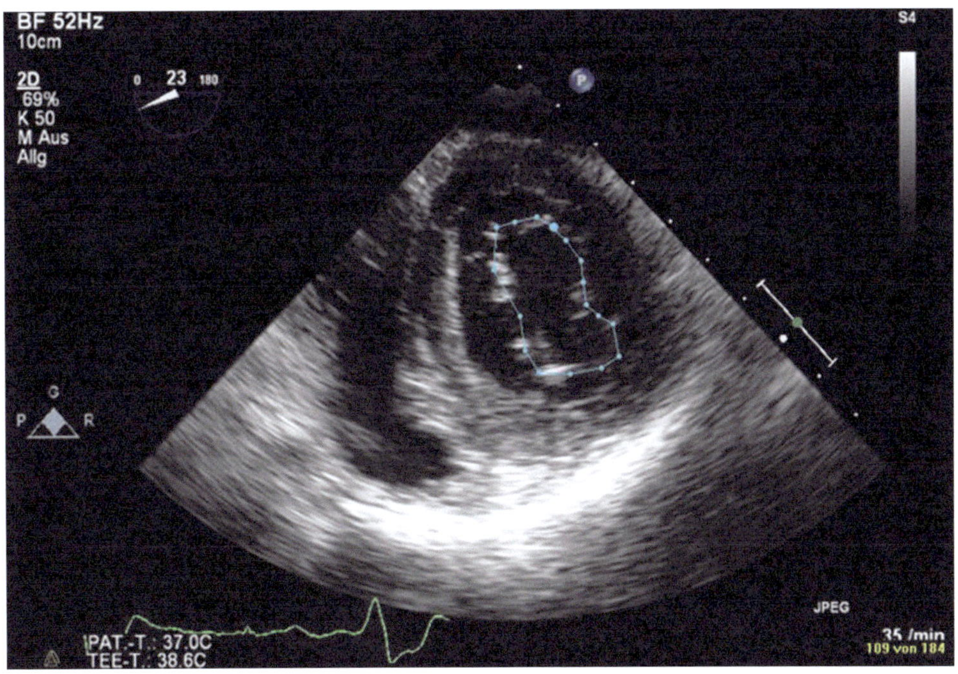

Fig. 44.6 TEE transgastric view with a mitral surface area 4.1 cm^2

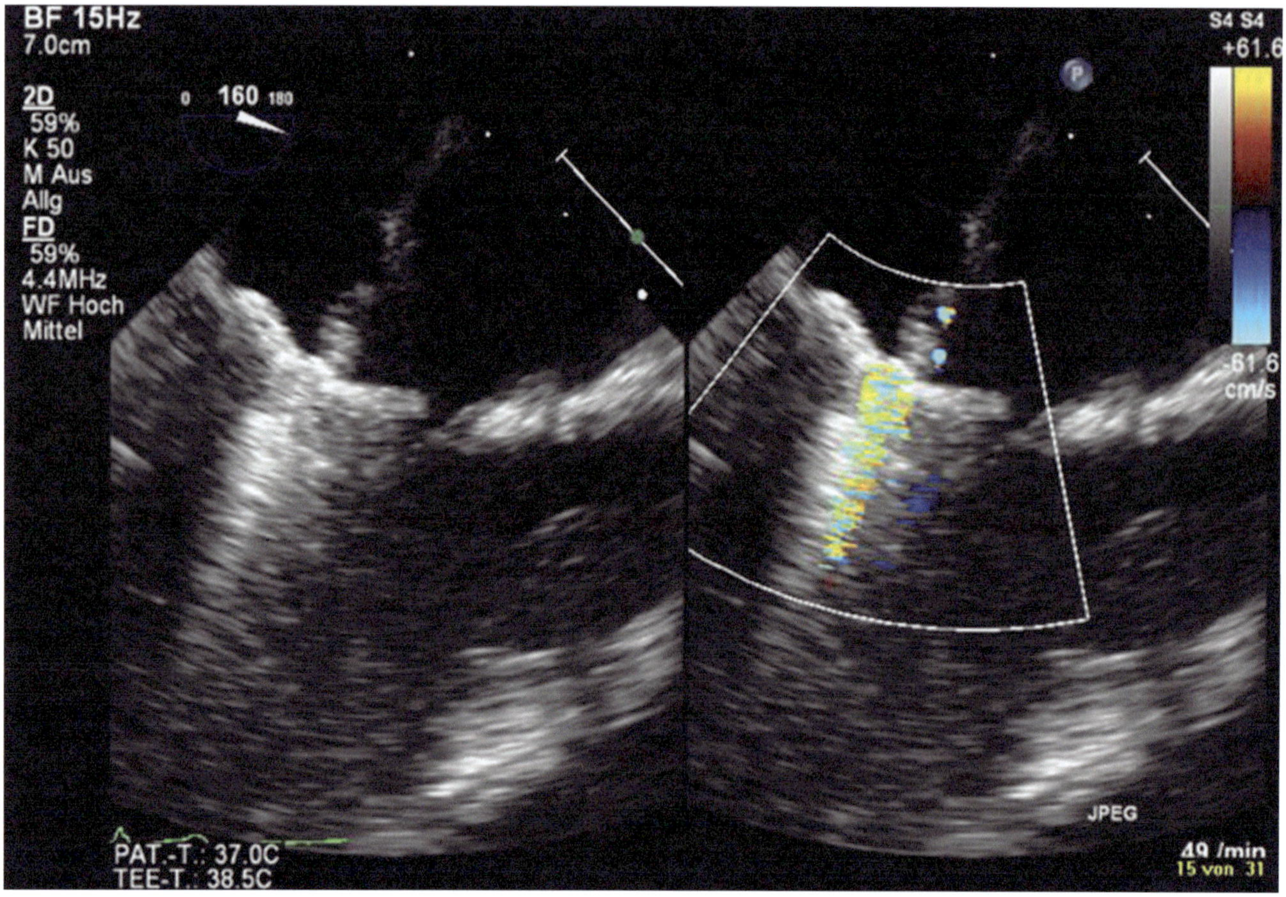

Fig. 44.7 TEE LVOT view with MitraClip oriented on the atrial site before first grasp

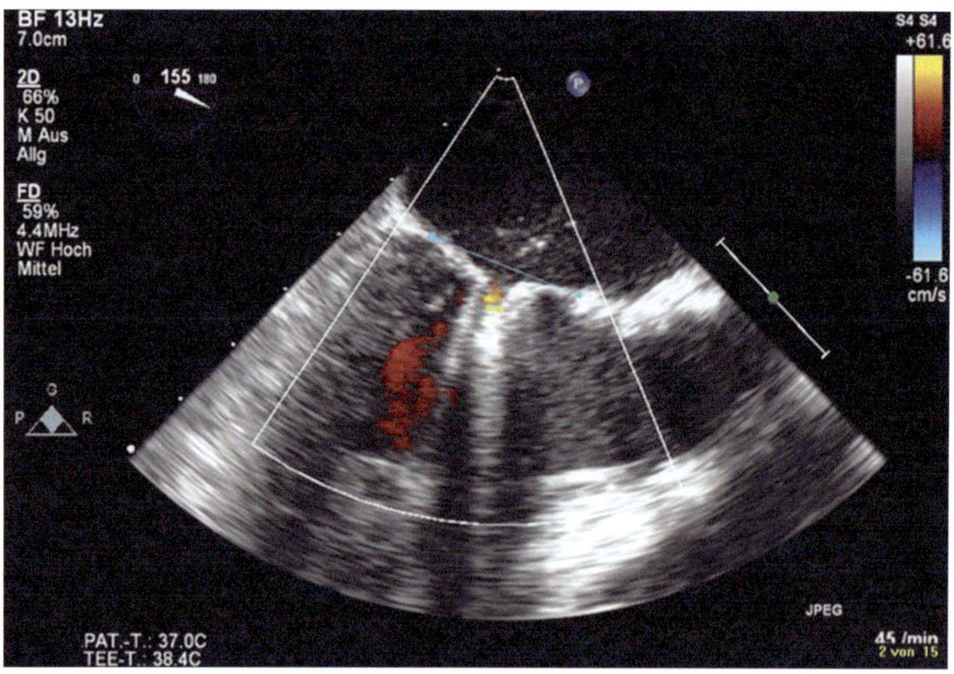

Fig. 44.8 TEE color Doppler with LVOT view after first grasp (note the shortening of the anterior–posterior diameter by 5 mm, now 2.1 mm and before 2.6 mm)

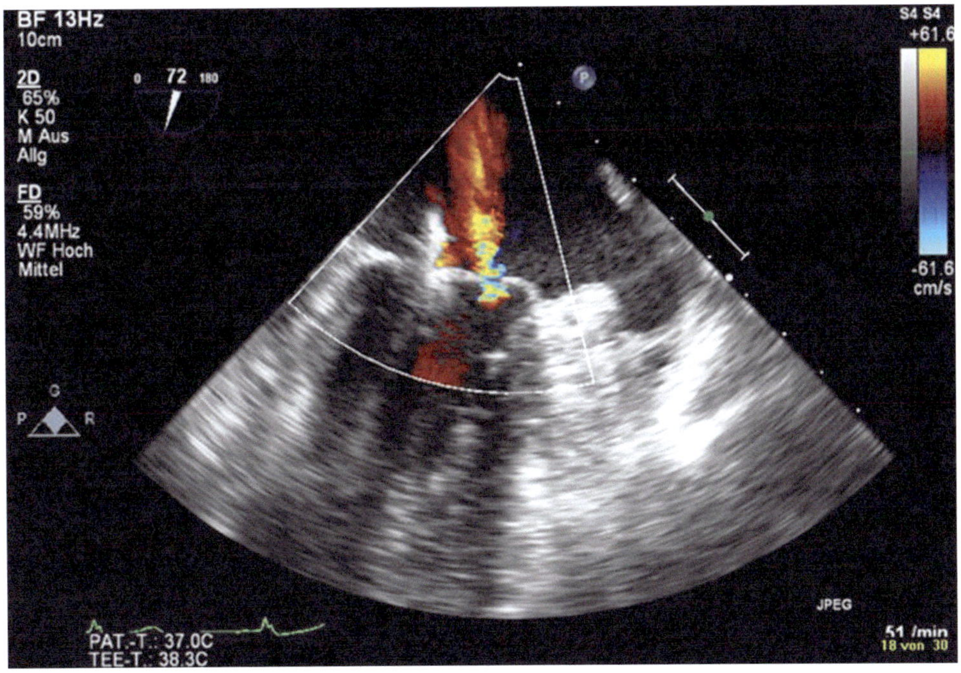

Fig. 44.9 TEE color Doppler with intercommissural view after first grasp

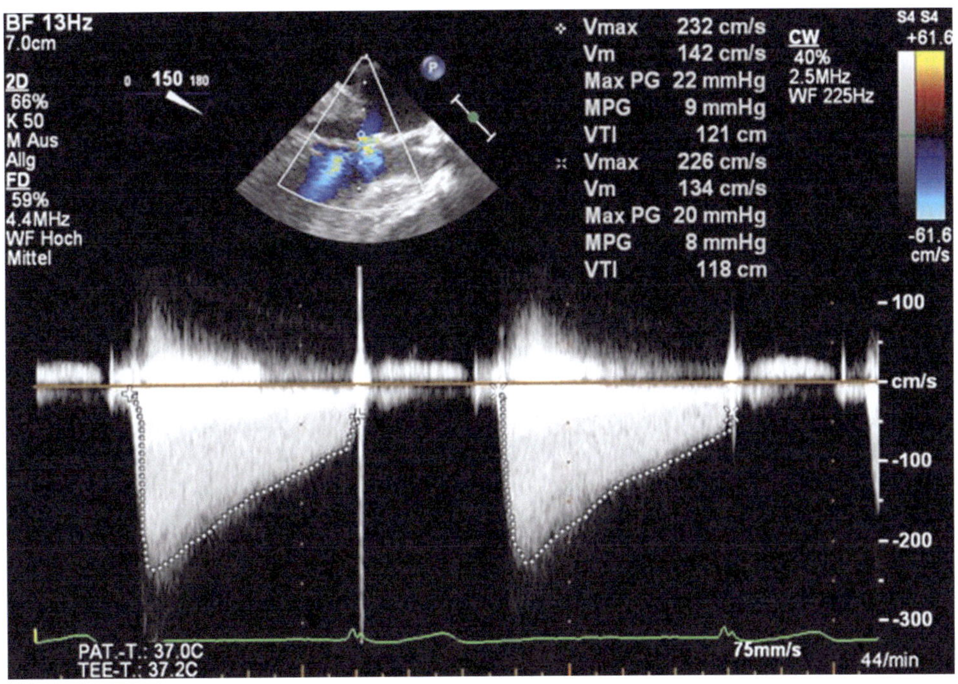

Fig. 44.10 TEE CW Doppler with significant gradient across mitral valve

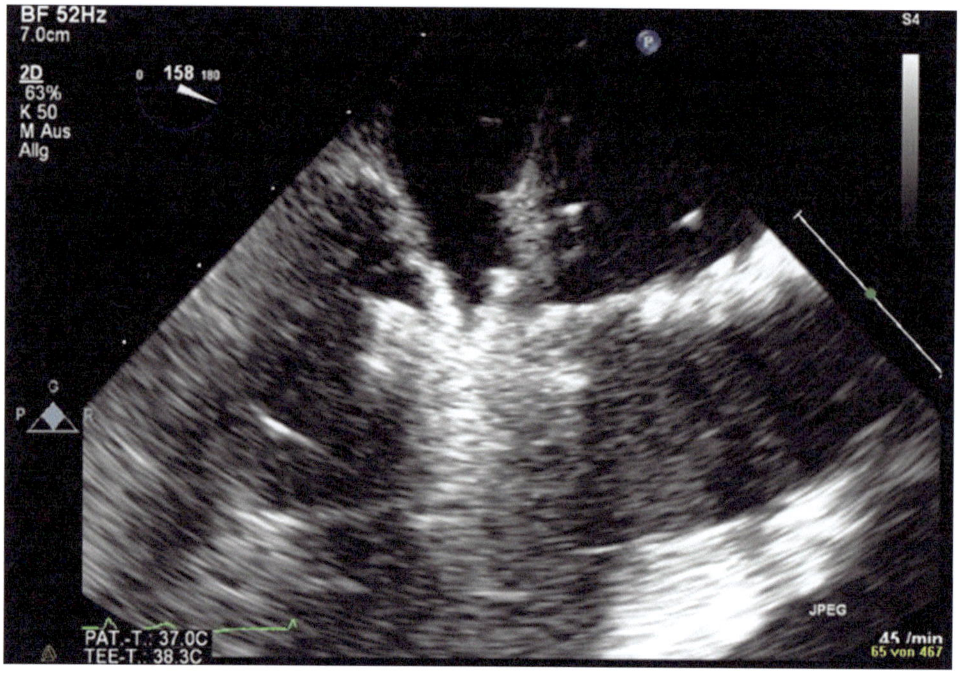

Fig. 44.11 TEE LVOT view with MitraClip before second grasp deeper inside LV

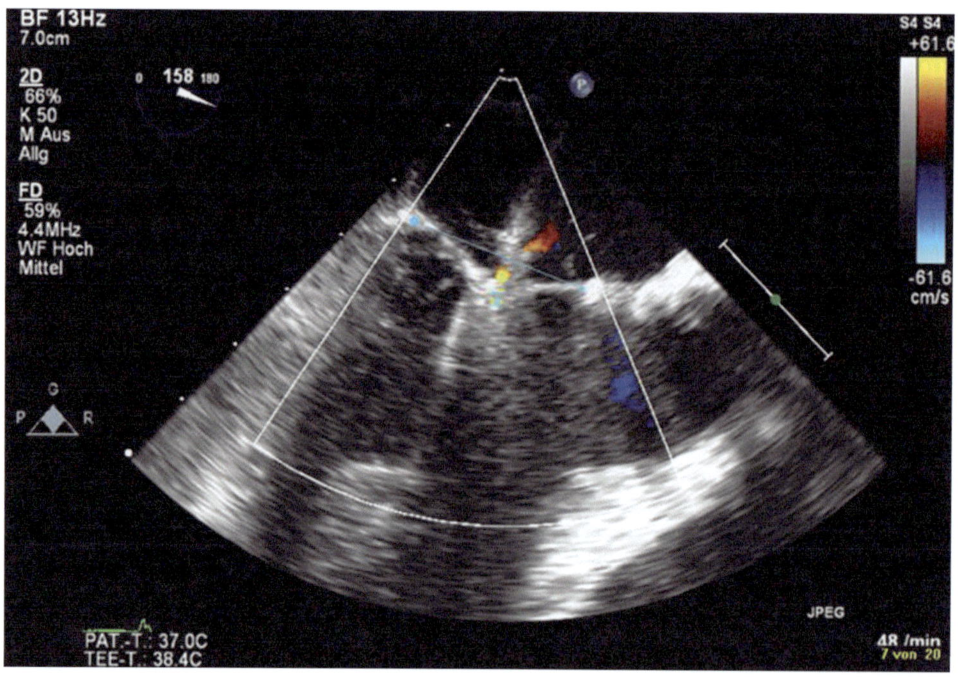

Fig. 44.12 TEE color Doppler with LVOT view after second grasp (note the shortening of the anterior–posterior diameter is now less, i.e., 2 mm, now 2.4 mm and before 2.6 mm)

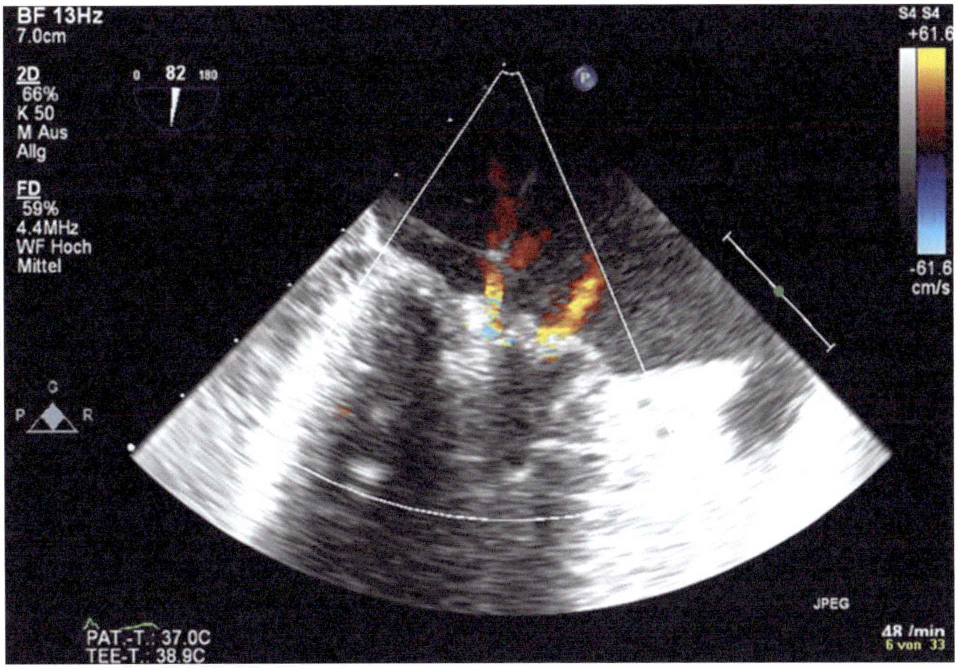

Fig. 44.13 TEE color Doppler with intercommissural view after second grasp

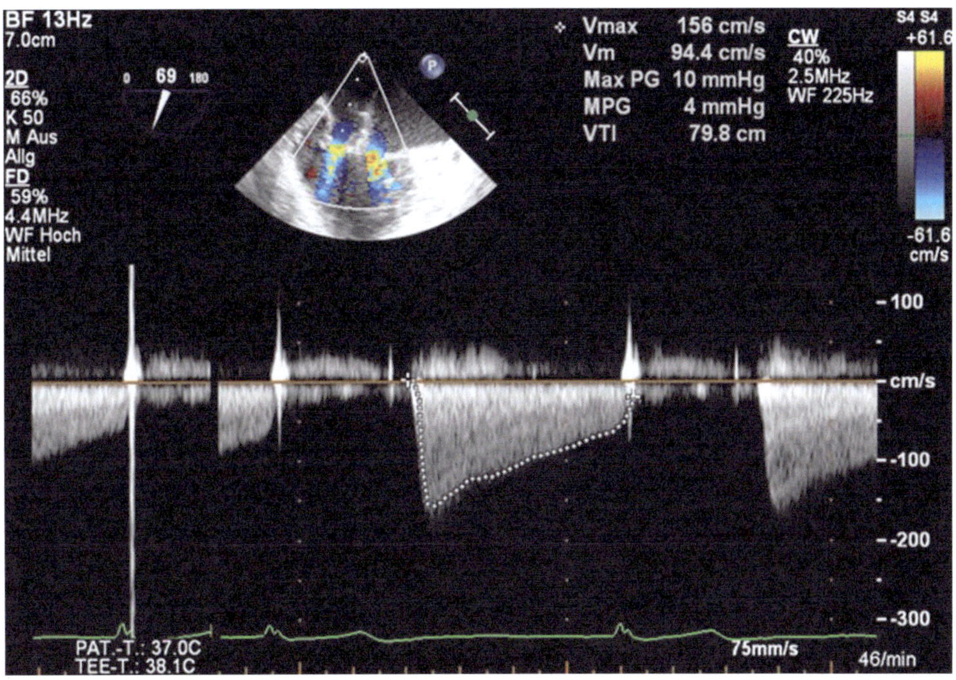

Fig. 44.14 TEE CW Doppler with reduced gradient across mitral valve (mean 4 mmHg, max 10 mmHg)

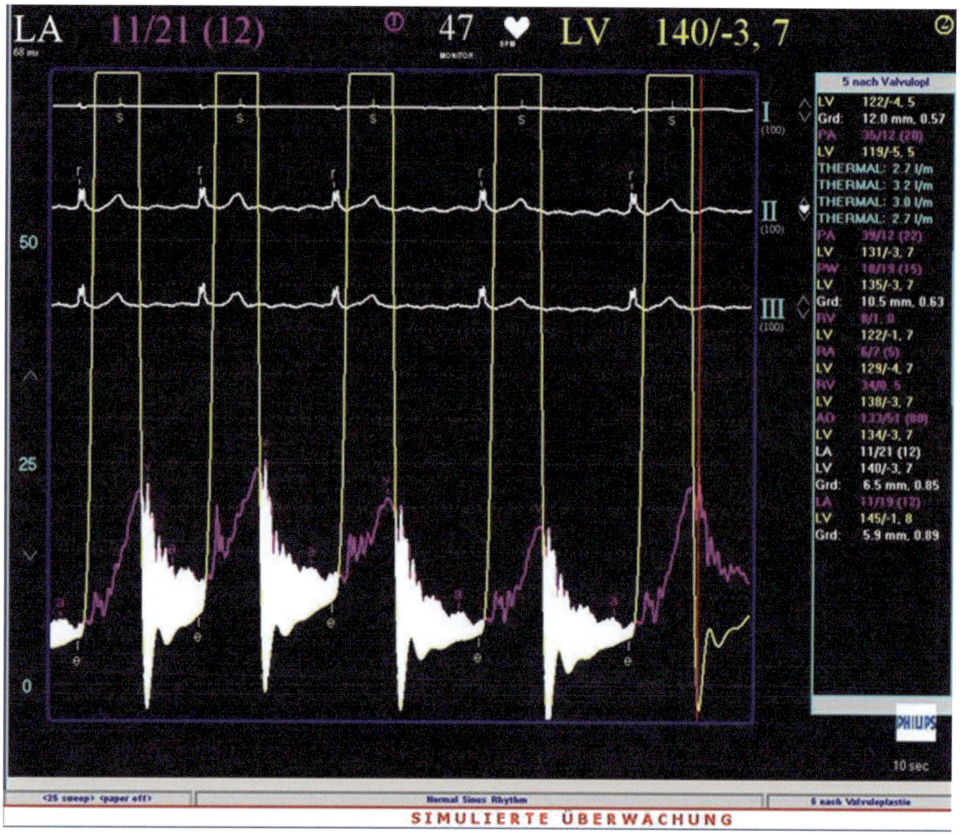

Fig. 44.15 Invasive transmitral gradient recording (LA vs. LV; mean 6.5 mmHg, max. 11 mmHg)

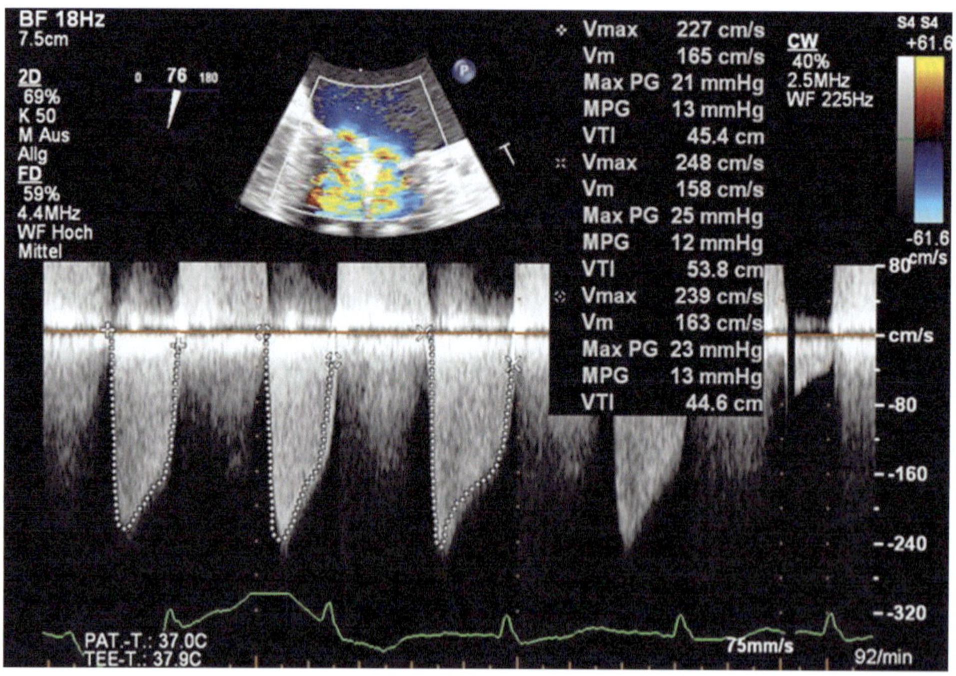

Fig. 44.16 TEE CW Doppler with severe gradient across mitral valve after 1 week (mean 12–13 mmHg, max 21–25 mmHg)

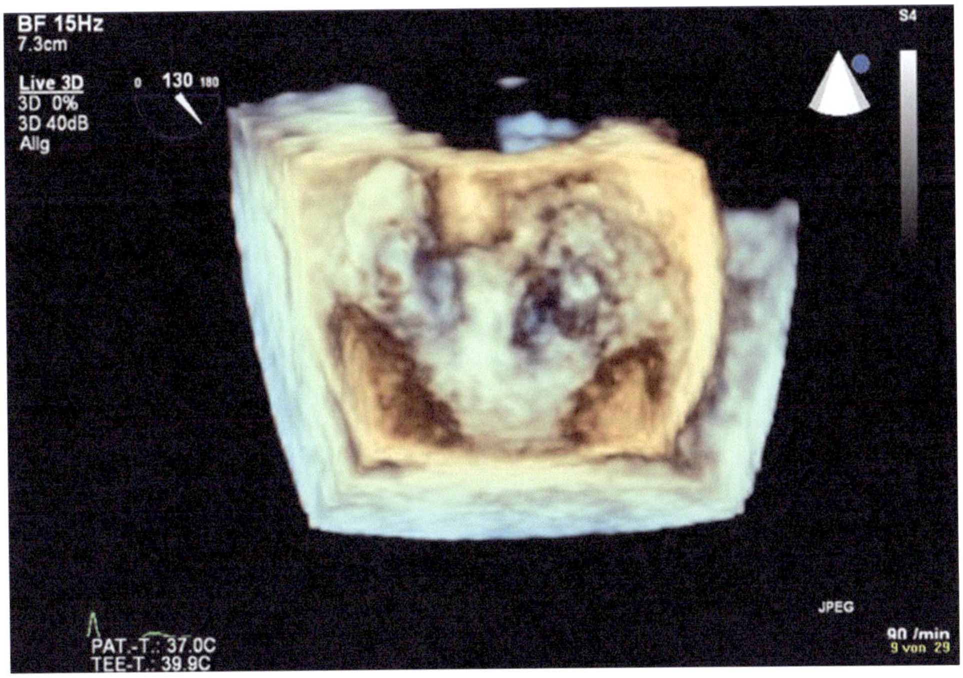

Fig. 44.17 TEE 3-D surgical view with broad tissue bridge (A2P2) after 1 week

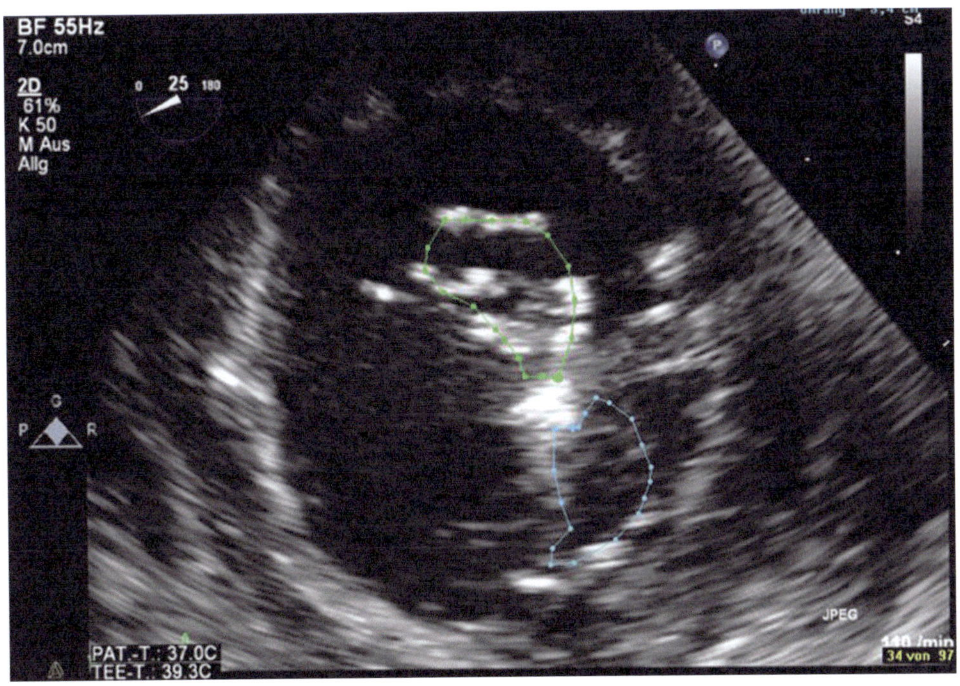

Fig. 44.18 TEE transgastric view with two small openings of the mitral valve after 1 week (MSA1 0.88 cm² and MSA2 0.64 cm²)

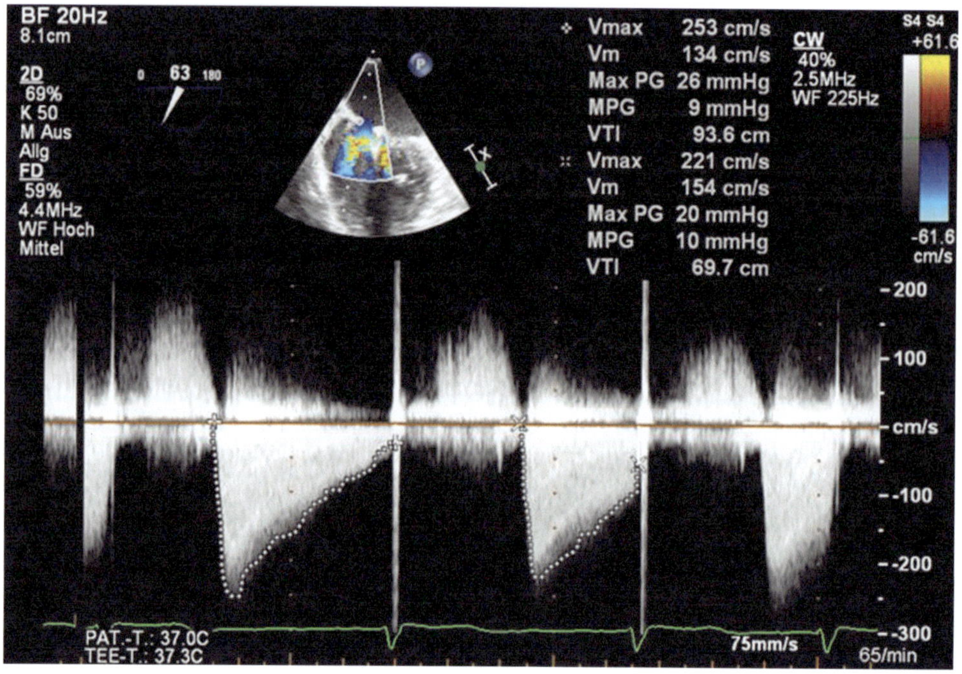

Fig. 44.19 TEE CW Doppler with severe gradient (mean 9–10 mmHg, max 20–26 mmHg) across mitral valve after 3 months

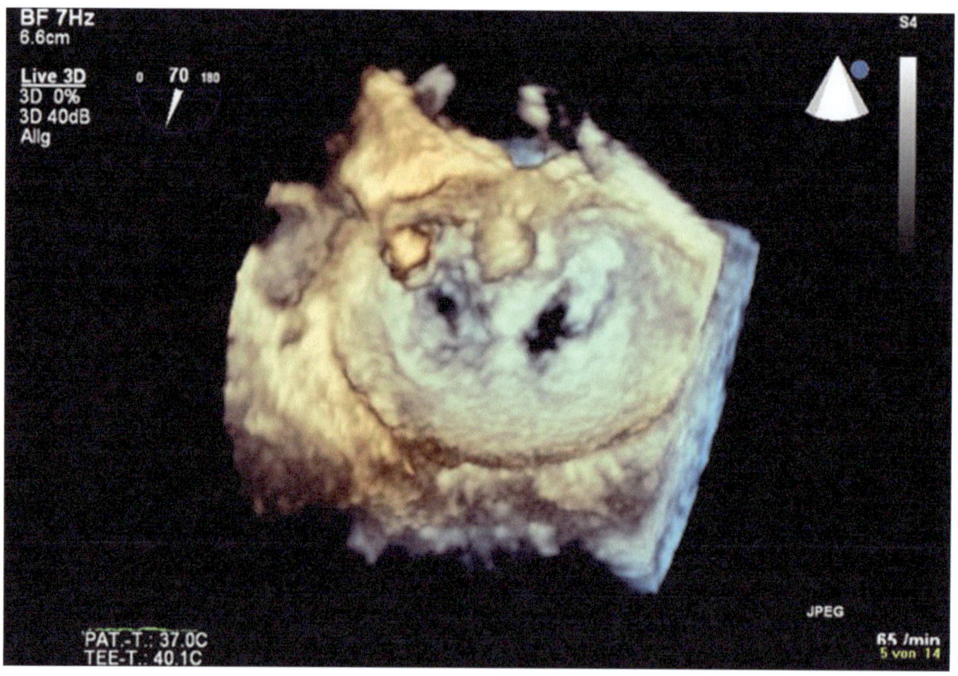

Fig. 44.20 TEE 3-D surgical view with a further reduced opening of the mitral valve after 3 months

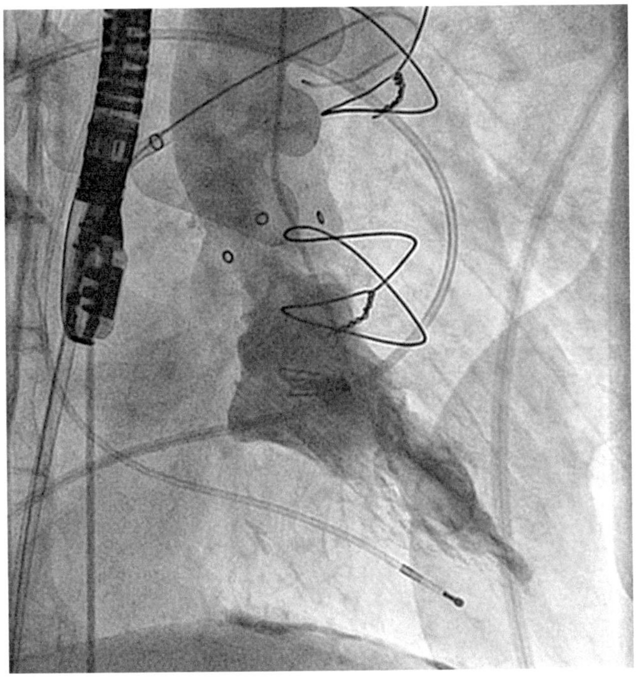

Fig. 44.21 LV angiography before sequential valvuloplasty of the mitral valve

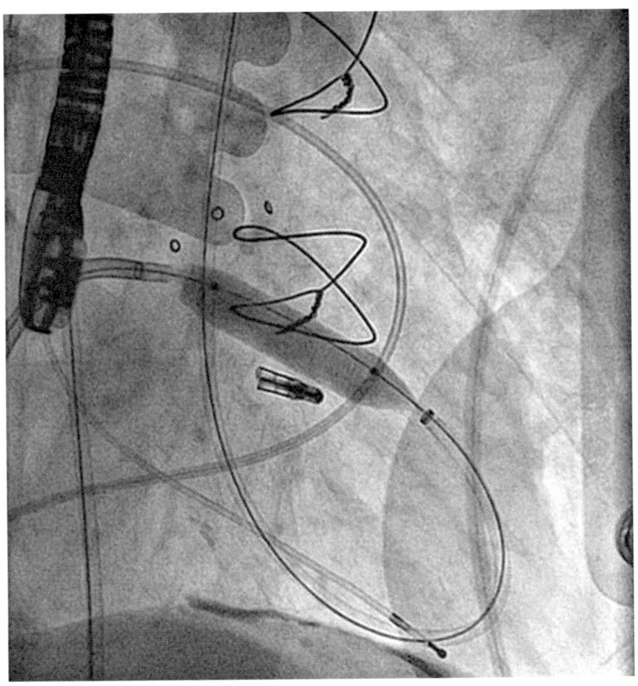

Fig. 44.22 Fluoroscopy with sequential valvuloplasty (balloon 12×40 mm) of the lateral orifice

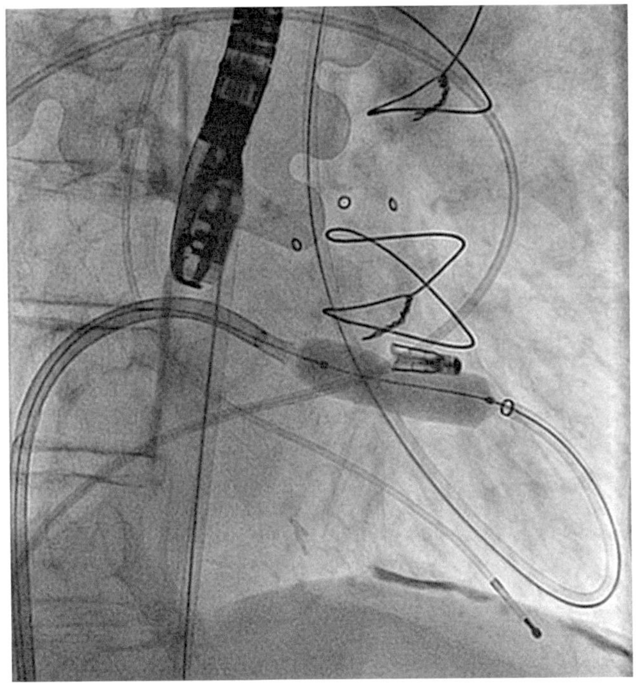

Fig. 44.23 Fluoroscopy with valvuloplasty (balloon 12×40 mm) of the medial orifice

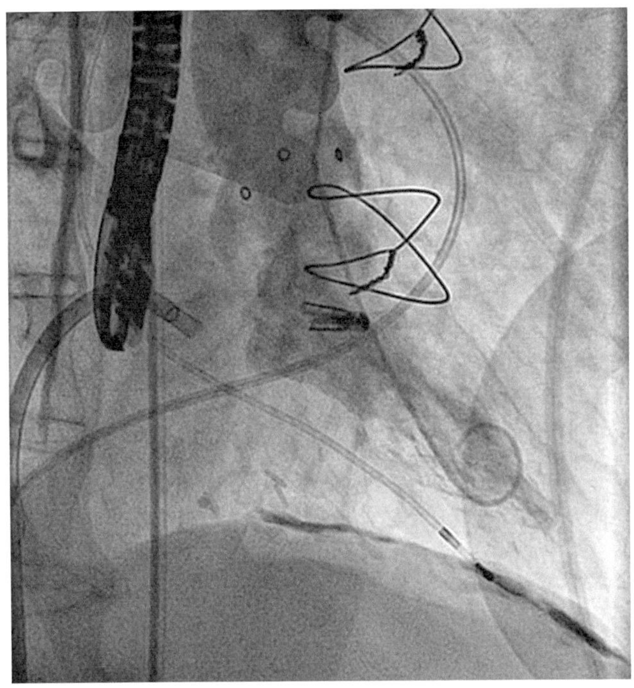

Fig. 44.24 LV angiography after sequential valvuloplasty of the mitral valve

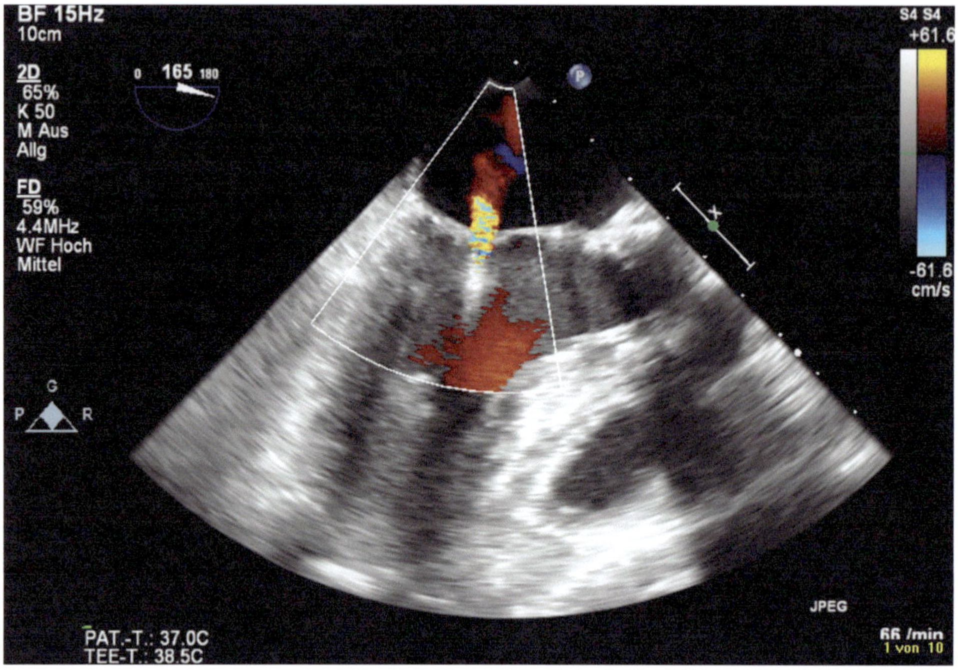

Fig. 44.25 TEE color Doppler with LVOT view after mitral valvuloplasty

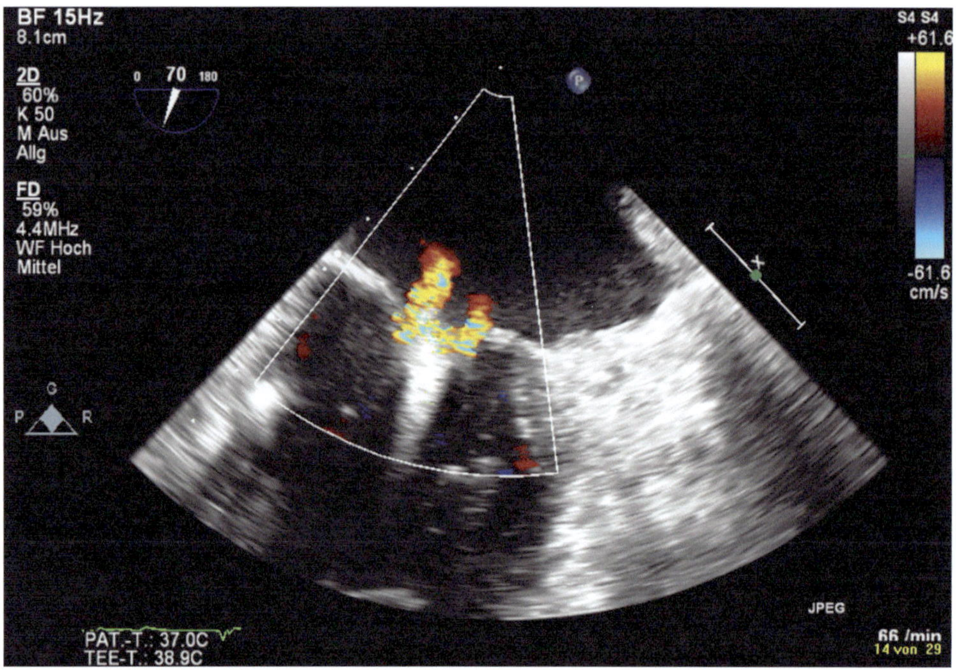

Fig. 44.26 TEE color Doppler with intercommissural view after mitral valvuloplasty

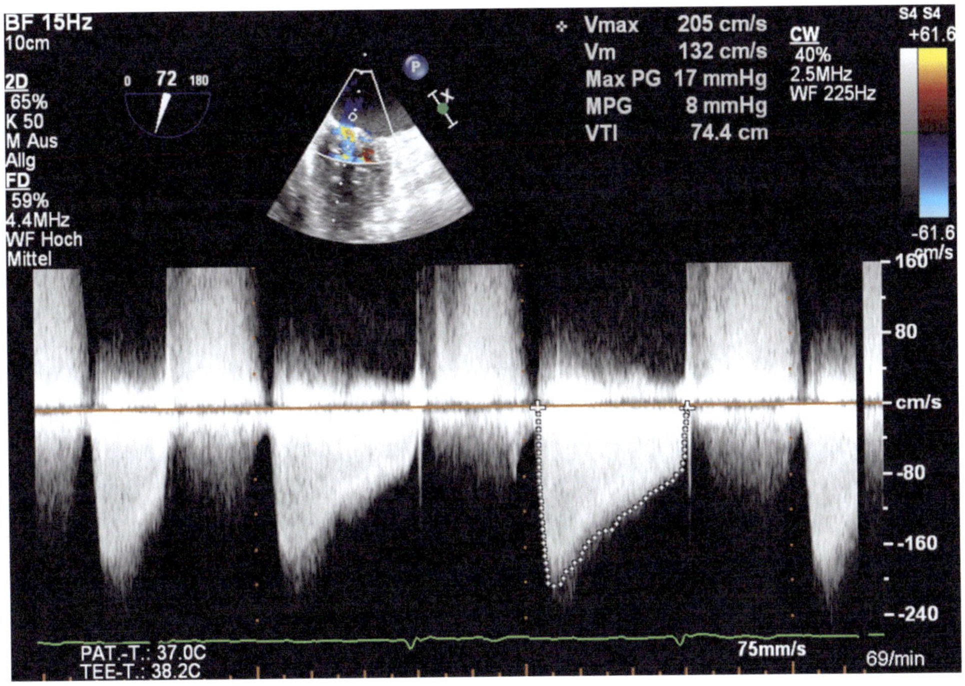

Fig. 44.27 TEE CW Doppler with a slightly reduced gradient across the mitral valve (mean 8 mmHg, max 17 mmHg) after mitral valvuloplasty

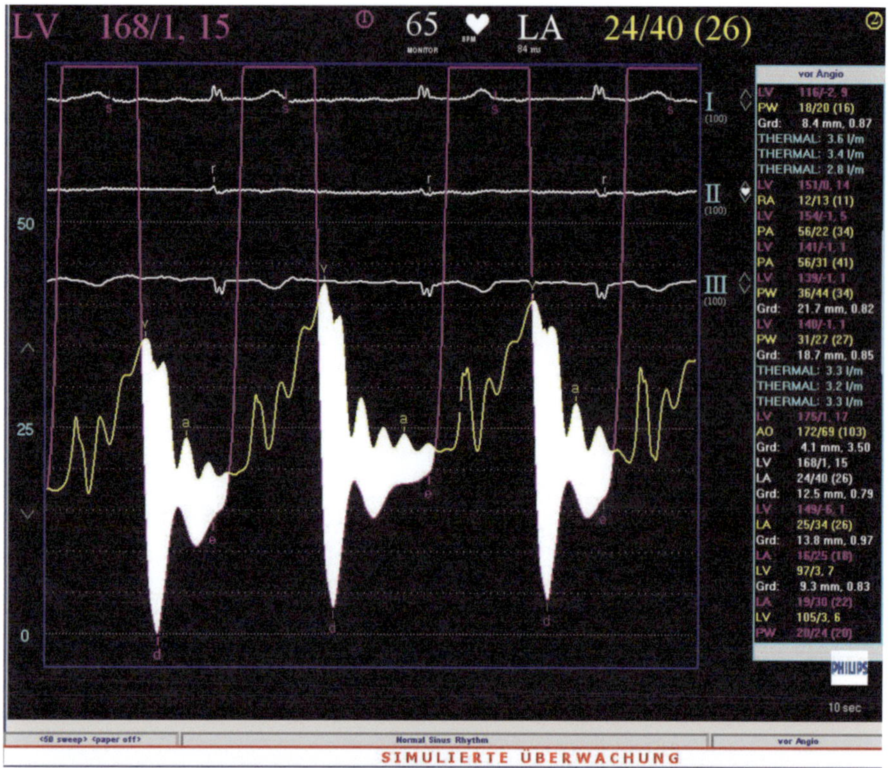

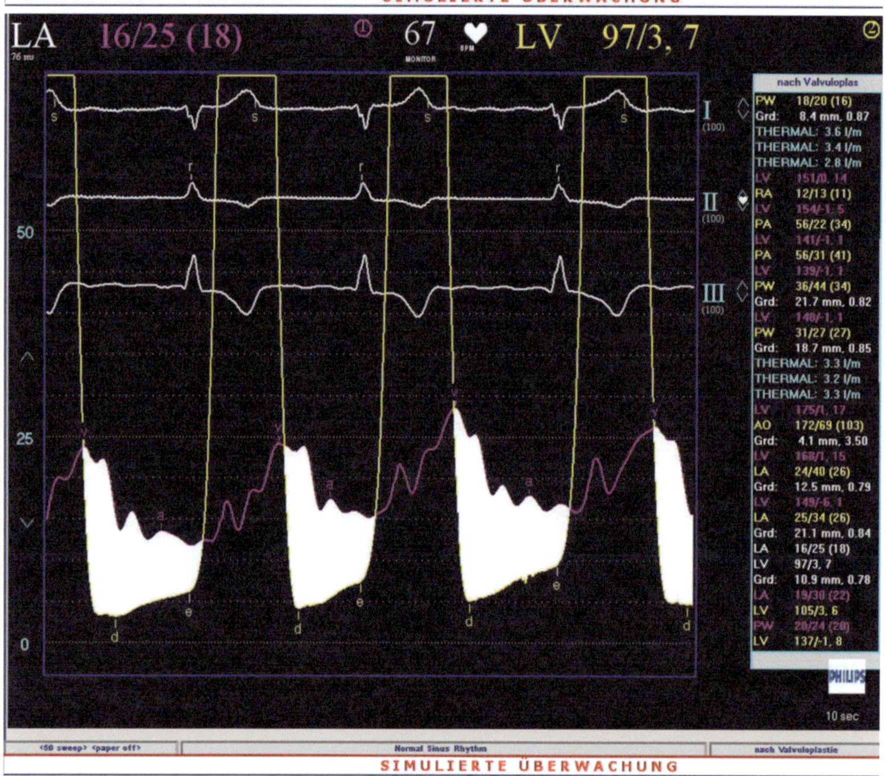

Figs. 44.28 and 44.29 Invasive transmitral gradient recording (*LA* vs. *LV*) before (*upper*; i.e., 12.5 mmHg) and after mitral valvuloplasty (*lower*; i.e., 10.9 mmHg)

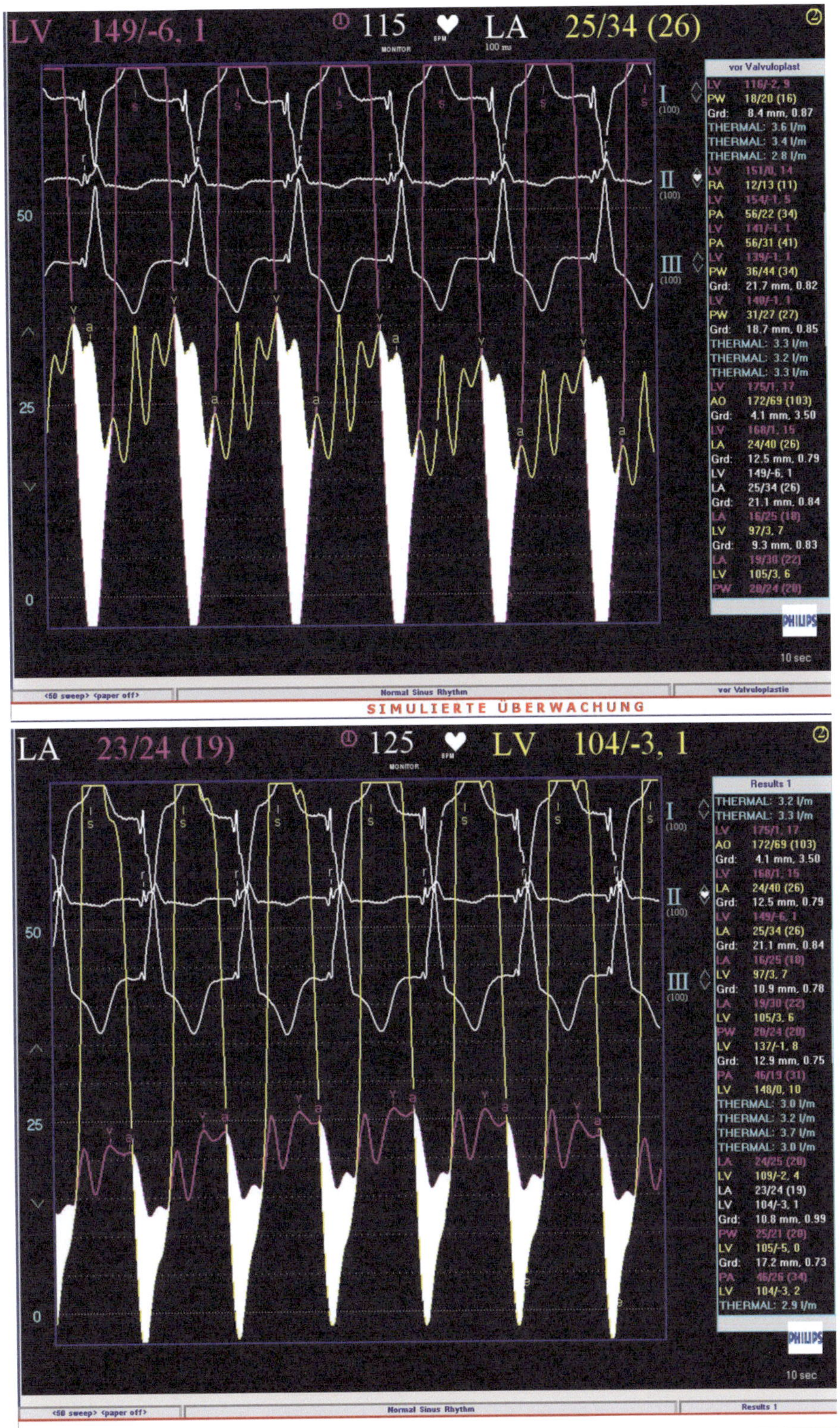

Figs. 44.30 and 44.31 Invasive transmitral gradient recording (*LA* vs. *LV*) with rapid pacing (120 bpm) before (*upper*) and after mitral valvuloplasty (*lower*), note: the transmitral gradient increases with pacing from 12.1 mmHg (at rest) to 21 mmHg (pacing) before mitral valvuloplasty and is lower after valvuloplasty (i.e., 17.2 mmHg but still high)

MitraClip Therapy for Functional Mitral Regurgitation: Importance of Jet Localization to Direct MitraClip Placement

45

Mamta Buch, Saqib Chowdhary, Anita Macnab, and Jaydeep Sarma

Abstract
This case highlights the use of the MitraClip to treat a patient with severe functional mitral regurgitation. Of note, TEE imaging, especially 3-D imaging, showed that the maximal mitral regurgitation jet was from a restricted P2 scallop with a slight medial bias. This allowed targeted placement of the MitraClip with dramatic results.

Keywords
Mitral regurgitation • MitraClip • Functional mitral regurgitation • Restricted posterior leaflet

Clinical History

A 72-year-old female patient with a significant history of coronary artery disease presented to our institution with worsening dyspnea and reduced exercise tolerance. Her past medical history included coronary artery bypass grafting in 1990 and then repeat coronary grafting in 2003.

She had echocardiographic evidence of an ischemic cardiomyopathy with severe mitral regurgitation but no angiographic evidence of major epicardial graft failure. Initial management was conservative, with optimization of vasodilator drugs and diuretics. However, her symptomatic status remained at NYHA class IV, and she required successive hospital admissions with congestive cardiac failure. Because of her short QRS duration, she was not a candidate for cardiac resynchronization therapy. She was discussed with cardiac surgical colleagues with regard to open surgical valve repair but was deemed too high a peri- and postoperative risk.

Despite optimal medical therapy, her condition deteriorated. She was readmitted for the sixth time in 9 months, confined to bed, and dependent on intravenous infusions of loop diuretics and nitrates. She was assessed for suitability for percutaneous mitral valve repair with the MitraClip.

A transesophageal echocardiographic (TEE) study showed severe mitral regurgitation (MR) secondary to tethering of the middle scallop of the posterior leaflet of the mitral valve, P2 (see Fig. 45.1). The key jet on color flow emanated from an eccentric posteromedial position. There was reversal of pulmonary vein flow.

The posterior leaflet tethering was due to infero-posterior wall akinesia. Left ventricular function was moderately impaired, with an estimated ejection fraction of 45 %.

Mild dilatation of the right heart was present with moderate tricuspid regurgitation and an estimated pulmonary artery pressure of 65 mmHg.

A targeted MitraClip strategy was adopted, with placement of a single MitraClip in the posteromedial position at the point of greatest regurgitation on color flow mapping (Fig. 45.2).

The resultant reduction in mitral regurgitation was from grade 3+ to 1+ by echo criteria. Only a small residual lateral MR jet was visible after clip placement (Fig. 45.3) with immediate resolution of pulmonary vein flow reversal.

Following procedural completion, the patient was extubated and returned to the cardiac ward. Increases in urine

M. Buch, MBChB, Ph.D., MRCP
S. Chowdhary, M.B.B.S., Ph.D., MRCP • A. Macnab, MBChB, FRCP
J. Sarma, M.A., MB, BChir, Ph.D., FRCP (✉)
Department of Cardiology, North West Heart Centre, University Hospital of South Manchester NHS Foundation Trust, Southmoor Road, Manchester, Lancashire M23 9LT, UK
e-mail: mamta.buch@uhsm.nhs.uk; saqib.chowdhary@uhsm.nhs.uk; anita.macnab@uhsm.nhs.uk; jaydeep.sarma@uhsm.nhs.uk

T. Feldman et al. (eds.), *Atlas of Percutaneous Edge-to-Edge Mitral Valve Repair*,
DOI 10.1007/978-1-4471-4294-2_45, © Springer-Verlag London 2013

output and decreases in serum urea and creatinine were noted within 48 h. Intravenous diuretics and nitrates were discontinued. The patient mobilized independently and was fit for discharge home within 5 days of the procedure.

Outpatient follow-up and feedback from primary care physicians confirmed a marked clinical improvement with a reduction in symptoms to NYHA class II and significant improvement in quality of life. An absolute reduction in diuretic requirements continued, with further improvement in renal function.

To date, the patient has had no further hospital admissions in the 15 months following MitraClip procedure.

Learning Points

- This case emphasizes the importance of correct steering and positioning of the MitraClip to ensure axial alignment and splitting of the mitral regurgitant jet.
- An appreciation of the asymmetric nature of the MR jet was crucial to optimal clip positioning and enabled a simple single clip strategy to produce an excellent echocardiographic and clinical result.
- The transgastric and 3-D views confirm this position clearly (Fig. 45.4a, b) and are highly valuable in ensuring procedural success.

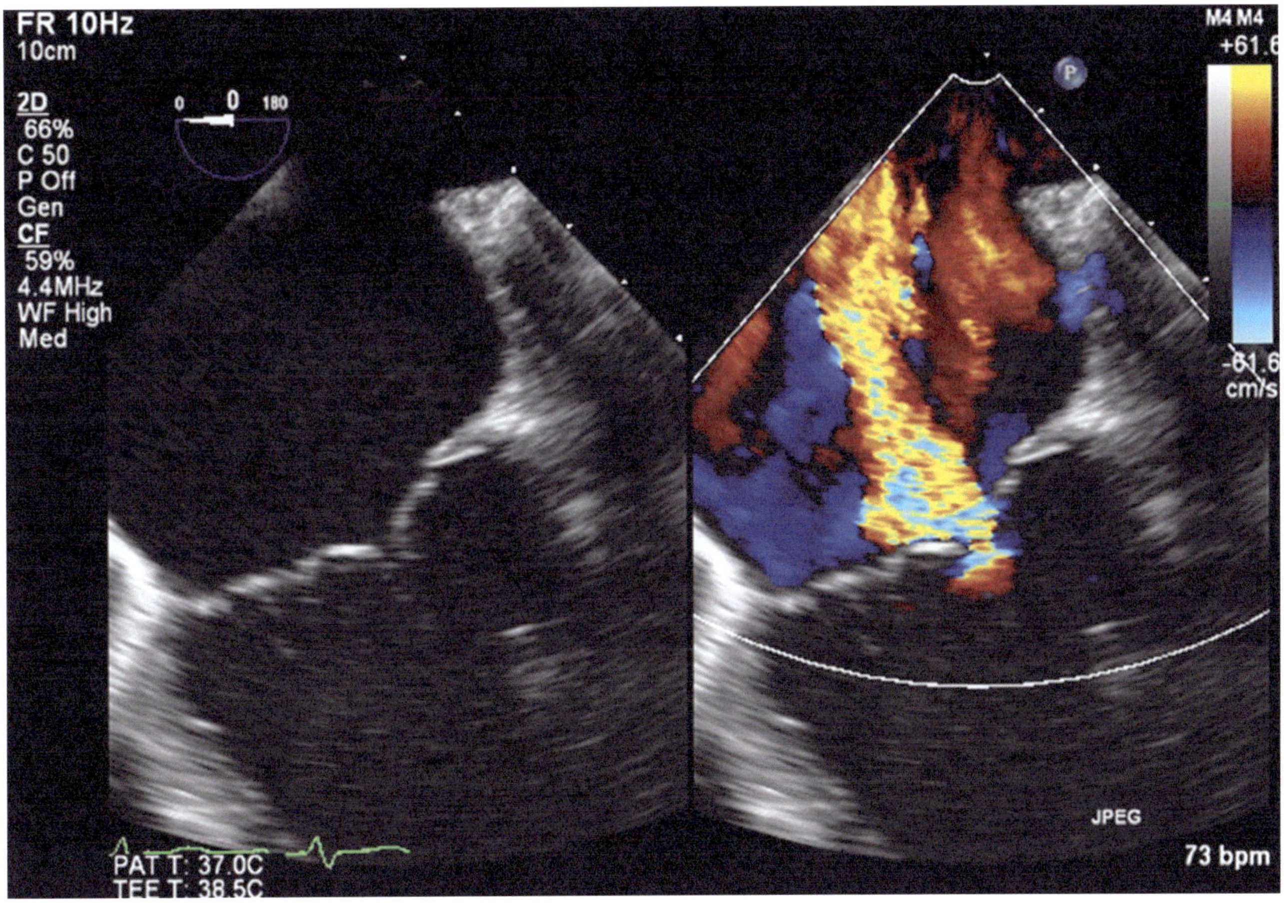

Fig. 45.1 Severe mitral regurgitation secondary to tethering of P2

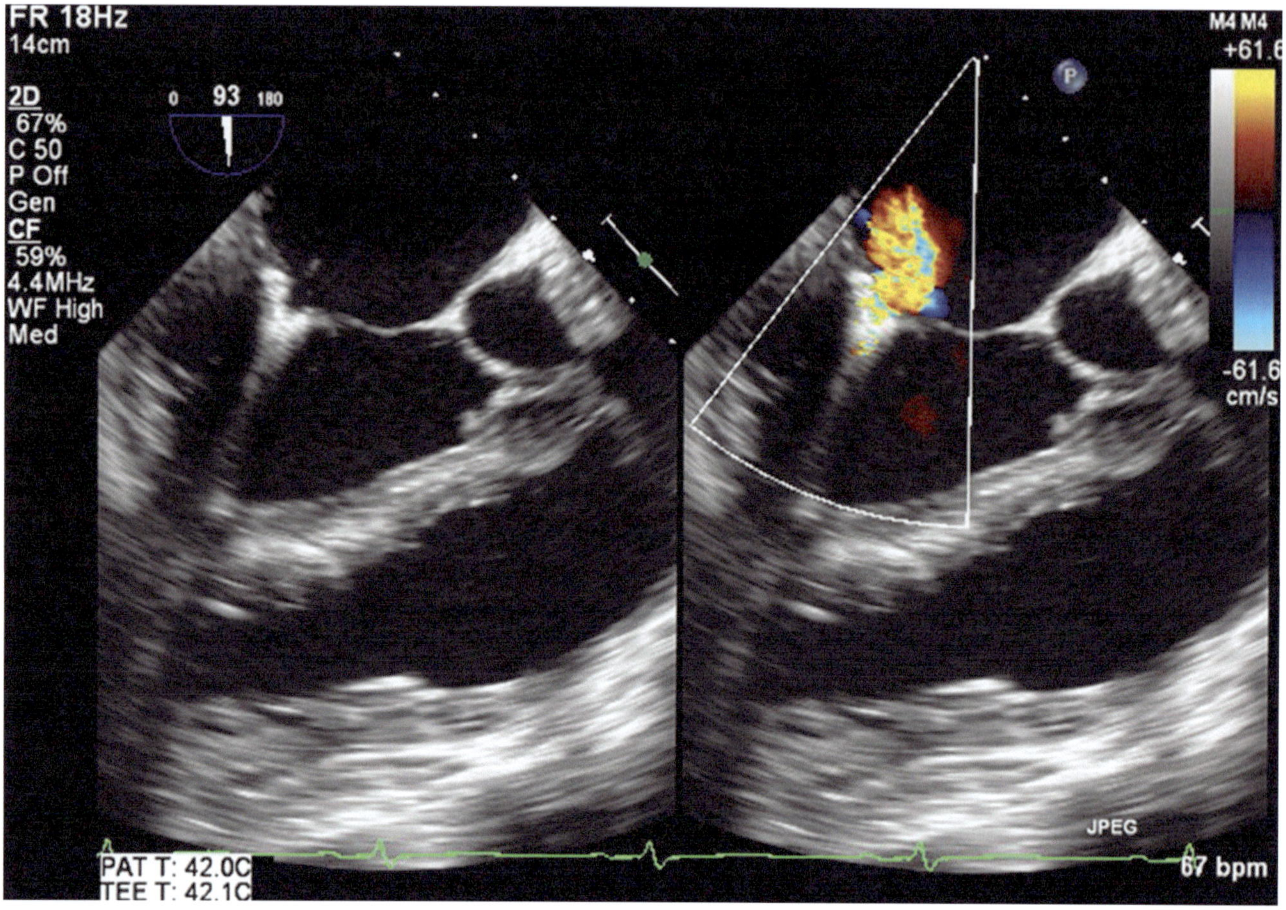

Fig. 45.2 Positioning of MitraClip to split MR jet

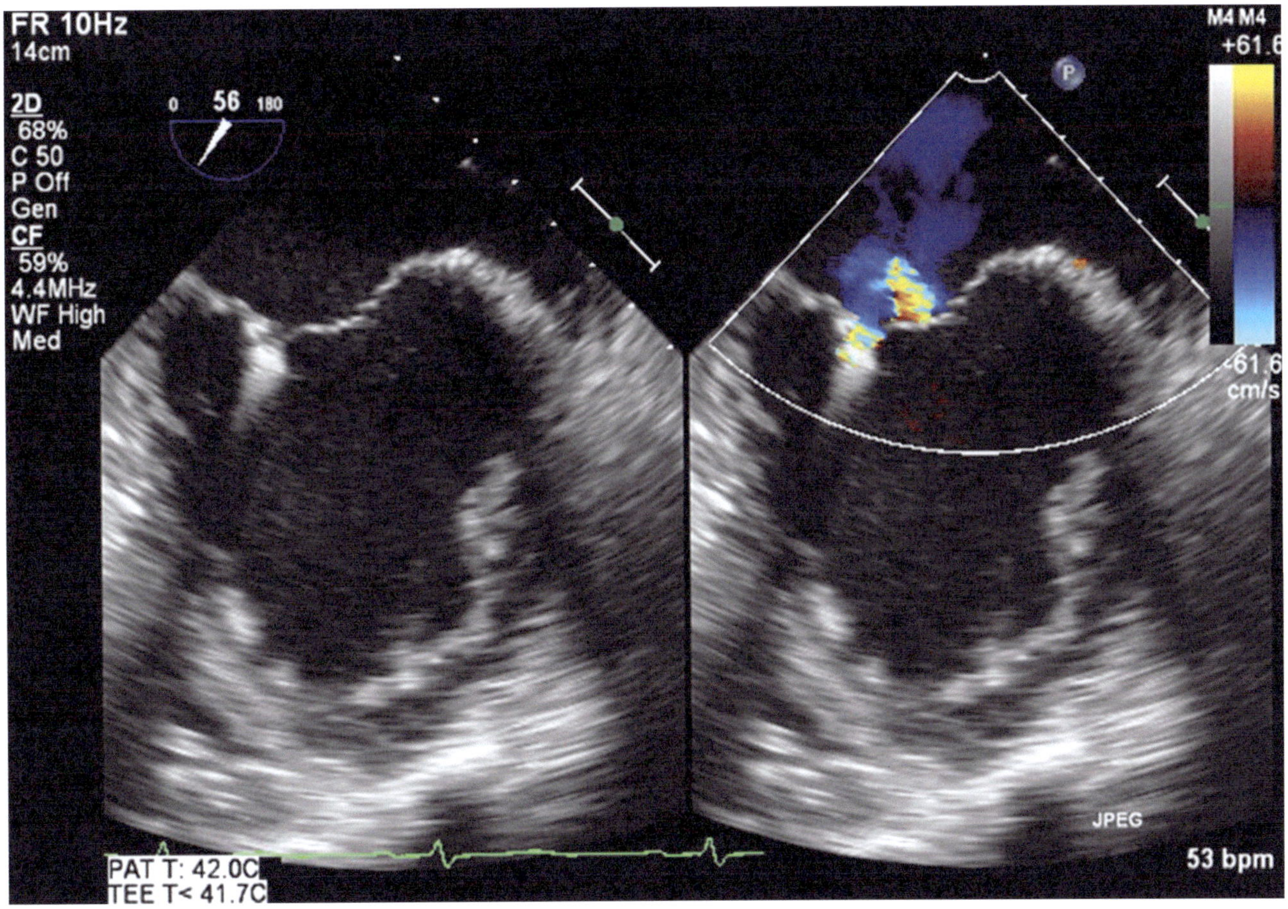

Fig. 45.3 Marked reduction in MR following single MitraClip implantation. Residual small lateral MR jet

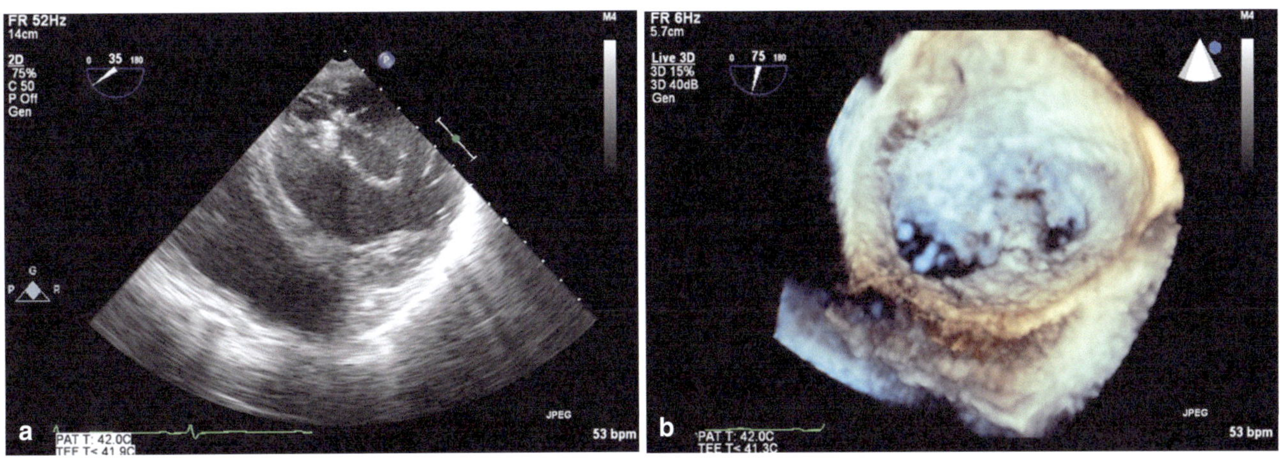

Fig. 45.4 Asymmetric clip position toward the posteromedial aspect of the mitral valve. (**a**) Transgastric view of "bow tie" double-orifice mitral valve conformation. (**b**) 3-D left atrial surgical view

MitraClip: Acute Thrombus Formation During Guide Insertion

46

Edgar L.W. Tay, Kian Keong Poh, Raymond Wong, and James Wei Luen Yip

Abstract

Thrombus formation can occur during the mitraclip procedure and predispose patients to significant complications from thromboembolism. This case illustrates the need to be vigilant despite anticoagulation. The entire system had to be removed and re-prepared to remove the thrombus and prevent complications. In addition, increased anticoagulation had to be administered.

Keywords

Mitral regurgitation • MitraClip • Thrombus • Anticoagulation

Clinical History

A 51-year-old Malay man with a known history idiopathic dilated cardiomyopathy presented with two separate admissions for congestive heart failure. He was in NYHA class II. He was previously referred to the cardiac surgeons but had been turned down for open heart surgery due to morbid obesity. His transthoracic and transesophageal echo showed a dilated left ventricle with reduced LV ejection fraction of 30 % with severe centrally directed mitral regurgitation (MR). The estimated pulmonary systolic pressure was 42 mmHg. During the MitraClip procedure, a thrombus was seen on the steerable guide despite having an ACT of 270 s (Figs. 46.1, 46.2, and 46.3). This device had to be removed, and higher doses of heparin was administered to achieve an ACT of >350 s. The procedure was successful with 1 clip eventually deployed (Figs. 46.4 and 46.5).

E.L.W. Tay, M.B.B.S. (✉) • K.K. Poh, MBBChir (Camb)
R. Wong, M.B.B.S. • J.W.L. Yip, M.B.B.S.
Department of Cardiology, National University Heart Centre Singapore, NUHS Tower Block Level 9, 1E Kent Ridge Road, Singapore 119228, Singapore
e-mail: edgar_tay@nuhs.edu.sg; kian_keong_poh@nuhs.edu.sg; raymond_cc_wong@nuhs.edu.sg; james_yip@nuhs.edu.sg

Summary

This is a case of functional mitral regurgitation. A thrombus can form on the devices despite achieving ACTs of >250 s. The delivery system had to be removed and re-flushed, and heparin doses had to be increased.

Learning Points

This case illustrates the need to be conscious of thrombus formation during the procedure. Strict adherence to monitoring of ACT is needed. In addition, strategies for dealing with thrombus formation need to be considered.

T. Feldman et al. (eds.), *Atlas of Percutaneous Edge-to-Edge Mitral Valve Repair*, DOI 10.1007/978-1-4471-4294-2_46, © Springer-Verlag London 2013

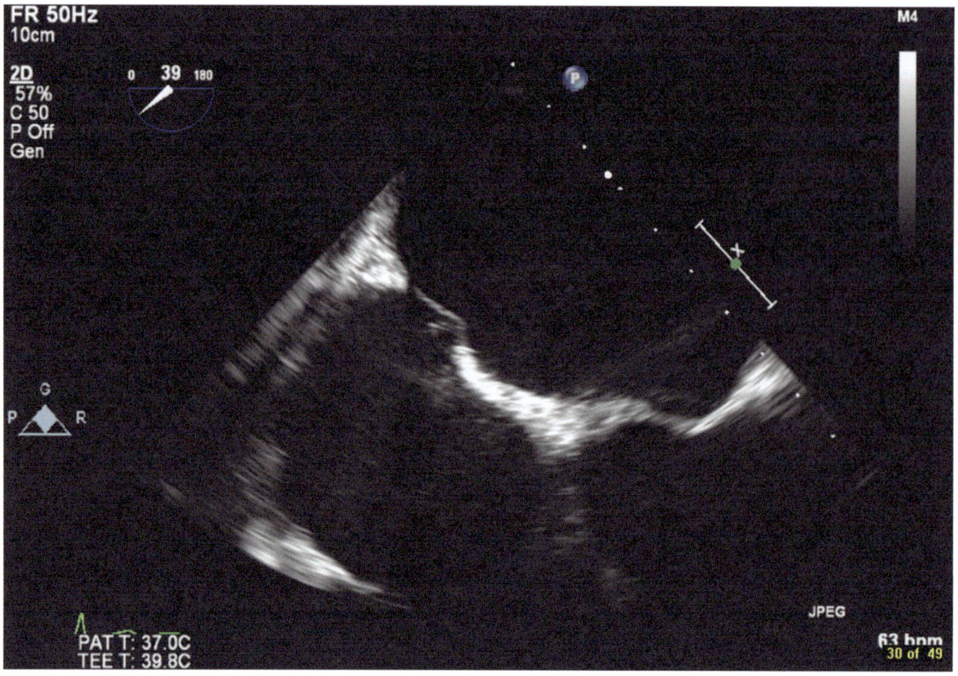

Fig. 46.1 Transesophageal echocardiographic guidance during transseptal puncture

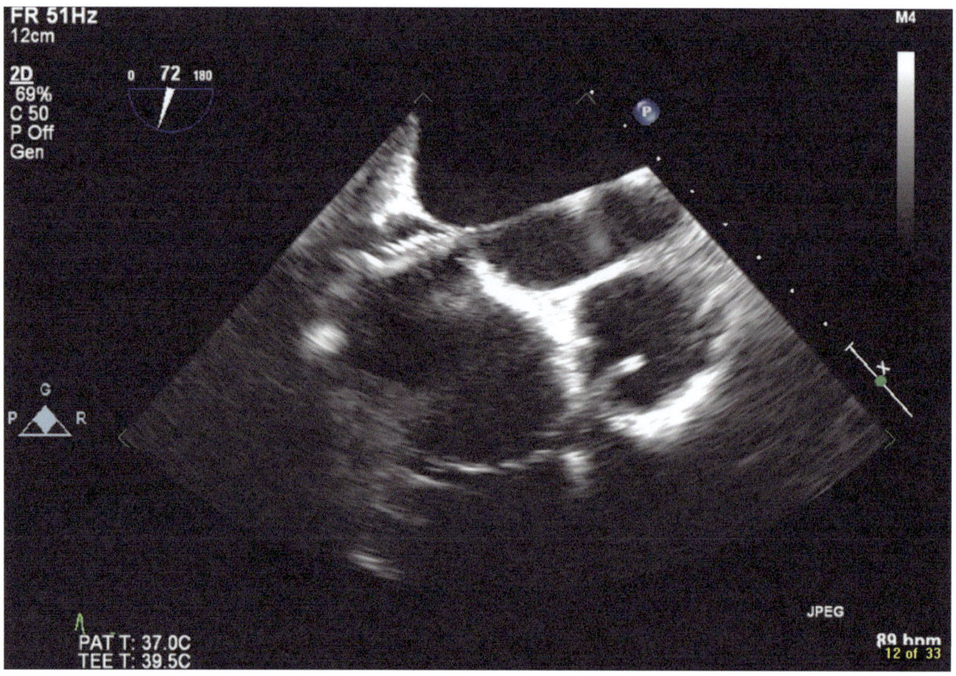

Fig. 46.2 Introduction of the steerable guide across the atrial septum

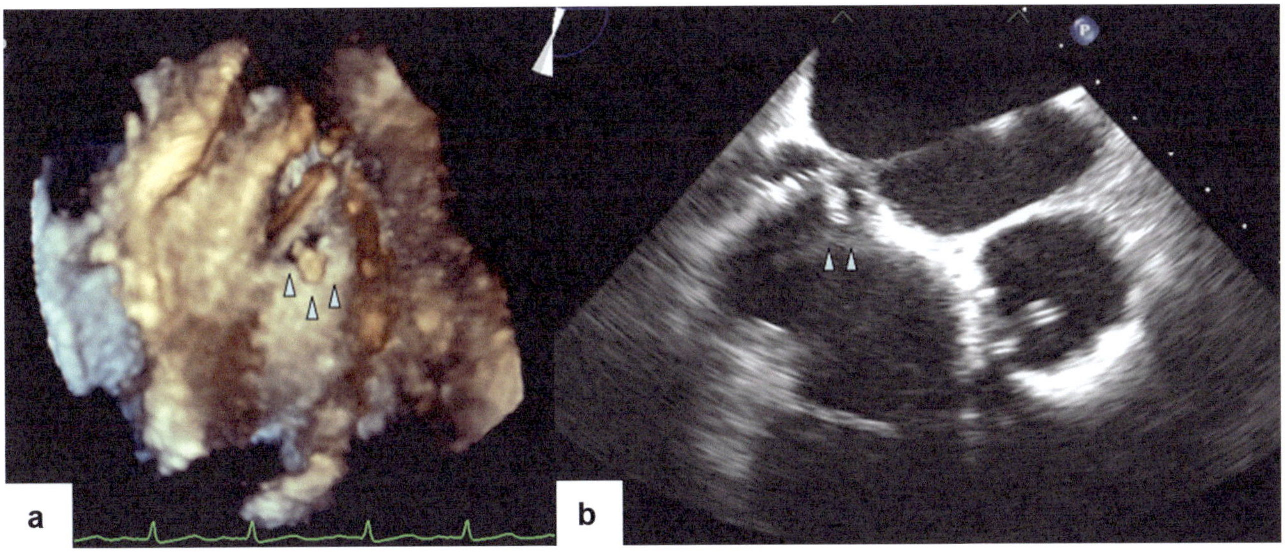

Fig. 46.3 Thrombus seen on the right atrial side attached to the steerable guide. (**a**) 3-D transesophageal images (*arrows heads* show thrombus). (**b**) 2-D transesophageal imaging showing the thrombus

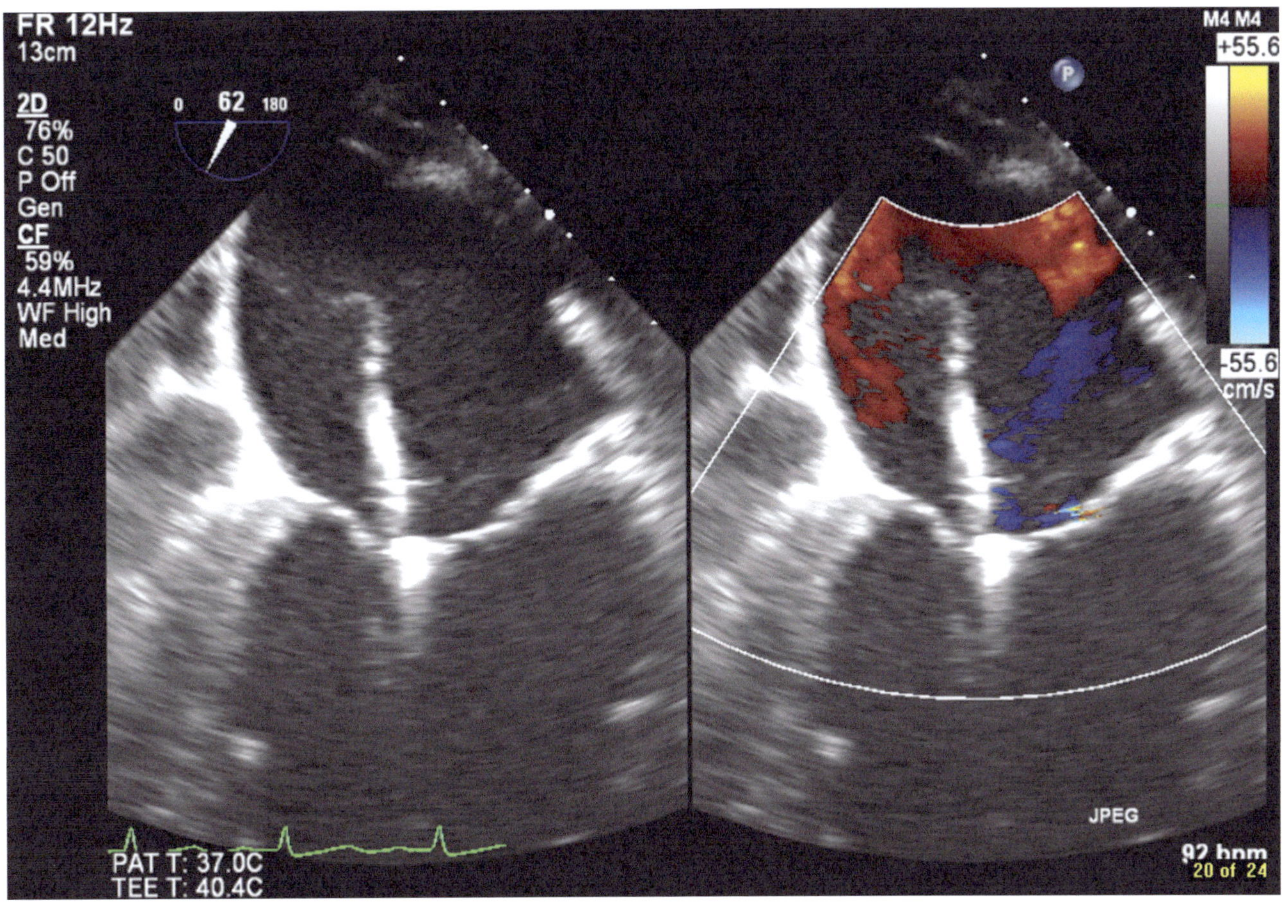

Fig. 46.4 Clip delivery system in place with mitral valve leaflets captured

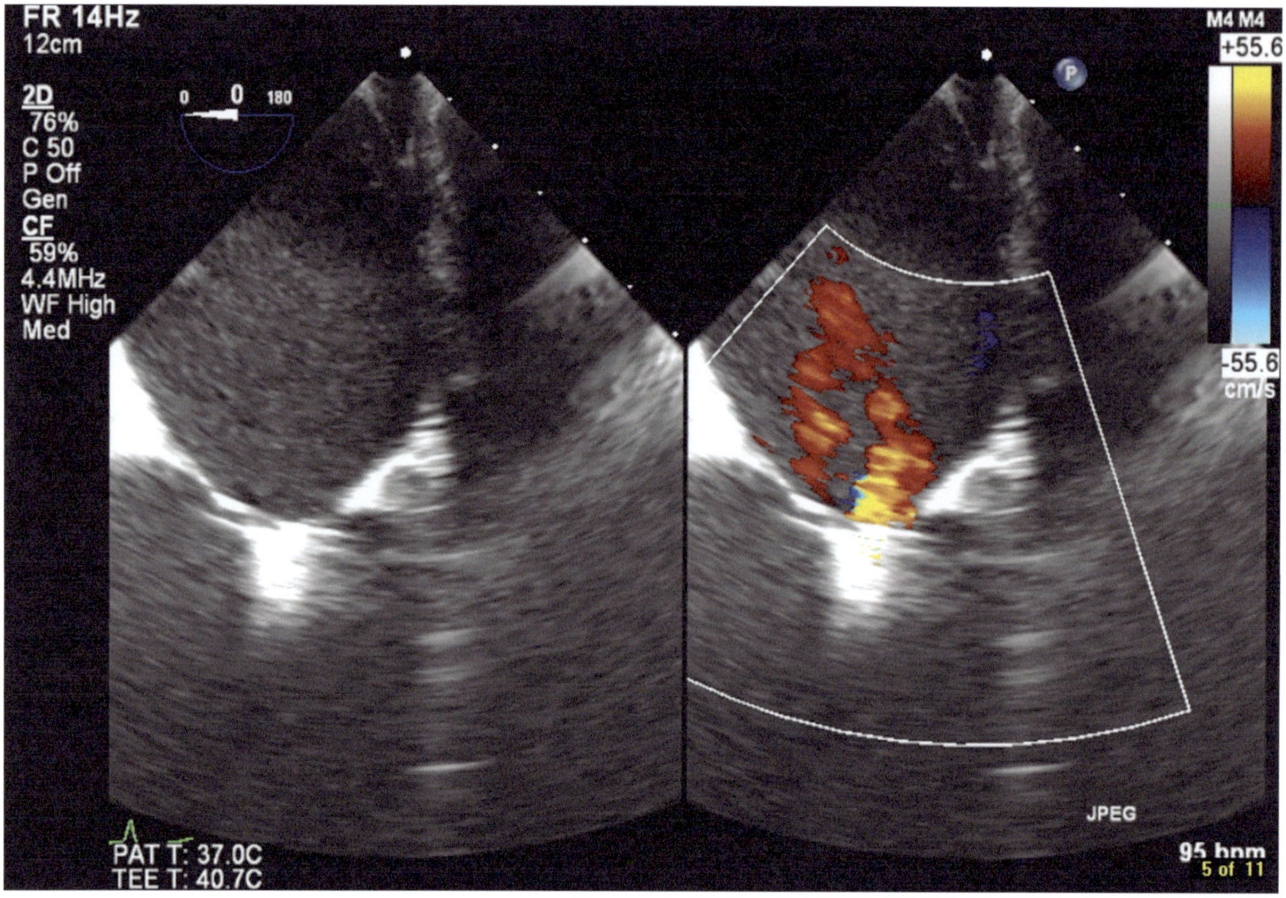

Fig. 46.5 Final result showing 1+ mitral regurgitation after the clip was released

47 MitraClip Placement in a Patient with Severe Kyphoscoliosis and Bileaflet Prolapse

Ehrin J. Armstrong and Jason Rogers

Abstract
This case highlights successful MitraClip implantation in a patient with severe kyphoscoliosis. The associated anatomic rotation made MitraClip placement extremely challenging.

Keywords
Mitral regurgitation • Mitral valve prolapse • MitraClip • Transseptal puncture

Clinical History

A 65-year-old man with a history of childhood polio requiring iron lung therapy and tracheostomy until adulthood presented with shortness of breath and severe mitral regurgitation due to bileaflet and severe P2 prolapse. He was not a surgical candidate due to his multiple comorbidities. Due to his severe kyphoscoliosis and cardiac rotation, transseptal puncture and MitraClip implantation were technically challenging and required the use of additional devices, including a "buddy wire" technique to straighten the inferior vena cava, and an Agilis catheter to facilitate transseptal puncture. Device implantation was very challenging due to unusual cardiac rotation, and 3-D TEE guidance was critical for device orientation. The procedure was ultimately successful with implantation of one MitraClip with reduction of MR from 3–4+ to 2+. A second MitraClip could not be implanted due to technical complexity and fear of dislodging the first clip. Nonetheless, the patient reported significantly improved symptoms on clinical follow-up.

E.J. Armstrong, M.D., M.Sc.
Division of Cardiovascular Medicine,
University of California, Davis Medical Center,
4860 Y Street, Suite 2820, Sacramento, CA 95817, USA
e-mail: ehrin.armstrong@ucdmc.ucdavis.edu

J. Rogers, M.D., FACC, FSCAI (✉)
Department of Cardiovascular Medicine, University of California,
Davis Medical Center,
4860 Y Street, Suite 2820, Sacramento, CA 95817, USA
e-mail: jason.rogers@ucdmc.ucdavis.edu

Summary

In this case, the patient's anatomic rotation complicated all steps of the MitraClip procedure. This case demonstrates the feasibility of performing MitraClip implantation in patients with significant anatomic abnormalities.

Learning Points

Use of an Agilis catheter and multiple support wires may facilitate orientation for transseptal puncture in cases of cardiac rotation. 3-D TEE is essential for MitraClip device orientation and positioning in distorted anatomies where catheter movements may not be predictable. MitraClip placement is feasible even in anatomically complex situations.

Electronic supplementary material The online version of this chapter (doi:10.1007/978-1-4471-4294-2_47) contains supplementary material, which is available to authorized users.

T. Feldman et al. (eds.), *Atlas of Percutaneous Edge-to-Edge Mitral Valve Repair*,
DOI 10.1007/978-1-4471-4294-2_47, © Springer-Verlag London 2013

Screening Transthoracic Echocardiogram

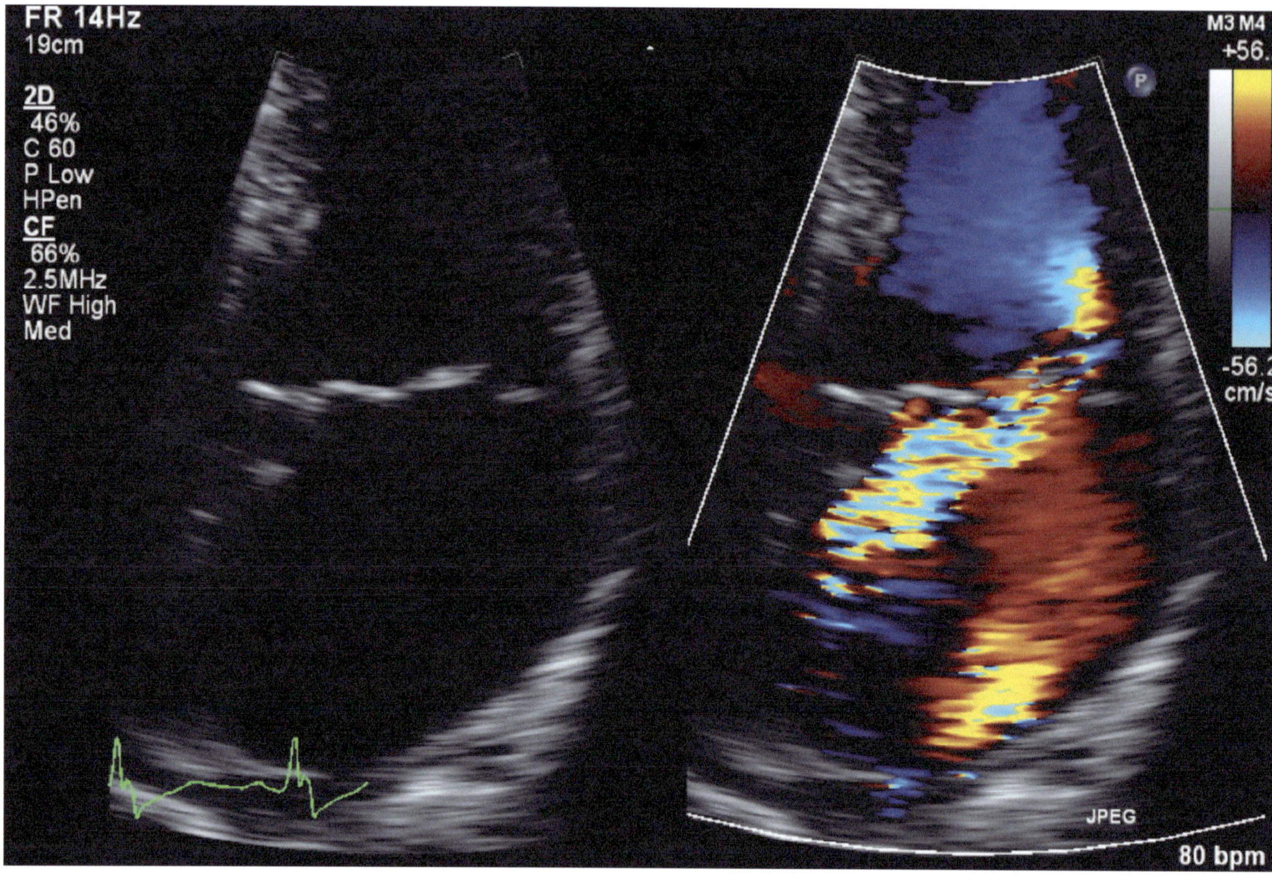

Fig. 47.1 TTE: Apical 4C with and without Doppler. Transthoracic imaging in this patient was technically difficult due to his cardiac rotation, and adequate parasternal images could not be obtained. In this apical four-chamber view, the thickened leaflets can be appreciated. There is an eccentric jet of severe mitral regurgitation

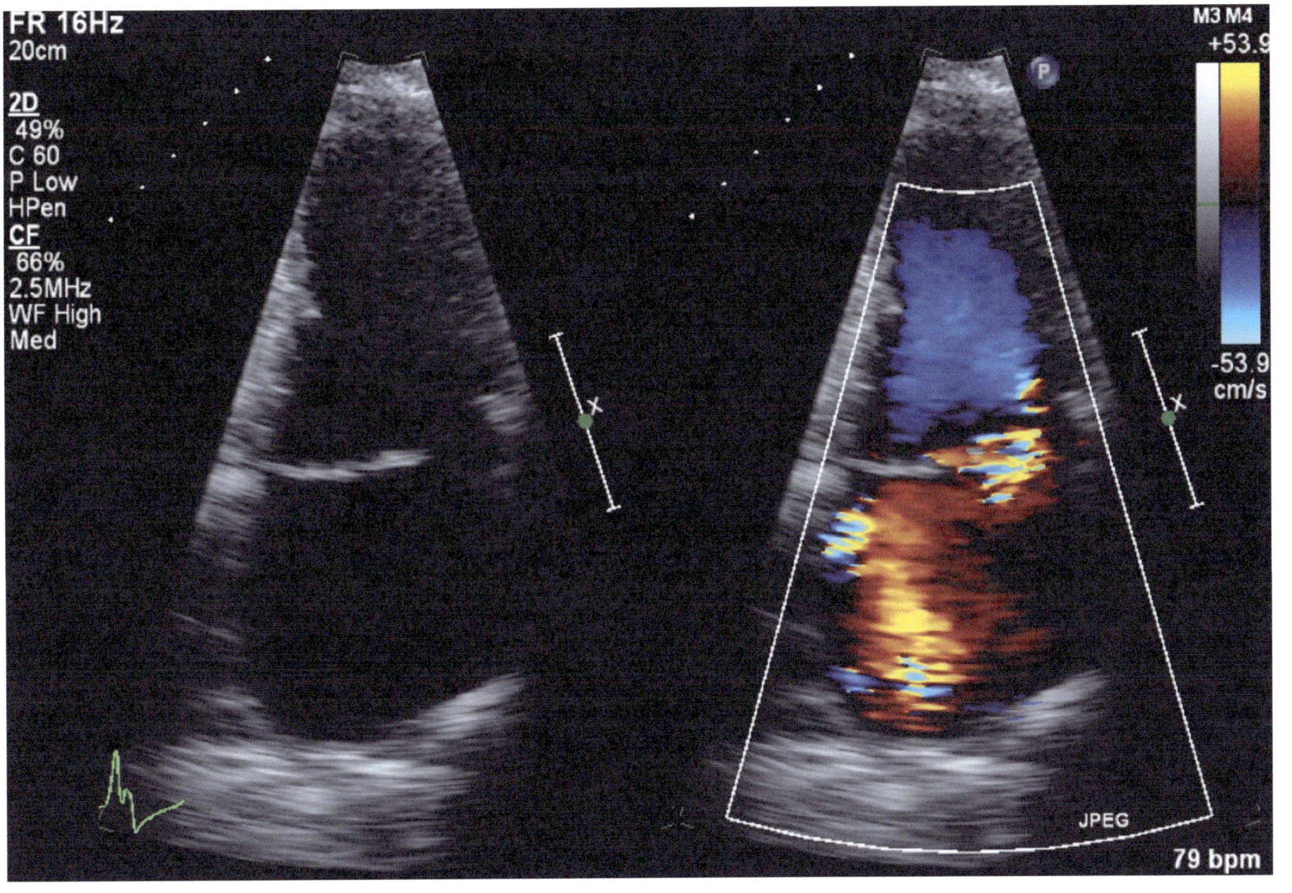

Fig. 47.2 TTE: Apical 2C with and without Doppler: In the apical two-chamber view, the Doppler jet of mitral regurgitation can be seen throughout most of the left atrium, consistent with severe mitral regurgitation

Screening Transesophageal Echocardiogram

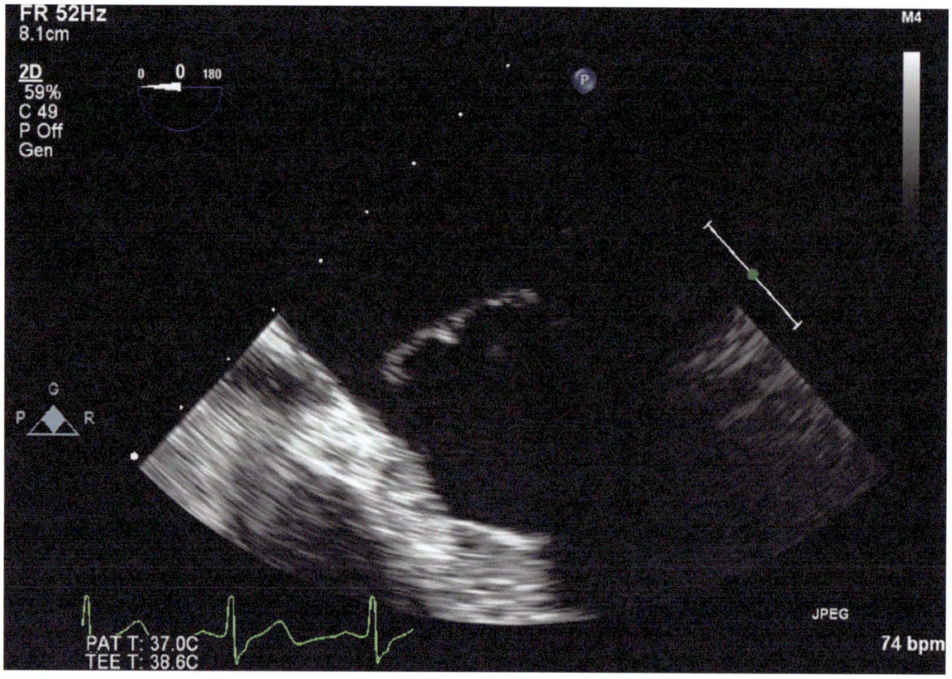

Fig. 47.3 TEE: 4C view without color: There is bileaflet prolapse with a central area of coaptation

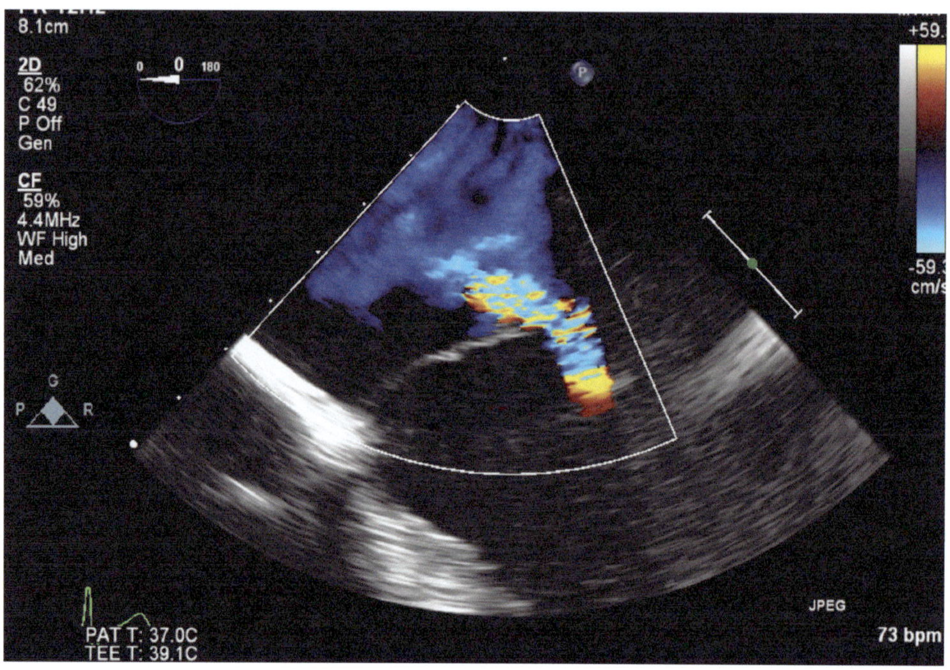

Fig. 47.4 TEE: 4C view with color: The regurgitant jet originates from the A2-P2 interface but has an eccentric course

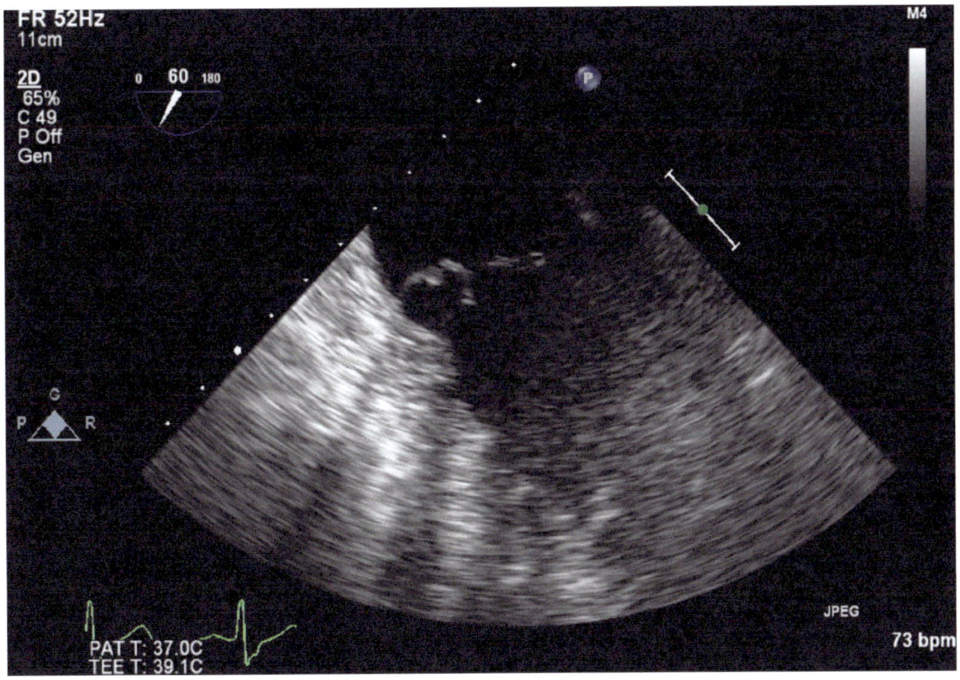

Fig. 47.5 TEE: Bicom view without color: The anterior leaflet has significant prolapse along its lateral border. Due to the patient's rotation, bicommisural imaging was challenging

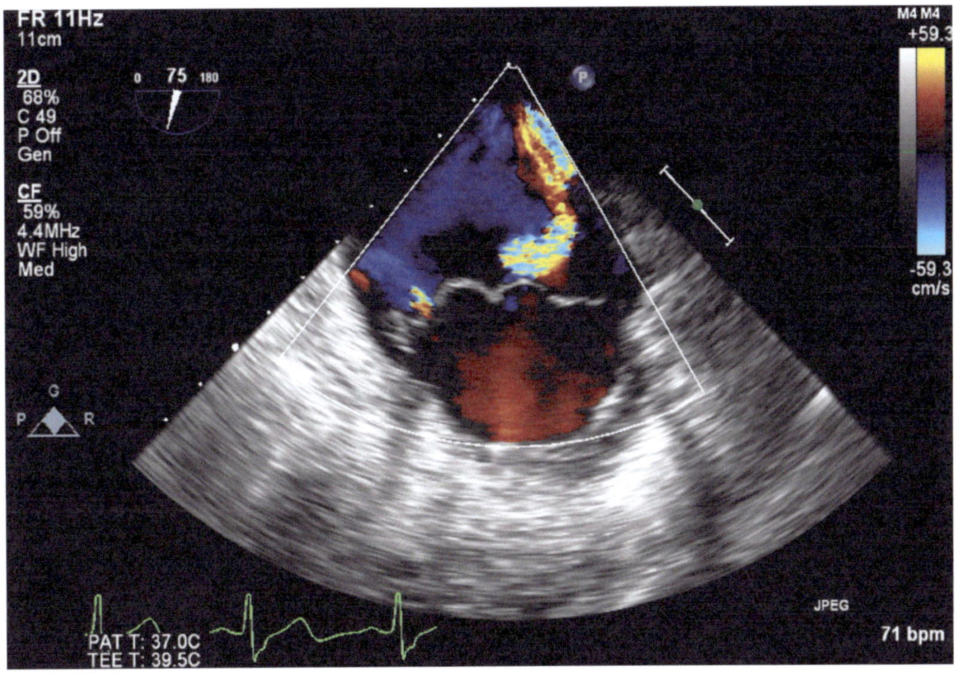

Fig. 47.6 TEE: Bicom view with color: The regurgitant jet appears to have a single central origin

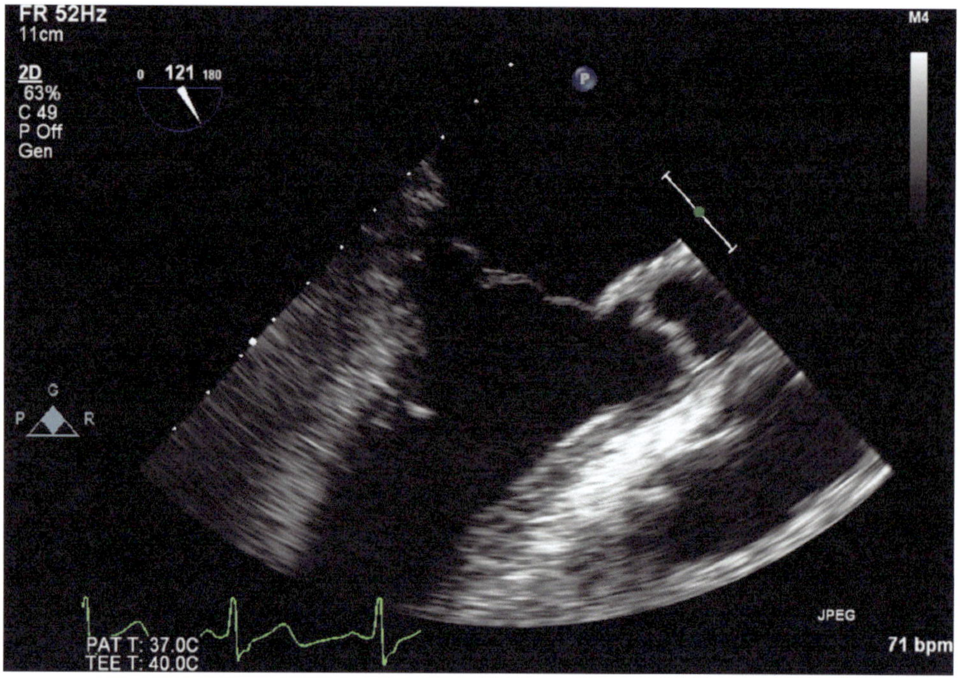

Fig. 47.7 TEE: 3C without color: The leaflets appear thickened, but there is no evidence of chordal rupture

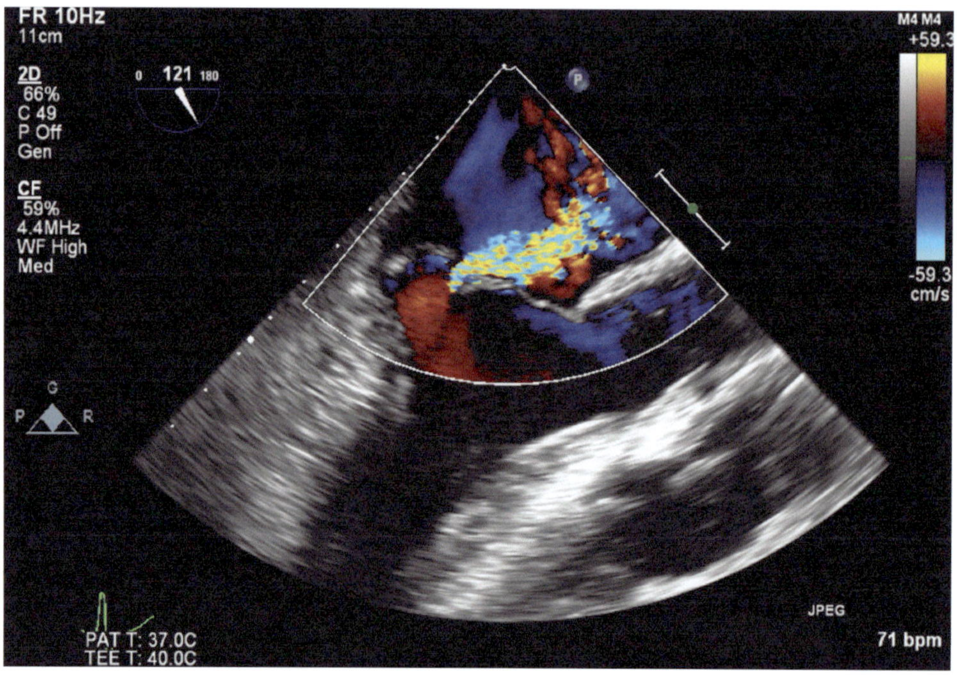

Fig. 47.8 TEE: 3C with color: The regurgitant jet has a central origin with a jet that is directed anteriorly

Intra-procedural Echocardiography and Fluoroscopy

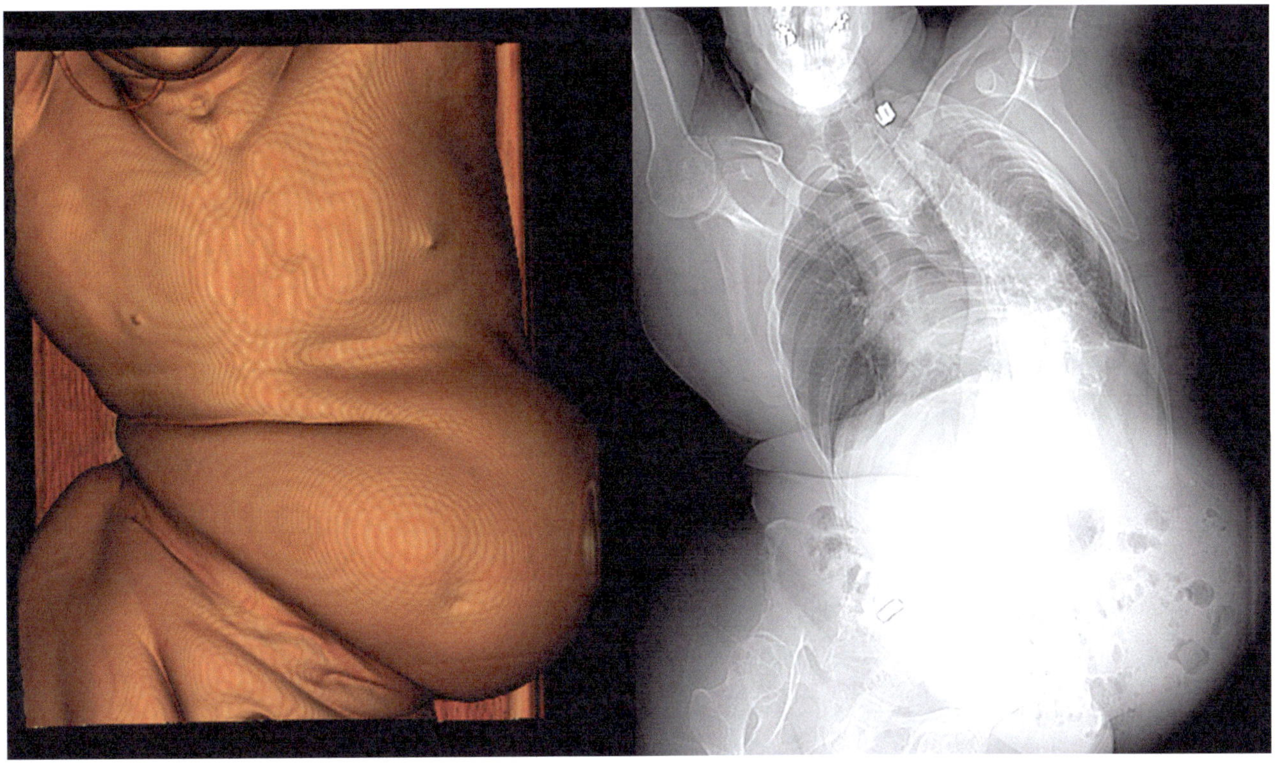

Fig. 47.9 X-Ray: A surface reconstruction and scout film from the patient's chest CT demonstrate the severe angulation of the patient's abdomen and cardiac rotation

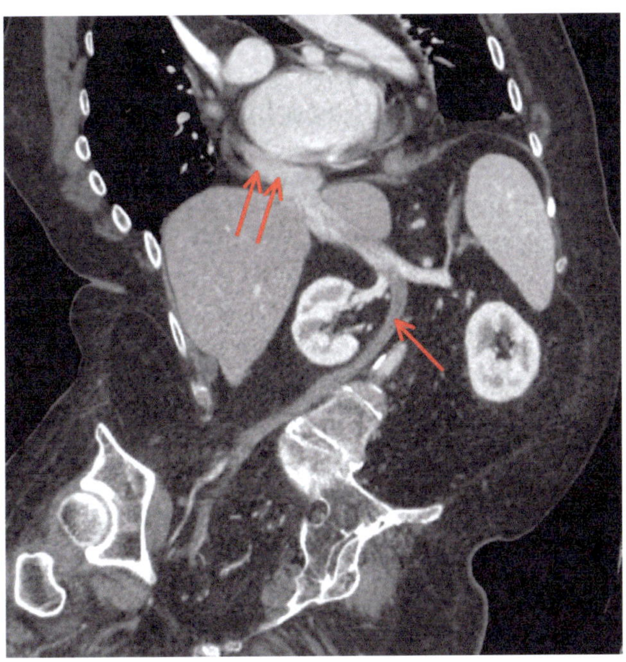

Fig. 47.10 Abdominal CT: The inferior vena cava (*arrow*) is severely angulated in the mid-abdomen. Note also the somewhat small horizontal right atrium and horizontal interatrial septum (*double arrow*)

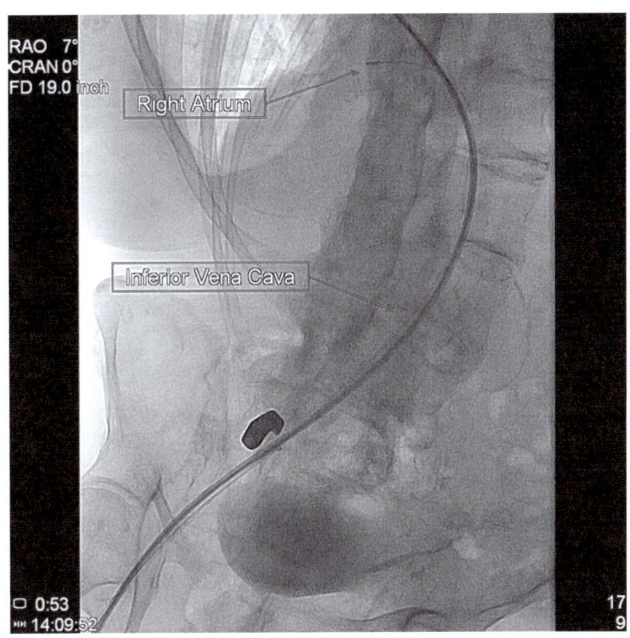

Fig. 47.11 Fluoroscopy: The angulation of the inferior vena cava is apparent with a sheath in place from the right femoral vein to the right atrium

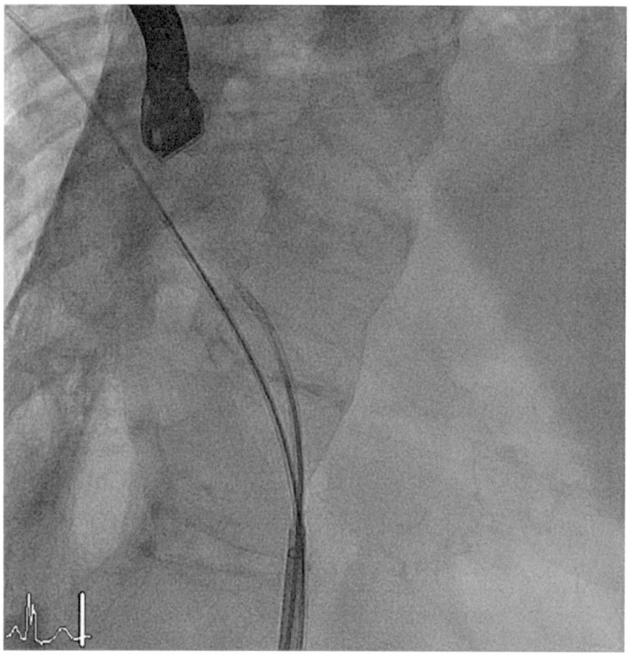

Fig. 47.12 Fluoroscopy: There was inadequate catheter stability with a Mullins sheath and Brockenbrough needle to allow stable engagement of the interatrial septum. In order to improve the IVC angulation and make a transseptal puncture feasible, an Amplatz super-stiff "buddy wire" was directed from the right femoral vein into the superior vena cava. A multipurpose catheter was advanced over the wire to prevent laceration. This provided some straightening of the approach angle

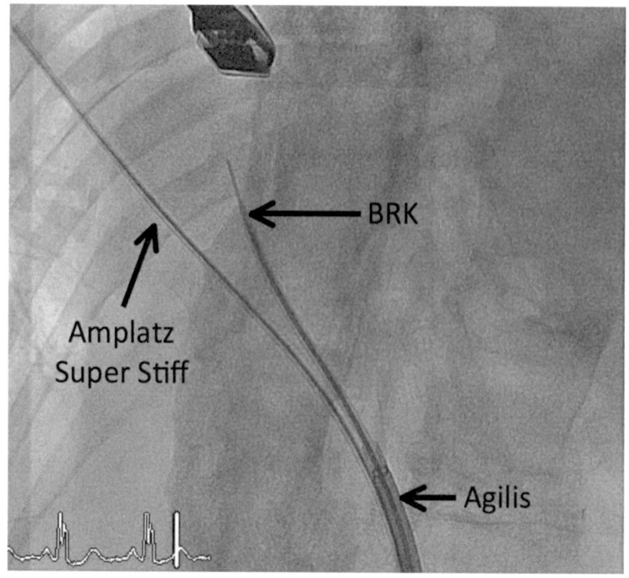

Fig. 47.13 Fluoroscopy: With the Amplatzer wire in place in the SVC, a medium-curl Agilis catheter was advanced into the right atrium and allowed controlled direction of the transseptal catheter toward the interatrial septum. A BRK needle and Mullins sheath were advanced through the Agilis catheter, and transseptal puncture was performed under TEE guidance

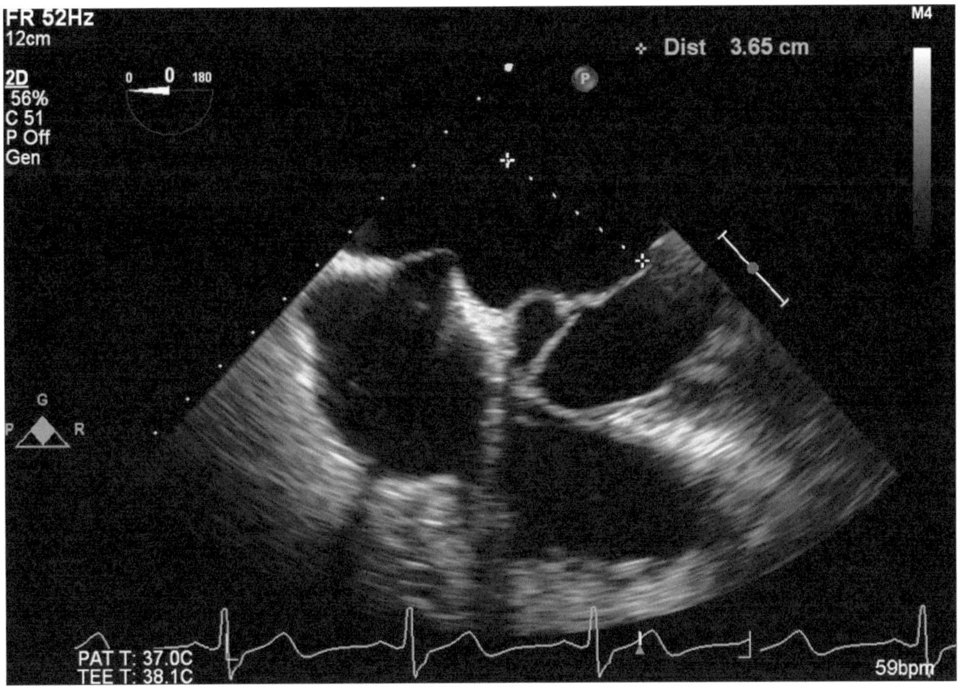

Fig. 47.14 TEE: The transseptal puncture site is confirmed at 3.65 cm above the site of leaflet coaptation. This height provided height to allow angulation of the MitraClip delivery system toward the leaflets

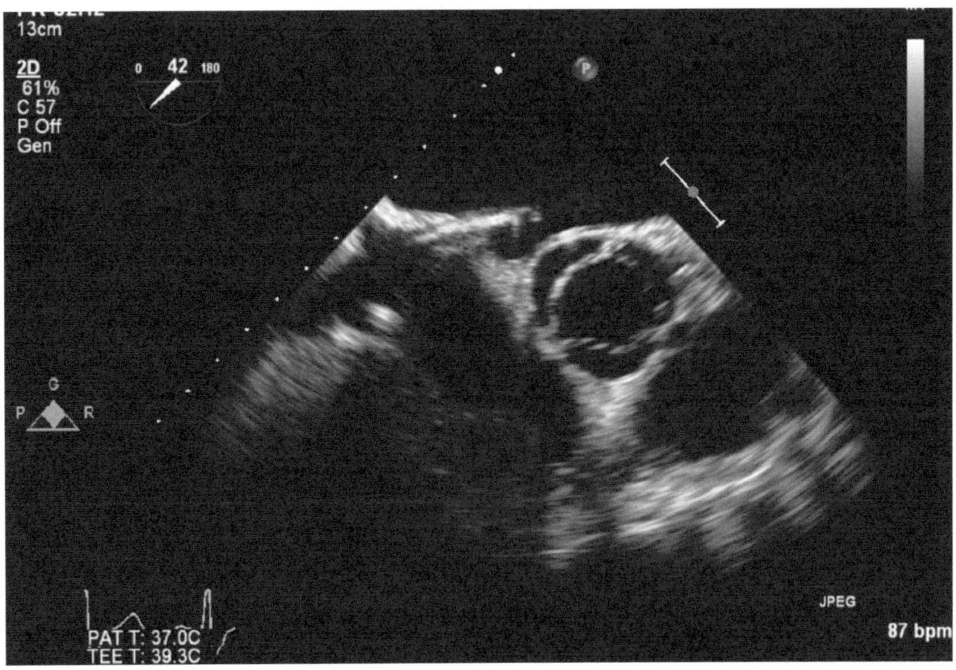

Fig. 47.15 TEE: Short axis views show that the puncture site is somewhat anterior but acceptable for device orientation relative to the mitral valve

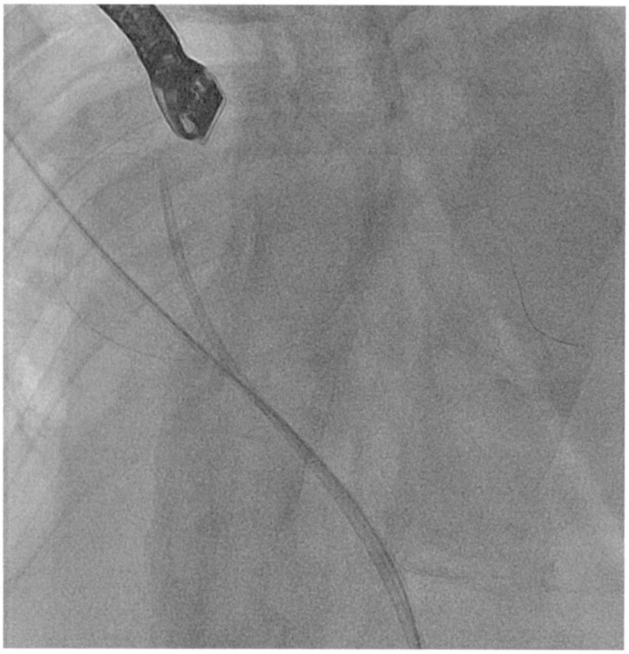

Fig. 47.16 Fluoroscopy: A 0.014 extra-support wire was looped in the left atrium to provide support while removing the Agilis catheter and advancing the Mullins sheath across the interatrial septum

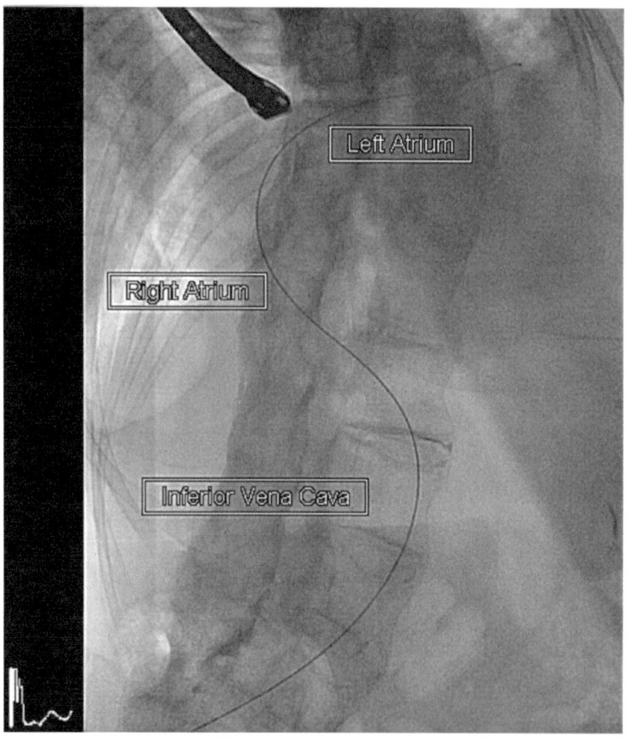

Fig. 47.17 Fluoroscopy: An Amplatz super-stiff wire is across the interatrial septum. This provides some straightening and support for the MitraClip guiding catheter

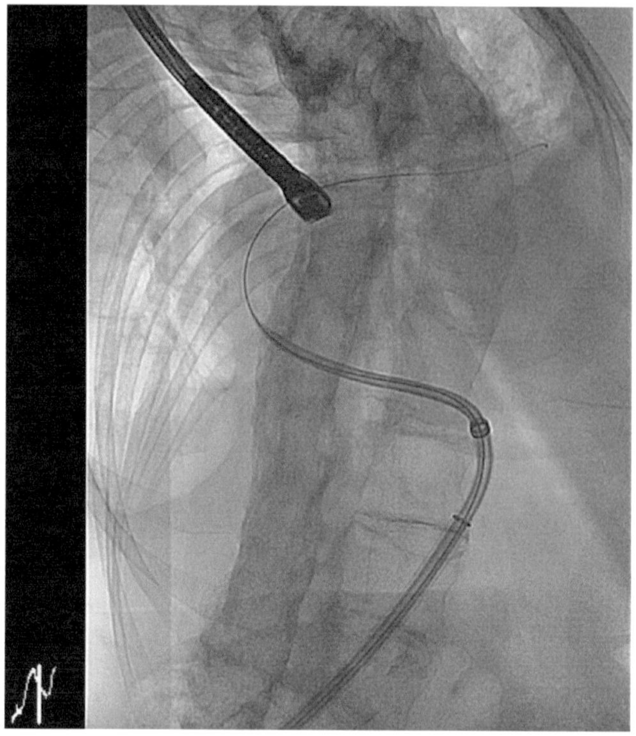

Fig. 47.18 Fluoroscopy: The MitraClip guiding catheter is directed around the angulation of the inferior vena cava to the interatrial septum. The dilator was maximally extended to facilitate tracking the tortuosity. Patience was required as the MitraClip guiding catheter was advanced across the interatrial septum to avoid prolapsing the wire back into the right atrium

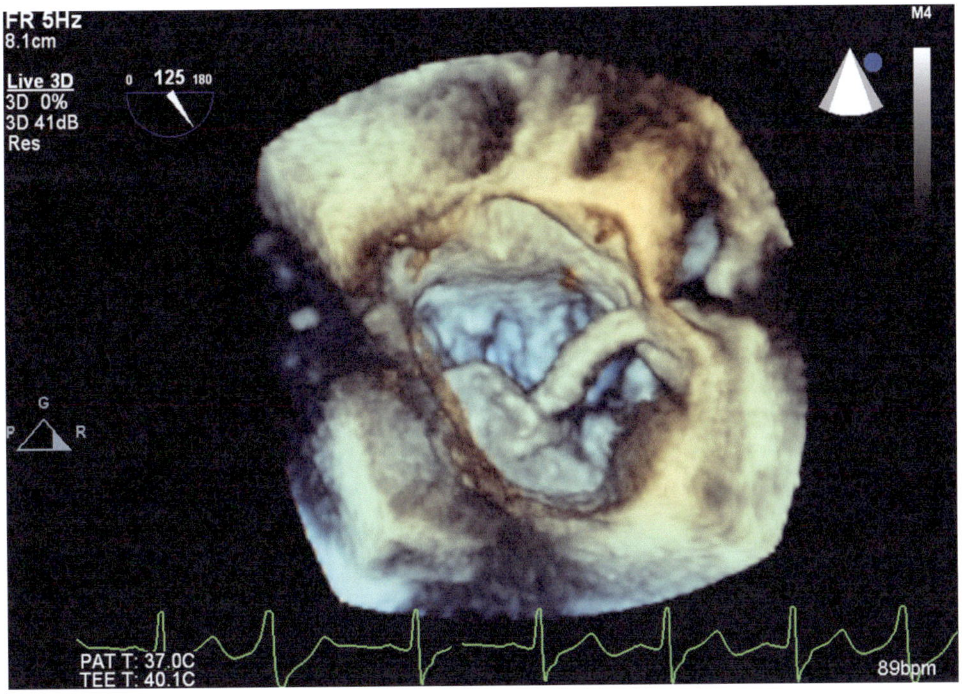

Fig. 47.19 3-D TEE: Three-dimensional TEE shows the orientation of the MitraClip device across the interatrial septum toward the leaflets. Because of severe cardiac rotation and IVC angulation, control of the MitraClip was not predictable and did not follow the anticipated movements that would usually occur with adjustments of the guide and clip delivery system. 3-D TEE was indispensable for determining proper orientation

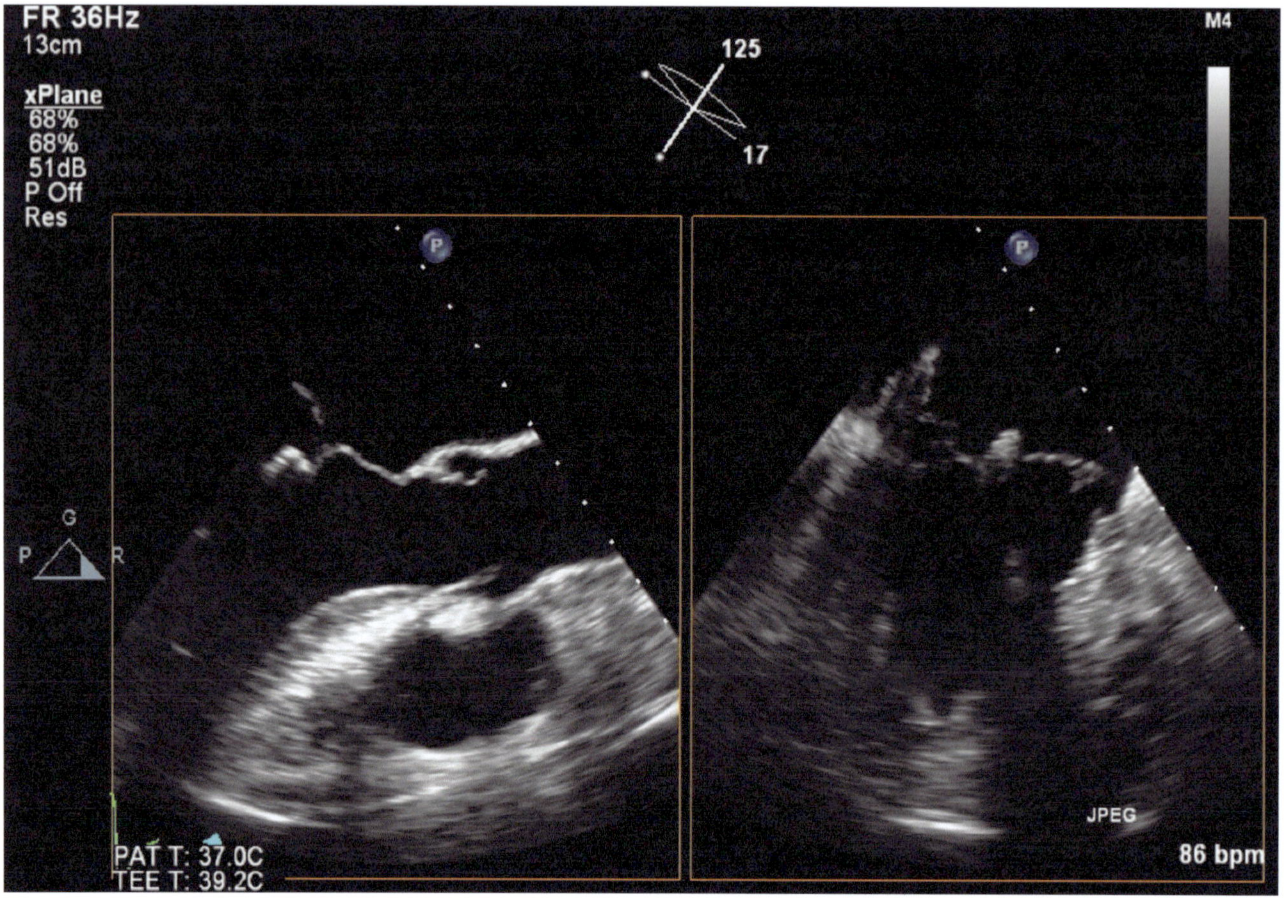

Fig. 47.20 Biplane TEE: Biplane views show the MitraClip device across the central zone of coaptation with good orientation. Note that because of lack of sufficient height, the MitraClip guide was brought back into the right atrium to allow the MitraClip to be retracted sufficiently for leaflet grasping

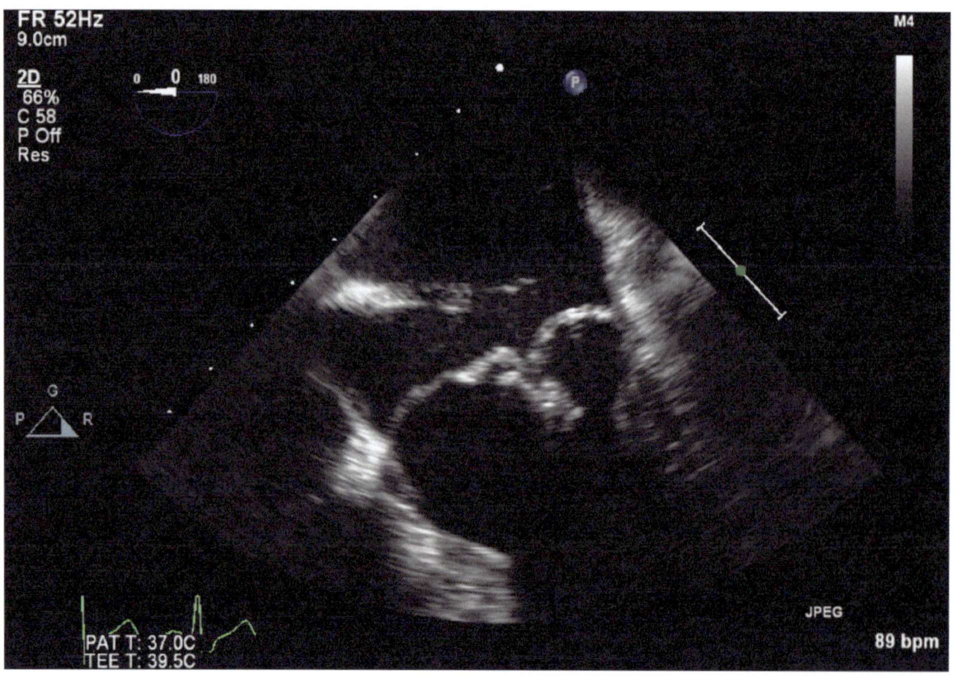

Fig. 47.21 TEE: Post deployment, the MitraClip appears well seated at the central A2-P2 interface

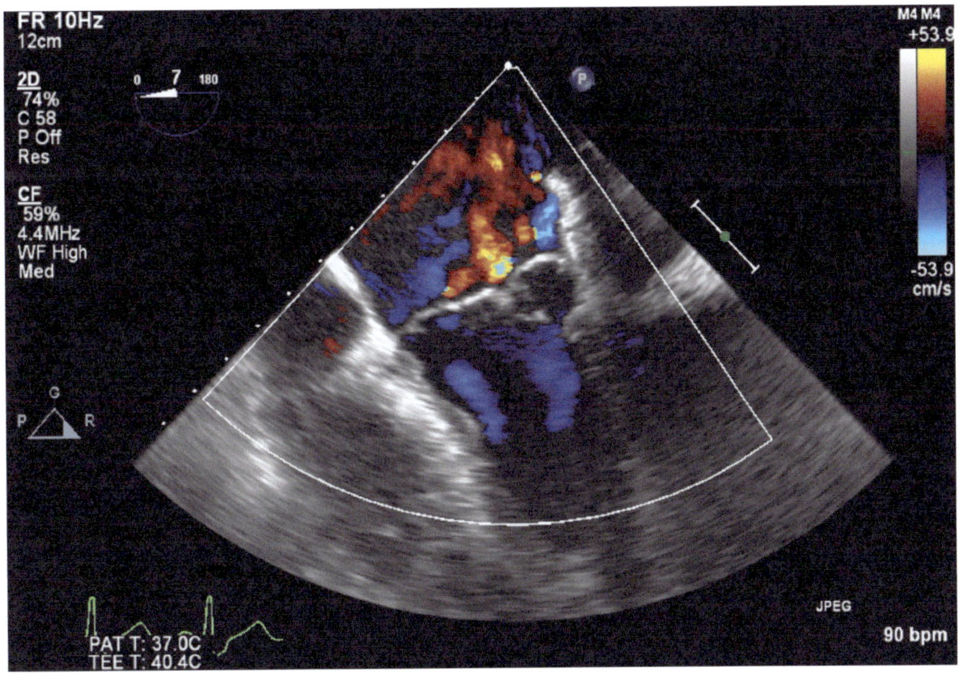

Fig. 47.22 TEE w/color: Doppler echocardiography reveals mild residual MR around the site of device deployment

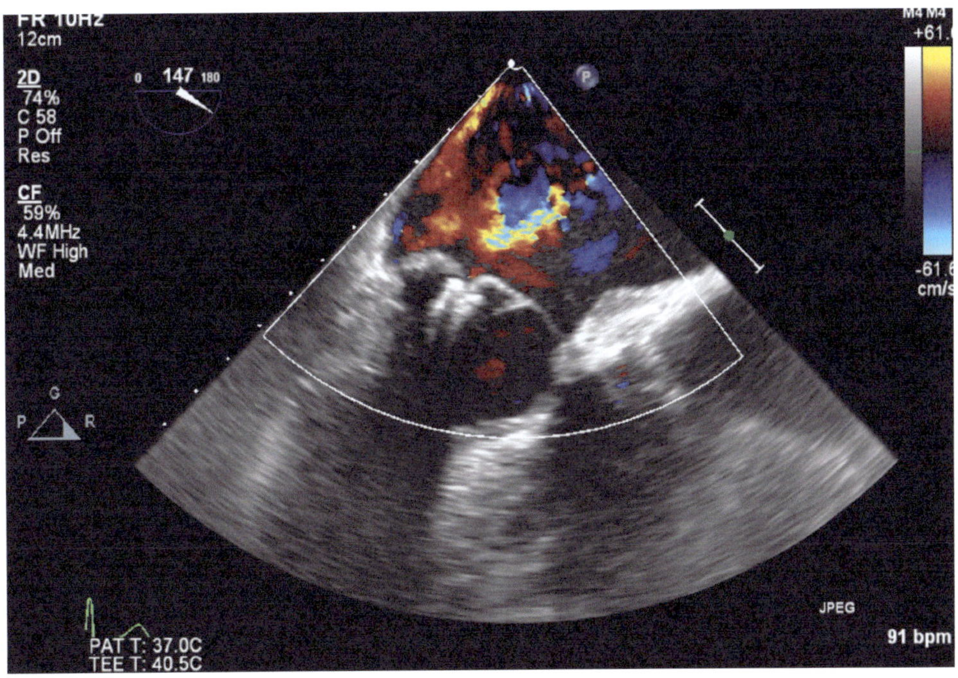

Fig. 47.23 TEE w/color: On three-chamber views, there is a persistent mild jet of mitral regurgitation

Post-procedure Transthoracic Echocardiogram

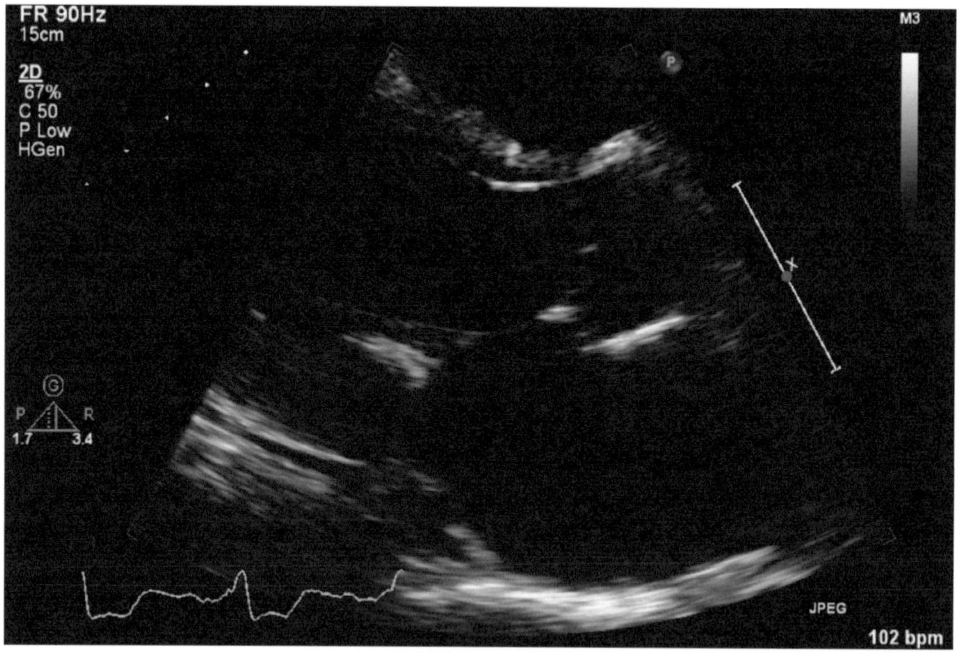

Fig. 47.24 TTE: On parasternal long axis views, the device appears well seated in a central location

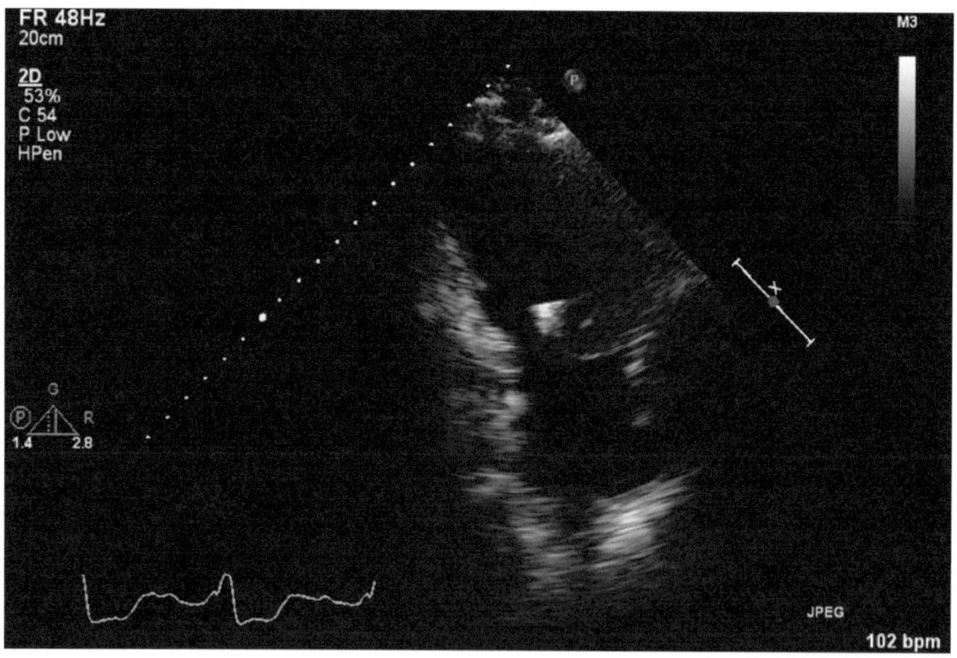

Fig. 47.25 TTE: Two-chamber views also confirm a central location of the device

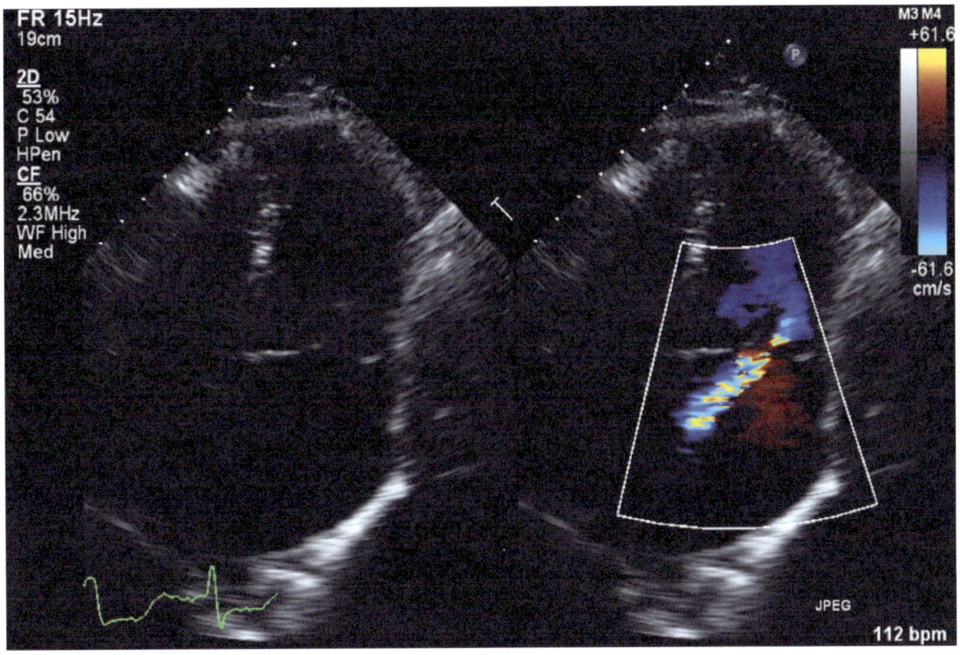

Fig. 47.26 TTE: On four-chamber views with and without Doppler, the mitral regurgitation is eccentric and mild (1–2+)

Index

T. Feldman et al. (eds.), *Atlas of Percutaneous Edge-to-Edge Mitral Valve Repair*,
DOI 10.1007/978-1-4471-4294-2, © Springer-Verlag London 2013

N

P

MIX
Papier aus verantwortungsvollen Quellen
Paper from responsible sources
FSC® C105338

If you have any concerns about our products,
you can contact us on
ProductSafety@springernature.com

In case Publisher is established outside the EU,
the EU authorized representative is:
Springer Nature Customer Service Center GmbH
Europaplatz 3, 69115 Heidelberg, Germany

Printed by Libri Plureos GmbH
in Hamburg, Germany